Textbook of Men's Health and Aging

Textbook of Men's Health and Aging

Second Edition

Editors in Chief

Bruno Lunenfeld MD FRCOG FACOG (Hon)
Professor Emeritus, Reproductive Endocrinology
Bar-Ilan University, Ramat Gan
Israel

Louis JG Gooren MD
Professor, Vrjie Universiteit Medical Center
Amsterdam
The Netherlands

Alvaro Morales MD
Queen's University General Hospital
Kingston, ON
Canada

John E Morley MB MCh
St Louis University
St Louis, MO
USA

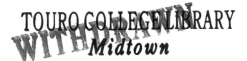

informa
healthcare

First published in the United Kingdom in 2007 by Informa Healthcare, Telephone House, 69–77 Paul Street, London EC2A 4LQ. Informa Healthcare is a trading division of Informa UK Ltd. Registered Office: 37/41 Mortimer Street, London W1T 3JH. Registered in England and Wales number 1072954.

Tel: +44 (0)20 7017 6000
Fax: +44 (0)20 7017 6699
Email: info.medicine@tandf.co.uk
Website: www.informahealthcare.com

A CIP record for this book is available from the British Library.

Library of Congress Cataloging-in-Publication Data

Data available on application

ISBN-10: 0 415 42580 8
ISBN-13: 978 0 415 42580 3

Distributed in North and South America by
Taylor & Francis
6000 Broken Sound Parkway, NW, (Suite 300)
Boca Raton, FL 33487, USA
Within Continental USA
Tel: 1 (800) 272 7737; Fax: 1 (800) 374 3401
Outside Continental USA
Tel: (561) 994 0555; Fax: (561) 361 6018
Email: orders@crcpress.com

Distributed in the rest of the world by
Thomson Publishing Services
Cheriton House
North Way
Andover, Hampshire SP10 5BE, UK
Tel: +44 (0)1264 332424
Email: tps.tandfsalesorder@thomson.com

Composition by C&M Digitals (P) Ltd, Chennai, India
Printed and bound in India by Replika Press Pvt Ltd

08/25/08

Contents

Contents

Contents

Contributors

Angela Marie Abbatecola
*Department of Geriatric Medicine
and Metabolic Diseases
University of Naples
Italy*

Peter Alexandersen MD
*Center for Clinical and Basic Research
Vejle
Denmark*

HJ Armbrecht MD PhD
*Professor of Biochemistry and Molecular Biology
Geriatric Research
Education and Clinical Center
St Louis VA Medical Center
St Louis, MO
and
St Louis University
School of Medicine, MO
USA*

Nikiforos Ballian
*Johns Hopkins University
School of Medicine
USA*

William A Banks MD
*GRECC
VA Medical Center
St Louis, MO
and
Division of Geriatric
Department of Internal Medicine
St Louis University School of Medicine
St Louis, MO
USA*

Martin Bergmann
*Institut fur Veterinär-Anatomie
Histologie und Embryologie
der Justus-Liebig-Universität Giessen
Germany*

Marc R Blackman MD
*National Center for Complementary and
Alternative Medicine
National Institutes of Health
Bethesda, MD
USA*

Laurent Boccon-Gibod MD PhD
*Professor
CHU BICHAT
University of Paris VII
Paris
France*

Steven Boonen MD PhD
*Leuven University Center for
Metabolic Bone Diseases
Katholieke Universiteit Leuven
Belgium*

Simon RJ Bott FRCS
*Trustees of the London Clinic Ltd
London
UK*

Alberto Briganti
*Department of Urology
Vita-Salute University
Milan
Italy*

Gerald B Brock MD FRCSC
St Joseph's Health Centre
London, ON
Canada

Emiro Caicedo MD
University of Minnesota
Minneapolis, MN
USA

Christopher P Cardozo MD
VA Medical Center
Bronx, NY
and
Associate Professor of Medicine
Mount Sinai School of Medicine
New York, NY
USA

Shanon Casperson DTR
Professor
University of Texas Medical Branch
Eralveston, TX
USA

Oscar A Cepeda MD
Fellow, Division of Geriatric Medicine
Department of Internal Medicine
St Louis University School of Medicine
and
GRECC VA Medical Center
St Louis, MO
USA

Richard YT Chen
Associate Consultant (Endocrinology)
Department of Medicine
Changi General Hospital
Singapore

Xi Chen MD PhD
Department of Neurology
St Louis University School of Medicine
St Louis, MO
and
St Louis VA Medical Center
St Louis, MO
USA

Peter Collins MD FRCP FESC
National Heart and Lung Institute
London
UK

David Crook PhD
Senior Research Methodologist
Clinical Investigations and Research Unit
Brighton amd Sussex Universities
Hospital Trust
Brighton
UK

Federico Dehò
Department of Urology
Vita-Salute University
Milan
Italy

Thorsten Diemer
Poliklnik für Urologie und Kinderurologie
Zentrum für Chirurgie
Anästhesiologie und Urologie
Universitätsklinikum Giessen
und
Marburg GmbH
Standort Giessen
Justus-Liebig-Universität Giessen
Germany

Ali R Djalilian MD
National Eye and Health Institute
Bethesda, MD
USA

Hamid R Djalilian MD
UCI Medical Center
University of California
Irvine, CA
USA

Isaak Effendy MD
Department of Dermatology
Municipal Hospital of Bielefeld
Germany

Dariush Elahi MD
Johns Hopkins University
School of Medicine
USA

Andrea Gallina
Department of Urology
Vita-Salute University
Milan
Italy

Spas V Getov
Academic F2 SHO in Stroke Medicine
Brighton and Sussex University Hospitals
UK

Sidney Glina MD PhD
Head of Department of Urology
Hospital Ipiranga
and
Director of Instituto H Ellis
São Paulo
Brazil

Ian F Godsland PhD
Faculty of Medicine
Imperial College London
St Mary's Hospital
London
UK

Louis JG Gooren MD
Professor, Vrjie Universiteit Medical Center
Amsterdam
The Netherlands

George Harris BS

Axel Heidenreich MD
Klinikum der Philipps
Universitat Marburg
Germany

Jerome M Hershman MD
Distinguished Professor of Medicine
David Geffen School of Medicine UCLA
VA Greater Los Angeles
Healthcare System
Los Angels, CA
USA

Rolf Hoffmann MD
Dermaticum
Freiburg
Germany

Michael Horowitz
University of Adelaide
Department of Medicine
Royal Adelaide Hospital
Adelaide
Australia

Seema Joshi MD
St Louis University Medical Center
St Louis, MO
USA

Hosam K Kamel MD MPH
Director, Geriatrics and Extended Care
St Joseph's Mercy Health Center
Hot Springs National Park
Hot Spring, AR
USA

Pierre I Karakiewiz
Cancer Prognostics and Health Outcomes Unit
University of Montreal
Quebec
Canada

Rafi T Kevorkian MD
Assistant Professor
Division of Geriatic Medicine
Department of Internal Medicine
St Louis University School of Medicine
and
GRECC VA Medical Center
St Louis, MO
USA

Roger S Kirby MA MD FRCS (UROL) FEBU
Professor, the Prostate Centre
London
UK

Walter Krause MD
Philipps University Marburg Medical Center
Marburg
Germany

Karen Kuschela
Department of Dermatology
Municipal Hospital of Biekfeld
Biekfeld
Germany

Charles P Lambert PhD
Assistant Professor
University of Arkansas for Medical Sciences
Little Rock, AR
USA

Richard W Lee
Academic F2 SHO in Stroke Medicine
Brighton and Sussex University Hospitals
UK

Kok Bin Lim
Singapore General Hospital
Singapore

Guy Lloyd MD FRCP
East Sussex NHS Trust
UK

Bruno Lunenfeld MD FRCOG FACOG **(Hon)**
Professor Emeritus, Reproductive Endocrinology
Bar-Ilan University
Ramat Gan
Israel

Mahmoud Malas
Johns Hopkins University
School of Medicine
Baltimore, MO
USA

Francesco Montorsi MD
Professor
Department of Urology
Vita-Salute University
Milan
Italy

Alvaro Morales MD
Queen's University General Hospital
Kingston, ON
Canada

John E Morley MB BCH
Divison of Geriatric Medicine
St Louis University School of Medicine
St Louis, MO
and
VA GRECC Medical Center
St Louis, MO
USA

Sergio Musitelli
School of Urology
University of Pavia
Pavia
Italy

Michael Oettel
Professor Dr Med Vet Habil
Jena
Germany

Frank Ondrey MD PhD
University of Minnesota
School of Medicine
Minneapolis, MN
USA

Feliztas Pannier
Dermatology Clinic and Polyclinic
Rheinischen Friedrich Wilhelms Universitat
Bonn
Germany

Giuseppe Paolisso MD
Department of Geriatric Medicine and
Metabolic Diseases
University of Naples
Italy

Michaël Peyromaure MD
Service d'Urologie
Hospital Cochin
Paris
France

Diego Preciado MD PhD
Assistant Professor
George Washington University
School of Medicine
Children's National Medical Center
Washington, DC
USA

Eberhard Rabe MD PhD
Professor of Dermatology
Klinik und Poliklinik für Dermatologie
University of Bonn
Bonn
Germany

C Rajkumar
Chair in Geriatrics and
Stroke Medicine
Brighton and Sussex Medical School
UK

Vincent Ravery MD PhD
Professor
Hospital Bicat
Paris
France

Christopher K Rayner
University of Adelaide
Department of Medicine
Royal Adelaide Hospital
Adelaide
Australia

Andrea Salonia MD
Department of Urology
Vita-Salute University
Milan
Italy

Mary H Samuels MD
Oregon Health and Science University
Portland, OR
USA

Fred Sattler MD
Professor of Medicine and Biokinesiology
Keck School of Medicine
University of Southern California
Los Angeles, CA
USA

Claude C Schulman MD
University Clinics Brussels
Belgium

Dirk Schultheiss

Weiru Shao MD
Director, Division of Otology and Neurotology
Tufts – New England Medical Center
Boston, MA
USA

Melinda Sheffield-Moore PhD
Associate Professor
University of Texas Medical Branch
Galveston, TX
USA

Shirley Shidu Yan MD PhD
Department of Pathology and Surgery
Tranub Institute for Research of
Alzheimer's Disease and Aging Brain
Columbia University
New York, NY
USA

Ann M Spungen PhD
Associate Professor of Medicine and
Rehabilitation Medicine
Mount Sihai School of Medicine
New York, NY
and
Co-chair VA
Cooperative Study
VA Medical Center
Bronx, NY
USA

Syed H Tariq MD FACP
Assistant Professor of Medicine
Division of Geriatic Medicine
St Louis University Medical Center
St Louis, MO
and
GRECC Veterans Affairs Medical Center
St Louis, MO
USA

David R Thomas MD FACP AGSF
Division of Geriatric Medicine
St Louis University Health Sciences Center
St Louis, MO
USA

Ralph Trüeb MD
Department of Dermatology
University of Zurich
Switzerland

Randall J Urban MD
Professor
University of Texas Medical Branch
Galveston, TX
USA

Dirk Vanderschueren MD PhD
Katholieke Universiteit Leuven
Belgium

Alex Vermeulen MD
Professor Emeritus
University Hospital Ghent
Belgium

Adrian Wagg FRCP
Senior Lecturer in Geriatric Medicine
University College London Hospital
UK

Carolyn M Webb PhD
Cardiac Medicine
National Heart and Lung Institute
Imperial College School of Medicine
London
UK

Wolfgang Weidner MD
Direktor der Klinik und Poliklnik
für Urologie und Kinderurologie
Zentrum für Chirurgie
Anästhesiologie und Urologie
Universitätsklinikum Giessen und
Marburg GmbH
Standort Giessen
Justus-Liebig-Universität Giessen
Germany

Michael John Wheeler
Professor
Department of Chemical Pathology
Guy's and St Thomas Foundation Trust
St Thomas Hospital
London
UK

Margaret-Mary G Wilson MD MRCP
Division of Geriatric Medicine
St Louis University
St Louis, MO
USA

Gary A Wittert
Mortlock Professor of Medicine and Head
Department of Medicine
University of Adelaide
Royal Adelaide Hospital
Adelaide
Australia

Giuseppe Zanni
Department of Urology
Vita-Salute University
Milan
Italy

Foreword

This a long road knows no turning (Sophokles: Ajax)

In the 'sleepwalkers' (1964) Arthur Koestler remarks that 'I mistrust the word progress and much prefer the word evolution simply because progress, by definition, can never go wrong, whereas evolution constantly does and so does the evolution of the ideas'. Indeed, it is fascinating to observe throughout history the evolution of quite a few 'ruling' ideas, moving from gradual acceptance, to popularization, vulgarization, overextension, collapse and disappearance. At the height of their importance, some of them are so generally accepted, that they become the *spirit of the time* (the famous *'Zeitgeist'* in German) with all of its societal consequences, masterfully characterized by Virginia Woolf (1929) saying that 'what is amusing now had to be taken in desperate earnest once'. Other ideas may show a markedly different evolution; as Jean Monnet (1978) emphasized in his Mémoires, 'When an idea corresponds to the necessity of an epoch, it ceases to belong to those who invented it and it becomes stronger than those who are in charge of it'. In fact, such an idea may become stronger than political power by developing into the common property of humankind; it may deeply influence the spiritual content of an entire era and may resist the historical forces of destruction for a long time. In a few, rare, cases a new idea becomes exceptionally strong, when – in addition – it is generated as a response to powerful historical challenges by some new realities. The aging of populations presents such a challenge. It is a fundamentally new and unique problem in our history, with no previous analogies. Hence, people and their governments have not had yet enough time (and/or courage?) to consider the necessary – and in part fundamental – socioeconomical and political adjustments needed to meet one of the greatest challenges of the 21st century, which will profoundly affect many aspects of our life, social institutions and perhaps even ethical values. The Population division of the United Nations Secretariat estimates that last year (2006) some 11% of the global population (688 million persons) were aged 60 years or more and 13% of these persons were aged 80 years and over. The sex ratio of those aged 60 and over was 82 men for 100 women and among those aged 80 years and more it was 55 men for 100 women. Life expectancy at the age of 60 was 17 years for men and 21 years for women. The Population division projects that by the year 2050, 22% of the world population (or almost 2 billion people) will be aged 60 years and over and that 20% of these 2 billion persons will be aged 80 years or more. The United Nations also point out that, by the year 2050 – for the first time in our history – the population of persons older than 60 years will be larger than the population of children (0 to 14 years of age). Humankind is growing rapidly and it is aging very rapidly... Fortunately, scientific knowledge is growing even more rapidly. In 1830, Alfred Tennyson still could say with some justification that 'Science moves, but slowly slowly, creeping on from point to point'. However, by the mid-1950s it was recognized, that science progresses in proportion to the mass of knowledge that is left to it by preceding generations, that is under the most ordinary circumstances in geometrical proportion (F. Engels, 1963). The same year Derek John de Solla Price has put this progress in a proper perspective: 'Using any reasonable definition of a scientist, we can say that between 80 and 90 per cent of all scientists that have ever lived are alive now. Now depending on what one measures and how, the crude size of science in manpower or in publications tends to double within a period of 10 to 15 years'. This was 44 years ago and nowadays it is often said that today the amount of new information tends to double every 6 to 7 years.... And when the amount of new information increases so rapidly, the perimeter between the known and unknown also increases and opens new avenues for fruitful investigation. If I am allowed to quote another foreword written more than 400 years ago, in the Preface to De La Sagesse, Pierre Charron remarks that '*La vraye science et le vray étude de l'homme c'est l'homme*' (The true science and study of mankind is man). This will particularly be true in the world of tomorrow, where the octagenarian populations will grow most rapidly of all groups and lots of new information will be required on their pathophysiology and optimal medical care. It is said that Leonardo da Vinci was the last scientist in history, who still could grasp the entire body of knowledge of his epoch. I doubt very much that there exists any medical scientist today, who could claim to grasp all medical knowledge, or even that of any major discipline, the Study of the Aging Male being no exception. It is sufficient to look at a few of the almost 60 excellent articles of the present textbook to be convinced. *Science is organized knowledge*, said Herbert Spencer; therefore, a textbook will always represent an important contribution to the body of contemporary knowledge, particularly, when it contains so many carefully selected articles, as the present textbook. In fact, when the perimeter between the known and unknown rapidly increases, it inevitably results in increasing specialization and in the establishment of new disciplines. The establishment of a new discipline for the Study of the Aging Male slightly more than a decade ago, was considered then by some medical scientists as a courageous innovation with a somewhat uncertain future. Few, if any of them would doubt today that this discipline has come to stay and for a long time, since more and more evidence is forthcoming to indicate that many aspects of aging are gender specific, like the localization of certain receptors in different tissues or the functions of the blood–brain barrier. Therefore, an in-depth study of the various aspects of gender specificity is likely to lead to improved diagnostic and therapeutic methods for aging populations. Therefore, as Shakespeare says '*What is past is prologue*'. Last, but not least, I feel that the scientific community ought to be grateful to the editors and contributors of this textbook. Their effort should remind us that the acquisition, critical evaluation, systematization and dissemination of positive knowledge are the only human activities which are truly cumulative and progressive (George Sarton, 1930, paraphrased).

Egon Diczfalusy MD PhD
Professor Emeritus, Karolinska
Institutet, Stockholm, Sweden

Preface

This second edition of Textbook of Men's Health and Aging breaks new ground in the medical care and management of men, particularly as they progress through the inevitable aging process. Whilst women's health care has been specific focus of scientific and clinical attention for more than a century, comparatively little attention has been given to the gender-specific needs of men. Of course, certain specialties-urology in particular- have focused on men, but there has been very little recognition that the bodily, endocrinological, psychological and changes that take place in male physiology throughout life have an impact on men's health that warrants and requires an integrated understanding and approach to medical management.

The International Society for the Study of the Aging Male was formed in 1998 to increase clinical awareness of this need and to encourage gender-specific research and practice designed to improve the medical care of men from maturity to old age. Since its foundation more than 8 years ago, the development of the Society has been meteoric. It has established a peer-review journal for the field and has organized a series of Regional, Local and World Congresses. In addition, not only has it attracted a rapidly growing world-wide membership but it has encouraged the development of a number of local, national societies affiliated to it – and this process if continuing apace.

This new edition of our textbook is the latest initiative of the International Society for the Study of the Aging Male. It represents an attempt to draw together relevant gender-specific knowledge across the whole field of men's health and to establish the outline of a curriculum for those clinicians concerned to develop their knowledge of, and expertise in, the subject. The range of topics covered by the textbook is wide; musculoskeletal disorders, cardiovascular disease, conditions related to testosterone deficiency, endocrine disease, the metabolic syndrome, obesity, central nervous system and cognitive disorders, genitourinary problems, sensory organ degeneration, gastroenterology, dermatology and other age-realted conditions are all discussed by an impressive international team of expert contributors. The book does, therefore, provide a unique overview of male health as an entity and offers valuable insights for improved management and clinical care.

Of course, this is only the start of an ongoing process of education and development but it is very important start. It is hoped that this volume will provide a foundation from which clinicians in many parts of the world can develop their own studies and which will also provide a basic framework from which specialist courses and learning programs can be planned and developed.

New and expanded editions of this textbook are envisaged on a regular basis and with each edition we hope to expand it coverage and depth, based on the practical experience gained from the use of each new volume. In due course we hope to provide a fully tested and truly comprehensive clinical guide that will serve the ongoing needs of all clinicians anxious to expand their knowledge of this gender-specific field. This second edition does, therefore, represent a major milestone in the important road that lies ahead.

Bruno Lunenfeld

History of research on the aging male – selected aspects

Michael Oettel, Sergio Musitelli, and Dirk Schultheiss

Doubtless, in all periods of the history of mankind the possibility of prolonging the life of the man including the preservation of his masculinity has claimed more attention than the treatment and/or cure of, e.g., specific infectious, cardiovascular, mental, or tumor diseases. This interest was also often greater than the impetus to find new ways for the treatment of women's diseases – at least in patriarchal periods. In early primitive civilizations, erotic matters including those of aging males were of prime importance and became an integral part of life. According to Hippocrates, old men suffer from difficulty in breathing, catarrh accompanied by coughing, strangury, difficult micturition, pains at the joints, kidney diseases, dizziness, apoplexy, cachexia, pruritus of the whole body, sleeplessness, watery discharges from the bowels, eyes and nostrils, dullness of sight, cataract, and hardness of hearing.[1]

The history of research on elderly men's health reflects most parts of the broad cultural history and, therefore, an attempt to press this field into only one chapter of a textbook is at the beginning an act of despair. Additionally, the story of the 'fountain of youth' for males is also the story of wrong ways, blind alleys, hasty speculations, and of charlatanism. Christian Wilhelm Hufeland (1762–1836) characterized the unsuccessful attempts to prolong life simply as 'gerontokomic'. Furthermore, describing our item in ancient times we are often unable to distinguish between historic facts, mysticisms, and mythologic or religious interpretations.

Here we can discuss and reflect only selected historic aspects pronouncing the endocrinologic background of hypogonadism and testosterone therapy. For more historic details, see references 1 to 14.

Obviously, the highly sophisticated molecular pharmacology of androgen action substantially improved our knowledge of the molecular biology of endogenous signal systems in the second half of the last century. Nevertheless, there is still a certain suspicion in some quarters about androgen therapy. Why should that be so? A look at the history of testosterone therapy in aging men shows remarkable scientific achievements, but often, however, also a great deal of speculation and many dubious practices. Already John Hunter (1728–1793) performed testicular transplantation experiments while studying tissue transplantation techniques in 1767 and, almost a century later, Arnold Berthold (1801–1863) linked the physiologic and behavioral changes of castration to a substance secreted by the testes. He wrote in 1849[15] 'Da nun aber an fremden Stellen transplantierte Hoden mit ihren ursprünglichen Nerven nicht mehr in Verbindung stehen können, und da es, …, keine specifischen, der Secretion vorstehenden Nerven giebt, so folgt, dass der fragliche Consensus durch das productive Verhältnis der Hoden, d.h. durch deren Einwirkung auf das Blut, und dann durch entsprechende Einwirkung des Blutes auf den allgemeinen Organismus überhaupt, …, bedingt wird.' Summarizing transplanted testes affect behavioral and sexual

1

characteristics by secreting a substance into the bloodstream.

Aging as an endocrine disorder?

The earliest contribution of modern medicine to the understanding of the clinical features of a disorder related to the beginning of aging was the article 'On the climacteric disease' by Sir Henry Halford, which was read at the Royal College of Physicians in London in 1813:[16] '... I will venture to question, whether it be not, in truth, a disease rather than a mere declension of strength and decay of the natural powers.' He seems to be the first to connect the term climacteric with the symptoms observed in some men between the ages of 50 and 75: 'Sometimes the disorder comes on so gradually and insensibly, that the patient is hardly aware of its commencement. He perceives that he is sooner tired than usual, and that he is thinner than he was; but yet he has nothing material to complain of. In process of time his appetite becomes seriously impaired: his nights are sleepless, or if he gets sleep, he is not refreshed by it. His face becomes visibly extenuated, or perhaps acquires a bloated look. His tongue is white, and he suspects that he has fever.' Halford pointed out that this disease had been overlooked so far: 'We find it generally complicated with other complaints, assuming their character, and accompanying them in their course, and perhaps this may be the reason why we do not find the climacteric disease described in books of nosology as a distinct and particular distemper.' Interestingly, concerning the etiology of this climacteric disease, he drew no connection to the testes: 'It is not very improbable that this important change in the condition of the constitution is connected with a deficiency in the energy of the brain itself, and an irregular supply of the nervous influence to the heart.' The therapeutic options were rather limited. 'In fact, I have nothing to offer with confidence, in that view, beyond a caution that the symptoms of the disease be not met by too active a treatment.' And, after suggesting 'local evacuations' and 'warm purgatives', Halford came to the conclusion: 'For the rest, "the patient must minister to himself".'

'To be able to contemplate with complacency either issue of a disorder which the great Author of our being may, in his kindness, have intended as a warning to us to prepare for a better existence, is of prodigious advantage to recovery, as well as to comfort, and the retrospect of a well-spent life is a cordial of infinitely more efficacy than all resources of the medical art.' And this was just the opinion of the 90-year-old Cephalus at the very beginning of the dialogue 'The Republic' of Plato (428–348 BC).

For unknown reasons, the term climacteric was not used again in relation to the aging male for more than 100 years, although the problem in general was discussed by other scientists, as demonstrated, for example, in the studies of Charles Edouard Brown-Séquard (see below). The French physician Maurice de Fleury reactivated the topic in 1909 with his contribution 'Sur le retour d'âge de l'homme,' a condition detected in males 'de quarante et quelques années.'[17] In addition to the clinical symptoms, he found significant changes in the genital organs of women. The thyroid gland was the main cause of the disease in men: 'Pourtant, il est une autre glande à secretion interne qui me paraît jouer un role dans la genèse de ce faux retour d'âge: je veux parler de la thyroid'.

In July 1910, Archibald Church, professor of nervous and mental diseases in Chicago, Illinois, USA, published his article on 'Nervous and mental disturbances of the male climacteric', not citing any of the above-mentioned works.[18] On the other hand, he gave a detailed review of the literature dealing with the issue of certain symptoms that might occur in a 'monthly rhythm in men', e.g. variations in weight and temperature, frequency of nocturnal emissions, hemorrhoidal flux, or attacks of cardiac asthma. He even refers to the earlier 'Selected papers on hysteria' of Sigmund Freud, who wrote 'There are men who show a climacterium like woman, and merge into an anxiety neurosis at the time when their potency diminishes.' Church continues with his own description of symptoms observed over 10 years at the 'involutional or climacteric period' of his patients between the ages of 50 and 65: 'the particular interest of my subject does not pertain to the insanities, but to minor psychoses and neurotic disturbances. These, one and all, however, have mental background.'

In October 1910, the German physician Kurt Mendel[19] and, in response to Mendel's article, Bernard Hollander[20] from England both published articles entitled 'Die Wechseljahre des Mannes (Climacterium virile),' claiming that they were also aware of this clinical entity and had treated patients over the last decade. Mendel's father, a well-known university professor of neurology, had already used the term when dealing with such in his lectures. Although Mendel and Hollander approached the problem from the point of view of neurologists, they both agreed that the involution of the testes is the main pathomechanism responsible for the climacteric disease that can then be influenced by other factors:[19] 'Sehe ich somit die Hypofunktion der Keimdrüsen als Grundursache des beschriebenen Krankheitsbildes an, so können daneben aber andere Momente in Betracht kommen, die als mitwirkende Faktoren bei Auslösung und Entwicklung des Leidens anzusprechen sind.' Despite organotherapy with 'Spermin' and unspecific treatments like cold showers and faradization of the body, Mendel suggested psychotherapy as the preferable and most successful therapeutic modality. Furthermore, he discussed some forensic aspects of the climacteric in males. As is the case with women, a higher rate of criminal acts – mainly consisting of insults towards others – is to be expected in the sixth decade of man's life and this circumstance should be kept in mind by medical experts who are asked for their professional opinion in court.

In 1916, the dermatologist and sexologist Max Marcuse from Berlin drew a connection between the 'climacterium virile' and some urosexual disturbances or changes of the prostate making his work of special interest to urologists.[21] In most of his patients he detected an involuted small and soft prostate, a status he called 'Prostata-Atonie'. In several cases, he successfully applied either organotherapy with 'Testikulin', 'Testogan', and 'Hormin', or faradization of the prostate.

Two examples of comprehensive monographies on the topic written in German are 'Über den Mann von 50 Jahren' by FK Wenckebach[22] in 1915 and 'Die Wechseljahre des Mannes' by A Hoche[23] in 1928. According to Hoche, in the sixth decade of life a deep decline in psychic and physical fitness occurs in men. In this period, for example, poets, writers, and musicians have passed their zenith. Well known exceptions are Joseph Haydn, who composed 'The Creation' at 66 and 'The Seasons' at 68 years of age, and Konrad Ferdinand Meyer and Theodor Fontane, who in their sixth and seventh decades, respectively, reached the top of their artistic work. Hoche concluded that a true male climacteric doesn't exist, but men aged between 40 and 60 years show many typical natural as well as pathologic changes, which need mainly psychologic or psychiatric care. According to Diepgen (cited by Hoche[23]) the term 'Wechseljahre' (changing years for turn of life) is exemplified in German literature in the 17th and 18th centuries.

August Werner from St Louis, USA, re-introduced the term male climacteric (from the Greek for 'rung of a ladder') in the late 1930s and today his name is still associated with it by most authors. In 1939, Werner suggested the following theoretic background for this clinical condition:[24] 'it seems reasonable to believe that many if not all men pass through a climacteric period somewhat similar to that of women, usually in a less severe but perhaps more prolonged form … . The endocrine dysfunction, plus the imbalance of equilibrium between the two divisions of the autonomic nervous system, with evidence at times of disturbance in psychic centres, is the climacteric. The true climacteric is due primarily to decline of function of the sex glands. Decline of sex function is not limited to women but is also a heritage of all men.'[25,26]

Testosterone and the aging male

Throughout history, many concepts have been suggested and practiced to achieve eternal youth, longevity, and rejuvenation. To point out only one example, one might think of the biblical case (Kings, III, 1, 3 ff) of King David, who was old in years and showed a significant loss of 'heat'. A young virgin was chosen to compensate this deficit: … 'and let her lie in thy bosom, that my lord the king may get heat'. As the name of this virgin was Abhisag the Sunamite, the method of bringing an aged man in close contact with a young woman was, henceforth, called 'sunamitism' and this idea was kept up among many others until recent centuries and is still an attractive option of machismo for the future of mankind.[27]

Tales and myths about aphrodisiacs and rejuvenation extracts from testicular tissue or blood were reported from ancient times up to the present. As early as 140 BC Suçruta of India advocated the ingestion of testis tissue for the cure of impotence. A vague foreshadow of the endocrine function of the testis was speculated by Aretaeus of Cappadocia (2nd to 3rd century AD) and more vigorously in 1775 by de Bordeu. They proposed that each organ of the body produced a substance, which was secreted into the blood to regulate bodily function.[28]

With the birth of modern endocrinology in the 19th century, the testes and, later, their identified hormonal product testosterone increasingly attracted the interest of scientists who were investigating the aging process. The first considerations regarding the relationship between hormone production and the aging process stemmed from the French neurologist Charles Edouard Brown-Séquard (1817–94), the son of a Philadelphia seaman, giving rise to the field of organotherapy. In 1869 he suggested injecting semen into the blood of old men in order to increase mental and physical strength and performed the first animal experiments 6 years later. His famous self-experiment at the age of 72 with several subcutaneous injections of a mixture of blood from the testicular veins, semen, and juice extracted from crushed testicles of young and vigorous dogs and guinea pigs in 1889 was one of the first milestones for androgen therapy in the aging male. He reported an increase in his physical and mental abilities, a better stream of urine and the relief of constipation. Brown-Séquard had inspired physicians around the world to investigate the nature of this compound, and by the end of 1889 over 12 000 physicians were administering this new 'elixir of life'.[29] Nevertheless, Brown-Séquard's 'pharmaceutic' prescription must have been equivalent to a placebo.[27,30,31] The following passage on 'seminal losses', a condition Brown-Séquard also called 'spermatic anemia', and which was generally better known as 'spermatorrhea', reveals the limited understanding of testicular endocrinology at that time:[30] 'Besides, it is well known that seminal losses, arising from any cause, produce a mental and physical debility which is in proportion to their frequency. These facts and many others have led to the generally admitted view that in the seminal fluid, as secreted by the testicles, a substance or several substances exist which, entering the blood by resorption, have a most essential use in giving strength to the nervous system and to other parts.' Arthur Biedl,[32] the author of the first textbook on internal secretory organs in 1910 categorically states that: 'The date of birth of "the science of internal secretion" is that memorable meeting of the Société de Biologie of Paris of June 1st 1889, where Brown-Séquard, then 72 years of age reported on his experiments undertaken to prove his hypothesis by means of subcutaneous injections of testicular juice into himself.'

In 1902, Ancel and Bouin in France ligated the ductus deferens in rabbits and noted atrophy of the seminal epithelium. However, the Leydig cells remained unchanged, and many of the animals appeared to have increased sexual activity.[33] This paved the way for Eugen Steinach (1861–1944) in Vienna. This physiologist started conducting experiments with testicular transplantation in animals at the turn of the century in order to study the sexual differentiation and the hormonal function of the gonads. In this theory of 'autoplastic' treatment of aging, he postulated an increased increatory hormonal production following the cessation of the secretory output of the gonads after surgical ligation of the seminal ducts.[34] The basic idea was that ligature of the spermatic ducts leads to an atrophy of the seminal epithelium and (hopefully) to hypertrophy of the Leydig cells. The first operation was performed in 1918 and resulted in a worldwide vasoligation boom over the next two decades. Steinach nicely summarized the results of his scientific life in his late biography:[35] 'It has frequently been said that a man is as old as his blood vessels. One may have greater justification for saying that a man is as old as his endocrine glands.'

Early in his career, the Russian Serge Voronoff (1866–1951), working in Paris and elsewhere, discussed the life expectancy and signs of aging in castrates. He was one of the first to transplant testicular tissue from a monkey into a human testicle in 1920. He later became the world's leading surgeon to transplant testicular tissue from ape to man.[36] But AS Parkes remembered as follows: 'This attractive idea was naturally exploited in dubious ways, and early in the period under review Voronoff, working in Algiers, became notorious for his so-called rejuvenation experiments on man and farm animals. His claims were such that an international deputation visited his establishment in Algiers in 1927 to make a critical review of the work. The report of the British contingent to the Ministry of Agriculture was very cautious.'[37]

At the same time, several American surgeons performed testicular transplantations (or rather, implantations), such as Victor D Lespinasse, Robert T Morris, Leo L Stanley, John R Brinkley, and George F Lydston.[38] Victor Lespinasse, Professor of Genitourinary Surgery at North-Western University, treated impotence by oral glandular extracts. When this failed, Lespinasse grafted slices of human testicles taken from fresh cadavers into the rectus muscle of impotent men. He believed that most cases of impotence in middle-aged men were caused by a failure of hormone secretion, and reported positive results after several weeks, athough these were transient.[39]

Leo Stanley, a physician working at the San Quentin Prison in California, performed 1000 testicular substance implantations into 656 prisoners under his care. Unlike Lespinasse, Stanley used the testicles of goats, rams, boars, or deer. He cut the testicles into strips of such a size that he could put them into a pressure syringe for injection under the skin of the abdomen. He reported a marked improvement in impotence.[40]

A rejuvenation boom took place in the early 1920s with both vasoligation and testis implantation, which were performed by many doctors in Europe and America.[4,27] The Swiss genito-urinary surgeon Paul Niehans (1882–1971) claimed to have performed more than 50 000 'cellular therapy' treatments. He envisioned the replacement of organ transplantation by the injection of viable cells.[4,41]

All these hormonal approaches to rejuvenation were made before the discovery of testosterone or the supply of suitable androgen products by the pharmaceutic industry. Is it true, that they are all completely out of date now? Machluf and co-workers[42] reported on the microencapsulation of Leydig cells as a system for testosterone supplementation in the future. And could stem cell technology be the modern version of 'organotherapy' or 'cellular therapy'?

The identification and chemical synthesis of testosterone and other steroid hormones was achieved in the 1930s.[43] This was a 'condition sine qua non' for the further development of modern endocrinology and the basis for a rational therapy with sexual hormones. Only with the introduction of high-quality testosterone preparations did it become possible to provide a scientific basis for androgen therapy.

As defined traditionally, an androgen is a substance that stimulates the growth of the male reproductive tract. It is important to realize that this is a biologic and not a chemical definition. Nonetheless, the most potent androgens are steroids. It has been proved to be a difficult challenge in steroid chemistry to isolate, characterize, and synthesize the male hormones.[44]

Pezard, in 1912, reported that aqueous extract of pig testes maintained the comb and wattles of the capon.[28] Eighteen years later, Gallagher and Koch developed the response in the capon into a quantitative assay procedure, which was adopted with minor modifications by most laboratories as the standard assay procedure for male hormone activity.[45]

As early as 1927, Lemuel Clyde McGee[46] demonstrated the isolation of a biologically active extract of the lipid fraction of bull testicles. In 1933 McCullagh and co-workers[47] reported in a very elegant paper, using the chick comb assay for measuring androgenic activity, that extracts from blood, urine, or spinal fluid of men are useful for the treatment of male hypogonadism. The authors called the substance which is produced in the testes 'androtin'. The magnitude of the problem faced by steroid chemists has been illustrated by the fact that labor-intensive extracts from up to 100 g of testes were required for a positive result in the so-called chick comb bioassay.[2,48] It is not surprising, therefore, that 15 mg of the first known androgen – androsterone – was isolated under the leadership of Adolf Butenandt, at the age of 28 years, from 15 000–25 000 liters of policemen's urine in 1931.[49,50] The name of this relatively weak urinary 5α-reduced androgen comes from 'andro' = male, 'ster' = sterol, and 'one' = ketone. The chemical synthesis of androsterone was performed by Leopold Ruzicka and co-workers 3 years later.[51] The Japanese workers Ogata and Hirano,[52] not sufficiently acknowledged by the Europeans and Americans, found in 1934 that the androgen from the urine (Butenandt's androsterone) was not identical with the androgen extracted from boar testes. The androgenic properties of this crystal hormone were more active than any of the testicular preparations previously reported. One year later, Karoly David, Elizabeth Dingemanse, Janos Freud, and Ernst Laqueur[53] reported the isolation of testosterone, the main secretory product from the testes and the main androgen in the blood, from several tonnes of bull testes. The term 'testosterone', coined by this Dutch group, combines 'testo' = testes, 'ster' = sterol, and 'one' = ketone. In the same year, the chemical synthesis of testosterone was published by three groups from Germany, the Netherlands, and Switzerland, led by Adolf Butenandt,[54] Ernst Laqueur,[53] and Leopold Ruzicka.[55] Ruzicka and Butenandt were offered the 1939 Nobel Prize for chemistry for their work, but Butenandt was forced by the Nazi government to decline the honor.

Adolf Butenandt wrote in 1941:[56] 'Die heute synthetisch zubereiteten Hormone sind den natürlichen Wirkstoffen nicht nur ähnlich, sondern mit ihnen … identisch; sie stellen demnach keine Kunstprodukte dar im Sinne körperfremder Pharmaka mit hormonartiger Wirkung, sondern natürliche, körpereigene Wirkstoffe. Daher bedeutet die Behandlung eines Kranken mit den heute von der pharmazeutischen Industrie dargebotenen Hormonen eine Therapie auf natürlicher Basis.' [The hormones synthesized today are not only similar to the naturally occurring drug substances, but are identical with … them; they are therefore not artificial products in the sense of exogenous pharmaceuticals with hormone-like action, but rather natural, endogenous substances. Thus, the treatment of a patient with the hormones now offered by the pharmaceutical industry means a treatment on a natural basis.] Is this point of view still applicable today? Is the administration of

testosterone to men an effective natural form of treatment without serious side-effects? This question will be answered by some of the authors of this textbook.

Heller and Myers[57] demonstrated that climacteric symptoms of men could be reversed by testosterone propionate therapy. They utilized a quasi-placebo trial to demonstrate this effect. Using the rat ovary-weight assay the authors demonstrated elevated gonadotropin concentrations in the urine of climacteric men.

In 1946 Werner[25] presented detailed results of the evaluation of 273 climacteric male patients. The most prominent symptoms were nervousness, decreased potency, decreased libido, irritability, fatigue, depression, memory problems, sleep disturbances, numbness, tingling, and hot flushes. Of these patients, 177 were treated with intramuscular testosterone propionate injections, only four of whom did not benefit from the treatment. Werner's summary is convincing: 'Men are subject to the hypogonadal or climacteric syndrome, just as women, when there is decrease of function or a function of the sexual glands. Testosterone propionate is as effective in relieving the subjective symptoms of this syndrome in men as estrogen is in relieving the symptoms of similar origin in women. Sex hormones should not be administered to men and women of climacteric age with the idea of stimulating increased sexual potency; if this is the object of treatment, disappointment will result in the great majority of instances.'

One of the earliest long-term experiences with testosterone therapy came from the writer Ernest Hemingway. He took testosterone for the last decade of his life, providing us with one of the longest patient histories for testosterone administration.[58]

In the first years after testosterone became available, an overgenerous application of this new therapeutic option to the problem of the 'climacteric in the aging male', was hinted at by an editorial in the *Journal of the American Medical Association* in 1942:[59] 'Recently many reports have appeared in medical journals claiming that a climacteric occurs in middle aged men. Brochures circulated by pharmaceutical manufacturers depict the woeful course of aging man. None too subtly these brochures recommend that male hormonal substance, like a veritable elixir of youth, may prevent or compensate for the otherwise inevitable decline. What of the postulated occurrence of a climacteric in men?'. The answer came from the author in the same editorial: 'Androgens exert a tonic and stimulating action, associated perhaps with their metabolic effects. Male hormones provide replacement therapy in castrates but are also active in normal middle aged men beset by aging processes which are in some large proportion irrespective of testicular function. Androgens may influence quite harmfully the physiologic and psychologic condition of previously well adjusted elderly men, as has been observed incidental to the trial use of male hormone substances in the treatment of benign hypertrophy of the prostate. Actual evaluation of androgenic treatment cannot be avoided by glib explanation that men normally undergo a spontaneous climacteric, an abruptly occurring state of primary testicular insufficiency in which male hormones act as substitutional therapy'.

The problem of hypogonadism of the aging man starts with the definition. A lot of synonyms often represent a certain unsteadiness in the scientific community. At present, we have the following synonyms:

- changing years, or change of life, or (in German) 'Wechseljahre'
- andropause
- male climacteric or climacterium virile
- androgen decline in aging males (ADAM)
- partial androgen decline in aging males (PADAM)
- acquired male hypogonadism
- late onset hypogonadism.

For a critical statement about testosterone therapy see reference 60. The story of testosterone is unending. Astonishingly, the first paper describing the conversion of testosterone to the powerful key metabolite 5α-dihydrotestosterone (DHT) in vitro and in vivo was not submitted until 32 years after the identification of testosterone.[48] It was not until two decades later that the groups led by Liao,[61,62] Wilson,[63,64] Brinkmann,[65] and McPhaul,[66] succeeded in characterizing and expressing a cDNA encoding the human androgen receptor.

It is also interesting to note that the indications and contraindications for testosterone change with time, and that in some cases the opinions of the old pioneers are reappearing in new clothes. For example, by 1937 testosterone therapy was being recommended for the treatment of benign prostatic hyperplasia (BPH)[67] and was also state of the art in the 1950s.[68] Thereafter, BPH – at least in the obstructive stages – was to become one of the contraindications for androgens.[69] Today, testosterone administration for BPH treatment is being revisited.[70] Also, it is well accepted that prostate cancer is an absolute contraindication for testosterone treatment.[71] Nevertheless, recent papers show that low levels of androgens in serum or prostate are correlated with higher prostate cancer aggressiveness.[72,73] Richmond Prehn speculated about the prevention and therapy of prostate cancer by androgen administration.[74] The treatment of erectile dysfunction (ED) by testosterone is another example. After initial euphoria in the middle of the last century, testosterone administration later became a malpractice. Now, the combination therapy of ED by PDE5 inhibitors together with testosterone is step by step and in some circumstances preferred.[75]

Outlook

To summarize, the scientific work on aging and the accompanying sexual and reproductive aspects often led to breakthroughs in medicine, as can be seen in original approaches in genetics, molecular biology, biochemistry, endocrinology, andrology, urology, pharmaceutic developments, and gerontology as well as in geriatrics. Therefore the basic idea of Vergil (70–19 BC), which was pronounced by the Russian writer Iwan S Turgenjew (1818–83) to be 'finding the future by discovery of the past'[76] can also be used for research on the aging male. However it is astonishing that research work on the aging male from antiquity until the first half of the 20th century was for a long time more or less forgotten, with the result that today the highlights from the past pioneering age have to be defended in comparison to modern 'trendy' approaches – and unfortunately not vice versa!

References

1. Musitelli S. The aging male in the literature. Aging Male 2001; 4: 170–87.
2. Tausk M. The emergence of endocrinology. In: Parnham MJ, Bruinvels J, eds. Discoveries in Pharmacology, Vol 2. Haemodynamics, Hormones and Inflammation. London: Elsevier Science Publishers, 1984: 219–49, 307–20.
3. Kochakian CD. How it was. Anabolic action of steroids and remembrances. The University of Alabama School of Medicine, 1984.
4. Schultheiss D, Denil J, Jonas U. Rejuvenation in the early 20th century. Andrologia 1997; 29: 351–5.
5. Schultheiss D, Bloom DA, Wefer J, Jonas U. Tissue engineering from Adam to the zygote: historical reflections. World J Urol 2000; 18: 84–90.
6. Schultheiss D, Jonas U, Musitelli S. Some historical reflections in the ageing male. World J Urol 2002; 20: 40–4.
7. Schultheiss D, Musitelli S, Stief CG, Jonas U, eds. Classical Writings on Erectile Dysfunction. An Annotated Collection of Original Texts from Three Millennia. Berlin: ABW Wissenschaftsverlag, 2005.
8. Isidori A. Storia dell'andrologia moderna. Medicina nei secoli arte e scienza. 2001; 13: 255–68.
9. Musitelli S, Gerokomikón. A brief survey of the history of geriatrics from creation to the 16th century. Aging Male 2002; 5: 181–98.
10. Musitelli S. The aging male in the Old Testament. Aging Male 2003; 6: 110–18.
11. Musitelli S. History and philosophy. Senility, illness and death on Açvaghosa's 'Buddhacárăta' (The Feats of Buddha). Aging Male 2003; 6: 264–74.
12. Musitelli S. History and philosophy. Welcome born-again Dr Faust! Aging Male 2004; 7: 170–83.
13. Marandola P, MusitelliS, Noseda R et al. Love and sexuality in aging. Aging Male 2002; 5: 103–13.
14. Morley JE. A brief history of geriatrics. J Gerontology 2004; 59A: 1132–52.
15. Berthold AA. Transplantation der Hoden. Arch Anat Physiol Wiss Med 1849; 16: 42–6.
16. Halford H. On the climacteric disease. Med Transact 1813; 4: 316–28.
17. De Fleury. Sur le retour d'àge de l'homme. Bull Acad Med Paris 1909; 62: 311–19.
18. Church A. Nervous and mental disturbances of the male climacteric. JAMA 1910; 55: 301–3.
19. Mendel K. Die Wechseljahre des Mannes (Climacterium virile). Neurol Zentralbl 1910; 29: 1124–46.
20. Hollander B. Die Wechseljahre des Mannes (Climacterium virile). Neurol Zentralbl 1910; 29: 1282–6.
21. Marcuse M. Zur Kenntnis des Climacterium virile, insbesondere über urosexuelle Störungen und Veränderungen der Prostata bei ihm. Neurol Zentralbl 1916; 35: 577–91.
22. Wenckebach FK. Über den Mann von 50 Jahren. Perles, Wien, 1915.
23. Hoche A. Die Wechseljahre des Mannes. Springer, Berlin, 1928.
24. Werner AA. The male climacteric. JAMA 1939; 112: 1441–3.
25. Werner AA. The male climacteric: report of two hundred and seventy-three cases. JAMA 1946; 132: 188–94.
26. Morley JE, Perry HM. Androgen treatment of male hypogonadism in older males. J Steroid Biochem Mol Biol 2003; 85: 367–73.
27. Trimmer EJ. Rejuvenation: the history of an idea. Robert Hale, London, 1967.
28. Kochakian CD. History, chemistry and pharmacodynamics of anabolic-androgenic steroids. Wien Med Wschr 1993; Heft 14/15: 359–63.
29. Hansen B. New images of a new medicine: visual evidence for the widespread popularity of therapeutic discoveries in America after 1885. Bull Hist Med 1999; 73: 629–78.
30. Brown-Séquard CE. The effects produced on man by subcutaneous injection of a liquid obtained from the testicles of animals. Lancet 1889; 137: 105–7.
31. Cussons AJ, Bhagat CI, Fletcher SJ, Walsh JP. Brown-Séquard revisited. A lesson from history on the placebo effect of androgen treatment. Med J Aust 2002; 177: 678–9.
32. Biedl A. Innere Sekretion. Urban und Schwarzenberg, Berlin, Wien, 1910.
33. Massaglia AC. The internal secretion of the testis. Endocrinology 1920; 4: 547–66.
34. Steinach E. Verjüngung durch experimentelle Neubelebung der alternden Pubertätsdrüse. Springer, Berlin, 1920.
35. Steinach E. Sex and Life: Forty Years of Biological and Medical Experiments. Faber and Faber, London, 1940.
36. Voronoff S. Testicular Grafting from Ape to Man. Brentanos, London, 1920.
37. Parkes AS. The rise of reproductive endocrinology 1926–1940. J Endocrinol 1965; 34: xx–xxxii.
38. Schultheiss D, Engel RM. G. Frank Lydston (1858–1923) revisited: androgen therapy by testicular implantation in the early twentieth century. Worl J Urol 2003; 21: 356–63.
39. Lespinasse VD. Transplantation of the testicle. JAMA 1913; 61: 1869–70.
40. Stanley LL. An analysis of one thousand testicular substance implantations. Endocrinology 1922; 6: 787.
41. Freeman ER, Bloom DA, McGuire EJ. A brief history of testosterone. J Urol 2001; 165: 371–3.
42. Machluf M, Orsola A, Boorjian S, Kershen R, Atala A. Microencapsulation of Leydig cells: a system for testosterone supplementation. Endocrinology 2003; 144: 4975–9.
43. Hobermann JM, Yesalis CE. The history of synthetic testosterone. Sci Am 1995; 272: 76–81.

44. Oettel M. The endocrine pharmacology of testosterone therapy in men. Naturwissenschaften 2004; 91: 66–76.
45. Gallagher TF, Koch FC. The quantitative assay for testicular hormone by comb growth reaction. J Pharmacol Exper Ther 1930; 40: 327–34.
46. McGee LC. The effect of an injection of a lipoid fraction of bull testicle in capons. Proc Inst Med Chicago 1927; 6: 242–54.
47. McCullagh EP, McCullagh DR, Hicken NF. Diagnosis and treatment of hypogonadism in the male. Endocrinology 1933; 17: 49–63.
48. Bruchovsky N, Wilson JD. The conversion of testosterone to 5α-androstan-17β-ol,3-ome by rat prostate in vivo and in vitro. J Biol Chem 1968; 243: 1314–24.
49. Butenandt A. Über die chemische Untersuchung der Sexualhormone. Z Angew Chem 1931; 44: 905–8.
50. Butenandt A, Tscherning K. Über Androsteron. II. Seine chemische Charakterisierung. Z Angew Chem 1934; 229: 167–84.
51. Ruzicka L, Goldberg MW, Meyer J, Brüngger H, Eichenberger E. Zur Kenntnis der Sexualhormone II. Über die Synthese des Testikelhormons (Androsteron) und Stereoisomere desselben durch Abbau hydrierter Sterine. Helv Chim Acta 1934; 17: 1395–406.
52. Ogata A, Hirano S. Study on the male hormone (VI). Study on the male hormone from boar testes (III). A new crystal male hormone. J Pharm Soc Jpn 1934; 54: 199–211.
53. David K, Dingemanse E, Freud J, Laqueur E. Über kristallinisches männliches Hormon aus Hoden (Testosteron), wirksamer als aus Harn und Cholesterin bereitetes Androsteron. Hoppe-Seylers Z Physiol Chem 1935; 233: 281–2.
54. Butenandt A, Hanisch G. Über Testosteron. Umwandlung des Dehydro-Androsterons in Androstendiol und Testosteron; ein Weg zur Darstellung des Testosterons aus Cholesterin. Hoppe Seyler's Z Physiol Chem 1935; 237: 89–92.
55. Ruzicka L, Wettstein A. Sexualhormone VII. Über die künstliche Herstellung des Testikelhormons Testosteron (Androsten-3-on-17-ol). Helv Chim Acta 1935; 18: 1264–75.
56. Butenandt A. Aufgaben und Ziele der Hormonforschung. Pharmazeutische Industrie 1941; 8: 43–5.
57. Heller CG, Myers GB. The male climacteric: its symptomatology. JAMA 1944; 126: 472–7.
58. Morley JE, Perry HM. Andropause: an old concept in new clothing. Clin Geriatr 2003; 19: 507–28.
59. Editorial. Climacteric in aging men. JAMA 1942; 118: 458–60.
60. Handelsman DJ. Testosterone: use, misuse and abuse. Med J Aust 2006; 185: 436–9.
61. Chang C, Kokontis J, Liao S. Structural analysis of complementary DNA and amino acid sequences of human and rat androgen receptors. Proc Natl Acad Sci USA 1988; 85: 7211–15.
62. Chang C, Kokontis J, Liao S. Molecular cloning of human and rat complementary DNA encoding androgen receptors. Science 1988; 240: 324–6.
63. Lubahn DB, Joseph DR, Sar M et al. The human androgen receptor: complementary deoxyribonucleic acid cloning, sequence analysis and gene expression in prostate. Mol Endocrinol 1988; 2: 1265–75.
64. Lubahn DB, Joseph DR, Sullivan PM, Willard HF, French FS, Wilson EM. The human androgen receptor: complementary deoxyribonucleic acid cloning, sequence analysis and gene expression in prostate. Mol Endocrinol 1988; 2: 1265–75.
65. Trapman J, Klaassen P, Kuiper GG et al. Cloning, structure and expression of a cDNA encoding the human androgen receptor. Biochem Biophys Res Commun 1988; 153: 241–8.
66. Tilley WD, Marcelli M, Wilson JD, McPhaul MJ. Characterization and expression of a cDNA encoding the human androgen receptor. Proc Natl Acad Sci USA 1989; 86: 327–31.
67. Laroche G, Marsan F, Bompard E, Corcos A. L'hypertrophie de la prostate. Essais de traitement hormonal par les sels de testosterone. Presse Médicale 1937; 45: 932–6.
68. Banzer G. Arzneitherapie des praktischen Arztes, Dritte Auflage. Berlin and München: Urban & Schwarzenberg, 1949; 119.
69. Gooren L. Risks of androgen therapy. J Men's Health Gender 2006; 3: 404–9.
70. Kaplan SA. Male pelvic health: a urological call for arms. J Urol 2006; 176: 2351–2.
71. Qoubaitary A, Swerdloff RS, Wang C. Advances in male hormone substitution therapy. Expert Opin Pharmacother 2005; 6: 1493–506.
72. San Francisco IF, Regan MM, DeWolf WC, Olumi AF. Low age adjusted free testosterone levels correlate with poorly differentiated prostate cancer. J Urol 2006; 175: 1341–6.
73. Nishiyama T, Ikarashi T, Hashimoto Y, Suzuki K, Takahashi K. Association between the dihydrotestosterone level in the prostate and prostate cancer aggressiveness using the Gleason score. J Urol 2006; 176: 1387–91.
74. Prehn RT. On the prevention and therapy of prostate cancer by androgen administration. Cancer Res 1999; 59: 4161–4.
75. Yassin AA, Saad F, Diede HH. Testosterone and erectile function in hypogonadal men unresponsive to tadalafil: results from an open-label uncontrolled study. Andrologia 2006; 38: 61–8.
76. von Albrecht M. 'Vergil'. Bucolica, Georgica, Aeneis. Eine Einführung. Universitätsverlag Carl Winter, Heidelberg, 2006.

Biology of aging

CHAPTER 1

The biology of gender differences in animal models of aging

HJ Armbrecht

Introduction

One of the hallmarks of human aging is the gender difference. Across many different cultures and genetic backgrounds, women on the average outlive men by 7 years (see Chapter 2). Along with this, women seem more resistant to certain types of diseases than men. The fact that this gender difference is so robust would lead one to believe that it has, at least in part, a biologic basis. Gender differences are also seen in animal models of aging such as fruit flies, mice, and rats. The study of these animal models has shown that they mimic aspects of human aging in important ways. It is becoming apparent that common biochemical pathways modulate aging in these organisms and that these pathways have their counterparts in humans.[1] Thus, the study of gender differences in the aging of these organisms may give some insight into the marked gender differences seen in human aging.

This review is divided into four parts. First, we will discuss the aging process from a biologic perspective. Next, we will summarize the characteristics of the aging process at the organs/systems level, the cellular level, and the subcellular level. Then, we will discuss gender differences in the aging of flies, mice, and rats. Finally, we will discuss the relevance of the findings in animal models to human gender differences.

The biology of aging

What is aging?

Miller has proposed a definition that captures the basic elements of aging: 'A process that converts healthy adults into frail ones, with diminished reserves in most physiological systems and an exponentially increasing vulnerability to most diseases and to death.'[2] Aging is not merely the passage of time. It focuses on changes in adulthood rather than on developmental changes, and it is characterized by a decreasing ability to adapt to a changing environment in a physiologic way. These changes may involve nutrition, temperature, disease, and even societal changes. A hallmark of most aging organisms is an increase in the incidence of disease and the risk of death. This definition then makes the distinction between the aging process and disease. It assumes that there are fundamental aging processes that are not just the sum of all of the diseases of aging. These processes predispose the aging organism to a greater likelihood of disease.

Why do we age?

The question of why we age can be approached from many different perspectives – psychologically, sociologically, spiritually, and biologically. There have been a number of different biologic perspectives. Each species appears to have a well-defined lifespan and pattern of aging. Therefore, it has been proposed that there is a biologic clock or genetic program that controls the aging of an organism.[3] This was thought to be analogous to the well-characterized developmental program of higher animals that is under tight genetic control. A number of 'clocks' have been proposed for the regulation of the aging process – the pituitary, the immune system, cellular senescence, etc. Upon closer investigation, most of these clocks, although they regulate important aspects of the aging process, are the result of aging rather than driving the aging process itself.

A more recent biologic perspective on why we age has been articulated by Martin et al:[4] 'There is no aging program, nor is there an aging gene. Instead, we age because evolution has no reason to protect us against unwelcome actions of multiple genes late in life.' In terms of our genes, there are two processes potentially working against increased longevity.[5,6] First, there is selective pressure *for* genes with beneficial effects early in the lifespan. Second, there is a lack of selective pressure *against* genes which have negative effects late in the lifespan. On the other hand, the idea that aging is programmed for the benefit of the species as a whole has been recently re-examined.[1]

How do we age?

There has been a tendency in aging research to find the *one* theory that accounts for all that we see in terms of the biology of aging. Perhaps this thinking is a holdover from looking for *the* biologic clock or pacemaker of aging. Thus, there was the neuroendocrine theory of aging, the cell senescence theory of aging, and the free radical theory of aging. The early proponents of these theories tended to regard them as universal theories, explaining all of aging. However, it may be that aging is not something that is programmed but rather something that happens because it is not selected against. Then the aging process becomes much more difficult to generalize. Aging may vary by species and within the organs in a given species. It may also happen at multiple levels in a given species – at the organ/systems level, at the cellular level, and at the subcellular level.

Table 1.1 *Components of the aging process*

At the organ/systems level
- Neuroendocrine component
- Immune system component

At the cellular level
- Genetic component
- Cell senescence component

At the subcellular level
- Free radical component
- DNA damage component
- Glycation component

One way to think about how we age is shown in Table 1.1. This structure for thinking about biologic aging has been followed by Robert Arking[7] and Weinert and Timiras.[8] Aging takes place at three major levels of biologic organization – at the organ/systems level, at the cellular level, and at the subcellular level. At each of these levels there are components of the aging process – changes that contribute to the aging process we observe. However, they are not, in themselves, the whole picture. Previously, each of these components would be seen as competing *theories* of aging.

At the organ/systems level we have a neuroendocrine component and an immune component. There are also other systems that 'age', but these are some well-studied examples. At the cellular level, there is the cell senescence component and the genetic component. In reality, the genetic component can profoundly affect all three levels, but it is put here for convenience. Finally, there is the subcellular level, which has the free radical component, the DNA damage component, and the glycation component.

What is the relationship of aging to disease?

What is the relationship of these three levels to each other and to age-related diseases? The effects of aging can manifest themselves independently at any level of biologic organization. However, they also affect the other levels. For example, free radical production at the subcellular (mitochondrial) level may ultimately lead to effects at the cellular level. These cellular effects could include cell senescence, premature cell death, or uncontrolled cell growth (cancer). These cellular effects could cause deleterious effects at the organ/system level, as in the case of tumors caused by uncontrolled cell growth. However, there can also be independent changes at the organ/systems level, such as the build-up of plaque with time in the circulatory system. There is some evidence, though, that even plaque build-up is the result of cellular changes in the endothelial cells lining the circulatory system. With regard to disease, disease and death are the outcomes of the basic biologic processes that occur during aging. Aging is not just the sum of all age-related diseases. According to Arking, 'the common age-related diseases … highlight the weak points of the evolved anatomical and physiological design of the organism.' [7]

The components of aging

Aging at the organ/systems level
The neuroendocrine component

The neuroendocrine system is an integral part of the body's homeostatic mechanisms. It regulates reproduction, growth, and response to stress among many other things. Modulation of this system can markedly affect longevity and the expression of age-related diseases. There are three major hormonal systems whose function changes with age.[9] These are the reproductive system, the growth regulatory system, and the stress response system.

In terms of reproduction, women undergo the rapid loss of estrogens at menopause. Men undergo a slower loss of testosterone that has been termed the andropause. Many of the gender differences in longevity and age-related diseases have been attributed to these two hormones (see Chapter 2). In some cases, these hormones may work indirectly to modulate the aging process. For example, some of the beneficial effects of estrogen may be due to its stimulation of antioxidant defenses.

A second important system is the growth hormone/insulin/insulin-like growth factor (IGF) system. In terms of circulating hormones, there is a decrease in growth hormone and IGF-1 with age. This may partly explain the decreased muscle mass and increase in frailty seen in the elderly. This has been termed the somatopause. In mice, perturbation of this system can markedly increase lifespan, although it usually results in a dwarf appearance as well.[10] This system has been implicated in the gender differences seen in the aging of fruit flies and mice.

Steroid hormone production by the adrenal gland is a third neuroendocrine system that undergoes major age-related changes. The production of dehydroepiandrosterone (DHEA), an important steroid hormone precursor, declines with age. This occurs despite normal levels of ACTH and cortisol, and it has been termed the adrenopause. In humans, differences in the cortisol/ACTH ratio may contribute to gender differences in aging (Chapter 2).

These neuroendocrine changes with age have been well documented and are important characteristics of the aging process. Their effects can be reversed or moderated by hormone replacement therapy in appropriate situations. However, these neuroendocrine changes do not direct the aging process, and hormone replacement therapy does not necessarily extend maximal lifespan.[11]

The immune component

Age-related changes in the immune system have been well documented in humans and experimental animals. These changes include the involution of the thymus gland and a decrease in the number and function of specific immune cell types.[12] These physiologic changes may account for the increase in a number of diseases seen in the elderly. The altered T-cell number and function may result in a greater incidence of infection. Altered B-cell response to stimuli may result in increased autoimmune disease. The increased risk for cancer in the elderly has also been attributed to decreased immune surveillance. However, other risks for cancer include increased free radical damage and altered regulation of cell division (see below).

Age-related changes in the human immune system have been studied with regard to gender differences in aging (Chapter 2). Age-related changes in immune function are an important manifestation of the aging process. However, like the neuroendocrine changes, they do not drive the aging process. Even organisms with poorly developed immune systems age.

Aging at the cellular level
The genetic component

Aging clearly has a genetic component as demonstrated by 'twins' studies. In addition to more subtle effects, even single gene mutations can produce catastrophic phenotypes that seem to mimic the aging process in a very compressed lifespan. Two of these diseases are Werner's syndrome and Hutchinson–Gilford progeria. The defect in Werner's syndrome was found to be single-base mutations in the gene coding for a DNA helicase.[13] Helicases are enzymes that are involved in the unraveling of double-stranded DNA for transcription or replication. The defect in Hutchinson–Gilford progeria was found to be in lamin A.[14] This protein is a structural component of the cell nucleus.

The potential for genetic modification of the lifespan in mammals has been shown by a number of spontaneous and engineered modifications of the growth hormone/insulin/IGF system.[10] Although such modifications result in markedly increased lifespans, they usually result in undesirable phenotypic characteristics as well. These include stunted growth and decreased reproductive function. More recently, other strategies have been used to increase the mouse lifespan. These include deleting the insulin receptor from adipose tissue[15] and overexpressing mitochondrial catalase, an important antioxidant enzyme.[16] As interesting as these transgenic mouse models are, it is not clear whether humans have a similar potential for lifespan extension. It is also not clear whether such extension could be achieved without undesirable side-effects.

The cell senescence component

The fact that cells senesce was originally observed by Leonard Hayflick.[17] Hayflick found that human skin fibroblasts would only divide a finite number of times despite optimal growth conditions. Initially, there were a number of experimental correlations that suggested that limits on cell replication might be related to aging of the whole organism. The correlations included the fact that the number of population doublings correlated inversely with donor age, correlated directly with the longevity of donor species, and was decreased in Werner's and progeric patients.

Because of these correlations there was an intense effort to determine what regulated the number of cell divisions. It was found that telomeres, structures found on the tips of chromosomes that serve a protective function, play a major role in determining the number of cell divisions.[18] With each cell division, the telomeres shorten, and eventually they reach a point where cell division is halted. The importance of telomeres was further underscored with the discovery of telomerase, an enzyme found in germ line and immortalized cells. Telomerase repairs the telomere shortening that takes place after each cell division and so delays cell senescence.[19]

However, with additional research it has become clear that telomeres and telomerase are not the sole regulatory factors. It has been shown that cells undergo stress-induced as well as replicative senescence.[20] There are also a number of different factors and cellular pathways that interact to induce cell senescence.[21] Some of these other factors are oxidative stress and DNA damage (see below). These factors may affect telomere length directly, as well as work through other mechanisms to induce senescence.

Telomere length and cell senescence may play a role in certain tissues in human aging. They may contribute to gender differences (see Chapter 2). However, telomere shortening with age has been difficult to observe in rodents, except in some circumstances. In addition, cell senescence would not be expected to play a role in the aging of organs comprised mostly of non-dividing cells, such as the brain.

Aging at the subcellular level
The free radical component

The link between free radicals, which are highly reactive chemical compounds, and aging was first proposed by Harmon.[22] The free radical theory states in general terms that free radicals within the body cause oxidative damage to cellular molecules – proteins, DNA, lipids, etc.[23] This molecular damage eventually causes cellular dysfunction such as cell death (necrosis), premature cell senescence (see above), premature programmed cell death (apoptosis), and uncontrolled cell growth (cancer). These cellular changes then lead to decreased organ function, decreased regulatory systems function, and ultimately death. Initially, it was felt that most free radical production in the body came from external sources such as ionizing radiation or environmental pollutants. However, recently the focus has been on free radicals produced by normal cellular functions such as energy production by mitochondria and the reaction mechanisms of certain enzymes.

There are several lines of evidence supporting the importance of the free radical component of aging. First, oxidative damage to DNA, proteins, and lipids has been shown to increase with age in experimental animals.[24] Because free radical damage results mostly in oxidative damage, the free radical theory is sometimes referred to in more general terms as the 'oxidative stress' theory. Second, longer lived species are less susceptible to oxidative stress than shorter lived species[25] and have more efficient repair mechanisms.[26] Third, a high metabolic rate, which generates more free radicals, is associated with a shorter lifespan. This correlation formed the basis for the 'rate of living' theory of aging which was proposed a number of years ago.[27] Fourth, organisms engineered to have higher antioxidant defenses live longer. This has been shown in a number of organisms including fruit flies,[28] roundworms,[29] and mice.[16]

A final piece of evidence supporting the importance of free radicals in aging comes from dietary restriction studies. Dietary restriction is feeding animals less food than they would normally eat.[30] It has been demonstrated to increase mean and maximal lifespan in a diverse number of organisms, including worms, flies, yeast, mice, and rats. The increased longevity induced by dietary restriction is associated with decreased oxidative damage.[24]

Since mitochondria generate much of the free radical load of the cell, as well as producing energy for cellular metabolism, these subcellular organelles have been extensively studied for their role in biological aging. These observations are sometimes referred to as the 'mitochondrial theory of aging'.[31] Mitochondria in older aerobic tissue such as skeletal muscle tend to be fewer in number and have an altered appearance. They produce less energy and more free radicals as the energy-producing reactions become less efficient. Oxidative damage to mitochondrial proteins and DNA has been shown to increase with age.[32] Mitochondrial DNA codes for some of the proteins involved in energy production. It has been suggested that this leads to a downward spiral as far as mitochondrial function is concerned. Increased free radical production leads to increased damage to mitochondrial DNA and proteins, which, in turn, leads to decreased energy production and more free radical production.

Because free radicals can cause so much disruption of cellular function, it has become increasingly clear that there are extensive cellular mechanisms for the neutralization of free radicals. Oxygen free radicals generated by mitochondria and enzymatic reactions are converted to hydrogen peroxide by the enzyme superoxide dismutase (SOD). Hydrogen peroxide is then converted to water by two pathways. One pathway is via the enzyme catalase. The second pathway is via the glutathione cycle. Glutathione is constantly reduced (via glutathione reductase) and then re-oxidized (via glutathione peroxidase). In the process it converts hydrogen peroxide to water. The protein components of these free radical defense pathways are under genetic control.

The free radical component of aging plays a major role in other subcellular components of aging – the DNA damage component and the glycation component (see below). Together they play an important role in the biology of aging. However, it is still not clear whether oxidative damage accounts for all of the features of aging.[8] The fact that the free radical defenses are under genetic control underscores the potential importance of other mechanisms. Nevertheless, many of the gender differences in animal models of aging are explained in terms of differences in free radical production and free radical defense pathways (see below).

The DNA damage component

One of the molecular structures most sensitive to free radical damage is DNA. This includes the DNA found in nuclear chromosomes as well as the circular DNA found in mitochondria. The damage to chromosomal DNA includes strand breaks, covalent modifications, and chromosomal rearrangements. It has been proposed that such damage may result in altered gene expression and contribute to the aging process.[33] It is not clear how much these events contribute to the global aging process. Much DNA damage is in the form of chromosomal rearrangements. Such rearrangements are usually associated with diseases such as cancer rather than with aging. As mentioned above, damage to mitochondrial DNA has been most thoroughly studied as a manifestation of free radical damage. It may be in this context that DNA damage is most important. Alteration of mitochondrial DNA replication leads to a premature aging phenotype in mice.[34]

The glycation component

The glycation component of aging arises from the non-enzymatic combining of glucose with proteins. A common example of this is the high amount of hemoglobin that is glycosylated in the blood of diabetics. This non-enzymatic glycosylation results in the formation of AGEs (advanced glycation end products). This process increases with age because the glycation reaction is accelerated by free radicals. This ties glycation in with the free radical component of aging. Glycation again is not a universal explanation but may play an important role in the aging of certain tissues. Proteins which have been shown to be glycosylated include collagen, vascular proteins, and lens crystalline proteins. The glycosylation of these proteins could play a role in the aging of connective tissue, blood vessels, and the lens of the eye, respectively.

Gender differences in animal model longevity

Fruit fly

The fruit fly has many advantages as a model organism for the study of aging in general and gender differences in particular.[35] It has a short lifespan, it is easy to manipulate genetically, and it has distinct male and female sexes. The female of several species lives longer than the male.[36,37] In addition, the females show a much greater response to dietary restriction in terms of increased lifespan.[36]

Several factors have been cited as contributing to these gender differences. First, there may be intrinsic genetic differences in the way that longevity is regulated in male and female flies. A genome-wide screen for regions of DNA (quantitative trait loci) that affect longevity found that these regions had sex-specific effects.[38]

Second, there may be gender differences in the insulin/IGF signaling (IIS) pathway.[39] Mutation of this pathway increases the lifespan of female flies much more than male flies. In fact, very strong mutations in this pathway decrease male longevity while increasing female longevity. This suggests that the IIS pathway is more active in normal female flies compared to males. Differences in the IIS system may also explain the fact that females show a greater response to dietary restriction.[36]

Finally, the greater female response to dietary restriction may reflect the fact that female flies have a higher nutrient demand than male flies due to egg production.[36] Dietary restriction reduces egg production and this may increase longevity. There is generally an inverse relationship between reproduction and longevity.

These gender differences in the effect of dietary restriction have been generalized to other longevity-extending manipulations in flies. In a survey of the literature, Burger and Promislow[40] found that these manipulations tended to favor females over males in reports where both sexes were studied. In addition to the factors mentioned above (genetic, IIS pathway, and reproductive needs), the authors also cite the fact that females have two X chromosomes while males have an X and a Y. In male flies, most genes on the X chromosome are overexpressed to offset the fact that there is only one X chromosome. Anything that modifies this process could lead to gender effects affecting longevity.

In summary, gender differences in fruit fly longevity could be due to sex-linked genetic differences, differences in the insulin/IGF signaling pathway, the greater

Table 1.2 *Biologic basis of gender differences*

Fruit flies
- Sex-linked genetic differences
- Insulin/IGF signaling pathway
- Female reproductive needs
- Sex chromosome differences (XX vs XY)

Mice
- Insulin/IGF signaling pathway
- Reduced glucose tolerance in males
- Elevation of antioxidant pathways by estrogen
- Telomere length (?)

Rats
- Greater free radical production in males
- Elevation of antioxidant pathways by estrogen
- Telomere shortening

Humans (from Chapter 2)
- Sex chromosome differences (XX vs XY)
- Elevation of antioxidant pathways by estrogen
- Telomere length
- Stress hormones (cortisol/ACTH)
- Immune function

reproductive needs of females, and differences in sex chromosomes (Table 1.2).

Mice

In general, female mice tend to live longer than male mice, but the magnitude of this effect is dependent on the strain.[41] In some strains the relationship is reversed.[42] A number of mice have been characterized that have either a spontaneously occurring or targeted mutation that interferes with the growth hormone/IGF system.[10] In some cases these mutations show gender effects and in some cases not. In mice where the IGF-1 receptor was partially inactivated, female mice showed a significant increase in lifespan while males did not.[42] The authors discuss these gender differences in terms of reduced glucose tolerance and decreased resistance to oxidative stress in males. In another study, deleting the growth hormone receptor significantly

increased both male and female lifespan.[41] However, the shorter-lived males showed a greater percentage increase to the point that their lifespan was now equal to the females'. In a third study, the insulin receptor in fat tissue was deleted.[15] This modification produced similar increases in longevity in both sexes.

One study in mice has looked at the interaction between estrogen and insulin in regulating resistance to oxidative stress in males and females.[43] Insulin action was reduced by making mutant mice with reduced levels of the insulin receptor. When subjected to oxidative stress, mutant female mice survived significantly longer than males. Relative to this, the mitochondrial superoxide dismutase (SOD) activity in the liver was elevated in the female mutant mice relative to the normal animals. There was no elevation of SOD activity in the mutant male mice. These studies also indicated a role for estrogen in these gender differences. When estrogen was administered to mutant mice, it increased their resistance to oxidative stress. Conversely, ovariectomy reduced resistance to oxidative stress. Both these changes correlated with changes in mitochondrial SOD activity. One limitation of these studies is that they were performed in 4-month-old mice and longevity itself was not measured.

In terms of mechanisms, several studies have reported that the antioxidant pathways in female mice are more robust than in male mice. The glutathione content of most tissues declines with age more rapidly in male mice than in female mice, due to decreased synthesis.[44] In the mouse brain, catalase and glutathione activity are higher in old female mice compared to male mice, which correlates with higher levels of lipid peroxidation in male mice.[45] The increased activity of female antioxidant pathways may underlie the finding that the hearts of old female mice are more tolerant of ischemic insult than are the hearts of old males.[46]

Finally, in humans it has been proposed that differences in telomere length may underlie gender differences (see Chapter 2). In mice, telomeres are much longer than in humans, and it has been difficult to relate telomere shortening to the aging of individual organs or longevity in general. However, in one study using a strain of mice with short telomeres, female mice had significantly longer telomeres than males over the whole lifespan in a number of tissues.[47]

In summary, factors that could contribute to gender differences in mouse longevity include differences in the insulin/IGF signaling pathway, such as is seen in fruit flies. However, they also include hormonal factors such as reduced glucose tolerance in males, and elevation of antioxidant pathways by estrogen, leading to increased resistance to oxidative stress (Table 1.2). The longer telomeres in female mice may also be a factor, but this is difficult to interpret, since the regulation of telomere length and its relationship to aging is markedly different in the mouse compared to humans.

Rats

Gender differences in the longevity of Wistar rats have been studied extensively by Vina and colleagues.[31,48] The female Wistar rat lives longer, and they have studied this in terms of free radical production and free radical defenses.[48] Mitochondrial hydrogen peroxide production is less and free radical defenses are elevated in female livers.[49] The concentration of glutathione in males is about half that of females in mitochondria. The activity of mitochondrial SOD in females is about twice that of males,[49] and others have shown that glutathione peroxidase activity is also elevated.[50] Finally, mitochondrial cytochrome c oxidase activity, an important component of the respiratory chain, is higher in females than males.[48]

The net result of these gender differences is that male mitochondria produce more free radicals. At the same time, they have less efficient mechanisms for getting rid of them than do female mitochondria.[31] One evidence of this is that oxidative damage to mitochondrial DNA has been found to be 4-fold higher in males than in females.[48]

The gender differences in the aging Wistar rat have been pursued in more detail by looking specifically at the aging kidney.[51] Studying the kidney is important, since kidney disease is a major cause of death in rats. As reported above for the liver, significantly higher levels of antioxidant enzymes were seen in the older female kidney compared to the male. In addition, a greater degree of telomere shortening was seen in the male with age. This shortening was associated with an increase in the cellular

pathway that leads to cell senescence. These changes correlated with age-related changes in renal function, which were much more severe in the male.

What is the source of these gender differences in mitochondrial antioxidant defenses? These investigators make the case that estrogen is responsible for the increased expression of antioxidant enzymes.[48] They have shown that in a mammary gland tumor cell line estrogen can increase expression of SOD and glutathione peroxidase and reduce hydrogen peroxide concentrations.[52] To show the relevance of this in intact rats, they have used ovariectomized rats with and without estrogen treatment. Ovariectomy significantly increased mitochondrial hydrogen peroxide production while estrogen treatment reduced it back to normal.[48] Thus, the gender differences seen in rat longevity may involve differences in the expression of free radical defenses as modulated by estrogen.

In summary, factors that could contribute to gender differences in rat longevity focus on free radical damage and its modulation by estrogen. These factors include increased free radical production in males, increased antioxidant activities in females, and a positive effect of estrogen in decreasing free radical production and increasing antioxidant pathways (Table 1.2). Increased oxidative damage may also contribute to the telomere shortening reported in the rat kidney. The gender differences in the insulin/IGF pathway seen in fruit flies and mice have not been studied in the rat due to the difficulty of performing genetic manipulation in the rat.

Relevance to human longevity

What is the relevance of these studies to human gender differences? The biologic basis of human gender differences is discussed in Chapter 2. Some of the factors contributing to human gender differences are listed in Table 1.2 (bottom). Many of these factors have also been identified in the model systems discussed in this chapter. These include differences in sex chromosome expression, elevation of antioxidant defenses by estrogen, and perhaps telomere length. Other factors that may play a role in human longevity differences include stress hormone levels and immune function. Stress hormones and immune function have been well studied in rats and mice as a function of age. Therefore, these rodents would be excellent model systems in which to study the contribution of the neuroendocrine and immune systems to gender differences in longevity.

As we stated in the beginning of this chapter, recent comparative studies of aging in model organisms indicate that they have many characteristics of aging in common. At the biologic level, there appear to be common biochemical pathways that modulate aging in these organisms. These pathways regulate growth, glucose metabolism, and resistance to oxidative damage.[1] As we have outlined in this chapter, gender effects in model organisms can be understood in terms of gender differences in these pathways. These pathways have their counterparts in humans. However, further work is needed to determine the degree to which these pathways modulate human aging and the marked gender differences that characterize it. There is every reason to expect that as we learn more about the biologic basis of aging, we will be able to better understand gender differences. Likewise, the gender differences themselves will give insight into which mechanisms are important in terms of modulating the aging process.

References

1. Longo VD, Mitteldorf J, Skulachev VP. Opinion: programmed and altruistic ageing. Nat Rev Genet 2005; 6: 866–72.
2. Miller RA. The biology of aging and longevity. In: Hazzard WR, Blass JP, Ettinger WH, Halter JB, Ouslander JG, eds. Principles of Geriatric Medicine and Gerontology. New York: McGraw-Hill, 1998: 3–19.
3. Hayflick L. How and Why We Age. New York: Ballantine, 1994.
4. Martin GM, Austad SN, Johnson TE. Genetic analysis of ageing: role of oxidative damage and environmental stresses. Nat Genet 1996; 13: 25–34.
5. Kirkwood TBL. Comparative and evolutionary aspects of longevity. In: Finch CE, Schneider EL, eds. Handbook of the Biology of Aging. New York: Van Norstrand Reinhold, 1985: 27–44.
6. Austad SN. What evolution explains about aging. In: Austad SN, ed. Why We Age. New York: John Wiley, 1997: 94–122.
7. Arking R. Biology of Aging: Observations and Principles, 3rd edn. Oxford: Oxford University Press, 2006.
8. Weinert BT, Timiras PS. Invited review: theories of aging. J Appl Physiol 2003; 95: 1706–16.
9. Lamberts SWJ, van den Beld AW, van der Lely AJ. The endocrinology of aging. Science 1997; 278: 419–24.
10. Bartke A. Minireview: role of the growth hormone/insulin-like growth factor system in mammalian aging. Endocrinology 2005; 146: 3718–23.
11. Olshansky SJ, Hayflick L, Carnes BA. Position statement on human aging. J Gerontol A Biol Sci Med Sci 2002; 57: B292–7.
12. Ernst DN, Hobbs MV. Age-related changes in cytokine expression by T cells. In: Morley JE, Armbrecht HJ, Coe RM, Vellas B, eds. The Science of Geriatrics. Paris: Serdi Publisher, 2000: 541–54.
13. Yu CE, Oshima J, Fu YH et al. Positional cloning of the Werner's syndrome gene. Science 1996; 272: 258–62.
14. Eriksson M, Brown WT, Gordon LB, Glynn MW, Singer J, Scott L, Erdos MR, Robbins CM, Moses TY, Berglund P, Dutra A, Pak E, Durkin S, Csoka AB, Boehnke M, Glover TW, Collins FS. Recurrent de novo point mutations in lamin A cause Hutchinson–Gilford progeria syndrome. Nature 2003; 423: 293–8.
15. Bluher M, Kahn BB, Kahn CR. Extended longevity in mice lacking the insulin receptor in adipose tissue. Science 2003; 299: 572–4.
16. Schriner SE, Linford NJ, Martin GM, Treuting P, Ogburn CE, Emond M, Coskun PE, Ladiges W, Wolf N, Van RH, Wallace DC, Rabinovitch PS. Extension of murine life span by overexpression of catalase targeted to mitochondria. Science 2005; 308: 1909–11.
17. Hayflick L, Moorehead PS. The serial cultivation of human diploid cell strains. Exp Cell Res 1961; 25: 585–621.
18. Campisi J. Cancer, aging and cellular senescence. In Vivo 2000; 14: 183–8.
19. Bodnar AG, Ouellette M, Frolkis M, Holt SE, Chiu C, Moran GB, Harley CB, Shay JW, Lichsteiner S, Wright WE. Extension of life span by introduction of telomerase into normal human cells. Science 1998; 279: 349–52.
20. Marcotte R, Wang E. Replicative senescence revisited. J Gerontol A Biol Sci Med Sci 2002; 57: B257–69.
21. Campisi J. Senescent cells, tumor suppression, and organismal aging: good citizens, bad neighbors. Cell 2005; 120: 513–22.
22. Harmon D. Aging: a theory based on free radical and radiation chemistry. J Gerontol 1956; 2: 298–300.
23. Finkel T, Holbrook NJ. Oxidants, oxidative stress and the biology of ageing. Nature 2000; 408: 239–47.
24. Sohal RS, Weindruch R. Oxidative stress, caloric restriction, and aging. Science 1996; 273: 59–63.

25. Agarwal RS, Sohal RS. Relationship between susceptibility to protein oxidation, aging, and maximum life span potential of different species. Exp Gerontol 1996; 31: 365–72.

26. Hart RW, Setlow RB. Correlation between deoxyribonucleic acid excision repair and lifespan in a number of mammalian species. Proc Nat Acad Sci USA 1974; 71: 2169–73.

27. Pearl R. The Rate of Living. London: University of London Press, 1928.

28. Orr WC, Sohal RS. Extension of life-span by overexpression of superoxide dismutase and catalase in *Drosophila melanogaster*. Science 1994; 263: 1128–30.

29. Melov S, Ravenscroft J, Malik S, Gill MS, Walker DW, Clayton PE, Wallace DC, Malfroy B, Doctrow SR, Lithgow GJ. Extension of life-span with superoxide dismutase/catalase mimetics. Science 2000; 289: 1567–9.

30. Masoro EJ. Overview of caloric restriction and ageing. Mech Ageing Dev 2005; 126: 913–22.

31. Vina J, Sastre J, Pallardo F, Borras C. Mitochondrial theory of aging: importance to explain why females live longer than males. Antioxid Redox Signal 2003; 5: 549–56.

32. Mandavilli BS, Santos JH, Van HB. Mitochondrial DNA repair and aging. Mutat Res 2002; 509: 127–51.

33. Vijg J, Gossen JA. Somatic mutations and cellular aging. Comp Biochem Physiol 1993; 104B: 429–37.

34. Kujoth GC, Hiona A, Pugh TD, Someya S, Panzer K, Wohlgemuth SE, Hofer T, Seo AY, Sullivan R, Jobling WA, Morrow JD, Van RH, Sedivy JM, Yamasoba T, Tanokura M, Weindruch R, Leeuwenburgh C, Prolla TA. Mitochondrial DNA mutations, oxidative stress, and apoptosis in mammalian aging. Science 2005; 309: 481–4.

35. Partridge L, Piper MD, Mair W. Dietary restriction in *Drosophila*. Mech Ageing Dev 2005; 126: 938–50.

36. Magwere T, Chapman T, Partridge L. Sex differences in the effect of dietary restriction on life span and mortality rates in female and male *Drosophila melanogaster*. J Gerontol A Biol Sci Med Sci 2004; 59: 3–9.

37. Davies S, Kattel R, Bhatia B, Petherwick A, Chapman T. The effect of diet, sex and mating status on longevity in Mediterranean fruit flies (*Ceratitis capitata*), Diptera: Tephritidae. Exp Gerontol 2005; 40: 784–92.

38. Nuzhdin SV, Pasyukova EG, Dilda CL, Zeng ZB, Mackay TF. Sex-specific quantitative trait loci affecting longevity in *Drosophila melanogaster*. Proc Natl Acad Sci USA 1997; 94: 9734–9.

39. Clancy DJ, Gems D, Harshman LG, Oldham S, Stocker H, Hafen E, Leevers SJ, Partridge L. Extension of life-span by loss of CHICO, a *Drosophila* insulin receptor substrate protein. Science 2001; 292: 104–6.

40. Burger JM, Promislow DE. Sex-specific effects of interventions that extend fly life span. Sci Aging Knowl Environ 2004; e30: 2004.

41. Coschigano KT, Holland AN, Riders ME, List EO, Flyvbjerg A, Kopchick JJ. Deletion, but not antagonism, of the mouse growth hormone receptor results in severely decreased body weights, insulin, and insulin-like growth factor I levels and increased life span. Endocrinology 2003; 144: 3799–810.

42. Holzenberger M, Dupont J, Ducos B, Leneuve P, Geloen A, Even PC, Cervera P, Le BY. IGF-1 receptor regulates lifespan and resistance to oxidative stress in mice. Nature 2003; 421: 182–7.

43. Baba T, Shimizu T, Suzuki Y, Ogawara M, Isono K, Koseki H, Kurosawa H, Shirasawa T. Estrogen, insulin, and dietary signals cooperatively regulate longevity signals to enhance resistance to oxidative stress in mice. J Biol Chem 2005; 280: 16417–26.

44. Wang H, Liu H, Liu RM. Gender difference in glutathione metabolism during aging in mice. Exp Gerontol 2003; 38: 507–17.

45. Sobocanec S, Balog T, Sverko V, Marotti T. Sex-dependent antioxidant enzyme activities and lipid peroxidation in ageing mouse brain. Free Radic Res 2003; 37: 743–8.

46. Willems L, Zatta A, Holmgren K, Ashton KJ, Headrick JP. Age-related changes in ischemic tolerance in male and female mouse hearts. J Mol Cell Cardiol 2005; 38: 245–56.

47. Coviello-McLaughlin GM, Prowse KR. Telomere length regulation during postnatal development and ageing in *Mus spretus*. Nucleic Acids Res 1997; 25: 3051–8.

48. Vina J, Borras C, Gomez-Cabrera MC, Orr WC. Part of the series: from dietary antioxidants to regulators in cellular signalling and gene expression. Role of reactive oxygen species and (phyto)oestrogens in the modulation of adaptive response to stress. Free Radic Res 2006; 40: 111–19.

49. Borras C, Sastre J, Garcia-Sala D, Lloret A, Pallardo FV, Vina J. Mitochondria from females exhibit higher antioxidant gene expression and lower oxidative damage than males. Free Radic Biol Med 2003; 34: 546–52.

50. Pinto RE, Bartley W. Changes in glutathione reductase and glutathione peroxidase activities in rat liver related to age and sex. Biochem J 1968; 109: 34P.

51. Tarry-Adkins JL, Ozanne SE, Norden A, Cherif H, Hales CN. Lower antioxidant capacity and elevated p53 and p21 may be a link between gender disparity in renal telomere shortening, albuminuria, and longevity. Am J Physiol Renal Physiol 2006; 290: F509–16.

52. Borras C, Gambini J, Gomez-Cabrera MC, Sastre J, Pallardo FV, Mann GE, Vina J. 17Beta-oestradiol up-regulates longevity-related, antioxidant enzyme expression via the ERK1 and ERK2[MAPK]/NFkappaB cascade. Aging Cell 2005; 4: 113–8.

CHAPTER 2

The biologic basis for longevity differences between men and women

Rafi T Kevorkian and Oscar A Cepeda

Introduction

In the modern world much has changed over the last 50 years. Lifestyles have become healthier with emphasis on regular exercise, healthy diets, and a declining dependence on tobacco. As a result, life expectancy has also changed, rising slowly but in a steady manner year after year. In the Western world, the average lifespan is 73.7 years for men and 83.8 years for women. People of both sexes live longer, but every year women have outpaced men. Life expectancy is roughly 7 years longer for women than for men. Although women live longer than men, they do so with greater time spent with disability. This chapter will examine the biologic reasons why women outlive men.

Aging could be defined as a normal process of every living cell, arising from metabolic changes leading to a functional decline, and is associated with structural impairment of somatic tissues. Aging and gender have been studied for several decades and it is clear that gender accounts for important differences in the incidence and prevalence of many age-related diseases. Potentially preventable environmental causes, such as smoking, alcohol, and dietary behavior, have played an important role in the large gender differential in some countries. However, several theories for the longevity gender gap support a biologic basis for aging, making it a source of endless debate due to the complex interaction of environmental, historic, and genetic factors playing an important role in determining the gender-specific probability of achieving longevity.[1]

Epidemiology

The gender gap in human beings tends to change depending on biologic and socio-cultural issues. Life expectancy is different across countries and it is related in some way to the level of development in each region of the world.[2] Nations struggling with poverty and underdevelopment have a limited life expectancy for women, mainly because of a high maternal mortality, making the difference between genders less evident. The opposite situation is observed in developed countries such as Sweden, Canada, Western Europe, and the United States, where great improvements in public health and maternal and infant mortality have been made, leading to a substantially higher life expectancy and a marked difference in the gender gap of longevity that favors women, resulting in a larger number of women surviving the age of 65. The ratio of women to men at age 65 is close to 120:100 and by age 85 is 250:100. This longevity gap persists to very old age, even beyond the age of 85, when the average woman outlives the average man by 1.2 years.[3]

The basis for this gender difference in longevity between men and women is thought to be a complex interaction of environmental, behavioral, and biologic factors. Major causes of mortality and death rates are higher in men. Mortality from cardiovascular disease is more likely to occur in men than in women (173.1 per 100 000 vs 95.4 per 100 000);[1,3] whereas the rate of stroke is 20% higher in men. However, cardiovascular disease remains the leading cause of death in older women, exceeding the number of deaths in older men in terms of absolute number of cardiovascular deaths.

The incidence of cancer is higher in men compared to women, and this difference is most evident after 64 years of age. There is a sharp rise in cancer incidence after the age of 64 for both men and women, but it is higher for men (559.6 per 100 000 men vs 420.1 per 100 000 women). Among elderly men, three cancers account for 50% of all malignancies: prostate, lung, and colon cancer. Lung cancer is the most common malignant entity in both men and women over age 60 and is responsible for 30% of all cancer deaths in this group. The second and third highest rates of incidence for cancer are breast and colorectal cancer for women, and colorectal and prostate for men.[4] Although far less common as a cause of death than either cardiovascular disease or malignancy, mortality from trauma, as a result of accidents or violence, contributes significantly to the total loss of anticipated life years.

Life expectancy varies throughout the lifespan and actually the gap between men and women is greatest at younger ages and becomes smaller with increasing age. However, the biggest increase in the ratio of females to males occurs at the extremes of age. Nevertheless, at all ages, women have better survival than do men. At birth the gap is about 6 years; at age 65 it decreases to about 3 years; and at age 75 it is even lower at about 2 years. Nowadays women have an excellent chance to reach the eighth decade, and for those who reach age 85, the remaining average life expectancy is an additional 6 years. Demographic trends have shown that at very old age mortality in human beings begins to decelerate. These trends are based on European calculations from a database of 70 million people who reached the age of 80 and of 200 000 who lived to at least 100. Research has shown that there is an observed deceleration in mortality rate as age 100 is approached, and it is maintained through age 105 for men and 107 for women.[5] One acceptable theory

is that frailer individuals drop out of the population, leaving behind a more robust cohort that continues to survive.[6]

Genetic differences in human longevity

Aging could be considered a result of the interaction between genes and environment, in which genetics becomes a powerful tool to understand the fundamental mechanisms of aging since it deals with the blueprints for life that we inherit. The rate of aging and maximum lifespan vary among species, and therefore must be at least partly under genetic control.[7] Variation in human longevity has a very strong genetic basis. A Scandinavian study of monozygotic and dizygotic twins calculated the heritability of life expectancy to be 20 to 30%,[8] and this could in some way be the reason why cases of exceptional longevity tend to cluster in families. The familial contribution (some combination of shared genes and environment) to exceptional longevity has been explored with centenarian pedigrees. The survival of siblings of 102 centenarians was compared with the survival of siblings of a control group (n = 77) who were from a similar birth cohort born in 1896 but whose parents had died 27 years earlier at the age of 73.[9] The relative risk of survival steadily increased with age for siblings of the centenarians to the point that they had four times the probability of surviving to age 91. The relative risk for survival to older age continued to rise beyond age 91, although these larger differences were not statistically significant because of the small numbers of siblings at these extreme ages.

Clinical syndromes that have features of accelerated aging, such as Werner's syndrome and Hutchinson–Gilford progeria, are characterized by mutations in two of the genes involved in the metabolism and repair of DNA. Werner's syndrome is characterized by mutations in the WRN gene, which is thought to be involved in maintaining genomic stability. Hutchinson–Gilford disease is caused by a mutation in the LMNA gene, which codes for a group of nuclear membrane proteins called *lamins* that affect nuclear morphology, chromatin structure, DNA synthesis, and gene expression.[10] Another factor related to longevity and genetic differences is the apolipoprotein (apo) ε-4 allele dropout seen with extreme age as an example of a polymorphism with an influence powerful enough to have a noticeable effect upon survival in the general population and across various ethnic lines. Hyman et al[11] noted that the frequency of the ε-4 allele decreases markedly with advancing age. Results from the Italian centenarian study showed an association between specific variations in the locus for the apo-B allele and extreme longevity.[12] One of its counterparts, the ε-2 allele, becomes more frequent with advanced age among Caucasians. Presumably the drop-out at earlier age of the ε-4 allele is because of its association with 'premature' mortality secondary to Alzheimer's disease and heart disease.[13] In another study, nonagenarian subjects had an extremely low frequency of histocompatibility locus antigen (HLA)-DRw9 and an increased frequency of DR1. A high frequency of DRw9 and a low frequency of DR1 are associated with autoimmune or immune-deficiency diseases, which can cause premature mortality.[14]

Genes that reduce the risk of atherosclerosis may be more common in centenarians, and two such genes have been identified. In the first case, a mutation in the cholesteryl ester transfer protein (CETP) gene leads to larger lipoproteins and a reduced prevalence of cardiovascular disease,[15] and the second gene has variations for microsomal transfer protein (MTP) – the rate-limiting step in lipoprotein synthesis.[16] Although such genes may have substantial effects on longevity, they do not appear to modulate the aging process.

Regulation of telomere length

The telomere and its potential role in cellular senescence has generated excitement in the field of genetics of aging. Telomeres are tandem repeat sequences (TTAGGG) of DNA that cap the ends of linear chromosomes. Because typical DNA polymerases cannot fully duplicate these sequences, telomeres shorten with each cell division in somatic cells. Eventually the chromosomes become unstable

and the cell is no longer able to replicate. The progressive shortening of telomeres acts as an inherent replicative clock in which the somatic cell has a finite capacity for division (proliferating germ line cells, lymphocytes, and cancer cells do not undergo telomeric shortening). Thus, telomere length may be an important determinant of replicative capacity, leading to apoptosis or neoplastic transformation.[17]

Multiple cross-sectional population analyses of telomere length in white blood cells have been the main source of information regarding human telomere dynamics in vivo. Telomere length is highly heritable,[18] and inversely correlated with age, longer in adult women than men, and yet equivalent in newborn boys and girls. Two factors have been identified as responsible for the observed longer telomeres in women, namely estrogen and somatic cell selection. Gender and age considerably influence reactive oxygen species (ROS) metabolism. While the exact mechanisms whereby age modifies ROS metabolism are poorly defined, the sex effect is largely related to ovarian steroid hormones, particularly estrogen. Estrogen and its derivatives exert an antioxidant effect via a number of mechanisms, including scavenging free radicals, inhibiting free radical formation, and stimulating enzymes which are crucial for free radical detoxification.[19] Estrogens also stimulate the transcription of the gene encoding the telomerase reverse transcriptase enzyme that adds telomere repeats to chromosome ends, thereby slowing down the rate of telomere erosion as a result of the oxidative stress. This upregulation of telomerase and reduced oxidative damage could be a reasonable explanation for the longer telomeres observed in women as compared with men. Estrogen also stimulates nitric oxide production in vascular endothelial cells, and a study has shown that nitric oxide stimulates telomerase in these cells.[20] The antioxidant effect of estrogens tends to disappear with advancing age in old women. However, its premenopausal influence could set telomere attrition at a trajectory that maintains longer telomeres in women throughout the entire cycle of life.

The relationships between telomere length and indicators of vascular aging and cardiovascular risks in humans have been examined. Two studies found that telomere length in white blood cells is inversely correlated with pulse pressure, and one of these studies showed that this relationship is modified by sex.[21] Since pulse pressure increases with age and is an indicator of the biologic aging of central arteries, and given that cardiovascular risks are increased with age, it is logical to propose that biologic aging of individuals with relatively short telomeres may be more advanced than their chronologic age would indicate, and also telomere length is shorter in patients with atherosclerotic coronary heart disease than in their age-matched peers.[22] Vascular dementia, which leads to a progressive intellectual impairment resulting from cerebrovascular disease, is frequently observed with essential hypertension and diabetes mellitus,[23] and is associated with relatively short telomeres.

The skewed X-linked selection theory of somatic cells, as a function of aging, is another factor that might explain longer telomeres in women as compared with men. This has been observed primarily in women older than 60 years. Ninety-six percent of the combined length of telomeres in a newly formed zygote is contributed by autosomal telomeres, which suggests that factors on the X chromosome influence telomere length considerably, modulating the functional activity of telomerase or other telomere length-influencing factors. As women get older, the two somatic cell populations would be redistributed toward the population that has comparatively longer telomeres, not only because telomere length appears to be influenced by an X-linked gene or genes, but also for the reason that longer telomeres denote resistance to oxidative stress.[24]

Role of sex hormones controling aging and longevity

The role that sex hormones play, estrogen in females and testosterone in males, in terms of lifespan differences is widely accepted as a factor for longevity differences.[25] The role of testosterone in a decreased lifespan has been explained on the basis of the characteristics which are particular to the male gender, such as competitiveness and aggression. Also testosterone decreases blood concentrations of high-density

lipoproteins (HDLs), and increases low-density lipoproteins, increasing the risk of cardiovascular morbidity and mortality.[25] On the other hand, estrogens have demonstrated effective reductions in LDL cholesterol and increases in HDL, thus having beneficial effects on the cardiovascular system, lowering morbidity and mortality from cardiovascular diseases in women.[26] Due to their phenolic structure, estrogens exhibit marked antioxidant properties, but not as a direct chemical antioxidant, since the amount of estrogens needed for this action exceeds that observed in normal blood. It seems that estrogens exert an antioxidant effect rather than upregulating the expression of the genes encoding antioxidant enzymes through estrogen receptors and cell signaling pathways.[26]

The primary estrogen produced by the ovaries is estradiol, and its antioxidant activity relies on the activation of mitogen-activated protein kinases (MAPKs) ERK1 and ERK2, that subsequently activate the signaling pathway for the nuclear factor kappa B (NFκB), thus behaving as double transgenics leading to increased expression of antioxidant enzymes glutathione peroxidase and manganese-superoxide dismutase (MNSOD).[26] Glutathione is a major intracellular antioxidant, with concentrations similar to those of glucose, and it constitutes a major low molecular weight thiol in cells.[27] Glutathione levels have been considered a biologic marker of aging, and its level inside the mitochondria is directly related to the damage associated with the aging process. Mitochondrial concentrations of glutathione in males are approximately half those found in females. The degree of DNA oxidation increases with aging and the level of 8-oxo-deoxyguanosine (8-oxo-dG) is an excellent marker of oxidative damage to the DNA. Levels of 8-oxo-dG are 4-fold higher in males than in females.[28]

Phytoestrogens, natural products that exert an estrogen-like effect, could mimic the favorable effect of estrogens as an upregulator of antioxidant longevity-related genes without the substantial postmenopausal drawbacks of estrogens. Phytoestrogens constitute an interesting alternative with very few detrimental effects.[29] Genistein is a phytoestrogen present in soy and is able to decrease oxidative stress at nutritionally relevant concentrations. As demonstrated by Viña and co-workers,[30] the beneficial effects of genistein are mediated by its interactions with estrogen receptors, and the cell signaling pathways of MAPKs and NFκB.

Mitochondrial theory of aging

Mitochondria are the intracellular organelles responsible for oxidative metabolism. More than 90% of the oxygen used by aerobic cells is consumed in mitochondria. Mammalian cells have several hundred mitochondria, all of which were inherited from those in the maternal egg. Each mitochondrion has a few identical copies of its own circular DNA, which codes for 13 mitochondrial enzymes involved in cellular respiration (using a slightly different genetic code than does nuclear DNA), and a few ribosomal and transfer RNA molecules.[31] The rate of mutation of mitochondrial DNA in somatic cells is about 10 to 20 times faster than nuclear DNA, and this could in part be explained because mitochondria are an important source of free radicals, particularly hydrogen peroxide; hydroxyl radicals cause oxidative damage to proteins, lipids, and DNA.[25]

These mutations accumulate with age in postmitotic tissues such as neurons, and in cardiac and skeletal muscle. The mitochondrial theory of aging is based on the cellular changes that occur at the level of mitochondrial DNA related to the balance between the load of age-related mutations and the healthy inherited DNA. The damage to mitochondrial DNA prevents the regeneration of new mitochondria from postmitotic cells, reducing the level of adenosine triphosphate and consequently cell death.[32] Studies by Sohal and co-workers[33] have shown that shorter-lived species produce higher amounts of hydroperoxide than the longer-lived species. Females live longer than males in many mammalian species, including humans. Mitochondria from males produce significantly more hydrogen peroxide (approximately 50%) than those from females and have a reduced level of mitochondrial reduced glutathione, manganese, superoxide dismutase, and glutathione peroxidase than females. Oxidative damage to mitochondrial DNA is also

4-fold less in females than in males. These differences may be explained by estrogens. Ovariectomy abolishes the gender differences between males and females, and estrogen replacement rescues the ovariectomy effect in animal models.[25]

Stress resistance

Early in their history, invertebrates appear to have evolved systems for recognizing environmental conditions, such as food shortages or adverse temperatures, which favored differentiation into long-lived stress-resistant forms rather than into more vulnerable breeding forms. These stress-resistance systems may have been adopted as developmental controls, for aging pathways by more advanced organisms. Several of these genes have human homologs. There is a good correlation between resistance to cytotoxic stress and maximal lifespan in a variety of mammals, from hamsters to humans, whose lifespan varies 40-fold. Fibroblasts from small, long-lived mice are more resistant to cytotoxic stress than those from normal mice.[34] The phenomenon of aging, which is characterized by a reduction in the capability to respond to situations that endanger life and survival, could be paralleled to the progressive increase in the level of plasma catecholamines, inadequate cortisol secretion, decrease in peripheral adrenoreceptor sensitization, reduction in the activity of the insulin growth factor-1 (IGF-1) axis, and decreased secretion of sex steroids as a result of a global dysfunction at the level of the hypothalamo–pituitary–adrenal axis in response to stress challenges.[35]

The response to stress has a clear sexual pattern of differentiation, and it has been attributed to the opposite effects on the cortisol/ACTH balance, caused by estrogens and androgens. Troiano and co-workers[36] showed the sex-related dimorphism is evident until the extreme limits of the human lifespan, and that cortisol and ACTH levels at different ages show different rates of change depending on sex. So it is not surprising that sex-related differences in the regulation of stress response mediators could play a causative role in differing male and female life expectancy and longevity.[35] Other reports have

27

shown that the genetic variability of tyrosine hydroxylase (TH), when compared between centenarians and younger persons, showed a considerable sex-specific TH locus/longevity association.[37] A more recent investigation was able to prove that the variability in the mitochondrial genome (mtDNA) has a sex-specific impact on longevity. The mtDNA variant was represented at an expectedly high frequency among centenarian males.[38]

Immunology and longevity

The process of aging imposes changes at all levels in human beings, and the immune system is no exception. Human immunosenescence is the consequence of chronic antigenic overload; some of the most important features of age-related immune cell remodeling are: clonal expansion of memory and effector T-lymphocytes, reduction of naive T cells, and shrinkage of T-cell repertoire. In most elderly subjects there is an increased plasmatic level of pro-inflammatory cytokines, despite the lack of clinical signs of inflammatory disease,[39] which is associated with a concomitant alteration of the lipid profile and an increased capability of activated mononuclear cells to produce pro-inflammatory cytokines (IL-1, IL-6, TNFα) in comparison with younger individuals. Elevated levels of pro-inflammatory cytokines are predictors of mortality and morbidity in the elderly. In particular, 'high producer' alleles of pro-inflammatory cytokines have been shown to be associated with inflammatory age-related diseases,[40–44] such as Alzheimer's dementia, and disability,[45] and with a decreased probability to reach extreme longevity.[46] Gene polymorphisms involving hemochromatosis,[47] and interferon-γ[48] have been associated with longevity in women but not in men.

Human leukocyte antigen (HLA) is the general name of a group of genes in the human major histocompatibility complex (MHC) region on human chromosome 6 (mouse chromosome 17) that encodes the cell-surface antigen-presenting proteins. HLA, besides antigen presentation, is responsible for the T-cell repertoire and target cell recognition in cytotoxicity. An excess of the 8.1AH haplotype has been reported in a group of elderly males when compared to young males and also elderly females.[49] Further research is needed in this field to confirm this association between male longevity and 8.1AH, which is associated with a variety of immune dysfunctions and autoimmune diseases. Lagaay et al[50] HLA typed 964 Dutch subjects (278 males and 686 females) over 85 years, who were compared with a group of 2444 young adults. A decrease in B40 and an increase in DR-11 (DR5split) in women over 85 years were observed with an association for longevity for women. Ivanova et al[51] studied a group of French centenarians and compared them to an adult control group. Three differences were noted in three alleles, DR-7, DR-11, and DR-13, that were statistically significant in the older group; DR-11 was higher in women.

Conclusions

The components of different pathways in women and men by which they achieve longevity with and without major age-related disabilities are not completely defined yet. Several biologic mechanisms could be responsible for the difference between men and women. It is clear that estrogens play a pivotal role, making women live longer than men, since estrogens have effects at the level of cellular oxidation and telomere length, and it has also been shown that estrogens induce a reduction in LDL cholesterol and hence in cardiovascular morbidity. Also immune function has some different genetic determinants that increase women's resistance to external aggressors. However, aging and extreme longevity are not only determined by biologic markers; complex socio-cultural factors are involved in this process. It has been demonstrated that poor socioeconomic conditions are important factors in determining length of survival; careful comparison of data from different countries is necessary to ascertain the roles of nature and nurture in this phenomenon which plays a complementary role in the aging process. Since changes in the environment could trigger changes at the molecular-genetic level by inducing mutations, it is possible that this could result in conditions favoring a shorter lifespan.

Changes and manipulation of the aging process will affect the overall risk of developing conditions seen in older people and perhaps will delay the onset of several diseases. The maximal lifespan appears to be 120 years and the average in developed nations is about 80 years. Incapacitating conditions particular to old people appear at about age 70 or later, and if the human lifespan were increased to 150 years, it is likely that debilitating diseases such as Alzheimer's disease would not be noted until age 100, allowing more patients to be free from chronic debilitating illnesses.

References

1. Newman A, Brach J. Gender gap in longevity and disability in older persons. Epidemiol Rev 2001; 23(2): 343–50.

2. Bonita R, Howe AL. Older women in an aging world: achieving health across the life course. World health statistics. Quarterly Rappaport Trimestriel de Statistiques Sanitaires Mondiales 1996; 29: 134–41.

3. Kramarow E, Lentzner H, Rooks R et al. Health and aging chartbook. Health, United States, 1999. Hyattsville, MD: National Center for Health Statistics 1999: 1–177.

4. Hajar R. Cancer in the elderly: is it preventable? Clin Geriatr Med 2004; 20: 293–316.

5. Perls T, Kumkel L, Puca A. The genetics of exceptional longevity. J Am Geriatr Soc 2002; 50(2): 359–68.

6. Vaupel JW, Carey JP, Christensen K et al. Biodemographic trajectories of longevity. Science 1998; 280: 855–60.

7. Hekimi S, Guarente L. Genetics and specificity of the aging process. Science 2003; 299: 1351–4.

8. McGue M, Vaupel JW, Holm N et al. Longevity is moderately inheritable in a sample of Danish twins born 1870–1990. J Gerontol A Biol Med Sci 1993; 48: B237–44.

9. Perls T, Wager C, Bubrick E et al. Siblings of centenarians live longer. Lancet 1998; 351: 1560.

10. Yu CE, Oshima J, Fu YH et al. Positional cloning of the Werner's syndrome gene. Science 1996; 272: 258–62.

11. Hyman BT, Gomez-Isla T, Rebeck GW et al. Epidemiological, clinical, and neuropathological study of apolipoprotein E genotype in Alzheimer's disease. Ann N Y Acad Sci 1996; 862: 1–5.

12. Tan Q, De Benedictis G, Ukraintseva SV et al. A centenarian-only approach for assessing gene–gene interaction in human longevity. Eur J Hum Genet 2002; 10: 119–24.

13. Gerdes LU, Jeune B, Ranberg KA et al. Estimation of apolipoprotein E genotype-specific mortality risks from the distribution of genotypes in centenarians and middle aged men: apolipoprotein E gene is a frailty gene not a longevity gene. Genet Epidemiol 2000; 19: 202–10.

14. Takata H, Suzuki M, Ishi T et al. Influence of major histocompatibility complex region genes on human longevity among Okinawan-Japanese centenarians and nonagenarians. Lancet 1997; 2: 824–6.

15. Barzilai N, Atzmon G, Schechter C et al. Unique lipoprotein phenotype and genotype associated with exceptional longevity. JAMA 2003; 290: 2030–40.

16. Gesaman BJ, Benson E, Brewster SJ et al. Haplotype-based identification of a microsomal transfer protein marker associated with the human life span. Proc Natl Acad Sci USA 2003; 100: 14115–20.

17. Marciniak R, Guarente L. Human genetics. Testing telomerase. Nature 2001; 413: 370–1, 373.

18. Nawrot TS, Staessen JA, Gardner JP et al. Telomere length and possible link to X chromosome. Lancet 2004; 363: 507–10.

19. Aviv A, Shay J, Christensen K et al. The longevity gap: are telomeres the explanation? Sci Aging Knowl Environ 2005; 23: 8–12.

20. Vasa M, Breitschopf K, Zeiher AM, Dimmeler S. Nitric oxide activates telomerase and delays endothelial cell senescence. Circ Res 2000; 87: 540–2.

21. Benetos A, Okuda K, Lajemi M et al. Telomere length as an indicator of biologic aging: the gender effect and relation with pulse pressure and pulse wave velocity. Hypertension 2001; 37: 381–5.

22. Samani NJ, Boultby R, Butler R et al. Telomere shortening in atherosclerosis. Lancet 2001; 358: 472–3.

23. Butler RN, Ahronheim J, Fillit H et al. Vascular dementia: how to make the diagnosis in office practice. Geriatrics 1993; 48: 39–42, 47.

24. Harley CB, Vaziri H, Counter M et al. The telomere hypothesis of cellular aging. Exp Gerontol 1992; 27: 375–82.

25. Viña J, Sastre J, Pallardo F et al. Mitochondrial theory of aging: importance why females live longer than males. Antioxidants and Redox Signaling 2003; 5(5): 549–56.

26. Viña J, Borras C, Gambini J. Why females live longer that males: control of longevity by sex hormones. Sci Aging Knowl Environ 2005; 23: 17.

27. Viña C, Borras C, Gambini J. Why do females live longer than males? Importance of the upregulation of longevity associated genes by oestrogenic compounds. FEBS Lett 2005; 579: 2541–5.

28. Borras C, Sastre J, Garcia-Sala D. Mitochondria from females exhibit higher antioxidant gene expression and lower oxidative damage than males. Free Rad Biol Med 2003; 5: 549–56.

29. Park D, Huang T, Frishman WH. Phytoestrogens as cardioprotective agents. Cardiol Rev 2005; 13: 13–17.

30. Borras C, Gambini J, Gomez-Cabrera MC et al. Genistein, a soy isoflavone, up-regulates expression of antioxidant genes: involvement of estrogen receptors, ERK 1/2, and NFkappaB. FASEB J 2006; 20: 2136–8.

31. Shoffner JM, Wallace DC. Mitochondrial genetics: principles and practice. Am J Hum Genet 1992; 51: 1179–86.

32. Merriwether Da, Clark AG, Ballinger SW et al. The structure of human mitochondrial DNA variation. J Mol Evol 1991; 33: 543–55.

33. Sohal RS, Muller A, Koletzko B, Sies H. Effect of age and ambient temperature on n-pentane production in adult housefly, Musca domestica. Mech Ageing Dev 1985; 29: 317–26.

34. Mukarami S, Salmon A, Miller RA. Multiplex stress resistance in cells from long lived dwarf mice. FASEB J 2003; 17: 1565–6.

35. Franceschi C, Motta L, Rapisarda R. Do men and women follow different trajectories to reach extreme longevity? Aging Clin Exp Res 2000; 12: 77–84.

36. Troiano L, Pini G, Petruzzi E et al. Evaluation of adrenal function in aging. J Endocrinol Invest 1999; 105: 74–5.

37. De Benedicts G, Carotenuto L, Carrieri G et al. The Sardinia study of extreme longevity. Eur J Hum Genet 1998; 6: 534–41.

38. De Benedicts G, Rose G, Carrieri G et al. Mitochondrial DNA inherited variants are associated with successful aging and longevity in humans. FASEB J 2003; 13: 1532–6.

39. Baggio G, Donazzan S, Monti D et al. Lipoprotein(a) and lipoprotein profile in healthy centenarians: a reappraisal of vascular risk factors. FASEB J 1998; 12: 433–7.

40. Bhojak J, Dekosky ST, Ganguli M, Kamboh MI. Genetic polymorphisms in the cathepsin D and interleukin-6 genes and the risk of Alzheimer's disease. Neurosci Lett 2000; 288: 21–4.

41. Grimaldi LM, Casadei VM, Ferri C et al. Association of early onset Alzheimer's disease with an interleukin-1 alpha gene polymorphism. Ann Neurol 2000; 47: 361–5.

42. Hobson EE, Ralston SH. Role of genetic factors in the pathophysiology and management of osteoporosis. Clin Endocrinol 2001; 54: 1–9.

43. Franceschi C, Valnesin S, Lescai et al. Neuroinflammation and the genetics of Alzheimer's disease: the search for a pro-inflammatory phenotype. Aging 2001; 13: 163–70.

44. McCusker SM, Curran MD, Dynan KB et al. Association between polymorphism in regulatory region of gene encoding tumour necrosis factor alpha and risk of Alzheimer's disease and vascular dementia: a case controlled study. Lancet 2001; 357: 436–9.

45. Ferruci L, Harris TB, Guralnik JM et al. Serum IL-6 level and the development of disability in older persons. J Am Geriatr Soc 1999; 47: 639–46.

46. Bonafe M, Olivieri F, Cavallone L et al. A gender-dependent genetic predisposition to produce high level of IL-6 is detrimental for longevity. Eur J Immunol 2001; 31: 2357–61.

47. Lio D, Balsteri CR, Colonna-Romano G et al. Association between the MHC class I gene HFE polymorphisms and longevity: a study in Sicilian population. Genes Immun 2002; 3: 20–4.

48. Lio D, Scola L, Crivello A et al. Allele frequencies of +874T→A single nucleotide polymorphism at the first introns of Interferon-γ gene in a group of Italian centenarians. Exper Gerontol 2002; 37: 315–19.

49. Rea IM, Middleton D. Is the phenotypic combination A1B8Cw7DR3 a marker of male longevity? J Am Geriatr Soc 1994; 42: 978.

50. Lagaay AM, D'Amaro J, Ligthart V et al. Longevity and heredity in humans. Association with the human leucocyte antigen phenotype. Ann NY Acad Sci 1991; 621: 78–89.

51. Ivanova R, Fhenon N, Lepage V et al. HLA-Dr alleles display sex-dependent effects on survival and discriminate between individual and familial longevity. Hum Mol Genet 1998; 7: 187–94.

CHAPTER 3

The biology of the aging brain

Xi Chen and Shirley Shidu Yan

Introduction

Aging brings about characteristic changes in brain functions, which can present in such diverse aspects as alterations in cognitive function, motor coordination, and sleep pattern. Although there is a general trend towards functional decline during aging, the degree of these changes can vary widely between individuals and generally they do not seriously compromise the quality of life. However, some age-related alterations might increase a person's vulnerability to some neurodegenerative disorders, such as Alzheimer's disease (AD). Recent advances in molecular biology, neurophysiology, and functional brain imaging have made significant progress in understanding some aspects of the biological mechanisms underlying the aging process.

Age-associated cognitive and behavioral changes

The most consistent behavioral change in the elderly observed in neuropsychologic studies is a general slowing of mental processing. Some studies have even suggested that psychomotor slowing and slowed cognitive processing can account for most of the aging-associated performance decline. Further analyses of performance slowing in the elderly have indicated that the slowing tends to occur at decision points. An increased cautiousness of many elderly persons may also add to their slow performance. The intelligence quotient (IQ) test in the elderly usually reveals a 'classic aging pattern,' in which there is a greater decline in the speed-dependent performance IQ as compared to the vocabulary IQ, and a greater decline in 'fluid' (novel solutions) versus 'crystallized' (old solutions) intelligence. The elderly are not as efficient at integrating unfamiliar information or using novel approaches as they are in employing old information in old solutions, strategies, or templates (wisdom). Thus, overlearned, well-practiced, and familiar skills, ability, and knowledge are 'crystallized' and continue to be fully operative and even show gains into the seventies and eighties; while activities requiring 'fluid' intelligence, which involves reasoning and problem solving for unfamiliar solutions, follow the typical pattern of relatively slow decline through the middle years until the late fifties or early sixties, when decline proceeds at an increased rate.[1]

Most elderly individuals show decreased engagement, risk-taking, and goal-oriented behaviors, and become more conventional, cautious, and routine-bound, which is generally attributed to changes in frontal lobe executive functions. Reasoning about familiar material holds up well with aging. In contrast, when reasoning is brought to solving unfamiliar or complex problems, and to those requiring the subject to distinguish relevant from irrelevant or redundant elements, then older persons tend to do increasingly poor with advancing age. Concept formation and abstraction also suffer with aging, as older persons tend to think in more concrete terms. Mental flexibility for making new abstractions and forming new conceptual links diminishes with age, with an increasingly steep decline after age 70. Mental inflexibility appears as difficulty in adapting to new situations, solving novel problems, or changing the mental set in many studies of elderly persons. It is suggested that reduced flexibility may occur when the task becomes more difficult, as when memory load or task complexity increases beyond the subject's capacity for efficient processing. Perseveration and difficulty in withstanding distractions also contribute to older subjects' poorer performances.[1]

Age-associated memory impairment (AAMI) is one of the most common geriatric neuropsychologic complaints. Most elderly persons experience mildly increased difficulty to recall the names of people and places due to decreased retrieval of information. During neuropsychologic testing, while short-term retention of simple span is resistant to the age effect, the declines are noted when the task requires mental manipulation such as reversing a string of digits, with distraction or when the amount of material exceeds the normal primary storage capacity of six or seven items. Almost all studies report that learning ability diminishes with aging and that losses are particularly prominent when learning is measured by recall. Visual, auditory, and tactile memory tends to be compromised at an earlier age than verbal memory. Decreased ability to retrieve information can also impede the verbal fluency tests: elderly subjects show slowed reaction times and, on tests of confrontation naming, are more likely to require phonetic or semantic cues to aid retrieval, and to make more errors due to misperceptions. A standardized memory test such as the Wechester Memory Scale–Revised helps to differentiate AAMI from mild cognitive impairment (MCI): subjects with AAMI only show a statistically lower score when they are compared to younger controls (i.e., not age-adjusted) and subjects with an MCI score 1.5 standardized deviations or more below the mean when compared to education and age-adjusted controls.[2] MCI is considered as a potential early stage or precursor of AD. The conversion rates of MCI to AD average about 12 to 17% compared to 1 to 7% for the normal elderly.[3]

Decline in motor coordination is a well-recognized phenomenon in aging. The gait of an elderly person is slower, with a shorter stride, and less erect posture. Postural reflexes are often sluggish, making the individuals more susceptible to losing their balance and falling. These motor changes involve both central nervous system mechanisms, such as performance slowing and poor coordination, and peripheral alterations, such as reduced position sense, muscle weakness, and skeletal changes. Beginning at age 30, simple reaction time follows a pattern of gradual slowing and typically continues at about the same steady rate over the lifespan. In contrast, speed in the performance of complex activities in which mental processing is involved shows a rapid rate of slowing after age 60. Diminished dexterity and coordination tend to compromise fine motor skills. Motor strength also decreases a little around age 40, with accelerated losses thereafter. In the test for idiomotor apraxia, older persons are much more likely to use a body part as object (e.g., hand and fingers as comb, rather than shaping and moving hand and arm as if holding a comb). All sensory modalities, such as vision, hearing, tactile, odor, and olfaction, decline in sensitivity and acuity during aging and may contribute significantly to age-related functional impairments.[1]

The sleep pattern changes with age. Elderly individuals awaken more frequently after falling asleep and have less total sleep time. Stage I slow-wave sleep is increased in the elderly while stage III, stage IV, and rapid eye movement (REM) sleep are reduced. Sleep spindles may show decreased frequency, amount, and amplitude. Sleep becomes fragmented with increased daytime somnolence. The prevalence of sleep disorders such as sleep apnea and periodic limb movements in sleep become more prevalent with aging.[4]

Electroencephalographic changes in old age include slowing of the posterior dominant frequency from 11 to 12 Hz in the young to 8 to 9 Hz in the aged. There is also an increase in intermittent fast activities, diffuse slow activity, or focal slow waves.[4] Intermittent focal slow waves in the temporal regions (particularly in the middle and anterior temporal regions and greater on the left side) are noted in 17–59% of healthy elderly individuals. Some studies suggest that intermittent temporal slowing is associated with white matter hyperintensity found on MRI scan, but not with either blood pressure levels or cognitive functioning.[5] Alpha blocking and photic driving response to intermittent photic stimulation are also diminished in old age.[6]

Age-associated structural and biochemical changes

Underlying the cognitive and behavioral changes mentioned above, there are also significant structural changes in aging brain. The brain size remains essentially unchanged from the early adult years until 40 to 50 years of age, after which a much greater rate of shrinkage begins. Cortical atrophy first appears in the forties, with increasingly widened sulci, narrowed gyri, and thinning of the cortical mantle. Ventricular size follows a similar pattern of slow enlargement into the fifties, with increasingly greater dilatation through the seventies for both sexes, with rapid changes beginning in the forties for men but not until the fifties for women. Subcortical structures showing a reduction in volume on MRI scan include the anterior diencephalon involved in the cholinergic system, and basal ganglia, but there is little loss of volume in the thalamus.[7] More than one-third of persons over age 65 show areas of increased signal intensity in the deep white matter (leukoaraiosis). At least some shrinkage in brain tissue appears to be due to neuronal loss, which occurs in both the cortex and subcortical structures. The hippocampus and anterior dorsal frontal lobe, including the frontal poles, are the areas most susceptible to neuronal loss. For example, for every decade after age 40, the hippocampus loses approximately 5% of its cells. Other areas lose fewer neurons and the occipital lobes virtually none. Among subcortical structures, the thalamus, the locus coeruleus, and Purkinje cells in the cerebellum are particularly vulnerable to neuronal loss. White matter loss may also account for significant amounts of brain shrinkage. Some studies have suggested that neuron counts remain relatively stable over the years while cell sizes shrink; while large neurons ($>90\,\mu m$) decrease in number in midfrontal, superior temporal, and inferior parietal areas of the neocortex, the small neurons and glial cells increase in number with aging.[8]

Astrocytic hyperactivity, cerebrovascular arteriosclerosis and mild amyloid β peptide ($A\beta$) accumulation are common even in healthy aging brain. There is a 10–30% increase in astrocyte volume with advancing age. Cerebrovascular arteriosclerosis is ubiquitous in the aging brain and the microvasculature shows increased hyalinization and PAS staining even in normal human brain. These changes may alter regional blood flow as well as local microperfusion.[9] Neuropathologic studies in the unimpaired normal elderly disclose changes similar to but not as extensive as those for AD, with neurofibrillary tangles and diffuse plaques detected in the hippocampal CA1 region and entorhinal cortex.[10]

Given the many structural brain alterations that take place with aging, it is not surprising that biochemical changes also occur, although most biochemical systems remain intact with aging. Loss of neurons in the subcortical structures and reduction in the enzyme activities may result in deficiencies in neurotransmitters such as dopamine, norepinephrine, and acetylcholine in aging brain. For example, there is a decrease with age in the number of neurons in the substantia nigra, a major dopaminergic center in the midbrain, and in the locus ceruleus, a noradrenergic nucleus in the pons. There are also reductions in the receptors for dopamine, norepinephrine, and acetylcholine. Both ligand binding and PET imaging have demonstrated a progressive reduction of dopamine D2 receptors in the striatum. These declines can be detected during midlife and appear to be progressive, reaching net decreases of 20–40% by the end of the lifespan. Generally speaking, aging changes in neurotransmitters and their receptors are mild and inconsistent in neurologically normal humans, unlike the major loss of basal ganglia dopaminergic neurons in Parkinson's disease (PD) and the variable loss of choline acetyltransferase (ChAT) and other cholinergic markers in AD. Age-related alterations in the synthesis and degradation of neurotransmitters and their receptors could explain some of the characteristics of aging, such as alterations in sleep pattern, mood, appetite, neuroendocrine functions, motor activity, and memory.

Resting brain metabolism during aging has been characterized. In neurologically normal individuals, basal cerebral glucose and oxygen consumption show modest declines of 10–30% over the lifespan. These decreases are correlated with the decreases in cerebral blood flow and parenchymal atrophy. Overall, age contributes much less to the total variance than intersubject variations. However, correlations in metabolism between cortical regions may be stronger in young adults than in the elderly, which implies an aging-associated decrease in the integration of cortical functions, which could contribute to the subtle age-related alterations in cognitive functions.[9]

Age-associated functional alterations in specific regions of the brain include loss of synaptic connection, loss of dendritic spines (the lateral protrusions on the shafts of dendrites that are specialized to receive excitatory synaptic input), and calcium dyshomeostasis. One of the most intensively studied areas is the relationship between the hippocampus and the learning process. The hippocampus of the temporal lobe plays an important role in memory storage and the neurons in the hippocampus show plastic capability, which is required for associative learning. The hippocampus has three major excitatory pathways running from the subiculum to the CA1 region in this sequence: (1) the perforant pathway runs from the subiculum to the granule cells in the hilus of the dentate gyrus; (2) the mossy fiber pathway that runs from the granule cells in the dentate gyrus to the pyramidal cells lying in the CA3 region of the hippocampus; and (3) the Schaffer collaterals (excitatory collaterals) run from the pyramidal cells in the CA3 region to the pyramidal cells in CA1. In 1973, Timothy Bliss and Terje Lomo[11] demonstrated that a brief high-frequency train of stimuli to any one of the three afferent pathways to the hippocampus produces an increase in the excitatory synaptic potential in the postsynaptic hippocampal neurons, which can last for hours, and in the intact animal for days and even weeks. They called this facilitation long-term potentiation (LTP), which is considered as an example for mammalian brain learning at the neuronal level.[12] With respect to aged neurons, there is no deficit in inducing LTP when robust induction parameters are used.

However, synaptic strength decays more rapidly in aged neurons, which is correlated with increased rates of forgeting in the aged animals. Conversely, long-term depression (LTD) is more easily induced in aged animals than in young animals, implying the mechanisms for information storage might be compromised in older animals. The underlying mechanism is considered to be due to dysregulation of Ca^{2+} homeostasis in the aging brain, with Ca^{2+} influx through N-methyl-D-aspartate (NMDA) receptors reduced and through L-type voltage-gated Ca^{2+} channels increased. The Ca^{2+} dysregulation also contributes to decreased cell excitability, altered synaptic function, and increased susceptibility to neuron loss in the aging hippocampus.[13] Another feature of learning-related neuronal plasticity changes is the expression of immediate-early genes (IEG), a diverse group of proteins including transcription factors, structural and scaffolding proteins, signal transduction proteins, growth factors, proteases, and enzymes. They are called IEGs since their corresponding mRNAs can be transcribed in the presence of protein synthesis inhibitors in response to the neural activity associated with learning and they have been studied as potential mediators of long-lasting plasticity. Induction of c-fos mRNA in dorsal hippocampus following LTP induction has been observed to be greater in aged animals as compared to young animals.[14]

Mitochondrial dysfunctions in the brain have been hypothesized to be responsible for some aspects of the aging process. One of the examples is the accumulation of somatic mitochondrial DNA (mtDNA) mutations in the postmitotic tissues, including muscle and brain. When the level of mtDNA rearrangements was quantitated by the analysis of a common 5-kb mtDNA deletion, mtDNA deletion was found to accumulate to the highest levels in the basal ganglia, followed by the cerebral cortex, with the least being found in the cerebellum. As a predominant species of mtDNA rearrangement, the highest level of the common 5-kb deletion was estimated in approximately 0.1% of the total mtDNA when the total tissue DNA was analyzed.[15] The actual proportion of mutated mtDNA in the individual cells or individual mitochondrium can be much higher considering the compartmentalized clonal expansion of deleted mtDNA within the individual organelle.[16,17] Since mtDNA encodes multiple subunits of the mitochondrial respiratory chain, these mutations can contribute to respiratory chain failure and oxidative damage observed in the specific brain regions during aging.[18] The importance of mtDNA mutations in causing aging was also demonstrated by the knock-in mouse models with a mutant form of the mtDNA polymerase γ (POLG) subunit A in which the proofreading function was inactivated by the mutation D257A. These mice had a shortened lifespan and developed premature aging phenotypes involving weight loss, reduction of subcutaneous fat, hair loss (alopecia), curvature of the spine (kyphosis), osteoporosis, anemia, reduced fertility, and heart enlargement. This was associated with an age-related decline in respiratory chain complexes I and IV activities and ATP production rates. Analysis of the mtDNA revealed that the knock-in animals had a 3- to 5-fold increase in mtDNA base substitution mutations in brain, heart, and liver, with the highest number of mutations in the cytochrome b coding region.[19]

Alzheimer's disease is an age-related neurodegenerative disorder

The increased life expectancy brought by medical advances has unmasked a new epidemic: dementia due to age-related deterioration of brain functions. Among them, AD affects about 5% of people over the age of 65 years, and about 30% over the age of 85 years. It has an estimated worldwide prevalence of 15 million people, making it the most common cause of dementia in adults. The patients present progressive loss of memory, disturbances of emotion, and behavior and general cognitive deterioration. Autopsy of the brain reveals loss of neurons associated with the formation of amyloid plaques and neurofibrillary tangles. Neuronal loss and neurofibrillary tangles in the nucleus basalis of Meynert of the frontal forebrain contribute to cholinergic abnormalities. The nucleus basalis manufactures ChAT that is distributed in a diffuse cholinergic projection system to the cerebral cortex. In the presynaptic terminals within the cerebral cortex, ChAT catalyzes synthesis of acetylcholine for release into the synapse. Neuronal death and dysfunction in the nucleus basalis leads to a reduction in ChAT and a subsequent deficiency in presynaptic acetylcholine production. In the AD brain, cholinergic activity is reduced 80 to 90% in affected cortical regions of the hippocampus, midtemporal gyrus, parietal cortex, and frontal cortex.[2]

Genetic factors have been suggested to play a role in the pathogenesis of AD. Both the familial, early-onset form and the more common sporadic form of AD have been recognized clinically. The clinical and pathologic features are identical in the two forms, but early-onset disease is sometimes Mendelian transmitted and autosomal dominantly inherited, whereas late-onset AD is non-Mendelian transmitted and shows only modest familial clustering. In dominant, early-onset families, genetic linkage analysis allowed mapping and subsequent cloning of three genes, amyloid β peptide precursor (APP) at chromosome 21q21, preseniline-1 (PS1) at chromosome 14q24, and presenilin-2 (PS2) at chromosome 1q42. These mutations account for about 10% of early-onset AD cases. In late-onset cases, apolipoprotein E (APOE, located at chromosome 19q13.2) has been identified as a 'susceptibility factor.' In cross-sectional studies of people over the age of 65, people with the APOE ε3/ε4 isoform have about three times the risk of developing AD and ε4 homozygotes have about 14 times the risk of developing AD, as compared to ε3 homozygotes. The population attributable risk associated with APOE ε4 was calculated to be approximately 20%.[20]

Consistent with the role of 'mitochondrial failure' in aging, there is also a large amount of evidence implicating an important role in AD for impaired energy metabolism and oxidative stress due to mitochondrial dysfunction. Metabolic impairment in AD patients has been demonstrated through functional imaging with PET and SPECT scans, which show hypometabolism, especially in the temporoparietal cortex of patients with AD, even at an early clinical stage of the disease.[21–23] Respiratory chain enzyme cytochrome c oxidase activity was found to be markedly decreased in brain[24] and platelets of AD as compared to control subjects.[25] Mitochondrial dysfunction also leads to reactive oxygen species (ROS) production causing neuronal oxidative stress. Recent studies further demonstrated that Aβ peptide might gain access to the intramitochondrial matrix and bind to β-amyloid binding alcohol dehydrogenase (ABAD), which may further impair the mitochondrial integrity and function. An animal model study demonstrated that binding of Aβ and ABAD can mediate reduced glucose utilization and ATP production, decreased respiratory chain activity, and increased oxidative stress, leading to memory impairment.[26] However, the direct link between Aβ accumulation and neuronal dysfunction/loss in humans remains missing.

In parallel with the aging-associated alterations of the endocrine system, the role of hormonal changes in the pathogenesis of AD is supported by epidemiologic data showing a predisposition of postmenopausal women to AD. Large epidemiologic studies have indicated that AD affects women 1.5 times as often as men, and remains more common in women even after adjusting for greater longevity among women and shorter disease survival among men.[27,28] When the cognitive function was correlated to AD pathology in the autopsy brain, it was found that AD pathology is more likely to be clinically expressed as dementia in women than in men.[29] The role of estrogen deficiency following the menopause remains inconclusive, and a recent Women's Health Initiative Memory Study[30] even demonstrated that estrogen plus progestin therapy could increase the risk for probable AD. Possible pathogenic effects of elevated gonadotropin levels[31] and testosterone depletion in brain[32] are also suggested by recent reports.

Acknowledgments

This work was supported by grants from the NIH (National Institute on Aging, AG16736, PO1 AG17490, P50 AG08702), the Michael J Fox Foundation, and the Alzheimer's Association to SSY. The authors thank Mr John S Luddy for critical reading of the manuscript.

References

1. Lezak MD. Neuropsychological Assessment, 3rd edn. New York: 1995.
2. Mendez MF, Cummings JL. Dementia: A Clinical Approach, 3rd edn. Philadelphia, PA: Butterworth Heinemann, 2003.
3. Petersen RC, Stevens JC, Ganguli M et al. Practice parameter: early detection of dementia: mild cognitive impairment (an evidence-based review). Report of the Quality Standards Subcommittee of the American Academy of Neurology. Neurology 2001; 56(9): 1133–42.
4. Chokroverty S. Sleep Disorders Medicine: Basic Science, Technical Considerations, and Clinical Aspects, 2nd edn. Boston, MA: Butterworth Heinemann, 1999.
5. Oken BS, Kaye JA. Electrophysiologic function in the healthy, extremely old. Neurology 1992; 42(3 Pt 1): 519–26.
6. Kelley J, Reilly E, Beller S. Photic driving and psychogeriatric diagnosis. Clin Electroencephalogr 1983; 14(2): 78–81.
7. Jernigan TL, Archibald SL, Berhow MT, Sowell ER, Foster DS, Hesselink JR. Cerebral structure on MRI, Part I: Localization of age-related changes. Biol Psychiatry 1991; 29(1): 55–67.
8. Terry RD, DeTeresa R, Hansen LA. Neocortical cell counts in normal human adult aging. Ann Neurol 1987; 21(6): 530–9.
9. Siegel GJ, Agranoff BW, Albers RW, Molinoff PB. Basic Neurochemistry, 5th edn. New York: Raven Press; 1994.
10. Davis DG, Schmitt FA, Wekstein DR, Markesbery WR. Alzheimer neuropathologic alterations in aged cognitively normal subjects. J Neuropathol Exp Neurol 1999; 58(4): 376–88.
11. Bliss TV, Lomo T. Long-lasting potentiation of synaptic transmission in the dentate area of the anaesthetized rabbit following stimulation of the perforant path. J Physiol 1973; 232(2): 331–56.
12. Kandel ER, Schwartz JH, Jessell TM. Principles of Neural Science, 3rd edn. Norwalk, CT: Appleton & Lange; 1991.
13. Foster TC, Kumar A. Calcium dysregulation in the aging brain. Neuroscientist 2002; 8(4): 297–301.
14. Lanahan A, Lyford G, Stevenson GS, Worley PF, Barnes CA. Selective alteration of long-term potentiation-induced transcriptional response in hippocampus of aged, memory-impaired rats. J Neurosci 1997; 17(8): 2876–85.
15. Simonetti S, Chen X, DiMauro S, Schon EA. Accumulation of deletions in human mitochondrial DNA during normal aging: analysis by quantitative PCR. Biochim Biophys Acta 1992; 1180(2): 113–22.

16. Bender A, Krishnan KJ, Morris CM et al. High levels of mitochondrial DNA deletions in substantia nigra neurons in aging and Parkinson disease. Nat Genet 2006; 38(5): 515–17.

17. Kraytsberg Y, Kudryavtseva E, McKee AC, Geula C, Kowall NW, Khrapko K. Mitochondrial DNA deletions are abundant and cause functional impairment in aged human substantia nigra neurons. Nat Genet 2006; 38(5): 518–20.

18. Wallace DC. A mitochondrial paradigm of metabolic and degenerative diseases, aging, and cancer: a dawn for evolutionary medicine. Annu Rev Genet 2005; 39: 359–407.

19. Trifunovic A, Wredenberg A, Falkenberg M et al. Premature ageing in mice expressing defective mitochondrial DNA polymerase. Nature 2004; 429(6990): 417–23.

20. Strachan T, Read AP. Human Molecular Genetics, 3rd edn. London: Garland Science; 2004.

21. Minoshima S, Giordani B, Berent S, Frey KA, Foster NL, Kuhl DE. Metabolic reduction in the posterior cingulate cortex in very early Alzheimer's disease. Ann Neurol 1997; 42(1): 85–94.

22. Vander Borght T, Minoshima S, Giordani B et al. Cerebral metabolic differences in Parkinson's and Alzheimer's diseases matched for dementia severity. J Nucl Med 1997; 38(5): 797–802.

23. Hoffman JM, Welsh-Bohmer KA, Hanson M et al. FDG PET imaging in patients with pathologically verified dementia. J Nucl Med 2000; 41(11): 1920–8.

24. Cottrell DA, Blakely EL, Johnson MA, Ince PG, Turnbull DM. Mitochondrial enzyme-deficient hippocampal neurons and choroidal cells in AD. Neurology 2001; 57(2): 260–4.

25. Parker WD Jr, Filley CM, Parks JK. Cytochrome oxidase deficiency in Alzheimer's disease. Neurology 1990; 40(8): 1302–3.

26. Lustbader JW, Cirilli M, Lin C et al. ABAD directly links Abeta to mitochondrial toxicity in Alzheimer's disease. Science 2004; 304(5669): 448–52.

27. Heyman A, Peterson B, Fillenbaum G, Pieper C. The consortium to establish a registry for Alzheimer's disease (CERAD). Part XIV: Demographic and clinical predictors of survival in patients with Alzheimer's disease. Neurology 1996; 46(3): 656–60.

28. Fratiglioni L, Viitanen M, von Strauss E, Tontodonati V, Herlitz A, Winblad B. Very old women at highest risk of dementia and Alzheimer's disease: incidence data from the Kungsholmen Project, Stockholm. Neurology 1997; 48(1): 132–8.

29. Barnes LL, Wilson RS, Bienias JL, Schneider JA, Evans DA, Bennett DA. Sex differences in the clinical manifestations of Alzheimer disease pathology. Arch Gen Psychiatry 2005; 62(6): 685–91.

30. Shumaker SA, Legault C, Rapp SR et al. Estrogen plus progestin and the incidence of dementia and mild cognitive impairment in postmenopausal women: the Women's Health Initiative Memory Study: a randomized controlled trial. JAMA 2003; 289(20): 2651–62.

31. Webber KM, Casadesus G, Marlatt MW et al. Estrogen bows to a new master: the role of gonadotropins in Alzheimer pathogenesis. Ann NY Acad Sci 2005; 1052: 201–9.

32. Rosario ER, Chang L, Stanczyk FZ, Pike CJ. Age-related testosterone depletion and the development of Alzheimer disease. JAMA 2004; 292(12): 1431–2.

CHAPTER 4

The blood–brain barrier: age and gender differences

William A Banks

Introduction

The blood–brain barrier (BBB) forms the interface between the central nervous system (CNS) and the peripheral circulation. It is capable of virtually excluding from the CNS many substances and controls the entry of most others and so is responsible for the nutritive and homeostatic environment of the CNS.[1] In addition, the BBB is increasingly recognized to play a role in communication between the CNS and peripheral tissues through its ability to control the exchange of regulatory and informational molecules such as peptides and proteins.[2]

The BBB changes with regard to its membrane composition, the rate at which it transports amino acids, glucose, and regulatory substances, and its effect on the cerebrospinal fluid (CSF)/blood ratio of serum proteins throughout the life cycle. Most of these changes reflect the response of the BBB to the variable needs of the CNS and so are adaptive changes. With aging however, it is unclear to what extent the changes in BBB function are also pathologic.

Although the BBB remains intact to serum proteins with healthy aging, it is more vulnerable to insults. Aging is also associated with an increase in the incidence of disease states that can alter the function of the BBB regardless of age. Stroke, diabetes, and Alzheimer's disease are examples of conditions in which the BBB has been proposed or shown to be disrupted or its functions altered.

This review will examine the changes which occur with aging in the morphology, membrane composition, and permeability of the endothelial cell and the BBB.

Basis of the blood–brain barrier

Experiments done at the end of the 19th century which found that many basic dyes and acids would stain the brain and CSF or affect CNS function when given centrally but not peripherally gave rise to the concept of the BBB.[3] These substances were found to be prevented from entering the CNS by barriers formed by the endothelial cells of the vasculature and by the epithelial cells of the choroid plexus. These cells are modified when compared to endothelial cells from most non-CNS tissues in that they are joined together by tight junctions which eliminate intercellular pores, have a paucity of intracellular fenestrations, and have a low rate of pinocytosis. These modifications mean that the oncotic and hydrostatic forces of Starling are not operational in the CNS and so no plasma ultrafiltrate is produced to nourish the CNS.

Because of the lack of formation of a plasma ultrafiltrate, circulating proteins are largely excluded from the CNS. Instead, substances enter the CNS by one of two major mechanisms. Small lipid-soluble substances can easily diffuse through the membranes which comprise the

Table 4.1 *Morphologic changes in the aging BBB vasculature*

Decreased number of pericytes

Decreased number of endothelial cells

Decreased cytoplasm in endothelial cells

Decrease in the number of mitochondria per endothelial cell

Increased length of endothelial cells

Increased density of mitochondria in endothelial cells

Increased thickness of basement membrane

Altered diameter of capillary lumen

Thinning of capillary wall

BBB.[4] Nicotine, heroin, and ethanol are examples of substances that cross by membrane diffusion. Larger peptides and proteins can also use this pathway, but their entry by this pathway is correspondingly reduced.[5] Second, many substances are transported across the BBB by saturable systems. Essential amino acids, glucose, thyroxine, and some regulatory substances such as insulin and leptin cross by saturable transport systems.[6] The transporters usually are highly specific for a class or type of molecule. The Glut-1 transporter, for example, transports other hexoses in addition to glucose and there are distinguishable transporters for large neutral, acidic, and basic amino acids.

Efflux systems are as important to normal CNS functioning and the prevention of disease as are influx systems. For example, efflux of potassium prevents CSF levels from becoming too high during hyperkalemia,[7] the dysfunction of the peptide transport system (PTS)-1 with alcohol withdrawal is associated with seizures,[8] and an efflux system for nicotine in the tobacco hornworm allows it to ingest tobacco without suffering nicotine poisoning of the CNS.[9]

Morphologic changes with aging

Table 4.1 is a summary of a previous review that examined the aging brain for changes in its vasculature.[10] As reported in the literature, these changes are regional and variable.[11–13] For example, the capillary lumen diameter has been reported to be decreased in the hippocampus, increased in the frontal cortex, and unaltered in other areas.

The BBB remains intact with normal aging despite morphologic changes in the brain vasculature. Albumin, sucrose, and horseradish peroxidase are substances used to assess the BBB for increased leakiness and studies with them have failed to find any disruption,[14–16] even though peripheral vascular beds do appear to become more leaky.[17] The vascular space of the brain is unchanged with aging, a finding that is consistent with maintenance of BBB integrity. However, the changes that do occur in the vasculature with aging may make the BBB more susceptible to subsequent pathologic insults.

The vessels in the aging brain show increased tortuosity, kinking, looping, spiraling, and corkscrewing. Such angioarchitectural distortions are even more pronounced in Alzheimer's disease. The resulting hemorheologic aberrations have been proposed to interfere with the passage of oxygen, glucose, and other substances across the BBB.[18–20] Retinal capillaries, which have blood–brain barrier properties, show increased glycogen deposits, pinocytotic vesicles, and cellular debris.[21]

Changes in aged endothelial cells

Although few studies have been done on aged brain endothelial cells, ones that used aged endothelial cells derived from peripheral vascular beds showed alterations in function with aging that may be associated with disease. Endothelial cells derived from rat aorta have a decreased basal and stimulated prostacyclin production.[22] Endothelial cells from the wounds of aged animals have an increased proliferative capacity[23] but a decreased chemotactic response to platelet-derived growth factor.[24] Other studies have shown aging endothelial cells to have a decrease in mRNA[25] and altered location of centrosomes.[26] Aged endothelial

Table 4.2 *BBB transport systems in senescent animals*

Transport system	Ligand studied	Findings
Peptide Transport System-1	Tyr-MIF-1	Dec Km; Dec Vmax
LH system	LH	Increased inhibition with unlabeled material
Thyroid hormone	T3	Dec transport
Hexose	Glucose	Dec transport; dec Vmax, no change in Km, decreased efflux
Large neutral amino acid	Tyr/Val	No change
	Tryptophan	Dec Km; dec Vmax
	Phe-analog	No change in influx, increased efflux
Free fatty acid	Palmitate	Increased uptake in selected regions
	Arachidonate	No change
Choline	Choline	Dec Vmax; dec Km

cells produce less basal and stimulated nitric oxide, which may lead to increases in blood pressure.[27–29]

Studies specifically of aging brain cells are more rare. Stewart et al[30] reported that endothelial cells lose cytoplasm with aging, especially those in white matter. The number of mitochondria per endothelial cell was reported to be decreased in aged Macaque monkeys but not in aged rats. Most authors have found a decreased number and increased length of endothelial cells (Table 4.1). The numbers of tight junctions, vesicles, and gap junctions per endothelial cell are unchanged in brain endothelial cells.

Age-related changes in protein concentrations in the CSF

The choroid plexus produces the majority of fluid found within the brain. Therefore, increases in the CSF concentration of serum proteins have often been used to argue for a disruption in the barrier at the choroid plexus. Increases in CSF levels or CSF/serum ratios have been reported for albumin, total protein, and various serum proteins with aging.[31] CSF production, however, is decreased and the brain ventricular space is increased with aging. These changes suggest that the increase in CSF protein concentrations could be due to a reduced turnover rate of CSF.

Permeability of the blood–brain barrier in aging

Diffusion and saturable transport are the two major mechanisms by which substances can cross the BBB.[4,6] Membrane diffusion has not been rigorously investigated for changes with aging, but two studies do suggest a 25–33% reduction in passage through this pathway for thiourea and sucrose and a third study found decreased uptake of calcium channel blockers.[32]

Saturable transport systems have been studied in aged rodents, humans, and dogs by a variety of methods, including magnetic resonance imaging and PET scanning. Most transporters have been found to be decreased (Table 4.2) in the range of 20–40%. Km and Vmax are often proportionately decreased, producing unaltered Km/Vmax ratios. Unaltered Km/Vmax ratios suggest an uncompetitive form of inhibition, an effect not mediated through changes in transporter number or ligand affinity.

Some transporters have been shown to be reduced by more than 20–40%. The Vmax for glucose is reduced by about 75% and the Vmax and Km for choline transport are each reduced by over 95%.[33] Decreases in glucose transport begin in midlife for some brain regions and continue for other regions into senescence.

Unlike other substances, the transport of the free fatty acid palmitate increases with age in some regions of the brain. The uptake of palmitate is directly related to the regional brain synthesis of phosphatidylcholine and is especially incorporated into structural lipids.[34] Therefore, the decreased transport of palmitate with aging likely reflects age-related changes in membrane remodeling and synthesis or myelination. The free fatty acid arachidonate, which has a turnover rate in brain related to signal transduction, has a transport rate unaffected by age.[35]

Efflux, or brain to blood, systems are less uniformly affected than are the influx systems. PTS-1, which transports Tyr-MIF-1 and met-enkephalin out of the brain, has proportionate reductions in Km and Vmax. Both phenylalanine and glucose efflux rates are increased with aging. Daniel et al[36] have suggested that glucose efflux is decreased in aging because the lower rate of influx leaves less unmetabolized glucose available for re-entry into blood. A lesser amount of unmetabolized brain glucose could reduce the safety margin for the brain in the case of hypoglycemia.

Altered composition of brain endothelial cells with aging

Several studies have examined the composition of the BBB with aging. Unlike the membranes of other cell types, the brain endothelial cell does not appear to have an increase in membrane cholesterol or changes in lipid composition.[37] Phospholipid base exchange in brain endothelial cells is unchanged with aging.[38] Others, however, have suggested that there may be changes in membrane protein content. Lectin-binding studies are consistent with an increase in glycoprotein content. With the exception of an N-ethylmaleimide inhibitable component, ATPase activity, including oubain-sensitive ATPase activity, does not change with aging.

No change occurs in saturated fatty acids, but an increase in monounsaturated fats and a decrease in polyunsaturated fats do occur. Brain endothelial cell activity of glutathione peroxidase and glutathione reductase, alpha 1 adrenergic receptor number, and manganese content do not change with aging, whereas superoxide dismutase (SOD) activity and copper and zinc contents increase and catalase activity decrease. The changes in antigens associated with the BBB have been reviewed elsewhere.[39] The choroid plexus shows a different pattern with aging, with no change in catalase activity but an increase in glutathione peroxidase and SOD activity.

Autoregulation of cerebral blood flow

Cerebral blood flow (CBF) delivers oxygen and glucose to the brain and, because these substances are nearly maximally extracted from blood as it passes through the brain, an increase in the metabolic demand of the CNS must be met by increasing blood flow. Many drugs are also highly extracted from blood so that the amount of the drug entering the brain is a function of CBF.

CBF clearly declines with aging. Whether this decline is caused by a response of the cerebral vasculature to a decreased demand for oxygen and glucose by the CNS or by pathology of autoregulatory mechanisms is unanswered. Evidence suggests that at least part of the decrease in CBF is related to decreased blood levels of hormones such as growth hormone and insulin-like growth factors. The implication of a decrease in CBF in the healthy elderly for drug delivery to the brain is poorly explored.

In comparison to changes in baseline CBF, evidence suggests that the reactivity of the cerebral vasculature to vasoconstrictive and vasodilatory stimuli is largely intact. Although vasoconstriction in response to 100% oxygen and vasodilatation in response to hypercapnia occur to a normal or near normal degree, selected aspects of cerebrovascular reactivity may be impaired. Vasodilatation, for example, in response to TRH is impaired. Vasodilatation in response to hypercapnia is reduced in postmenopausal women and can be partially restored with estrogen replacement therapy; this again suggests important interactions between circulating hormones and the brain vasculature in aging. Several studies have found that the increase in regional CBF seen with mental activity or other types of CNS stimulation still occurs in the elderly, but is attenuated compared to younger individuals.

Implications for aged-related changes in the blood–brain barrier

The general picture of the aging BBB that emerges is one of subtle changes in morphology and composition with preservation of integrity and modest alterations in function. Of these various changes and adaptations, most are minimal compared to those that occur with aging in the rest of the CNS or that occur in the BBB with disease states such as Alzheimer's disease or stroke. It is likely that many of the changes seen in the aging BBB are adaptive to the altered demands of the aging CNS.

A conclusion often reached by many authors is that the changes seen with aging in the BBB make it more susceptible to pathologic insults. For example, it has been postulated that the decreased transport rate of glucose across the aging BBB may place the CNS at greater risk during hypoglycemia. The aged BBB is more susceptible to disruption from seizures[40] and alterations in permeability from haloperidol treatment. Decreases in CBF and cerebrovascular reactivity may make the aging CNS more susceptible to other conditions as well, such as stroke, vasculitides, and multiple sclerosis.

Changes in transport rates, membrane diffusion, and enzymatic activity could underlie many aspects of the aging CNS. The CNS is entirely dependent on the BBB's selective permeability for the adequate delivery of supplies of vitamins, minerals, amino acids, electrolytes, free fatty acids, nucleic acids, and in some cases hormones, peptides, and regulatory proteins. The delivery of these substances depends mainly on saturable transport systems. Impairment of transport capabilities has been implicated in alcohol withdrawal seizures (methionine enkephalin efflux), mental retardation (glucose

influx), and obesity (leptin and pancreatic polypeptide influx). Impaired transporter function could underlie many aspects of the aging CNS.

The neurovascular hypothesis

The amyloid hypothesis states that amyloid β protein plays a causal role in Alzheimer's disease. Whereas all Alzheimer's patients have elevated amyloid β protein levels in their brains, only about 1% of Alzheimer's patients overproduce this substance. Therefore, the majority of Alzheimer's patients must be clearing amyloid β protein poorly. One mechanism of clearance from the brain is by brain-to-blood transport. Amyloid β protein has such an efflux pump, low-density lipoprotein receptor-related protein-1 (LRP). The LRP protein is underexpressed in patients with Alzheimer's disease and efflux of amyloid β protein from brain is impaired in mice which overexpress amyloid β protein.[41–43] This has led Zlokovic to propose the neurovascular hypothesis of Alzheimer's disease,[44] which states that defective brain-to-blood transport of amyloid β protein leads to its accumulation and contributes to the development of Alzheimer's disease.

Sex steroids and blood–brain barrier function

The effects of gender and sex steroids on BBB function are perhaps one of the least studied areas in the field. Although it is well known that the BBB changes with maturation, the degree to which those changes are mediated directly or indirectly by changes in sex hormones is unknown. However, there are tantalizing clues that sex steroids play an important role in BBB regulation. For example, female rats are more susceptible to disruption of the BBB by osmotic insult than are male rats.[45] The effect of estrogen on edema formation in ovariectomized rats may be dependent on age.[46,47] Estrogen also likely controls expression of adhesion molecule expression and immune cell penetration into the brain;[48] these effects could underlie the gender difference in the development of multiple sclerosis. Androgens control other aspects of BBB function, including expression and function of organic ion efflux systems.[49]

Conclusions

The aging BBB remains intact to serum proteins during healthy aging. Many of the changes that are seen in BBB function may be adaptive to the changing demands of the aging CNS. The aged BBB is, however, likely to be increasingly vulnerable to insults from other diseases, such as hypertension and stroke. The role of sex steroids and gender differences remains a relatively understudied, but important, topic. In addition, some changes in BBB function may underlie diseases of the CNS, as has been postulated for glucose and amyloid β protein transport in Alzheimer's disease.

Acknowledgments

This work was supported by VA Merit Review.

References

1. Davson H, Segal MB. Physiology of the CSF and Blood–Brain Barriers. Boca Raton, FL: CRC Press, 1996.
2. Banks WA, Kastin AJ. Passage of peptides across the blood–brain barrier: pathophysiological perspectives. Life Sci 1996; 59: 1923–43.
3. Bradbury M. The Concept of a Blood–Brain Barrier. New York: John Wiley and Sons, 1979.
4. Oldendorf WH. Lipid solubility and drug penetration of the blood–brain barrier. Proc Soc Exp Biol Med 1974; 147: 813–16.
5. Banks WA, Kastin AJ. Peptides and the blood–brain barrier: lipophilicity as a predictor of permeability. Brain Res Bull 1985; 15: 287–92.
6. Davson H, Segal MB. Special aspects of the blood–brain barrier. In: Davson H, Segal MB, eds. Physiology of the CSF and Blood–Brain Barriers. Boca Raton, FL: CRC Press, 1996: 303–485.
7. Davson H, Segal MB. Blood–brain–CSF relations. In: Davson H, Segal MB, eds. Physiology of the CSF and Blood–Brain Barriers. Boca Raton, FL: CRC Press, 1996: 257–302.
8. Banks WA, Kastin AJ. Inhibition of the brain to blood transport system for enkephalins and Tyr-MIF-1 in mice addicted or genetically predisposed to drinking ethanol. Alcohol 1989; 6: 53–7.
9. Murray CL, Quaglia M, Arnason JT, Morris CE. A putative nicotine pump at the metabolic blood–brain barrier of the tobacco hornworm. J Neurobiol 1994; 25: 23–34.
10. Banks WA, Kastin AJ. Aging, peptides, and the blood–brain barrier: implications and speculations. In: Crook T, Bartus R, Ferris S, Gershon S, eds. Treatment Development Strategies for Alzheimer's Disease. Madison, CT: Mark Powley Associates, 1986: 245–65.
11. Bar T. Morphometric evaluation of capillaries in different laminae of rat cerebral cortex by automatic image analysis. Adv Neurol 1978; 20: 1–9.
12. Burns EM, Buschmann MBT, Kruckeberg TW, Gaetano PK, Meyer JM. Blood–brain barrier, aging, brain blood flow, and sleep. Adv Neurol 1981; 30: 301–6.
13. Hicks P, Rolsten C, Brizzee D, Samorajski T. Age-related changes in rat brain capillaries. Neurobiol Aging 1983; 4: 69–75.
14. Rapoport SI. Blood–brain barrier permeability in senescent rats. J Gerontol 1978; 34: 162–9.
15. Rudick RA, Buell SJ. Integrity of blood–brain barrier to peroxidase in senescent mice. Neurobiol Aging 1983; 4: 283–7.
16. Sankar R, Blossom E, Clemons K, Charles P. Age-associated changes in the effects of amphetamine on the blood–brain barrier of rats. Neurobiol Aging 1983; 4: 65–8.
17. Belmin J, Corman B, Merval R, Tedgui A. Age-related changes in endothelial permeability and distribution volume of albumin in rat aorta. Am J Physiol 1993; 264(3 Part 2): H679–85.
18. Ravens JR. Vascular changes in the human senile brain. Adv Neurol 1978; 20: 487–99.
19. Pickworth FA. Cerebral ischemia and mental disorder. J Mental Sci 1937; 83: 512–33.
20. de la Torre JC, Mussivand T. Can disturbed brain microcirculation cause Alzheimer's disease? Neurol Res 1993; 15: 146–53.
21. Schellini SA, Gregorio EA, Padovani CR, Spadella CT, Moraes-Silva MA. Ultrastructural and morphometric aspects of ageing in the retinal capillaries of rats. J Submicrosc Cytol Pathol 1997; 29(2): 275–80.
22. Nakajima M, Hashimoto M, Wang F et al. Aging decreases the production of PG12 in rat aortic endothelial cells. Exp Gerontol 1997; 32(6): 685–93.
23. Phillips GD, Stone AM, Scholtz JC, Jones BD, Knighton DR. Proliferation of wound derived capillary endothelial cells; young versus aged. Mech Ageing Devel 1994; 77(2): 141–8.
24. Phillips GD, Stone AM. PDGF-BB induced chemotaxis is impaired in aged capillary endothelial cells. Mech Ageing Devel 1994; 73(3): 189–96.

25. Sun L. Age-related changes of RNA synthesis in the lungs of aging mice by light and electron microscopic radioautography. Cell Mol Biol 1995; 41(8): 1061–72.

26. Kiosses BW, Kalnis VI. Age-related changes in the position of centrosomes in endothelial cells of the rabbit aorta. Exp Gerontol 1993; 28(1): 69–75.

27. Amrani M, Goodwin AT, Gray CC, Yacoub MH. Ageing is associated with reduced basal and stimulated release of nitric oxide by the coronary endothelium. Acta Physiol Scand 1996; 157(1): 79–84.

28. Cernadas MR, Sanchez de Miguel L, Garcia-Duran M et al. Expression of constitutive and inducible nitric oxide synthases in the vascular wall of young and aging rats. Circ Res 1998; 83(3): 279–86.

29. Higashi Y, Oshima T, Ozono R, Matsuura H, Kajiyama G. Aging and severity of hypertension attenuate endothelium-dependent renal vascular relaxation in humans. Hypertension 1997; 30(2 Part 1): 252–8.

30. Stewart PA, Magliocco M, Hayakawa K, Farrell CL, Del Maestro RF, Girvin J et al. A quantitative analysis of blood–brain barrier ultrastructure in the aging human. Microvasc Res 1987; 33(2): 270–82.

31. Tibbling G, Link H, Ohman S. Principles of albumin and IgG analyses in neurological disorders. I. Establishment of reference values. Scand J Clin Lab Invest 1977; 37: 385–90.

32. Waki H, Kon K, Tanaka Y, Ando S. Age-related changes in the uptake of calcium channel blockers by brain capillary endothelial cells and synaptosomal fractions. Neurosci Lett 1990; 116(3): 367–71.

33. Mooradian AD, Morin AM, Cipp LJ, Haspel HC. Glucose transport is reduced in the blood–brain barrier of aged rats. Brain Res 1991; 551: 145–9.

34. Banks WA, Kastin AJ, Rapoport SI. Permeability of the blood–brain barrier to circulating free fatty acids. In: Yehuda S, Mostofsky DI, eds. Handbook of Essential Fatty Acid Biology: Biochemistry, Physiology, and Behavioral Neurobiology. Totowa, NJ: Humana Press, 1997: 3–14.

35. Strosznajder J, Chalimoniuk M, Strosznajder RP, Albanese V, Alberghina M. Arachidonate transport through the blood–retina and blood–brain barrier of the rat during aging. Neurosci Lett 1996; 209(3): 145–8.

36. Daniel PM, Love ER, Pratt OE. The effect of age upon the influx of glucose into the brain. J Physiol (London) 1978; 274: 141–8.

37. Mooradian AD, Smith TL. The effect of age on lipid composition and order of rat cerebral microvessels. Neurochem Res 1992; 17: 233–7.

38. Terracina L, De Medio GE, Trovarelli G, Gaiti A. Phospholipid base-exchange in brain microvessels. Ital J Biochem 1994; 43(4): 151–6.

39. Shah GN, Mooradian AD. Age-related changes in the blood–brain barrier. Exp Gerontol 1997; 32: 501–19.

40. Oztas B, Kaya M, Camurcu S. Age related changes in the effect of electroconvulsive shock on the blood brain barrier permeability in rats. Mech Ageing Devel 1990; 51: 149–55.

41. Shibata M, Yamada S, Kumar SR et al. Clearance of Alzheimer's amyloid-β_{1-40} peptide from brain by LDL receptor-related protein-1 at the blood–brain barrier. J Clin Invest 2000; 106: 1489–99.

42. Deane R, Wu Z, Sagare A et al. LRP/amyloid beta-peptide interaction mediates differential brain efflux of Abeta isoforms. Neuron 2004; 43: 333–44.

43. Banks WA, Robinson SM, Verma S, Morley JE. Efflux of human and mouse amyloid ß proteins 1–40 and 1–42 from brain: impairment in a mouse model of Alzheimer's disease. Neuroscience 2003; 121: 487–92.

44. Zlokovic BV. Neurovascular mechanisms of Alzheimer's neurodegeneration. Trends Neurosci 2005; 28: 202–8.

45. Oztas B, Kucuk M, Kaya M. Sex-dependent changes in blood–brain barrier permeability in epileptic rats following acute hyperosmotic exposure. Pharmacol Res 2001; 43: 469–72.

46. O'Connoer CA, Cernak I, Vink R. Both estrogen and progesterone attenuate edema formation following diffuse traumatic brain injury in rats. Brain Res 2005; 1062: 171–4.

47. Bake S, Sohrabji F. 17Beta-estradiol differentially regulates blood–brain barrier permeability in young and aging female rats. Endocrinology 2004; 145: 5471–5.

48. Dietrich JB. Endotheial cells of the blood–brain barrier: a target for glucocorticoids and estrogens? Frontiers Biosci 2004; 9: 684–93.

49. Ohtsuki S, Tomi M, Hata T et al. Dominant expression of androgen receptors and their functional regulation of organic anion transporter 3 in rat brain capillary endothelial cells: comparison of gene expression between the blood–brain and –retinal barriers. J Cell Physiol 2005; 204: 896–900.

Diagnostics & Primary Assessment

CHAPTER 5

Aging men – the challenge ahead

Bruno Lunenfeld

An aging world

> First we were obsessed with the challenge of 'population explosion', then we shifted our concern to the problems of global ageing, and only now do we start to grasp the future consequences of a rapid fertility decline.
>
> E Diczfalusy, 2000

When Emperor Augustus died in the year AD 14 and was followed by Tiberius, the world population known at that time was less than 300 million people. Survival of individuals, clans, and nations was very difficult in those times, so that there was little, if any, increase in global population during the subsequent millennium and the world population of the year AD 1000 was still below 300 million people. Then the second millennium brought about dramatic changes in the world population; it is estimated that by the year 1500, the global population was around 400 million people. Population showed more rapid growth in the 17th and 18th centuries. It stood at 1 billion at the start of the 19th century, then 1.6 billion at the beginning of the 20th century, and now, in the first decade of the 21st century, it has reached 6 billion.

The estimates and projections of the United Nations indicate that between 1900 and 2100, world population will increase 7-fold, from 1.65 billion to 11.5 billion: an increase of almost 10 billion people. Better hygiene and public sanitation in the 19th century led to expanded life expectancies and quicker growth, primarily in developed countries. Demographic transition in the 19th and 20th centuries was the result of shifts from high to low mortality and fertility. The pace of change varies with culture, level of economic development, and other factors. Not all countries follow the same path of change. The reproductive revolution in the mid-20th century and modern contraception led to greater individual control of fertility and the potential for rapid fertility decline.

In 1970, there were 22 countries with a total fertility rate at or below the replacement of 2.1. In the year 1999 there were 68 countries, and it is projected that by 2020, 121 countries representing 75% of the global population will have birth rates below the replenishment level.

The European Union's overall population is projected to decrease between 2006 and 2050 by 9%, despite a net migration rate of 2/1000. The natural increase (the ratio of births over deaths) will turn negative for the EU in 2010, and the vast majority of Europe's countries – including Belgium, the Czech Republic, Germany, Italy, Poland, and Russia – are projected to lose population in the next 25 years.[1] Japan will have a population decrease of 25% between 2006 and 2050.[2]

Fertility rate and life expectancy at birth are the most important factors in population growth. Political and cultural barriers that limit access to fertility regulation affect the pace of decline. Population change is also affected by migration. Migration contributes to population growth but has

Table 5.1 *Demographic data 2006*

Region	Population 1950	Population 2006	Population 2025	Population 2050	Fertility rate	Life expectancy M	Life expectancy F	Net migration/ 1000	Population change %
World	2520	6555	7940	9243	2.7	65	69	0	41
Africa	224	924	1355	1994	5.1	51	53	0	116
N America	166	332	387	462	2.9	75	81	4	39
S America	111	378	465	525	2.4	69	76	−1	40
Asia	1437	3968	4739	5277	2.4	66	70	0	33
(China)	563	1311	1476	1437	1.6	70	74	0	10
(Japan)	84	127	121	100	1.3	79	86	0	−21
Europe	547	732	717	665	1.4	71	79	2	−9

Table 5.2 *Population aged 60 years or older (millions and % of total population)*

Region	Year 2006		Year 2050	
World	688	11%	1964	22%
North America	57	17%	118	27%
Asia	375	9%	1227	24%
Europe	151	21%	225	34%
Africa	48	5%	192	10%

Adapted from United Nations Publication, ST/ESA/SER.A/245 and International Updates (through September 2005).

the largest effect on the distribution of population and demographic changes in regions and countries (Table 5.1).

The aging population

Importantly, it is expected that the biggest increase in population will occur in those over 65 years of age. In 1950, less than 5% of the population were older than 65 years, by 2006 it was 11% and by 2025 this percentage is expected to increase to over 15%. Overall, it has been predicted that the world population aged over 65 years will double in the next 50 years[2] (Table 5.2). With all the rhetoric surrounding the impending

'age quake' produced by the 'graying of the world,' there has been surprisingly little serious analysis of the social and economic implications of increased longevity and the doubling of the number of elderly people that will occur over the next 30 years.

Humans had a life expectancy at birth of about 30 years for about 99.9% of the time we have inhabited this planet. In 1900 it increased to 47 years and it is expected to reach 85 years in 2010, varying according to continent.[1] In 2005 more than 75% of all human deaths in developed countries occurred after the age of 75.

The last century was marked by the triumph of partially preventing the premature termination of life. During the past 50 years infant mortality rates have declined from 155/1000 to 52/1000 live births in the world and from 72/1000 to 11/1000 in Europe.[3] During the same time frame a significant decline in overall mortality rates has also been seen. This decline can be attributed to the developments of modern medicine that have occurred in the 20th century, mainly the development of antibiotics, vaccines, safer water, pesticides, and improved sanitation and personal hygiene.[4] These events were responsible for the decrease in the number of epidemics and the control of most infectious diseases. Acute disease is no longer the major cause of death. Today one dies from or with chronic illnesses, degenerative diseases, metastatic cancer, immune deficiencies, and other diseases which prolong disability, immobility, and dependency. Dying has

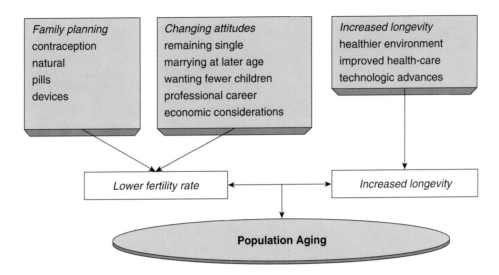

Figure 5.1 *Factors contributing to a global increase in aging populations.*

become in most instances a long, painful, and expensive procedure.[4]

The worldwide prolongation of the mean life expectancy and the drastic reduction in the fertility rate has resulted in a rapidly aging world population (Figure 5.1). Populations are aging even faster in the developing world, as fertility rates there have declined more rapidly and more recently than in the developed world. Table 5.3 demonstrates the effect of the decrease in fertility rate and increase in life expectancy in selected Asian countries on the increase of its population above the age of 65.

It is projected that, in general, the elderly (above 65) will increase within the next 25 years by 82%, whereas the newborn will increase only by 3%. The working age population will increase by only 46%. The UN projects (in their 2004 revision 1)[2] that, by 2050, the proportion of people above 60 will exceed for the first time the proportion of children below 15, and 13 countries will have more than 10% of the oldest old (> 80 years old) in their population. Italy will be leading with 14%.

In 1950, more than 34% of the world's population consisted of children, i.e. people aged less than 15 years; today it is only 28% and it is expected to diminish to some 20% by the year 2050. The decline in their numbers in Asia is also impressive: from 36.5% (in 1950) it was reduced to 27.8% (in 2005), and it is projected to diminish further to 18.3% by the year 2050. Today, the population of European children constitutes only 16% of the total population and is expected to decline further to 15%. In Italy, by the year 2050, the population of children will be 13%, i.e. less than that of the population of octagenarians. The same consideration applies also to Japan.[1]

By the year 2050 Asia will be inhabited by almost 1 billion people aged 65 and over. China, Japan, Singapore, Hong Kong, and Macao will have become members of the 'club of 14' with more then 10% of their population aged 80 and above.

Since the last years of life are accompanied by an increase in disability and sickness, the demands for the social and health services will increase immensely. The high cost in relation to these services will strain to the limit the potential ability of health, social, and even political infrastructures. Hence the marked increase of the elderly population in relation to the working age population will be compounded by a simultaneous decrease in the population of children who comprise the working age

Table 5.3 *The effect of the decrease in fertility rate and increase in mean life expectancy in selected Asian countries on their rising population (> 65 years)*

Country	Fertility rate		Life expectancy (years)		Percentage >65 years	
	2000	2025	2000	2025	2000	2025
Singapore	1.2	1.5	80.1	82.5	9.7	18.4
Japan	1.4	1.6	80.7	82.9	17.1	27.6
S Korea	1.7	1.7	74.4	79.2	10.8	23.4
China	1.8	1.8	71.4	77.4	10.2	19.7
Taiwan	1.8	1.7	76.4	80.4	12.6	24.1
Thailand	1.9	1.7	68.6	75.3	9.7	19.9
Vietnam	2.0	2.0	69.3	75.8	7.6	13.1
Burma	2.4	1.7	54.9	63.4	7.1	12.6
India	3.1	2.2	62.5	70.9	7.0	11.8
Malaysia	3.3	2.6	70.8	76.9	6.5	12.2
Philippines	3.5	2.4	67.5	74.6	5.7	10.1

Table 5.4 *Potential support ratio (number of persons aged 15 to 64 years per one person aged 65 or older)*

	Year	
Region	2006	2050
World	9	4
North America	5	3
Africa	16	10
Asia	11	4
Europe	4	2

population of the next generation. Thus a declining labor force will have to support an increasing number of elderly.[5]

In 2002 there were worldwide some 9 people in the working age group per 1 person aged 65 years; their number in Africa was 17, in Asia 11, but in Europe only 4. It is projected by the UN that, by 2050, these figures will be reduced to 4 worldwide, and to 9 in Africa, and to ratios as low as 2 (in Europe) and even 1 (in Italy) (Table 5.4). ... Hence, for the brave new world of future Italy, it is projected that – by the year 2050 – there will only be one person in the working-age group for each person aged 65 years, or older.

There is no historical precedent for such low potential support ratios. How will a society function with such an age distribution?[6]

Although the mean life expectancy at birth has been prolonged by more then 25 years within the last century, life expectancy at the age of 65 increased by less then 3 years during the same time frame (Table 5.5). Moreover, despite the enormous medical progress during the past few decades, 25% of life expectancy after age 65 is spent with some disability, and the last years of life are accompanied by a further increase in incapacity and sickness.

For a long time, life expectancy, the rate of infant mortality, and causes of death were sufficient data to assess a population's health status and to determine national public health priorities. These indicators remain indispensable, as important mortality inequalities remain between different countries, populations, and socio-economic categories. With the lengthening of life expectancy at birth, non-communicable diseases and associated disability receive increasing importance. Consequently, the need for a new type of indicator, namely 'health expectancies: disability-free life expectancy, healthy life expectancy, or active life expectancy' became necessary. The introduction of the concepts of the International Classification of Impairments, Disabilities and Handicaps[7] allowed the efficient use

Table 5.5 *Life expectancy of men at different ages*

		Expected number of years remaining at age (total lifespan)		
Year of birth	Life expectancy at birth (years)	15 years	45 years	65 years
1888	43.9	43.9 (58.9)	22.6 (67.6)	10.8 (75.8)
1988	70.5	56.4 (71)	28.2 (73.2)	13.0 (78)

Table 5.6 *Disability-free life expectancy in the developing world*

Country	Life expectancy at birth (years)	Years of disability-free life expectancy at birth	Disability (years)
1 Japan	81	74.5	6.5
2 Australia	79.5	73.2	6.3
30 Singapore	78	69.3	8.7
51 S Korea	72.8	65	7.8
59 Brunei	77.2	64.4	12.8
81 China	69.7	62.3	7.4
89 Malaysia	68.8	61.4	7.4
99 Thailand	68.2	60.2	8.0
113 Philippines	66.7	58.9	7.8
134 India	60.4	53.2	7.2
145 N Guinea	55	47	8
148 Cambodia	53.8	45.7	8.1

of health expectancy indicators. The Jakarta Declaration on leading health promotion into the 21st century confirms that 'the ultimate goal is to increase health expectancy and to narrow the goal in health expectancy between countries and groups.'[8] Today the first estimate of health expectancy (in most cases 'disability-free life expectancy') is available in most developed countries and increasingly also in developing countries (Table 5.6). Calculations on gains, differences, or losses in health expectancy (disability-free life expectancy, disease-free life expectancy, and dementia-free life expectancy) make it possible to define public health priorities and assess health strategies, social inequalities, lifestyles, and therapeutic interventions. This kind of indicator demonstrates that not only do the poorest and least educated live less long, but they also experience a greater part of their life affected by disability or disease. In Canada, for example, the difference in life expectancy between the highest and lowest income levels was estimated to be 6.3 years; the difference in disability-free life expectancy was 14.3 years (Table 5.7).[9]

The majority of older men today reside in developing countries. As the demographic transition gathers pace in the poorer regions of the world, an even greater proportion of the world's older men will live in countries and regions that have the least resources to respond to their needs. The communication revolution with globalization as its consequence, which started at the end of the last century, will peak during this century. However, if we do not learn to share the resources and wealth of the earth,

Table 5.7 *Difference between the highest and lowest income levels in disability-free life expectancy in Canada*

Income level	Life expectancy (years)	Health expectancy (years)
Lowest	67.1	50
Second	70.1	57.9
Fourth	72.0	62.6
Highest	73.4	64.3
Total	70.8	59.5
Difference between richest and poorest	6.3	14.3

poverty will remain the biggest threat to mankind. It must be our aim that every human being on this earth should be able to age in reasonable health and with dignity.

The cost of caring for the increasing population of senior citizens will become prohibitive with its attendant socio-economic consequences. Less developed countries – which have much lower levels of economic development and access to adequate health-care than more developed countries – will be hard pressed to meet the challenges of more elderly people, especially as traditional family support systems for the elderly are breaking down. Policymakers in the developing world need to invest soon in formal systems of old-age support to be able to meet these challenges in the coming decades. Although population aging presents major challenges for even the most developed countries, developing countries face particular issues in constructing policies that address increasing elderly populations.

To the prudent health-care administrators, the establishment of preventive measures, rather than concentration on interventive care, is an important strategic thrust in overall management of the aging population.[10] Frailty, disability, and dependency will increase immensely the demand for the social and health services. The very high cost to these services may strain to the limit the capacity of health, social, and even political infrastructures, not only of developing but also of the most developed and industrialized nations. The ability for men to age gracefully and maintain independent living, free of disability,

for as long as possible is a crucial factor in aging with dignity and would furthermore reduce health service costs significantly. To achieve this objective, a holistic approach to the management of aging has to be adopted.[10]

The promotion of healthy aging and the prevention or drastic reduction of morbidity and disability of the elderly must assume a central role in the formulation of the health and social policies of many, if not all, countries in the next century. It must emphasize an all-encompassing life-long approach to the aging process, beginning with preconceptual events and focusing on appropriate interventions at all stages of life. Life-history studies of childhood and adolescence demonstrate clearly that social factors probably operate in a cumulative fashion. There are significant social class differences in attainment of height, growth, and other aspects of physical development, as well as in the incidence of infectious and other diseases and risk of injury. For example, the nutritional status of the mother is now known to influence intrauterine growth rates, birth weights, and the later life risks of several important health problems. In addition, a whole host of factors influence growth and development and in turn these factors influence the health status of men in the latter decades of their lives. Vulnerability to physical ill health in childhood and later adult life is associated with poor parental socio-economic circumstances and low levels of parental education and concern. Cross-sectional studies show differences in mortality and morbidity as a function of socio-economic status, across various disease categories throughout the lifespan. Poverty has a significant impact on both life and health expectancy. It should not only be measured in terms of property, employment, wages, and income, but also in terms of basic education, health-care, nutrition, water, and sanitation. Educational attainment and marital status have also been shown in several longitudinal studies to be powerful predictors of morbidity, health expectancy, and mortality. In addition, age, gender, and socio-economic status influence disability-free life expectancy. The economic consequences of retirement place many older citizens in positions of financial vulnerability. As populations age, in both the developing and the developed worlds, the issue becomes how to keep older people economically viable within their respective societies. No community is exempt from the financial hardships experienced by aging populations.

The life course perspective leads to important policy and strategy decisions. Firstly, it is clearly possible and desirable to improve the health status of men when they are old, although this approach is still not fully implemented. Secondly, a complementary approach to improving the health of older men would focus on appropriate interventions at all stages of their lives. The determinants of 'aging' and of 'life expectancy' extend from genetic and molecular determinants to the increasingly powerful forces of environmental, economical, technologic, and cultural globalization. Specific measures for the promotion of healthy aging should include:

1. the promotion of a safe environment
2. healthy lifestyle including proper nutrition
3. appropriate exercise
4. avoidance of smoking
5. avoidance of drug and alcohol abuse
6. social interactions to maintain good mental health
7. medical health-care, including the control of chronic illnesses.

If the program is implemented effectively, it should result in a significant reduction in the costs of health and social care, reduce pain and suffering, increase the quality of life of the elderly, and enable them to remain productive and contribute to the well-being of society. The medical and socio-economic implications of the demographic reality of this new world will be very different from all preceding epochs in history, indeed so new that most people, governments, national and private pension funds, as well as most health insurers, and pharmaceutic and health industries are not yet prepared for the emerging markets. An increase in the quality of life with a delay, decrease, or prevention of disabilities will increase the length of the productive life of aging populations, will decrease dependency, and will decrease health costs related to expensive curative and palliative services.

Men, aging, and health

Before a thing has made its appearance; order should be secured before this order has begun

Lao Tzu

It is impossible to understand aging and health without a gender perspective. Both from a physiologic and from a psychosocial point of view, the determinants of health as we age are intrinsically related to gender. There is increasing recognition that unless research and programs – on both clinical science and public health – acknowledge these differences, they will not be effective. While women experience greater burdens of morbidity and disability, men die earlier, yet the reasons for such premature mortality are not fully understood. The rapidity with which the global population is aging will require a sharp focus on gender issues if meaningful policies are to be developed. Yet so often gender in the health context is taken as being synonymous only with women's issues.[11] In contrast to the recent and much needed attention to the social position and health status of women, male health concerns have been relatively neglected. Men continue to have a higher morbidity and mortality rate,[10] and differences in lifespan, in favor of women, exist in various regions of the world with a mean difference of 4.2 years, and this is projected to increase to 4.8 years by the year 2050.[6]

The added burden of deleterious mutations on the Y chromosome may in part explain the reduced average lifespan of males versus females. The advantage of having two X-chromosomes is also apparent.[11] Moreover, oxidative damage to mitochondrial DNA is 4-fold higher in males than in females,[12] further contributing to the difference in lifespan between men and women. Many more factors which influence lifespan are due to lifestyle-related causes such as smoking, and alcohol-related mortality (aggression, accidents, suicide).

The course of disease, response to disease, and public response to illness exhibit gender differences and often result in different treatments and different access to health-care. The conventional approach of the medical, behavioral, and social sciences to the problem of male aging has been for a long time subject to oversight, disconnection, and lack of interdisciplinary collaboration.

The major causes of morbidity and mortality all take effect over extended periods. For example, DNA is constantly being damaged and repaired, bones are in a constant process of cellular loss and replacement, and atheromas are constantly accumulating inside arteries, which may or may not be removed. If the rate of decay is faster than the rate of repair, healthy tissue will be lost until the damage produces symptoms and finally results in disease. Therefore, primary prevention strategies will be most effective when initiated at the earliest opportunity. Ischemic heart disease, hypertension, stroke, and lung cancer are diseases whose primary prevention needs to be addressed. When diseases are more prevalent at older ages (e.g. prostate and colorectal cancers, or osteoporosis) early diagnostic tests (e.g. PSA) and screening procedures play an important role in secondary prevention and self-care strategies.

A significant number of male-related health problems, such as changes in body constitution, fat distribution, muscle weakness, urinary incontinence, loss of cognitive functioning, reduction in well-being, depression, and sexual dysfunction, could be detected and treated at an earlier stage if both physicians' and public awareness of these problems were more pervasive. This could effectively decrease morbidity, frailty, and dependency, increase quality of life, and reduce health service costs. Women visit the doctor 150% as often as men, enabling the detection of health problems in their early stages. However, usually men cost the health services more than women since they seek medical services at a more advanced stage of disease. While women are geared to preventive care, men generally come for 'reparation'.

When discussing age-related problems, it is often difficult to separate and to distinguish between (1) the natural aging process, primarily genetically determined (which today cannot be changed), (2) aging amplifiers determined by environmental and developmental factors (which can be modified), and (3) an acute or chronic illness or intercurrent diseases (which can be prevented, delayed, or cured). It must not be forgotten that aging by itself is associated with reduced productivity and decreased general vigor, as well as with increased incidence of defined diseases. These include:

1. cardiovascular disease (CVD)
2. malignant neoplasm
3. chronic obstructive pulmonary disease
4. degenerative and metabolic diseases (arthrosis, diabetes, osteoporosis)
5. visual loss (macular degeneration, cataract)
6. hearing loss
7. anxiety, mood, depression, and sleep disorders
8. sexual dysfunction
9. various dementias (e.g. Alzheimer's disease)
10. endocrine deficiencies.

Five out of six men in their sixties have one or more of these diseases. The chronic degenerative diseases have a long latency period before symptoms appear and a diagnosis is finally made. Once the diagnosis is made, drugs may alleviate symptoms, but are not very effective in altering the underlying disease, which unfortunately usually continues to deteriorate.

Cardiovascular disease

Heart disease and stroke are the major causes of death and disability in aging men. Approximately 52 million deaths occur worldwide each year, 39 million occurring in developing countries. About one-quarter of all deaths in developing countries and half of all deaths in developed countries are attributed to CVD. Globally, there are more deaths from coronary heart disease (5.2 million) than from stroke (4.6 million). Death rates from CVD increase dramatically with age. Within each country, age-specific death rates for all CVD increase at least 2-fold between the age groups 65–74 years and 75–84 years in both sexes, with at least 50% higher rates for elderly men than for women. Morbidity and disability from these diseases are also high; for example, the Global Burden of Disease project[13] estimates that, by 2020, coronary heart disease and stroke will be the first and second leading causes of death. Lack of exercise, smoking, and obesity are recognized risk factors for CVD. A significant relationship exists between body fat mass and both CVD and overall mortality in men. The increased mortality as observed in obese men is inversely related with physical fitness. For a full discussion see Section VIII.

Malignancy

Although malignant tumors occur at all ages, cancer disproportionately strikes individuals in the age group 65 years and older. Data from the National Cancer Institute Surveillance, Epidemiology, and End Results Program[14] (USA) for the most recent 5-year period, 1998–2002, reveal that 56% of all newly diagnosed cancer patients and 71% of cancer deaths are in this age group. Median ages of cancer patients at death for the major tumors common to both males and females, all races (lung, colorectal, lymphoma, leukemia, pancreas, stomach, urinary bladder) range from 71 to 77 years. The median age for prostate cancer is 79 years. As the proportion of elderly people has increased in most countries during the last few decades, and will increase further in the coming years, the incidence of cancer is expected to increase.[15] Cancer is the most common cause of death in people over 60 years of age, and the second most common cause of death in people over 80 years of age. Thus, age is the single most important risk factor for cancer.[16]

The International Agency for Research on Cancer (IARC) has calculated the incidence rates of cancer per 100 000 elderly persons based on data from cancer registries in 51 countries across five continents. The overall incidence of any cancer in elderly men is 61%. The frequency of any cancer except non-melanoma skin cancer is almost 7-fold more among elderly men (2158 per 100 000 person-years), and 4-fold more among elderly women (1192 per 100 000 person-years) than among younger persons (30–64 years old).[17] The incidence of cancer is higher in men than in women, and this difference is most evident after 64 years of age.

Worldwide, more than 9 million people developed cancer in 1997 and more than 6 million died of cancer. Cancer deaths increased from 6% to 9% of total deaths from 1985 to 1997 in developing countries, but remained constant at about 21% of total deaths in developed countries. The highest mortality rate was observed for lung cancer, with approximately 790 000 deaths in 1997, followed by stomach, liver, colorectal, esophageal, and prostate cancer.

In Europe and the USA, prostate carcinoma represents the most common cancer in males. Its incidence has rapidly increased since the 1970s because of the aging population and better diagnosis methods.[18] In 1990, worldwide, there were 193 000 deaths from prostate cancer, with 127 000 of those deaths occurring amongst men aged 70 years and over and 51 000 amongst those aged 60–69 years. Since prostate cancer is primarily a disease affecting men over 50, the global trend towards an aging population means that the number of prostate cancer deaths is predicted to increase markedly. In the year 2020, a global increase of 393 000 deaths is expected, with 359 000 of those deaths among men >70 years.

Chronic obstructive pulmonary diseases and lung cancer are not only among the most frequent problems in men, but are the most preventable. In men, 90% of all cases are attributable to cigarette smoking. These data suggest that almost every male lung cancer patient could have prevented his disease. Strategies to promote smoking cessation should be a top public priority, especially in those developing countries where aggressive marketing by the tobacco industry is not counterbalanced by adequate public health information advertisements.

These cancer statistics, when cast against the demographic changes occurring in the population, take on urgency and importance for cancer treatment and care in health-care systems.

In older men, a careful approach using the comprehensive geriatric assessment to identify functional deficits, frailty, and comorbidity is critical before embarking on cancer screening or a plan of cancer treatment.[19] The approach to cancer in this group should always be viewed in the context of the state of health of the patient: strive for an early diagnosis when a survival benefit is likely, implement curative treatments when the patient is functional, use less toxic or palliative regimens when the patient is frail or has a high burden of comorbidity, and always focus on maintaining the best quality of life possible.[17]

Osteoporosis

With the increase in lifespan, osteoporotic fractures are also becoming more frequent in men. It has been estimated that 19% of men over the age of 50 in the United States will have one or more fragility fractures in their lifetime, moreover more than 4 million men in the United States have low bone mass and are at risk for fractures.[20] A major portion of the morbidity, mortality, and social cost due to fall injuries is associated with age-related fractures, especially hip fractures. The risk of such injuries rises as the intensity of trauma increases and as bone resistance to fracture decreases. Both osteoporosis and trauma appear to be necessary but not sufficient causes of most age-related fractures.[21]

There is a great need to identify persons at risk for osteoporosis, it would be useful to obtain a quantitative evaluation of rates of bone loss to identify 'fast bone losers' at an early stage in order to target interventions to decrease further rapid loss of bone. Population studies have shown that biochemical measurements may predict rates of bone loss and occurrence of fractures.[20] Skeletal fractures diminish quality of life, advance dependency, and constitute an important public health problem. Hip fractures in men result in a higher morbidity and mortality than in women. Secondary causes such as gastrointestinal diseases with malabsorption, alcoholism, and malignant diseases are common. Etiologies such as hypogonadism and/or decrease of growth hormone (GH) are frequently not diagnosed, as clinical signs are subtle. The first sign of osteoporosis is often a spontaneous fracture of the lumbar spine,

proximal femur, or distal forearm after a fall. Elderly persons are at a higher risk of falling, which can be attributed to use of certain medications, alterations in balance, poor vision, loss of muscle strength, and prolonged reaction times. Preventive measures should target reducing bone loss and factors that contribute to falling. One of the most cost-effective prevention strategies is an adequate intake of calcium and vitamin D, and a physical exercise program which maximizes bone mass and muscle strength.[22] Hormone therapy (HT) together with proper nutrition and targeted physical activity may postpone the appearance of osteoporosis and delay or prevent bone fractures. The loss of vision, hearing, and other senses should be recognized as more than physical problems. Such conditions have profound effects on social and personal interactions, economic viability, and the mental health of those affected, and should be treated seriously. For further reading please refer to Section XI.

Depression

Depression is the most common functional mental disorder affecting aging males, and is underdiagnosed and undertreated.[23] While there appears to be some divergence of statistics on its prevalence in the elderly population, most studies have found prevalence rates of depression of between 5 and 15%. Depression has a high rate of recurrence and is associated with significantly increased mortality. Depression is closely linked in this group with physical illness and atypical or disguised altered presentations can make diagnosis difficult. Thorough holistic assessment and good communication skills are of the utmost importance. Nurses and medical professionals can improve the mental health of these patients with therapeutic attitudes and actions. It must be remembered that about 90% of older men who attempt or complete suicide have had depression either undiagnosed or inadequately treated. If men continue to underreport depression, the morbidity of this condition will continue to increase. Proper identification and treatment of depression will have significant public health implications. For a detailed discussion of diagnosis and management of depression see Chapter 42.

Cognitive decline

Cognitive decline with age is inevitable but the overall global impairment of the higher cortical functions can be delayed. Estrogen specifically maintains verbal memory in women and may prevent or forestall the deterioration in short- and long-term memory that occurs with normal aging. There is also evidence that estrogen decreases the incidence of Alzheimer's disease, delays its onset, or both.[11] The delayed onset of Alzheimer's disease in men may be due to the fact that estrogen levels are significantly higher in aging men than in postmenopausal women. In women HRT has been shown to delay the onset of Alzheimer's disease and there is an urgent need to obtain equivalent information in men. Dementia is a major public health issue accounting for significant morbidity, loss of independence, loss of dignity, and eventual institutionalization. The prevalence of severe dementia increases from 1% at age 65–74, to 7% at age 75–84, up to 25% after the age of 85. Thirty-seven percent of patients with Alzheimer's disease live in institutions compared with 1.7% of subjects without dementia.

Sexual dysfunction

Sexual desire, arousal, performance, and activity decrease significantly with age with a striking increase in the prevalence of impotence in men over 50 years. Reasons for decreased sexual activities include loss of libido (partially due to decreased androgen production), lack of partner, chronic illness, and/or various social and environmental factors, as well as erectile dysfunction (ED). It has been shown that sex education significantly and independently contributes to sexual enjoyment and satisfaction. Persistent interest in sexual activity results in positive mental and physical health benefits. The frequency, duration, and degree of nocturnal penile tumescence decreases significantly with age. These events are concomitant with a significant decrease in bioavailable testosterone and a compensatory increase in luteinizing hormone, showing that aging is associated with decreased gonadal activity.

Worldwide more than 100 million men are estimated to have some degree of ED. Erection is a neurovascular phenomenon under hormonal control and includes arterial dilatation, trabecular smooth muscle relaxation, and activation of the corporeal occlusive vein mechanism. Some of the major etiologies of ED are hypertension, diabetes, depression, and heart disease. It should also be remembered that genitourinary and colon surgery very often cause ED. Nerve-sparing surgery, which may reduce the incidence of ED, should be used whenever possible. Patients should be counseled prior to such interventions. Many drugs, particularly antihypertensive, antidepressant, and psychotropic drugs, may cause various degrees of ED. Therefore the treatment/therapy should be carefully considered, weighing the cost and benefit for each product and each individual patient. When focusing on the maintenance of quality of life among aging men, efforts to maintain, restore, or improve sexual function should not be neglected. Recent advances in basic and clinical research have led to the development of new treatment options for ED, including new pharmacologic agents for intracavernosal, intraurethral, and oral use. Orally acting preparations with either central action (apomorphine) or peripheral action (PDE5 inhibitors) alone or in concert with androgens have significantly improved the fate of men with erectile and/or sexual dysfunction. The management of ED should only be performed following proper evaluation of the patient and only by physicians with basic knowledge and clinical experience in diagnosis and treatment of ED. (See Chapter 10 for a detailed discussion on ED.)

Endocrine deficiencies

With prolonged life expectancy, men and women live one-third of their life with some hormone deficiency. Hormone deficiencies reduce the quality of life (Section V discusses this subject in detail). In cases of endocrine deficiency, irrespective of age, traditional endocrinology aims to supplement the deficient hormones or substances with hormone-like action. The decision to start hormone treatment (HT) in men should only be taken after obtaining objective evidence of hormone deficiency, with exclusion of secondary causes of endocrine dysfunction and after making the balance of risks and expected benefits of the replacement therapy. When data from long-term well-controlled studies become available, long-term therapy with one or more hormonal preparations will most probably, if used correctly, improve the quality of life of aging men and may even delay the aging process. It has been demonstrated that interventions, such as HT, the use of antioxidant drugs, proper and personally tailored nutrition, with vitamin supplements whenever necessary, as well as individually adjusted regular physical activity (aerobic, anaerobic, and stretching), have significant physiologic, psychologic, and social benefits for the elderly and may favorably influence some of the symptoms of aging as well as some of the pathologic conditions in aging men.

Strategies to improve and maintain aging men's health

Das Altwerden kann kein Arzt verhindern. Aber er kann – ist er gut – viel dazu beitragen die Beschwerdlichkeiten zu mildern.

Johann Wolfgang von Goethe

(Aging no physician can stop. But he can if he is good do a lot to reduce the suffering and aches of aging.)

With all the rhetoric surrounding the impending 'entitlement crisis' produced by the 'graying world,' there has been surprisingly little serious analysis of the social and economic implications of increased longevity and the doubling of the number of elderly people that will occur over the next 30 years. Patterns of work life and labor-force participation will almost inevitably change. Government expenditure will increase, intrafamily care-giving patterns will necessarily change.

The level of disability and dependence of older people, for which the rate of change is inherently unpredictable, will have a major effect on all these and other phenomena. Whether one views the net effect of all these changes as a positive or a negative, it is necessary to begin thinking a lot harder and more systematically about all of them.

The correct strategies in the management of aging should permit men to age in health and dignity, improving their quality of life by preventing

the preventable, and delaying and decreasing the pain and suffering of the inevitable.

Educating both the public and health-care providers about the importance of early detection of male health problems will result in reduced rates of morbidity and mortality, as well as health costs, for many age-related diseases. Many men are reluctant to visit their health center or physician through fear, lack of information, and for psychologic reasons. For more than 100 years, gynecologists have been specialized physicians for the medical care of the woman. About 50 years ago, gynecologists understood that the woman's health physician is more than an obstetrician and an 'oncology oriented surgeon,' and slowly the medically oriented gynecologist evolved, trained in reproductive endocrinology, perineonatology, ultrasound, family planning, and recently in assisted reproductive procedures. The training curricula (especially in the USA and UK) are constantly modified and adapted to the needs of 'women's health.' The modern gynecologist is not only cure-oriented, but has been trained in preventive strategies and in the maintenance of health and well-being, from adolescence to menopause.

The present day surgically oriented urologist has also arrived at the same crossroad gynecologists reached 50 years ago. Urologists today are highly specialized surgeons for the prostate, kidney, bladder, and the urinary tract. They have become highly specialized oncologists and diagnosticians and many have also specialized in the diagnosis and treatment of ED. Others have become nephrologists or specialists in transplantation, or andrologists specializing in gonadal physiology and pathology, and in the treatment of infertility, in collaboration with gynecologists, extracting sperm from testis or epididymis or diagnosing and managing varicoceles. Training in urology is extremely long. With surgical procedures decreasing and being replaced by medical interventions the idea of medical urologists has evolved. The number of urologists worldwide today is far too low to take care of all men. To become the 'man's health physician' they will have to receive sufficient training in endocrinology, internal medicine, especially cardiology, and psychology/psychiatry; they will have to be trained to give guidance on nutrition and exercise and have a solid understanding of gerontology. The International Society for the Study of the Aging Male (ISSAM) is working together with the diverse urologic and andrologic associations to obtain this goal.

However, until this goal is achieved and sufficient urologists/andrologists have been trained, a 'gate keeper' will be required to serve and manage male health. Those who aspire to take the role of 'gate keeper' for male health will depend on the specific training, culture, and the medical services of each geographic area and country.

Male health could be managed by an interdisciplinary group practice or by the primary health worker, the family physician, the endocrinologist, or a specialist in internal medicine or gerontology. Each member of this profession can be trained to become a 'gate keeper' for male health and learn to screen men for their most probable risk factors, advise them on lifestyle, and, whenever necessary, refer them to the specialist they need. When a man attends his family doctor for a common cold, a gastrointestinal disorder, or any other acute infection the physician should, on the basis of the family history, body constitution, lifestyle, and risk factors, advise the patient on preventive strategies or refer him to consult the correct specialist.

Conclusions

Men who are educated about the value of preventative health-care in prolonging their lifespan, quality of life, and their role as productive family members will be more likely to participate in health screening. To obtain this goal it will be necessary:

1. To make available a group of trained medical professionals who can understand, guide, educate, and manage the problems of aging men.
2. To provide more information about the normal male aging process and to advertise and promote aging in a positive and active way. Men should receive education and be prompted to take on teaching roles themselves, leading self-help groups and advocating on behalf of their aging communities.

3. To establish programs empowering men to become well-informed, active managers of their own health and the health of their surrounding society.
4. To obtain essential epidemiologic data and to intensify basic and clinical research on aging men.
5. To assess age-related nutritional needs.
6. To develop strategies for physical exercise (aerobic for maintaining cardiac function, anaerobic, targeted to specific muscle groups, and stretching).
7. To develop and assess new and improved drugs for the prevention and treatment of pathologic changes related to aging.

To this end, the efforts of all governmental and non-governmental organizations to promote aging men's health at local, national, and international levels must be strongly encouraged. A holistic approach to this new challenge of the 21st century will necessitate a quantum leap in multidisciplinary and internationally coordinated research efforts, supported by a new partnership between industry and governments, philanthropic and international organizations. This collaboration we hope will enrich us with a better understanding of male health and aging, permit us to help to improve the quality of life, prevent the preventable, and postpone and decrease the pain and suffering of the inevitable.

References

1. Lutz W. European Demographic Data Sheet 2006. Vienna and Washington, DC: Vienna Institute of Demography, International Institute for Applied Systems Analysis, and Population Reference Bureau, 2006.
2. Population Division, Department of Economic and Social Affairs, United Nations Secretariat. Population Prospects. The 2004 Revision. Population Database. New York: United Nations, 2005.
3. United Nations Secretariat, Department of Economic and Social Affairs Population Division. World Population Prospects, The 1998 Revision. ESA/P/WP 150. New York: United Nations, 1998.
4. Lunenfeld B. Aging male. Aging Male 1998; 1: 1–7.

5. Lunenfeld B. The aging male: demographics and challenges. World J Urol 2002; 20: 11–16.
6. Diczfalusy E. Our common future: a rapidly growing and rapidly aging humankind. Aging Male 2006; 9: 125–34.
7. World Health Organization. International Classification of Impairments, Disabilities and Handicaps. Geneva: WHO, 1980.
8. World Health Organization. Jakarta Declaration on Leading Health Promotion into the 21st Century. Geneva: WHO, 1997.
9. Wilikins R, Adams OB. Health expectancy in Canada, demographic, regional and social dimensions. Am J Public Health 1983; 73: 1073–80.
10. Kalache A, Lunenfeld B. Health and the aging male. Aging Male 2000; 3: 1–36.
11. Smith DW, Warner HR. Does genotypic sex have a direct effect on longevity? Exp Gerontol 1989; 24: 277–88.
12. Viña J, Borrás C, Gambini J et al. Why females live longer than males: control of longevity by sex hormones. Sci Aging Knowledge Environ 2005; 23: 7.
13. Lopez AD. Global Burden of Disease and Risk Factors. New York: Oxford University Press; 2006.
14. US Department of Health and Human Services. Healthy People 2010: Understanding and Improving Health. Washington, DC: US Department of Health and Human Services, 2000.
15. Balducci L. New paradigms for treatment of elderly patients with cancer: the comprehensive geriatric assessment and guidelines for supportive AO care. J Support Oncol 2003; 1(Suppl 2): 30–7.
16. Cepeda OA, Gammack JK. Cancer in older men: a gender based review. Aging Male 2006; 9: 149–59.
17. Hansen J. Common cancers in the elderly. Drugs Aging 1998; 13(6): 467–78.
18. McDavid K, Lee J, Fulton JP et al. Prostate cancer incidence and mortality rates and trends in the United States and Canada. Public Health Rep 2004; 119: 174–86.
19. Balducci L. New paradigms for treatment of elderly patients with cancer: the comprehensive geriatric assessment and guidelines for supportive care. J Support Oncol 2003; 1(Suppl 2): 30–7.
20. Melton LJ 3rd, Cummings SR. Heterogeneity of age-related fractures: implications for epidemiology. Bone Min 1987; 2(4): 321–31.
21. Melton LJ 3rd, Riggs BL. Risk factors for injury after a fall. Clin Geriatr Med 1985; 1(3): 525–39.
22. Rudman D, Drinka PJ, Wilson CR et al. Relations of endogenous anabolic hormones and physical activity to bone mineral density and lean body mass in elderly men. Clin Endocrinol 1994; 40: 653–61.
23. Ganguli M, Du Y, Dodge HH, Ratcliff GG, Chang CC. Depressive symptoms and cognitive decline in late life: a prospective epidemiological study. Arch Gen Psychiatry 2006; 63(2): 153–60.

CHAPTER 6

Screening of the aging male

Louis JG Gooren, Alvaro Morales, and Bruno Lunenfeld

The traditional role of the physician is to diagnose, treat, and manage disease processes. Preventive medicine has been largely the domain of public health. But over recent decades subjects have experienced increasingly a need for preventive medicine in their individual lives. So an additional role for the physician emerges: the screening and counseling of subjects who are asymptomatic, who have not (yet) signs or symptoms of disease. The motivation of individuals to seek medical screening may vary: some will have a family history of disease, others like to make a calculated risk before making major decisions in their lives and feel that they have thus more control over their lives. These subjects expect that medical examination will reveal their propensity to develop a particular disease and they are prepared to take early measures to prevent or ameliorate its course. Examples are cardiovascular disease and its risk factors hypertension, lipid disorders, and diabetes mellitus type 2. Others expect that early diagnosis of conditions such as cancer promise a better outcome, or even cure of the disease. Some subjects will feel that information on a health risk profile permits them to plan their life better, enabling them to take important decisions before it is too late. By contrast, there are others who do not wish to have this information since it would now sap the joy of their life. This group will avoid screening opportunities.

Screening usually implies physical examination, laboratory tests, and basic radiologic tests but sometimes more extensive investigations like a CT scan or a colonoscopy, with the aim to discover or to reasonably exclude (sub)clinical disease. A positive result usually leads to a more extensive diagnostic work-up. It is impossible to screen a person for all ailments, even if this would lead to early and meaningful preventive interventions. Screening will be more or less guided by the probability of certain risks in this particular subject's life.

Preventive medicine can be categorized as primary, secondary, and tertiary. Primary prevention refers to general measures to prevent disease such as cessation of smoking, and dietary and exercise recommendations in non-diseased subjects. It is non-individualized. Secondary prevention is the (early) detection of pathology in individual subjects so as to reverse or slow the course and improve the prognosis of (highly prevalent) diseases (routine measurement of blood pressure or lipid profile). Tertiary prevention covers efforts to minimize the future negative health effects of factors operating in disease already present, e.g., improving lipid profiles in patients with cardiovascular disease.

Value of screening tests

Interpretation of the results of diagnostic tools in screening requires an understanding of some basic principles of epidemiology.

The sensitivity and specificity of a test are important principles of diagnostic work-ups of patients and of screening of asymptomatic subjects. The sensitivity of a test represents the proportion of patients actually having the disease who will test positive in this test (true-positive rate). The specificity of a test equals the proportion of non-diseased patients who will have a negative outcome on testing (true-negative rate); in every day parlance: will the test miss patients who actually have the disease? In the medical practice of screening there is a great interest in the predictive value of a test. This does not refer so much to the ability of a test to confirm a disease but the ability of that test to predict the disease. Similar to the sensitivity and specificity of a test there is a positive predictive value: the proportion of patients with a positive test who actually (will) have the disease; the negative predictive value of a test equals the proportion of patients with a negative test result who indeed do not have the disease, and are unlikely to develop it; again, in everyday parlance: what is the chance that an actual case will be overlooked? The predictive value of a test is influenced by the prevalence of the disease or condition of concern.

Guiding principles of screening

It goes without saying that screening never can cover all diseases and conditions from which a human being can suffer. The resources to screen for all potential diseases are simply not available. So, the question arises what principles should guide the physician in the decision to screen. Naturally, a person's age, medical history, and family history provide information on their health risks. There are a number of general principles directing the decisions. Are the morbidity and mortality of the condition serious? Does the condition screened for have an important impact on the health and life expectancy of the subject in question? Will it save years of life and will these years have a reasonable quality of life? The disease should be common enough. It is not cost-effective to screen for very rare conditions. The disease should also have a long enough preclinical duration before it becomes clinically manifest. Diseases with a rather sudden onset, such as certain forms of leukemia, are difficult to screen for. For screening to be meaningful, there should be a certain outlook for an available and efficacious treatment, which can positively change the outcome and course of the disease. The screening procedure should have a very reasonable sensitivity, specificity, and predictive value. The screening tests must be acceptable to the subject. Painful and tedious diagnostic procedures are less acceptable. The procedures should also be reasonably safe, and the costs of the screening should be affordable.

Interpretation of results of screening

As indicated earlier, for the interpretation of the results of screening, an understanding of the epidemiology and the natural course of disease, with and without therapeutic intervention, is required. The basic tenet of screening is to do more good than harm. The test result can be a reason to refer the subject to the relevant medical specialty, but the person in question will always receive an initial evaluation of the screening results from the physician who performed the screening. The implications of specificity, sensitivity, and predictive value have been indicated above. How certain can the subject be that he does not suffer from the disease if he tests negative? If tested positive, how sure is the patient that he actually suffers from the disease and how much reason is there to undergo additional testing? Needless to say a positive result of screening is anxiety provoking. It is difficult to cope emotionally with statistical data of disease probability and disease course once one has tested positive in a screening procedure. The physician who embarks on screening of subjects should have a sound understanding of the diseases these subjects are screened for so as to counsel the patients if they test positive.

General screening tests

It is difficult to make a fair assessment of the infirmity associated with the aging process. Part of it will be due to 'natural aging' and part of it to emerging disease processes, which will be increasingly part of life with aging. 'Natural aging' and emerging diseases affect an individual subject to varying degrees. For instance, hormone deficiencies do not affect all men to the same degree, and hypertension and diabetes mellitus range from mild to severe. Therefore it is useful to have tools that provide a 'grip' on signs and symptoms of aging. Such an instrument also facilitates assessment of the successes of interventions in these populations.

The development of rates scales is a difficult venture. The validation of questionnaires is an arduous process. Translation into another language implies a new validation in that language to test whether questions are understood and interpreted linguistically and culturally in the same way as in the original language. A recently developed instrument is the 'Aging Males' Symptoms' (AMS) rating scale.[1, 2] The rating scale measures somatic, sexual, and psychologic aspects of an aging male's life. Originally developed in the German language it has now been validated for English[1] (Appendix 1) while validations for other European languages are now available.[3,4] Validations in other languages and in other geographic areas are welcomed. Another scale, developed by Morley et al,[5] tests whether certain symptoms are more likely to be present in aging men with declining levels of bioavailable testosterone (Appendix 6.2).

Urologic screening

Lower urinary tract symptoms

Many aging men will experience urinary problems ranging from nocturia, increased frequency of micturition, urgency, hesitancy, poor stream, postmicturition dribbling, loss of bladder control resulting in incontinence, and retention. Many of these complaints were previously referred to as 'prostatism'. However, these complaints may not be caused by prostatic disease and, therefore, now the term 'lower urinary tract symptoms' (LUTS) is preferred to describe these voiding problems. A correct nomenclature may avoid premature conclusions as to the etiology of the symptoms as being prostatic in origin. Polyuria may, for instance, be a symptom of diabetes mellitus.

LUTS may have a considerable impact on quality of life of the patient. The degree of bothersomeness rather than the objective magnitude of LUTS is the indication for diagnostic and therapeutic

interventions. LUTS may be subdivided into voiding and storage problems. Voiding problems are usually due to bladder outlet obstruction or detrusor dysfunction. The storage capacity of the bladder and the detrusor contractility decrease with age. In many cases storage complaints are related to detrusor instability. Population studies show a frequency of moderate-to-severe LUTS from 8 to 31% in men in their fifties, increasing to 27–44% of men in their seventies. But many men experience symptoms of LUTS much earlier in life!

Several symptom scores have been developed as tools to quantify LUTS. The best known are the symptom index[6] and the international prostate symptoms score (IPSS),[7–9] both produced by task forces of the American Urological Association. The specificity is rather low because of the non-specificity of LUTS itself as a complaint. The IPSS has therefore been criticized as lacking specificity, lacking usefulness for screening, and for not including symptoms such as dribbling and incontinence. Therefore, bothersomeness and disease-specific or non-specific quality of life indices have been added as a tool in the management of LUTS and benign prostate hypertrophy in Barry's impact index (BII).[10,11]

Patient screening for LUTS

Physicians screening for LUTS must be aware of the heterogeneity of the condition but the first responsibility of the physician is to exclude serious life-threatening conditions such as prostate carcinoma or carcinoma in situ of the bladder. Patients with LUTS usually show few signs of disease on inspection. Palpation of the abdomen may disclose a renal mass, and palpation of the suprapubic area may reveal bladder dilatation.

Digital rectal examination

Digital rectal examination provides clues as to whether there are signs of prostate cancer, but it only examines the posterior aspect of the prostate. Nodularity, induration, or asymmetry of the prostate may be indications of cancer. But small tumors and those deep in the prostate gland may go unnoticed. It also provides information on the size of the prostate, though digital rectal examination tends to underestimate prostate volume.[12,13]

Urine analysis

A simple urine dipstick test to rule out urinary tract infection and hematuria is recommended. It has a low predictive value but it is simple and cheap. Also a urine sediment may provide valuable information on the presence of leukocytes, erythrocytes, and protein cylinders.

Measurement of serum creatinine is indicated to rule out renal insufficiency which may be secondary to LUTS.

Prostate-specific Antigen

Prostate-specific antigen (PSA) is a serine protease released by prostatic tissue. Healthy prostate tissue produces low levels, but prostatic conditions with elevated cellular proliferation, such as BPH and cancer, are associated with higher levels. Also inflammatory conditions of the prostate may be associated with (even strong) elevations of PSA values. Since it is also produced by normal and benign hyperplastic prostatic tissue it lacks specificity as a prostate cancer marker.

Various assays of PSA are available and the (arbitrary!) cutoff for normal values is above 4 ng/ml. Temporary elevations of PSA occur after prostate biopsy or prostate surgery as a result of an outpouring of PSA into the circulation. Digital rectal examination of the prostate or ejaculation has, however, a limited effect on blood levels of PSA.[14] This is pertinent information. Usually blood sampling for PSA takes place after physical examination of the patient which may have included a digital rectal examination.

PSA values increase with age due to an age-related increase in prostate cellular growth. Further, race is a factor in the distribution of normal PSA values. Therefore age- and race-specific normal ranges have been proposed but their clinical usefulness has not been validated.

Unfortunately, PSA characteristics lack specificity, sensitivity, and predictive value, particularly when they are mildly elevated, for instance between 4 and 10 ng/ml. In men with PSA values above 10 ng/ml approximately, one in three will have a false positive result. In men with PSA values between 4 and 10 ng/ml, the positive predictive value is only 28–35%. Consequently, about two-thirds of men tested will have false positive results. There are also (mainly small) prostate cancers associated with PSA values below 4 ng/ml.[15,16]

Usefulness of PSA measurement to detect prostate cancer

Whether men should be screened for prostate cancer is presently hotly debated (for review see references 17 and 18). Points in case are:

- PSA values lack sensitivity, specificity, and predictive value. Men with small prostate tumors may still have normal PSA values. Conversely, the likelihood that a man with an elevated PSA value has indeed prostate cancer is relatively low, but increases with the value of PSA.
- Digital rectal examination has only a limited capacity to diagnose cancers. Small tumors and those deep in the gland are not recognized. So a negative digital rectal examination of the prostate is not a ground for reassurance. If the tumor is readily palpable, it is less likely to be confined to the prostate capsule and has already an unfavorable prognosis. In other words 'this tumor has been detected too late to be of great value for preventive medicine and belongs already to the domain of curative medicine.' On the positive side, digital rectal examination sometimes discovers tumors associated with normal PSA values.
- Men with elevated PSA will undergo additional testing. In a large proportion of these men, particularly when PSA levels are only mildly elevated, this testing will be redundant since PSA values above normal have a high percentage of false positives. Prostate biopsies carry a certain risk of bleeding and infection. The prostate volume, the measurement of the free/total PSA ratio, the PSA velocity over time, and the age and general health of the individual are all factors that must be taken into consideration prior to deciding on further testing or treatment.
- If a cancer diagnosis is made, what will the next step be? Can the patient and/or his urologist

accept a wait-and-see policy, justified in many cases, or will the patient be treated with one of the available treatment modalities which are associated with potential considerable morbidity, such as incontinence and erectile dysfunction, with frequently an enormous impact on quality of life.

- The conclusion must be that, presently, there is absolutely no consensus among experts that the benefits outweigh the harm, which is the basic tenet of screening.

Practical recommendations

Screening of the aging male should include a digital examination of the prostate and most men will expect to have their PSA value measured. Discovery of a prostate nodule should lead to urologic examination. Subjects who have an elevated PSA should be monitored and followed up by digital rectal examination and PSA measurements. There is evidence that in the normal range of PSA level the rate of change of PSA level over time provides useful information. An annualized rate of change of > 0.75 ng/ml/year (or the so-called PSA velocity) for 2 years should lead to urologic evaluation and prostate biopsy. If the first value of PSA was > 4.0 ng/ml then an annualized rate of 0.4 ng/ml should be taken as a guideline.[15,19,20] Such guidelines allow administration of androgens to individual hypogonadal aging men, with due concern for adverse effects on the prostate. When aging men receive androgens and/or growth hormone it is thought to be reasonable to screen PSA levels every 3 months for the first 12–18 months and once a year thereafter.

Assessment of body mass index and fat distribution

Body mass index (BMI) (body weight in kilograms divided by the square of height in meters) provides a better index than body weight itself to describe the degree of obesity. There is now solid evidence that fat distribution (a large visceral fat depot) is a strong predictor of cardiovascular disease and of the development of diabetes mellitus type II. Visceral fat is quantitatively most reliably assessed with computerized tomography or magnetic resonance imaging, which is too costly to become a method of mass screening and probably redundant in assessing an individual case. A number of studies document that surrogate measures provide a reasonable indication of the amount of visceral fat accumulation. A waist/hip ratio > 0.95, a waist circumference of more than 101 cm, and a sagittal diameter > 23 cm (measured with the patient supine) are all indications of visceral obesity. These patterns of body fat distribution are also linked to a negative biochemical cardiovascular risk profile.[21] Thus, it is possible, by simple means, to determine overweight and fat distribution patterns. The above values have typically been obtained in a Caucasian population. However, in Chinese subjects the waist/hip ratio also provides additional information on cardiovascular risks,[22] but different criteria apply to Asians.[23] In Asians a BMI of 23–25 indicates overweight and > 25 indicates obesity, a waist circumference > 90 cm means abdominal obesity.

Screening for cardiovascular disease

Cardiovascular disease continues to be a leading cause of death, with coronary heart disease accounting for more than 50% of the mortality. One in six deaths is explained by stroke. If patients survive stroke there is usually an impaired functional capacity. A large number of risk factors for cardiovascular disease have been identified. It has sometimes been difficult to establish whether the given variable constitutes a risk factor in itself or whether the identified risk factor is merely a marker of cardiovascular risk (for an extensive review see reference 24). In the first instance modification of that variable may reduce a person's cardiovascular risk, in the second instance interventions to modify the surrogate marker do not benefit the individual. Intervention aimed at modifying surrogate markers of cardiovascular risks may be useless as long as the underlying risk is not modified. Many intervention studies in cardiovascular disease have assessed their impact on risk factors (lipid levels, blood pressure values) without measuring their effects on clinical endpoints such as cardiovascular morbidity, its disease burden, and its mortality. Admittedly, studies assessing cardiovascular morbidity and mortality are difficult and expensive, but the true value of interventions can only be convincingly demonstrated if and when this intervention reduces morbidity and/or mortality.

Unless present to an extreme degree, cardiovascular disease is rarely explained by one single risk factor. It is mostly multifactorial. Risk factors are additive in their effects and many risk factors are interdependently clustered, such as visceral obesity, insulin insensitivity, hypertension, and hyperlipidemia (metabolic syndrome).[25,26] Not all risk factors carry equal weight in their potential harm to the cardiovascular system. Variables, such as elevated blood pressure or hypercholesterolemia, are continuous or graded, and therefore some risk factors cannot be treated as a category, simply present or absent. Sometimes the absolute value is less significant than the ratio of two variables, as is the case with the ratio of total cholesterol to high-density lipoprotein (HDL) cholesterol. Most risk factors have been identified in epidemiologic studies and carry a higher predictive value for populations than for individual subjects. In other words, it is often difficult to attribute the right weight to the presence of risk factors in individuals unless the magnitude of that risk factor is extreme, but most subjects will have moderate magnitudes of risk factors such as a mildly elevated blood pressure and mild hypercholesterolemia.

Risk factors for cardiovascular disease

There are several risk factors whose control has been shown to reduce the risk of cardiovascular disease; of others it is likely that their control contributes to cardiovascular health. Non-modifiable risk factors such as age, sex, and family history will not be addressed, or only indirectly. Risk factors whose control reduces cardiovascular risk will be discussed in the following sections.

Smoking

Cigarette smoking is a serious threat for cardiovascular disease, stroke, and peripheral arterial disease in a dose-dependent fashion. Smoking is linked to myocardial infarction and sudden cardiac death.[27]

Hypertension

The relationship between hypertension and cardiovascular disease is graded; in other words, there is no cut-off value below which there is no increased risk. Therefore it is desirable to diagnose and treat mild-to-moderate hypertension as well. Since mild hypertension is much more prevalent in the general population than serious hypertension, many more people die of mild hypertension than of grossly elevated blood pressure. It is estimated that 35% of all cardiovascular events are related to hypertension. The protective effect of lowering blood pressure values in hypertensive subjects is well established. Obesity, particularly visceral obesity, is a major risk factor for hypertension. The notion that 'white coat hypertension' does not reflect a person's 'true' blood pressure, and is innocent, is no longer held by experts. The fact that the blood pressure rises to abnormally high values in situations of stress is not without significance for a person's cardiovascular health. It often forebodes 'fixed' hypertension.

There is a reasonable degree of consensus as to what values of blood pressure constitute hypertension. There are different schools of thought with regard to interventions. Some will deem the need for treatment more pressing if an elevated blood pressure in a person is associated with other risk factors, such as lipid disorders and/or diabetes mellitus. Others will take the value of blood pressure in itself as the guiding principle. There is a trend to regard lower values of blood pressure as criteria for hypertension and targets of treatment. The blood pressure is considered to be elevated when systolic values above 140 mmHg and/or diastolic values above 90 mmHg are found.[28] When additional risk factors are present the upper level of the systolic value considered acceptable is 130/80 mmHg.[28]

The blood pressure is assessed during normal medical consultations. It may require three measurements during a couple of weeks or up to five measurements over 6 months before a verdict on the presence of hypertension can be made. Twenty-four-hour monitoring is recommended in cases where measurements do not provide the necessary information on whether to treat or not to treat. Self-monitoring of blood pressure adds significantly to better compliance.

Thrombogenic factors

Endothelial function is of the utmost importance for maintaining a non-thrombogenic state. Inhibition of platelet clotting and of fibrinogenesis is of great significance in the prevention of thrombosis. A large number of thrombogenic factors has been identified. It has been established that circulating levels of fibrinogen impact on the occurrence of cardiovascular disease.[29] Low-dose aspirin inhibits thrombogensis and therewith cardiovascular events.

Diabetes mellitus

Diabetes is associated with both macrovascular and microvascular disease through a multitude of pathogenetic mechanisms. In all likelihood strict glycemic control is helpful in slowing the development of atherosclerosis. Many risk factors of cardiovascular disease are cumulatively present in diabetics (insulin resistance, hypertension, dyslipidemia). The presence of diabetes is a reason for aggressive treatment of other risk factors. Diabetes mellitus is certainly a modifiable disease and therefore well worth early diagnosis. The guidelines are straightforward. If fasting glucose levels are between 6 and 7 mmol/l there is an impaired glucose tolerance, warranting follow-up every 6 months. Values above 7 mmol/l represent clinical diabetes mellitus, requiring treatment. A 2-hour glucose tolerance test provides a more reliable diagnostic criterion: if the serum glucose is >11 mmol/l after 2 hours then the diagnosis diabetes mellitus is certain.

Physical inactivity

The impact that lack of physical fitness has on cardiovascular disease is now well established. Even moderate levels of physical activity are beneficial. It leads to an improvement of virtually all known risk factors (body weight, blood pressure, glucose tolerance, lipid profile). A consensus meeting of the National Institute of Health in the USA has recommended regular, moderately intense exercise (at least 30 minutes on most or all days of the week).[30,31]

Cholesterol

The causal relationship between total cholesterol, and even more so of LDL cholesterol and cardiovascular disease is well established. It is a graded relation. Levels normally present in certain Western populations might already be in the danger zone. Reduction of cholesterol and particularly of LDL cholesterol reduces the occurrence of cardiovascular disease, including stroke. Therefore, determination of cholesterol is pivotal.

High-density lipoprotein cholesterol

There is a graded, continuous, inverse relationship between the level of HDL cholesterol and cardiovascular risk. Several studies document that drug treatment to improve levels of HDL cholesterol has a beneficial effect on cardiovascular mortality. Smoking, overweight, and physical inactivity all have negative effects on HDL cholesterol levels.

Triglycerides

Hypertriglyceridemia is often intertwined with other risk factors such as low HDL cholesterol, visceral obesity with its associated insulin resistance, and a prothrombotic state. Therefore, hypertriglyceridemia deserves attention but often requires a more comprehensive diagnostic work-up and therapy modifying the associated risk factors as well.

Measurement of lipids

An assessment of a lipid profile consists of total cholesterol, HDL cholesterol, a calculated value of low-density lipoprotein (LDL) cholesterol, and triglycerides. There is a reasonable degree of consensus that total cholesterol should be <5 mmol/l (<200 mg/dl), HDL >1.0 nmol/l (>35 mg/dl), calculated LDL <4.0 mmol/l (<130 mg/dl), and triglycerides <1.4 mmol/l (<150 mg/dl). The LDL/HDL ratio should be <4. For recommendations see reference 32. In their clinical significance and in the decisions to undertake interventions, these results should be set against other cardiovascular risk factors such as hypertension, diabetes mellitus, and family history.

Lipoprotein(a)

Lipoprotein(a) is an LDL particle linked to apoliprotein(a). The gene for apolipoprotein(a) has a high degree of homology with the gene for plasminogen, which has led to the theory that lipoprotein(a) may displace plasminogen from its sites of action, thereby reducing its antithrombotic capacity. It is also similar in structure to LDL and may impair endothelial function. There are no known methods of modulating lipoprotein(a) levels.

Homocysteine

Homocysteine levels have been linked to cardiovascular disease; it is probably an independent risk factor. Its pathogenetic mechanism is likely interference with endothelial nitric oxide production. Its levels can be reduced by folic acid and vitamins B_6 and B_{12}, but the clinical efficacy of a reduction has not been demonstrated.

Screening for coronary artery disease

The exercise electrocardiogram for detection of coronary artery disease is the cornerstone. Ischemia manifests itself by ST segment depression. Its accuracy is greater when the ST segment depression is associated with angina pectoris in the test. Its accuracy is less for the posterior wall of the heart. The accuracy of the test ranges between 70 and 75%. Its cost is acceptable but its value in people at low risk is arguable.

There are a number of screening procedures such as stress nuclear perfusion imaging, the use of electron-beam computed tomography, measurement of intima media thickness, and determination of brachial artery reactivity. They can only be done in specialized centers and are beyond the scope of this contribution.

Primary hemochromatosis

Primary hemochromatosis is a genetically determined disease occurring in approximately 1 in 360 men and women. (For a review see reference 33.) The disorder is characterized by excessive storage of iron in tissues, leading to tissue damage. Its clinical manifestations may vary. The symptoms are chronic fatigue, arthralgia, infertility, erectile dysfunction, cardiac disease, diabetes mellitus, and an abnormal profile of liver enzymes, a series of complaints not rare in aging men. Patients have a normal hemoglobin level but an increased serum ferritin and transferrin saturation.

Osteoporosis

Few men under the age of 60–70 will suffer from osteoporosis. If a man presents with severe osteoporosis a number of diseases should be ruled out. Alcohol abuse, glucocorticoid treatment, and hypogonadism account for 40–50% of cases of male osteoporosis. Other causes important to rule out are hyperthyroidism (either as a disease or as an overdose of thyroid hormone replacement), multiple myeloma (Kahler's disease) and other malignancies, anticonvulsants, past or present chemotherapy, and gastrointestinal disorders impairing calcium absorption. The latter may be subtle in their clinical manifestations, like gluten enteropathy. Long-term hypogonadism, rheumatic disease, chronic use of corticosteroids, alcoholism, intestinal malabsorption, renal disease, dietary factors, and heavy smoking may lead to premature loss of bone. A decrease in height and vertebral kyphosis, mostly occurring in men over 60 years of age, may be a sign of vertebral osteoporosis. The history and clinical evaluation are factors in the decision to have the patient undergo bone densitometry.

The most widely used techniques to measure bone mineral density are dual-photon absorptiometry (DPA), dual-energy X-ray absorptiometry (DEXA), and quantitative computed tomography. Bone mineral density is measured usually at one or more of the following sites: lumbar spine (L_{2-4}), femoral neck, proximal femur, and forearm. The values are absolute values but, for a more meaningful interpretation, values are often expressed as T-scores (the number of statistical standard deviations of the mean of a general young population of that sex) or as Z-scores (the number of statistical standard deviations of the mean of a population of that sex of similar age).

By definition, a bone mineral density more than 2.5 SD below the mean indicates osteoporosis, requiring treatment and frequent follow-up at intervals of 6–12 months. Values between 1 and 2.5 SD below the mean represent osteopenia. Elimination of risk factors and preventive treatment are indicated. In the laboratory serum calcium plus serum albumin (to which it is largely bound) must be measured. Serum alkaline phosphatase (if possible bone-specific) and osteocalcin provide insight in the degree of bone turnover. Excretion of calcium in the urine indicates whether an abnormal amount of calcium is being lost. Hydroxyproline or deoxypyrolidine or collagen cross-links N telopeptide are metabolic products of bone resorption. Calcium and hydroxyproline or deoxypyrolidine can be measured in a 24-hour urine sample, but a reasonably good impression is also obtained from a 2-hour sample if levels are related to creatinine levels in this 2-hour sample.

Functionality and functional dependency

Screening of the aging male will be performed across a large age range of men. For men in their fifties functional dependency is almost never an issue; with aging it becomes, however, increasingly relevant. Several scales have been developed to measure independent functioning. They may be divided into basic, intermediate, and advanced activities. Both the scales developed by Katz et al[34] and by Gill et al[35] are widely used to assess basic activities of daily living (ADL), and whether a person needs help with the following activities:

1. bathing
2. dressing
3. transferring within the home
4. toileting
5. maintaining continence
6. feeding.

Less basic, intermediate ADL are usually measured by the instrumental ADL scale developed by Carey et al[36] which assesses the person's ability to perform the following activities:

1. shopping
2. transportation
3. using the telephone
4. preparing meals
5. taking medications
6. managing money
7. performing work around the house
8. doing laundry.

Advanced ADL can be measured by the scale developed by Reuben et al:[37]

1. strenuous physical activity (such as hiking, bicycling)
2. heavy work around the house
3. number of times walks one mile or more without rest
4. number of times walks one quarter of a mile or more without rest.

These scales may impress as simple tools but several studies have documented that they are highly predictive of mortality, providing better indications than most laboratory-based tests.

Intervening variables in the actual performance of ADL are muscle weakness, particularly lower extremity weakness, and cognitive impairment. Lower extremity performance can be investigated with rather simple tests:[38]

1. Chair stands: how often can a person stand up from a chair within 30 seconds, with the arms crossed over the chest?
2. The tandem stand: can a person maintain balance for at least 3 seconds with one foot placed behind the other on a straight line?
3. The timed walk: a subject is asked to walk approximately 3 meters, turn 180°, and walk 3 meters back in a straight line without staggering or stumbling, within 90 seconds.

These rather simples procedures have been validated as reliable measures of functionality.

Cognitive status

The prevalence of dementia at age 65 is approximately 5–10%, rising progressively to 40–50% at age

85; it is worthwhile to have an assessment of the cognitive status. The medical interview itself, probing into the patient's medical history, may already reveal defects in short-term memory. For more elaborate testing the Mini-Mental State Examination[39] is available, and if the performance is poor on this test the Short Portable Mental Status Questionnaire[40] may be used. Age and education influence the performance of these tests. For a review of tests of mental functioning see reference 41.

Visual impairment

Age-related visual changes affect central visual acuity, peripheral vision, contrast sensitivity, and color vision. Two common conditions, cataract and glaucoma, are essentially preventable causes of blindness. Degeneration of the macula, which reveals itself by loss of central vision, is the leading cause of poor vision in elderly men. The medical history inquires whether the patient has an impairment of vision. The Snellen eye chart, which patients read from 5 meters using their corrective lenses, provides an impression of visual acuity. Handheld cards, such as the Rosenbaum pocket vision screener, are useful alternatives for near and distant vision. Inability to read better than 20/50 with correction is an indication for a specialist assessment. The Amsler grid can be used to discover visual field defects which may be related to macular degeneration or glaucoma.

Hearing impairment

Hearing impairment is present in 24% of subjects between 65 and 74 years old, and increases to 40% in those older than 75 years. Hearing loss is associated with social dysfunction and is to a large degree underdiagnosed. Hearing aids are, strangely enough, more negatively perceived as a sign of aging than corrective eye lenses. The whisper test is simple and provides a first indication of hearing loss. The examiner stands 5 meters behind the patient, who covers alternate the left and right ear. Three words are whispered which are to be repeated by the patient. Naturally, the acoustics of the room influence the result of the test.

Depression in old age

Poor sleep, decreased appetite, lethargy, fatigue, and difficulty concentrating may be symptoms of depression. If accompanied by suicidal thoughts this depression is to be taken very seriously. Depression is often, by the patient or his environment, related to a recently experienced unhappy but trivial event, which is thought to account for the depressed mood, and this may lead to a delay in diagnosis. Naturally, in old age organic factors may be responsible for depressed mood, such as impairment of brain function, cardiovascular disease, metabolic factors (diabetes mellitus, renal dysfunction, hypercalcemia), use of medical drugs, and their side-effects on biologic systems. As a rating scale Beck's depression inventory[42] may be helpful. Internet tests are available.[43]

Sexual functioning in old age

It is common knowledge that sexual functioning declines with aging. The latter is now substantiated by several population surveys. The inter-individual differences in degree of sexual problems encountered varies strongly. So does the willingness to ask for help. In aging men it is primarily erectile function which shows a decline with aging. Normal sexual functioning including erectile capacity presupposes an integrity of the vascular, nervous, and hormonal/metabolic systems, as well as a mindset ready to engage in sexual activity. So in the work-up of aging men these factors must be considered. Some drugs interfere with the above factors. A widely used multidimensional self-administered scale, validated cross-culturally, assesses five domains of human sexuality: erectile function, orgasmic function, sexual desire, intercourse satisfaction, and overall satisfaction.[44]

Physical examination includes cardiovascular assessment, simple neurologic testing (bulbocavernosus reflex, anal sphincter tone, testicular and penile sensitivity, perineal sensation), and primary and secondary sexual characteristics (testicular volume, sexual hair, gynecomastia).

Hormonal deficiencies in old age

Growth hormone

It is difficult to establish growth hormone (GH) deficiency in adulthood or at an advanced age. The pulsatile nature of GH secretion and the large number of factors determining circulating levels of GH complicate the matter considerably in the sense that a single measurement of GH does not provide meaningful information. A single measurement of IGF-1 is a reasonable first indicator of one's GH status. In subjects under the age of 40 years a normal level of IGF-1 almost excludes GH deficiency. In subjects over the age of 40 years things are more complicated. However, an IGF-1 value of 15 nmol/l or higher excludes a deficiency of GH. So, the problem lies with patients with values below this level. It is amazing that some patients with proven GH deficiency (on the basis of extensive endocrine testing such as insulin-hypoglycemia, growth hormone releasing hormone (GHRH), and L-dopa stimulation tests) still have normal IGF-1 levels. IGF-binding protein-3 is another useful index of GH status. For the time being, the combination of signs and symptoms potentially attributable to GH deficiency, and an IGF-1 level and IGF-binding protein-3 level in the lowest third provide a first reasonable indication of (relative) GH deficiency. To confirm the diagnosis, a provocation test with GHRH in combination with arginine or synthetic growth hormone releasing substance (GHS) is highly desirable.[45]

Once a patient is placed on GH administration, individual dose titration must be done on the basis of the IGF-1 levels resulting from GH administration and the occurrence of side-effects. It is desirable to produce IGF-1 levels in the normal or only slightly above normal (0–1 standard deviation above the mean level of IGF-1) range. Secondly, if side-effects occur (flu-like symptoms, myalgia, arthralgia, carpal tunnel syndrome, edema, impairment of glucose homeostasis) GH dosage is reduced in steps of 25%. Contraindications for GH use are type 1 diabetes mellitus, active or a history of cancer, intracranial hypertension, diabetic retinopathy or carpal tunnel syndrome, or severe cardiac insufficiency.

Dehydroepiandrosterone

There is an impressive decline in the adrenal androgens with aging: plasma levels are at their peak in the twenties. They subsequently decline at 10% per decade. By age 60 years plasma levels may be down to 30–40% of young adult levels, and by age 80 years levels are prepubertally low again, for which the term 'adrenopause' has been coined. There is a considerable interindividual difference in plasma levels, up to 3-fold or more, persisting with increasing age. There is no consensus on what levels of dehydroepiandrosterone (DHEA) represent a deficiency. Levels of DHEA-sulfate found in patients with primary adrenal failure are in the order of 1.0–1.5 μmol/l. Reference values of DHEA-sulfate for adults are not established, but values reported in the literature for aging populations lie in the order of 2-8-7 mmol/l. Most studies that have established beneficial effects of DHEA (usually 50 mg/day) have not defined cut-off values for inclusion in the study. (For a review see reference 46.)

Testosterone

There is no consensus on normal decreased values of testosterone in old age. Therefore we are left with arbitrary criteria. On the basis of their large samples of healthy men, young, middle-aged, and old, Vermeulen and colleagues have proposed accepting the same range of normal testosterone values for elderly men as for younger men. The proposed cut-off point for low testosterone values is arbitrarily 11 nmol/l for total testosterone and 0.255 nmol/l for free testosterone, but these criteria should be set against local reference values of testosterone.[20,47] Until more data are collected this is for the moment a reasonable approach to the vexing question of who is testosterone-deficient in old age.

Another variable that might be significant to assess the androgen status in old age is plasma levels of SHBG. Its levels increase with aging, possibly due to a decrease in growth hormone production and an increase in the ratio of free estradiol over free testosterone.[47] The same authors demonstrated that the free testosterone value calculated by total testosterone/SHBG as determined by immunoassay appears to be a rapid, simple, and reliable indicator of bioavailable testosterone, comparable to testosterone values obtained by equilibrium dialysis. So, without much in the way of solid criteria for testosterone deficiency in old age, determination of testosterone values together with SHBG might provide a reasonable index of the androgen status of an aging person.

Hypothyroidism

Hypothyroidism may be overlooked in the elderly since the symptoms are often attributed to the aging process with its associated asthenia, effects of drug use, and loss of agility. The symptoms range from weakness, chronic fatigue, and decreased heart rate, to dry skin, hoarseness, and slower tendon reflexes. Intolerance to cold and weight gain may be less pronounced in the elderly. Hypothyroidism should be suspected if there are occurrences of unexplained high levels of cholesterol and creatinine phosphokinase, severe constipation, congestive heart failure with cardiomyopathy, and unexplained macrocytic anemia. The best diagnostic test for primary hypothyroidism is an increased serum TSH level, although TSH levels in the elderly who have hypothyroidism are lower than in younger patients with the same disease, so determination of T_4 is also required. (For review see reference 48.)

Hyperthyroidism

Hyperthyroidism in the elderly may have a different presentation than in younger hyperthyroid subjects. Symptoms of hyperthyroidism in the young are signs of a hyperadrenergic state: nervousness, sweating, diarrhea, tremor, tachycardia, and hyperactive reflexes. In elderly subjects, cardiac symptoms (atrial fibrillation, cardiac insufficiency), bone loss, or mental symptoms (confusion, anorexia) may be the manifestations of thyroid hyperfunction. Weight loss with anorexia is more prevalent than increased eating. Treatment with amiodarone or iodine-containing radiocontrast agents may also evoke hyperthyroidism in the elderly. The diagnosis is based essentially on elevated levels of T_4 and free T_3 and suppressed levels of TSH. (For review see reference 48.)

Dysfunction of the thyroid may severely impact on sexual functions.[49]

Summary

Screening of the aging male has definite benefits. Early diagnosis and early intervention may delay morbidity and increase the health span of aging subjects. Early detection of visual and hearing impairment will contribute to the quality of life. There are also a number of difficulties which may arise with screening. The interpretation of the findings requires an understanding of epidemiologic principles on the side of the physician. What is the prognostic value of a positive finding? In which cases should it lead to intervention? Is the intervention warranted and meaningful in that it slows the course of the disease?

The information of positive findings of screening may become a psychologic burden to the patient. It may induce a form of hypochondria and may evoke a quest for redundant medical tests and interventions. A wait-and-see policy usually does not appeal to the kind of patient who seeks screening. Alternatively, a negative outcome of the screening may produce a false sense of good health, or at least of an absence of pathology. The patient usually underrates the complexity of disease processes and overrates the comprehensiveness and predictive power of the screening. The patient or his family may react with hostility if, shortly after the screening, a serious ailment befalls the patient. He may interpret this occurrence as negligence on the side of the physician. This is particularly true if risk factors for the disease in question were screened for (for instance, a myocardial infarction in the absence of serious risk factors, a small prostate carcinoma without an elevation of PSA levels). So each patient, having undergone screening tests, must receive a thorough evaluation of the results and of the relativity of negative tests.

Another aspect is health economics. Who is financing the costs of screening? The patient himself, or his health insurance? In the latter case the policy does not necessarily cover screening (tests not motivated by a reasonable suspicion of pathology) and it may be a breach of the contract to charge these costs to the insurance.

References

1. Heinemann LA, Saad F, Zimmermann T et al. The Aging Males' Symptoms (AMS) scale: update and compilation of international versions. Health Qual Life Outcomes 2003; 1: 15.

2. Daig I, Heinemann LA, Kim S et al. The Aging Males' Symptoms (AMS) scale: review of its methodological characteristics. Health Qual Life Outcomes 2003; 1: 77.

3. Myon E, Martin N, Taieb C et al. Experiences with the French Aging Males' Symptoms (AMS) scale. Aging Male 2005; 8: 184.

4. Valenti G, Gontero P, Sacco M et al. Harmonized Italian version of the Aging Males' Symptoms scale. Aging Male 2005; 8: 180.

5. Morley JE, Charlton E, Patrick P et al. Validation of a screening questionnaire for androgen deficiency in aging males. Metabolism 2000; 49: 1239.

6. Barry MJ, Fowler FJ Jr, O'Leary MP et al. The American Urological Association symptom index for benign prostatic hyperplasia. The Measurement Committee of the American Urological Association. J Urol 1992; 148: 1549.

7. Abrams P. Benign prostatic hyperplasia. Poorly correlated with symptoms. BMJ 1993; 307: 201.

8. Thomas AW, Abrams P. Lower urinary tract symptoms, benign prostatic obstruction and the overactive bladder. BJU Int 2000; 85(Suppl 3): 57.

9. Griffiths CJ, Harding C, Blake C et al. A nomogram to classify men with lower urinary tract symptoms using urine flow and noninvasive measurement of bladder pressure. J Urol 2005; 174: 1323.

10. Barry MJ, Fowler FJ, Jr, O'Leary MP et al. Measuring disease-specific health status in men with benign prostatic hyperplasia. Measurement Committee of The American Urological Association. Med Care 1995; 33: AS145.

11. Welch G, Weinger K, Barry MJ. Quality-of-life impact of lower urinary tract symptom severity: results from the Health Professionals Follow-up Study. Urology 2002; 59: 245.

12. Roehrborn CG, Girman CJ, Rhodes T et al. Correlation between prostate size estimated by digital rectal examination and measured by transrectal ultrasound. Urology 1997; 49: 548.

13. Bosch JL, Bohnen AM, Groeneveld FP. Validity of digital rectal examination and serum prostate specific antigen in the estimation of prostate volume in community-based men aged 50 to 78 years: the Krimpen Study. Eur Urol 2004; 46: 753.

14. Crawford ED, Schutz MJ, Clejan S et al. The effect of digital rectal examination on prostate-specific antigen levels. JAMA 1992; 267: 2227.

15. Morales A. Testosterone treatment for the aging man: the controversy. Curr Urol Rep 2004; 5: 472.

16. Riffenburgh RH, Amling CL. Use of early PSA velocity to predict eventual abnormal PSA values in men at risk for prostate cancer. Prostate Cancer Prostatic Dis 2003; 6: 39.

17. Burack RC, Wood DP, Jr. Screening for prostate cancer. The challenge of promoting informed decision making in the absence of definitive evidence of effectiveness. Med Clin North Am 1999; 83: 1423.

18. Klotz L. Active surveillance for prostate cancer: for whom? J Clin Oncol 2005; 23: 8165.

19. Morales ALB. Androgen replacement therapy in aging men with secondary hypogonadism. Draft of Recommendations for Endorsement by ISSAM. Aging Male 2001; 4: 151.

20. Nieschlag E, Swerdloff R, Behre HM et al. Investigation, treatment and monitoring of late-onset hypogonadism in males. Aging Male 2005; 8: 56.

21. Zhu S, Heymsfield SB, Toyoshima H et al. Race-ethnicity-specific waist circumference cutoffs for identifying cardiovascular disease risk factors. Am J Clin Nutr 2005; 81: 409.

22. Wildman RP, Gu D, Reynolds K et al. Are waist circumference and body mass index independently associated with cardiovascular disease risk in Chinese adults? Am J Clin Nutr 2005; 82: 1195.

23. Misra A, Wasir JS, Vikram NK. Waist circumference criteria for the diagnosis of abdominal obesity are not applicable uniformly to all populations and ethnic groups. Nutrition 2005; 21: 969.

24. Frolkis JP. Screening for cardiovascular disease. Concepts, conflicts, and consensus. Med Clin North Am 1999; 83: 1339.

25. Wannamethee SG, Lowe GD, Shaper AG et al. The metabolic syndrome and insulin resistance: relationship to haemostatic and inflammatory markers in older non-diabetic men. Atherosclerosis 2005; 181: 101.

26. Nigam A, Bourassa MG, Fortier A et al. The metabolic syndrome and its components and the long-term risk of death in patients with coronary heart disease. Am Heart J 2006; 151: 514.

27. Twardella D, Rothenbacher D, Hahmann H et al. The underestimated impact of smoking and smoking cessation on the risk of secondary cardiovascular disease events in patients with stable coronary heart disease: prospective cohort study. J Am Coll Cardiol 2006; 47: 887.

28. Choi KL, Bakris GL. Hypertension treatment guidelines: practical implications. Semin Nephrol 2005; 25: 198.

29. Lip GY, Blann AD. Thrombogenesis, atherogenesis and angiogenesis in vascular disease: a new 'vascular triad'. Ann Med 2004; 36: 119.

30. Physical activity and cardiovascular health. NIH Consensus Development Panel on Physical Activity and Cardiovascular Health. JAMA 1996; 276: 241.

31. Bensimhon DR, Kraus WE, Donahue MP. Obesity and physical activity: a review. Am Heart J 2006; 151: 598.

32. www.nhlib.nih.gov/guidelines/cholesterol/atglance.htm.

33. Franchini M. Hereditary iron overload: update on pathophysiology, diagnosis, and treatment. Am J Hematol 2006; 81: 202.

34. Katz S, Ford AB, Moskowitz RW et al. Studies of illness in the aged. The index of Adl: a standardized measure of biological and psychosocial function. JAMA 1963; 185: 914.

35. Gill TM, Williams CS, Tinetti ME. Assessing risk for the onset of functional dependence among older adults: the role of physical performance. J Am Geriatr Soc 1995; 43: 603.

36. Carey EC, Walter LC, Lindquist K et al. Development and validation of a functional morbidity index to predict mortality in community-dwelling elders. J Gen Intern Med 2004; 19: 1027.

37. Reuben DB, Laliberte L, Hiris J et al. A hierarchical exercise scale to measure function at the Advanced Activities of Daily Living (AADL) level. J Am Geriatr Soc 1990; 38: 855.

38. Ostchega Y, Harris TB, Hirsch R et al. Reliability and prevalence of physical performance examination assessing mobility and balance in older persons in the US: data from the Third National Health and Nutrition Examination Survey. J Am Geriatr Soc 2000; 48: 1136.

39. Folstein MF, Folstein SE, McHugh PR. 'Mini-mental state'. A practical method for grading the cognitive state of patients for the clinician. J Psychiatr Res 1975; 12: 189.

40. Pfeiffer E. A short portable mental status questionnaire for the assessment of organic brain deficit in elderly patients. J Am Geriatr Soc 1975; 23: 433.

41. http://trans.nih.gov/CEHP/hbpcog-list.htm.

42. Beck AT, Ward CH, Mendelson M et al. An inventory for measuring depression. Arch Gen Psychiatry 1961; 4: 561.

43. http://www.med.nyu.edu/psych/screens/depres.html.

44. Rosen RC, Riley A, Wagner G et al. The international index of erectile function (IIEF): a multidimensional scale for assessment of erectile dysfunction. Urology 1997; 49: 822.

45. Giordano R, Aimaretti G, Lanfranco F et al. Testing pituitary function in aging individuals. Endocrinol Metab Clin North Am 2005; 34: 895.

46. Cameron DR, Braunstein GD. The use of dehydroepiandrosterone therapy in clinical practice. Treat Endocrinol 2005; 4: 95.

47. Kaufman JM, Vermeulen A. The decline of androgen levels in elderly men and its clinical and therapeutic implications. Endocr Rev 2005; 26: 833.

48. Stan M, Morris JC. Thyrotropin-axis adaptation in aging and chronic disease. Endocrinol Metab Clin North Am 2005; 34: 973.

49. Carani C, Isidori AM, Granata A et al. Multicenter study on the prevalence of sexual symptoms in male hypo- and hyperthyroid patients. J Clin Endocrinol Metab 2005; 90: 6472.

Appendix 6.1

Office procedures

Personal data
Name
Date of birth
Occupation
Marital status
Employment status

Habits affecting health
Smoking
Alcohol consumption
Non-medical drug use
Balanced diet
Self-medication (painkillers/sleeping pills)
Sleep patterns
Mobility and exercise/recreation
Depressive feelings
Stress levels and coping mechanisms/relaxation

Medical history
Past medical conditions
Present medical conditions and their follow-up
Prescription drugs/continued use warranted?

Family history
Cardiovascular disease (hypertension/stroke/myocardial infarction/lipid disorders)
Parents alive? Age at death? Cause of death?
Diabetes mellitus
Prostate cancer
Other cancers

Accidents
Accident prone
Drunken driving
Risk taking

Psychosexual situation
Depressions?
Married?
In a relationship?
Sex life satisfactory?

Any specific concerns of the patient himself?

Specific history with regard to diseases of the aging male

Prostate disease
Frequency of micturition? Increased?
Nycturia
Dysuria/dribbling

Osteoporosis
Previous fractures
Family history
Rheumatic disease
Calcium intake
Thyroid disease
Intestinal disease
Corticosteroid use
Alcohol consumption
Risk factors warranting bone density measurement?

Cardiovascular disease
History of a cardiac event
Diagnosis/follow-up/medication
Hypertension/medication
Lipid profiles ever assessed
Smoking
Exercise tolerance/dyspnea
Cardiac arrhythmia
Angina pectoris
Nycturia/edema
Signs of peripheral arterial disease

Impaired vision and hearing

Erectile function
Morning erections
Libido
Erectile problems (always/when tired/after alcohol consumption)

Physical examination
Routine
Special attention to the following:
- Height/weight and calculation of body mass index (BMI)
- BMI 25–30 = obesity/30–35 obesity requiring intervention/> 35 grossly obese
- Waist circumference: if > 102 cm obesity
- Sagittal diameter of the abdomen: if > 24 cm: visceral obesity

Assessment of muscle strength: ask the patient to get up 5 times from his chair without using hands
Blood pressure
Rectal examination

Laboratory work-up
Hemoglobin/ESR
Creatinine
Fasting glucose/total cholesterol/triglycerides/high-density lipoprotein
PSA
Urine: glucose/protein
Testosterone

Simple office procedures
Peak expiratory flow rate
Hand-held dynamometer

More advanced procedures
Electrocardiogram/stress electrocardiogram
Prostate ultrasound
Bone densitometry

Appendix 6.2

Individual items of International Index of Erectile Function Questionnaire and response options (US version)[44]

Question	Response options
How often were you able to get an erection during sexual activity? When you had erections with sexual stimulation, how often were your erections hard enough for penetration?	0 = No sexual activity 1 = Almost never/never 2 = A few times (much less than half the time) 3 = Sometimes (about half the time) 4 = Most times (much more than half the time) 5 = Almost always/always
When you attempted sexual intercourse, how often were you able to penetrate (enter) your partner? During sexual intercourse, how often were you able to maintain your erection after you had penetrated (entered) your partner?	0 = Did not attempt intercourse 1 = Almost never/never 2 = A few times (much less than half the time) 3 = Sometimes (about half the time) 4 = Most times (much more than half the time) 5 = Almost always/always
During sexual intercourse, how difficult was it to maintain your erection to completion of intercourse?	0 = Did not attempt intercourse 1 = Extremely difficult 2 = Very difficult 3 = Difficult 4 = Slightly difficult 5 = Not difficult
How many times have you attempted sexual intercourse?	0 = No attempts 1 = One to two attempts 2 = Three to four attempts 3 = Five to six attempts 4 = Seven to ten attempts 5 = Eleven + attempts
When you attempted sexual intercourse, how often was it satisfactory for you?	0 = Did not attempt intercourse 1 = Almost never/never 2 = A few times (much less than half the time) 3 = Sometimes (about half the time) 4 = Most times (much more than half the time) 5 = Almost always/always

Question	Response options
How much have you enjoyed sexual intercourse?	0 = No intercourse 1 = No enjoyment 2 = Not very enjoyable 3 = Fairly enjoyable 4 = Highly enjoyable 5 = Very highly enjoyable
When you had sexual stimulation or intercourse, how often did you ejaculate? When you had sexual stimulation or intercourse, how often did you have the feeling of orgasm or climax?	0 = No sexual stimulation/intercourse 1 = Almost never/never 2 = A few times (much less than half the time) 3 = Sometimes (about half the time) 4 = Most times (much more than half the time) 5 = Almost always/always
How often have you felt sexual desire?	1 = Almost never/never 2 = A few times (much less than half the time) 3 = Sometimes (about half the time) 4 = Most times (much more than half the time) 5 = Almost always/always
How would you rate your level of sexual desire?	1 = Very low/none at all 2 = Low 3 = Moderate 4 = High 5 = Very high
How satisfied have you been with your overall sex life? How satisfied have you been with your sexual relationship with your partner?	1 = Very dissatisfied 2 = Moderately dissatisfied 3 = About equally satisfied and dissatisfied 4 = Moderately satisfied 5 = Very satisfied
How do you rate your confidence that you could get and keep an erection?	1 = Very low 2 = Low 3 = Moderate 4 = High 5 = Very high

Katz et al 1963

Appendix 6.3

Index of Independence in Activities of Daily Living

The Index of Independence in Activities of Daily Living is based on an evaluation of the functional independence or dependence of patients in bathing, dressing, going to toilet, transferring, continence, and feeding. Specific definitions of functional independence and dependence appear below the index.

A. Independent in feeding, continence, transferring, going to toilet, dressing, and bathing
B. Independent in all but one of these functions
C. Independent in all but bathing and one additional function
D. Independent in all but bathing, dressing, and one additional function
E. Independent in all but bathing, dressing, going to toilet, and one additional function
F. Independent in all but bathing, dressing, going to toilet, transferring, and one additional function
G. Dependent in all six functions

Other: Dependent in at least two functions, but not classifiable as C, D, E, or F

Independence means without supervision, direction, or active personal assistance, except as specifically noted below. This is based on actual status and not on ability. A patient who refuses to perform a function is considered as not performing the function, even though he is deemed able.

Bathing (sponge, shower, or tub)
Independent:
Assistance only in bathing a single part (as back or disabled extremity) or bathes self completely
Dependent:
Assistance in bathing more than one part of body; assistance in getting in or out of tub or does not bathe self

Dressing
Independent:
Gets clothes from closets and drawers; puts on clothes, outer garments, braces; manages fasteners; act of tying shoes is excluded
Dependent:
Does not dress self or remains partly undressed

Going to toilet
Independent:
Gets to toilet; gets on and off toilet; arranges clothes; cleans organs of excretion (may manage own bedpan used at night only and may or may not be using mechanical supports)
Dependent:
Uses bedpan or commode or receives assistance in getting to and using toilet

Transfer
Independent:
Moves in and out of bed independently and moves in and out of chair independently (may or may not be using mechanical supports)
Dependent:
Assistance in moving in or out of bed and/or chair; does not perform one or more transfers

Continence
Independent:
Urination and defecation entirely self-controlled
Dependent:
Partial or total incontinence in urination or defecation: partial or total control by enemas, catheters, or regulated use of urinals and/or bedpans

Feeding
Independent:
Gets food from plate or its equivalent into mouth (precutting of meat and preparation of food, as buttering bread, are excluded from evaluation)
Dependent:
Assistance in act of feeding (see above); does not eat at all or parenteral feeding

Evaluation form

Name .... Date of evaluation ....
For each area of functioning listed below, check description that applies. (The word 'assistance' means supervision, direction of personal assistance)

Bathing
Either sponge bath, tub bath, or shower

❐ Receives no assistance (gets in and out of tub by self if tub is usual means of bathing)
❐ Receives assistance in bathing only one part of the body (such as back or a leg)
❐ Receives assistance in bathing more than one part of the body (or not bathed)

Dressing
Gets clothes from closets and drawers, including underclothes, outer garments, and using fasteners (including braces if worn)

❐ Gets clothes and gets completely dressed without assistance
❐ Gets clothes and gets dressed without assistance except for assistance in tying shoes
❐ Receives assistance in getting clothes or in getting dressed, or stays partly or completely undressed

Toileting
Going to the 'toilet room' for bowel and urine elimination; cleaning self after elimination, and arranging clothes

❐ Goes to 'toilet room', cleans self, and arranges clothes without assistance (may use object for support such as cane, walker, or wheel chair and may manage night bedpan or commode, emptying same in morning)
❐ Receives assistance in going to 'toilet room' or in cleansing self or in arranging clothes after elimination or in use of night bedpan or commode
❐ Doesn't go to room termed 'toilet' for the elimination process

Transfer

- ☐ Moves in and out of bed as well as in and out of chair without assistance (may be using object for support such as cane or walker)
- ☐ Moves in or out of bed or chair with assistance
- ☐ Doesn't get out of bed

Continence

- ☐ Controls urination and bowel movement completely by self
- ☐ Has occasional 'accidents'
- ☐ Supervision helps keep urine or bowel control; catheter is used, or is incontinent

Feeding

- ☐ Feeds self without assistance
- ☐ Feeds self except for getting assistance in cutting meat or buttering bread
- ☐ Receives assistance in feeding or is fed partly or completely by using tubes or intravenous fluids

Reuben et al 1990

Self-assessed current advanced social activities health status, and mental health score at entry, by group

Social activities

Entertain at home:

1. At least weekly
2. At least monthly
3. At least yearly
4. Less than yearly or never

Visit others at their homes:

1. At least weekly
2. At least monthly
3. At least yearly
4. Less than yearly or never

Go out to eat:

1. At least weekly
2. At least monthly
3. At least yearly
4. Less than yearly or never

Work at a hobby:

1. At least weekly
2. At least monthly
3. At least yearly
4. Less than yearly or never

Travel out of town:

1. At least weekly
2. At least monthly
3. At least yearly
4. Less than yearly or never

Do you take longer trips?

1. Without help
2. With some help
3. Do not take longer trips

Health status

1. Excellent
2. Good
3. Fair
4. Poor

Pfeiffer (1975)

Appendix 6.4

Short portable mental status questionnaire (SPMSQ)

Instructions: Ask questions 1–10 in this list and record all answers. Ask question 4A only if patient does not have a telephone. Record total number of errors based on 10 questions.

+	–

1. What is the date today? _____
   Month   Day   Year

2. What day of the week is it? _____

3. What is the name of this place? _____

4. What is your telephone number? _____

4A. What is your street address? _____

5. How old are you? _____

6. When were you born? _____

7. Who is the President of the US now? _____

8. Who was President just before him? _____

9. What was your mother's maiden name? _____

10. Subtract 3 from 20 and keep subtracting 3 from each new
    number, all the way down

_____ Total number of errors

To be completed by interviewer

Patient's Name:_____Date_____

        Sex: 1. Male   Race: 1. White

               2. Female   2. Black

        Other:

Years of education: _____   1. Grade School

        High School

        Beyond High School

Interviewer's name: _____

Folstein et al 1975

Appendix 6.5

Patient ....

Examiner ....

Date ....

'MINI-MENTAL STATE'

Maximum score
Score

Orientation
5 ( )   What is the (year) (season) (date) (day) (month)?
5 ( )   Where are we: (state) (county) (town) (hospital) (floor)

Registration
3 ( )   Name 3 objects:1 second to say each. Then ask the patient all 3 after you have said them.
        Give 1 point for each correct answer. Then repeat them until he learns all 3.
        Count trials and record.
Trials

Attention and calculation
5 ( )   Serial 7s. 1 point for each correct. Stop after 5 answers. Alternatively spell 'world' backwards.

Recall
3 ( )   Ask for the 3 objects repeated above. Give 1 point for each correct.

Language
9 ( )   Name a pencil, and watch (2 points)
        Repeat the following 'No ifs, ands or buts' (1 point)
        Follow a 3-stage command:
        'Take a paper in your right hand, fold it in half, and put it on the floor'
        (3 points)
        Read and obey the following:
        Close your eyes (1 point)
        Write a sentence (1 point)

_____Copy design (1 point)
            Total score
            ASSESS level of consciousness
            along a continuum

_____
            Alert Drowsy Stupor Coma

Instructions for administration of mini-mental state examination

Orientation
1. Ask for the date. Then ask specifically for parts omitted, e.g., 'Can you also tell me what season it is?' One point for each correct.
2. Ask in turn: 'Can you tell me the name of this hospital? (town, county, etc.).' One point for each correct.

Registration
Ask the patient if you may test his memory. Then say the names of 3 unrelated objects, clearly and slowly, about one second for each. After you have said all 3, ask him to repeat them. This first repetition determines his score (0–3), but keep saying them until he can repeat all 3, up to 6 trials. If he does not eventually learn all 3, recall cannot be meaningfully tested.

Attention and calculation
Ask the patient to begin with 100 and count backwards by 7. Stop after 5 subtractions (93, 86, 79, 72, 65). Score the total number of correct answers. If the patient cannot or will not perform this task, ask him to spell the word 'world' backwards. The score is the number of letters in correct order. E.g. dlrow = 5, dlorw = 3.

Recall
Ask the patient if he can recall the 3 words you previously asked him to remember. Score 0–3.

Language
Naming: Show the patient a wrist watch and ask him what it is. Repeat for pencil. Score 0–2. Repetition: Ask the patient to repeat the sentence after you. Allow only one trial. Score 0 or 1. Three-stage command: Give the patient a piece of plain blank paper and repeat the command. Score 1 point for each part correctly executed.

Beck et al 1961

Appendix 6.6

Depression Inventory

A. (Mood)

0   I do not feel sad.
1   I feel blue or sad.
2a I am blue or sad all the time and I can't snap out of it.
2b I am so sad or unhappy that it is very painful.
3   I am so sad or unhappy that I can't stand it.

B. (Pessimism)

0   I am not particularly pessimistic or discouraged about the future.
1a I feel discouraged about the future.
2a I feel I have nothing to look forward to.
2b I feel that I won't ever get over my troubles.
3   I feel that the future is hopeless and that things cannot improve.

C. (Sense of failure)

0   I don't feel like a failure.
1   I feel I have failed more than the average person.
2a I feel I have accomplished very little that is worthwile or that means anything.
2b As I look back on my life all I can see is a lot of failures.
3   I feel I am a complete failure as a person (parent, husband, wife).

D. (Lack of satisfaction)

0   I am not particularly dissatisfied.
1a I feel bored most of the time.
1b I don't enjoy things the way I used to.
2   I don't get satisfaction out of anything anymore.
3   I am dissatisfied with everything.

E. (Guilty feeling)

0   I don't feel particularly guilty.
1   I feel bad or unworthy a good part of the time.
2a I feel bad or unworthy practically all the time now.
3   I feel as though I am very bad or worthless.

F. (Sense of punishment)

0   I don't feel I am being punished.
1   I have a feeling that something bad may happen to me.
2   I feel I am being punished or will be punished.
3a I feel I deserve to be punished.
3b I want to be punished.

G. (Self hate)

0   I don't feel disappointed in myself.
1a I am disappointed in myself.
1b I don't like myself.
2   I am disgusted with myself.
3   I hate myself.

H. (Self accusations)

0   I don't feel I am any worse than anybody else.
1   I am very critical of myself for my weaknesses or mistakes.
2a I blame myself for everything that goes wrong.
2b I feel I have many bad faults.

I. (Self-punitive wishes)

0   I don't have any thoughts of harming myself.
1   I have thoughts of harming myself but I would not carry them out.
2a I feel I would be better off dead.
2b I have definite plans about committing suicide.
2c I feel my family would be better off if I were dead.
3   I would kill myself if I could.

J. (Crying spells)

0   I don't cry any more than usual.
1   I cry more now than I used to.
2   I cry all the time now. I can't stop it.
3   I used to be able to cry but now I can't cry at all even though I want to.

K. (Irritability)

0   I am no more irritated now than I ever am.
1   I get annoyed or irritated more easily than I used to.
2   I feel irritated all the time.
3   I don't get irritated at all at the things that used to irritate me.

L. (Social withdrawal)

0   I have not lost interest in other people.
1   I am less interested in other people now than I used to be.
2   I have lost most of my interest in other people and have little feeling for them.
3   I have lost all my interest in other people and don't care about them at all.

M. (Indecisiveness)

0   I make decisions about as well as ever.
1   I am less sure of myself now and try to put off making decisions.
2   I can't make decisions any more without help.
3   I can't make any decisions at all any more.

N. (Body image)

0   I don't feel I look any worse than I used to.
1   I am worried that I am looking old or unattractive.
2   I feel that there are permanent changes in my appearance and they make me look unattractive.
3   I feel that I am ugly or repulsive looking.

O. (Work inhibition)

0   I can work about as well as before.
1a   It takes extra effort to get started at doing something.
1b   I don't work as well as I used to.
2   I have to push myself very hard to do anything.
3   I can't do any work at all.

P. (Sleep disturbance)

0   I can sleep as well as usual.
1   I wake up more tired in the morning than I used to.
2   I wake up 1–2 hours earlier than usual and find it hard to get back to sleep.
3   I wake up early every day and can't get more than 5 hours' sleep.

Q. (Fatigability)

0   I don't get any more tired than usual.
1   I get tired more easily than I used to.
2   I get tired from doing anything.
3   I get too tired to do anything.

R. (Loss of appetite)

0   My appetite is no worse than usual.
1   My appetite is not as good as it used to be.
2   My appetite is much worse now.
3   I have no appetite at all any more.

S. (Weight loss)

0   I haven't lost much weight, if any, lately.
1   I have lost more than 5 pounds.
2   I have lost more than 10 pounds.
3   I have lost more than 15 pounds.

T. (Somatic preoccupation)

0   I am no more concerned about my health than usual.
1   I am concerned about aches and pains *or* upset stomach *or* constipation *or* other unpleasant feelings in my body.
2   I am so concerned with how I feel or what I feel that it's hard to think of much else.
3   I am completely absorbed in what I feel.

U. (Loss of libido)

0   I have not noticed any recent change in my interest in sex.
1   I am less interested in sex than I used to be.
2   I am much less interested in sex now.
3   I have lost interest in sex completely.

Lawton & Brody 1969

Physical self-maintenance scale

A. *Toilet*

1. Cares for self at toilet completely, no incontinence.
2. Needs to be reminded, or needs help in cleaning self, or has rare (weekly at most) accidents.
3. Soiling or wetting while asleep more than once a week.
4. Soiling or wetting while awake more than once a week.
5. No control of bowels or bladder.

B. *Feeding*

1. Eats without assistance.
2. Eats with minor assistance at meal times and/or with special preparation of food, or help in cleaning up after meals.
3. Feeds self with moderate assistance and is untidy.
4. Requires extensive assistance for all meals.
5. Does not feed self at all and resists efforts of others to feed him.

C. *Dressing*

1. Dresses, undresses, and selects clothes from own wardrobe.
2. Dresses and undresses self, with minor assistance.
3. Needs moderate assistance in dressing or selection of clothes.
4. Needs major assistance in dressing, but cooperates with efforts of others to help.
5. Completely unable to dress self and resists efforts of others to help.

D. *Grooming* (neatness, hair, nails, hands, face, clothing)

1. Always neatly dressed, well groomed, without assistance.
2. Grooms self adequately with occasional minor assistance, e.g. shaving.
3. Needs moderate and regular assistance or supervision in grooming.
4. Needs total grooming care, but can remain well groomed after help from others.
5. Actively negates all efforts of others to maintain grooming.

E. *Physical ambulation*

1. Goes about grounds or city.
2. Ambulates within residence or about one block distant.

3. Ambulates with assistance of (check one) a ( ) another person, b ( ) railing, c ( ) cane, d ( ) walker, e ( ) wheel chair.
    1. ( ) Gets in and out without help.
    2. ( ) Needs help in getting in and out.
4. Sits unsupported in chair or wheelchair, but cannot propel self without help.
5. Bedridden more than half the time.

F. *Bathing*

1. Bathes self (tub, shower, sponge bath) without help.
2. Bathes self with help in getting in and out of tub.
3. Washes face and hands only, but cannot bathe rest of body.
4. Does not wash self but is cooperative with those who bathe him.
5. Does not try to wash self and resists efforts to keep him clean.

Instrumental activities of daily living scale

A. *Ability to use telephone*

1. Operates telephone on own initiative. Looks up and dials numbers, etc.
2. Dials a few well-known numbers.
3. Answers telephone but does not dial.
4. Does not use telephone at all.

B. *Shopping*

1. Takes care of all shopping needs independently.
2. Shops independently for small purchases.
3. Needs to be accompanied on any shopping trip.
4. Completely unable to shop.

C. *Food preparation*

1. Plans, prepares, and serves adequate meals independently.
2. Prepares adequate meals if supplied with ingredients.
3. Heats and serves prepared meals, or prepares meals but does not maintain adequate diet.
4. Needs to have meals prepared and served.

D. *Housekeeping*

1. Maintains house alone or with occasional assistance (e.g. 'heavy work – domestic help').
2. Performs light daily tasks such as dish washing, bedmaking.
3. Performs light daily tasks but cannot maintain acceptable level of cleanliness.
4. Needs help with all home maintenance tasks.
5. Does not participate in any housekeeping tasks.

E. *Laundry*

1. Does personal laundry completely.
2. Launders small items: rinses socks, stockings, etc.
3. All laundry must be done by others.

F. *Mode of transportation*

1. Travels independently on public transportation or drives own car.
2. Arranges own travel via taxi, but does not otherwise use public transportation.
3. Travels on public transportation when assisted or accompanied by another.
4. Travel limited to taxi or automobile with assistance of another.
5. Does not travel at all.

G. *Responsibility for own medications*

1. Is responsible for taking medication in correct dosages at correct time.
2. Takes responsibility if medication is prepared in advance in separate dosages.
3. Is not capable of dispensing own medication.

H. *Ability to handle finances*

1. Manages financial matters independently (budgets, writes checks, pays rent, bills, goes to bank), collects and keeps track of income.
2. Manages day-to-day purchases, but needs help with banking, major purchases, etc.
3. Incapable of handling money.

CHAPTER 7

Laboratory tests in the endocrine evaluation of aging males

Michael John Wheeler

Introduction

In the routine investigation of a male presenting with low libido, perhaps with tiredness, obesity, and erectile dysfunction, a wide range of hormones may be investigated, depending on the clinical presentation and history of the patient. These may include the investigation of pituitary, testicular, thyroid, and adrenal function depending on patient presentation and clinical history.

Much information presented in this chapter, relating to method comparisons and method performance, is drawn from recent data from the UK National External Quality Assessment Schemes (NEQAS). These schemes are well known internationally and include many laboratories from outside the UK. Detailed discussion of assays will be limited to those that have a clear role in the initial investigations of erectile dysfunction and low libido in the male.

Thyroid function

Any patient presenting with symptoms associated with lack of drive and lethargy should be investigated for hypothyroidism. Hypothyroidism is common, particularly in the elderly. Population studies report an incidence of about 3–5% in men overall, rising to about 16% in those over 65 years.[1]

TSH

TSH is the most sensitive test for hypothyroidism. There is some dispute about the upper limit of the reference range. Population studies carried out by laboratories usually give an upper limit for the reference range of about 5.5 mIU/l. However, within such a population mildly hypothyroid subjects might be hidden. The American Thyroid Association (www.thyroid.org) suggests that a TSH >2.5 mIU/l indicates a patient at risk of hypothyroidism, a TSH between 4.0 and 10.0 mIU/l indicates subclinical hypothyroidism, and a TSH above 10.0 mIU/l indicates overt hypothyroidism. This may be too simplistic an approach and the TSH result should be considered along with free thyroxine (FT_4) and thyroid antibody results. Clinicians should consider these factors when interpreting TSH results and ensure conformity with their colleagues.

TSH is measured by immunometric assay and the greatest improvements in assay sensitivity and quality have been achieved with TSH assays. Sensitivity of commercial assays is now at least 0.01 mIU/l, i.e. below the lower limit of the reference range. In a UK NEQAS recovery experiment in 2005, using the International Standard 80/558, all but one of the automated third generation assays gave a recovery between 96% and 108%. Imprecision between methods was between 10% and 12% and between-laboratory imprecision was as low as 5% for some methods.

Free thyroxine

While many laboratories measure TSH and FT_4 as the routine thyroid screen, other laboratories measure only TSH. TSH is a sensitive indicator of primary hypothyroidism but the TSH concentration is often normal in cases of secondary hypothyroidism. Secondary hypothyroidism is rare and an incidence of 9 new adult cases per million population per year has been reported.[2] However, Wardle et al[3] reported an incidence of 55 cases per million population per year of which 32 per million per year might be undiagnosed if TSH is the only test performed in a thyroid screen. Clinicians should bear this in mind when investigating hypothyroidism. In those laboratories where TSH alone is the first line screening test, men with a normal TSH and with a low or inappropriately low LH and FSH should have a repeat TSH with an FT_4 measurement requested.

FT4 is measured on automated immunoassay analyzers by competitive analog methods in most laboratories. Significant differences exist between these FT_4 methods, since no reference method has been developed. These differences can be between 4 and 5 pmol/l in the reference range. It is therefore not possible to compare results from one method with another. A change of method by a laboratory is likely to lead to significant changes in reference ranges and clinicians should be aware of this when interpreting a patient's FT_4 concentrations over an extended period.

Androgens and sex-hormone binding globulin

Total testosterone

Early methods for measuring testosterone involved column chromatography,[4] solvent extraction, and radioimmunoassay.[5] These methods were very specific and, when adjusted for losses, were very accurate. However, they were not suited to the routine analysis of large numbers of samples and later methods excluded the chromatography. These latter methods removed conjugates and displaced steroids from the binding proteins but were less specific. 5α-Dihydrotestosterone (DHT) was the main cross-reactant and could contribute up to 1.5 nmol/l to the testosterone result in some assays. As antisera became more specific, the contribution from DHT was only 0.3 to 0.5 nmol/l and was insignificant at normal male concentrations; female reference ranges usually reflected this contribution. The use of highly flammable solvents and radioactive tracers made these assays unsuitable for automation and they were eventually replaced with direct (non-extraction) assays using non-radioactive labels. These are now used in most routine clinical laboratories. These assays have introduced a number of problems to the measurement of testosterone and some laboratories have continued to use an extraction assay, particularly for the measurement of testosterone in female samples. More recently, methods using tandem mass spectrometry have been developed.[6] These methods are simple, fast, and, potentially, highly accurate. However until more methods have been developed and validated against the reference method, isotope dilution gas chromatography mass spectrometry (IDMS), it is too early to say how specific and comparable these methods are or whether more experience will reveal significant methodologic problems.

There are currently about eight direct testosterone assays on fully automated immunoassay platforms. An evaluation of eight testosterone assays[7] showed that five of them had been calibrated against the reference method IDMS.[8] However, there was a 3 nmol/l difference between the median of these methods for a serum pool with results from 9 to 16 nmol/l (Figure 7.1). At lower levels of testosterone, differences between methods were proportionally even greater. There is no information available on the calibration procedure with IDMS and so it is unclear why these differences exist. One problem may be that companies calibrate their calibrators against IDMS but do not use precalibrated serum samples. Calibrators are only serum-like and can behave immunologically significantly differently from serum. More recently others[9,10] have also reported on the large differences between methods as well as the poor agreement with mass spectrometric methods.

A reference range specific for each method is, therefore, essential. There are important issues that need to be considered in setting up a reference

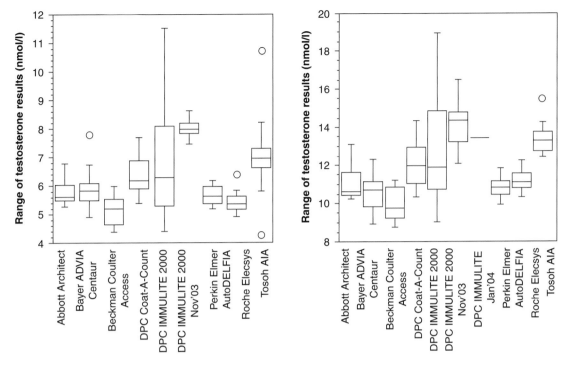

Figure 7.1 *Comparison of results for two serum pools analyzed by commercial automated testosterone methods (from Lamph et al 2004[7]).*

range.[11] Commercial companies provide reference ranges for their methods but these are only guides and should not be used as the laboratory reference range. Unfortunately, due to lack of time and sufficient relevant samples, some laboratories do adopt the manufacturer's quoted range. A large number of normal subjects are required to derive a statistically sound reference range (at least 100 subjects). In addition, testosterone levels, as well as the other hormones like LH and FSH, have a skewed distribution. Data should, therefore, be log transformed to achieve a more accurate reference range. Figure 7.2 is derived from the paper of Sikaris et al[11] and shows that a company's quoted reference range is usually quite different from that derived from a normal population, in this case of over 124 subjects. Also the transformed data gave a reference range that had a lower limit 2 nmol/l higher than the lower limit of the arithmetically derived reference range. This was true for all the methods investigated. The

findings reported here for testosterone relate to most hormone reference ranges.

Testosterone concentrations also show a marked circadian rhythm both in young and elderly men.[12,13] Samples collected throughout the day will give a much wider reference range than one derived from morning samples only. Where a reference range has been established using morning samples, testosterone concentrations can be below the reference range at 4 pm in both young and elderly healthy males (Figure 7.3). Hence blood samples should be drawn ideally in the early morning between 9 and 10 am. A repeat sample collected in the early morning should always be requested when a result below the reference range is reported for a sample collected in the afternoon.

It is now well established that testosterone levels fall from the fourth decade of life.[14–16] Although there is no consensus on whether age-related ranges should be used to assess testicular function there is

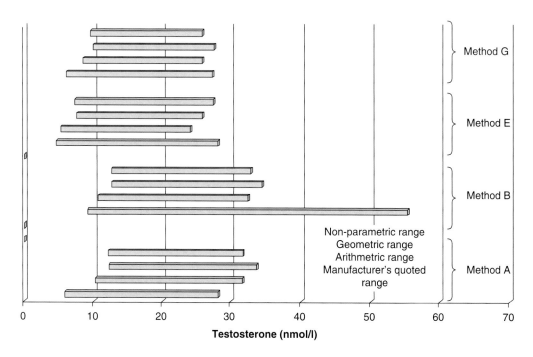

Figure 7.2 *The reference ranges (a) quoted by the manufacturer, (b) by arithmetic calculation, (c) by geometric calculation, and (d) by non-parametric calculation, for four different commercial kits (from Sikaris et al[11]).*

a trend to use younger males (20–40 years) as the reference population.[17]

Figure 7.3 shows data for 10 healthy young men and 10 healthy older men. The laboratory's reference range for men aged 20–50 years was 10.0 to 35 nmol/l and for older men 9.0 to 30 nmol/l. These ranges were derived arithmetically. Using these reference ranges all but one older male had normal testosterone concentrations at 9 am. At 4 pm there were 3 subjects in each group that were below their appropriate reference ranges. Taking the observation from the paper of Sikaris et al[11] that log transformed data increase the reference range by about 2 nmol/l, and using the data for the younger men, the figure shows that four older men are now below the reference range at 9 am and 7 younger men and 8 older men are below the reference range at 4 pm. This exercise shows the importance of constructing a well-defined reference range using log transformed data. Until there is more research and a consensus

on whether to use age-related reference ranges or not, the author suggests age-related reference ranges may avoid unnecessary treatment of the older male. However, some clinicians may suggest that some of these older patients had subclinical primary hypothyroidism due to low testosterone at 9 am (using the log transformed younger male range) but no apparent symptoms of androgen deficiency.

The subjects used for constructing the reference range should also reflect the local population since ethnic variation has also been reported. Heald et al[18] found that total and free testosterone concentrations were lower in Parkistani men than in white European and Afro-Caribbean men. Lookingbill et al[19] found no significant difference between Caucasian and Chinese males and Wang et al[20] found no significant difference between young white men and young Asian men for either the metabolic clearance rate or the production rate of testosterone, although the number of subjects was

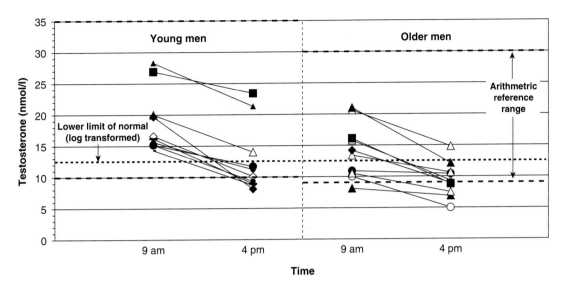

Figure 7.3 *Testosterone concentrations for 10 young men (20–35 years) and 10 older men (>50 years) at 9 am and 4 pm. The laboratory's arithmetic reference ranges for the two age groups are shown along with the assumed lower limit of normal after log transformation (extrapolated from Sikaris et al[11]).*

low. Santer et al,[21] however, found a lower production rate of testosterone in Chinese subjects living in China. Care should be taken when interpreting results in Asian males.

Therefore, blood sampling should be consistent with the data collected for the reference range. That is it should be carried out preferably between 9 and 10 am. This is not always practical as clinics may be held in the late afternoon. Samples collected outside of these times should be regarded as screening samples. It may be helpful to the clinician should consider a testosterone concentration above which they consider the result to be normal e.g. above −1 SD of the mean. Patients with results below this can then have a further blood sample taken between 9 and 10 am. Since testosterone secretion is episodic a low result may also be due to collecting a trough sample and a second sample may show normal testosterone concentration. It has been reported that men have a significant day-to-day variation that can be as much as 49%.[12,22] Therefore, diagnosis of hypogonadism should never be based on a single testosterone result.

The sample type, which is acceptable for different methods, varies. Some methods recommend only serum and state that plasma may give lower results.

Other methods state that both serum and plasma, even EDTA plasma, is acceptable. Serum would appear to be the safest blood sample to use as it is suitable for all methods. The evaluation report from the UK indicated that methods can be very sensitive to sample matrix. Clinicians should always use the sample type required by the laboratory.

Extended exercise, both acute and chronic, sleep, and sexual intercourse have all been reported to alter testosterone concentrations. These factors are unlikely to be a major issue for most men attending the male clinic since effects are of relatively short duration. The exception may be the body builder taking anabolic steroids, although LH and testosterone results should indicate steroid abuse.

Some problems with testosterone measurement are out of the hands of the clinician and depend on the laboratory's vigilance. These include the reported effect of surfactant present in SST or 'gel' tubes[23] and prolonged storage. However, the clinician should be aware that testosterone increases in unseparated blood[24] although this only affects low testosterone concentrations. This is due to conversion of androstenedione to testosterone by red cell enzymes and is most significant when the testosterone is low.

For male samples it should be a minor problem but, if blood cannot be sent to the lab within a couple of hours, it should be stored at 4°C until it is transferred to the laboratory. Blood can be kept for up to 6 hours at room temperature without any significant change in the testosterone level.

Free testosterone

Equilibrium dialysis is usually considered to be the 'reference' method for free testosterone (FT) measurement.[25] The method is not without criticism with purity of tracer, disturbance of the equilibrium between bound and free hormone, and the dilution effects being cited. Other methods on a par with equilibrium dialysis are ultracentrifugation and steady-state gel filtration. The latter method has been used in the author's laboratory for a number of studies and does not have the problems of dilution or disturbance of the equilibrium, but for all these methods purity of the label is paramount.[26] These methods are lengthy and complex and unsuited to the routine laboratory. There have been a number of different approaches to try to provide a more convenient indicator of FT. These involve some form of calculation of the FT concentration. Calculated measurement of FT ranges from a simple ratio of T/SHBG[26] to quite complex formulae.[27] Several formulae exist although probably the most common one now used is that of Vermeulen.[25]

An alternative approach is to measure non-sex-hormone-binding globulin (SHBG) bound testosterone.[28,29] This is a relatively simple procedure but, since there is no automated method available, few routine laboratories offer the assay. This measurement arose from the suggestion that as the binding affinity of testosterone to albumin was low some of this testosterone might be available to tissues. It is debatable whether this is true given the fast transit time of blood through most tissues.

There are currently two commercial kits purported to measure free testosterone. These methods have been heavily criticised as their correlation with equilibrium dialysis is poor[30,31] and it has been recommended that these methods should not be used as a measure of true FT concentration.

Is any indirect method for the measurement of FT better than the others? The most useful study to date is that of Vermeulen et al[25] who compared different methods for FT and non-SHBG bound testosterone (nsbT) measurement with an equilibrium dialysis (ED) method. The conclusion from their study was that the measures that correlated best with the ED method were the calculated FT (using Vermeulen's formula) and nsbT. They also reported that, for relatively normal levels of albumin, calculated FT only required the measurement of total testosterone and SHBG, conveniently both automated methods. The website of the International Society for the Study of the Aging Male (www.issam.ch) has a calculator for FT and bioavailable testosterone. Albumin, testosterone, and SHBG concentrations can be entered after choosing the units of measure. Clinicians will benefit in clinical diagnosis by encouraging their laboratory to use one of these indicators if currently unavailable.

Limitations

Since the direct measurement of FT is complex and is unsuited to routine clinical investigations it will not be discussed further. Further information can be found in the review of Wheeler.[33] Most laboratories will use a calculated value or the androgen index. Although both are helpful clinically they are both dependent upon the reliability of two measures, total testosterone and SHBG. Fortunately SHBG methods appear to be very robust and there is good agreement between methods (see below). Most variation therefore comes from the total testosterone method and the most precise methods will give the most reliable calculated FT results. As discussed above there are significant differences between testosterone methods and each testosterone method will give rise to different reference ranges for FT. The different formulae that have been published also give different values and are not transferable.[34] It is important that each laboratory establishes its own reference range for FT.

As well as the differences that exist between total testosterone methods and between the formulae for calculating FT, all the problems discussed above for the measurement of total testosterone regarding cut-off values, circadian rhythms, and inter-individual variation also hold for FT. There is no UK NEQAS for FT.

Sex hormone-binding globulin

Early methods for this protein used competitive protein binding of tritiated DHT. Eventually these methods were replaced by immunometric methods and most laboratories found good agreement between the competitive binding assays and the immunometric assays. The UK NEQAS for SHBG is comprised mainly of four methods, DPC Immulite, DPC Immulite 2000, Roche Elecsys, and the Wallac DELFIA methods. Until recently the DPC Immulite methods used to dominate the scheme and were used by about 80% of participants. Roche has recently introduced a method on their popular automated system and now about 30% of participants use this method. The latter method is slightly higher than the DPC Immulite method by about 4% and about 13% higher than the DPC Immulite 2000 method. This difference means that the Roche method gives a result for calculated FT concentration about 9% higher than the DPC Immulite 2000 method. For example, a testosterone concentration of 10 nmol/l would result in a calculated FT concentration of 161 nmol/l by the DPC method and 175 nmol/l by the Roche method. Clinically these differences are small but, depending on cut-offs, they could make a difference in interpretation at some concentrations. It is important that there is good communication between clinicians and the laboratory so that method changes are notified, recorded, and the consequences of method changes fully discussed. Of course, the laboratory should prepare a new reference range whenever there is a method change but this may not be done if differences are considered small (no more than about 10%). It is hoped that agreement between SHBG methods will improve further with the use of the WHO 1st International Reference Preparation 95/560 for calibration.

Data from UK NEQAS show that the assays are very stable. The overall imprecision between all methods is about 13% from 10 to 100 nmol/l; this includes the normal male range of about 10 to 60 nmol/l. Also the agreement between users of the same method is very good and is about 5% for the Roche and Immulite 2000 methods. This indicates that the imprecision of FT calculation comes mostly from the testosterone method when investigating healthy men.

Limitations

SHBG is affected by a number of pathologic conditions.[34] It is increased when testosterone is low and is also increased by estrogen therapy. It is also increased in cirrhosis of the liver and in patients taking anticonvulsant therapy. In the latter case hypogonadal men can have a normal testosterone although an elevated LH and SHBG will indicate the true clinical condition. SHBG is also raised in thyrotoxicosis with increased testosterone concentrations, but the FT will be normal or low.

There are few technical problems with the measurement of SHBG but a careful clinical history is important for the interpretation of the SHBG result.

Androstenedione

The measurement of androstenedione is not clinically helpful in the investigation of low libido and erectile dysfunction in men. It is used mostly in the investigation of hirsutism in women and monitoring treatment of congenital adrenal hyperplasia.

Androstenedione has always been measured by competitive immunoassay and direct methods are now available. As its clinical use is limited there are currently few automated procedures and it is an assay that is mostly carried out in specialist steroid laboratories or laboratories in teaching hospitals. Reviewing current usage in UK NEQAS shows that 60% of laboratories use manual assays, with the DPC Immulite and Immulite 2000 assays being the only automated methods used by participants. Agreement between methods is just under 20% down to a concentration of about 5 nmol/l, below which agreement worsens. Within-method agreement is about 10%. The relationship between the manual methods and the automated methods is concentration dependent, with the automated methods demonstrating a marked positive bias at low concentrations.

Dehydroepiandrostenedione

No clinical requirement has been established for the measurement of dehydroepiandrostenedione (DHEA) as the role of DHEA in the body, and the benefit of DHEA therapy, are controversial. Most of the studies indicating a beneficial effect of DHEA are based on animal studies in which the normal levels are very low. Human studies have tended to use pharmacologic doses of the steroid. The benefits of DHEA therapy have included maintenance of the immune system, cancer, heart disease, and cognitive function. The latter case has attracted much interest because of the fall in DHEA concentrations from the fourth decade of life and the very low levels encountered in the elderly. The steroid is available as a dietary supplement in many Western countries. At the moment there are insufficient data to define a clear clinical role for this steroid.[36]

Measurement of DHEA is confined to a few specialized steroid laboratories and there is no EQA scheme for the steroid in the UK.

Dehydroepiandrosterone sulfate

The measurement of dehydroepiandrosterone sulfate (DHEAS) is not helpful in the investigation of low libido and erectile dysfunction in men. It may be measured in the investigation of hirsutism in women to establish the adrenal contribution to high androgen levels in the blood.

DHEAS is essentially an adrenal steroid and has a concentration about a thousand times greater than other androgens. It shows the same decline with age as DHEA. Because of the high concentrations some investigators have felt that it must have a role in the body and hence the interest in DHEA therapy.[36]

Pituitary hormones

LH and FSH

These two peptide hormones are discussed together as many laboratories measure both at the same time on their automated systems. The two hormones are now measured by immunometric assay and are available on all automated systems. The development of immunoassays to immunometric assays did not significantly change FSH results but there was a fall of about 30% in LH results. As immunoassays are no longer used for clinical purposes this is not a problem.

LH and FSH are standard assay requests in any investigation of infertility in men and women. FSH is useful in the investigation of spermatogenesis and early testicular failure. In the male FSH can be raised when the LH and testosterone levels are normal. Many males then go on to develop general testicular failure with raised LH and low testosterone. LH may not be particularly helpful in the aging male with mild testicular failure. It has been shown that, although LH levels increase with age as testosterone levels fall, the extent of this rise is less than that of testosterone. It has been demonstrated that this is due to an increased sensitivity of the hypothalamus to testosterone feedback in the older male.[37] Therefore the LH concentration may still be in the upper normal range when the testosterone is low and care must be taken in interpreting LH results in the older male.

There are over 12 different assay platforms used in the UK with the Bayer, Centaur, DPC Immulite 2000, and the Roche Elecsys systems being the most popular. UK NEQAS data for 2005 show an overall between-method agreement of about 10% for FSH and about 12% for LH. For both assays, taking the mean results of methods, there is about a 30% difference between the lowest method mean and the highest method mean. All methods are calibrated against the same reference preparations and it is not known at this time whether these method differences are due to differences in calibration. Therefore clinicians should be aware of changes of method in their laboratories and great care should be taken when interpreting results from another center using a different methodology. However, clinicians can have more confidence in the consistency of a single method.

Limitations

LH and FSH assays have the same potential interference problems as all immunometric assays, namely the hook effect and interference from heterophilic antibodies and rheumatoid factor. The hook effect is not a problem in the investigation of male fertility as the concentrations encountered for these two hormones are never very high. Interference from the presence of heterophilic antibodies and rheumatoid factor is well recorded. Marks[38] sent out samples from 10 donors, 8 of whom tested positive for rheumatoid factor; 1 also had high levels of human anti-mouse antibodies (HAMAs). In 12 laboratories, using 11 different assay systems, 9 of the assays gave erroneous results for LH and FSH for a patient with high rheumatoid factor. Clinically inconsistent results for LH and FSH were obtained in 9 out of 11 systems for the donor sample with high levels of HAMAs. Ismail et al.[39] examined retrospectively 5310 results for TSH, LH, and FSH and found 28 (0.53%) analytically incorrect results. Not all the assays were simultaneously affected, which itself could lead to clinical confusion. Of the 28 cases, 22 of them were corrected by treating for heterophilic antibodies. The other 6 were not corrected in this way, suggesting that other proteins or antibodies were causing interference. It is important that if a result does not fit the clinical picture the clinician should discuss this with the laboratory. The laboratory may re-analyze the sample although it is usually more efficient to take another sample to exclude a mix-up of patient names and blood bottles occurring, either at the time of blood collection or when the sample was received in the laboratory.

Prolactin

Immunoassays have been replaced by immunometric assays and are available on all automated systems. Again prolactin should be a routine request in the investigation of infertility in both men and women to exclude the presence of a prolactinoma. Unlike the female, where high levels of prolactin are normally associated with disruption of the menstrual cycle, the male has no such early indicators. Males with large prolactinomas usually present with headaches and visual field defects.

Laboratories will use the same analytic platform as they use for LH and FSH assays. However, agreement between methods is not as good as the other two assays. About 9 years ago agreement in UK NEQAS between methods was about 10% but over recent years agreement has deteriorated so that now between-method agreement is about 20%. Also the difference between the mean method results ranges from −15% to 40% of the target value, i.e. there are significant method differences.

Limitations

Prolactin assays are susceptible to the same interference seen in LH and FSH assays. However, the hook effect can be a problem. Recently our laboratory found a prolactin concentration of 1 million mIU/l in a female patient. This patient had a large cranial tumor that had grown up from the pituitary. Surprisingly the patient had normal adrenal, reproductive, and thyroid function. Her prolactin was later measured in another hospital, to which she had been transferred, where a prolactin result of 3567 mIU/l was reported. The patient was operated on and rendered hypopituitary. It became evident that the second assay system suffered from a 'hook' effect and gave an erroneously low result. This suggests that a normal or modestly raised prolactin concentration <5000 mIU/l in a male with symptoms associated with a pituitary tumor should have a repeat measurement with the sample analyzed at several dilutions.

Although interference from heterophilic antibodies is also possible, Marks[38] found no clear evidence of such interference. He did report 16 false high results but they all remained within the reference range.

The major interference encountered in prolactin assays is with macroprolactin or 'big big' prolactin.[40] This is monoprolactin bound to an immunoglobulin. All assays appear to cross-react with this molecule but to varying extents. Presumably this is due to recognition of different epitopes. The presence of macroprolactin can lead to false high results that are frequently mildly raised (1000–5000 mIU/l), but may be grossly high. Figure 7.4 shows an example of a Sephacryl chromatography profile of a sample with significant macroprolactin. In this case the situation was further complicated by antipsychotic therapy raising the prolactin concentration. Table 7.1 shows how changing the therapy from risperidone and

Table 7.1 *Hyperprolactinemia in a patient caused by antipsychotic therapy and the presence of macroprolactin. Recovery of monoprolactin after PEG precipitation with the calculated monoprolactin is shown. The patient showed true hyperprolactinemia, as shown by the concentration of monoprolactin, when on, and due to, risperidone and amisulpride but not on clozapine*

Date	Therapy	Total prolactin (mIU/l)	Recovery (%)	Monoprolactin (mIU/l)
16.05.04	Risperidone	21 257	9.0	2584
24.06.04	Amisulpride	31 388	10.4	4417
22.07.04	Amisulpride	38 835	9.2	4829
12.09.04	Clozapine	7376	9.9	986
15.10.04	Clozapine	392	20.4	108

Reference range ≤ 500 mIU/l.

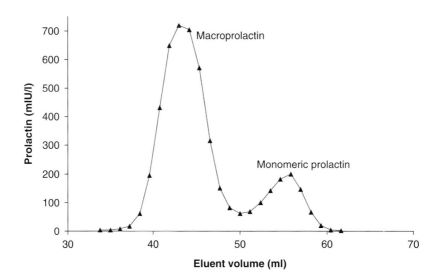

Figure 7.4 *A profile from a Sephacryl gel column of a serum sample containing macroprolactin. The total prolactin concentration was measured as 1840 mIU/l; the monoprolactin concentration was in the normal range.*

amisulpride to clozapine reduced the level of prolactin to normal. During therapy the prolactin concentration was elevated to very high levels due to the presence of macroprolactin. The presence of macroprolactin is easily tested and should be a routine procedure on all samples with a raised prolactin.[41,42] Clinicians should ensure that samples with a raised prolactin result have been tested for the presence of macroprolactin before acting upon the result.

Growth hormone and insulin-like growth factor 1

The measurement of growth hormone (GH) has no place in the initial investigation of low libido and erectile dysfunction and is no longer used in the routine investigation of the GH axis since insulin-like growth factor 1 (IGF-1) is a superior assay.

GH used to be measured in the investigation of acromegaly and GH deficiency. However, a random GH measurement is frequently unhelpful and misleading. GH increases with stress and anxiety and so a raised result is not confirmatory of acromegaly. Equally some acromegalics have only mildly elevated GH concentrations and so low GH results do not exclude acromegaly. Also undetectable results are found in normal people during the day so that the method is unsuitable for detecting GH deficiency. Acromegaly and GH deficiency, using GH measurement, can only be confirmed with dynamic tests.

IGF-1 concentrations are more stable and are not affected by anxiety. High levels of IGF-1 indicate acromegaly[43,44] or overtreatment with GH, but GH deficiency may be accompanied by low normal IGF-1 results. In a patient with suspected pituitary insufficiency dynamic tests of the GH axis should be carried out.

IGF-1 has no place in the initial investigation of erectile dysfunction or low libido in men.

Summary

There have been significant improvements in the delivery of hormone results over recent years due to the automation of routine hormone assays. These assays are faster and use less serum. However, this has come with a cost. The development of direct steroid assays has led to loss of sensitivity, deterioration in precision, and poor agreement between methods. There have been more problems of interference in some assays. Although LH and FSH assays have good precision the agreement between prolactin assays is less good and interference from the presence of macroprolactin is a significant problem. Tandem mass spectrometry gives some hope for the future as it has the potential for precise, accurate assays leading to better between-method agreement. To date there has been no interlaboratory comparison of results from tandem mass spectrometry methods.

The quality of the result also depends on the correct sample being taken at the correct time into the correct tube and sent as quickly as possible to the laboratory. If these parameters are not addressed the quality of the assay is irrelevant. This is very much the responsibility of the clinician.

Finally good communication between clinician and the laboratory is essential so that the clinician is aware of assay problems and changes of method as they happen. The clinician has the perfect bioassay, namely the patient, and if results do not appear to fit with the clinical picture, the clinician should have no hesitation in either sending a second sample or discussing the results with a senior person in the laboratory. A quality service to the patient requires a partnership between the clinician and the laboratory.

Acknowledgments

My sincere thanks to colleagues at the UK NEQAS centers in Birmingham and Edinburgh for reviewing and updating the data from their schemes. Also to Sophie Barnes for the prolactin data.

References

1. Roberts CGP, Ladenson PW. Hypothyroidism. Lancet 2004; 363: 793–803.
2. Lamberts SWJ, De Herder WW, van der Lely AJ. Pituitary insufficiency. Lancet 1998; 352: 127–34.
3. Wardle CA, Fraser WD, Squire CR. Lancet 2001; 357: 1013–14.
4. Davison SL, Bell R, Monalto JG et al. Measurement of total testosterone in women: comparison of a direct radioimmunoassay versus radioimmunoassay after organic solvent extraction and celite partition chromatography. Fertil Steril 2005; 84: 1698–704.
5. Wheeler MJ. Measurement of androgens. In: Wheeler MJ, Hutchinson J, eds. Hormone Assays in Biological Fluids. New Jersey, USA: Humana Press, 2006.
6. Cawood ML, Field HP, Ford CG et al. Tesosterone measurement by isotope-dilution liquid chromatography–tandem mass spectrometry: validation of a method for routine clinical practice. Clin Chem 2005; 51: 1472–9.
7. Lamph S, Wheeler M, Halloran S. Eight testosterone assays. MHRA Evaluation report. MHRA 03127.
8. Thienpont LM. Standardization of steroid immunoassays – in theory an easy task. Clin Chem Lab Med 1998; 36: 349–352.
9. Taieb J, Mathian B, Millot F et al. Testosterone measured by 10 immunoassays and isotope-dilution gas chromatography–mass spectrometry in sera from 116 men, women and children. Clin Chem 2003; 49: 1381–95.

10. Wang C, Catlin DH, Demers LM, et al. Measurement of total serum testosterone in adult men: comparison of current laboratory methods versus liquid chromatography–tandem mass spectrometry. J Clin Endocrinol Metab 2004; 89: 534–43.

11. Sikaris K, MacLachlan R, Kazlauskas R. et al. Reproductive hormone reference intervals for healthy fertile young men: evaluation of automated platform assays. J Clin Endocrinol Metab 2005; 90: 5928–36.

12. Ahokoski O, Virtanen A, Huupponen R et al. Biological day-to-day variation and daytime changes of testosterone, follitropin, lutropin and oestradiol-17beta in healthy men. Clin Chem Lab Med 1998; 36: 485–91.

13. Diver MJ, Imtiaz KE, Ahmadt AM et al. Diurnal rhythms of serum total, free and bioavailable testosterone and of SHBG in middle-aged men compared with those in young men. Clin Endocrinol 2003; 58: 710–17.

14. Leifke E, Gorenoi V, Wichers C et al. Age-related changes of serum sex hormones, insulin-like growth factor-1 and sex-hormone binding globulin in men: cross-sectional data from a healthy male cohort. Clin Endocrinol 2000; 53: 689–95.

15. Feldman HA, Longcope C, Derby CA et al. Age trends in the level of serum testosterone and other hormones in middle-aged men: longitudinal results from the Massachusetts male aging study. J Clin Endocrinol Metab 2002: 589–98.

16. Allan CA, McLachlan RI. Age-related changes in testosterone and the role of replacement therapy in older men. Clin Endocrinol 2004; 60: 653–70.

17. Vermeulen A. Declining androgens with age: an overview. In: Oddens B, Vermeulen A, eds. Androgens and the Aging Male. New York: Parthenon Publishing Group, 1996: 3–14.

18. Heald AH, Ivison F, Anderson SG et al. Significant ethnic variation in total and free testosterone concentration. Clin Endocrinol 2003; 58: 262–6.

19. Lookingbill DP, Demers LM, Wang C et al. Clinical and biochemical parameters of androgen action in normal and healthy Caucasian versus Chinese subjects. J Clin Endocrinol Metab 1991; 72: 1242–8.

20. Wang C, Catlin DH, Starcevic S et al. Testosterone metabolic clearance and production rates determined by stable isotope dilution/tandem mass spectrometry in normal men: influence of ethnicity and age. J Clin Endocrinol Metab 2004; 89: 2936–41.

21. Santer SJ, Albertson B, Zhang GY et al. Comparison of androgen production and metabolism in Caucasian and Chinese subjects. J Clin Endocrinol 1998; 83: 2104–9.

22. Diver MJ. Variability in day-to-day concentration of total testosterone in men. Aging Male 2006; 9: 15.

23. Medical and Healthcare Products Regulatory Agency. Medical Device Alert for BD vacutainer® SST™, and SST II™ Advance™ blood collection tubes (glass and plastic). MDA/2004/048.

24. Hammer EJ, Astley JP. Increase in serum testosterone following contact with blood cells. Ann Clin Biochem 1985; 22: 539–40.

25. Vermeulen A, Verdonck L, Kaufman J M. A critical evaluation of simple methods for the estimation of free testosterone in serum. J Clin Endocrinol Metab 1999; 84: 3666–72.

26. Wheeler MJ, Nanjee MN. A steady-state gel filtration method on micro-columns for the measurement of percentage free testosterone in serum. Ann Clin Biochem 1985; 22: 185–9.

27. Nanjee MN, Wheeler MJ. Plasma testosterone – is an index sufficient? Ann Clin Biochem 1985; 22: 387–90.

28. Södergard R, Bäckström T, Shanbhag V, Carstensen H. Calculation of free and bound fractions of testosterone and estradiol-17β to human plasma protein at body temperature. J Steroid Biochem 1982; 16: 801–10.

29. Cumming DC, Wall SR. Non-sex-hormone-binding globulin-bound testosterone as a marker of hyperandrogenicity. J Clin Endocrinol Metab 1985; 61: 873–6.

30. Blight LF, Judd SJ, White GH. Relative diagnostic value of serum non-SHBG-bound testosterone, free androgen index and free testosterone in the assessment of mild to moderate hirsutism. Ann Clin Biochem 1989; 26: 311–16.

31. Winters SJ, Kelley DE, Goodpater B. The analog free testosterone assay: are the results in men clinically useful? Clin Chem 1998; 44: 2178–82.

32. Rosner W. An extraordinary inaccurate assay for free testosterone is still with us. J Clin Endocrinol Metab 2001; 86: 2903.

33. Wheeler MJ. The determination of bio-available testosterone. Ann Clin Biochem 1995; 32: 345–57.

34. De Ronde W, van der Schouw YT, Pols HA et al. Calculation of bioavailable and free testosterone in men: a comparison of five published algorithms. Aging Male 2006; 9: 14.

35. Anderson DC. Sex-hormone-binding globulin. Clin Endocrinol 1974; 3: 69–96.

36. Arlt W. Dehydroepiandrosterone and ageing. J Clin Endocrinol Metab 2004; 18: 363–80.

37. Veldhuis JD. Recent insights into neuroendocrine mechanisms of aging of the human male hypothalamic–pituitary–gonadal axis. J Androl 1999; 20: 1–17.

38. Marks V. False-positive immunoassay results: a multi-center survey of erroneous immunoassay results from assays of 74 analytes in 10 donors from 66 laboratories in seven countries. Clin Chem 2002; 48: 2008–16.

39. Ismail AAA, Walker PL, Barth JL et al. Wrong biochemistry results: two case reports and observational study in 5310 patients on potentially misleading thyroid-stimulating hormone and gonadotropin immunoassay results. Clin Chem 2002; 48: 2023–9.

40. Lindtstedt G. Endogenous antibodies against prolactin – a 'new' cause of hyperprolactinaemia. Euro J Endocrinol 1994; 130: 429–32.

41. Fahie-Wilson MN, Soule SG. Macroprolactinaemia: contribution to hyperprolactinaemia in a district general hospital and evaluation of a screening test based on precipitation with polyethylene glycol. Ann Clin Biochem 1997; 43: 252–8.

42. Olukoga AO, Kane JW. Macroprolactinaemia: validation and application of the polyethylene glycol precipitation test and clinical characterisation of the condition. Clin Endocrinol 1999; 51: 119–26.

43. Sneppen SB, Lange M, Pedersen LM et al. Total and free insulin-like growth factor 1, insulin-like growth factor binding protein 3 and acid labile subunit reflect clinical activity in acromegaly. Growth Hormone IGF Res 2001; 11: 384–91.

44. Kim HJ, Kwon SH, Kim SW et al. Diagnostic value of serum IGF-I and IGFBP-3 in growth hormone disorders in adults. Horm Res 2001; 56: 117–23.

The Genitourinary System

CHAPTER 8

Genitourinary system: an introduction

Claude C Schulman

Genitourinary diseases increase in prevalence with aging, and with the significant increase in life expectancy, the majority of men will probably be affected by a genitourinary disease during their lifetime. This has a major impact on public health resources.

In most Western countries men live an average of 5.8 years less than women. Education and awareness of male health problems for both the public and health-care providers, and early detection of these problems, will eventually result in reduced rates of morbidity and mortality, as well as reduced health costs for these diseases. Indeed, men visit the doctor 150% less than women for a variety of reasons, including fear, lack of information, a greater emphasis on performance rather than longevity, and a natural tendency to be a 'risk taker'. Significant numbers of male health problems, such as prostate cancer (the most frequent cancer in men), benign prostatic hypertrophy, testicular cancer, incontinence, erectile dysfunction and various endocrine problems could be diagnosed and treated if men's awareness of these problems was greater.

Prostate cancer is the most common malignancy affecting men beyond middle age, and is the second most common cause of cancer death after lung tumors. This type of cancer usually has a slow growth rate; the lifetime risk of developing clinical cancer is about 16% and the risk of dying from the disease is about 3%. One out of 11 men will present with clinical prostate cancer. The widespread early detection programs during the past decade have led to an absolute increase in the incidence of prostate cancer diagnosed at an earlier age and earlier stage. Hence, it is projected that more than one million men will be diagnosed with prostate cancer in the USA during the next 3 years. Age is the strongest predictor of the development of prostate cancer, and as a result of the world-wide trend towards an aging population, the incidence of clinical prostate cancer is predicted to increase very significantly. *Benign prostatic hypertrophy* is one of the most common conditions affecting men after the age of 60 years, with about 40% of men showing symptomatic disease. Of these, about 17% between 50 and 59 years, 27% between 60 and 69 years, and 35% between 70 and 79 years will need some form of treatment.

Erectile dysfunction has been shown in the last 20 years to be predominantly of organic etiology with a strong psychological impact. The probability of complete erectile dysfunction almost triples between the fifth and the seventh decade of life, affecting 5% of men over the age of 40, 10% of men in their sixties and 20% of men in their seventies. These figures suggest that some 20 million men in the USA may suffer from erectile dysfunction, with a similar prevalence among men in Europe. In the last few years, the treatment of erectile dysfunction has been revolutionized by new pharmacologic approaches offering a simple and effective treatment for the vast majority of these men.

Testicular cancer is the most common cancer in men aged between 25 and 34 years. It is estimated that one man in 500 may develop testicular cancer by the age of 50. Provided that they are diagnosed at an early stage and treated adequately, the majority of these affected men will survive this disease due to successful combinations of different forms of treatment.

Incontinence, which affects between 20–30% of women over the age of 60 years, also affects men significantly after their seventies, and can be a severely debilitating condition.

In conclusion, education of both patients and health-care providers on the importance of the early detection of male health problems, and more specifically of urologic diseases, will result in reduced morbidity and mortality, as well as in a reduction of health-care costs and the impact on the community.

CHAPTER 9

Benign prostatic hyperplasia

Simon RJ Bott and Roger S Kirby

Introduction

Benign prostatic hyperplasia (BPH) is the most common benign human neoplasm. Most men will live to an age where they have an 88% chance of developing histologic BPH and a more than 50% chance of being symptomatic from benign prostatic obstruction (BPO).[1] BPH seldom reduces the duration of a man's life, but it may impact heavily on his quality of life and on those closest to him.

The demand for medical intervention in BPH is increasing. The population of the Western world is aging such that, at birth, a man now has a life expectancy of over 73 years. Furthermore, the media and the Internet have heightened the awareness of BPO as a treatable condition, rather than an inevitability of old age as previously presumed.

While surgery remains the mainstay of treatment for symptomatic BPH, medical therapies are increasingly used, with proven effect. Patients often favor a tablet over an operation. Likewise, those who control the purse-strings perceive medical treatment as a cheaper alternative. This may or may not be true for two reasons. First, more men receive treatment than if surgery was the only treatment option. Second, some men start medical therapy that subsequently fails and then require a definitive surgical procedure, such as transurethral resection of the prostate (TURP). This phenomenon is termed the therapeutic cascade. Cost for medical treatment and the TURP must then be met rather than the cost of the TURP alone. From a health-care point of view, more men receiving treatment should reduce the incidence of lower urinary tract symptoms (LUTS) in the community as a whole. Furthermore, the therapeutic cascade is often favored by the patient who appreciates the stepwise approach to his care.

Prostate research is at an all-time high. Both the prevalence of BPH and its impact on men's quality of life have fueled the public's demand for newer, better treatments.

Etiologic factors

Inherited and environmental factors are implicated in the etiology of BPH. Prostatic enlargement appears to run in families, which suggests it is to some degree inherited.[2] Asian people have a lower incidence than white individuals, unless they migrate to the Western world where the incidence of BPH closely matches that of their white compatriots.[3] Furthermore, the incidence of BPH in Japan is rising as the Western diet becomes more popular there.

A large number of dietary components have been examined as causative agents for BPH. High-fat diets increase serum prolactin, which has a proliferative effect on the prostatic epithelium. Alcohol consumption of 25 oz or more per month may reduce the risk of surgery, as alcohol reduces serum testosterone.[3]

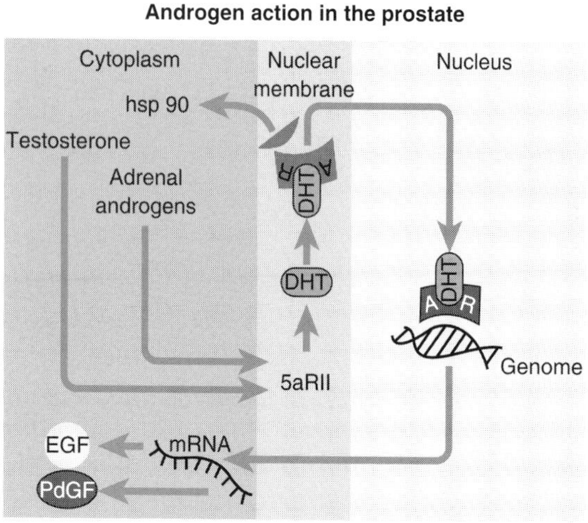

Androgen action in the prostate

![Figure 9.1 diagram showing androgen action in the prostate]

Figure 9.1   *Androgen action in the prostate.*

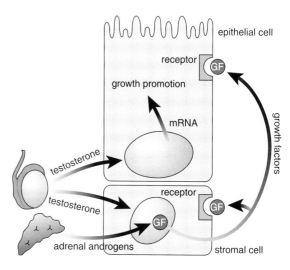

Figure 9.2   *Growth factors promoting benign prostatic hyperplasia (BPH).*

Pathogenesis

The development of BPH is a complex process that is not fully understood. What is clear is that aging and the hormone dihydrotestosterone (DHT) play a key role.

Dihydrotestosterone is a metabolite of the male sex hormone testosterone (Figure 9.1). Serum free testosterone levels fall with aging, whereas estrogen levels remain the same. This acquired endocrine imbalance may trigger BPH. What is interesting is that if a man is castrated before puberty he will not develop BPH. However, if a man with BPH is castrated, the BPH does not necessarily regress, implying androgens have a role in initiating but not maintaining BPH.

The role of DHT in prostate development is elegantly demonstrated by a small population of men living in the village of Salinas in the Dominican Republic.[4] They have a congenital deficiency of the enzyme 5α-reductase that converts testosterone into DHT. They are capable of all the testosterone-dependent functions, such as the development of normal secondary sexual characteristics, but without DHT their prostates remain vestigial and they retain their hairline. Furthermore, they never develop BPH, unless DHT is administered.

Dihydrotestosterone binds to androgen receptors and stimulates the production of local growth factors (Figure 9.2). These include epidermal growth factor (EGF), fibroblast growth factor (FGF), and transforming growth factor (TGF). The precise role these factors play in BPH remains elusive. However, they normally control cell division and cell death (apoptosis); when an imbalance occurs, the rate of cell division exceeds the rate of cell death and this may lead to hyperplasia.

Pathophysiology

The prostate lies between the neck of the bladder and the urogenital diaphragm, and in man (and in dogs) it surrounds the urethra. It is normally the size of a walnut but may grow 100–200% larger in BPH. It consists of three zones: the transition zone in which BPH develops, the peripheral zone where 70% of prostate cancers originate, and the central zone (Figure 9.3).

The first histologic sign of BPH may be evident in men in their twenties. Microscopic nodules appear in the periurethral glands around the verumontanum. These nodules are composed of varying amounts of fibrous and smooth muscle cells as well

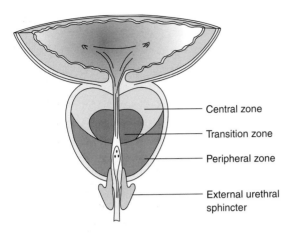

Central zone

Transition zone

Peripheral zone

External urethral sphincter

Figure 9.3 *Anatomical zones of the prostate.*

as glandular hyperplasia, and may be a few millimeters to a few centimeters in diameter. As the prostatic adenoma enlarges it encroaches on the urethra, increasing resistance to urine flow by mechanical, or 'static', obstruction.

Interestingly, the overall size of the prostate does not correspond well with the degree of obstruction for two reasons. First, enlargement of the middle lobe of the prostate obstructs the bladder outflow but does not significantly affect the overall size of the prostate. Second, there is a 'dynamic' component to BPO exerted by the smooth muscle cells, contracting in response to sympathetic stimulation. The sympathetic nerves release norepinephrine (noradrenaline), which binds to receptors on the smooth muscle cells, initiating contraction.

The increased resistance exerted by the enlarged prostate causes the bladder muscle to undergo hypertrophy. Eventually, the detrusor muscle decompensates as collagen is deposited among the smooth muscle cells; this reduces the bladder compliance and renders the detrusor muscle atonic.

Furthermore, the bladder becomes 'irritable'. Recent research indicates that bladder irritability is due to transient ischemia of the autonomic nerves in the bladder at the time of voiding. A high intravesical pressure is required to expel the urine through the obstructing prostate; this pressure impedes blood flow. The impaired blood supply

reduces oxygen delivery, damaging the nerves in the bladder wall. As the nerves are irreparably damaged, the bladder relies on its inbuilt myogenic, or muscle-generated, stimulation for bladder contraction. Myogenic stimulation is not under the control of higher nerve centers, and leads to more frequent bladder contraction as the bladder starts to fill. This gives rise to the symptoms of frequency, nocturia, and urgency. The obstructing prostate impedes the flow of urine such that the patient observes a reduced stream. The bladder detrusor muscle taking longer to generate the higher pressure required to expel the urine results in hesitancy. This high pressure may be unsustainable, and the bladder tires before recovering and contracting again, giving rise to intermittency. Incomplete emptying occurs if the detrusor is unable to recover in a short time and residual urine remains in the bladder.

Benign prostatic hyperplasia progresses slowly with time, but patients' symptoms do not necessarily deteriorate. In one study looking at the symptoms of men with BPH in whom surgery was not warranted, 27% remained stable, 15% improved, and 58% deteriorated over 3 years without any other treatment.[5]

Presentation

Lower urinary tract symptoms are so common in the aging male that they are considered by many as part of growing older. Media coverage, heightened awareness of health-care professionals, and the availability of medical therapy have meant that now more and more men are seeking treatment for their bothersome symptoms. Furthermore, as the profile of prostate cancer rises, patients are requesting assessment of their prostate to exclude malignancy; this inevitably draws attention to their outflow symptoms.

History
When assessing a man with LUTS, it is important to confirm that the symptoms arise from the BPH rather than another pathology (Table 9.1), particularly prostate cancer. Second, it is essential to ensure the obstructing prostate has not given rise to complications including bladder stones (Figure 9.4),

117

Table 9.1 *Differential diagnosis of a man with lower-urinary-tract symptoms*

Malignancy
Prostate cancer
Carcinoma in situ (bladder)
Infection
Bacterial
Tuberculosis/bilharzia
Inflammation
Bladder stone
Interstitial cystitis
Neurological
Parkinson's disease
Cerebrovascular event
Multiple sclerosis
Bladder neck dysynergia
Mechanical
Urethral stricture
Severe phimosis
Drug-induced
Antidepressants, e.g. amitriptyline
Anticholinergics, e.g. oxybutynin
Diuretics, e.g. furosemide

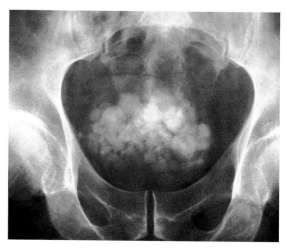

Figure 9.4 *Pelvic radiograph showing multiple bladder stones.*

urinary tract infection, or renal failure. A comprehensive history, a focused examination, and the relevant preliminary investigation enable an accurate diagnosis to be made in the vast majority of cases. Those in whom uncertainty still exists can undergo further evaluation by transrectal ultrasound and biopsy, flexible cystoscopy, and urodynamic studies.

Assessment of a man's LUTS is best achieved using a symptom score sheet (Figure 9.5); the most widely employed is the International Prostate Symptom Score (IPSS). This is used to assess the 'obstructive' and 'irritative' symptoms, and also asks how these symptoms affect the individual's quality of life. A score is given for each symptom, and these scores are totalled to give a value that indicates whether a patient has mild, moderate, or severe symptoms. These scores enable a quantitative assessment of symptoms; they do not enable the diagnosis of BPH to be made. Poor urinary flow and incomplete emptying are the most reliable indicators of prostatic obstruction, but this may be due to prostate cancer rather than BPH.

The irritative symptoms of frequency, nocturia, and urgency are common in BPO. However, other pathologies give rise to an irritative picture: either as a complication of BPH such as a urinary tract infection or bladder stones, or as a separate bladder pathology such as carcinoma in situ of the bladder.

Medical conditions including diabetes mellitus and insipidus as well as treatment with diuretic agents can cause polyuria. The volumes of urine passed as well as the frequency are excessive. A time–volume chart in these men distinguishes polyuria from frequency. Neurologic conditions can cause irritative bladder symptoms; Parkinson's disease, a history of strokes, and multiple sclerosis can all alter bladder function.

A drug history especially pertaining to antidepressants such as amitriptyline or anticholinergic agents such as oxybutynin may be relevant, and a brief family history is prudent as a first-degree relative with prostate cancer increases the patient's chance of acquiring the disease by 2–3-fold.

Clinical examination

A routine clinical examination should be performed. Abdominal examination may reveal a palpable bladder, indicating chronic retention of urine. A focused neurologic examination will exclude neurologic conditions that give rise to urinary

	Not at all	Less than 1 time in 5	Less than half the time	About half the time	More than half the time	Almost always	Patient score
• Incomplete emptying Over the past month, how often have you had a sensation of not emptying your bladder completely after you finished urinating?	0	1	2	3	4	5	
• Frequency Over the past month, how often have you had to urinate again less than 2 hours after you finished urinating?	0	1	2	3	4	5	
• Intermittency Over the past month, how often have you found you stopped and started again several times when you urinated?	0	1	2	3	4	5	
• Urgency Over the past month, how often have you found it difficult to postpone urination?	0	1	2	3	4	5	
• Weak stream Over the past month, how often have you had a weak urinary stream?	0	1	2	3	4	5	
• Straining Over the past month, how often have you had to push or strain to begin urination?	0	1	2	3	4	5	
• Nocturia Over the past month, how many times did you most typically get up to urinate from the time you went to bed at night until the time you got up in the morning?	0	1	2	3	4	5+	
Total IPSS							

Figure 9.5 *International Prostate Symptom Score (IPSS).*

symptoms. The digital rectal examination (DRE) is an essential component of the clinical examination of a man with LUTS. This includes assessment of the anal sphincter tone, palpation of the anal canal and rectal mucosa, and, finally, examination of the prostate. Prostate examination should concentrate on the size, shape, and consistency of the gland (Table 9.2).

Although the DRE is not very sensitive (fewer than 50% of cancers can be felt on DRE), together with a prostate-specific antigen (PSA) result it can be used to improve detection of prostate cancer (Table 9.3).

Table 9.2 *Prostate examination*

	Benign prostatic hyperplasia	Prostatitis	Prostate cancer
Size	Enlarged	Enlarged	Enlarged or normal
Shape	Smooth, symmetrical, central sulcus	Smooth, symmetrical	Nodular, asymmetrical loss of central sulcus, lateral and cranial extension
Consistency	Rubbery	Tender, firm or boggy, warm	Hard

Table 9.3 *Incidence of prostate cancer detected by prostate-specific antigen (PSA) and digital rectal examination (DRE)*

	Incidence (%)		
	PSA < 4 ng/ml	PSA 4–10 ng/ml	PSA > 10 ng/ml
Normal DRE	9	20	31
Abnormal DRE	17	45	77

Investigation

Urinalysis

Urinalysis may identify whether a patient's symptoms are as a result of another pathology, for example urinary tract infection or bladder cancer. Microscopic hematuria requires further investigation with urine culture and cytology. Upper-tract imaging and cystoscopy may also be requested to exclude conditions such as stones and bladder or renal tumors. If these investigations do not yield a diagnosis, there may be a 'medical' cause for microscopic hematuria. Glomerulonephritis, endocarditis, and vasculitis can all produce dipstick-positive hematuria and require specialist investigation.

The presence of leukocytes implies infection, requiring formal urine microscopy and culture.

Blood tests

Serum creatinine levels are elevated in 10% of patients who present with LUTS. This is not always due to outflow obstruction, leading to back-pressure on the kidneys, but partly reflects the degree of comorbidity in the aging population tested.

However, if the creatinine level is elevated further, investigation with upper-tract imaging may be required. Patients who have renal insufficiency have an increased risk of postoperative complications, and the mortality increases 6-fold.[6]

Acute and chronic retention can both impair renal function; overcoming the obstruction with a catheter or a TURP will improve the serum urea and electrolyte levels. Clearly, without relief of the obstruction, the renal function will continue to deteriorate; consequently, these cases are managed on an urgent basis.

PSA

The use of PSA testing as a screening tool remains controversial, and will continue to be until the results of large trials in Europe and North America are available. PSA testing in the symptomatic man is, however, recommended in the majority of cases. Patients should be counseled before undergoing the test. The merits and the drawbacks of the test, the possible need for a prostate biopsy, and the therapeutic options if prostate cancer is diagnosed should be discussed. While PSA lacks specificity, it remains the most sensitive, simple test available to diagnose prostate cancer, especially when combined with DRE.

Attempts have been made to refine PSA testing to improve its sensitivity and specificity in detecting prostate cancer. Age-specific PSA correlates advancing age with increasing PSA; PSA velocity charts PSA over time to look at the rate of PSA rise; PSA density compares the PSA value with that expected for the size of the patient's prostate; and the free/total ratio relies on patients with BPH having a higher concentration of PSA in the free form. Patients with prostate cancer tend to have a free/total ratio of less than 0.19, although they frequently have concomitant BPH that may distort the result.

Flow rate and residual volume

The urine flow test and post-void residual urine volume provide an objective assessment of a patient's symptoms. When performing a flow test, at least 150 ml must be passed to obtain an accurate result. For volumes smaller than 150 ml the bladder does not generate its maximum pressure, and therefore the achievable maximum flow rate is never reached. A maximum flow rate of less than 15 ml/s is considered significant for obstruction, although it is often helpful to repeat the test as a single result may not be representative. It should be remembered that factors other than BPH reduce the maximum flow rate, for example poor detrusor contractility or urethral strictures (Figure 9.6).

A significant residual volume, over 150 ml, is predictive of acute urinary retention and is a good indicator of whether a patient will ultimately require surgery for their LUTS. Again, more than one reading should be taken to minimize individual variation.

Urodynamics

Where the diagnosis is still in doubt, urodynamic studies can be undertaken. This involves passing a pressure transducer into the rectum and one into the bladder. The transducers record the change in pressure as the bladder is filled. The patient voids into a flow meter, and the pressures generated are again recorded (Figure 9.7). The rectal transducer

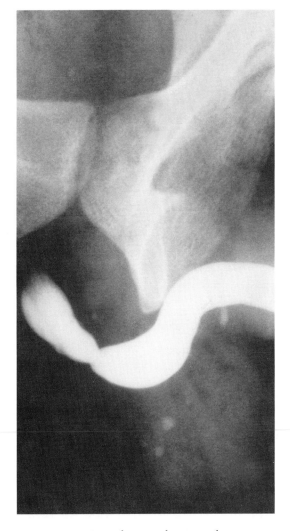

Figure 9.6 *Ascending urethrogram demonstrating stricture in the bulbar urethra.*

records a change in abdominal pressure when the patient performs tasks, such as coughing, as this will also affect the intravesical pressure. The rectal pressure is subtracted from the intravesical pressure to give the pressure generated by the detrusor muscle: the detrusor pressure. This enables the specialist to distinguish between detrusor hypocontractility, where the detrusor muscle is weak, dysynergia, where the detrusor contracts satisfactorily but the sphincter fails to relax appropriately, and outflow obstruction.

121

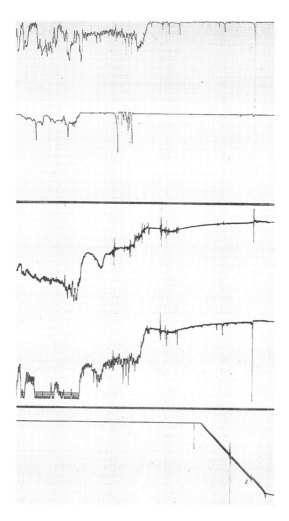

Figure 9.7 *Urodynamic study (filling and voiding). Curve 1, bladder filled with saline; curve 2, intravesical pressure; curve 3, detrusor pressure: high pressure (>100 cmH2O) is required to overcome the obstruction; curve 4, intra-abdominal pressure, subtracted from intravesical pressure to give detrusor pressure: this patient is straining to overcome the obstruction; curve 5, urine flow rate: poor maximum flow with interruption (intermittency).*

Treatment

The choice of treatment for a man with BPH depends on a number of issues: first, the degree to which he finds the symptoms bothersome; second, the symptom score; and finally, the objective assessments of flow rate and residual volume.

Medical

Medical therapies offer a safe and effective treatment for patients who are troubled by their symptoms, and in whom complications have been excluded. Currently, the gold standard treatment for BPH is transurethral resection of the prostate (TURP); however, increasingly, medical options are used either as first-line treatment or as a definitive treatment over the longer term. The symptom score and flow rate improvements are less dramatic with oral medication; nevertheless, patients suffer less from side-effects.

Two classes of drugs are used: α-blockers reduce the dynamic component, and 5α-reductase inhibitors reverse the static component of BPO (Table 9.4). Using these together gives no significant advantage over monotherapy.[7]

α-Blockers

α_1-Receptors are situated on smooth muscle cells found in the prostatic stroma, urethra, and capsule, as well as the bladder neck. The stroma consists of smooth muscle and fibrous connective tissue. In normal individuals the stromal to epithelial component is 2:1; in BPH this becomes 5:1. Norepinephrine from sympathetic nerves binds to α-receptors and stimulates smooth muscle contraction, leading to outflow obstruction (Figure 9.8).

Development   Marco Caine and colleagues[8] first introduced α-blockers as a treatment for symptomatic BPH in 1978. They demonstrated an improvement in patient symptoms and voiding using the α-blocker phenoxybenzamine. Phenoxybenzamine binds non-selectively to both α_1- and α_2-receptors; the former are found in the lower urinary tract, and the latter are in nerve endings and are involved in the re-uptake of norepinephrine. As a result of this non-selective α-blockade, a third of their patients suffered side-effects including dizziness, postural hypotension, tiredness, and nasal congestion.

In 1978, the α_1-selective blocker prazosin, used as an antihypertensive agent, was shown to cause urinary incontinence.[9] Further studies identified the α-receptor subtype α_1-adrenoceptor in prostate tissue.[10] Hedlund and colleagues[11] presented prazosin

Table 9.4 *Alpha-blockers vs. finasteride*

	Alpha-blockers	Finasteride
Onset of action	Few hours	6–12 weeks
Symptom score improvement	40–60%	15%
Flow-rate improvement	1.0–4.0 ml/s	1.3–1.6 ml/s
Urinary retention/surgery	May reduce incidence	Reduces incidence
Side-effects	Postural hypotension drowsiness and headache, retrograde ejaculation	Impotence, decreased libido, breast tenderness
Treatable prostate size	Any	>40 g
Effects on PSA	None	Halves

PSA, prostate-specific antigen

as the first selective α_1-adrenoceptor blocker to be used to treat BPO. They reported that prazosin improved symptoms and urine flow rate as well as reducing the post-void residual volume. Prazosin does not antagonize α_2-receptors; consequently, the side-effects were limited to 10–15% of cases. This resulted in the development of second-generation α-blockers, which include doxazosin, alfuzosin, terazosin, and indoramin (Figure 9.9).

More recent research has uncovered further sub-classes of α_1-adrenoceptors,[12] and these are now the target of further pharmaceutic research. Drugs that reduce BPO with minimal side-effects, by selectively inhibiting the subtype of α_1-adrenoceptor found predominantly in the lower urinary tract, are termed 'uroselective'. Tamsulosin is an α_{1A}-adrenoceptor antagonist and, as such, is uroselective.

Efficacy The α-blockers all have similar efficacy, despite the differing incidence of side-effects. Placebo-controlled trials have reported that symptom scores improve by 40–60%, and flow rates by 30–50%.[13] What is more, they have a rapid onset of action; alfuzosin produces an optimal flow rate improvement after a single dose, symptom improvement after 1 week, and full therapeutic benefit after 3 months.[14] Furthermore, these improvements are maintained in open-label studies for at least 4 years. The risk of developing acute urinary retention and the need for surgical intervention is probably also

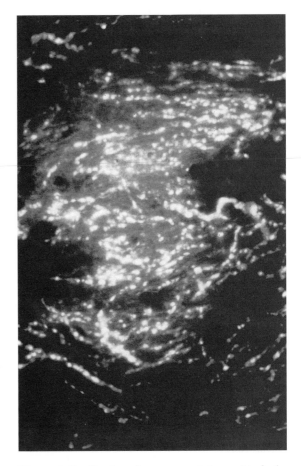

Figure 9.8 *Section of prostate staining positively for norepinephrine.*

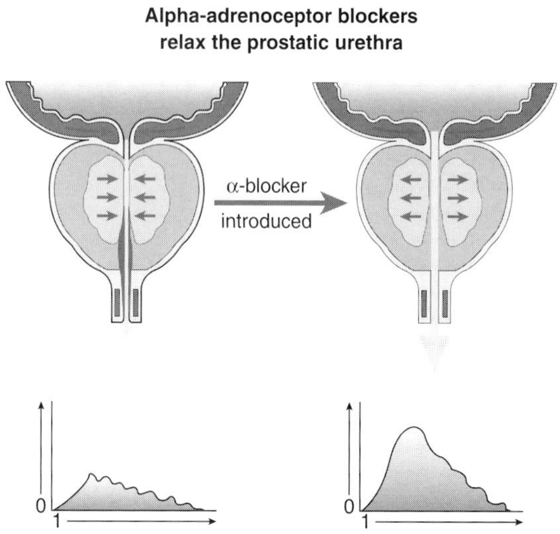

**Alpha-adrenoceptor blockers
relax the prostatic urethra**

Figure 9.9 *Effect of alpha-blockers on the prostate and corresponding flow rate.*

reduced, although data from long-term, randomized, placebo-controlled trials are not yet available.

Side-effects   α-Blockers are generally well tolerated. The main side-effects occur as a result of α_1-blockade in the brain and cardiovascular system. The most common adverse effects include tiredness, dizziness, and headaches, which occur in 10–15% of patients. Less common side-effects (1–2%) include asthenia, palpitations, and gastrointestinal disturbance such as nausea, vomiting, diarrhea, and constipation.

Care is taken when prescribing these drugs for patients with orthostatic hypotension and in those using antihypertensive therapy, as they are prone to hypotensive collapse. The first and second generation of α_1-blockers may also give rise to hypotension after the first dose: the 'first dose effect'; therefore, a low initial dose is given and then subsequent doses are increased, titrating the therapeutic effect against any unwanted symptoms.

The hypotensive effect of α_1-blockers can be used to treat hypertensive patients with BPO. Normotensive men do not experience a clinically significant fall in their blood pressure with doxazosin; however, hypertensive men achieve a significant reduction in mean arterial pressure.[15] One drug can therefore be given to improve compliance, limit drug interaction, and reduce cost. Where the hypotensive effects would be detrimental, tamsulosin is a safer alternative. Tamsulosin may, however, cause retrograde ejaculation by relaxing the smooth muscle of the bladder neck.

5α-Reductase inhibitors

These act by blocking the enzyme-driven conversion of testosterone to dihydrotestosterone (DHT), and in doing so reverse the process of BPH. The enzyme responsible is 5α-reductase, which is also found in hair follicles of the skin. DHT plays a role in male-pattern balding, and patients taking a 5α-reductase inhibitor may notice some reversal of the balding pattern.

Background   John Hunter, the Scottish surgeon, noted in 1786 that prostatic enlargement was related to the aging process and was dependent on normal testicular function.[16] JW White proposed bilateral orchidectomy as a treatment for BPH in the 19th century,[17] and, although effective in 100 of his patients, not surprisingly castration was never popularized.

In 1963 it was reported that testosterone was metabolized in the prostate to DHT,[18] and less than a decade later researchers identified DHT as the main androgen modulating prostate growth.[19] A frenetic search by the pharmaceutic industry resulted in the development of one drug: finasteride, which inhibits 5α-reductase and thereby reduces both prostate DHT levels by 90% and prostate size by an average of 30%.[20] Moreover, it does not affect the testosterone-dependent functions and is therefore better tolerated than the earlier anti-androgen treatments. Research is ongoing with dutasteride (GI198745), which inhibits two isoenzymes of 5α-reductase; this may in the future prove faster and more effective than finasteride.

Efficacy   Finasteride, Proscar® 5 mg once daily, has been extensively investigated in a number of placebo-controlled trials. The SCARP trial (Scandinavian Reduction of the Prostate),[21] a large, double-blind, multicenter trial, compared the efficacy of finasteride with that of placebo over a 24-month period. The symptom score improved in the finasteride arm by 15%, compared with a 2% improvement in the placebo group, at 2 years. Likewise, the flow rate improved by 1.5 ml/s compared with a reduction of 0.3 ml/s in the controls. In the Proscar long-term efficiency and safety study (PLESS),[22] another randomized, placebo-controlled trial involving 3000 men in North America, finasteride was compared with placebo. This study showed that finasteride reduced the risk of urinary retention from 2.7% in the placebo group to 1.1% in the finasteride arm, and the need for surgical intervention from 6.5 to 4.2%.

It should be noted, however, that finasteride has been shown to be of little benefit over placebo for patients with smaller prostates (<40 mg). Furthermore, as finasteride acts by reversing the disease process, it may take 3–6 months before an improvement in symptoms is seen. However, it has proven efficacy for at least 7 years.

Side-effects Finasteride is well tolerated. Approximately 3% of patients will suffer impotence, loss of libido, and reduced ejaculatory volume, and patients should be warned of this before starting treatment. This is reversible if the treatment is discontinued. Breast enlargement or tenderness occurs in 1% of cases.

Proscar reduces serum PSA levels by 50% in patients with BPH, with or without prostate cancer. When evaluating the PSA of a patient who has been taking finasteride for 6 months or more, the PSA level should be doubled, to compare with the normal range for untreated men.

Phytotherapy

Phytotherapeutic agents are chemicals derived from plant extracts, and men have been taking a variety of these substances for their LUTS over many centuries. The fact that these 'natural remedies' have endured the test of time, and despite their expense are increasingly popular, is testament to their therapeutic potential, be this real or placebo. Evidence that these 'medicinal botanicals' are either safe or

efficacious is difficult to obtain. Phytotherapies vary enormously, different plant extracts are incorporated into different tablets, the extraction process is not standardized, and there is even variation within the same plant species.[23] The active ingredients are often not known; therefore, combining the appropriate substances at a therapeutic, but non-toxic, dose is haphazard.

Trials that have been undertaken are either small or not placebo-controlled, or do not show a statistically significant difference from placebo. *Serenoa repens* (saw palmetto) is the most widely used phytotherapeutic for BPO. Its mechanism of action is probably similar to that of finasteride, i.e. it inhibits 5α-reductase, although it may have other effects. In a placebo-controlled trial, Permixon®, an extract of the American dwarf palm tree berry (*Serenoa repens*), improved symptom and flow rate scores compared with placebo; however, at the end of the trial neither patient nor clinician could show a difference in satisfactory response between Permixon and placebo.[24] Another trial compared Permixon with finasteride in over 1000 men; both treatments improved symptom scores by nearly 40% and peak flow improved in the finasteride group by 3.2 ml/s and by 2.7 ml/s in the Permixon group, a significant difference.[25] The trial was not placebo-controlled and lasted only 6 months, and therefore has less impact.

Undoubtedly though, in in vivo and in vitro studies,[26,27] histologic changes including prostate epithelial contraction and gland atrophy occur in response to Permixon treatment; furthermore, the incidence of side-effects is low. *Serenoa repens* may yet prove, in randomized placebo-controlled trials, to be a safe and effective treatment for BPO.

Other phytotherapies used for BPH include *Pygeum africanum* (African plum), *Urtica dioica* (stinging nettle), and *Secale cereale* (rye pollen). To date, no long-term, placebo-controlled, double-blind trials have been performed to prove their efficacy and safety.

Surgical

Surgical treatments for BPH have been used since White performed bilateral orchidectomy on over 100 patients at the latter end of the 19th century. The first endoscopic prostatectomies were carried out in the 1930s, when the mortality from the procedure was 25%.[28] Since then, newer techniques have evolved: newer energy sources such as ultrasound, microwaves, and lasers; newer modes of delivering the energy such as loops, bands, needles, and transrectal probes, and, with the advent of fiberoptics, an improved light source. Despite these more recent developments, transurethral resection of the prostate (TURP) remains the gold standard with which all new technologies are compared.

TURP

In the National Health Survey of 1986, 96% of surgical procedures for BPH performed under the Medicare system in the USA were TURPs, and 350 000 TURPs were carried out that year. Despite an 80% increase in the diagnosis of BPH, fewer than 200 000 TURPs were performed a decade later.[29] This is because new guidelines were issued in the USA, recommending watchful waiting for patients with minimal symptoms, greater information for patients of the possible harmful effects of surgery, and a greater role for the patient in the decision-making process of which treatment modality should be adopted. Furthermore, alternative surgical treatments including vaporization, microwave, and laser prostatectomies were under development, and newer, safer, and more effective medical therapies became available. In Europe, although the number of TURPs performed is declining, the reduction is less dramatic. TURP can be performed under spinal, epidural, or general anesthesia, and involves passing a resectoscope up the urethra. A diathermy loop is used to cut and cauterize the hyperplastic tissue, while irrigating fluid maintains a clear surgical field. The prostatic chips are flushed out and sent for histologic examination.

Currently, 20% of patients with an obstructing prostate undergo TURP. TURP achieves a reduction in symptom score of 75%, an increased flow rate of 125% (absolute mean improvement of 9.7 ml/s), and a reoperation rate in the order of 2% per annum.[30]

Morbidity and mortality of TURP   The mortality from the procedure has improved from 25% in Alcock's paper of 1932[28] to virtually zero today.[30]

The morbidity likewise has decreased with advances in technology and experience. The transfusion rate is less than 8%[31] and frequency of surgery for urethral strictures and bladder neck stenoses is less than 5%. The transurethral resection syndrome remains a rare, but important complication. It is caused by absorption of irrigating fluid via the prostatic veins, and leads to hyponatremia and fluid overload resulting in fitting, coma, and, ultimately, death. During an average TURP lasting 40 minutes, 1–2 l of irrigant is absorbed, but for larger prostates or in inexperienced hands the operating time is prolonged, increasing the amount of fluid absorbed and the risk of developing the syndrome.

Retrograde ejaculation occurs in 65% of men after TURP.[30] This is because the bladder neck sphincter is resected during TURP and so semen is able to reflux into the bladder during ejaculation, rather than pass down the urethra. TURP, however, does not affect potency: in a large study of American war veterans, potency was no different after TURP when compared with an age-matched population.[32]

Open prostatectomy

Open prostatectomy is reserved nowadays for patients with large prostates in whom sufficient resection would not be achieved in the time available to perform a TURP. Likewise, patients who have a large bladder stone may also undergo this procedure, as the stone and BPH can be treated under one anesthetic. Open prostatectomy is an effective treatment, reducing the symptom score by 88% and increasing the flow rate by 230%. However, the morbidity and mortality associated with an open procedure and the prolonged hospital stay mean this is now used only for men with very large prostates (>100 ml).

Transurethral vaporization of the prostate

Transurethral vaporization of the prostate was developed in an attempt to reduce blood loss. Vaporization employs a rollerball through which electric current passes to heat the prostate to over

100°C. This high temperature vaporizes intracellular water, and the cells explode leaving an immediate tissue defect. Blood loss and the incidence of transurethral resection syndrome are reduced, and it has follow-up symptom and flow rate scores equivalent to those of TURP in moderate-sized glands, after 3 years.[33] Some men suffer with prolonged irritative symptoms, particularly dysuria. Attempts are being made to combine the hemostatic properties of the electrovaporizing technique with the cutting abilities of the TURP loop – 'adding more gold to the gold standard'.[34] A resecting loop with similar cutting abilities to the TURP loop but with an increased contact area for coagulation is being developed. However, to date, the results of this band loop have failed to meet expectations, with no significant reduction in blood loss[35] when compared with TURP.

Lasers

Lasers are used more and more and in a greater variety of ways in the urinary tract, whether to treat ureteric stones, to resect bladder tumors or in surgery for BPH. They offer a precise cutting tool that is hemostatic; this makes them ideal for prostate surgery. They are used to heat the prostatic adenoma either under direct vision (visual laser ablation, VLAP) or with ultrasound guidance (transurethral laser incision of the prostate, TULIP). In both these prostate-ablating procedures the BPH undergoes coagulative necrosis and then sloughs off; tissue is not excised at the time of the procedure. Patients may therefore have prolonged periods of catheterization and frequently suffer from perineal and urethral pain.

Lasers are also used to excise prostatic tissue. Holmium laser resection and enucleation (HoLRP and HoLEP) involve cutting the prostate into wedges like the segments of an orange. The wedges are flushed into the bladder, fragmented with a tissue morcellater, and removed. As the whole adenoma is excised, the symptom and flow rate improvements are even better than with TURP; furthermore, the hemostatic property of the laser not only reduces blood loss but also allows patients on anticoagulant therapy to continue their

treatment. Although some fine-tuning is required before this kit is optimized, HoLEP is likely to replace TURP as the gold standard surgical treatment for BPH within the next decade.

High-intensity focused ultrasound

High-intensity focused ultrasound is a technique that, without any direct contact, ablates the prostate. A probe is passed into the rectum, and ultrasound waves are focused to heat the prostate to 80–200°C without damaging adjacent structures. There is no direct urethral trauma; this limits postoperative dysuria and theoretically urethral strictures. Early data were promising; significant improvements in both symptom score and flow rates were reported in the short term. The longer-term results, however, were disappointing; the symptoms and flow rate improvements were not sustained.[36] Consequently, this technique is no longer used in the treatment of BPH.

However, it is being adapted for use in prostate cancer for patients in whom radical treatment is inappropriate.

Transurethral microwave thermotherapy

Low- and high-energy microwave thermotherapy has been employed to heat the prostate either transurethrally or via a probe inserted through the rectum. The advantage of this technique is that it can be performed under local anesthesia as a day case, as there is minimal blood loss. It is therefore preferred for patients with significant comorbidity. The symptom score improvements are reasonable over the short term; however, two-thirds of patients require supplementary BPH treatment, the flow rate improvements are small, and the duration of catheterization is often prolonged.[30]

Transurethral needle ablation

Transurethral needle ablation (TUNA) involves inserting two antennae into the prostate transurethrally; these emit radiofrequency waves that heat the prostate to 60–90°C, without heating adjacent structures. As a result the pain-sensitive prostatic urethra is preserved, intraoperative pain is reduced, and the procedure can be performed under local anesthesia. Moreover, postoperative irritative symptoms and retention are also reduced.

The blood loss is negligible, although some patients complain of irritative symptoms; these usually resolve in a matter of a few weeks after surgery. Roehrborn and colleagues[37] demonstrated that TUNA improved urodynamic parameters, although these improvements did not predict the degree of symptomatic response in either their TUNA or their TURP group. In an earlier study from the same institution, the authors demonstrated that TUNA was well tolerated, and provided substantive and lasting improvements in symptom score, flow rates, and quality of life over 1 year.[38]

Summary

Benign prostatic hyperplasia has a significant effect on men's quality of life in middle and old age. For some men the symptoms are of minor inconvenience, for others BPO and its complications have a profound effect on their own lives and the lives of those around them.

In the future, research will improve our understanding of the pathophysiology, and with this knowledge will come progress in our pharmacologic management of BPH. Advances in surgical techniques will reduce the incidence of complications and further improve symptom and flow rate scores. Improved patient education and a greater role for patients in the decision-making process will enable more men to obtain a better quality of life.

References

1. Carter HB, Coffey DS. The prostate: an increasing medical problem. Prostate 1990; 16: 39–48.
2. Abrams P, Schulman C, Vaage S, and the European Tamsulosin Study Group. Tamsulosin, a selective α_{1C}-adrenoceptor antagonist; a randomised controlled trial in patients with benign prostatic 'obstruction' (symptomatic BPH). Br J Urol 1995; 76: 325–36.
3. Chyou PH, Nomura AM, Stemmermann GN, Hankin JH. A prospective study of alcohol, diet and other lifestyle factors in relation to obstructive uropathy. Prostate 1993; 22: 253–64.
4. Imperato-McGinley J, Guerrero L, Gautler T et al. Steroid 5α-reductase in man: an inherited form of pseudohermaphroditism. Science 1974; 186: 1213–15.
5. Birkoff J, Wiederhorn A, Hamilton M, Xinsser H. Natural history of benign prostate hypertrophy and acute urinary retention. Urology 1976; 7: 48–52.
6. Holtegrewe HL, Valk WL. Factors influencing the mortality and morbidity of transurethral prostatectomy: a study of 2015 cases. J Urol 1962; 87: 450–9.
7. Lepor H, Williford WO, Barry MJ et al. The efficacy of terazosin, finasteride or both in benign prostatic hyperplasia. Veterans Affairs Co-operative Studies Benign Prostatic Hyperplasia Study Group. N Engl J Med 1996; 335: 533–9.
8. Caine M, Perlberg S, Meretyk S. A placebo controlled double-blind study of the effect of phenoxybenzamine in benign prostatic obstruction. Br J Urol 1978; 50: 551–6.
9. Thien T, Delaere KP, Debruyne FM, Koene RA. Urinary incontinence caused by prazosin. BMJ 1978; 2: 622–3.
10. Caine M, Raz S, Ziegler M. Adrenergic and cholinergic receptors in the human prostate capsule and bladder neck. Br J Urol 1975; 47: 193–202.
11. Hedlund H, Andersson K-E, Ek A. Effects of prazosin in patients with benign prostatic obstruction. J Urol 1983; 130: 275–8.
12. McGrath JC. Evidence for more than one type of postjunctional-adrenoceptor. Biochem Pharmacol 1982; 31: 467–84.
13. Chapple CR. Pharmacotherapy for benign prostatic hyperplasia – the potential for α_1-adrenoceptor subtype specific blockade. Br J Urol 1998; 81(Suppl 1): 34–47.
14. Jardin A, Bensadoun H, Delauche Cavallier MC, Attali P. Alfuzosin for treatment of benign prostatic hypertrophy. The BPH-ALF Group. Lancet 1991; 337: 1457–61.
15. Kirby RS. Doxazocin in benign prostatic hyperplasia: effects on blood pressure and urinary flow in normotensive and hypertensive men. Urology 1995; 46: 182–6.
16. Hunter J. Observations on Certain Parts of the Animal Oeconomy, 1st edn. London: Biblioteche Osteriana, 1786: 38–9.
17. White JW. Results of double castration on hypertrophy of the prostate. Ann Surg 1895; 25: 1–59.
18. Farnsworth WE, Brown JR. Testosterone metabolism in the prostate. Natl Cancer Inst Monogr 1963; 12: 323–5.
19. Andersen KM, Liao S. Selective retention of dihydrotestosterone by prostatic nuclei. Nature (London) 1968; 219: 227–79.
20. Stoner E and the Finasteride Study Group. The clinical effects of a 5 alpha-reductase inhibitor,

finasteride, on benign prostatic hyperplasia. J Urol 1992; 147: 1298–302.

21. Andersen J-T, Ekman P, Wolff H et al, and the Scandinavian BPH Study Group. Can finasteride reverse the progress of benign prostatic hyperplasia? A two-year placebo-controlled study. Urology 1995; 46: 631–7.

22. McConnell JD, Bruskewitz R, Walsh PC et al. The effect of finasteride on the risk of acute urinary retention and the need for surgical treatment among men with benign prostatic hyperplasia. Finasteride Long-Term Efficacy and Safety Study Group. N Engl J Med 1998; 338: 557–63.

23. Dreikorn K, Borkowski A, Braeckman J et al. Other medical therapies. In: Denis L, Griffiths K, Murphy G, eds. Proceedings of the Fourth International Consultation on Benign Prostatic Hyperplasia (BPH), July 1997. Plymouth, UK: Health Publications, 1998: 635–59.

24. Descotes JL, Rambeaud JJ, Deschaseaux P et al. Placebo-controlled evaluation of the efficacy and tolerability of Permixon® in benign prostatic hyperplasia after exclusion of placebo responders. Clin Drug Invest 1995; 9: 291–7.

25. Carraro JC, Raynaud JP, Koch G et al. Comparsion of phytotherapy (Permixon®) with finasteride in the treatment of benign prostatic hyperplasia: a randomised international study of 1089 patients. Prostate 1996; 29: 231–40.

26. Marks LS, Partin AW, Epstein JI et al. Effects of saw palmetto herbal blend in men with symptomatic benign prostatic hyperplasia. J Urol 2000; 163: 1451–6.

27. Bayne CW, Donnelly F, Ross M, Habib FK. Serenoa repens (Permixon): a 5 alpha-reductase type I and II inhibitor – new evidence in a coculture model of BPH. Prostate 1999; 40: 232–41.

28. Alcock NG. Ten months' experience with transurethral prostate resection. J Urol 1932; 28: 545–60.

29. Mebust WK. Transurethral surgery. In: Walsh PC, Retik AB, Vaughan ED, Wein AJ, eds. Cambell's Urology, 7th edn. Philidelphia, PA: WB Saunders Co, 1998: Ch 49.

30. Madersbacher S, Marberger M. Is transurethral resection of the prostate still justified? Br J Urol 1999; 83: 227–37.

31. Horninger W, Unterlechner H, Stasser H, Bartsch G. Transurethral prostatectomy: mortality and morbidity. Prostate 1996; 28: 195–200.

32. Wasson JH, Reda DJ, Bruskewitz RC et al. The Veterans Affairs Co-operative Study Group on transurethral resection of the prostate. A comparison of transurethral surgery with watchful waiting for moderate symptoms of benign prostatic hyperplasia. N Engl J Med 1995; 332: 75–9.

33. Hammadeh MY, Madaan S, Singh M, Philp T. A 3-year follow-up of a prospective randomised trial comparing transurethral electrovaporization of the prostate with standard transurethral prostatectomy. Br J Urol Int 2000; 86: 648–51.

34. Patal A, Fuchs GJ, Gutierrez-Aceves J, Andrade-Perez F. Transurethral electrovaporization and vapour-resection of the prostate: an appraisal of possible electrosurgical alternatives to regular loop resection. Br J Urol Int 2000; 85(Suppl 2): 202–10.

35. Cynk M, Woodhams H, Mostafid H et al. A prospective randomised controlled trial comparing Vaportome prostatic resection with TURP. Br J Urol Int 1999; 83(Suppl 4): 6.

36. Madersbacher S, Schatzl G, Djavan B et al. Long-term outcome of transrectal high intensity focused ultrasound therapy for benign prostatic hyperplasia. Eur Urol 2000; 37: 687–94.

37. Roehrborn CG, Burkhard FC, Bruskewitz RC et al. The effects of transurethral needle ablation and resection of the prostate on the pressure flow urodynamic parameters: analysis of the United States randomised study. J Urol 1999; 162: 92–7.

38. Roehrborn CG, Issa MM, Bruskewitz RC et al. Transurethral needle ablation for benign prostatic hyperplasia: 12-month results of a prospective, multicenter US study. Urology 1998; 51: 415–21.

CHAPTER 10

Prostate cancer

Michaël Peyromaure, Vincent Ravery, and Laurent Boccon-Gibod

Introduction

Prostate cancer is the most common malignancy and the second leading cause of cancer mortality in males. Traditionally, prostate cancer was considered as a disease of the aging male, and this may be partly responsible for the delay in diagnosis and management. With the use of prostate-specific antigen (PSA) testing in screening programs, prostate cancer is being diagnosed at an earlier age and stage.

The increasing number of low-staged cancers in young men has led to the development of curative treatments. In males whose life expectancy is above 10 years, radical prostatectomy is the standard curative therapy when the tumor is organ-confined. However, impotence is a frequent long-term complication of surgery that impairs the patient's quality of life. Therefore, attention is focused on decreasing morbidity related to surgical treatment and developing alternative therapies such as external radiotherapy and brachytherapy. For locally advanced tumors various approaches, including combination treatments, are available. In metastatic disease the management remains palliative, and is based on hormonal therapy and chemotherapy. In elderly men whose survival is not expected to be improved by curative therapy, watchful waiting and deferred treatment if necessary is the standard approach for localized tumors.

Epidemiology

In Europe and the USA, prostate carcinoma represents the most common cancer in males. Its incidence has rapidly increased since the 1970s because of the aging population and better diagnosis methods.[1] There are national and racial differences in the incidence of prostate cancer. In Asia, the incidence and mortality rates of prostate cancer are much lower than in Western countries.[2]

The geographic differences in the incidence of prostate neoplasia may be explained by genetic factors. Heredity seems to be the most important risk factor. Indeed, men with a family history of prostate cancer have a 4-fold increased risk of developing prostate cancer, and the risk is higher when two or more relatives are affected or when the affected relative is a brother.[3] Nevertheless, other findings suggest that prostate carcinogenesis depends partly on exogenous factors. When Asiatics move to the USA, their risk of having prostate cancer becomes similar to that of Americans after one generation.[4] Some lifestyle factors are believed to play a role in the occurrence of prostate cancer, but only few data, to date, are available in the literature. A high animal fat content in the diet may be one of the most important environmental factors related to prostatic carcinoma.[5] Other food components have been suggested to protect men from the risk of prosrate cancer, including soy, carotenoids, tomatoes, pumpkin, spinach, watermelon, citrus, and green tea.

Even though only 3% of patients will die of their prostate cancer, the overall mortality of the disease is very important because of its high prevalence. After lung cancer, prostate carcinoma is the second leading cause of death by cancer in males. Since the 1990s, the mortality rate of prostate cancer has been tending to decrease in Europe and the USA due to the detection of early stage tumors and to the improvement of curative treatments.

Detection

Since the 1980s, the wide use of the digital rectal examination (DRE) and PSA testing has resulted in an increased detection of prostate cancer. A DRE abnormality leads to prostate carcinoma diagnosis in more than 20% of cases, regardless of the physician's specialty. When performed in a population of asymptomatic men, DRE allows the detection of prostate cancer in 0.1–4% of males submitted to screening.[6]

The PSA level is a better independent predictor of prostate cancer than the DRE. Using a monoclonal antibody assay, the overall predictive value of PSA testing is approximately 30% when the PSA level is between 4 and 10 ng/ml, and more than 50% when the level is greater.[7] However, the threshold of PSA level to indicate a prostate biopsy remains uncertain. Some investigators suggest performing a prostate biopsy for a PSA level lower than 4 ng/ml. Recently, a 14.3% rate of prostate cancer detection has been reported among patients with PSA levels between 2 and 3.9 ng/ml when systematic prostate biopsies were performed regardless of DRE findings.[8]

Other PSA variables have been tested in an attempt to increase the predictive value of PSA, such as PSA density, PSA velocity, PSA doubling time, free PSA ratio, complexed PSA, BPSA ('benign PSA'), and pro PSA, the precursor form of PSA. Free PSA ratio is of particular interest when PSA is between 4 and 10 ng/ml.[9] Indeed, free PSA ratio has been proved to be significantly lower in prostate cancer than in benign prostatic hyperplasia. The use of free PSA ratio is recommended when PSA is in the intermediate range (4–10 ng/ml) and when the DRE is normal. However, the threshold value of free PSA ratio that may optimize the specificity of total PSA testing remains unknown.[10] Complexed PSA, BPSA, and pro PSA seem to optimize the sensitivity and specificity of PSA for the detection of prostate cancer. However, only few data are available regarding their clinical impact, and these markers are still under investigation.

Performing a prostate biopsy is the standard way to prove the presence of cancer and to obtain a cytologic grading. Biopsy cores are guided by ultrasound, and can be carried out without anesthesia in an outpatient setting. Bleeding complications occur in approximatively 70% of patients.[11] Hematuria, hematospermia, and rectal bleeding are the most common complications. The rate of acute prostatitis is less than 2% when an antibiotic and a rectal enema are given prior to the biopsy. Major complications requiring hospital admission are exceptional. The optimum number of biopsy cores for cancer detection is controversial. The standard number of cores is six, but several studies indicate that performing 10 or 12 core biopsies may improve the detection rate of prostate cancer by 6–35%, without increasing the biopsy-related morbidity.[12–14]

Recently, attention has been focused on the potential role of prostate saturation biopsy, which consists in performing an extended number of biopsy cores (up to 36). This technique may be useful in patients with previous negative biopsies and with a persistent suspicion of prostate cancer. It can be also used to improve the characterization of low volume, well-differentiated tumor in patients with a diagnosis of potentially insignificant microfocal prostate cancer, as defined by 1 single focus positive core with less than 5 mm of Gleason score ≤ 6 tumor on primary biopsy.

Staging

Local staging (T-staging) of prostate carcinoma is of particular interest in patients with a life expectancy of 10 years or more. Indeed, the intent of treatment in these patients is curative only in the case of organ-confined disease. Although serum PSA level increases with local stage, its ability to predict the final pathologic stage is limited when used as an individual parameter. In contrast, the combination of PSA, DRE, cytologic grade (Gleason score), and percentage of positive biopsy cores has been proved to be predictive of local extension.[15] Some nomograms can be used to predict the risk of extracapsular extension. These nomograms include various parameters, the most significant being clinical stage of cancer, PSA, and Gleason score on biopsy. Endorectal ultrasonography and/or endorectal magnetic resonance imaging (MRI) may be useful in addition to clinical and cytologic parameters to assess local invasion, particularly in cases of seminal vesicle involvement and significant capsular effraction. The sensitivity of endorectal MRI for the detection of extracapsular extension varies between 60 and 75%.

Nodal staging (N-staging) should be performed only when curative treatment is planned. The combination of PSA and biopsy findings has a predictive value for N-staging. Other useful factors to detect nodal metastases are computed tomography (CT) scan and endorectal MRI. The accuracy of endorectal MRI is at least equivalent to that of CT scan for N-staging. High-resolution endorectal MRI with magnetic nanoparticles has been reported to have a 100% sensitivity and a 96% specificity for the detection of nodal metastases.[16] Nodal metastases can also be detected by surgical open or laparoscopic lymphadenectomy. Regarding the risk of nodal involvement, three groups of patients have been identified: low risk (no biopsy core with Gleason > 3), moderate risk (≥ 1 core with Gleason > 3), and high risk (≥ 4 cores with Gleason > 3).[17] In the opinion of most authors, preoperative imaging by CT and/or MRI is not necessary in the low risk group.

Metastasis staging (M-staging) is important in patients whose disease is suspected to be advanced. The gold standard for M-staging is bone scintigraphy, since bone metastases are the most frequent occurrence. The presence of bone metastases is associated with poor prognosis, and can generate skeletal complications that impair quality of life. Serum PSA level is the best predictive parameter of bone metastases. A PSA level greater than 100 ng/ml has been reported to have a positive predictive value of 100%.[18] In contrast, the negative predictive value of a PSA level below 20 ng/ml is approximately 99%.[19] Bone scintigraphy is considered by most authors to be unnecessary when the pretreatment PSA level is <10 ng/ml and when the Gleason score of tumor is < 8.

Localized prostate cancer

Definitions and general considerations

'Clinically localized prostate cancers' are stage T1 and T2 cancers. Stage T1a and T1b cancers are incidental histologic findings after transurethral resection or open prostatectomy for benign prostatic hyperplasia. Stage T1a is defined as 5% or less of prostatic tissue involved in the cancer, while stage T1b is defined as more than 5% of tissue involved. The risk of tumor progression of untreated T1a prostate cancer is only 5% after 5 years, but increases up to 50% after 10 years.[20] The risk of tumor progression of untreated T1b is more than 80% after 5 years. Stage T1c cancers are clinically undetectable, and diagnosed by needle biopsy for PSA abnormality. The incidence of T1c prostate cancer has increased since PSA testing has become widely used. One study showed that 30% of T1c prostate cancers had an extraprostatic extension (locally advanced cancers).[21] Stage T2 cancers are clinically palpable and confined to the prostate. Stage T2a is defined as one abnormal lobe of the prostate, while T2b involves both lobes. Disease progression rates of untreated T2a and T2b carcinomas after 5 years are 40% and 75%, respectively.[22]

Three treatments have been proved to be efficient in eradicating localized prostate cancer: surgical removal of the prostate and vesical vesicles (radical prostatectomy), external beam radiotherapy, and interstitial radiotherapy. It is admitted that patients who will benefit from these treatments are those whose life expectancy exceeds 10 years. No benefit is expected in older patients who are likely to die from another disease.

Radical prostatectomy

Indications for radical prostatectomy are presumably curable tumors in patients whose life expectancy is above 10 years: localized tumors (T1, T2), PSA level < 10 ng/ml, Gleason score < 8, tissue core invaded by cancer ≤ 20%, and percentage of positive biopsies ≤ 50%.

Many experts consider radical prostatectomy to be the gold standard treatment in young patients having organ-confined disease. Open radical prostatectomy can be performed with a transperineal or a retropubic approach. Compared with the perineal approach, the retropubic approach is associated with a lower rate of positive surgical margins, especially in stage T2 cases.[23] Moreover, the retropubic approach allows simultaneous removal of pelvic lymph nodes. In recent years the laparoscopic approach for radical prostatectomy has been developed in most of the institutions. Although long-term data are lacking regarding the results of the laparoscopic approach, this technique seems to provide similar results to the open approach.

The complication rates of radical prostatectomy have considerably decreased over the last decade. Perioperative mortality, which is reported to be less than 1% in most series, is usually due to medical complications rather than surgical complications.[24] Major bleeding complications requiring blood transfusion and rectal injuries occur in less than 5% of patients. Urinary incontinence is common during the first weeks after intervention, but it decreases with time. The rates of persistent urinary incontinence depend on the definition of continence and the method of assessment. Moreover, they vary among institutions. However, those rates are usually inferior to 10% 2 years after surgery.[25] The most common and worrisome complication at long-term follow-up is impotence. At 12 months, the rates of erectile dysfunction vary between 30 and 70%.

Nerve-sparing techniques have been described to decrease the rate of postoperative impotence, leading to impotence rates inferior to 30% after 12 months.[26] However, a great proportion of 'potent' patients still need to use medical therapies to improve their sexual function. For some authors, the risk for local recurrence after nerve-sparing surgery is higher than after the standard procedure. Therefore, candidates for nerve-sparing radical prostatectomy should have low-staged and low-graded tumors. Other experts have reached opposite conclusions, and the impact of the nerve-sparing technique on the oncologic outcome remains a matter of debate.

Since the early 1990s, laparoscopic radical prostatectomy has been commonly performed in most of the urologic centers. The main difficulty of the laparoscopic procedure is its long learning curve. Compared with open surgery, the laparoscopic procedure has been reported to result in less morbidity, without increasing positive surgical margins and impotence.[27] However, further follow-up is needed to assess postoperative results. Recently, the use of a surgical robot has been shown to be feasible for laparoscopic radical prostatectomy. This technique may decrease the learning curve of laparoscopy. Moreover, for some authors the robot-assisted approach could improve the functional outcome.

Many studies have evaluated the results of radical prostatectomy, but only a few have been performed prospectively with a long follow-up. In most reports, surgical removal of the prostate has been shown to be curative in localized cancer, with an overall disease-free survival rate of greater than 60% within 10 years. For example, Han and colleagues from the Johns Hopkins Medical Institution reported the oncologic results of radical retropubic prostatectomy in 2091 patients.[28] The actuarial 15-year PSA recurrence-free survival was 61%, and the actuarial 15-year cancer-specific survival rate was 89%. More recently, Roehl reported a series of 3478 radical prostatectomies performed between 1983 and 2003.[29] Mean follow-up was 65 months. The 10-year progression-free survival was 79% for patients with pathologically localized tumors.

Follow-up after radical prostatectomy is based on PSA monitoring. PSA is expected to be undetectable within 3 weeks after radical prostatectomy. An increasing PSA level may indicate local recurrence or systemic recurrence. When PSA is still detectable, three parameters will help to distinguish between local recurrence and distant metastases: pathology, time to PSA elevation, and PSA doubling time. Positive surgical margins and/or undifferentiated tumors increase the risk of residual cancer and pelvic disease recurrence. A delayed and slowly increasing PSA level is generally due to residual local disease, while a rapidly increasing PSA rather indicates distant metastases.

Neoadjuvant hormonal therapy prior to radical prostatectomy

To improve the results of radical prostatectomy alone in prostate cancer, some authors have proposed giving hormonal therapy prior to prostate removal. Most of the published studies report a lower rate of positive surgical margins after surgery associated with androgen suppression than after surgery alone. However, the rate of PSA failure at long-term follow-up seems to be the same in both groups. Comparing radical prostatectomy alone with neoadjuvant complete androgen blockade followed by surgery for T2b tumors, Soloway and colleagues[30] found rates of PSA failure at 24 months of 21% in both groups. Similarly, Aus et al prospectively compared surgery alone with neoadjuvant hormone therapy followed by surgery in 126 patients with clinically localized prostate cancer.[31] Neoadjuvant therapy significantly reduced the rate of positive surgical margins, but not the PSA progression free survival. One study showed better local disease control achieved by neoadjuvant therapy. Evaluating the effects of a 3-month neoadjuvant treatment prior to radical prostatectomy, Schulman and associates[32] reported a decreased rate of positive surgical margins in the neoadjuvant hormonal therapy group, in T2 tumors as well as in T3 tumors. Moreover, when evaluating the local control rate at 4 years in T2 tumors, the local recurrence rate was significantly lower in the neoadjuvant therapy group than in the control group (3% versus 11%). This was not the case for T3 tumors. Even though local control may be, in the opinion of some authors, improved by neoadjuvant androgen deprivation, the question remains whether or not survival may be increased. To date, it remains impossible to answer this question because of insufficient published data. To date, neoadjuvant hormonal therapy prior to radical prostatectomy is not recommended in routine practice.

External radiation therapy

The curative indication of external radiotherapy is similar to that of radical prostatectomy: organ-confined cancer in patients with a life expectancy above 10 years. Radiotherapy is considered to result in lower rates of incontinence and erectile dysfunction than with radical prostatectomy. In a study comparing both treatments, some authors found a statistically lower rate of impotence related to external radiation than after surgery (41–55% versus 80–91%).[33] However, studies comparing sexual dysfunction after radiotherapy and nerve-sparing prostatectomy are lacking.

The major side-effects of conventional external radiotherapy are urinary irritative symptoms and bowel complications. Quality of life related to urinary problems seems to be worse after radiation at

2 years of follow-up than after radical prostatectomy.[34] One year after external radiotherapy, the rates of rectal urgency and bowel incontinence are 40% and 10%, respectively.[35]

To improve tumor targeting and to increase radiation intensity, three-dimensional conformal radiotherapy (3D-CRT) was developed in the mid-1990s. Bowel toxicity related to this technique has been reported to be significantly lower than that related to conventional radiotherapy. One year after radiation therapy, the rates of rectal urgency and bowel incontinence are 22% and 0%, respectively.[35] Although intestinal complications occur less frequently, quality of life and urinary symptoms do not seem to be improved by 3D-CRT.[35]

Oncologic results of external radiotherapy are similar to those of radical prostatectomy. After radiation or radical prostatectomy, the survival rate depends on clinical stage, initial PSA level, and Gleason score. For clinically localized cancer, the overall rate of disease-free survival after 10 years ranges between 43 and 70%.[36,37] Evaluating tumor response after 3D-CRT, Zelefsky and colleagues[38,39] reported that 93% of patients had no biochemical recurrence (PSA > 1 ng/ml) after 5 years, when the initial PSA level had been ≤ 10 ng/ml. This rate was 60% in patients with an initial PSA level between 10 and 20 ng/ml and 40% in those with a PSA level > 20 ng/ml. In some reports, results of 3D-CRT have been proved to be dose-dependent, especially for an initial level of PSA < 10 ng/ml.

After radiation therapy, PSA monitoring is more difficult than after prostatectomy, because of residual PSA levels related to residual prostatic tissue. The DRE cannot distinguish between local disease recurrence and radiation-induced fibrosis. The level of PSA nadir seems to be of particular importance. It has been reported that a better negative value of tumor progression was obtained with a PSA nadir below 0.5 ng/ml. Hanlon and colleagues showed that the predictors of improved cause-specific survival are a lower PSA nadir and a longer interval to nadir from the start of treatment.[40] In their study, the 8-year metastases-free survival rate was 96%, 89%, and 61% for PSA nadir values of ≤ 1 ng/ml, 1.1–2.0 ng/ml, and > 2.0 ng/ml, respectively.[40] The PSA nadir threshold remains controversial. For some authors, a PSA nadir below 1 ng/ml is associated with a low rate of disease recurrence within 5 years. Regardless of the actual PSA level, the kinetics of PSA levels seems to be informative. Most authors consider that three consecutive rises of PSA level after radiation are predictive of disease progression. In a study including 1650 patients subjected to external radiotherapy for prostate cancer, men with a PSA doubling time of 0 to 3 and 3 to 6 months demonstrated a 7.0 and 6.6% increased hazard of developing metastases or death, respectively, compared with patients with a PSA doubling time of more than 12 months.[41]

Interstitial radiotherapy (brachytherapy)

Interstitial radiotherapy consists of placing radioactive sources within the prostate, to deliver higher radiation doses without damaging surrounding tissues. Under anesthesia, radioactive seeds are placed using ultrasound guidance. Brachytherapy can be performed either with a high dose rate (HDR) for a short time or with a permanent low dose rate (LDR). HDR brachytherapy is usually used in combination with external radiotherapy in locally advanced tumors, while LDR brachytherapy may be indicated in organ-confined tumors (T1, T2). LDR brachytherapy is indicated in a curative intent. The most commonly used isotopes in LDR brachytherapy are iodine-125 and palladium-103. In some centers, the procedure is commonly performed on an outpatient basis. The operative time is about 2 hours. Compared with radical prostatectomy, the major advantage of brachytherapy is its low morbidity rate. Although irritative bladder symptoms are frequent within the first week, major complications are exceptional. Rectal toxicity (diarrhea, urgency, bleeding) depends on dosimetric parameters. Major rectal complications occur in less than 5% of patients.[42] At 12 months of follow-up, the urinary incontinence rate is reported to be 1%.[43] In high-volume institutions, the impotence rate varies between 50 and 80%.[43,44]

Previous transurethral surgery is a contraindication of interstitial radiotherapy because of an increased risk of postoperative incontinence.

Intermediate-term oncologic results of brachytherapy are similar to those of other curative treatments.

Potters and colleagues reported the results of prostate brachytherapy for clinically localized tumors in a series of 1449 patients.[45] In this study the median follow-up was 82 months. Overall and disease-specific survival at 12 years were 81% and 93%, respectively. Some studies have compared the oncologic results of permanent brachytherapy, radical prostatectomy, and external radiotherapy for localized prostate cancer. Most of these studies have shown similar results in terms of tumor recurrence and progression. Therefore, brachytherapy may be an alternative treatment to radical prostatectomy and external beam radiation. However, this therapy must be evaluated with longer follow-up. Today, some urologists remain cautious, and brachytherapy is not recommended when the PSA level is above 10 ng/ml and/or the Gleason score is above 7.

PSA monitoring after brachytherapy is difficult because of the long half-life of the isotopes. Using iodine-125, the PSA nadir may be expected after 4 years. A PSA threshold of 0.5 ng/ml is considered by most experts to be acceptable, but this threshold is still debated.

Watchful waiting

Watchful waiting/deferred treatment consists of a standpoint strategy until an active treatment may be required. Only patients with good compliance and easy access to health-care should be candidates for watchful waiting. The support for such management is based on the natural course of prostate cancer progression, which has been proved to be slow. Commonly, deferred treatment is indicated in asymptomatic old patients (life expectancy < 10 years because of age or debilitating conditions) with localized or locally advanced cancer. However, it is now suggested by some experts that watchful waiting can also be indicated in younger patients in very selected cases. Only patients with stage T1a and well or moderately differentiated tumors can benefit from deferred treatment. It is prudent to perform rebiopsy to avoid understaging of the tumor.

Chodak and colleagues[46] studied the results of watchful waiting in patients with clinically localized prostate cancer. The authors reported a correlation between survival rate and tumor grade. The overall 10-year disease-specific survival rate was 87% for grade 1 tumors, while it was 34% for grade 3 tumors. The 10-year metastasis-free survival rates for grade 1 and grade 3 tumors were 81% and 26%, respectively. When analyzing the outcome of T1a patients, Chodak and colleagues found cancer-specific 10-year survival rates with grade 1 and grade 2 tumors to be 96% and 94%, respectively.

More recently, Albertsen and co-workers reported the outcome of 767 men with clinically localized prostate cancer treated with either observation or immediate or delayed hormone therapy, with a median observation of 24 years.[47] In this study, the prostate cancer mortality rate was 33 per 1000 person-years during the first 15 years of follow-up, and 18 per 1000 person-years after 15 years. The mortality rates for these two follow-up periods were not statistically different, after adjusting for differences in tumor histology. Men with low-grade prostate cancers had a minimal risk of dying from prostate cancer during 20 years of follow-up (Gleason score of 2–4, 6 deaths per 1000 person-years). Men with high-grade prostate cancers had a high probability of dying from prostate cancer within 10 years of diagnosis (Gleason score of 8–10, 121 deaths per 1000 person-years). Men with a Gleason score of 5 or 6 had an intermediate risk of prostate cancer death. The authors concluded that the annual mortality rate from prostate cancer remains stable after 15 years from diagnosis, which does not support aggressive treatment for localized low-grade prostate cancer.

Although conservative treatment is admitted to be advantageous in elderly patients without symptoms, its indication in younger men remains controversial.

Prostatic intra-epithelial neoplasia and 'clinically insignificant' prostate cancer

Performing prostate biopsies for PSA elevation among patients with a clinically unapparent tumor has led to the identification of premalignant abnormalities: prostatic intra-epithelial neoplasia (PIN).[48] Although patients with high-grade PIN have a high risk of developing a carcinoma within 5 years, PIN is not considered to be an indication for radical treatment. Most authors recommend a rebiopsy in males presenting with PIN because of its

frequent association with prostate carcinoma. Indeed, in autopsy series, high-grade PIN is reported to be associated with prostate cancer in more than 40% of cases.[49,50]

The wide use of prostate biopsy has also resulted in the discovery of small and low-grade tumors (less than 3 mm in only one biopsy core and Gleason score ≤ 6), considered by some authors to be 'clinically insignificant'. In the opinion of these experts, the treatment of such tumors should be curative in young patients but should be deferred in asymptomatic patients whose life expectancy is less than 10 years. The significance of such 'clinically insignificant' prostate neoplasms is still a matter of debate. Indeed, it has been shown that approximately 30% of prostate carcinomas are understaged by biopsy.[51] Therefore, it seems dangerous to defer treatment in patients whose tumor may contain pathologic features more pejorative than those revealed by the biopsy. For some authors, the detection of a clinically insignificant prostate cancer by standard biopsy could represent an indication for saturation biopsy. Saturation biopsy consists in performing a repeat biopsy with an extended number of cores. This procedure could help to better determine the characteristics of the tumor (percentage of positive cores, cytologic grade).

Locally advanced prostate cancer

Definitions and general considerations
Locally advanced carcinomas are stage T3 and T4 cancers. Stage T3a is defined as capsular perforation and T3b as invasion of the seminal vesicles. T4 cancer is defined as extension to the surrounding organs (bladder and rectum). In the past, locally advanced cancers were more frequent than today and commonly treated by surgery. To date, it is universally admitted that patients with T4 tumors require palliative treatment. The management of T3 tumors is more controversial and may be curative in some patients without pejorative pathologic features.

Radical prostatectomy for T3 tumors
Compared with prostatectomy for T1–T2 prostate cancer, surgical removal of T3 carcinoma is associated

with an increased risk of positive surgical margins and local recurrence. A recent study has analyzed the outcome of 176 men who underwent radical retropubic prostatectomy for clinical stage T3 prostate cancer from 1983 to 2003.[52] Of the patients, 36% received neoadjuvant hormonal therapy. At a mean follow-up of 6.4 years, 48% of patients had disease recurrence with a median time to biochemical recurrence of 4.6 years. The actuarial 10-year probability of freedom from recurrence was 44%. Neoadjuvant hormonal therapy was not a significant predictor of biochemical recurrence. Overall the 5-, 10, and 15-year probabilities of death from prostate cancer were 6%, 15%, and 24%, respectively. In fact, some T3 prostate cancers are clinically overstaged, and pathologic examination of the radical specimen shows organ-confined tumor (pT2 stage). In the literature, the rate of clinical stage T3 tumors that are overstaged varies between 8 and 27%.[53] These findings support the curative intent of treatment in young patients with T3 cancer.

Radical prostatectomy may be an option for patients with locally advanced cancer, but a selected group needs to be individualized. Until further reports are available, it seems reasonable in the opinion of some authors to limit indications to T3aN0 tumors with PSA levels < 10 ng/ml.[54]

As for localized cancer, neoadjuvant hormonal therapy prior to radical prostatectomy in T3 cancer has been recently proposed, but no advantage of such combined therapy has been noted.

Postoperative radiotherapy for T3 tumors

After radical prostatectomy for organ-confined cancer, approximately 30% of specimens are found to contain foci of capsular effraction.[55] The risk of local recurrence without adjuvant therapy is considered to be 25–68%.[56] In such cases, postoperative radiotherapy has been proved to improve local disease control. In a study comparing radical prostatectomy alone and surgery plus adjuvant radiotherapy for T3 tumors, Valicenti and colleagues[57] reported rates of 5-year freedom from PSA relapse of 55% and 89%, respectively. Ansher and colleagues recently reported a series of 159 patients who underwent radical prostatectomy and were found to have

positive surgical margins, extracapsular extension, and/or seminal vesicle invasion.[58] Of these, 46 received adjuvant radiotherapy and 113 did not. The median time to failure in the surgery alone group was 7.5 versus 14.7 years in the radiotherapy group. Late recurrences were less common in the surgery alone group than in the radiotherapy group (9 and 1% at 10 and 15 years, respectively, versus 17 and 9%).

In the opinion of some authors, radiation therapy should be delayed until the PSA level rises and becomes >1 ng/ml.[55] Other authors consider that early adjuvant radiotherapy is more effective than salvage therapy for a rising PSA. To date, no benefit at long-term follow-up has been shown in published series. Further data are required to assess the benefit of postoperative radiation therapy in terms of survival.

Hormonal manipulation alone

Hormonal manipulation is the standard therapy for T4 tumors and T3 tumors with high risk of recurrence (elevated PSA and/or unfavorable histologic features). Many studies evaluating hormonal therapy alone in metastatic disease are available, but only a few with regard to locally advanced tumors. Consequently, the effectiveness of endocrine monotherapy in this latter indication remains unknown.

External radiotherapy combined with hormonal manipulation

In the past, radiation therapy alone was proposed not only for localized tumors but also for T3–T4 tumors. In stage T3 cancer, the overall 10-year survival rate and 10-year disease-free survival rate after radiotherapy alone have been reported to be 42% and 38%, respectively.[59] It is now admitted that radiation therapy alone is not the optimal treatment for locally advanced prostate cancer. Some authors suggest that hormonal therapy administered before and/or after radiation may improve the tumor response.

Bolla and associates[60] showed that 79% of patients with locally advanced prostate cancer treated by radiotherapy alone were local recurrence-free within 5 years, versus 97% of those treated by adjuvant hormonal blockade. The 5-year survival rate was 62% in the radiotherapy-alone group versus 78% in the combined group. In this study, the authors reported no increased morbidity when combination treatment was administered, even though hot flushes occurred in 33% of patients in the combined-treatment group.

More recently, the same team analyzed 415 patients treated with radiotherapy alone or radiotherapy plus immediate androgen suppression.[61] Five-year clinical disease-free survival was 40% in the radiotherapy-alone group and 74% in the combined-treatment group. Five-year overall survival was 62% and 78%, respectively, and 5-year specific survival 79% and 94%.

There is concern regarding the time when hormone therapy should be initiated. In another randomized study, Bolla and co-workers[62] compared the results of radiation therapy plus 3 years of adjuvant hormonal therapy with those of radiation therapy initially plus hormonal therapy only at disease recurrence, and found a better 5-year survival rate in the first group.

Deferred treatment

In the opinion of some experts, watchful waiting may be proposed in asymptomatic patients with locally advanced cancer and short life expectancy. This choice of therapy requires careful follow-up because of early occurrence of symptoms due to local disease progression.

Prostate cancer with nodal involvement or distant metastases

Hormonal therapy as first-line treatment

In the case of nodal involvement or distant metastases at diagnosis, treatment is palliative and comprises hormone therapy. Watchful waiting should be proposed only in exceptional cases of asymptomatic patients with very short life expectancy. Supported by the endocrine dependence of prostate cancer, hormonal therapy involves decreasing the level of testosterone. Hormonal manipulation is administered to reduce the tumor volume and the risk of progression, but it is not indicated for curative intent. Indeed, most prostate carcinomas become refractory to endocrine therapy after a median delay of 2 years. The mechanism of such hormonal resistance is not well known. Mutations of the androgen receptor gene may be responsible for the development of hormone independence.[63]

Surgical castration (bilateral orchiectomy) is an efficient way to eliminate the circulating level of testosterone and cause the prostate to atrophy. Surgical castration used to be the gold standard of hormonal therapy before medical castration became available. To date, orchiectomy is still widely performed because of its simplicity and reduced cost. A benefit in terms of time to tumor progression is obtained in approximately 80% of patients, with a mean duration of 2.5 years.[64] The main complications of bilateral orchiectomy are hot flushes, decreased libido, and erectile dysfunction, which occur in more than 70% of patients. Long-term adverse effects of androgen blockade are muscle atrophy, osteoporosis, gynecomastia, depression, and anemia.[65]

Luteinizing hormone releasing hormone analogs (LHRHas) have also been proved to be efficient in advanced prostate cancer. LHRHas decrease the secretion of luteinizing hormone (LH) and follicle stimulating hormone (FSH) from the pituitary via a biofeedback mechanism, and thereby reduce the level of testosterone. However, the initial rise in LH and FSH results in a transient (3–5 days) increase of circulating testosterone levels. In patients with potential bone metastasis, this 'flare-up phenomenon' may worsen symptoms, and should be prevented by the administration of an anti-androgen during the first weeks of therapy. In practice, LHRHas are administered every 3 months or monthly by injection. The results for survival and complications of LHRHas have been shown to be similar to those reported after bilateral orchiectomy.[66]

Estrogens represent an alternative hormone therapy. Estrogens block the secretion of LH and FSH by a feedback mechanism, and achieve medical castration. In the opinion of some investigators, decreased androgen synthesis may also be a direct effect of estrogen administration. In one of the largest series evaluating the effects of estrogen therapy on advanced prostate cancer, 5-year progression-free survival was 68%.[67] At a follow-up exceeding 60 months, the survival rate was 31%, and similar to that reported following orchiectomy. Estrogens can be administered either orally or parenterally. The major disadvantage of estrogen therapy is cardiovascular toxicity (venous thrombosis, pulmonary embolism, stroke, and heart attack).[68] The combined use of acetyl salicylic acid may reduce the rate of cardiovascular complications.

Anti-androgens block the action of androgens within intraprostatic cells. Anti-androgens can be administered either alone or in combination with surgical or medical castration (complete androgen blockade). Non-steroidal anti-androgens act only upon androgen receptors in cells, while steroidal androgens also have effects upon the pituitary gland. Non-steroidal androgens tend to increase the serum testosterone level, whereas steroidal anti-androgens lower levels of testosterone and LH, which may induce loss of libido and erectile dysfunction.[69] In patients with locally advanced cancer, there are no published data that support the advantage of complete androgen blockade compared with anti-androgen monotherapy. There are differences in side-effects with various anti-androgens when taken alone.[70] Flutamide induces mainly diarrhea, hepatic dysfunction, and breast tenderness. The main side-effects of nilutamide are visual disturbances, respiratory disturbance, and hepatic dysfunction. Gynecomastia and breast pain are noted using bicalutamide.[70]

Few studies have evaluated results of androgen blockade with long-term follow-up. Because of the outcome of hormonal independence, progression-free survival rates at 5 years are estimated to be less than 70%. According to the literature, approximately one-third of patients with advanced prostate cancer are still alive 5 years after the beginning of hormonal manipulation.[67]

To prevent early androgen independence, some authors propose beginning hormonal therapy at the time of symptom presentation instead of at the time of diagnosis. To date, no randomized study has shown any benefit in terms of survival and quality of life from delayed versus early treatment.

Intermittent hormonal therapy

The goals of intermittent hormonal manipulation are to prolong survival by delaying progression to androgen independence and to improve quality of life by avoiding the side-effects of continuous androgen deprivation. Intermittent hormonal therapy has been evaluated in a few studies, either with LHRHa alone or with complete androgen blockade. Unfortunately, prospective randomized studies with long-term follow-up have not, to date, been published. This lack of data is responsible for controversies regarding intermittent androgen suppression. In the opinion of experts who recommend such intermittent treatment, periods of 6–9 months on therapy are usually necessary, and the mean off-therapy intervals are approximately 50% of this duration.

De Leval and colleagues compared the efficacy of total intermittent androgen deprivation with total continuous androgen deprivation in 68 patients with advanced prostate cancer.[71] Median cycle length and percentage of time off therapy were 9 months and 59.5, respectively. The estimated 3-year progression rate was significantly lower in the intermittent therapy group (7.0%) than in the continuous therapy group (38.9%).

Sato and co-workers analyzed the effect of intermittent androgen suppression on the changes in quality of life in 49 patients with locally advanced or metastatic prostate cancer.[72] They found that quality of life remarkably improved during the off-treatment periods. However, only few data are available regarding the oncologic and functional results of intermittent hormonal therapy. To date, the benefit of such therapy remains unknown. Moreover, the optimal treatment and the PSA threshold to stop and start hormonal treatment have not been determined.

After radical prostatectomy

In the opinion of most urologists, adjuvant treatment by androgen suppression may be advocated in patients who are found to have nodal involvement after radical prostatectomy. Although no prospective randomized study to date has evaluated the impact upon survival of such a treatment, it seems reasonable to propose androgen suppression when disease is found to have nodal involvement. Indeed, it has been proved that nodal involvement is associated with a high risk of local recurrence and distant metastases. Immediate adjuvant surgical castration has shown a 10-year cancer-specific survival rate of 80%.[73] Conflicting data exist regarding the time to initiate neoadjuvant hormonal therapy: some authors suggest that early hormone therapy should be advantageous, while others recommend delayed treatment.

Androgen-independent cancer

About 10% of prostate cancers are androgen-independent at diagnosis, and more than 80% become androgen-independent after a mean hormonal treatment period of 2 years.[68] When tumor progression occurs despite endocrine deprivation, it is essential to document the castration levels of testosterone.

If the serum testosterone level is not decreased, optimized hormonal therapy is indicated to improve castration. Incomplete androgen blockade should be completed by the combination of LHRHa or surgical castration and an anti-androgen. The dose of anti-androgen should be increased when using an anti-androgen that achieves a dose-dependent response.

If the serum testosterone is at a minimal level, there is evidence that the cancer has become hormone-independent and requires a second-line treatment. Some clinical and biochemical responses have been described with discontinued anti-androgen therapy. The mechanism of this phenomenon, called the 'anti-androgen withdrawal syndrome,' remains unknown, but androgen receptor mutations are suspected.[74] There are no published data dealing with the efficacy of discontinued anti-androgens. What is known is that a few patients with hormone-independent cancer will show a brief response when stopping anti-androgens. This suggests that discontinued treatment should be tested before proposing chemotherapy. Secondary hormonal therapy using estrogens with corticosteroids or anti-androgens at high dose is an alternative.

Chemotherapy is indicated when prostate cancer becomes refractory to other treatments. No single chemotherapeutic agent has been demonstrated to provide a survival benefit, but several studies have suggested a synergy effect when chemotherapy is combined with other drugs.[75]

In recent years, attention has been focused on a new agent for the treatment of advanced prostate cancer, docetaxel. Several trials have shown that docetaxel improves survival of patients with hormone-refractory cancer. For example, Petrylak and colleagues compared the effectiveness of docetaxel and estramucine with that of mitoxantrone and prednisone for advanced refractory prostate cancer.[76] Each specimen was given in 21-day cycles: 280 mg of estramustine three times daily on days 1 through 5, 60 mg of docetaxel per square meter of body surface area on day 2, and 60 mg of dexamethasone in three divided doses before docetaxel, or 12 mg of mitoxantrone per square meter on day 1 plus 5 mg of prednisone twice daily; 338 patients were assigned to receive docetaxel and estramustine, and 336 to receive mitoxantrone and prednisone. The median overall survival was longer in the group given docetaxel and estramustine (17.5 months versus 15.6 months). The median time to progression was 6.3 months in the group given docetaxel and estramustine, versus 3.2 months in the other group. In another study, 130 patients were randomly assigned to receive docetaxel and estramustine or mitoxantrone.[77] All patients received prednisone. Overall survival was better in the docetaxel arms (18.6 and 18.4 months) compared with the mitoxantrone arm (13.4 months). Over the last decade, docetaxel demonstrated clinical benefit in androgen-independent prostate cancer. It is now admitted that docetaxel represents the new standard of care for hormone-refractory prostate cancer.[78]

Attention is also focused on new cytotoxic agents. Growth factor inhibitors have been proved to decrease the proliferation of prostate cancer cells in vitro, but further evaluation by clinical trials is required. For example, the combination of suramin plus hydrocortisone has been shown to be advantageous when compared with placebo plus hydrocortisone in a multicenter, double-blind phase III study.[79]

Radioisotopes such as strontium-89 and samarium-153 may be useful in decreasing pain related to bone metastases. The use of parenteral radioisotopes is reported to achieve a clinical response in approximately 70% of patients. The use of zoledronic acid, a new bisphosphonate, decreases bone pain and the risk of skeletal complications in patients with bone metastases.[80]

Prostate cancer and the aging male

General considerations

In the opinion of most authors, it is not suitable to perform prostate biopsies when localized cancer is suspected (PSA < 10 ng/ml) in elderly men, because the natural course of the disease without treatment is expected to be longer than the patient's life expectancy. Patients over 75 years old are considered to have a life expectancy below 10 years, and therefore to receive no benefit from curative therapies.

However, randomized studies dealing with quality of life and survival in elderly patients, comparing watchful waiting or hormonal manipulation versus curative treatment, have not been performed. With increasing longevity, it should be questioned whether elderly men should be diagnosed and treated like younger patients.

Deferred treatment

Deferred treatment is widely accepted, as it is felt that this approach may not compromise survival. Gronberg and colleagues[81] reported a direct influence of age on the loss of life expectancy. These authors also underlined the difference between relative survival and loss of life expectancy, the latter signifying the absolute effect of prostate cancer. In their series, relative survival was the same for all age groups if adjusted for cancer grade. However, the loss of life expectancy varied among age groups. For grade 1 tumors, the loss was 11 years for the younger group and only 1.2 years for the older group.[82] These authors suggest that patients with well and moderately differentiated clinically localized prostate cancer, with a life expectancy of 10 years or less, can be safely monitored and treatment deferred until progression. Early treatment, usually hormonal, at the time of local or systemic progression results in a better quality of life than delaying treatment until symptomatic progression.

Analysis of the literature suggests that deferred treatment may be appropriate in elderly patients with PSA < 10 ng/ml, Gleason score ≤ 6, good performance status, and reasonable life expectancy, in whom the risk for having disease-related symptoms is particularly low.

Radical prostatectomy

Kerr and Zincke[83] investigated the benefits of radical prostatectomy in men over 75 years old, by comparing two groups of patients (≤ 55 years and ≥ 75 years old) treated for clinically localized prostate cancer. In this series, elderly patients had higher-pathologic-stage and higher-grade tumors. Significant urinary incontinence occurred in 16% of the elderly compared with 3% of the younger patients at 1 year. This study confirmed that if well selected, these patients can have excellent survival, but that it is difficult to recommend such a surgical procedure owing to the high rate of incontinence, which significantly impairs quality of life.

A recent study compared health-related quality-of-life and survival of elderly men (aged 75 to 84 years) with localized prostate cancer who received aggressive treatment with those receiving conservative management.[84] At 2 years following diagnosis, aggressively treated men were significantly more likely to report daily urinary leakage and to be bothered by urinary problems and sexual problems. The adjusted disease-specific mortality hazard ratio was 0.43, favoring aggressive treatment. However, the absolute 5-year disease-specific survival difference was only 6% (98% versus 92%). Over 80% of all deaths were from other causes. The authors concluded that elderly patients who were aggressively treated for localized cancer had a minimally reduced risk of dying from prostate cancer. Therefore, physicians and old patients should consider these outcomes in making decisions about screening and treatment.

Andropause

Andropause, a syndrome in aging men, consists of physical, sexual, and psychologic symptoms that include weakness, reduced muscle and bone mass, sexual dysfunction, depression, anxiety, insomnia, and reduced cognitive function.[85] Andropause is associated with a low testosterone level. The free testosterone level begins to decline at a rate of 1% per year after age 40 years. It is estimated that 20% of men aged 60–80 years have levels below the lower limit of normal. Epidemiologic studies point toward an association with increased morbidity and mortality, with low testosterone states in aging males. For example, there is a higher prevalence of coronary heart disease, osteoporosis, fracture rates, frailty, and even dementia with low testosterone states.

The administration of testosterone results in clinical improvements. Most studies to date have focused on the physical benefits of testosterone replacement, and have failed to assess psychologic symptoms rigorously. Preliminary data suggest that therapy may benefit elderly men with new-onset depression. It remains unclear at what age such therapy should start and what monitoring should be performed.

Testosterone prescriptions have increased in recent years, partly because of the introduction of newer delivery systems that are topical, and have good bioavailability. In the USA alone, approximately 2 million prescriptions for testosterone were written in 2002.[86] This represents a 30% increase from 2001 and a 170% increase from 1999. There has also been a 500% increase in prescription sales in the past 10 years. The rise in prescriptions may be in part due to the increasing recognition of hypogonadism in aging males or andropause. Recently, there have been some concerns regarding the long-term safety of testosterone replacement therapy. The most worrisome problem of testosterone replacement is the potential risk for increased prostate cancer occurrence. According to some studies, there is no causal relationship between prostate cancer and physiologic dosing of testosterone, especially with careful selection and monitoring of patients. Further clinical investigations are necessary to evaluate the long-term risk for developing prostate cancer in men submitted to testosterone therapy.

References

1. McDavid K, Lee J, Fulton JP et al. Prostate cancer incidence and mortality rates and trends in the United States and Canada. Public Health Rep 2004; 119: 174–86.
2. Sim HG, Cheng CW. Changing demography of prostate cancer in Asia. Eur J Cancer 2005; 41: 834–45.
3. Negri E, Pelucchi C, Talamini R et al. Family history of cancer and the risk of prostate cancer and benign prostatic hyperplasia. Int J Cancer 2005; 114: 648–52.
4. Cook LS, Goldoft M, Scwhartz SM et al. Incidence of adenocarcinoma of the prostate in Asian immigrants to the United States and their descendants. J Urol 1999; 161: 152–5.
5. Denis L, Morton MS, Griffiths K. Diet and its preventive role in prostatic disease. Eur Urol 1999; 35: 377–87.
6. Pedersen KV, Carlsson P, Varenhorst E et al. Screening for carcinoma of the prostate by digital rectal examination in a randomly selected population. BMJ 1990; 300: 1041–4.
7. Haas GP, Montie JE, Pontes JE. The state of prostate cancer screening in the United States. Eur Urol 1993; 23: 337–47.
8. Raaijmakers R, Blijenberg BG, Finlay JA et al. Prostate cancer detection in the prostate specific antigen range of 2.0 to 3.9 ng/ml: value of percent free prostate specific antigen on tumor detection and tumor aggressiveness. J Urol 2004; 171: 2245–9.
9. Morote J, Encabo G, De Torres IM. Use of free prostate-specific antigen as a predictor of the pathological features of clinically localized prostate cancer. Eur Urol 2000; 38: 225–9.
10. Ravery V, Boccon-Gibod L. Free/total PSA ratio – hope and controversies. Eur Urol 1997; 31: 385–8.
11. Rodriguez LV, Terris MK. Risks and complications of transrectal ultrasound guided prostate needle biopsy: a prospective study and review of the literature. J Urol 1998; 160: 2115–20.
12. Levine MA, Ittman M, Melamed J, Lepor H. Two consecutive sets of transrectal ultrasound guided sextant biopsies of the prostate for the detection of prostate cancer. J Urol 1998; 159: 475–6.
13. Naughton CK, Ornstein DK, Smith DS, Catalona WJ. Pain and morbidity of transrectal ultrasound guided prostate biopsy: a prospective randomized trial of 6 versus 12 cores. J Urol 2000; 163: 168–71.
14. Ravery V, Goldblatt L, Royer B et al. Extensive biopsy protocol improves the detection rate of prostate cancer. J Urol 2000; 164: 393–6.
15. Partin AW, Yoo J, Pearson JD et al. The use of prostate specific antigen, clinical stage and Gleason score to predict pathological stage in men with localized prostate cancer. J Urol 1993; 150: 110–14.
16. Harisinghani MG, Barentsz J, Hahn PF et al. Noninvasive detection of clinically occult lymph-node metastases in prostate cancer. N Engl J Med 2003; 348: 2491–9.
17. Haese A, Epstein JE, Huland H et al. Validation of a biopsy-based pathologic algorithm for predicting lymph node metastases in patients with clinically localized prostate carcinoma. Cancer 2002; 95: 1016–21.
18. Rana A, Karamanis K, Lucal MG, Chisholm GD. Identification of metastatic disease by T category, Gleason score and serum PSA level in patients with carcinoma of the prostate. Br J Urol 1992; 69: 277–81.

19. Oesterling JE. Prostate-specific antigen: a critical assessment of the most useful tumour marker for adenocarcinoma of the prostate. J Urol 1991; 145: 907–23.

20. Lowe BA, Listrom MB. Incidental carcinoma of the prostate: an analysis of the predictors of progression. J Urol 1988; 140: 1340–4.

21. Oesterling JE, Suman VJ, Zincke H, Bostwick DG. PSA detected (clinical stage T1c or B0) prostate cancer: pathologically significant tumours. Urol Clin North Am 1993; 20: 687–93.

22. Graverson PH, Nielsson KT, Gasser TC et al. Radical prostatectomy versus expectant primary treatment in stages I and II prostatic cancer. A 15 year follow-up. Urology 1990; 36: 493–8.

23. Boccon-Gibod L, Ravery V, Vordos D et al. Radical prostatectomy for prostate cancer: the perineal approach increases the risk of surgically induced positive margins and capsular incisions. J Urol 1998; 160: 1383–5.

24. Konety BR, Allareddy V, Modak S et al. Mortality after major surgery for urologic cancers in specialized urology hospitals: are any better? J Clin Oncol 2006; 24: 2006–12.

25. Sacco E, Prayer-Galetti T, Pinto F et al. Urinary incontinence after radical prostatectomy: incidence by definition, risk factors and temporal trend in a large series with a long-term follow-up. BJU Int 2006; 97: 1234–41.

26. Gontero P, Kirby RS. Nerve-sparing radical retropubic prostatectomy: techniques and clinical considerations. Prostate Cancer Prostatic Dis 2005; 8: 133–9.

27. Touijer K, Guillonneau B. Laparoscopic radical prostatectomy: a critical analysis of surgical quality. Eur Urol 2006; 49: 625–32.

28. Han M, Partin AW, Zahurak M et al. Biochemical (prostate specific antigen) recurrence probability following radical prostatectomy for clinically localized prostate cancer. J Urol 2003; 169: 517–23.

29. Roehl KA, Han M, Ramos CG et al. Cancer progression and survival rates following anatomical radical retropubic prostatectomy in 3,478 consecutive patients: long-term results. J Urol 2004; 172: 910–14.

30. Soloway MS, Sharifi R, Wajsman Z et al. The Lupron Depot Neoadjuvant Prostate Cancer Study Group. Randomized prospective study comparing radical prostatectomy alone versus radical prostatectomy preceded by androgen blockade in clinical stage B2 (T2bNxM0) prostate cancer. J Urol 1995; 154: 424–8.

31. Aus G, Abrahamsson PA, Ahlgren G et al. Three-month neoadjuvant hormonal therapy before radical prostatectomy: a 7-year follow-up of a randomized controlled trial. BJU Int 2002; 90: 561–6.

32. Schulman CC, Debruyne F, Forster G et al. The European Study Group on Neoadjuvant Treatment of Prostate Cancer. 4-Year follow-up of a European prospective randomized study on neoadjuvant hormonal therapy prior to radical prostatectomy in T2–3N0M0 prostate cancer. Eur Urol 2000; 38: 706–13.

33. Madalinska JB, Essink-Bot ML, De Koning HJ et al. Health-related quality-of-life effects of radical prostatectomy and primary radiotherapy for screen-detected or clinically diagnosed localized prostate cancer. J Clin Oncol 2001; 19: 1587–8.

34. Lithin MS, Pasta DJ, Yu J et al. Urinary function and bother after radical prostatectomy or radiation for prostate cancer: a longitudinal, multi-variate quality of life analysis from the Cancer of the Prostate Strategic Urologic Research Endeavor. J Urol 2000; 164: 1973–7.

35. Hanlon AL, Natvinsbruner D, Peter R, Hanks GE. Quality of life study in prostate cancer patients treated with 3-dimensional conformal radiation therapy: comparing late bowel and bladder quality of life symptoms to that of the normal population. Int J Radiat Oncol Biol Phys 2001; 49: 51–9.

36. Fowler JE, Braswell NT, Pandey P, Seaver L. Experience with radical prostatectomy and radiation therapy for localized prostate cancer at a Veterans Affairs medical center. J Urol 1995; 153: 1026–31.

37. Krygiel JM, Smith DS, Homan SM et al. Intermediate term biochemical progression rates after radical prostatectomy and radiotherapy in patients with screen detected prostate cancer. J Urol 2005; 174: 126–30.

38. Zelefsky MJ, Wallner KE, Ling CC. Comparison of the 5-year outcome and morbidity of three-dimensional conformal radiotherapy versus transperineal permanent iodine-125 implantation for early-stage prostate cancer. J Clin Oncol 1999; 17: 517–22.

39. Zelefsky MJ, Lyass O, Fuks Z et al. Predictors of improved outcome for patients with localized prostate cancer treated with neoadjuvant androgen ablation therapy and three-dimensional conformal radiotherapy. J Clin Oncol 1998; 16: 3380–5.

40. Hanlon AL, Diratzouian H, Hanks GE. Posttreatment prostate-specific antigen nadir highly predictive of distant failure and death from prostate cancer. Int J Radiat Oncol Biol Phys 2002; 53: 297–303.

41. Zelefsky MJ, Ben-Porat L, Scher HI et al. Outcome predictors for the increasing PSA state after definitive external-beam radiotherapy for prostate cancer. J Clin Oncol 2005; 23: 826–31.

42. Shah JN, Ennis RD. Rectal toxicity profile after transperineal interstitial permanent prostate brachytherapy: use of a comprehensive toxicity scoring system and identification of rectal dosimetric toxicity predictors. Int J Radiat Oncol Biol Phys 2006; 64: 817–24.

43. Feigenberg SJ, Lee WR, Desilvio ML et al. Health-related quality of life in men receiving prostate brachytherapy on RTOG 98-05. Int J Radiat Oncol Biol Phys 2005; 62: 956–64.

44. Merrick GS, Butler WM, Galbreath AW et al. Erectile function after permanent prostate brachytherapy. Int J Radiat Oncol Biol Phys 2002; 52: 893–902.

45. Potters L, Morgenstern C, Calugaru E et al. 12-year outcomes following permanent prostate brachytherapy in patients with clinically localized prostate cancer. J Urol 2005; 173: 1562–6.

46. Chodak GW, Thisted RA, Gerber GS et al. Results of conservative management of clinically localized prostate cancer. N Engl J Med 1994; 330: 242–8.

47. Albertsen PC, Hanley JA, Fine J. 20-year outcomes following conservative management of clinically localized prostate cancer. JAMA 2005; 293: 2095–101.

48. Fowler JE Jr, Bigler SA, Lynch C et al. Prospective study of correlations between biopsy-detected high grade prostatic intraepithelial neoplasia, serum PSA concentration, and race. Cancer 2001; 91: 1291–6.

49. Netto GJ, Epstein JI. Widespread high-grade prostatic intraepithelial neoplasia on prostatic needle biopsy: a significant likelihood of subsequently diagnosed adenocarcinoma. Am J Surg Pathol 2006; 30: 1184–8.

50. Girasole CR, Cookson MS, Putzi MJ et al. Significance of apical and suspicious small cinar proliferations, and high grade prostatic intraepithelial neoplasia on prostate biopsy: implications for cancer detection and biopsy strategy. J Urol 2006; 175: 929–33.

51. Ravery V, Boccon-Gibod LI, Dauge-Geffroy MC et al. Systematic biopsies accurately predict extracapsular extension of prostate cancer and persistent/recurrent detectable PSA after radical prostatectomy. Urology 1994; 44: 371–6.

52. Carver BS, Bianco FJ Jr, Scardino PT et al. Long-term outcome following radical prostatectomy in men with clinical stage T3 prostate cancer. J Urol 2006; 176: 564–8.

53. Ward JF, Slezak JM, Blute ML et al. Radical prostatectomy for clinically advanced (cT3) prostate cancer since the advent of prostate-specific antigen testing: 15-year outcome. BJU Int 2005; 95: 751–6.

54. Van Poppel H, Goethuys H, Callewaert P et al. Radical prostatectomy can provide cure for well-selected clinical stage T3 prostate cancer. Eur Urol 2000; 38: 372–9.

55. Ravery V, Lamotte F, Hennequin C et al. Adjuvant radiation therapy for recurrent PSA after radical prostatectomy in T1–T2 cancer. Prostate Cancer Prostatic Dis 1998; 1: 321–5.

56. Zietman AL. Locally advanced or recurrent prostate cancer. In: Vogelzang NJ, Miles BJ, eds. Comprehensive Textbook of Genitourinary Oncology. Baltimore, MD: Williams & Wilkins, 1996: 782–90.

57. Valicenti RK, Gomella LG, Ismail M et al. The efficacy of early adjuvant radiation therapy for pT3N0 prostate cancer: a matched-pair analysis. Int J Radiat Oncol Biol Phys 1999; 45: 53–8.

58. Anscher MS, Clough R, Robertson CN et al. Timing and patterns of recurrences and deaths from prostate cancer following adjuvant pelvic radiotherapy for pathologic stage T3/4 adenocarcinoma of the prostate. Prostate Cancer Prostatic Dis 2006; 9: 254–60.

59. Perez CA, Hanks GE, Leibel SA et al. Localized carcinoma of the prostate (stages T1B, T1C, T2, and T3). Review of management with external beam radiation therapy. Cancer 1993; 72: 3156–73.

60. Bolla M, Gonzales D, Warde P et al. Improved survival in patients with locally advanced prostate cancer treated with radiotherapy and goserelin. N Engl J Med 1997; 337: 295–300.

61. Bolla M, Collette L, Blank L et al. Long-term results with immediate androgen suppression and external irradiation in patients with locally advanced prostate cancer (an EORTC study): a phase III randomised trial. Lancet 2002; 360: 103–6.

62. Bolla M, Collette L, Gonzales D et al. Long term results of immediate adjuvant hormonal therapy with goserelin in patients with locally advanced prostate cancer treated with radiotherapy (phase III EORTC study). Int J Radiat Oncol Biol Phys 1999; 45: 147.

63. Taplin ME, Rajeshkumar B, Halabi S et al. Androgen receptor mutations in androgen-independent prostate cancer: Cancer and Leukemia Group B Study 9663. J Clin Oncol 2003; 21: 2673–8.

64. Veterans Administration Cooperative Urological Research Group. Treatment and survival of patients with cancer of the prostate. Surg Gynecol Obstet 1967; 124: 1011–17.

65. Catalona WJ. Management of cancer of the prostate. N Engl J Med 1994; 331: 996–1004.

66. Peeling WB. Phase III studies to compare goserelin with orchidectomy and with diethylstilboestrol in treatment of prostatic carcinoma. Urology 1989; 33(Suppl 5): 45–52.

67. Haapiainen R, Ranniko S, Ruutu M. Orchiectomy versus oestrogen in the treatment of advanced prostate cancer. Br J Urol 1991; 67: 184–7.

68. Byar DP, Corle DK. Hormone therapy for prostate cancer: results of the Veterans Administration Cooperative Urological Research Group Studies. Natl Cancer Inst Monogr 1988; 7: 165–70.

69. Soloway MS, Matzkin H. Antiandrogenic agents as monotherapy in advanced prostatic carcinoma. Cancer 1993; 71: 1083–8.

70. Mason M. What implications do the tolerability profiles of antiandrogens and other commonly used

prostate cancer treatments have on patient care? J Cancer Res Clin Oncol 2006; 132(Suppl 13): 27–35.

71. De Leval J, Boca P, Yousef E et al. Intermittent versus continuous total androgen blockade in the treatment of patients with advanced hormone-naive prostate cancer: results of a prospective randomized multicenter trial. Clin Prostate Cancer 2002; 1: 163–71.

72. Sato N, Akakura K, Isaka S et al. Intermittent androgen suppression for locally advanced and metastatic prostate cancer: preliminary report of a prospective multicenter study. Urology 2004; 64: 341–5.

73. Zincke H. Hormonal treatment of stage D1 adenocarcinoma of prostate. Significant influences of immediate adjuvant hormonal treatment (orchiectomy) on outcome. Urology 1989; 33: 27–36.

74. Kelly WK, Scher HI. Prostate specific antigen decline after antiandrogen withdrawal syndrome. J Urol 1993; 149: 607–9.

75. Kamradt JM, Pienta KJ. Etoposide in prostate cancer. Expert Opin Pharmacother 2000; 1: 271–5.

76. Petrylak DP, Tangen CM, Hussain MH et al. Docetaxel and estramustine compared with mitoxantrone and prednisone for advanced refractory prostate cancer. N Engl J Med 2004; 351: 1513–20.

77. Oudard S, Banu E, Beuzeboc P et al. Multicenter randomized phase II study of two schedules of docetaxel, estramustine, and prednisone versus mitoxantrone plus prednisone in patients with metastatic hormone-refractory prostate cancer. J Clin Oncol 2005; 23: 3343–51.

78. Berry WR. The evolving role of chemotherapy in androgen-independent (hormone-refractory) prostate cancer. Urology 2005; 65: 2–7.

79. Small EJ, Meyer M, Marshall ME et al. Suramin therapy for patients with symptomatic hormone refractory prostate cancer: results of a randomized phase III trial comparing suramin plus hydrocortisone to placebo plus hydrocortisone. J Clin Oncol 2000; 18: 1440–50.

80. Ryan CW, Huo D, Demers LM et al. Zoledronic acid initiated during the first year of androgen deprivation therapy increases bone mineral density in patients with prostate cancer. J Urol 2006; 176: 972–8.

81. Gronberg H, Damber JE, Jonsson H, Lenner P. Patient age as a prognostic factor in prostate cancer. J Urol 1994; 152: 892–5.

82. Gronberg H, Berg HA, Damber JE et al. Prostate cancer in Northern Sweden. Incidence, survival and mortality in relation to tumour grade. Acta Oncol 1994; 33: 359–63.

83. Kerr LA, Zincke H. Radical retropubic prostatectomy for prostate cancer in the elderly and the young: complications and prognosis. Eur Urol 1994; 25: 305–12.

84. Penson DF, Hoffman RM, Barry MJ et al. Health outcomes in older men with localized prostate cancer: results from the Prostate Cancer Outcomes Study. Urol Oncol 2006; 24: 457.

85. Darby E, Anawalt BD. Male hypogonadism: an update on diagnosis and treatment. Treat Endocrinol 2005; 4: 293–309.

86. Tan RS, Salazar JA. Risks of testosterone replacement therapy in ageing men. Expert Opin Drug Saf 2004; 3: 599–606.

CHAPTER 11

Erectile dysfunction in the aging male

**Andrea Gallina, Alberto Briganti, Andrea Salonia, Federico Dehò,
Giuseppe Zanni, Pierre I Karakiewiz, and Francesco Montorsi**

Introduction

Erectile dysfunction (ED) is defined as the persistent inability to attain and/or maintain a penile erection sufficient to complete a satisfactory sexual intercourse. It was suggested that a 3-month minimum duration should be present for establishment of this diagnosis, except in some instances of trauma or surgically induced erectile dysfunction. The introduction of oral phosphodiesterase inhibitor therapy in 1998 was associated with a surge in resource use for erectile dysfunction (ED), as demonstrated by a 50% increase in physician office visits for ED in the last years.[1]

As the mean life expectancy is progressively increasing, we should expect a steady increase in the number of men reporting ED. However, ED becomes a matter of sufficient medical interest to lead to a search for an appropriate therapy only when it causes personal distress either to the patient himself or to the couple. This definition is critical when evaluations of the prevalence of ED are considered, especially in the aging man. In fact, even if it has been demonstrated that erectile function deteriorates progressively with aging, only a minority of patients who report some form of ED when questioned will request treatment.[2] The aim of this chapter is to review the data currently available on the epidemiology, pathophysiology, and management of ED.

Epidemiology of erectile dysfunction

In 1948 Kinsley et al provided the first description of the association between the aging male and ED.[3]

They demonstrated a decline in sexual activity and erectile function with aging. In that report the incidence of ED was 25% in 65-year-old men and 75% in men aged over 80 years. These historic findings have been confirmed in several recent studies. The National Health and Social Life Survey, which defined various types of sexual dysfunction in men and women, documented an ED incidence of 18% in men from 50 to 59 years old.[4] The initial report of the longitudinal Massachusetts Male Aging Study in 1290 men with ages ranging from 40 to 70 years old showed an incidence of ED in 52% of included subjects, with 10% of the study population experiencing severe ED.[5] Between subject ages of 40 and 70 years, the probability of complete ED tripled from 5.1 to 15%, while the probability of moderate ED doubled from 17 to 34%. Within the same age range, the probability of minimal ED remained constant at approximately 17%. An estimated 40% of the men included in the study were impotent at age 40 years, with an increase to 67% impotent men at age 70 years. Whenever age was tested by multivariate linear regression or multivariate analysis of variance in conjunction with another predictor of ED, age invariably proved to be an independent predictor.

More recently, in a large population-based study, Saigal et al found that, in men aged 20 and older, self-reported ED affected almost 1 in 5 respondents.[6] This prevalence dramatically increased with advanced age: 77.5% of men aged 75 or older reported some form of ED. In their multivariable analyses, addressing the presence of

ED, they found several associated medical conditions. Increasing age was the strongest predictor of ED. There was a constant increase in the odds of ED with each decade after the age of 40 years. After adjusting for other factors, men aged 60 to 69 years and men 70 years and older were, respectively, 9 and 30 times more likely to report ED, compared to young men, aged 20 to 29 years. Diabetes mellitus imparted the greatest increase in risk of all medical comorbidities included in the model. In addition, modifiable risk factors, such as obesity, hypertension, and smoking, were independently associated with ED. Similar results were obtained by Grover et al.[7] They analyzed a cross-sectional sample of 3921 men aged 40 to 88 years referring to primary care physicians. Using the International Index of Erectile Function (IIEF) questionnaire,[8] they recorded an overall prevalence of ED of 49%, defined as IIEF erectile function domain lower than 26. Moreover, they demonstrated that cardiovascular disease, diabetes, future coronary risk, undiagnosed hyperglycemia, metabolic syndrome, and impaired fasting glucose levels were independently associated with ED.

Currently, ED represents an important health problem both from the clinical as well as the public health perspective. Based on the projected aging of the population,[9] it may be anticipated that it will affect an even larger proportion of men in the 21st century.[10]

Pathophysiology of erectile dysfunction

Penile erection is a neurovascular phenomenon under psychologic control. Erections are usually classified as central, reflexogenic, and nocturnal erections. In central erections, an initial stimulus arising from supraspinal centers travels through the spinal cord and reaches the corpora cavernosa, traveling ultimately along the cavernous nerves. Terminal branches of the cavernous nerves release several neurotransmitters, which are involved in initiating the erectile process. In addition, endothelial cells lining the walls of the cavernous sinusoids release active mediators. Nitric oxide (NO), vasoactive intestinal polypeptide, acetylcholine, and a number of prostaglandins are considered the most important erectogenic neurotransmitters, which ultimately lead to relaxation of the smooth muscle cells within the walls of the penile arteries and sinusoids. Relaxation of the intracavernosal sinusoids leads to blood filling of the corpora cavernosa, with the subsequent compression of the subalbugineal venular plexus against the inner surface of the tunica albuginea, thus activating the veno-occlusive mechanism of the corpora cavernosa. When this mechanism is activated, blood is actually entrapped within the corpora cavernosa, which become an isovolumetric reservoir. Further arterial inflow then leads to an increase in intracorporeal pressure and to penile rigidity. When ejaculation and orgasm are achieved, norepinephrine is released by neural adrenergic fibers within the corpora cavernosa, and smooth muscle contraction is stimulated with subsequent penile detumescence.

The same cascade of events is also seen with reflexogenic erections, in which the triggering event is produced by mechanical stimulation of the dorsal nerve of the penis, which sends signals to the lumbosacral cord where synapses with parasympathetic fibers traveling back to the corpora cavernosa occur. The continuous stimulation of the penis occurring naturally during sexual intercourse contributes to maintain activation of the descending neural pathways to the corpora cavernosa, sustaining penile rigidity until ejaculation or cessation of stimulation.[11] Nocturnal erections occur during rapid eye movement (REM) sleep from intrauterine life to late senescence, and are still poorly understood. They are believed to represent a spontaneous mechanism for oxygenating the corpora cavernosa and maintaining the viability of cavernosal tissue.[12]

Abnormalities of erectile function have been traditionally classified as neurogenic (failure to initiate), arteriogenic (failure to fill), and venogenic (failure to store).[13] However, the term venogenic ED should be viewed as affecting the anatomy and histology of the corpus cavernosum, leading to alteration of the cavernous veno-occlusive mechanism. In addition, abnormalities of the sex hormone milieu may significantly affect the quality of penile erections, and this aspect has attracted much interest with regard to its role in the aging population. The process of aging may affect all the pillars of the erectile process including nerves, arteries, veins, cavernous tissue, and hormones. However, evidence in the literature of aging-induced damage to these structures has certainly been influenced by the availability of techniques for identifying certain types of damage, and this is why vascular and endocrinologic abnormalities affecting the male erectile system seem to play a leading role in this regard.

The process of aging is multifactorial in nature and dependent on several factors, including but not limited to metabolic rate, genetics, lifestyle, and environmental conditions.[14] Independently from the initiating factor, the ultimate common pathologic process is damage to smooth muscle cells and an increase in the accumulation of fibrosis, which decrease the vasodilator response. Age-related smooth muscle dysfunction has long been recognized in the respiratory,[15] gastrointestinal,[16] and cardiovascular[17] systems. Aging also affects the genitourinary tract and is associated with lower urinary tract symptoms (LUTS)[18] and sexual dysfunction[3–12] in both men and women.

The exact mechanism that links aging to smooth muscle dysfunction is not completely understood. Normal erectile function is a delicate balance between vasoconstricting and vasorelaxing mediators on corporal smooth muscle tone.[19] Endothelium-derived nitric oxide (NO) and endothelin-1 (ET-1) have been individuated as modulators of erectile function. Nitric oxide is a key regulator of cavernosal smooth muscle relaxation, whereas ET-1 is believed to maintain penile flaccidity.[20,21] Evidence suggests that there are age-related alterations in the levels of these modulators of erectile function in ED.[22–25] Garban et al demonstrated that a decreased NO synthase (NOS) activity and a reduction in NOS-containing nerve fibers within the corpus cavernosum occurs in the penis of aging male rats.[22] Rajasekaran et al, in 2002, recorded age-related impairments in the expression of NO and ET-1, and in the production of growth factors, such as transforming growth factor-beta1 (TGF-β1).[25] Defects in the production or release of neurotransmitters or the presence of antagonists could cause inhibition

of cavernosal smooth muscle relaxation, resulting in inhibition of erection.

However, another mechanism has been suggested by Chitaley et al,[26] who examined the role of the molecules involved in maintaining penile flaccidity. Besides the well-established noradrenergic contraction mechanisms in the penis, an additional mechanism involving increased sensitivity to ionic calcium has been proposed.[26,27] This pathway involves RhoA, a small monomeric G-protein that activates Rho-kinase. Activated Rho-kinase phosphorylates the regulatory subunit of smooth muscle myosin phosphatase (SMPP-IM). Inhibitory phosphorylation of SMPP-IM leads to the sensitization of myofilaments to Ca^{++},[28] which translates into smooth muscle contraction. An age-related increase in RhoA expression has been documented in rat vascular tissues and this overexpression has been suggested as responsible for age-associated vascular disorders.[29] This hypothesis has been tested and confirmed. Chitaley et al showed that a specific inhibitor of Rho-kinase is able to relax vascular and non-vascular smooth muscle, and intracavernosal injection of this inhibitor in rats has been shown to induce penile erection.[26] Moreover, hypertension, that has been recognized as a well-known vascular risk factor for ED,[30] is associated with elevated penile RhoA levels.[31] In turn, inhibition of Rho-kinase activity has been demonstrated to be beneficial in attenuating the decline in erectile function in hypertensive rats.[32] In addition, Rho-kinase inhibition has been shown to be effective in reversing ED in castrated hypogonadal rats.[33] In summary, the net result of the impairment of erection regulators, such as NO, ET-1, and Rho-kinase, would be an increased penile smooth muscle tone, which may be responsible for the impaired erectile response seen in the aging rats.

Another mechanism suggested as a potential cause of ED is pelvic atherosclerosis. Atherosclerosis-induced arterial insufficiency is a common clinical problem in the elderly, and remains the leading cause of death in the adult population.[34,35] The abdominal aorta and its branches, especially the bifurcation of the iliac arteries, are early and severely involved atherosclerotic lesions.[36] In animal models mimicking pelvic ischemia and hypercholesterolemia, Azadzoi et al demonstrated an evident similarity in the smooth muscle alterations of the detrusor and of the corpora. In their report, chronic ischemia resulted in fibrosis, smooth muscle atrophy, and non-compliance of the bladder.[37] Chronic ischemia is also involved in the deterioration of cavernosal smooth muscle and in the development of corporeal fibrosis, which in turn may lead to ED.[38,39] Moreover, pelvic atherosclerosis may damage the pudendal–cavernous–helicine arterial tree. In the early stages of atherosclerosis, this results in a decreased arterial blood flow to the corpora cavernosa and, in consequence, in ED.[40] However, in more advanced stages, the erectile tissue loses its capability of producing the sufficient quantity of NO needed for smooth muscle relaxation, due to the downregulation of the expression of the constitutive NOS.[39] In addition, elderly men are subjected to a decrease in smooth muscle content in the corpus cavernosum, which is associated with an impairment of the corpora expandibility. This phenomenon is responsible for the veno-occlusive dysfunction observed in the aging male.[41] Chronic ischemia is also responsible for the overexpression of TGF-β1. This protein is a pleotropic cytokine, demonstrated to be an essential mediator of tissue fibrosis.[30] Overproduction of TGF-β1 decreases the smooth muscle–connective tissue ratio by inducing the expression of collagen, fibronectin, and proteoglycans, while inhibiting the growth of smooth muscle cells and the activity of collagenase.[42] Azadzoi et al demonstrated in the rabbit that the level of TGF-β1 correlates with the severity of the fibrosis.[37]

Oxidative stress is another important mechanism recently suggested as a potential factor in the pathogenesis of ED in the elderly. Oxidative damage to the vasculature, caused by reactive oxygen species (ROS), plays a fundamental role in the natural aging process.[43] The interaction between ROS and NO has been indicated as crucial in the development of ED.[44] Specifically, NO interacts with superoxide to form peroxynitrite, which has been reported to play a central role in atherogenesis.[45] In the presence of peroxynitrite, the enzyme responsible for inactivating superoxide is inhibited. In turn, this results in a further increase of peroxynitrite and in a reduction of the available NO concentration.[46] Moreover, peroxynitrite and superoxide increase the incidence of apoptosis in the endothelium,

leading to a further decrease in available NO. Finally, the reduction in NO concentration increases the adhesion of platelets and leukocytes to the endothelial cells, which react with a vasoconstriction stimulus, mediated by thromboxane A2 and leukotrienes.[47] Since the reduced availability of NO and the long-term endothelial damage are the two most important causes of ED, the role of oxidative stress in the corpora cavernosa is critical in the pathophysiology of ED.

The endocrine status plays a significant role in the regulation of erectile function. Hypogonadism is a state of deficiency in gonadal function manifest by deficient secretion of gonadal hormones and/or gametogenesis.[48] In aging men, an alteration in androgen production has been described that has been defined as androgen decline in the aging male (ADAM) or late onset hypogonadism. The hormones affected by a decrease in androgen production include testosterone, dihydroepiandrosterone, thyroxine, melatonin, and growth hormone. Hypogonadism is associated with a decrease in sexual interest and a worsening in the erectile function. Moreover, it is characterized by a gradual decline in serum total and bioavailable testosterone, owing to a decrease in testicular Leydig cell number and in their secretory capacity, as well as an age-related decrease in episodic and stimulated gonadotropin secretion.[49] The prevalence of hypogonadism has been addressed in several longitudinal studies and it has been recorded in 2% of men younger than 50 years old, while it ranges from 34 to 70% in patients aged 70–79 years.[50–52]

The hypothalamic–pituitary–gonadal system is a closed loop of feedback control mechanisms modulating and maintaining reproductive function. The gonadal hormones have inhibitory effects on the secretion of luteinizing hormone (LH) and follicle stimulating hormone (FSH). Testosterone represents the major secretory product of the testis and it is the primary inhibitor of LH secretion in men.[53] However, other hormones are involved in LH suppression, such as estrogens and dihydrotestosterone (DHT).

In normal males, 2% of testosterone is free in the blood, 30% is bound to the sex-hormone-binding-globulin (SHBG), and the remainder is transported by albumin and other plasma proteins.[54] Since the affinity between testosterone and SHBG is very high, the bioavailable testosterone is the fraction of testosterone not bound to this protein. Bioavailable testosterone is the cornerstone of the androgen function and, in turn, changes in SHBG concentration are responsible for androgen function regulation. In healthy subjects, the normal testosterone range is 300–1000 ng/dl, corresponding to 10.4–34.7 nmol/l in most assays of serum total testosterone.[55] However, as previously mentioned, the levels of total and free testosterone decrease with age.[56] Therefore, it is still unclear whether the reference range of serum androgens derived from younger men is also appropriate for the elderly population. However, recently Mohr and colleagues have suggested age-specific thresholds for defining hypotestosteronemia: 251, 215, 196, and 156 ng/dl for men in their forties, fifties, sixties, and seventies, respectively.[56]

Testosterone is a key factor in sexual function and it is necessary for libido, ejaculation, and spontaneous erections. Animal data suggest that testosterone may play a role in the mechanism of NO-mediated vasodilation in the penis and in other organs.[57,58] In castrated rats, Chamness et al demonstrated that the activity of NOS is reduced by 45% and that testosterone replacement can recover its production.[57] Moreover, testosterone is implicated in the modulation of alpha-adrenergic vasoconstrictor activity[59,60] and, in turn, it can enhance erections by attenuation of vasoconstriction and by contributing to the venous occlusion mechanism that maintains erection.[60] Furthermore, testosterone is involved in central nervous system control of erections. In fact, animal studies demonstrate that testosterone may facilitate erection in the dopaminergic mesolimbic cortex, responsible for sexual arousal.[61] In human subjects with pharmacologically induced hypogonadism, the libido and the frequency of spontaneous erections decreased. These alterations were reversible after restoration of normal blood levels of testosterone.[62] Moreover, recent studies highlighted the interaction between testosterone and phosphodiesterase-5 (PDE5) inhibitors. Aversa et al showed that, in a small group of patients defined as non-responders to sildenafil with arteriogenic ED and low-normal androgen levels, short-term testosterone administration increases testosterone (T) and free testosterone (FT) levels

and improves the erectile response to sildenafil, likely by increasing arterial inflow to the penis during sexual stimulation.[63]

In summary, it seems reasonable to hypothesize that the ED of aging is the result of atherosclerosis-induced cavernosal ischemia, leading to cavernosal fibrosis and veno-occlusive dysfunction. Abnormalities in circulating levels of hormones controling sexual organs, especially testosterone, most probably play a significant role at least in some patients. As the ED of aging appears to be a slowly progressive disorder, it appears to be wise for the patient to seek medical intervention earlier rather than later, to minimize the development of veno-occlusive dysfunction.

Assessment of the patient with erectile dysfunction

As already mentioned in the introduction to this chapter, it is relevant to stress that many aging men (and their partners) experience a sexual dysfunction but do not want (or seek) any form of treatment because they are not bothered by the dysfunction itself or not willing to disclose their concern. This was investigated by de Boer and colleagues in an epidemiologic study in the Netherlands, where a representative sample of a city population ($n = 1481$) were interviewed about the prevalence of ED and its impact on quality of life. They recorded that 32.7% of patients reporting a certain extent of ED were not bothered by their condition and that the bother relative to ED decreased after the age of 60 years.[64] This study was corroborated by previous reports that demonstrated a decreasing trend in bother relative to ED, according to increasing age.[65,66]

During a medical visit, ED should be invariably explored, although treatment may not always be requested or immediately necessary. Moreover, ED should be investigated as it could be the initial presentation of an underlying cardiovascular disease or diabetes.[67] The wide availability of self-administered questionnaires designed to investigate the patient's sexual function[8,68] has rendered the evaluation of ED less time consuming and thereby has resulted in greater interest in the evaluation of the patient's sexual health.

The most important component of diagnosis of ED is obtaining a complete medical and sexual history. It is mandatory to identify the sexual problem (for example, erectile dysfunction versus premature ejaculation versus loss of libido), as the patient may be unaware of what represents a sexual problem. The duration of ED, time of onset, and degree of patient and partner concern should also be investigated and elucidated. The circumstances surrounding ED may be helpful in diagnosis since a sudden onset, maintenance of nocturnal erections, presence of psychologic problems, and concurrent major life events may be suggestive of non-organic ED.[69]

It is also important to identify ED risk factors, which include serious medical conditions such as ischemic heart disease, hypertension, diabetes, perineal–pelvic trauma, hyperlipidemia, depression, and previous pelvic surgery. Moreover, it is extremely important to identify the presence of reversible risk factors for ED, namely smoking, heavy drinking, and the use of recreational or medically indicated drugs.[70] Most of these risk factors are more frequently found in the aging population.

During the history taking, particular attention should be focused on the potential risk of cardiovascular disease.[67,71] There is a high prevalence of cardiovascular disease among patients consulting for ED and sexual activity has a strong relationship with cardiac risk.[67,72] Patients should be stratified into three risk categories: low, intermediate or indeterminate, and high risk. In low-risk patients, sexual activity is not associated with significant cardiac risk (they can perform exercise of modest intensity without symptoms). The intermediate-risk category includes men with an uncertain cardiac condition or patients whose risk profile needs further testing before the resumption of sexual activity. High-risk patients have a cardiac condition that is sufficiently severe or unstable that sexual activity may lead to potentially life-threatening cardiac events and they should be referred for further cardiologic evaluation.[67]

A psychosocial history is also important. It may provide information on the couple's relationship (if existing) and on the partner's health. This is of particular importance in the aging male, as the female partner may be menopausal or could be affected by a male-unrelated sexual dysfunction. Investigation,

diagnosis, and, eventually, treatment of female sexual dysfunction should be considered in patients consulting for ED in order to consider ED in the context of a couple's sexual dysfunction.[73] Female sexual dysfunctions in the aging woman may worsen a man's ability to achieve successful intercourse, despite only mild or moderate ED. Moreover, female sexual dysfunction is frequent.[74] Therefore, this field needs to be explored when assessing a patient with ED.

Physical examination should include an overall assessment as well as a focused urologic examination. Patient height and weight should be assessed and the body mass index calculated. The cardiovascular part should focus on the determination of blood pressure and the identification of the peripheral vascular pulses (carotid, aortic, femoral, and pedidial). The neurologic part should target the peripheral reflexes (knee reflex, Achilles tendon reflex, and bulbo-cavernosus reflex) and a brief evaluation of peripheral sensitivity. The genito-urinary examination should emphasize the genitals, specifically, the presence of penile deformities, phimosis, and/or signs of hypogonadism should be sought. Digital rectal examination of the prostate gland should always be performed in the aging man, as this population is, by definition, at higher risk of developing prostate cancer.

Laboratory tests should invariably include prostate specific antigen (PSA), testosterone, and prolactin.[70] Moreover, blood glucose and serum lipids should be investigated. Inclusion of further tests should be based on history, physical examination, and any clinical suspicion. The above laboratory values virtually invariably allow identification of one or several underlying causes of ED. This information may allow a more targeted and more specific approach to ED treatment.

Treatment of patients with erectile dysfunction

Erectile dysfunction treatment guidelines fit the aging population, which represents the bulk of ED patients. The objective of the guidelines is to treat ED using an integrated, multisystemic approach.

Modifiable and reversible factors should be addressed. The treatment of underlying causes of ED may at times improve or correct ED. For example, lifestyle changes may offer potential benefits when ED is associated with specific comorbidity, such as diabetes or hypertension.[75,76] A hypogonadal patient may obtain relief of his ED with testosterone supplementation. However, this therapy is contraindicated in patients with a history of prostate cancer and all patients should be strictly monitored for clinical response as well as the development of prostate cancer.[77] Patients diagnosed with a significant psychologic problem may benefit from a psychosexual therapy. Each of these treatments is associated with a specific success rate.[78,79] These should be communicated to the patient to ensure realistic expectations.

The introduction of new oral compounds has completely changed the therapeutic approach to ED. First-line therapy mainly consists of oral drug therapy.

Phosphodiesterase type 5 (PDE5) is a protein mainly situated in the trabecular smooth muscle and its function is to hydrolyze cyclic guanosine monophosphate (cGMP). The inhibition of PDE5 leads to an increase in intracellular cGMP, responsible for the local release of NO.[80] This results in decreased cytosolic Ca^{2+} concentration and, in turn, in smooth muscle relaxation, vasodilatation, and penile erection. Therefore, PDE5 inhibitors represent the cornerstone of oral therapy.

Sildenafil, the first commercialized selective PDE5 inhibitor, has certainly revolutionized ED management in the aging patient. Sildenafil is rapidly adsorbed and its half-life is approximately 4 hours.[81] Men aged 65 or older should be considered for a starting dose of 25 mg.[82] Several studies have shown that sildenafil is an effective and well-tolerated oral agent for treating ED in the general population of adult men with ED of broad spectrum etiology.[83] Wagner et al assessed the efficacy and tolerability of sildenafil in the elderly population using data from five major, double-blind, placebo-controlled studies.[84] Oral sildenafil was taken as required (but no more than once daily) over a 12-week to 6-month period. Data from the elderly (aged > 65 years) patients enrolled in four studies (two fixed dose and two flexible dose studies in

patients with broad-spectrum etiology ED) were pooled for analysis. The fifth study considered had enrolled only men with ED and a concurrent clinical diagnosis of diabetes of more than 5 years' duration for type I diabetes and more than 2 years' duration for type II diabetes. A total of 411 elderly patients with ED of broad spectrum etiology and 71 elderly patients with ED and diabetes were randomized to treatment in these studies. The patients in the broad spectrum ED studies were randomized to receive either fixed- or flexible-dose sildenafil (from 25 to 100 mg) or placebo. In all five studies, patients were instructed to take the study drug 1 hour before sexual activity but not more than once daily. At the end of treatment, 69% of the patients in the broad spectrum ED subgroup who received sildenafil reported that treatment had improved their erections, compared with 18% who had received placebo ($P < 0.001$). Similarly, a significant treatment effect was observed for the ED and diabetes subgroup patients who received sildenafil. Fifty percent of these patients reported improvements in their erections, compared with 10% of those who received placebo ($P < 0.001$). The most commonly experienced adverse events in the two subgroups were headache, flushing, and dyspepsia, which occurred in respectively 17%, 13%, and 8% of patients receiving sildenafil. Most of these adverse events were mild to moderate in nature. Twenty-two elderly patients enrolled in these studies experienced serious adverse events: 11 were patients receiving placebo and 11 were patients receiving sildenafil. None of these serious adverse events were considered to be related to treatment. The results of this combined analysis show that sildenafil is an effective therapy in elderly men with ED of various etiologies and with concomitant illnesses. More than two-thirds of the men in the broad-spectrum ED subgroup and one-half of the men in the ED and diabetes subgroup reported improved erections with sildenafil treatment.

Other oral drugs are available for the treatment of ED. Tadalafil is a PDE5 inhibitor, with a half-life of 17.5 hours, significantly longer than sildenafil,[85] and its efficacy is maintained up to 36 hours.[86] Tadalafil is effective in elderly men and its safety profile is comparable to sildenafil. In 11 studies involving

2102 patients affected with ED of heterogeneous etiology, tadalafil significantly improved the erectile function in 67 and 81% of men treated with respectively 10 or 20 mg of tadalafil.[85] Moreover, tadalafil showed good efficacy and tolerability in difficult to treat subgroups of patients.[87]

The latest PDE5 inhibitor which has entered the market is vardenafil. This molecule shows a pharmacologic profile similar to sildenafil, even if it is a 10-fold more potent inhibitor.[88] Vardenafil showed good efficacy and tolerability profiles both in pre- and post-marketing studies.[88–90]

Clinical trials and post-marketing studies have assessed the safety of PDE5 inhibitors. All three molecules have demonstrated no increase in the rate of myocardial infarction in either double-blind, placebo-controlled trials, or open-label studies.[91] However, organic nitrates and other nitrate preparations are absolute contraindications for the use of PDE5 inhibitors. Other drugs, such as antihypertensive or α-blocker compounds, can have interactions with PDE5 inhibitors. In consequence, the verdenafil should be used with caution when a patient is already being treated with those drugs.[71]

Other agents are available, including apomorphine, phentolamine, and yohimbine. Apomorphine is a centrally acting dopamine receptor agonist which ultimately activates the cascade of events leading to smooth muscle relaxation within the corpus cavernosum and penile erection. It is available as a small tablet to be administered sublingually, 20 minutes prior to sexual activity. Doses include 2 and 3 mg preparations; patients are instructed to take the 2 mg dose first and titrate to the higher dose if 2 mg is ineffective. Large randomized studies on apomorphine have been completed in the United States and Europe and showed conflicting results in patients with ED of broad-spectrum etiology.[92,93] Efficacy rates ranged from 28.5 to 55% for attempts to have sexual intercourse. Apomorphine was well tolerated and side-effects included nausea and vomiting in less than 2% of the cases. Syncope has been reported with higher doses but its rate of occurrence with the 2 and 3 mg doses was less than 0.5%.[92] However, comparative studies clearly show that apomorphine is associated with significantly lower efficacy and satisfaction rates than sildenafil.[94] Therefore the indication for

apomorphine is limited to patients with mild to moderate ED or psychogenic ED variants.[71]

Phentolamine is a rapidly acting, short-lived, non-selective α_1/α_2 adrenoreceptor antagonist. This drug is available for ED treatment only outside the United States. Studies in animal models indicate that phentolamine has a high potency of inducing cavernous smooth muscle relaxation, independently from the stimulated neurogenic system.[95] Yohimbine is the principal alkaloid of the bark of the West-African tree *Pausinystalia yohimbe*. This selective competitive α_2-adrenergic receptor antagonist is a potential option in men with mild or moderate ED. However, patients' response to treatment with yohimbine is not excellent. In a study involving 18 subjects, Guay et al demonstrated that yohimbine was able to improve the erectile function in 50% of the patients.[96]

Several vasoactive drugs have been considered as topical agents in the treatment of ED. Topical application of nitroglycerin, paverine, or minoxidil has been suggested. However, none of these topical agents have been formally approved.[71]

Finally, vacuum constrictor devices were extensively used in the pre-PDE5 inhibitor era. These devices provide passive engorgement of the corpora cavernosa when applied in conjunction with a constrictor ring placed at the base of the penis. Regardless of ED etiology, patient satisfaction is achieved in a proportion that ranges from 27 to 94%.[97] However, the use of vacuum devices has been dramatically reduced by the advent of oral treatments.

Although PDE5 inhibitors are clearly a reliable option for the majority of elderly patients with ED, other therapeutic options should be discussed. These should include intracavernous injection therapy, intraurethral drug therapy, and, if all else fails, placement of penile implants. These treatment options represent, respectively, second- and third-line alternatives in the management of ED. These treatment modalities may be of interest to patients who are not candidates for PDE5 inhibitor therapy or who have not achieved an adequate response rate/satisfaction with oral agents.

Intraurethral administration of alprostadil using the Medicated Urethral System for Erection (MUSE) system can be considered an attractive alternative in sildenafil non-responders.[98,99] A semi-solid pellet of prostaglandin E1 is inserted in the urethra, promoting erectile response in 70–83% of cases.[99,100]

Intracavernosal injection of alprostadil or vasoactive drug mixtures represents another valid option for ED treatment. The erectogenic effect of intracavernosal injections (in terms of penile rigidity) is usually superior to that of sildenafil[53] and it may be offered to oral therapy non-responders with high success rates.[101,102] Although some type of manual dexterity is needed to handle the intracorporal injection, new injection devices are now available that make this treatment readily usable by the elderly.

Placement of a penile implant is usually considered for patients who have not responded to other less invasive forms of therapy. However, it is uncommon to place a penile implant in patients older than 65 years, as the sexual needs of these patients are usually well addressed by other therapeutic alternatives.[103]

Hormonal replacement in the treatment of ED in the aging male remains controversial. The link between androgen deficiency and ED has not been fully elucidated.[104] However, although no studies can firmly link testosterone replacement with an increased incidence of prostate cancer,[105] it is not clear if the benefits of testosterone replacement outweigh the potentially increased risk of prostate cancer. In aging hypogonadal men, testosterone replacement therapy can improve libido, muscle mass, bone density, and mood.[106] However, some adverse sequelae may be associated with topical or transdermal testosterone administration such as erythrocytosis (polycythemia), skin reactions, testicular atrophy, and infertility.[107] Other adverse events, such as acne, hirsutism, flushing, fluid retention, benign prostatic hyperplasia, gynecomastia, hypertension, and lipid alterations, are less common.[107]

In summary, management of ED in the aging male is first based on extensive evaluation of the patient's sexual and medical history and on the assessment of the patient's and couple's needs and expectations. Although several therapeutic options are currently available to treat the patient's symptoms, it seems that, in most patients, oral pharmacotherapy plays the major role because of its high efficacy and safety.

References

1. US Renal Data System, USRDS 2006 Annual Data Report: Atlas of End-Stage Renal. Disease in the United States. Bethesda, MD: National Institutes of Health, National Institute of Diabetes and Digestive and Kidney Diseases, 2006.

2. Slob AK. Age, libido, and male sexual function. Prostate Suppl 2000; 10: 9–13.

3. Kinsey AC, Pomeroy PW, Martin CE. Age and sexual outlet. In: Kinsey AC, Pomeroy WB, Martin CE, eds. Sexual Behaviour in the Human Male. Philadelphia, PA: WB Saunders Co, 1948.

4. Laumann EO, Paik A, Rosen RC. Sexual dysfunction in the United States: prevalence and predictors. JAMA 1999; 281(6): 537–44.

5. Feldman HA, Goldstein I, Hatzichristou DG, Krane RJ, McKinlay JB. Impotence and its medical and psychosocial correlates: results of the Massachusetts Male Aging Study. J Urol 1994; 151(1): 54–61.

6. Saigal CS, Wessells H, Pace J, Schonlau M, Wilt TJ. Predictors and prevalence of erectile dysfunction in a racially diverse population. Arch Intern Med 2006; 166(2): 207–12.

7. Grover SA, Lowensteyn I, Kaouache M et al. The prevalence of erectile dysfunction in the primary care setting: importance of risk factors for diabetes and vascular disease. Arch Intern Med 2006; 166(2): 213–19.

8. Rosen RC, Riley A, Wagner G et al. The international index of erectile function (IIEF): a multidimensional scale for assessment of erectile dysfunction. Urology 1997; 49(6): 822–30.

9. United States Bureau of the Census. Statistical Abstract of the United States 1992. Washington, DC: USBC, 1992.

10. United States Bureau of the Census. Historical Statistics of the United States, Colonial Times to 1970. Bicentennial edn. Part 2 Washington, DC: USBC, 1975.

11. Andersson KE, Wagner G. Physiology of penile erection. Physiol Rev 1995; 75(1): 191–236.

12. Tarcan T, Azadzoi KM, Siroky MB, Goldstein I, Krane RJ. Age-related erectile and voiding dysfunction: the role of arterial insufficiency. Br J Urol 1998; 82(Suppl 1): 26–33.

13. Benet AE, Melman A. The epidemiology of erectile dysfunction. Urol Clin North Am 1995; 22(4): 699–709.

14. Schoneich C. Reactive oxygen species and biological aging: a mechanistic approach. Exp Gerontol 1999; 34(1): 19–34.

15. Rossi A, Ganassini A, Tantucci C, Grassi V. Aging and the respiratory system. Aging (Milano) 1996; 8(3): 143–61.

16. Bitar KN. Aging and neural control of the GI tract: V. Aging and gastrointestinal smooth muscle: from signal transduction to contractile proteins. Am J Physiol Gastrointest Liver Physiol 2003; 284(1): G1–7.

17. Al-Shaer MH, Choueiri NE, Correia ML, Sinkey CA, Barenz TA, Haynes WG. Effects of aging and atherosclerosis on endothelial and vascular smooth muscle function in humans. Int J Cardiol 2006; 109(2): 201–6.

18. McVary K. Lower urinary tract symptoms and sexual dysfunction: epidemiology and pathophysiology. BJU Int 2006; 97(Suppl 2): 23–8; discussion 44–5.

19. Taub HC, Lerner SE, Melman A, Christ GJ. Relationship between contraction and relaxation in human and rabbit corpus cavernosum. Urology 1993; 42(6): 698–704.

20. Saenz de Tejada I, Carson MP, de las Morenas A, Goldstein I, Traish AM. Endothelin: localization, synthesis, activity, and receptor types in human penile corpus cavernosum. Am J Physiol 1991; 261(4 Pt 2): H1078–85.

21. Burnett AL. Role of nitric oxide in the physiology of erection. Biol Reprod 1995; 52(3): 485–9.

22. Garban H, Vernet D, Freedman A, Rajfer J, Gonzalez-Cadavid N. Effect of aging on nitric oxide-mediated penile erection in rats. Am J Physiol 1995; 268(1 Pt 2): H467–75.

23. Carrier S NP, Morgan DM, Baba K, Nunes L, Lue TF. Age decreases nitric oxide synthase-containing nerve fibers in the rat penis. J Urol 1997; 157(3): 1088–92.

24. Dahiya R, Chui R, Perinchery G, Nakajima K, Oh BR, Lue TF. Differential gene expression of growth factors in young and old rat penile tissues is associated with erectile dysfunction. Int J Impot Res 1999; 11(4): 201–6.

25. Rajasekaran M, Kasyan A, Jain A, Kim SW, Monga M. Altered growth factor expression in the aging penis: the Brown–Norway rat model. J Androl 2002; 23(3): 393–9.

26. Chitaley K, Wingard CJ, Clinton Webb R et al. Antagonism of Rho-kinase stimulates rat penile erection via a nitric oxide-independent pathway. Nat Med 2001; 7(1): 119–22.

27. Wang H, Eto M, Steers WD, Somlyo AP, Somlyo AV. RhoA-mediated Ca2+ sensitization in erectile function. J Biol Chem 2002; 277(34): 30614–21.

28. Somlyo AP, Somlyo AV. Signal transduction by G-proteins, rho-kinase and protein phosphatase to smooth muscle and non-muscle myosin II. J Physiol 2000; 522 (Pt 2): 177–85.

29. Miao L, Calvert JW, Tang J, Parent AD, Zhang JH. Age-related RhoA expression in blood vessels of rats. Mech Ageing Dev 2001; 122(15): 1757–70.

30. Dusing R. Sexual dysfunction in male patients with hypertension: influence of antihypertensive drugs. Drugs 2005; 65(6): 773–86.

31. Lee DL, Webb RC, Jin L. Hypertension and RhoA/Rho-kinase signaling in the vasculature: highlights from the recent literature. Hypertension 2004; 44(6): 796–9.

32. Wilkes N, White S, Stein P, Bernie J, Rajasekaran M. Phosphodiesterase-5 inhibition synergizes rho-kinase antagonism and enhances erectile response in male hypertensive rats. Int J Impot Res 2004; 16(2): 187–94.

33. Wingard CJ, Johnson JA, Holmes A, Prikosh A. Improved erectile function after Rho-kinase inhibition in a rat castrate model of erectile dysfunction. Am J Physiol Regul Integr Comp Physiol 2003; 284(6): R1572–9.

34. Atherosclerotic disease of the aortic arch as a risk factor for recurrent ischemic stroke. The French Study of Aortic Plaques in Stroke Group. N Engl J Med 1996; 334(19): 1216–21.

35. Meissner I, Khandheria BK, Sheps SG et al. Atherosclerosis of the aorta: risk factor, risk marker, or innocent bystander? A prospective population-based transesophageal echocardiography study. J Am Coll Cardiol 2004; 44(5): 1018–24.

36. Hirsch AT, Haskal ZJ, Hertzer NR et al. ACC/AHA 2005 Practice Guidelines for the management of patients with peripheral arterial disease (lower extremity, renal, mesenteric, and abdominal aortic): a collaborative report from the American Association for Vascular Surgery/Society for Vascular Surgery, Society for Cardiovascular Angiography and Interventions, Society for Vascular Medicine and Biology, Society of Interventional Radiology, and the ACC/AHA Task Force on Practice Guidelines (Writing Committee to Develop Guidelines for the Management of Patients With Peripheral Arterial Disease): endorsed by the American Association of Cardiovascular and Pulmonary Rehabilitation; National Heart, Lung, and Blood Institute; Society for Vascular Nursing; TransAtlantic Inter-Society Consensus; and Vascular Disease Foundation. Circulation 2006; 113(11): 463–654.

37. Azadzoi KM, Tarcan T, Siroky MB, Krane RJ. Atherosclerosis-induced chronic ischemia causes bladder fibrosis and non-compliance in the rabbit. J Urol 1999; 161(5): 1626–35.

38. Montorsi F, Briganti A, Salonia A et al. The ageing male and erectile dysfunction. BJU Int 2003; 92(5): 516–20.

39. Azadzoi KM, Master TA, Siroky MB. Effect of chronic ischemia on constitutive and inducible nitric oxide synthase expression in erectile tissue. J Androl 2004; 25(3): 382–8.

40. Grein U, Schubert GE. Arteriosclerosis of penile arteries: histological findings and their significance in the treatment of erectile dysfunction. Urol Int 2002; 68(4): 261–4.

41. Nehra A, Azadzoi KM, Moreland RB et al. Cavernosal expandability is an erectile tissue mechanical property which predicts trabecular histology in an animal model of vasculogenic erectile dysfunction. J Urol 1998; 159(6): 2229–36.

42. Border WA, Noble NA. Transforming growth factor beta in tissue fibrosis. N Engl J Med 1994; 331(19): 1286–92.

43. Dugan LL, Quick KL. Reactive oxygen species and aging: evolving questions. Sci Aging Knowledge Environ 2005; 2005(26): 20.

44. Jones RW, Rees RW, Minhas S, Ralph D, Persad RA, Jeremy JY. Oxygen free radicals and the penis. Expert Opin Pharmacother 2002; 3(7): 889–97.

45. Beckman JS, Koppenol WH. Nitric oxide, superoxide, and peroxynitrite: the good, the bad, and ugly. Am J Physiol 1996; 271(5 Pt 1): C1424–37.

46. Zou M, Martin C, Ullrich V. Tyrosine nitration as a mechanism of selective inactivation of prostacyclin synthase by peroxynitrite. Biol Chem 1997; 378(7): 707–13.

47. Agarwal A, Nandipati KC, Sharma RK, Zippe CD, Raina R. Role of oxidative stress in the pathophysiological mechanism of erectile dysfunction. J Androl 2006; 27(3): 335–47.

48. American Association of Clinical Endocrinologists. Medical guidelines for clinical practice for the evaluation and treatment of hypogonadism in adult male patients – 2002 update. Endocr Pract 2002; 8(6): 440–56.

49. Vermeulen A. Clinical review 24: androgens in the aging male. J Clin Endocrinol Metab 1991; 73(2): 221–4.

50. Harman SM, Metter EJ, Tobin JD, Pearson J, Blackman MR. Longitudinal effects of aging on serum total and free testosterone levels in healthy men. Baltimore Longitudinal Study of Aging. J Clin Endocrinol Metab 2001; 86(2): 724–31.

51. Feldman HA, Longcope C, Derby CA et al. Age trends in the level of serum testosterone and other hormones in middle-aged men: longitudinal results from the Massachusetts male aging study. J Clin Endocrinol Metab 2002; 87(2): 589–98.

52. Morley JE, Kaiser FE, Perry HM 3rd et al. Longitudinal changes in testosterone, luteinizing hormone, and follicle-stimulating hormone in healthy older men. Metabolism 1997; 46(4): 410–13.

53. Morales A, Buvat J, Gooren LJ et al. Endocrine aspects of sexual dysfunction in men. J Sex Med 2004; 1(1): 69–81.

54. McClure RD. Endocrine investigation and therapy. Urol Clin North Am 1987; 14(3): 471–88.

55. Matsumoto AM, Bremner WJ. Serum testosterone essay – accuracy matters. J Clin Endocrinol Metab 2004; 89(2): 520–4.

56. Mohr BA, Guay AT, O'Donnell AB, McKinlay JB. Normal, bound and nonbound testosterone levels in normally ageing men: results from the Massachusetts Male Ageing Study. Clin Endocrinol (Oxf) 2005; 62(1): 64–73.

57. Chamness SL, Ricker DD, Crone JK et al. The effect of androgen on nitric oxide synthase in the male reproductive tract of the rat. Fertil Steril 1995; 63(5): 1101–7.

58. Chou TM, Sudhir K, Hutchison SJ et al. Testosterone induces dilation of canine coronary conductance and resistance arteries in vivo. Circulation 1996; 94(10): 2614–19.

59. Reilly CM, Stopper VS, Mills TM. Androgens modulate the alpha-adrenergic responsiveness of vascular smooth muscle in the corpus cavernosum. J Androl 1997; 18(1): 26–31.

60. Mills TM, Lewis RW, Stopper VS. Androgenic maintenance of inflow and veno-occlusion during erection in the rat. Biol Reprod 1998; 59(6): 1413–18.

61. Mitchell JB, Stewart J. Effects of castration, steroid replacement, and sexual experience on mesolimbic dopamine and sexual behaviors in the male rat. Brain Res 1989; 491(1): 116–27.

62. Bagatell CJ, Heiman JR, Rivier JE, Bremner WJ. Effects of endogenous testosterone and estradiol on sexual behavior in normal young men. J Clin Endocrinol Metab 1994; 78(3): 711–16.

63. Aversa A, Isidori AM, Spera G, Lenzi A, Fabbri A. Androgens improve cavernous vasodilation and response to sildenafil in patients with erectile dysfunction. Clin Endocrinol (Oxf) 2003; 58(5): 632–8.

64. de Boer BJ, Bots ML, Nijeholt AA, Moors JP, Verheij TJ. The prevalence of bother, acceptance, and need for help in men with erectile dysfunction. J Sex Med 2005; 2(3): 445–50.

65. Braun M, Wassmer G, Klotz T, Reifenrath B, Mathers M, Engelmann U. Epidemiology of erectile dysfunction: results of the 'Cologne Male Survey'. Int J Impot Res 2000; 12(6): 305–11.

66. Meuleman EJ, Donkers LH, Robertson C, Keech M, Boyle P, Kiemeney LA. [Erectile dysfunction: prevalence and effect on the quality of life; Boxmeer study.] Ned Tijdschr Geneeskd 2001; 145(12): 576–81.

67. Kostis JB, Jackson G, Rosen R et al. Sexual dysfunction and cardiac risk (the Second Princeton Consensus Conference). Am J Cardiol 2005; 96(12B): 85–93M.

68. Rosen RC, Cappelleri JC, Smith MD, Lipsky J, Pena BM. Development and evaluation of an abridged, 5-item version of the International Index of Erectile Function (IIEF-5) as a diagnostic tool for erectile dysfunction. Int J Impot Res 1999; 11(6): 319–26.

69. Montorsi F. Assessment, diagnosis, and investigation of erectile dysfunction. Clin Cornerstone 2005; 7(1): 29–35.

70. Lue TF, Basson R, Rosen R, Giuliano F, Khoury S, Montorsi F. Second International Consultation on Sexual Medicine: Sexual Dysfunctions in Men and Women. Paris: Health Publications; 2004.

71. Wespes E, Amar E, Hatzichristou D et al. EAU guidelines on erectile dysfunction: an update. Eur Urol 2006; 49(5): 806–15.

72. Roumeguere T, Wespes E, Carpentier Y, Hoffmann P, Schulman CC. Erectile dysfunction is associated with a high prevalence of hyperlipidemia and coronary heart disease risk. Eur Urol 2003; 44(3): 355–9.

73. Corona G, Petrone L, Mannucci E et al. Assessment of the relational factor in male patients consulting for sexual dysfunction: the concept of couple sexual dysfunction. J Androl 2006; 27: 795–801.

74. Greenstein A, Abramov L, Matzkin H, Chen J. Sexual dysfunction in women partners of men with erectile dysfunction. Int J Impot Res 2006; 18(1): 44–6.

75. Moyad MA, Barada JH, Lue TF, Mulhall JP, Goldstein I, Fawzy A. Prevention and treatment of erectile dysfunction using lifestyle changes and dietary supplements: what works and what is worthless, part I. Urol Clin North Am 2004; 31(2): 249–57.

76. Moyad MA, Barada JH, Lue TF, Mulhall JP, Goldstein I, Fawzy A. Prevention and treatment of erectile dysfunction using lifestyle changes and dietary supplements: what works and what is worthless, part II. Urol Clin North Am 2004; 31(2): 259–73.

77. Gaylis FD, Lin DW, Ignatoff JM, Amling CL, Tutrone RF, Cosgrove DJ. Prostate cancer in men using testosterone supplementation. J Urol 2005; 174(2): 534–8; discussion 538.

78. Morales A, Heaton JP. Hormonal erectile dysfunction. Evaluation and management. Urol Clin North Am 2001; 28(2): 279–88.

79. Rosen RC. Psychogenic erectile dysfunction. Classification and management. Urol Clin North Am 2001; 28(2): 269–78.

80. Burnett AL. Nitric oxide in the penis: physiology and pathology. J Urol 1997; 157(1): 320–4.

81. Boolell M, Allen MJ, Ballard SA et al. Sildenafil: an orally active type 5 cyclic GMP-specific phosphodiesterase inhibitor for the treatment of penile erectile dysfunction. Int J Impot Res 1996; 8(2): 47–52.

82. Seftel AD. From aspiration to achievement: assessment and noninvasive treatment of erectile dysfunction in aging men. J Am Geriatr Soc 2005; 53(1): 119–30.

83. Montorsi F, McDermott TE, Morgan R et al. Efficacy and safety of fixed-dose oral sildenafil in the treatment of erectile dysfunction of various etiologies. Urology 1999; 53(5): 1011–18.

84. Wagner G, Montorsi F, Auerbach S, Collins M. Sildenafil citrate (VIAGRA) improves erectile function in elderly patients with erectile dysfunction: a subgroup analysis. J Gerontol A Biol Sci Med Sci 2001; 56(2): M113–19.

85. Brock GB, McMahon CG, Chen KK et al. Efficacy and safety of tadalafil for the treatment of erectile dysfunction: results of integrated analyses. J Urol 2002; 168(4 Pt 1): 1332–6.

86. Porst H, Padma-Nathan H, Giuliano F, Anglin G, Varanese L, Rosen R. Efficacy of tadalafil for the treatment of erectile dysfunction at 24 and 36 hours after dosing: a randomized controlled trial. Urology 2003; 62(1): 121–5; discussion 125–6.

87. Montorsi F, Verheyden B, Meuleman E et al. Long-term safety and tolerability of tadalafil in the treatment of erectile dysfunction. Eur Urol 2004; 45(3): 339–44; discussion 344–5.

88. Hellstrom WJ, Gittelman M, Karlin G et al. Sustained efficacy and tolerability of vardenafil, a highly potent selective phosphodiesterase type 5 inhibitor, in men with erectile dysfunction: results of a randomized, double-blind, 26-week placebo-controlled pivotal trial. Urology 2003; 61(4 Suppl 1): 8–14.

89. Hellstrom WJ, Gittelman M, Karlin G et al. Vardenafil for treatment of men with erectile dysfunction: efficacy and safety in a randomized, double-blind, placebo-controlled trial. J Androl 2002; 23(6): 763–71.

90. Potempa AJ, Ulbrich E, Bernard I, Beneke M. Efficacy of vardenafil in men with erectile dysfunction: a flexible-dose community practice study. Eur Urol 2004; 46(1): 73–9.

91. Kloner RA. Novel phosphodiesterase type 5 inhibitors: assessing hemodynamic effects and safety parameters. Clin Cardiol 2004; 27(4 Suppl 1): I20–5.

92. Heaton JP. Apomorphine: an update of clinical trial results. Int J Impot Res 2000; 12(Suppl 4): S67–73.

93. Dula E, Bukofzer S, Perdok R, George M. Double-blind, crossover comparison of 3 mg apomorphine SL with placebo and with 4 mg apomorphine SL in male erectile dysfunction. Eur Urol 2001; 39(5): 558–63; discussion 564.

94. Eardley I, Wright P, MacDonagh R, Hole J, Edwards A. An open-label, randomized, flexible-dose, crossover study to assess the comparative efficacy and safety of sildenafil citrate and apomorphine hydrochloride in men with erectile dysfunction. BJU Int 2004; 93(9): 1271–5.

95. Sharabi FM, Daabees TT, El-Metwally MA, Senbel AM. Comparative effects of sildenafil, phentolamine, yohimbine and l-arginine on the rabbit

corpus cavernosum. Fund Clin Pharmacol 2004; 18(2): 187–94.

96. Guay AT, Spark RF, Jacobson J, Murray FT, Geisser ME. Yohimbine treatment of organic erectile dysfunction in a dose-escalation trial. Int J Impot Res 2002; 14(1): 25–31.

97. Lewis RW, Witherington R. External vacuum therapy for erectile dysfunction: use and results. World J Urol 1997; 15(1): 78–82.

98. Jaffe JS, Antell MR, Greenstein M, Ginsberg PC, Mydlo JH, Harkaway RC. Use of intraurethral alprostadil in patients not responding to sildenafil citrate. Urology 2004; 63(5): 951–4.

99. Padma-Nathan H, Hellstrom WJ, Kaiser FE et al. Treatment of men with erectile dysfunction with transurethral alprostadil. Medicated Urethral System for Erection (MUSE) Study Group. N Engl J Med 1997; 336(1): 1–7.

100. Williams G, Abbou CC, Amar ET et al. Efficacy and safety of transurethral alprostadil therapy in men with erectile dysfunction. MUSE Study Group. Br J Urol 1998; 81(6): 889–94.

101. Shabsigh R, Padma-Nathan H, Gittleman M, McMurray J, Kaufman J, Goldstein I. Intracavernous alprostadil alfadex (EDEX/VIRIDAL) is effective and safe in patients with erectile dysfunction after failing sildenafil (Viagra). Urology 2000; 55(4): 477–80.

102. Shabsigh R, Padma-Nathan H, Gittleman M, McMurray J, Kaufman J, Goldstein I. Intracavernous alprostadil alfadex is more efficacious, better tolerated, and preferred over intraurethral alprostadil plus optional actis: a comparative, randomized, crossover, multicenter study. Urology 2000; 55(1): 109–13.

103. Montorsi F, Rigatti P, Carmignani G et al. AMS three-piece inflatable implants for erectile dysfunction: a long-term multi-institutional study in 200 consecutive patients. Eur Urol 2000; 37(1): 50–5.

104. Mikhail N. Does testosterone have a role in erectile function? Am J Med 2006; 119(5): 373–82.

105. Morgentaler A. Testosterone and prostate cancer: an historical perspective on a modern myth. Eur Urol 2006; 50: 935–9.

106. Juul A, Skakkebaek NE. Androgens and the ageing male. Hum Reprod Update 2002; 8(5): 423–33.

107. Rhoden EL, Morgentaler A. Risks of testosterone-replacement therapy and recommendations for monitoring. N Engl J Med 2004; 350(5): 482–92.

CHAPTER 12

Infertility in the aging male

Wolfgang Weidner, Thorsten Diemer, and Martin Bergmann

Introduction

Spermatogenesis as well as the synthesis of testosterone in the human testis is a lifelong process that also persists in aging men. However, spermatogenic efficiency estimated by the number of spermatozoa produced per day per gram of testicular parenchyma (spermatogenic index) apparently declines with age. This decline is a result of an increase in germ cell degeneration throughout spermatogenesis as seen in all cell types of the germ cell line.

The clinical significance of these phenomena may be questioned since aging men appear to be still rare in infertility clinics although parental age increases in industrialized countries. In this context alterations in the endocrine system are of more significance since serum testosterone levels also appear to decrease with age. These alterations can be associated with clinical symptoms known as late-onset hypogonadism. Men suffering from late-onset hypogonadism can be successfully treated with testosterone; however, a broad discussion has started about the necessity, usefulness, cost, and risks of such a therapy in older men.

The most obvious and interesting finding in human males is the slow decrease of serum testosterone that appears to occur between the age of 40 and 70.[1–3] The terms ADAM (Androgen Decline of the Aging Male), PADAM (Partial Androgen Decline of the Aging Male), and lately late-onset hypogonadism have been designed to reflect this circumstance. Between 10 and 15% of males are believed to have significant decreases of testosterone already by around age 40 years and reveal symptoms that are typical of or similar to those of manifest hypogonadism.[4] The decrease in serum testosterone is a result of primary testicular changes, altered neuroendocrine regulation of Leydig cell function, and an increase in sex-hormone-binding globulin (SHBG). The testicular alterations include a reduced secretory response to Leydig cells under human chorionic gonadotropin (hCG) stimulation due to a reduction in Leydig cell number, and likely also due to changes in testicular steroid metabolism.[2,5,6] The decreased testicular activity is associated with a rise in luteinizing hormone (LH), but this modest increase is inadequate to compensate for the decreased testosterone levels in aging men. Furthermore, the circadian rhythmicity of LH is clearly disturbed in older men.[7] The main cause for this appears to be a reduced mean LH pulse amplitude due to altered hypothalamic GnRH secretion.[8]

There is also evidence of a *primary and general testicular deterioration* associated with a general decline in *fertility* due to aging.[9] The latter is documented by the decreasing concentration in blood of the Sertoli cell marker inhibin B, and the gradual lowering of the inhibin B/follicle-stimulating hormone ratio with age.[9]

Testicular alterations in aging males

Pathophysiology: alterations in spermatogenesis

Spermatogenesis is a lifelong process and testicular histology indicates ongoing spermatogenesis even in very old males. However, spermatogenic efficiency estimated by the number of spermatozoa produced per day per gram of testicular parenchyma apparently declines with age.[10] This decline is a result of an increase in germ cell degeneration throughout spermatogenesis as seen in spermatogonia, spermatocytes, and haploid round spermatids. These degenerating cells undergo phagocytosis by somatic Sertoli cells, resulting in typical morphologic alterations within the seminiferous epithelium. As a result of germ cell phagocytosis Sertoli cells typically already indicate an increased cytoplasmic storage of lipids after the fiftieth year (Figure 12.1). Sertoli cells may also show a re-expression of fetal characteristics such as cytokeratin 18 intermediate filaments.[11] Degenerative alterations of germ cells become obvious by the occurrence of (1) spermatogonia with large nuclei, (2) so-called 'megalospermatocytes', indicating a failure of the pairing of the homologous chromosomes, and (3) giant spermatids with numerous nuclei. In addition, maturation stops at the level of spermatogonia, primary spermatocytes, or early round spermatids, or the total loss of germ cells occurs, leaving only Sertoli cells within the seminiferous tubules (Sertoli cell-only). Apoptosis was found to be one mechanism of germ cell degeneration but is a somewhat rare event and does not seem to increase with age.[12,13] Concomitant with these alterations, seminiferous tubules show a reduction in the diameter and thickening of the lamina propria. After total atrophy of the seminiferous epithelium, only strands of fibrous tissue remain (tubular ghosts).[14]

Although these alterations are typical in elderly men, there is a great interindividual variation in degree. In addition, these alterations leading to the reduction of spermatogenic efficiency can also be observed in testes of adult young and middle-aged oligo- or azoospermic men.[14]

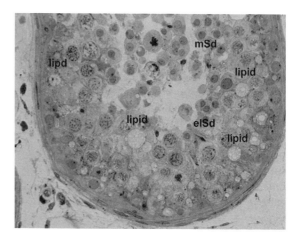

Figure 12.1 *Seminiferous tubule showing qualitatively intact spermatogenesis with few elongated spermatids (elSd) together with intraluminal multinucleated spermatids (mSd), and typical Sertoli cell lipid inclusions (lipid). (Semithin section, primary magnification × 40.)*

Sperm quality in aging males

The seminiferous tubules gradually become atrophic as a result of decreasing germinal epithelium, but these changes may not affect the entire testicular volume due to the focal character.[15] Comparing the daily sperm production of men aged 21 to 50 years with that of men aged 55 to 80 years, the younger group shows a 30% higher sperm production.[16] In contrast, men over 65 years show a highly significant decrease in daily sperm production.[17] This indicates a gradual decline of fertility with increasing age, although alterations in sperm quality may be minimal. In principle, spermatogenesis may be retained well into senescence. Although 50% of those over 80 have been reported to be completely infertile,[18] children have been fathered even by men over 90 years of age. When functional sperm parameters in older fathers were determined, no differences to those of younger men were found.[19] Another intriguing phenomenon with yet unknown clinical significance is represented by the fact that seminal leukocytes and PMN elastase appear to increase with age. It has not been elucidated if this just parallels decreasing sperm quality or if these alterations might provide an etiologic hint.

Fertility in aging males: clinical relevance and therapeutic considerations

Fertility usually persists well into old age. It is concluded that the age of the female partner, rather than the age of the husband, is the most important factor in determining the fertility chance of a couple presenting with infertility.[15] This opinion was published by Rolf and co-workers in 1996.[20] Interestingly, the number of pregnancies is not found to be different when comparing older males with a group of younger men with relatively old female partners.[20] Even where the male is of advanced age, the reduced conceptive facility of the female partner is a more important cause of low paternity than reduced sperm quality of the male.[21]

In our own experience, men of advanced age are still rare in infertility clinics. Specialized guidelines and specific therapies are not available for the treatment of infertility of older men.

ADAM/PADAM (late-onset hypogonadism) in human males

LH and FSH serum levels in males decrease with age, reflecting the reduction of Leydig cell steroidogenesis and alterations of the seminiferous epithelium with the reduction of Sertoli cells, respectively.[2,22] LH rhythmicity undergoes significant modulations in the elderly, likely due to altered secretion of GnRH in the hypothalamus, but molecular concepts to explain this phenomenon are lacking.[7,23] The reduction of steroidogenesis in Leydig cells is amplified by the slow enhancement of SHGB, resulting in an even sharper decrease in free testosterone (bioavailable) in the serum. Although there are technical problems concerning reliable techniques to estimate the free or non SHGB-bound testosterone, it is believed that bioavailable testosterone declines more steeply with increasing age than total serum testosterone due to an age-dependent increase in SHGB binding of testosterone.[3]

Patients with decreased levels of testosterone due to aging usually complain about a variety of symptoms. Erectile dysfunction is among the most mentioned symptoms of this clientele of men. The Massachusetts Male Aging Study (MMAS) found an incidence of erectile dysfunction in 5 to 15% of males between the ages of 40 and 70. Erectile dysfunction likely is not a direct consequence of the altered endocrine situation,[4] but is largely correlated with cofactors such as heart disease and medication. Loss of libido is an important symptom that correlates well with the loss of testosterone and is among those symptoms that respond well to hormone replacement therapy (HRT). Decline in bone density is another symptom that can be well explained by endocrine deficiency and might be a strong argument for HRT.[9] Loss of physical strength, reduction in muscle mass, and enhancement of body fat have their origin in the reduction of testosterone, but are also heavily dependent on conditions of lifestyle and physical training. Mood changes and other psychologic symptoms complete the picture of the variety of symptoms that are connected to the decline of testosterone in aging males.

Chronic illness in the aging: what is the impact on gonadal function?

In this context it seems to be important to focus the interest on the common determinants of aging that have to be considered also for reproductive health.[24] In particular, several forms of systemic chronic illness (Table 12.1[25]) may occur directly at the testicular level: reduced Leydig cell function will lead to androgen deficiency, while diseases affecting spermatogenesis may lead to male infertility. There is no doubt that testosterone decline may also significantly impair spermatogenesis. It is generally accepted that testicular volume is correlated with spermatogenetic quality. A decrease in testicular volume in the group of older men could not be observed in two studies,[21,26] although an influence of chronic disease status cannot be ruled out with 100% certainty.

Other factors influencing testicular function: disorders in the urogenital organs

Concerning decreasing gonadal function with age, infections have to be discussed etiologically.[25]

Table 12.1 *Chronic illness and reduced gonadal function[25]*

Metabolic	Organ-defined	Iatrogenic
Severe obesity	Chronic obstruction airway disease (COAD)	Hemodialysis
Diabetes mellitus	Pulmonary fibrosis	Renal transplantation
Hypothyroidism	Cystic fibrosis	Chemotherapy
Cushing's disease	Rheumatoid arthritis	Irradiation
Uremia	Systemic lupus erythematosus	
Severe liver cirrhosis	Celiac disease	

Orchitis may contribute to decreasing sperm quality; lymphocytic and plasmacytic infiltrates have been identified in biopsy specimens in the peritubular tissue, indicating an age-dependent exposition to recurrent urogenital infections. Others hypothesize that this effect may be blurred by a lower frequency of ejaculation in older men,[21] although disorders of ejaculation have not been evaluated in the literature with respect to age.[27] Besides typical congenital and acquired causes, functional seminal emission problems such as side-effects due to the intake of drugs (especially antidepressants and α-blockers) may play a special role in increasing age. In this context, the interference with sexual function caused by diseases of the prostate is of great importance for the urologist.[28] Undoubtedly, carcinoma of the prostate, untreated or under observation, has the greatest impact on sexual function, depending on the expectation of survival and treatment modalities. In benign prostatic hyperplasia (BPH), about two-thirds of patients scheduled for operation still have erections and ejaculation[29] that will be hampered by conventional BPH therapy.

Aging fathers and genetic risks for the offspring

The effects of genetic factors on various components of health in aging are poorly understood,[24] although in general the effect of hereditary influence on the incidence of chronic conditions seems to decrease with age.[16] There are many genetic syndromes that are associated with hypogonadism and which may consequently also influence the fertility status; examples are myotonic dystrophy, Kennedy's syndrome, some types of Down's syndrome, Prader–Willi syndrome, Kallmann's syndrome, and others.[25] All these syndromes affect primary androgen action and consequently also spermatogenetic capacity.

It seems to be accepted that structural chromosomal anomalies in sperm of aging men are detectable, but not significantly increased.[21] An age-dependent spontaneous mutation rate potentially promoted by aging fathers has to be discussed as a theoretic risk for future populations;[17] however, the real health risk was incalculable until now.[21]

Current opinion considers that the increased age of the female partner, not the age of the male, is an indication for dedicated prenatal diagnostic management.[21] Nevertheless, although a negative influence of paternal age on pregnancy rates cannot be demonstrated, an increase in structural abnormalities of aging spermatozoa has been reported and has to be kept in mind. Furthermore, the questionable higher risk of autosomal dominant diseases has been discussed in relation to increased paternal age.[30]

Conclusions

Sexual health includes 'normal' libido, sexuality, erectile function, and fertility. Sexual alternations in older men include libido disorders, decreasing sexual interest, and possibly a decline in intercourse frequency.

These findings are significantly associated with typical hormonal findings usually considered as ADAM/PADAM or late-onset hypogonadism. Although there are also characteristic alterations in gonadal function, with numerous indications of a significant decrease in steroidogenesis in the Leydig cell as the most important factor in aging, healthy men likely remain fertile during their lifetime.

Disturbed sperm parameters are frequently associated with chronic illness and concomitant diseases of the urogenital organs. Although a negative influence of paternal age on pregnancy cannot be demonstrated, the age of the female is the major factor in every infertile partnership. It is unclear whether increasing chromosomal abnormalities have to be discussed in relationship to the offspring.

Finally, it seems to be important not to view fertility problems in older men simply as a result of pathology while overlooking the effect of the natural process of aging.

References

1. Hermann M, Untergasser G, Rumpold H, Berger P. Aging of the male reproductive system. Exp Gerontol 2000; 35: 1267–79.
2. Kaufmann JM. Hypothalamo–pituitary–gonadal function in aging men. Aging Male 1999; 2: 157–65.
3. Vermeulen A. Androgens in the aging male – clinical review 24. J Clin Endocrinol Metab 1991; 73: 221–4.
4. Gray A, Feldman HA, McKinlay HB, Longcope C. Age, disease and changing sex hormone levels in middle-aged men: results of the Massachusetts Male Aging Study. J Clin Endocrinol Metab 1991; 73: 1016–25.
5. Zirkin BR, Chen H. Regulation of Leydig cell steroidogenic function during aging. Biol Reprod 2000; 63: 977–81.
6. Zirkin BR, Chen H, Luo L. Leydig cell steroidogenesis in aging rats. Exp Gerontol 1997; 32: 529–37.
7. Bremner WJ, Vitiello MV, Prinz PN. Loss of circadian rhythmicity in blood testosterone levels with aging in normal men. J Clin Endocrinol Metab 1983; 56: 1278–81.
8. Vermeulen A, Kaufmann JM. Role of the hypothalamo-pituitary function in the hypoandrogenism of healthy aging. J Clin Endocrinol Metab 1992; 74: 704–6.
9. Comhaire FH. Andropause: hormone replacement therapy in the aging male. Eur Urol 2000; 38: 655–62.
10. Johnson L, Varner DD, Roberts ME et al. Efficiency of spermatogenesis: a comparative approach. Anim Reprod Sci 2000; 60–61: 471–80.
11. Stosiek P, Kasper M, Karsten U. Expression of cytokeratins 8 and 18 in human Sertoli cells of immature and atrophic seminiferous tubules. Differentiation 1990; 43: 66–70.
12. Barnes CJ, Covington BW, Cameron IL, Lee M. Effect of ageing on spontaneous and induced mouse testicular germ cell apoptosis. Aging 1998; 10: 497–501.
13. Brinkworth MH, Weinbauer GF, Bergmann M, Nieschlag E. Apoptosis as a mechanism of germ cell loss in elderly men. Int J Androl 1997; 20: 222–8.
14. Holstein AF, Roosen-Runge EC, Schirren C. Illustrated Pathology of Human Spermatogenesis. Berlin: Grosse Verlag, 1988.
15. Schill W-B, Köhn FM, Haidl G. The aging male. In: Berg G, Hammar M, eds. The Modern Management of the Menopause. New York: Parthenon, 1993: 545–65.
16. Harris A, Cairns B. Health checks for people over 75. BMJ 1992; 305: 1437.
17. Crow JF. The high spontaneous mutation rate: is it a health risk? Proc Natl Acad Sci USA 1997; 94: 8380–6.
18. Harman SM. Clinical aspects of aging of the male reproductive system. In: Schneider EL, ed. The Aging Reproductive System. New York: Raven, 1978: 29–58.
19. Haidl G, Jung A, Schill WB. Aging and sperm function. Hum Reprod 1996; 11: 558–60.
20. Rolf C, Behre HM, Nieschlag E. Reproductive parameters of older compared to younger men of infertile couples. Int J Androl 1996; 19: 135–42.
21. Vermeulen A, Kaufmann JM, Giagulli VA. Influence of some biological indices on sex hormone binding globulin and androgen levels in the aging and obese male. J Clin Endocrinol Metab 1996; 81: 1821–7.
22. Veldhuis JD. Recent neuroendocrine facts of male reproductive aging. Exp Gerontol 2000; 35: 1281–308.
23. World Health Organization. Men, aging and health. Aging Male 2000; 3: 3–36.
24. Turner HE, Wass JAH. Gonadal function in men with chronic illness. Clin Endocrinol 1997; 47: 379–403.
25. Handelsman DJ, Staraj S. Testicular size: the effects of aging, malnutrition and illness. J Androl 1983; 6: 144–51.
26. Hendry WF. Disorders of ejaculation: congenital, acquired and functional. Br J Urol 1998; 82: 331–41.
27. Burger B, Weidner W, Altwein J. Prostate and sexuality: an overview. Eur Urol 1999; 35: 177–84.
28. Weidner W, Altwein J, Hauck E, Beutel M, Brähler E. Sexuality of the elderly. Urol Int 2001; 66: 181–4.
29. Bordson BL, Leonardo VS. The appropriate upper age limit for several semen donors. a review of the genetic effects of paternal age. Fertil Steril 1991; 56: 397–401.

CHAPTER 13

Urinary incontinence

Adrian Wagg

The prevalence of bladder problems in men is lower than that in women at all ages (Table 13.1), but as in women, the prevalence of bladder problems increases in association with older age. Chronic infections, bladder stones, bladder tumors, and primary bladder pathology such as detrusor overactivity may cause such problems in men, whether or not secondary to a neurologic lesion. Incompetence of the urethral sphincter occurs rarely in men, and where it does occur it is usually due to trauma, surgery, or nervous system disease. The elderly experience the same bladder problems as other adults. Where the elderly differ, though, is in their ability to respond and to compensate for problems which a younger adult may find trivial. Concomitant disease and drug therapy, in particular, may serve to render an elderly person incontinent.

The prevalence of incontinence also varies with the origin of the surveyed population (Table 13.1) and with the definition of incontinence employed in the study. In 1995, data from intensive testing of urinary tract function on normal, asymptomatic elderly people, half of them male, but without comparative controls were published, suggesting that normality was a rarity, only 18% of individuals falling into this category.[1] The problem with such research is that many 'age-related' studies have not used comparative samples of younger individuals and therefore it is difficult to ascribe their findings to age alone. However, it is certain that incontinence should never be viewed as a

Table 13.1 *Population estimates of prevalence of urinary incontinence in adults*

	Percentage incontinent
Community dwelling women	
15–44 years	5–7
45–64 years	8–15
65 + years	10–20
Community dwelling men	
15–64 years	3
65 + years	7–10
Residential homes (men/women)	25
Nursing homes (men/women)	40
Hospital care (elderly and elderly mentally infirm) (men/women)	50–70

Reproduced with permission from Royal College of Physicians. Incontinence: Causes, Management and Provision of Services. London: Royal College of Physicians, 1995.

normal consequence of aging and that, worldwide, the expanding proportion of the population in late life will place an increasing burden on services delivering continence care. This chapter will review current understanding of the changes in lower urinary tract function and incontinence in men in later life.

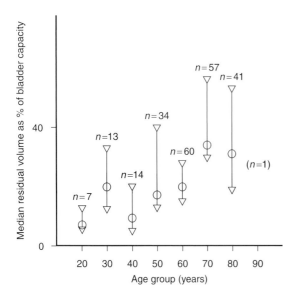

Figure 13.1 *Contractile function as measured by Q** *in association with greater age in men with lower urinary tract symptoms (n = 157). Reproduced with permission from reference 2.*

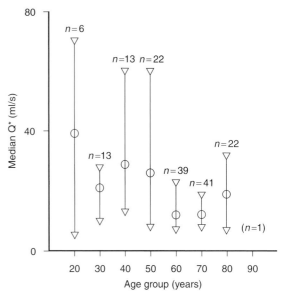

Figure 13.2 *Increased age is associated with a reduction in bladder capacity (median ± 95% CI). Reproduced with permission from reference 2.*

Age-related effects

Many of the data relating to changes in lower urinary tract function are derived from studies of individuals with lower urinary tract symptoms who have undergone urodynamic studies. Data from community-dwelling, continent individuals are sparse, but where they do exist, tend to confirm the associations identified by other means.

Detrusor contractile function (Figure 13.1), bladder capacity (Figure 13.2) and urinary flow rates (Figure 13.3) all appear to decline in association with greater age.[2] There is also an increase in the prevalence of incomplete emptying as demonstrated by the existence of a significant post-micturition residual volume of urine (Figure 13.4).[3] In men, the progressive enlargement of the prostate with age tends to dominate the behavior of the urinary outflow tract, with up to half of all men suffering from outflow tract obstruction.[4] The changes in the bladder associated with prostatic hypertrophy, significant detrusor muscle hypertrophy,[5] a reduction in the number of acetylcholinesterase-containing nerves,[6] and an increase in the collagen to smooth

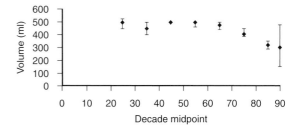

Figure 13.3 *Median (± 95% CI) maximum flow rate for men in relation to greater age (P < 0.001). Reproduced with permission from reference 2.*

muscle ratio[7] which causes the bladder to be less compliant have all been demonstrated in association with age alone.[8–10] Thus it is unclear to what extent prostatic hypertrophy alone may contribute to the observed changes. However, as obstruction increases, the bladder requires a greater contractile effort to overcome the effects of the obstruction. In a subgroup of men, this eventually leads to a chronically overdistended bladder, which fails to empty effectively; in others, acute urinary retention may develop.

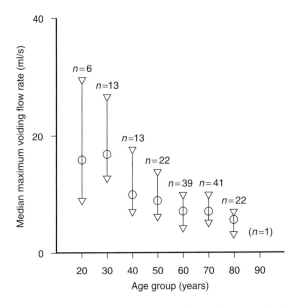

Figure 13.4 *Post-void residual volume of urine related to increasing age in men with lower urinary tract symptoms. Reproduced with permission from reference 2.*

The evolution of detrusor instability is conventionally thought to be associated with the development of significant outflow tract obstruction and is present in 43–86% of patients.[4] This viewpoint has been reinforced by the fact that relief of the obstruction leads to bladder stability in a significant proportion.[11] However, once again, the incidence of detrusor instability increases in association with age per se and is similar in females. In men with lower urinary tract symptoms, the likelihood of detrusor instability being the cause of these reaches 85% in the eighth decade, regardless of the presence of significant outflow tract obstruction.[2] Detrusor instability will be discussed in more detail below.

Conservative and lifestyle measures to address bladder problems in men

Smoking

One major study by Kosimaki and colleagues[12] has identified an association of bladder problems with cigarette smoking. The odds ratio of lower urinary tract symptoms was 1.47 for current smokers and 1.38 for former smokers when compared with men who had never smoked.[12] When adjusted for other risk factors associated with bladder problems, the risk associated with smoking still stood. As with other adverse effects of smoking, this association weakened following cessation of smoking and appeared to reach baseline after 40 years of abstinence. The association of smoking appeared to be strongest with the occurrence of detrusor instability. There are animal data which demonstrate an effect of nicotine upon the motor function of the bladder. There are, however, no prospective intervention trials of smoking cessation on improving bladder symptoms. However, there is little doubt that smoking should be discouraged in view of the cardiovascular risk, regardless of its effect upon lower urinary tract function.

Fluid advice

Fluid intake should be around 2–2.5 liters daily. Obviously an excessive fluid intake will lead to an increased urinary frequency. A daily average of 7–8 micturitions per 24 hours is considered the upper limit of normal. Limiting or reducing overall fluid intake is not effective for managing incontinence, and may lead to adverse effects, especially in the face of other medication, and particularly in the elderly, who already have a decrease in total body water. Judicious timing of fluid, especially at night, may be effective in reducing nocturnal urinary frequency.

The effect of caffeine on lower urinary tract function is hotly debated. Avoidance of excessive caffeine intake in teas, coffees, and colas may exacerbate urinary frequency. However, there have been several short-term urodynamic studies using oral caffeine which have shown no effect on the bladder.[13] Similarly in clinical trials no sustained benefit has been found.[14] However, a trial of caffeine reduction in a predominantly elderly group of women reported that a reduction in caffeine intake and maintenance of total fluid intake did lead to a reduction in urinary frequency.[15] Excess alcohol intake has a similar effect, in addition to the volume load, but there are no objective data from studies of alcohol reduction.

Weight reduction

In women, there is good evidence for a positive association of stress urinary incontinence and body mass, and some evidence that massive weight reduction (in a group of women who had undergone jaw wiring) reduces this.[14,16] Unfortunately, there is no such evidence for the male population and weight reduction should only be recommended as part of a management plan to maintain general health rather than for its putative effect upon continence status.

The 'lazy urethra'

Dribbling, which may occur late after micturition, is a significant problem in young men. The prevalence of this condition in one report ranged from 17% of men in their third decade to 27% in their sixth.[17] This phenomenon is due to the retention of a column of urine in the bulbus urethra after voiding. The urine is voided at a later time and is often a cause of considerable embarrassment, due to staining of garments. There have been some studies which have examined this problem. The recommended treatment is to perform perineal massage following micturition to 'milk' the urethra of all urine prior to leaving the lavatory. This is a successful intervention but is not acceptable to some individuals because of the manipulation required. An alternative approach to the problem has been recently reported. This study demonstrated efficacy of the application of voluntary pelvic floor contraction, following taught pelvic floor exercises, in controlling the problem.[18]

Overactive bladder (detrusor instability)

The overactive bladder is the commonest cause of urinary incontinence in the elderly regardless of gender. The conventional term for the condition, detrusor instability, fails to accurately reflect the true extent of the problem. This is because a diagnosis of detrusor instability, as defined by the International Continence Society, is based upon finding a spontaneous detrusor contraction whilst filling the bladder during urodynamic testing.[19] The difficulty with this definition is that 25% of people with the classic symptoms of urgency, frequency with or without urge incontinence, will potentially be excluded from effective treatment for their condition by this criterion. In addition, up to 60% of normal, asymptomatic individuals exhibit spontaneous detrusor contractions during urodynamic investigations.[20]

The true incidence of symptomatic detrusor instability is unknown due to the inherent difficulty of underreporting, but is estimated at between 10 and 15% of asymptomatic men and women between 10 and 50 years of age, rising to 35% of those aged over 75 years old.[21]

In the vast majority of cases, the cause of detrusor overactivity is unknown. However, as noted above, it is commonly associated with bladder outflow obstruction in men, pelvic surgery in women, and neurologic injury or disease, such as spinal cord injury, multiple sclerosis, cerebrovascular disease, Parkinson's, or Alzheimer's disease.

Patients' symptoms are extremely important in making a diagnosis of detrusor overactivity. Not all patients may experience all symptoms and many go to great lengths to avoid experiencing incontinence. Most often this is achieved either by restricting fluid intake or increasing urinary frequency. In addition to taking a relevant history, a patient-completed voiding diary is a useful aid.[22] The diary records urinary frequency and volumes passed as well as the number of incontinence episodes experienced.

Urinary tract infection and calculi may cause urinary urgency and urge incontinence, and should be excluded at an early stage. The simplest method to exclude infection is to use a rapid urinalysis dipstick. The leukocyte esterase and nitrite tests are an accurate method of assessing the absence of infection (combined negative predictive value 98%) and can enable early treatment. If recurrent infection or hematuria in the absence of infection is noted and subsequently confirmed then further investigation is needed.

Treatment interventions

The development of pharmacologic treatment for bladder problems has been slow and it is only recently that drugs designed specifically with the bladder in mind have been developed. Antimuscarinic drugs are still the most widely used treatment in the UK. Data suggesting that such drugs can inhibit contractions of the detrusor are conflicting,[23–25] however this does not appear to affect response to treatment. Trials which have utilized urodynamic studies to assess efficacy have normally shown that bladder capacity alone is significantly changed following treatment.[26] There are also data which suggest that those patients' symptoms respond as well to antimuscarinic agents regardless of the diagnosis being made by urodynamic or clinical characterization.[27] The chief drawback of these agents has been their side-effect profile, as the target receptor is ubiquitous in the body. Side-effects such as dry mouth, constipation, blurred vision, and esophageal reflux have limited the tolerability of these agents.

The most commonly prescribed treatment for the overactive bladder in the UK is oxybutynin. Oxybutynin is both antimuscarinic, a direct muscle relaxant, and a local anesthetic agent. Its chief metabolite, N-desethyl oxybutynin, is also pharmacologically active and occurs in higher concentrations than the parent compound. This metabolite is thought to be responsible for many of the adverse effects related to this drug. The efficacy of oxybutynin has been shown in both open and controlled trials.[28,29] The main drawback in trials of high dose oxybutynin (5 mg three times daily) has been the incidence of side-effects; the withdrawal rate has varied between 22 and 40%, with up to 80% of those withdrawing suffering significant adverse reactions. More recent work using lower doses of the drug has also shown efficacy with a concomitant reduction in the adverse effects and an enhanced level of tolerability.[30,31] However, only 10–30% of patients will still be taking the drug one year after initiation.[32] Oxybutynin has been found to add little to the clinical effectiveness of a prompted voiding regimen in a nursing home population.[33]

A modified release preparation with once daily administration has been approved for use in Europe. This preparation retains the efficacy of the standard release form but with up to 40% fewer reported side-effects.[34] Recent studies have concentrated upon comparing this compound to immediate release oxybutynin and have resulted in an equivalent efficacy in controlling urge incontinence. The incidence of dry mouth was similar, but with a reduced severity in one study by Versi and colleagues[35] and was reduced in incidence in a second study by

Anderson and co-workers.[36] Approximately two-thirds of the patients prescribed extended-release oxybutynin for detrusor instability were still taking the medication 6 months later.

The side-effect profile of oxybutynin is also improved by other alternative methods of administration; both the rectal and intravesical route have been assessed.[37,38] Winkler and Sand,[38] in a trial of 25 patients, found a 48% response rate using the rectal route and 58% of responders were able to use the drug in the longer term. However, 48% of all patients suffered from dry mouth. Clearly the intravesical route has a limited acceptability to patients who are not routinely practicing intermittent catheterization.

Tolterodine is a newer, non-selective antimuscarinic competitive antagonist, which in the anesthetized cat model appears to have some functional selectivity for bladder muscarinic receptors over those in the salivary glands.[39] This appears to explain the lower incidence of dry mouth and the reduction in withdrawals due to severe dry mouth seen with use of the drug. Like oxybutynin it too has an active metabolite which appears to be responsible for some of the observed therapeutic effect.[40] Several randomized, double-blind, placebo-controlled studies in patients with detrusor instability, detrusor hyperreflexia, overactive bladder, and specifically in the elderly have been performed.[41–43] In doses of 2 mg twice daily, tolterodine has consistently resulted in a reduction in urinary frequency and, in some trials, a reduction in the number of incontinence episodes. Where tolterodine has been compared to oxybutynin, the drug has been found equally efficacious. Tolterodine appears to have the advantage of greater tolerability and fewer withdrawals due to adverse effects, although there has been no direct comparison with the lower doses of oxybutynin used widely in UK practice. The proportion of patients continuing therapy for 6 months in one study comparing 500 patients taking either tolterodine or oxybutynin was statistically superior for tolterodine (32%) compared with oxybutynin (22%, $P < 0.001$). For those discontinuing either drug, oxybutynin was stopped significantly earlier.[44]

Although tolterodine is more costly than oxybutynin, its use may allow treatment of a greater number of patients. What is not known, and not yet tested, is whether tolterodine has any other advantages, such as its effect upon cognitive impairment, or other troublesome side-effects. In addition, the effect of bladder retraining with or without the drug has not been assessed.

The older antimuscarinic drug, imipramine, although not licensed for treatment of detrusor instability or overactive bladder, is commonly used for this indication. It is both a centrally and peripherally acting antimuscarinic agent, it blocks reuptake of serotonin (5-HT) and norepinephrine and has α-adrenergic agonist properties. There is also some evidence that the drug is an antidiuretic in mice. There is no evidence that imipramine can suppress unstable detrusor contractions but several small trials have shown the drug to be efficacious in the treatment of detrusor instability.[45] In the treatment of 10 elderly patients with detrusor instability the use of imipramine was efficacious in achieving continence (6/10 patients) in doses between 25 and 150 mg.[46] A commonly used antidepressant, doxepin, has also been assessed in a single-blinded cross-over study at a dose of either 50 mg at night or 50 mg nightly and 25 mg in the morning.[47] There was a significant decrease in nocturnal urinary frequency.

Propiverine hydrochloride has combined antimuscarinic and calcium channel blocking activity. It has several active metabolites and is rapidly absorbed orally where it undergoes significant first pass metabolism. There has been no cardiac toxicity associated with use of the drug to date. Clinical trials have demonstrated superiority to placebo in the treatment of detrusor hyperreflexia in a 2-week, double-blind, placebo-controlled trial of oral treatment.[48] In comparative trials against flavoxate and placebo and oxybutynin and placebo, propiverine has demonstrated a similar efficacy to oxybutynin.[49,50] Madersbacher and colleagues,[49] in a 4-week study comparing the use of propiverine against oxybutynin 5 mg twice daily and placebo, reported a similar efficacy in treatment of symptoms to oxybutynin, but with statistically significantly milder and less common incidence of dry mouth. Up to 20% of patients do, however, experience adverse effects which are mainly anticholinergic in nature. There are as yet no long-term data from

European trials of the drug and its use has been confined to patients with urodynamically confirmed detrusor instability, thus not including the 25% of patients with symptoms of bladder overactivity but normal urodynamics. In addition, there is no evidence regarding use of the drug in relation to behavioral intervention. The place of propiverine in the treatment of overactive bladder remains to be resolved, but given its equal efficacy and apparent milder incidence of side-effects it is likely to remain as an alternative second-line treatment.

Trospium chloride, an antimuscarinic agent derived from atropine, has also recently been approved for use in Europe. This drug has been shown to be effective in the treatment of detrusor instability in several randomized controlled trials using urodynamic measures of diagnosis and extent of disease as well as clinical and quality of life outcomes.[51,52]

The drug has been assessed in short-term studies versus placebo and standard release oxybutynin and has been found to be superior in effect to placebo and equivalent in efficacy to oxybutynin, when treating detrusor hyperreflexia, at doses of 5 mg three times daily. The number of withdrawals due to side-effects in the trospium group was lower than the oxybutynin group.[53]

The potential for antimuscarinic agents to cause a deterioration in cognition, especially in the elderly, has been well recognized in association with oxybutynin.[54,55] The effect of trospium chloride on electroencephalogram (EEG) activity has been assessed compared to oxybutynin administration in one study of 12 healthy volunteers. Trospium did not cause a significant reduction in EEG activity. The relationship of this to functional cognitive ability, however, is unknown and needs further study.[56]

The drug flavoxate has been widely promoted for the treatment of the overactive bladder. Its possible mechanism of action in the treatment of bladder problems is unclear but it appears to have no anticholinergic properties.[57] Studies of its efficacy versus placebo have failed to show any beneficial effect of flavoxate,[58,59] the reported reduction in urinary frequency ranging between 21 and 5%. In comparative, double-blind, cross-over studies versus emepromium or oxybutynin, flavoxate was found to be equally efficacious in achieving an improvement.[60,61] The use of flavoxate was associated with few side-effects. Given the lack of effect in placebo-controlled studies of flavoxate it is difficult to recommend its use.

Most drug therapy has conventionally been used in combination with bladder retraining. Bladder retraining was first described by Jeffcoate and Francis in 1966.[62] This technique involves the simple maxim 'hold on', which is simple to say but far from simple to perform, requiring much motivation and will-power. Even in the most motivated patient, bladder retraining can take months to achieve a lasting change in habit, and because of the difficulty and continual attention required there is a high relapse rate. The regimen involves a gradual increase in the voiding interval, using frequency–volume charts as an objective reinforcement and guide. Data from trials of this method alone are conflicting and there have been few of sufficient methodologic quality to allow firm conclusions to be drawn. Burgio and co-workers[63] showed that behavioral techniques alone may improve patients' experience of their disease to a similar extent to drug therapy when used alone, although the study was limited by its interpretation. There are data to suggest that a combination of pharmacotherapy and behavioral techniques may achieve results which are superior to either technique in isolation, although the number of patients in this study progressing to combination therapy was small. Where the patient is cognitively impaired or institutionalized, a progressive regular toiletting regimen may be employed.[64] There are no data to support the additional use of oxybutynin in this population,[65] but tolterodine does have efficacy data as a sole treatment modality. Care has to be taken when introducing antimuscarinic medication to those with pre-existing cognitive impairment and to those already taking anticholinergic medication, as this may be exacerbated.

Surgery

Surgery is most applicable for those with detrusor overactivity associated with other conditions, such as outflow tract obstruction where the overactivity resolves in two-thirds of patients. For those with intractable disease uncontrollable by other means, the technique of clam ileocystoplasty or detrusor myomectomy (bladder autoaugmentation) is used. Both of these techniques aim to create a high capacity, low pressure, and stable reservoir. The operation is effective, with abolition of the underlying instability in 50% of patients, in addition to an increase in bladder compliance and the functional capacity of the bladder. For between 15 and 75% of patients, the operation is associated with inefficient voiding so that self-catheterization is required to achieve complete bladder emptying. There is also concern about the metabolic effects due to the permeable endothelium of the small bowel being in contact with urine, the difficulty caused by intestinal mucus production, and urinary tract infection.

Good results from surgery have been reported with variable time of follow-up and in patients up to the age of 80 years.[66] There is no evidence that denervation procedures, such as trigonal phenol injection, are efficacious. Likewise, data on the efficacy of repeated cystodistension in alleviating symptoms of overactive bladder are lacking.

Stress and post-prostatectomy incontinence

Men seldom suffer from stress urinary incontinence due to urethral sphincter insufficiency in the absence of surgery or trauma. Studies estimate the prevalence of this condition to be 4.6–9.2% of men.[67,68]

There has been little, if any, systematic research of treatment of men with urethral incompetence. Two small studies of 20 and 7 men, 6 of whom in the latter were postoperative, have reported efficacy in terms of improvement of incontinence with ephedrine.[69,70]

The incidence of incontinence following prostatectomy varies between 1 and 15% depending on the procedure used. The highest incidence is associated with radical prostatectomy. Periurethral procedures are associated with rates reported at from 0 to 8%.[71,72]

The majority of these studies have followed patients in the short term and are retrospective reviews, rather than prospective studies with the express intent to examine the phenomenon. There are also few data available in the reports to allow

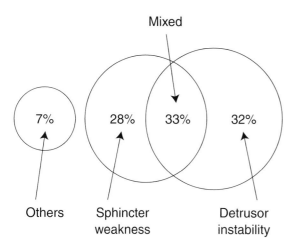

Mixed

7%   28%   33%   32%

Others   Sphincter   Detrusor
          weakness   instability

Figure 13.5 *Causes of post-prostatectomy incontinence in 203 patients identified by urodynamic study.*

underlying diagnosis of incontinence to be established. There is clearly a requirement for a prospective study in this population of men post-surgery that pays attention to the degree and type of incontinence and its resolution in the longer term.

In late life, pre-existing bladder problems may co-exist (Figure 13.5), accounting for the observed underlying pathology. The integrity of the striated muscle sphincter is compromised in approximately 25% of incontinent patients.[73] Underlying detrusor instability accounts for the majority of cases, either alone or in combination with sphincteric insufficiency. Factors that have been associated with an increased risk of incontinence following prostatectomy are an increased age,[74] associated neurologic disease, or cognitive impairment.[75,76] Patients with pre-existing cerebrovascular disease or Parkinson's disease are at an increased risk of becoming incontinent following prostatic surgery.[77] Likewise, patients who have received radiotherapy are more likely to suffer from postoperative incontinence.[78] Where the prostatectomy has been for malignant disease, the risk of incontinence has been reported at between 2 and 5%.[79,80]

When treated with artificial sphincters, the revision rate appears to be higher than when this technique is employed in patients who have not been exposed to radiotherapy, mostly due to a higher rate

of erosion. There is some debate about the influence of prior surgery in more recent series, and it appears likely that there is no additional risk attributable to a repeat procedure. Poorer results from prostatic surgery are reported if there is co-existent detrusor instability and there are some reports of symptomatic worsening.[81]

Treatment of post-prostatectomy incontinence should be targeted at the underlying pathology where appropriate. There is good evidence that the incidence of detrusor instability will rise in association with increasing age amongst the postoperative population and that this will lead to an increase in lower urinary tract symptoms which will require treatment.[82] There is good accumulating evidence that pelvic floor exercises should be the intervention of choice for post-prostatectomy incontinence, although there is an appreciable rate of spontaneous resolution. One short-term study of intensive pelvic floor therapy noted a significant reduction in incontinence.[83] Burgio and colleagues[84] reported the effective use of a combination of behavioral techniques to address this problem. There appears to be no additional benefit of electrostimulation.[85] Periurethral injectable materials such as collagen, teflon paste, and autologous fat have also been used in an attempt to treat stress incontinence in men. The reported results of this intervention have been contradictory and success in the short term is followed by relapse.[86,87] However, once again, data with which to make an informed decision with respect to this treatment for stress incontinence are lacking. For patients with persistent stress incontinence following medical management, the implantation of an artificial urethral sphincter is a successful option: more than 70% of men will be either cured or significantly improved following the procedure. The presence of co-existent detrusor instability leads to a reduction in the success rate. Failure is mainly due to infection, urethral erosion, or mechanical failure, although later devices are much less prone to this latter problem. In one report of long-term follow-up, 32.5% of patients required re-operation in the 3 years following the original operation.[88]

Clean intermittent catheterization

In combination with antimuscarinic drugs, many elderly men with co-existent voiding inefficiency who would not be candidates for surgical treatment can be successfully managed by this technique.[89] Where a patient's dexterity is not good, a voluntary or statutory carer may be successfully employed if the frequency of intermittent catheterization required is not too high. There is still considerable debate (and little evidence) at what volume to intervene. Empirically, if the patient is continent and asymptomatic, then many would treat conservatively, some up to volumes in excess of 250 ml.

Nocturnal frequency, polyuria, and enuresis

Nocturnal frequency is deemed to be excessive if greater than twice nightly. There is an increased incidence of frequent voiding in association with greater age. Prostatic hypertrophy and outflow tract obstruction is the commonest cause in men, the assessment and treatment of which is reviewed above. There are also several physiologic changes which lead to an increasing likelihood of developing nocturnal frequency. Normally, adults produce two-thirds of their 24-hour urine output by day and the other third by night. In older individuals this changes: renal concentrating ability falls and glomerular filtration rate increases in the supine position. There is a redistribution of fluid at night, particularly if the individual has venous insufficiency or is on medication, which predisposes to the development of peripheral edema. In addition, some older adults have a delayed diuresis in response to a fluid load and lose their diurnal rhythm of antidiuretic hormone (ADH) secretion.[90] When taken together, this means that the kidneys are working harder overnight to produce greater quantities of more dilute urine, the amount of which may be in excess of functional bladder capacity. All this is in the absence of any pathology, such as heart failure, which may exacerbate the situation. Other diseases which predispose to urinary incontinence are shown in Table 13.2. There is evidence for the efficacy of DDAVP[91] and early evening diuretic,[92] and limited evidence for daytime recumbence,[93] but these are not well tolerated by all. In particular, the usefulness of DDAVP may be limited to those individuals with true nocturnal polyuria – defined as producing

Table 13.2 *Concomitant diseases which may have an impact upon urinary incontinence*

Diseases affecting mobility
Arthritis hip fracture
Contractures
Peripheral vascular disease
Stroke
Parkinson's disease

Nervous system disorders affecting cognition and neural control mechanisms
Dementia
Stroke
Parkinson's disease

Other medical conditions
Diabetes mellitus; causing polyuria and autonomic neuropathy
Congestive heart failure (CHF); leading to excess nocturnal urinary production
Venous insufficiency; a similar mechanism as CHF
Chronic lung disease; exacerbation of stress incontinence

> 50% of total daily urine output at night – rather than urinary frequency,[94] and its use may be hampered by drug–drug interactions predisposing to hyponatremia or excessive secondary drinking habits.

Primary nocturnal enuresis may persist into adulthood. There is a genetic predisposition to primary nocturnal enuresis. In 1995, a Danish group reported finding a mutation on chromosome 13 that appeared to be partly responsible for nocturnal enuresis in some families.[95] Since then another gene, on chromosome 12, has been described.[96] These genes are known as *ENUR 1* and *2*, respectively. If both parents are enuretic then a child has a 70% chance of also being enuretic. This affects approximately 0.6–1% of all adults, 50% of whom will never seek help for the problem.[97] The majority of men with persistent nocturnal enuresis, up to the age of 65 years, appear to have underlying detrusor instability.[98–100]

Treatment with imipramine has shown a marked antidiuretic effect on patients with nocturnal polyuria; this appears to be a vasopressin-independent

Table 13.3 *Drug therapy which may potentially aggravate or predispose to urinary incontinence*

Drug	Effect
Diuretics	Increase urinary frequency and may precipiate urge incontinence in predisposed individuals
Calcium channel antagonists	Associated with polyuria, especially at night when fluid redistribution occurs. Constipation
Anticholinergics (including antihistamines, antipsychotics, antipasmodics, anti-Parkinsonian agents)	May precipitate confusion, especially in those with pre-existing cognitive inpairment
α-adrenoreceptor agonists	May predispose to stress incontinence, due to relaxant effect on the external urethral sphincter
Non-steroidal anti-inflammatory drugs	Salt and water retention
H_2 antagonists	Confusion
Benzodiazepines and neuroleptics	Any sedative medication with an appreciable hangover effect will exacerbate continence problems in those elderly people predisposed to problems

effect, mediated by α-receptors in the proximal convoluted tubule. DDAVP is used although there are few data to support the intervention in patients other than those with neurologic disease. A study comparing the use of DDAVP with the antimuscarinic medication oxybutynin showed no difference in improvement between the DDAVP group and combination treatment. For institutionalized, highly dependent men, the problem of nocturnal incontinence continues to require a major effort to manage effectively. The continuing developments in pad technology and the use of barrier creams can often minimize the disruption of sleep patterns. The use of electronic 'wet' alarms has also been advocated in the USA, but there has been little uptake in their use.

Containment

In most health economies, there is a massive expenditure on containment products. The most recent data for the UK suggest that in the region of £80 million is spent by the National Health Service annually. There is rationing of such products in many areas of England and Wales and, in addition, considerable spending on over-the-counter products. There are few up-to-date data on the efficacy of such products and even fewer comparative data upon which purchasing agencies may base their decisions; thus, for many, budgetary concerns dominate. However, a systematic comparison by the Continence Products Evaluation Network (all in one disposable bodywarm pads for heavy incontinence, 1998) demonstrated that the cheapest pads were not necessarily the most effective and, for that matter, neither were the most expensive. There has been a trend for single supplier contracts in many areas of the UK, which has been cost driven. This denies more useful products to some patient groups. Likewise there is a shift away from single-use pads to washable products.

Additional factors in the elderly male patient

Concomitant disease and drug therapy, in particular, may serve to push an elderly person over the edge and become incontinent. The treatments for many bladder problems do not differ in elderly people and there is evidence to show that the elderly do just as well with treatment.[101] However, attention has to be paid to other factors which may limit the application of routine treatments.

Drug therapy

Many commonly used drugs may, through a variety of mechanisms, have an adverse effect upon the function of the lower urinary tract or the physical ability of an elderly person to cope with pre-existing urinary symptoms (see Table 13.3). The elderly are more likely to be taking a number of different drugs; interactions between these and between any drug treatment for incontinence and pre-existing medication should be taken into account when prescribing for an elderly man.

Non-drug factors

Diabetes may certainly present incidentally as urinary incontinence in elderly people. Toxic confusional states and intercurrent illness may precipitate the problem, as can urinary retention. Whilst fecal impaction causes fecal incontinence and may cause urinary retention, the relationship between impaction and urinary incontinence is unclear, though often claimed. Other disease entities with an impact upon urinary problems are listed in Table 13.2.

Problems associated with physical disability

Physical problems with access to lavatory facilities and privacy also need to be considered, particularly in institutional settings. The provision of commodes or other urine collection devices, appropriate grab rails, and raised toilet seats may be essential in maintaining continence for some people. Strategies aimed at maintaining mobility of elderly individuals also have a positive effect upon urinary incontinence.[102]

Toileting schedules

For those patients who are cognitively impaired, where there is little chance of active participation in behavioral methods of treatment, drug treatment may help in reducing the burden of incontinence. However, there is little evidence that use of oxybutynin in this scenario is effective.[33] There is no direct evidence of efficacy for tolterodine, but there are data for its effectiveness as a sole modality of treatment.[103]

For many patients, strategies such as scheduled voiding (where patients are toileted at regular intervals), individualized toileting programs (where the toileting is titrated to the patient's known voiding habits), and prompted voiding programs (where the patient is prompted to visit the toilet at regular intervals) are effective treatment options. The latter requires staff ability to ascertain whether the patient is wet or not and depends upon the ability of the patient to request toileting. Neither regular nor individual toileting programs require this. All have been found to be effective in reducing incontinence episodes in nursing home patients.[104,105] All methods are very labor intensive, but there is evidence that, for regular toileting regimens, a 4-hourly interval is as effective as a 2-hourly one.[106] For some elderly males, the only option available for the treatment of their urinary incontinence is containment, whether this is by virtue of physical or cognitive impairment. The main aims of containment devices are the protection of skin and clothing and the prevention of malodor. Such devices include condoms, clamps, absorbent underwear, and single-use and reusable pads.

Conclusions

There is considerable debate about the contribution of outflow tract obstruction to the development of changes in bladder behavior leading to the development of detrusor instability. There is good evidence to suggest that this condition may develop in association with greater age alone. Detrusor instability accounts for the majority of cases of urinary incontinence in older males and can be successfully treated by behavioral techniques and pharmacotherapy. For men with post-prostatectomy incontinence, bladder overactivity accounts for over half of the observed cases of incontinence and thus is similarly amenable to treatment. There is much scope for further study of alterations in pathophysiology of the bladder in older men. This is especially pertinent given the increasing proportions of men who are likely to survive into late life.

References

1. Resnick NM, Elbadawi A, Yalla SV. Age and the lower urinary tract: what is normal? Neurourol Urodyn 1995; 14: 577–9.

2. Malone-Lee JG, Wahedna I. Characterisation of detrusor contractile function in relation to old age. Br J Urol 1993; 72: 873–80.

3. Bonde HV, Sejr D, Erdmann L et al. Residual urine in 75-year-old men and women. A normative population study. Scand J Urol Nephrol 1996; 30: 89–91.

4. Cockett ATK, Khoury S, Aso Y et al. The second international consultation on benign prostatic hyperplasia. Proceedings 2: The effects of obstruction and ageing on the function of the lower urinary tract. Scientific communication International. Jersey, CI, 1993.

5. Gilpin SA, Gosling JA, Barnard RJ. Morphological and morphometric studies of the human obstructed trabeculated urinary bladder. Br J Urol 1985; 57: 525–9.

6. Gosling JA, Gilpin SA, Dixon JS, Gilpin CJ. Decrease in the autonomic innervation of human detrusor muscle in outflow obstruction. J Urol 1986; 136: 501–3.

7. Cortivo R, Pagano F, Passerini G et al. Elastin and collagen in the normal and obstructed urinary bladder. Br J Urol 1981; 53: 134–7.

8. Holm NR, Horn T, Hald T. Detrusor in ageing and obstruction. Scand J Urol Nephrol 1995; 29: 45–9.

9. Gilpin SA, Gilpin CJ, Dixon JS et al. The effect of age on the autonomic innervation of the urinary bladder. Br J Urol 1986; 58: 378–81.

10. Lepor H, Sunaryadi I, Hartanto V, Shapiro E. Quantitative morphometry of the adult human bladder. J Urol 1992; 148: 414–17.

11. Abrams PH, Farrar DJ, Turner-Warwick R et al. The results of prostatectomy: a symptomatic and urodynamic analysis of 152 patients. J Urol 1979; 121: 640–2.

12. Kosimaki J, Hakama M, Huhtala H, Tammela TLJ. Association of smoking with lower urinary tract symptoms. J Urol 1998; 159: 1580–2.

13. Creighton SM, Stanton SL. Caffeine: does it affect your bladder? Br J Urol 1990; 66: 613–14.

14. Brown JS, Seeley DG, Fong J et al. Urinary incontinence in older women: who is at risk? Obstet Gynecol 1996; 87: 715–21.

15. Tomlinson BU, Dougherty MC, Pendergast JF et al. Dietary caffeine, fluid intake and urinary incontinence in older rural women. Int Urogynecol J Pelvic Floor Dysfunct 1999; 10: 22–8.

16. Bump RC, Sugerman JH, Fantl A, McClish DM. Obesity and lower urinary tract function in women: effect of surgically induced weight loss. Am J Obstet Gynecol 1992; 167: 392–8.

17. Furuya S, Ogura H, Tanaka M et al. Incidence of post-micturition dribble in adult males from their twenties through fifties. Acta Urol Japan 1997; 43: 407–10.

18. Paterson J, Pinnock CB, Marshall VR. Pelvic floor exercises as a treatment for post-micturition dribble. Br J Urol 1997; 79: 892–7.

19. Abrams PH, Blaivas JG, Stanton SL et al. Standardization of terminology of lower urinary tract function. Neurourol Urodyn 1988; 7: 403.

20. Robertson AS, Griffiths CJ, Ramsden PD, Neal DE. Bladder function in healthy volunteers: ambulatory monitoring and conventional urodynamic studies. Br J Urol 1994; 73: 242–9.

21. Abrams PH. Bladder instability: concept, clinical associations and treatment. Scand J Urol Nephrol 1984; 87: 7.

22. Abrams P, Klevmark B. Frequency volume charts: an indispensable part of lower urinary tract assessment. Scand J Urol Nephrol 1996; 179: 47–53.

23. Cardozo LD, Stanton SL. An objective comparison of the effects of parenterally administered drug in patients suffering from detrusor instability. J Urol 1979; 122: 58–9.

24. Blaivas JG, Labib KB, Michalik J, Zayed AAH. Cystometric response to propantheline in detrusor hyperreflexia: therapeutic implications. J Urol 1980; 124: 259–62.

25. Zorzitto ML, Jewett MAS, Fernie GR et al. Effectiveness of propantheline bromide in the treatment of geriatric patients with detrusor instability. Neurourol Urodyn 1986; 5: 133–40.

26. Jonas U, Hofner K, Madersbacher H, Holmdahl TH. Efficacy and safety of two doses of tolterodine versus placebo in patients with detrusor overactivity and symptoms of frequency, urge incontinence and urgency: urodynamic evaluation. The International Study Group. World J Urol 1997; 15: 144–51.

27. Hashimoto K, Ohnishi N, Esa A et al. Clinical efficacy of oxybutynin on sensory urgency as compared with motor urgency. Urologia Int 1999; 62: 12–16.

28. Cardozo LD, Cooper D, Versi E. Oxybutynin chloride in the management of idiopathic detrusor instability. Neurourol Urodyn 1987; 6: 256–7.

29. Moisey CU, Stephenson TP, Brendler CB. The urodynamic and subjective results of treatment of detrusor instability with oxybutynin chloride. Br J Urol 1980; 52: 472–5.

30. Bemelmans BL, Kiemeney LA, Debruyne FM. Low-dose oxybutynin for the treatment of urge incontinence: good efficacy and few side effects. Eur Urol 2000; 37: 709–13.

31. Malone-Lee JG, Lubel D, Szonyi G. Low dose oxybutynin for the unstable bladder. BMJ 1992; 304: 1053.

32. Kelleher CJ, Cardozo LD, Khullar V, Salvatore S. A medium-term analysis of the subjective efficacy of

treatment for women with detrusor instability and low bladder compliance. Br J Obstet Gynaecol 1997; 104: 988–93.

33. Ouslander JG, Schnelle JF, Uman G et al. Does oxybutynin add to the effectiveness of prompted voiding for urinary incontinence among nursing home residents? A placebo controlled trial. J Am Geriatr Soc 1995; 43: 610–17.

34. Birns J, Lukkari E, Malone-Lee JG. A randomized controlled trial comparing the efficacy of controlled release oxybutynin tablets (10 mg once daily) with conventional oxybutynin tablets (5 mg twice daily) in patients whose symptoms were stabilized on 5 mg twice daily of oxybutynin. Br J Urol Int 2000; 85: 793–9.

35. Versi E, Appell R, Mobley D et al. Dry mouth with conventional and controlled release oxybutynin in urinary incontinence. Obstet Gynecol 2000; 95: 718–21.

36. Anderson R, Mobley D, Blank B et al. Once daily controlled versus immediate release oxybutynin for urge urinary incontinence. J Urol 1999; 161: 1809–12.

37. Collas D, Malone-Lee JG. The pharmacokinetic properties of rectal oxybutynin – a possible alternative to intravesical administration. Neurourol Urodyn 1997; 16: 638–40.

38. Winkler HA, Sand PK. Treatment of detrusor instability with oxybutynin rectal suppositories. Int Urogynecol J 1998; 17: 100–2.

39. Nilvebrandt L, Hallen B, Larsson G. Tolterodine – a new bladder selective antimuscarinic agent. Eur J Pharmacol 1997; 327: 195–207.

40. Nilvebrandt L, Gillberg PG, Sparf B. Antimuscarinic potency and bladder selectivity of PNU-200577, a major metabolite of tolterodine. Pharmacol Toxicol 1997; 81: 169–72.

41. Abrams P, Freeman R, Anderstrom C, Mattiasson A. Tolterodine, a new antimuscarinic agent: as effective but better tolerated than oxybutynin in patients with an overactive bladder. Br J Urol 1998; 81: 801–10.

42. Millard R, Tuttle J, Moore K et al. Clinical efficacy and safety of tolterodine compared to placebo in detrusor overactivity. J Urol 1999; 161: 1551–5.

43. Malone-Lee JG. Proceedings of the International Continence Society. International Continence Society, Tokyo, Japan 1997; Abstract A188.

44. Lawrence M, Guay DR, Benson SR, Anderson MJ. Immediate-release oxybutynin versus tolterodine in detrusor overactivity: a population analysis. Pharmacotherapy 2000; 20: 470–5.

45. Diokno AC, Hyndman CW, Hardy DA, Lapides J. Comparison of action of imipramine (tofranil) and propantheline (propanthine) on detrusor contraction. J Urol 1972; 107: 42–3.

46. Castleden CM, Duffin HM, Gulati RS. Double blind study of imipramine and placebo for incontinence due to bladder instability. Age Ageing 1986; 15: 299–303.

47. Lose G, Jorgensen L, Thunedborg P. Doxepin in the treatment of female detrusor overactivity: a randomised double blind cross over study. J Urol 1989; 142: 1024–6.

48. Stohrer M, Madersbacher H, Richter R et al. Efficacy and safety of propiverine in SCI-patients suffering from detrusor hyperreflexia – a double-blind, placebo-controlled clinical trial. Spinal Cord 1999; 37: 196–200.

49. Madersbacher H, Halaska M, Voigt R et al. A placebo-controlled, multicentre study comparing the tolerability and efficacy of propiverine and oxybutynin in patients with urgency and urge incontinence. Br J Urol 1999; 84: 646–51.

50. Halaska M, Dorschner W, Frank M. Treatment of urgency and incontinence in elderly patients with propiverine hydrochloride. Neurourol Urodyn 1994; 13: 428–30.

51. Fuertes ME, Garcia Matres MJ, Gonzalez Romojaro V et al. Ensayo clinico para evaluar la eficacia y tolerancia del cloruro de trospio (Uraplex) en pacientes con incontinencia por inestabilidad del detrusor y su repercusion en la calidad de vida. Arch Esp Urol 2000; 53: 125–36.

52. Cardozo L, Chapple CR, Toozs-Hobson P et al. Efficacy of trospium chloride in patients with detrusor instability: a placebo-controlled, randomized, double-blind, multicentre clinical trial. Br J Urol 2000; 85: 659–64.

53. Madersbacher H, Stohrer M, Richter R et al. Trospium chloride versus oxybutynin: a randomized, double-blind, multicentre trial in the treatment of detrusor hyper-reflexia. Br J Urol 1995; 75: 452–6.

54. Donnellan CA, Fook L, McDonald P, Playfer JR. Oxybutynin and cognitive dysfunction. BMJ 1997; 315: 1363–4.

55. Katz IR, Sands LP, Bilker W et al. Identification of medications that cause cognitive impairment in older people: the case of oxybutynin chloride. J Am Geriatr Soc 1998; 46: 8–13.

56. Pietzko A, Dimpfel W, Schwantes U, Topfmeier P. Influences of trospium chloride and oxybutynin on quantitative EEG in healthy volunteers. Eur J Clin Pharmacol 1994; 47: 337–43.

57. Guarneri L, Robinson E, Testar R. A review of flavoxate: pharmacology and mechanism of action. Drugs Today 1994; 30: 91–8.

58. Chapple CR, Parkhouse H, Gardener C, Milroy EJG. Double-blind, placebo-controlled cross-over study of flavoxate in the treatment of idiopathic detrusor instability. Br J Urol 1990; 66: 491–4.

59. Dahm TL, Ostri P, Kristensen JK et al. Flavoxate treatment of micturition disorders accompanying benign prostatic hypertrophy: a double-blind, placebo-controlled multi-centre investigation. Urol Int 1995; 55: 205–8.

60. Stanton SL. A comparison of emepronium bromide and flavoxate hydrochloride in the treatment of urinary incontinence. J Urol 1973; 110: 529–32.

61. Milani R, Scalambrino S, Milia R et al. Double blind cross-over comparison of flavoxate and oxybutynin in women affected by urinary urge syndrome. Int Urogynecol J 1993; 4: 3–8.

62. Jeffcoate TNA, Francis WJA. Urgency incontinence. Am J Obstet Gynecol 1966; 94: 604.

63. Burgio KL, Locker JL, Goode PS et al. Behavioral versus drug treatment for urinary urge incontinence in older women. A randomized controlled trial. JAMA 1998; 280: 1995–2000.

64. Burgio K, Locher JL, Goode PS. Combined behavioural and drug therapy for urge incontinence in older women. J Am Geriatr Soc 2000; 48: 370–4.

65. Ouslander JG, Schnelle JF, Uman G et al. Does oxybutynin add to the effectiveness of prompted voiding for urinary incontinence among nursing home residents? A placebo controlled trial. J Am Geriatr Soc 1995; 43: 610–7.

66. Chapple CR. Surgery for detrusor overactivity. World J Urol 1998; 16: 268–73.

67. Kondo A, Saito M, Yamada Y et al. Prevalence of hand washing urinary incontinence in healthy subjects in relation to stress and urge incontinence. Neurourol Urodyn 1992; 11: 519–23.

68. Malmsten UG, Milsom I, Moklander U, Norlen LJ. Urinary incontinence and lower urinary tract symptoms: an epidemiological study of men aged 45 to 99 years. J Urol 1997; 158: 1733–7.

69. Diokno AC, Taub M. Ephedrine in the treatment of urinary incontinence. Urology 1975; 5: 624–5.

70. Awad SA, Downie JW, Kiruluta HG. Alpha adrenergic agents in urinary disorders of the proximal urethra. Part 1. Sphincter incompetence. Br J Urol 1978; 50: 332–5.

71. Doll HA, Black NA, McPherson K et al. Mortality, morbidity and complications following transurethral resection of the prostate for benign prostatic hypertrophy. J Urol 1992; 147: 1566–73.

72. Kaplan SA, Laor E, Fatal M, Te AE. Transurethral resection of the prostate versus transurethral electrovapourisation of the prostate: a blinded, prospective comparative study with one year follow up. J Urol 1998; 159: 454–8.

73. Fitzpatrick JM, Gardina RA, Worth PHL. The evaluation of 68 patients with post prostatectomy incontinence. Br J Urol 1979; 51: 552–5.

74. Steiner MS, Morton RA, Walsh PC. Impact of anatomical radical prostatectomy on urinary incontinence. J Urol 1991; 145: S12–15.

75. Hammerer P, Dieringer J, Schuler J et al. Urodynamic parameters to predict continence after radical prostatectomy. J Urol 1991; 145: 292A.

76. Barkin M, Dolfin D, Herschorn S et al. Voiding dysfunction in institutionalised elderly men: the influence of previous prostatectomy. J Urol 1983; 130: 258–9.

77. Staskin DS, Vardi Y, Siroky MB. Post-prostatectomy continence in the Parkinsonian patient: the significance of poor voluntary sphincter control. J Urol 1988; 140: 117–8.

78. Rainwater LM, Zincke H. Radical prostatectomy after radiation therapy for cancer of the prostate: feasibility and prognosis. J Urol 1988; 140: 1455–9.

79. Green N, Treible D, Wallack H. Prostate cancer: post irradiation incontinence. J Urol 1990; 144: 307–9.

80. Lee WR, Schultheiss TE, Hanlon AL, Hanks GE. Urinary incontinence following external beam radiotherapy for clinically localised prostate cancer. Urology 1996; 48: 95–9.

81. Cote RJ, Burke H, Schoenberg HW. Prediction of unusual postoperative results by urodynamic testing in benign prostatic hyperplasia. J Urol 1981; 125: 690–2.

82. Thomas AW, Cannon A, Bartlett E et al. The natural history of voiding dysfunction in men: the long term follow up of TURP. Br J Urol 1998; 81: 22.

83. Van Kampen M, De Weerdt W, Van Poppel H et al. Effect of pelvic-floor re-education on duration and degree of incontinence after radical prostatectomy: a randomised controlled trial. Lancet 2000; 355: 98–102.

84. Burgio KL, Stutzman RE, Engel BT. Behavioural training for post prostatectomy urinary incontinence. J Urol 1989; 141: 303–6.

85. Opsomer EJ, Castille Y, Abi Aad AS, van Cangh PJ. Urinary incontinence after radical prostatectomy: is professional pelvic floor training necessary. Neurourol Urodyn 1994; 13: 382–4.

86. Politano VA. Transurethral polytef injection for post prostatectomy incontinence. Br J Urol 1992; 69: 26–8.

87. Deane AM, English P, Hehir M et al. Teflon injection in stress incontinence. Br J Urol 1985; 57: 78–80.

88. Herschorn S, Radomski S, Fleschner N. Durability of the artificial sphincter in the management of urinary incontinence. J Urol 1996; 155: 456A.

89. Webb RJ, Lawson AL, Neal DE. Clean intermittent catheterisation in 172 adults. Br J Urol 1990; 65: 20–3.

90. Asplund R, Aberg H. Diurnal variation in the levels of antidiuretic hormone in the elderly. J Intern Med 1993; 229: 131.

91. Hilton P, Stanton SL. The use of desmopressin (DDAVP) in nocturnal frequency in the female. Br J Urol 1982; 54: 252–5.

92. Reynard J. A novel therapy for nocturnal polyuria: a double-blind randomized trial of furosemide against placebo. Br J Urol 1998; 82: 215–18.

93. O'Donnell PD, Beck C, Walls RC. Serial incontinence assessment in elderly inpatient men. J Rehab Res Dev 1990; 27: 1–9.

94. Asplund R, Sundberg B, Bergtsson P. Oral desmopressin for nocturnal polyuria in elderly subjects: a double blind, placebo-controlled randomised exploratory study. Br J Urol 1999; 83: 591–5.

95. Norgaard JP, Djurhuus JC, Watanabe H et al. Experience and current status of research into the pathophysiology of nocturnal enuresis. Br J Urol 1997; 79: 825–35.

96. Arnell H, Hjalmas K, Jagervall M et al. The genetics of primary nocturnal enuresis: inheritance and suggestion of a second major gene on chromosome 12q. J Med Genet 1997; 34: 360–5.

97. Hirasing RA, van Leerdam FJM, Bolk-Benink L, Janknegt RA. Enuresis nocturna in adults. Scand J Urol Nephrol 1997; 31: 533–6.

98. Torrens MJ, Collins CD. The urodynamic assessment of adult enuresis. Br J Urol 1975; 47: 433–40.

99. McGuire EJ, Savastano JA. Urodynamic studies in enuresis and the non-neurogenic, neurogenic bladder. J Urol 1984; 132: 299–302.

100. Fidas A, Galloway NTM, McInnes A, Chisholm GD. Neurophysiological measurements in primary adult enuretics. Br J Urol 1985; 57: 635–40.

101. Szonyi G, Collas DM, Ding YY, Malone-Lee JG. Oxybutynin with bladder retraining for detrusor instability in elderly people: a randomized controlled trial. Age Ageing 1995; 24: 287–91.

102. O'Donnell PD. Special considerations in elderly individuals with urinary incontinence. Urology 1998; 51: 20–3.

103. Appell RA. Clinical efficacy and safety of tolterodine in the treatment of overactive bladder: a pooled analysis. Urology 1997; 50: 90–6.

104. Engel BT, Burgio LD, McCormick KA et al. Behavioural treatment of incontinence in the long term care setting. J Am Geriatr Soc 1990; 38: 361–3.

105. Jilek R. Elderly toiletting: is two hourly too often? Nursing Standard 1993; 7: 25–6.

106. Ouslander JG, Schnelle JF, Uman G et al. Predictors of successful prompted voiding among incontinent nursing home residents. JAMA 1995; 273: 1366–70.

CHAPTER 14

Testicular cancer

Axel Heidenreich

Introduction

Although testicular cancer accounts for only about 1% of all human neoplasms, it represents the most common malignant tumor in young men in the age group of 20–40 years. In 1994, approximately 6800 new cases of testicular cancer were diagnosed.[1] The peak incidence is at age 32; this compares with a median age at diagnosis of 68 years for all other tumors.

Epidemiology

Testicular cancer demonstrates two incidence peaks, at the age of under 2 years and among men aged 25–34 years, with rates declining rapidly after the age of 40. There are striking differences in testicular cancer incidences around the world, with the highest incidence of 12–14 per 100 000 person-years in Switzerland and Denmark, and the lowest incidence of less than one per 100 000 person-years among the African-American and the Chinese populations.[2]

Although some risk factors have been identified as being associated with the development of testicular cancer, there are still a number of unknown parameters accounting for the increase in incidence.

Etiology

Cryptorchidism is the best-known risk factor and, according to case–control studies, the relative risk

for testicular cancer is 2.5–8.8.[3] However, an undescended testis accounts for only about 10% of all testicular cancer cases. According to some investigations, there seems to be an association between the age at correction of cryptorchidism and the risk of developing testicular cancer: patients undergoing orchidopexy prior to age 11 had a 3-fold increased risk, compared to a 7-fold increased risk in subjects never having undergone orchidopexy.

Familial and genetic factors have been suggested to be involved in the development of testicular cancer, since first-degree relatives of testicular cancer patients have a 6- to 10-fold higher risk of developing this form of cancer.[4-6] Furthermore, family members with testicular cancer have a significantly higher risk of cryptorchidism and bilateral disease and present at a younger age, indicating genetic factors already present at the time of embryologic development of the testis. With regard to predisposing genetic events, the Testicular Linkage Consortium[7] has recently identified the locus Xq27 to be predisposing for bilateral testicular cancer and bilateral cryptorchidism. Other studies have reported the loci 1p36, 4p14–13, 5q21–21, 14q13–q24.3, and 18q21.1–21.3 to be highly associated with testicular cancer.[8] Recently, it has been demonstrated that somatic mutations of exons 10, 11, and 17 of KIT occur significantly more often in patients with bilateral testicular cancer as compared to patients with unilateral disease.[9] The results indicate that KIT might be involved in the development of familial and a minority of sporadic germ cell

Table 14.1 *World Health Organization (WHO) classification of testicular germ-cell tumors (GCTs) and the relative frequency of histological subtypes[11–13]*

WHO classification of GCT	Relative frequency (%)	
	Pure histology	More than one histology
Tumors of one histological subtype		
Classical seminoma	43 (35–51)	12 (7–15)
Spermatocytic seminoma	2 (1–4)	0
Embryonal carcinoma	7 (3–11)	36 (28–44)
Yolk-sac tumor	1 (1–2)	25 (10–39)
Polyembryoma	< 1	0
Choriocarcinoma	< 1	17 (7–40)*
Pure teratoma	4 (3–5)	37 (22–44)
mature teratoma	4 (3–5)	37 (22–44)
immature teratoma	0	0
teratoma with malignant transformation	0	0
Tumors of more than one histological subtype		
Teratocarcinoma	11.5	—
Mixed GCT	—	7
Combined GCT	—	10.6

*Includes choriocarcinoma and the presence of syncytiotrophoblasts

tumors and that KIT mutations primarily take place during embryogenesis such that primordial germ cells with KIT mutations are distributed to both testes.

Prenatal exposure to estrogens might be associated with the development of testicular cancer, since excessive nausea during the first trimester is attributable to the rapid rise in endogenous estrogens, and the embryologic testicular development, highly sensitive to hormonal imbalances, starts at that time.[10,11]

No association between vasectomy, testicular trauma and torsion, infertility, inguinal hernia, and testicular cancer has been confirmed in case–control studies. Furthermore, there are no consistent occupational exposures predisposing to testicular cancer.

Pathology of testicular germ-cell tumors

About 90% of all testicular tumors are malignant germ-cell tumors, and the rest comprise benign tumors deriving from Leydig and Sertoli cells and other interstitial components.[12–14]

The classification of the World Health Organization (WHO) has become widely accepted in recent years (Table 14.1). With regard to the classification of a given testicular tumor, it is of major importance to identify each histologic pattern present, since the percentages of the various histologic subtypes have direct prognostic significance and might be applied for the stratification of further therapy.[15,16] Although the terminology of tumors of a single histologic type is straightforward, the classification of tumors consisting of more than one cell type is more controversial. However, mixed germ-cell tumors consist of multiple non-seminomatous elements, whereas combined germ-cell tumors consist of non-seminomatous and seminomatous components.

In many cases it might be possible to identify the major germ-cell tumor component macroscopically from the appearance of the sectioned surface of the tumor (Table 14.2).

As it is of the utmost importance to identify accurately the various histologic subtypes of germ-cell

Table 14.2 *Clinical characteristics of various histological subtypes of testis cancer*

Tumor	Frequency (%)	Macroscopy	Tumor marker	Average age (years)
Seminoma	35–55	homogeneous, white, pale	hCG in 5–15%	35–40
Spermatocytic seminoma	2	yellow–gray, cysts, mucoid or clear fluid	none	55–60
Embryonal carcinoma	3–10	gray–white, soft, necrosis, hemorrhage	AFP, hCG rare	20–35
Yolk-sac tumor	2–5	solid, soft, gray–white, mucoid	AFP	20–35
Choriocarcinoma	< 1	necrosis, hemorrhage	hCG	20–35
Teratoma	< 5	cystic	none	20–35

hCG, human chorionic gonadotropin; AFP, α-fetoprotein.

Table 14.3 *Immunohistochemical marker expression by testicular cancer subtypes used for pathohistological differentiation*

Marker	Seminoma	Spermatocytic seminoma	Embryonal carcinoma	Yolk-sac tumor	Choriocarcinoma	Teratoma	TIN
AFP	0	0	+	+++	0	0	0
hCG	+	0	+	0	+++	0	0
PLAP	+++	0/+	+++	+++	++	+	++
hPL	0	0	0	0	+++	0	0
EMA	0	0	0/+	0/+	++	+++	0
CEA	0	0	0	+	+	++	0
NSE	+++	0	+++	++	++	++	0
43-9F	++	+	+++	+++	+	+	++
Vimentin	+	0	++	+/+++	0/+	+/+++	0

AFP, α-fetoprotein; hCG, human chorionic gonadotropin; PLAP, placental alkaline phosphatase; hPL, human placental lactogen; EMA, epithelial membrane antigen; CEA, carcinoembryonic antigen; NSE, non-specific enolase; TIN, testicular intraepithelial neoplasia.

cancer in the primary tumor, a number of immuno-histochemical markers have been utilized in the diagnosis of germ-cell cancer. Table 14.3 summarizes the staining patterns of the most commonly used markers for each of the germ-cell tumor subtypes.[14] Alpha-fetoprotein (AFP) is most commonly associated with yolk-sac tumors, and is consistently negative in seminoma and choriocarcinoma; embryonal carcinoma expresses AFP only focally. Human chorionic gonadotropin (hCG) is specific for syncytiotrophoblasts, and therefore is highly expressed in choriocarcinomas; hCG,

however, is also expressed in seminomas and embryonal carcinomas to a lower extent. Placental alkaline phosphatase (PLAP) lacks specificity and is found in basically all types of testicular germ-cell tumors; it is most useful in the detection of testicular intraepithelial neoplasia (TIN) cells and in the differentiation of TIN from normal germinative cells, which do not stain positive. The marker 43-9F has been thought to be specific for embryonal carcinoma; however, follow-up studies demonstrated a common expression of 43-9F in all subtypes of germ-cell tumors and in TIN.[17,18]

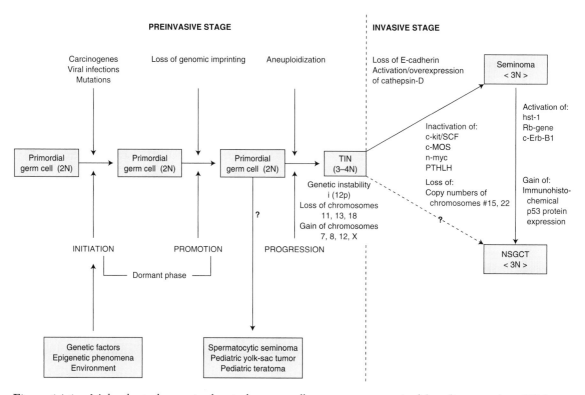

Figure 14.1 *Molecular pathogenesis of testicular germ-cell tumors, as summarized from literature data. TIN, testicular intraepithelial neoplasia; PTH/LH, parathyroid hormone/luteinizing hormone; NSGCT, non-seminomatous germ-cell tumor.*

Pathogenesis of testicular germ-cell tumors

Testicular germ-cell tumors originate from totipotent primordial germ cells, which undergo neoplastic transformation as a result of a number of endogenous, exogenous, hormonal, and genetic, as well as environmental, events (Figure 14.1). The neoplastic process results in the development of preinvasive carcinoma *in situ* (CIS) or TIN representing the common precursor for all testicular germ-cell tumors, except spermatocytic seminoma.[19–22]

Some 70% of all patients with TIN will develop an invasive testicular germ-cell tumor within 7 years, based on the data of Skakkebaek and colleagues[21] in cryptorchid testes. Histologically, TIN cells are larger than normal spermatogonia, and

have an enlarged and hyperchromatic nucleus, prominent nucleoli, and glycogen-rich cytoplasm (Figure 14.2a). Immunohistochemically, TIN will be detected by the abundant expression of PLAP (Figure 14.2b). After the initial observation by Skakkebaek,[20] a number of groups have demonstrated that approximately 5% of all patients with a unilateral germ-cell tumor will harbor TIN in their remaining testicle.[13]

The pathogenetic events resulting in the malignant transformation of atypical spermatogonia to TIN are not well characterized. Furthermore, it is still unclear whether differentiation from TIN to embryonal carcinoma might occur directly or whether seminoma always represents the intermediate stage of differentiation. However, based on literature data, an oncogenetic model can be defined, elucidating the pathogenetic events leading to

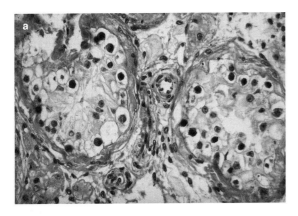
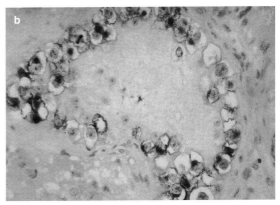

Figure 14.2 *Testicular intraepithelial neoplasia (TIN) exhibiting large cells with enlarged and hyperchromatic nuclei, prominent nucleoli and glycogen-rich cytoplasm (a); TIN and placental alkaline phosphatase (PLAP) staining: TIN cells are depicted by the abundant expression of PLAP at the cell surface (b).*

malignant transformation of spermatogonia to TIN and the progression of TIN to invasive germ-cell tumors (Figure 14.1). According to Damjanov,[24] the three stages of initiation, promotion, and progression result in the invasive phase of the germ-cell tumor. Pathogenetic events leading to local progression and metastases have been adapted (Figure 14.1) according to data available in the literature (for a more detailed summary see reference 25).

Diagnostic procedures and management of testicular cancer

Most patients present with a painless, solid testicular mass of varying size and duration; however, about 30% of patients present with scrotal pain. Therefore, any testicular tumor detected in young men 20–40 years of age should be regarded as malignant until proven otherwise.

Whereas the duration of symptoms does not correlate with survival and stage in classical seminoma, Moul[26] demonstrated a direct relationship between the mean symptomatic interval and clinical stage I–IIB, compared to clinical stages IIC and III, with intervals of 8.5–9.7 weeks and 26.4 weeks, respectively. In another study, Oliver[27] reported that delay in diagnosis was only 2 months in patients who were free of disease during follow-up, 4 months in

patients who relapsed but were salvaged, and 7 months in patients who died of their disease.

Physical examination should include bimanual palpation of the tumor-bearing and the contralateral testicle, and palpation of the inguinal lymph nodes, especially if the patient has had any prior scrotal or inguinal surgery. Scrotal ultrasonography usually reveals a hypoechoic mass within the tunica albuginea as suspicious for malignancy. Differential diagnosis between benign and malignant testicular tumors usually can only be made in the presence of simple testicular cysts and epidermoid cysts presenting either as smooth-lined, hypoechoic masses with a dorsal shadowing, or a well-demarcated cystic mass and an echogenic center caused by multiple acoustic reflections from the keratinous debris.[28]

Primary management of the testicular mass

Inguinal exploration and scrotal orchiectomy with early clamping of the spermatic cord is the therapy of choice for testicular cancer, revealing accurate information with regard to histopathology and pathological stage classification.[29,30] However, any testicular mass of uncertain ranking must be explored by the inguinal approach to verify or exclude malignancy. Since benign testicular lesions are recognized with increasing frequency, frozen section analysis should be considered intraoperatively, which accurately differentiates malignant from benign testicular lesions[31,32] with high sensitivity and specificity.

About 5% of all patients with a unilateral testicular germ-cell tumor will harbor TIN in their contralateral testicle, which will be detected by an immunohistochemical evaluation of a randomly taken testis biopsy at the time of orchiectomy.[22] In a recent prospective trial it has been shown that a systematic tow-site biopsy of the testis improved sensitivity of TIN detection and the diagnostic extra yield imparted was 18%.[33] Currently, there exists controversy about the clinical utility of the contralateral biopsy, supposedly unnecessary for 95% of patients.[34] An evidence-based meta-analysis of all studies concerned with the detection of TIN suggests that it is justified to recommend contralateral biopsy for men with a testis volume < 12ml and age < 30 years at the time of diagnosis, since their risk for contralateral TIN is > 34%.[22,30,33] It must be emphasized that the biopsy specimen should be fixed in Bouin's or Stieve's solution to preserve TIN cells for diagnosis.

Only in cases of a second metachronously or synchronously occurring testicular cancer, a testicular tumor developing in a solitary testis, or a benign testis tumor might an organ-sparing approach be considered, to maintain endogenous testosterone synthesis, to preserve fertility, and to improve quality of life in these long-term survivors. Guidelines identified by the German Testicular Cancer Intergroup based on results from more than 73 patients with a testicular germ-cell tumor and a mean follow-up of 91 months are outlined in Table 14.4.[35] However, it must be emphasized that tumor enucleation for testicular germ-cell tumors should be the exception for the very few patients presenting with bilateral testicular cancer.

Pathohistologic diagnosis

Meticulous pathologic work-up of the orchiectomy specimen should be performed according to the WHO recommendations, to identify all histologic

Table 14.4 *Guidelines for tumor enucleation in testicular germ-cell tumors as outlined by the German Testicular Cancer Intergroup based on 72 cases*

Tumor diameter less than 20 mm
Tumor must be organ confined
Multiple biopsies from the tumor bed to prove tumor-free resection rims
Normal preoperative testosterone and luteinizing hormone serum levels
Close follow-up, high compliance of patient and physician
Treatment in centers experienced in the management of testicular cancer

subtypes present and to identify vascular invasion. Especially in clinical stage I non-seminomatous germ-cell tumor (NSGCT), it might also be useful to calculate the percentage of all testicular cancer subtypes present, to obtain prognostic information with regard to the probability of occult metastatic retroperitoneal lymph-node disease.[15,16,36] As has been shown in previous studies, a high percentage of embryonal carcinoma associated with the presence of vascular invasion identifies patients at high risk of lymph-node metastases in the retroperitoneum, thereby enabling a risk-adapted approach to these patients.

Radiologic staging

Following radical orchiectomy, further staging includes computed tomography (CT) of the abdomen, the chest, and the mediastinum, to detect metastatic lymph-node disease or visceral metastases.[30,37] Unlike other solid neoplasms, the lymphatic spread of testicular cancer follows an anatomically predictable route, with the primary landing zones of the right testis including the interaortocaval region and the primary landing zones of the left side including the para-aortic and pre-aortic lymph nodes. Micrometastases are present in up to 20% and in approximately 30% of clinical stage I seminomas and non-seminomas, respectively, which will not be detected by classic interpretation of abdominal CT scans owing to the inability of morphologic differentiation. Therefore, primary landing zones and the transverse diameter of the largest lymph node might be helpful, as demonstrated:[38] using the shortest transaxial lymph-node diameter, the probability of lymph-node metastases increased with increasing diameter. Based on uni- and multivariate logistic regression analysis, an accuracy of 84% was attained at 8 mm to find metastatic disease. Furthermore, the expected primary landing zones of right- and left-sided primaries should be considered in CT interpretation, increasing the predictive ability.

More caudal deposits of metastases usually reflect retrograde spread to the common, external, and inguinal lymph nodes; in particular in patients having undergone previous scrotal or inguinal surgery, or presenting with scrotal tumor infiltration, it is advisable to scan the iliac region because of atypical lymphatic spread.

Magnetic resonance imaging (MRI) of the abdomen using currently available techniques does not provide additional clinically useful information, and should be reserved for patients with contraindications to CT.[37] The introduction of new contrast agents for evaluation of the lymphatic system might improve the diagnostic accuracy of MRI to detect retroperitoneal micrometastases.

In addition, positron emission tomography (PET) scans are not helpful in the detection of retroperitoneal micrometastases in patients with clinical stage I testicular cancer, as has been demonstrated in a variety of studies.[39,40] In this context, a prospective study in clinical stage non-seminomas demonstrated an 88% sensitivity to detect small retroperitoneal lymph node metastases, which was superior to standard imaging techniques such as CT scans. Also, positive and negative predictive values for PET (92% and 100%) were significantly superior to CT scans, with a predictive value of 78%.[41]

Although a lateral and posteroanterior chest X-ray will detect pulmonary metastases in approximately 15% of patients, a chest CT should be obtained owing to the higher sensitivity to identify lesions as small as 2 mm in diameter.[30,42] However, one has to consider that many of these small lesions are benign and do not relate to metastases from testicular cancer.[43]

Brain CT and bone scintigraphy are only to be performed in cases of advanced testicular cancer with high-volume metastatic disease ([3]IIC), in patients with intermediate and poor prognosis according to the International Germ Cell Consensus Classification Group (IGCCCG) criteria, and in case of specific symptomatology.

Tumor markers

Tumor markers are clinically useful for diagnosis, clinical staging, prediction of prognosis (see IGC-CCG classification below), and monitoring the response of therapy.[15,30,44,45] The most commonly used markers applied in clinical practice are AFP, the β-subunit of hCG, and lactic acid dehydrogenase (LDH); in seminomas, PLAP might be of clinical use. Approximately 40–60% of all testicular cancer patients present with elevated tumor markers at the time of diagnosis.

Serum β-hCG levels might be elevated in 80% of all embryonal carcinomas, in all patients with choriocarcinoma, and in 5–20% of patients with classical seminoma. Serum AFP levels might be elevated in patients with yolk-sac tumors and with mixed germ-cell tumors; seminomas are always AFP-negative. LDH reflects primarily tumor burden, and does not represent a specific tumor marker for testicular cancer. There is a correlation with stage and LDH in that 8% of clinical stage I, 32% of clinical stage II, and 81% of clinical stage III testicular germ-cell tumors demonstrate elevated serum LDH concentrations.

Following the initiation of therapy, elevated tumor markers should decline according to their half-life, which is 24–36 hours for β-hCG and 5–7 days for AFP. Any plateau phase or any delay in decline is predictive for a poor outcome in terms of response to therapy.

The prognostic significance of tumor markers at the time of diagnosis becomes evident for advanced disease only, adhering to the IGCCCG classification.[45]

Clinical staging

The Lugano classification[46] represents the most widely used clinical staging system for testicular

Table 14.5 *Clinical staging of testicular germ-cell tumors according to the Lugano classification*

Clinical stage	Description
I	no evidence of metastases
IA	tumor limited to testis and epididymis
IB	infiltration of spermatic cord or tumor in cryptorchid testicle
IC	infiltration of the scrotum, trans-scrotal surgery, tumor developing after trans-scrotal or inguinal surgery
IX	extent of primary tumor cannot be evaluated
II	retroperitoneal lymph-node metastases
IIA	all lymph nodes > 2 cm
IIB	more than one lymph node 2–5 cm
IIC	lymph nodes > 5 cm
IID	abdominal tumor palpable, fixed inguinal tumor
III	mediastinal and supraclavicular lymph-node metastases, visceral metastases
IIIA	mediastinal and supraclavicular lymph-node metastases only
IIIB	pulmonary metastases only
IIIC	hematogenous metastases outside the lung
IIID	persistent elevated markers without evidence of metastases

cancer (Table 14.5), and describes approximately the extent of metastatic involvement of the lymph nodes and visceral organs. However, in recent years it has been demonstrated that the prognostic relevance of the Lugano classification for clinical stage III patients is too poor to be used for stratification of therapy. Therefore, the IGCCCG has introduced a new staging system[45] defining three prognostic risk groups with regard to therapeutic outcome (Table 14.6). According to characteristics of the primary testicular tumor, the metastatic involvment of lymph nodes and organs, and the serum tumor marker level, patients are classified to be at good risk (probability of cure 95%), intermediate risk (probability of cure 70%), or poor risk (probability of cure 50%). The IGCCCG classification gives high prognostic evidence and enables an individualized risk-adapted approach in patients with advanced testicular germ-cell tumor.

Management of testicular germ-cell tumors

Testicular intraepithelial neoplasia
Once TIN is diagnosed, therapeutic intervention is recommended, since 70% of patients will develop invasive germ-cell tumor within the next 7 years.[21]

Local radiation therapy with 18 Gy is the therapy of choice in patients with a contralateral invasive germ-cell tumor, resulting in a 100% cure rate as demonstrated by the eradication of all TIN cells and a Sertoli-cell-only syndrome in follow-up biopsies.[20,22] Only in patients wishing to father a child and having active spermatogenesis does a surveillance strategy with close follow-up seem to be justified. In patients undergoing inductive chemotherapy after orchiectomy, a control biopsy should be performed 6 months after discontinuation of therapy, since about 40% of TIN will be cured by the systemic approach.

In patients with unilateral TIN and a contralateral normal testis, inguinal orchiectomy appears to be the preferred management, since local radiation bears the risk of damaging the healthy testicle.

Non-seminomatous germ-cell tumors
Clinical stage I non-seminomatous germ-cell tumor (NSGCT) represents a troublesome entity concerning recommendations for optimal management. Approximately 30% of stage I NSGCTs will exhibit microscopic lymph-node disease by means of retroperitoneal lymph-node dissection (RPLND);[47–51]

Table 14.6 *Staging system for advanced testicular germ-cell tumors according to the International Germ Cell Consensus Classification Group (IGCCCG)[36]*

Good prognosis

Non-seminoma	primary testicular cancer or extragonadal retroperitoneal cancer, AFP < 1000 ng/ml, hCG < 5000 IU/ml, LDH < 1.5 ´ normal no extrapulmonary visceral metastases
Seminoma	all primary locations all elevated serum markers no extrapulmonary visceral metastases

Intermediate prognosis

Non-seminoma	primary testicular cancer or extragonadal retroperitoneal cancer, AFP 1000 – 10 000 ng/ml, hCG < 5000–50 000 IU/ml, LDH 1.5–10 ´ normal no extrapulmonary visceral metastases
Seminoma	all primary locations all elevated serum markers extrapulmonary visceral metastases (liver, bones, CNS)

Poor prognosis

Non-seminoma	extragonadal mediastinal germ-cell tumor primary testicular/retroperitoneal germ-cell tumor with extrapulmonary metastases AFP > 10 000 ng/ml, hCG > 100 000 IU/ml, LDH > 10 ´ normal

AFP, α-fetoprotein; hCG, human chorionic gonadotropin; LDH, lactate dehydrogenase; CNS, central nervous system.

Table 14.7 *Chemotherapy and surgery in options for clinical stage I non-seminomatous germ-cell tumor (NSGCT)*

Therapy	Surgical intervention (%)	Chemotherapy (%)	Long-term survival (%)
nsRPLND	100	15	> 98
Surveillance	< 10	30–40	> 98
Primary chemotherapy	0	100	> 98

nsRPLND, nerve-sparing retroperitoneal lymph-node dissection.

however, for the remaining 70% of patients, RPLND is only a staging procedure without therapeutic benefit. Therefore, several treatment options such as primary nerve-sparing retroperitoneal lymphadenectomy, primary chemotherapy, and active surveillance have been developed. Altogether, all three therapeutic options – RPLND,[49–51] surveillance,[52,53] and primary chemotherapy[54,55] – will result in the same high cure rates of 98% gaining an additional lifespan of about 50 years; however, the associated complications and side-effects differ significantly (Table 14.7).[30] Since quality-of-life issues

have assumed great importance for both the patient and the physician, with the attention now focusing on the reduction of potential long-term toxicity, classic therapeutic endpoints such as response and survival rates are thrust into the background and quality of life, protection of fertility, and avoidance of major toxicities of the chosen therapy come to the fore.[57] The current guidelines of the European Germ Cell Cancer Consensus Group recommend an individualized, risk-adapted approach based on the results of prospective randomized trials considering the presence or absence of the risk factors vascular invasion and percentage of embryonal carcinoma.[30]

To enable a more individualized therapeutic approach, prognostic risk factors for occult retroperitoneal lymph-node disease can be integrated in the pretherapeutic discussion: vascular invasion has been identified as the most powerful clinical predictor of lymph-node metastasis with 48% of NSGCTs with vascular invasion developing metastases, compared to 14–22% of tumors without vascular invasion.[16,52] A combination of vascular invasion and percentage of embryonal carcinoma might be even more powerful, as has been suggested in a prospective randomized trial by the German Testicular Cancer Study Group.[15,56] In this trial, 200 patients with CS I NSGCT were prospectively assigned to retroperitoneal lymph-node dissection and risk factor assessment was performed within a multicenter protocol. Vascular invasion was the most predictive factor of stage in multifactorial analysis. With the absence of vascular invasion low-risk patients had a negative predictive value of 86.5%, favoring active surveillance in highly compliant patients. With the presence of vascular invasion, the positive predictive value was only at the 59.6% level; a combination of vascular invasion and percentage of embryonal carcinoma ≥ 50% increased the positive predictive value to 63.6%; however, still more than one-third of patients predicted to have pathologic stage II disease would have been overtreated. Therefore, the current guidelines are in favor of active in low-risk patients and recommend all three therapeutic options based on an individual discussion and decision-making process due to the low reliability of prognostic markers.[30] For patients with clinical stage I pure mature teratoma, primary nerve-sparing RPLND still represents a viable option, since up to 20% of all teratomas will harbor occult retroperitoneal lymph-node metastases at the time of diagnosis.[58–60]

Currently, all molecular markers such as p53, Ki-67, bcl-2, cathepsin D, and E-cadherin have not been proven to be clinically useful prognosticators;[16] only the reverse transcriptase-polymerase chain reaction for AFP, hCG, and germ cell alkaline phosphate (GCAP) mRNA for the detection of circulating tumor cells appears to be an interesting approach, with 60% of clinical stage I testicular cancer patients exhibiting positive signals that turn into negative signals following adjuvant chemotherapy.[61]

Nerve-sparing retroperitoneal lymph node dissection

Nowadays, nerve-sparing (ns) RPLND, if performed as reported by Jewett[62] and Donohue and colleagues,[63] is regarded as the standard approach in clinical stage I NSGCT, using the surgical resection templates described by Donohue and associates[47] and by Weißbach and Boedefeld,[48] and depicted in Figure 14.3. For a right-sided tumor, the paracaval, retrocaval, interaortocaval, and pre-aortic lymphatic tissue superior to the superior mesenteric artery should be dissected. For a left-sided tumor, the para-aortic, interaortocaval, and pre-aortic lymphatic tissue superior to the superior mesenteric artery should be dissected. Up to 10% of patients will suffer from pulmonary relapse within the first 2 years, and will be cured by platinum-based chemotherapy. Even in low-volume lymph-node disease such as pathologic stage IIA, the nerve-sparing RPLND can be performed as bilateral radical surgery without compromising the therapeutic outcome. Recurrence and complication rates are low if nsRPLND is performed in experienced tertiary care centers, so that RPLND still has its place in the management of low-volume NSGCT.[49] The role of primary nsRPLND in high-risk clinical stage I NSGCT is discussed controversially, although the recommendations of the EGCCCG are in favor of primary systemic chemotherapy. Stephenson et al,[50,51] however, performed nsRPLND in 267 patients with embryonal carcinoma predominance and lymphovascular invasion; even in pathologic stage IIA systemic chemotherapy was only applied sporadically and the authors described a high 5-year relapse-free rate of 91%, with 72% of the patients with positive lymph-node disease having avoided chemotherapy. Furthermore, the authors demonstrated a 16% frequency of mature teratoma which would not have been cured by systemic chemotherapy anyhow. Based on these data, primary nsRPLND remains the treatment of choice in many centers in the US.

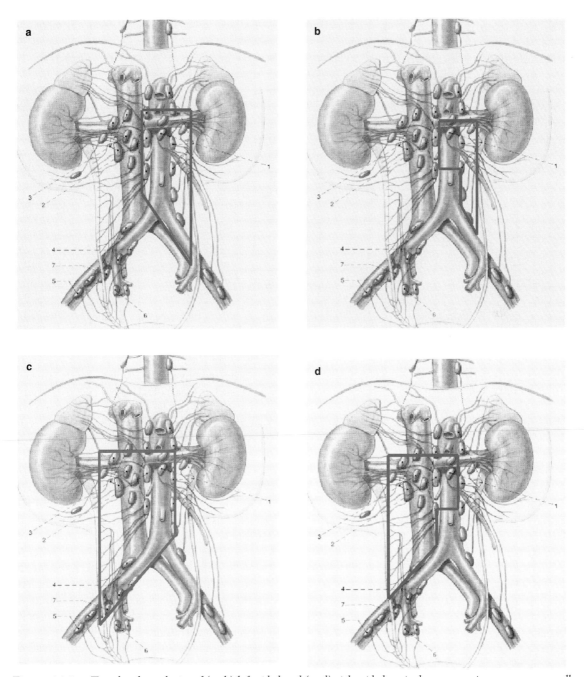

Figure 14.3 *Template boundaries of (a, b) left-sided and (c, d) right-sided testicular non-seminomatous germ-cell tumors as outlined by Donohue and colleagues[38] (a,c) and Weißbach and Boedefeld[39] (b,d).*

Primary chemotherapy or surveillance

In clinical stage I NSGCT, primary chemotherapy consisting of two cycles of cisplatin, etoposide, and bleomycin (PEB) results in the same high cure rate of 98% as with primary nerve-sparing RPLND.[29,30,53–55] Currently, a risk-adapted management of these

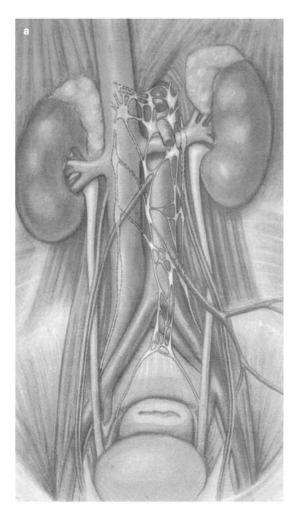
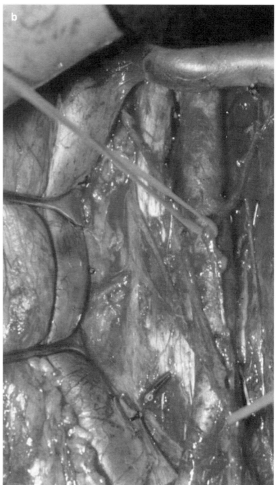

Figure 14.4 *(a) Schematic drawing of anatomic relationship of sympathetic nerve fibers and retroperitoneal lymph nodes. (b) Intraoperative situs of a nerve sparing RPLND resembling the schematic drawing.*

patients has been proposed, based on the presence of vascular invasion and the percentage of embryonal carcinoma in the primary orchiectomy specimen, which have been identified as significant prognosticators for occult retroperitoneal disease in a number of studies.[16,17,56] Prospective randomization to two cycles of PEB (presence of vascular invasion) or to surveillance (absence of vascular invasion) results in relapse rates of only 7% and 14%, respectively, compared to the initial observation series describing recurrence rates of 42%;[53–55] all relapsing patients can be salvaged by inductive platinum-based chemotherapy. In order to further reduce treatment-associated side-effects, current treatment protocols evaluate the role of a single course of PEB instead of the standard two cycles. Preliminary results suggest an equal therapeutic efficacy with reduced toxicity.[64] In summary, treatment decisions in CS I NSGCT can be based on the algorithm depicted in Figure 14.4.

Low-stage (IIA/B) NSGCT

Low-stage testicular disease comprises clinical stages IIA and IIB associated with a cure rate of

Table 14.8 *Advantages and disadvantages of therapeutic options in management of clinical stage IIA non-seminomatous germ-cell tumor (NSGCT)*

nsRPLND + adj. chemotherapy	nsRPLND + surveillance	Primary chemotherapy
Advantages	**Advantages**	**Advantages**
Accurate staging	Fewer associated side-effects owing to single therapy	RPLND necessary in only 10–15%
Risk for relapse 0–7%	Accurate staging revealing pathological stage I in up to 20%	Low relapse rate of 4–9%
Primary extraperitoneal recurrences		
Fewer CT scans for follow-up	Chemotherapy in only 20% of patients	
Disadvantages	**Disadvantages**	**Disadvantages**
Potential induction of secondary malignancies	Minimum of three cycles in case of relapse	Unnecessary chemotherapy in up to 20% owing to pathological stage I
Surgical morbidity of 10%	Surgical morbidity of 10%	Surgical morbidity due to secondary RPLND as high as 39%
Retrograde ejaculation in 5–15% operated in centers	Retrograde ejaculation in 5–15% operated in centers	Retrograde ejaculation as high as 15–20%
Higher incidence of associated morbidities	Risk for relapse is 20%, compared to 0–7% in first option	Higher frequency of follow-up CT scans
		Three cycles of chemotherapy, compared to two cycles in first option

nsRPLA, nerve-sparing retroperitoneal lymphadenectomy; adj., adjuvant; CT, computed tomography; nsRPLND, nerve-sparing retroperitoneal lymph-node dissection.

approximately 98%. Patients with low-volume disease and abnormal tumor marker levels of AFP, β-hCG, or LDH are treated according to the algorithm of the IGCCCG and the EGCCCG recommendations.[30] Patients with marker negative retroperitoneal lymph nodes suspected to be clinical stage IIA might be offered two treatment options: nsRPLND or surveillance. Primary RPLND is a viable approach in clinical stage IIA, since an overstaging is faced in about 20% of patients who would have been subjected to unnecessary chemotherapy otherwise; additional advantages of nsRPLND are preservation of sympathetic nerves in 80% of patients and accurate staging in all patients. Furthermore, adjuvant chemotherapy will only be necessary in patients with positive lymph node disease and unfavorable prognostic markers.[50,51,65,66]

Risk of relapse is only about 15% if fewer than three lymph nodes are involved, the maximum lymph node diameter is < 2 cm, and there is no extranodal extension, so not all patients must undergo adjuvant chemotherapy and a subgroup of patients might be followed by surveillance. If primary surveillance without nsRPLND is chosen, follow-up at 6-week intervals is indicated to document any growth or regression of the lesion. A growing mass indicates vital cancer and therapy can be initiated. A lesion decreasing in size usually does not harbor malignant disease and can be followed. As in clinical stage I disease, both therapeutic options should be intensively discussed with the patient, and parameters such as the wish to father a child, compliance of both patient and physician, and the need for safety must be integrated into the decision (Table 14.8).

Table 14.9 *Advantages and disadvantages of therapeutic options in management of clinical stage IIB non-seminomatous germ-cell tumor (NSGCT)*

nsRPLA + adj. chemotherapy	nsRPLND + surveillance	Primary chemotherapy
Advantages	**Advantages**	**Advantages**
Accurate staging	Fewer associated side-effects owing to single therapy	RPLA necessary in only 30–40%
Risk for relapse 0–7%	Accurate staging revealing pathological stage I in up to 20%	Low relapse rate of 11–15%
Primary extraperitoneal recurrences	Chemotherapy in only 50% of patients	
Fewer CT scans for follow-up		
Disadvantages	**Disadvantages**	**Disadvantages**
Potential induction of secondary malignancies	Minimum of three cycles in case of relapse	Unnecessary chemotherapy in up to 20% owing to pathological stage I
Surgical morbidity of 10%	Surgical morbidity of 10%	Surgical morbidity due to secondary RPLND as high as 39%
Retrograde ejaculation in up to 32%	Retrograde ejaculation in 32%	Retrograde ejaculation
Higher incidence of associated morbidities due to surgery and chemotherapy as high as 15–20%	Risk for relapse is 50%, compared to 0–7% in first option	Higher frequency of follow-up CT scans
		Three cycles of chemotherapy, compared to two cycles in first option

nsRPLA, nerve-sparing retroperitoneal lymphadenectomy; adj., adjuvant; CT, computed tomography; nsRPLND, nerve-sparing retroperitoneal lymph-node dissection.

The only exceptions are patients with elevated markers following radical orchiectomy but no visible metastases on CT scans, who should undergo primary chemotherapy with three cycles of PEB.

Patients with clinical stage IIB testicular cancer, however, will undergo primary chemotherapy depending on the serum concentrations of the markers AFP, β-hCG, and LDH with three or four cycles of PEB followed by secondary RPLND in about 30% of cases,[30] although basically the same three therapeutic options are available as for clinical stage IIA (Table 14.9).

Clinical stages IIC and III

Inductive chemotherapy represents the therapy of choice, with the number of cycles applied depending on the IGCCCG-based prognostic classification.[36]

Patients with a 'good prognosis' face a long-term survival rate of >90%, and are best managed by three cycles of PEB, whereas patients with a poor prognosis are best treated with four cycles.[30,45,67,68] If there are contraindications for the application of bleomycin, four cycles of platinol and etoposide should be administered. It appears to be crucial to give all agents without dose reduction at 22-day intervals. Only in the case of neutropenic fever or severe thrombocytopenia is dose reduction or prolongation of the next cycle justified.

Patients with an 'intermediate prognosis' face a survival rate of 70–80% and are managed by four cycles of PEB or cisplatin, etoposide, and ifosfamide (PEI); however, there are no prospective randomized trials defining a standard therapy.[30,45,69]

Table 14.10

Radiation therapy	Carboplatin	Surveillance
Advantages		
Mild to moderate acute side-effects	Mild side-effects	No therapy for 90% to 70% of patients following orchiectomy
Relapse rate as low as 3–4%	One-day, single treatment	
All relapses are outside the radiation field	Relapse rate as low as 3%	
Disadvantages		
Overtreatment in about 80%	Most relapses are in-field	Relapse rate of 12–30% with intensive salvage therapy
Potential risk of radiation-induced secondary malignancies	Relapses difficult to treat	Psychologic distress due to close follow-up
	Impact on fertility unknown	High intensity of follow-up CT scans

Patients with a 'poor prognosis' have a survival rate of only about 50%; standard therapy consists of four cycles of PEB or PEI.[30,45,70–73] A major advantage of primary high-dose chemotherapy has not been demonstrated, but this approach is currently being tested in prospective randomized trials.

Seminomatous germ-cell tumors

Clinical stage I seminoma

Despite negative CT scans, there is a risk of 12 to 32% of occult retroperitoneal lymph node metastases depending on the absence or presence of negative prognostic markers. The cure rate of clinical stage I seminomatous germ cell cancer is close to 100% and can be achieved by the three different therapeutic options active surveillance, radiation therapy, and carboplatin monochemotherapy (Table 14.10). Adjuvant retroperitoneal radiation therapy to the para-aortic or paracaval region is the most frequently used approach, resulting in a relapse-free long-term survival of 97%.[30,74,75] According to the results of recently published prospective randomized trials, a radiation dose of 20 Gy is sufficient to achieve high cure rates.[76] Active surveillance might represent the most reasonable approach to patients with good prognostic markers such as a tumor size < 4 cm and absence of rete testis invasion associated with a low recurrence rate of about 12%.[77] Most relapses develop in the retroperitoneum or in high iliac lymph nodes. Treatment of relapses is more intense with systemic chemotherapy of 3–4 cycles PEB in most cases. Adjuvant chemotherapy with 1 cycle carboplatin AUC 7 represents the third treatment alternative, resulting in a relapse-free rate of 97.7% according to recent prospective randomized clinical trials. Based on the results of current trials and recommendations, all three options result in an equally high cure rate of 100% associated with a different relapse pattern. The individual strategy should be based on the presence or absence of validated prognostic markers such as tumor size and rete testis invasion since a recent prospective randomized trial has demonstrated the feasibility of such a risk-adapted approach.[78]

Low-stage (clinical stage IIA/B) seminoma

Radiation therapy with 30 Gy (IIA) and 36 Gy (IIB), including the ipsilateral iliac and inguinal lymph nodes, is the standard therapeutic approach for low-stage seminomas.[30,79] The radiation field might be enlarged to the iliac and inguinal lymph nodes in the case of prior scrotal surgery. Relapse-free survival is as high as 92.5% in clinical stage IIA/B; relapse rates are about 5% in stage IIA and about 11% in stage IIB seminomas. Primary chemotherapy with two cycles of PEB can be an alternative to radiation in clinical stage IIB seminoma for patients not willing to undergo radiation therapy.[30] The clinical utility of three (IIA) and four (IIB) cycles of carboplatinum monotherapy in 108 patients with clinical stage IIA/B has been investigated in a prospective clinical trial.[80] A complete response rate of 81% was achieved whereas 17 patients (16%) and 2 patients (2%) demonstrated a partial response and no change, respectively. After a median follow-up of 48 months, 14 patients (13%) relapsed in the retroperitoneum, making up an overall failure rate of 18%. Since 3 and 4 cycles of single agent carboplatin do safely eradicate retroperitoneal disease, it cannot be recommended as alternative treatment to standard radiation therapy.

Clinical stage IIC and III

As pointed out for advanced non-seminomatous germ-cell tumors, therapy should be initiated according to the IGCCCG classification.[45] For patients with a good prognosis, 3 cycles of PEB chemotherapy are the treatment of choice. If there any contraindications against bleomycin, 4 cycles PE might be applied, resulting in a cure rate of 90%. Patients with an intermediate prognosis have a cure rate of about 80% and are best treated by 4 cycles PEB chemotherapy. Currently it is being investigated in prospective randomized trials whether the addition of taxol to PEB improves survival. For patients with a poor prognosis 4 cycles of PEB are the standard therapeutic approach, resulting in a 5-year progression-free and overall survival of 41% and 48%, respectively. It has not been proven that first-line high-dose chemotherapy plus autologous hematopoietic stem cell support is superior to standard chemotherapy in terms of survival. Therefore, high-dose chemotherapy should be applied in prospective clinical trials only.

Residual tumor resection following chemotherapy for advanced testicular cancer

Residual tumor resection (RTR) represents an integral part of the multimodality treatment of advanced testicular germ cell tumors.[30] The rationale for RTR is to completely resect mature teratoma and vital cancer which will be found in 30–40% and 20% of the patients, respectively; however, about 50–60% of all patients with residual masses following inductive chemotherapy harbor necrosis/fibrosis only. Within recent years there has been a significant change with regard to the indication of RTR following inductive chemotherapy for advanced testicular cancer.[30] Currently, all residual lesions independent of size should be resected in non-seminomatous germ cell cancer since even small lesions < 1 cm in diameter will harbor mature teratoma and vital cancer.[81,82] In order to enable a risk-adapted approach and to omit RTR several groups have tried to develop nomograms to predict necrosis and fibrosis.[83–85] Steyerberg and colleagues[83,84] have proposed several risk-adapted models for the prediction of final pathology in patients with residual masses, and claim a sensitivity and specificity of about 80%; this model, however, does allow a risk-adapted approach in an individual patient. Similar data have been reported by the German Testicular Cancer Study Group also demonstrating a sensitivity of only 80% to predict residual masses containing necrosis/fibrosis only.[85] If RTR is being performed, controversy exists on whether it is sufficient to resect the mass only, without respecting the boundaries of modified surgical templates during primary RPLND, or whether a formal modified RPLND has to be performed to achieve optimal oncologic control.[30,86] The extent of surgery depends on individual risk factors for relapse and quality of life issues. If the histology of the resected retroperitoneal masses is necrosis only, further resection of residual lesions in other organs might be omitted since there is concordance of histology in about 90% of the patients. RTR is a complex surgery associated with the necessity to resect adjacent organs or vascular structures in about 25% of the patients[82,87] and should, therefore, be performed in experienced tertiary cancer care centers only.

Whereas additional systemic chemotherapy is not indicated in patients with mature teratoma or necrosis/fibrosis, patients with vital tumor cells might undergo an additional 2 cycles of conventional polychemotherapy. According to one analysis of prognostic markers it has been shown that patients harboring a residual mass with > 10% vital cancer cells or those where the completeness of resection is in doubt might benefit from consolidation chemotherapy whereas all others do not benefit in terms of relapse-free and overall survival.[88]

Postchemotherapy or postradiotherapy RPLND in seminomas has only to be performed in lesions with a positive PET scan performed about 6 weeks after chemotherapy or radiation therapy in patients with residual lesions > 3 cm. A positive PET scan is a strong predictor of remaining vital cancer cells with a sensitivity and a positive predictive value of 100% and close to 100%, respectively.[89,90] It is recommended to perform a PET scan in all patients with seminomatous primaries and residual lesions > 3 cm in diameter prior to any decision with regard to RTR.

Salvage chemotherapy, high-dose chemotherapy

In seminomas relapsing after first-line radiation therapy a cure rate of > 90% can be achieved by cisplatin-based chemotherapy according to the IGC-CCG algorithm with regard to advanced seminomas. About 50% of relapsing seminomas following conventional chemotherapy can be salvaged with another combination chemotherapy consisting of PEI–etopside, ifosfamide, and platinol (VIP) or –vinblastine, ifosfamide, and platinol (VeIP). Currently, a 10% benefit of high-dose chemotherapy with regard to survival has been demonstrated; therefore, it seems advisable that all relapsing patients should be treated in a tertiary referral center.

With regard to non-seminomas relapsing following conventional chemotherapy, salvage rates are as low as 15–40% using standard salvage protocols such as PEI–VIP or PEI–VeIP.[71,72] In some institutions the addition of paclitaxel to ifosfamide and cisplatin has been favored due to a high response rate > 50%.[232] Conventional dose cisplatin-based salvage chemotherapy can achieve long-term remission in 15 to 40% of patients. Early consideration of high-dose chemotherapy seems advisable, according to a number of studies.[55,58] The trials reported from the Memorial Sloan Kettering Cancer Center suggest a benefit for the use of high-dose chemotherapy and autologous bone marrow transfer, with 46% and 50% of the patients being alive and disease-free after a median follow-up of 31 months and 30 months, respectively.[73] In another study including 35 patients, the progression-free survival rate for all patients was 44 months, and the 2-year survival rate was 65%.[30] However, one also has to consider that the results of high-dose chemotherapy combined with autologous bone marrow transfer are not superior to a combination therapy including paclitaxel, ifosfamide, and cisplatin as second-line therapy for relapsing germ-cell tumors. In the treatment of 30 patients, a complete response was achieved in 77% and all patients were without evidence of recurrent disease after a median follow-up of 30 months.[91] Therefore, high-dose chemotherapy is an option but not the standard for the management of relapsing testicular germ-cell tumors. Options for third-line chemotherapy are combinations such as paclitaxel and gemcitabine, gemcitabine and oxaliplatin, or paclitaxel, gemcitabine, and cisplatin, within clinical trials.[30]

Future directions in testicular cancer

Based on the excellent therapeutic outcome, there appear to be only a few developments possible that will have a further impact on the survival of testicular cancer patients. However, there might be many options to improve quality of life either due to reduction of acute toxicity associated with first-line therapy or due to the development of treatment regimens associated with a significantly reduced long-term toxicity.

Currently, the toxicity of adjuvant chemotherapy might be further decreased by applying only one cycle of PEB, as is currently being tested in a prospective randomized trial by the German Testicular Cancer Intergroup. Elucidation of those mechanisms involved in the development of chemo-refractoriness in testicular cancer will be a major issue in the future, to apply effective chemotherapeutic protocols and to save even more lives.

Despite the high cure rates, it will be necessary for testicular cancer to be treated by clinicians and institutions with sufficient experience in the diagnosis and management of germ-cell tumors. Specific problems such as extended tumor masses, relapsing tumors, or poor prognosis at initial diagnosis must be referred to tertiary centers having the facility of an interdisciplinary approach.

References

1. Boring CC, Squires TS, Tong T et al. Cancer statistics 1994. Cancer 1994; 44: 7–26.
2. Coleman MP, Esteve J, Damiecki P et al. Trends in Cancer Incidence and Mortality. IARC Science Publication No 121. Lyon, France: International Agency for Research on Cancer, 1993.
3. Pottern LM, Brown LM, Hoover RN et al. Testicular cancer risk among young men: the role of cryptorchidism and inguinal hernia. J Natl Cancer Inst 1985; 74: 377–81.
4. Forman D, Oliver RTD, Brett AR et al. Familial testicular cancer: a report of the UK family register; estimation of risk and HLA-class I sib-pair analysis. Br J Cancer 1992; 65: 255–62.
5. Heidenreich A, for the German Testicular Cancer Intergroup. Biological and clinical characteristics of familial, bilateral and sporadic germ cell tumors. J Urol 2000; 163(Suppl 1): 145.
6. Tollerud DJ, Blattner WA, Fraser MC et al. Familial testicular cancer and urogenital developmental abnormalities. Cancer 1985; 55: 1849–54.
7. Rapley E, Crockford GP, Teare D et al. Localization to Xq27 of a susceptibility gene for testicular germ-cell tumors. Nature Genet 2000; 24: 197–200.
8. Leahy MG, Tonks S, Moses JH et al. Candidate regions for testicular cancer susceptibility genes. Hum Mol Genet 1995; 4: 1551–5.
9. Rapley EA, Hockley S, Warren W et al. Somatic mutations of KIT in familial testicular germ cell tumors. Br J Cancer 2004; 90: 2397–401.
10. Brown LM, Pottern LM, Hoover RN. Prenatal and perinatal risk factors for testicular cancer. Cancer Res 1986; 46: 4812–16.
11. Depue RH, Pike MC, Henderson BE. Estrogen exposure during gestation and risk of testicular cancer. J Natl Cancer Inst 1983; 71: 1151–5.
12. Von Hochstetter AR, Hedinger CE. The differential diagnosis of testicular germ cell tumors in theory and practice. A critical analysis of two major systems of classifications and review of 389 cases. Virchow's Arch Pathol Anat 1982; 396: 247–77.
13. Jacobsen GK, Henriksen OB, von der Maase H. Carcinoma in situ of testicular tissue adjacent to malignant germ cell tumors: a study of 105 cases. Cancer 1981; 47: 2660–2.
14. Mostofi FK, Sesterhenn IA, Davis CJ. Immunopathology of germ cell tumours of the testis. Semin Diagn Pathol 1987; 4: 320–41.
15. Heidenreich A, Sesterhenn IA, Mostofi FK, Moul JW. Prognostic risk factors that identify patients with clinical stage I nonseminomatous germ cell tumors at low risk and high risk for metastasis. Cancer 1998; 83: 1002–11.
16. Moul JW, Heidenreich A. Prognostic risk factors in low stage nonseminomatous testicular cancer. Oncology 1996; 10: 1359–68.
17. Heidenreich A, Sesterhenn IA, Mostofi FK, Moul JW. Immunohistochemical expression of monoclonal antibody 43-9F in testicular germ cell tumors. Int J Androl 1998; 21: 283–8.
18. Visfeldt J, Giwercman A, Skakkebaek NE. Monoclonal antibody 43-9F: an immunohistochemical marker of embryonal carcinoma of the testis. Acta Pathol Microbiol Immunol Scand 1992; 100: 63–70.
19. Dieckmann KP, Skakkebaek NE. Carcinoma in situ of the testis: a review of biological and clinical features. Int J Cancer 1999; 83: 815–22.
20. Skakkebaek NE. Abnormal morphology of germ cells in two infertile men. Acta Pathol Microbiol Immunol Scand 1972; 80: 374–8.
21. Skakkebaek NE, Bertlesen JG, Giwercman A et al. Carcinoma in situ of the testis: possible origin from gonocytes and precursor of all types of germ cell tumours except spermatocytic seminoma. Int J Androl 1987; 10: 19–28.
22. Dieckmann KP, Loy V. Prevalence of contralateral intraepithelial neoplasia in patients with testicular germ cell neoplasms. J Clin Oncol 1996; 14: 3126–32.
24. Damjano V. Pathogenesis of testicular germ cell tumours. Eur Urol 1993; 23: 2–7.
25. Heidenreich A, Srivastava S, Moul JW, Hofmann R. Molecular genetic parameters in pathogenesis and prognosis of testicular germ cell tumors. Eur Urol 2000; 37: 121–35.
26. Moul JW. Early and accurate diagnosis of testicular cancer. Probl Urol 1994; 8: 58–66.
27. Oliver RTD. Factors contributing to delay in diagnosis of testicular tumours. BMJ 1985; 290: 356–60.
28. Heidenreich A, Engelmann UH, von Vietsch H et al. Organ preserving surgery in testicular epidermoid cysts. J Urol 1990; 153: 1147–50.

29. Souchon R, Krege S, Schmoll HJ et al. Interdisciplinary consensus on diagnosis and therapy of testicular germ cell tumors: results of an update conference based on evidence-based medicine. Strahlenther Onkol 2000; 176: 388–405.

30. Schmoll HJ, Souchon R, Krege S et al. European consensus on diagnosis and treatment of germ cell cancer: a report of the European Germ Cell Cancer Consensus Group (EGCCCG). Ann Oncol 2004; 15: 1377–99.

31. Tokuc R, Sakr W, Pontes JE, Haas GP. Accuracy of frozen section examination of testicular tumors. Urology 1992; 40: 512–16.

32. Elert A, Olbert P, Hegele A et al. Accuracy of frozen section examination of testicular tumors of uncertain dignity. Eur Urol 2002; 41: 290–3.

33. Dieckmann KP, Kulejewski M, Pichlmeyer U, Loy V. Diagnosis of contralateral testicular intraepithelial neoplasia (TIN) in patients with testicular germ cell cancer: systematic two-site biopsies are more sensitive than a single random biopsy. Eur Urol 2006; ahead of press.

34. Heidenreich A, Moul JW. Contralateral testis biopsy procedure in patients with unilateral testis cancer: is it indicated? Seminars Urol Oncol 2002; 20: 234–8.

35. Heidenreich A, Weißbach L, Höltl W et al. Organ sparing surgery for malignant germ cell tumor of the testis. J Urol 2001; 166: 2161–5.

36. Tumours of the testis and paratesticular tissue. In: Eble N, Sauter G, Epstein JI, Sesterhenn IA, eds. World Health Organization Classification of Tumors. Lyon: IARC Press, 2004: 217–78.

37. Krug B, Heidenreich A, Dietlein M, Lackner K. Lymph node staging in malignant testicular germ cell tumors. Fortschr Röntgenstr 1999; 171: 87–94.

38. Leibovitch I, Foster RS, Kopecky KK, Donohue JP. Improved accuracy of computerized tomography based clinical staging in low stage nonseminomatous germ cell cancer using size criteria of retroperitoneal lymph nodes. J Urol 1997; 154: 1759–63.

39. Albers P, Bender H, Ylmaz H et al. Positron emission tomography in the clinical staging of patients with stage I and II germ cell tumors. Urology 1999; 3: 808–11.

40. Cremerius U, Wildberger JE, Borchers H et al. Does positron emission tomography using 18-fluoro-2-deoxyglucose improve clinical staging of testicular cancer? Results of a study of 50 patients. Urology 1999; 54: 900–4.

41. Lassen U, Daugaard G, Eightved A, Hofgaard L, Damgaard K, Rorth M. Whole-body FDG-PET in patients with stage I nonseminomatous germ cell tumours. Eur J Nucl Med Mol Imaging 2003; 30: 396–402.

42. White PM, Howard GC, Best JJ et al. Imaging of the thorax in the management of germ cell testicular tumors. Clin Radiol 1999; 54: 207–11.

43. Fernandez EB, Moul JW, Foley JP et al. Retroperitoneal imaging with third and fourth generation computed axial tomography in clinical stage I nonseminomatous germ cell tumors. Urology 1994; 44: 548–52.

44. Bartlett NL, Freiha NS, Torti FM. Serum markers in germ cell neoplasms. Hematol Oncol Clin North Am 1991; 5: 1245–61.

45. International Germ Cell Consensus Classification Group. A prognostic factor-based staging system for metastatic germ cell cancers. J Clin Oncol 1997; 15: 594–603.

46. Cavalli F, Manfardini S, Pizzocaro G. Report on the international workshop on staging and treatment of testicular cancer. Eur J Cancer 1980; 6: 1367–72.

47. Donohue JP, Zachary JM, Maynard SD. Distribution of nodal metastases in nonseminomatous testicular cancer. J Urol 1982; 128: 315–20.

48. Weißbach L, Boedefeld E. Localization of solitary and multiple metastases in stage II nonseminomatous testis tumor as a basis for a modified staging lymph node dissection in stage I. J Urol 1982; 128: 77.

49. Heidenreich A, Albers P, Hartmann M et al. Complications of primary nerve-sparing lymph node dissection for clinical stage I nonseminomatous germ cell tumors of the testis: experience of the German Testicular Cancer Study Group. J Urol 2003; 169: 1710–14.

50. Stephenson AJ, Bosl GJ, Bajorin DF, Stasi J, Motzer RJ, Sheinfeld J. Retroperitoneal lymph node dissection in patients with low stage testicular cancer with embryonal carcinoma predominance and/or lymphovascular invasion. J Urol 2005; 174: 557–60.

51. Stephenson AJ, Bosl GJ, Motzer RJ et al. Retroperitoneal lymph node dissection for nonseminomatous germ cell testicular cancer: impact of patient selection factors on outcome. J Clin Oncol 2005; 23: 2781–8.

52. Peckham MJ, Barrett A, Husband JE, Hendry WF. Orchiectomy alone in testicular stage I nonseminomatous germ cell tumors. Lancet 1982; 2: 678–80.

53. Cullen MH, Stenning SP, Parkinson MC et al. Short course adjuvant chemotherapy in high risk stage 1 nonseminomatous germ cell tumors of the testis: a Medical Research Council report. J Clin Oncol 1996; 14: 1106–13.

54. Pont J, Höltl W, Kosak D et al. Risk adapted treatment choice in stage I nonseminomatous testicular germ cell cancer by regarding vascular invasion in the primary tumor: a prospective trial. J Clin Oncol 1990; 8: 16–20.

55. Studer UE, Burkhard FC, Sonntag RW. Risk adapted management with adjuvant chemotherapy in patients with high risk clinical stage I nonseminomatus germ cell tumors. J Urol 2000; 163: 1785–7.

56. Albers P, Siener R, Kliesch S et al. Risk factors for relapse in clinical stage I nonseminomatous testicular

germ cell tumors: results of the German Testicular Cancer Study Group Trial. J Clin Oncol 2003; 21: 1505–12.

57. Heidenreich A, Hofmann R. Quality of life issues in the treatment of testicular cancer. World J Urol 1999; 17: 230–8.

58. Heidenreich A, Moul JW, McLeod DG et al. The role of retroperitoneal lymphadenectomy in mature teratoma of the testis. J Urol 1997; 157: 160–3.

59. Leibovitch I, Foster RS, Ulbright TM, Donohue JP. Adult primary pure teratoma of the testis. Cancer 1995; 75: 2244–8.

60. Rabbani F, Farivar-Mohseni H, Leon A, Motzer RJ, Bosl GJ, Sheinfeld J. Clinical outcome after retroperitoneal lymphadenectomy of patients with pure mature teratoma. Urology 2003; 62: 1092–6.

61. Heidenreich A, Walter B, Hofmann R. RT-PCR for AFP, hCG, GCAP and PDGF-1a to detect circulating tumor cells in testicular germ cell tumors. Eur Urol 2000; 37(Suppl 2): 87.

62. Jewett MA. Retroperitoneal lymphadenectomy for testicular tumor with nerve-sparing for ejaculation. J Urol 1988; 139: 1220–4.

63. Donohue JP, Foster RS, Rowland RG et al. Nerve sparing retroperitoneal lymphadenectomy with preservation of ejaculation. J Urol 1990; 144: 287–92.

64. Albers P, Siener R, Krege S et al. One course of adjuvant PEB chemotherapy versus retroperitoneal lymph node dissection in patients with stage I nonseminomatous germ cell tumors: results of the German Prospective Multicenter Trial 01-94. Proc ASCO 2006; 24(Suppl): 220s–4512.

65. Pizzocaro G, Monfardini S. No adjuvant chemotherapy in selected patients with pathological stage II nonseminomatous germ cell tumors of the testis. J Urol 1994; 131: 677–80.

66. Weißbach L, Bussar-Maatz R, Flechtner H et al. RPLND or primary chemotherapy in clinical stage IIA/B nonseminomatous germ cell tumors? Results of a prospective multicenter trial including quality of life assessment. Eur Urol 2000; 37: 582–94.

67. Horwich A, Sleijfer DT, Fossa SD et al. Randomized trial of bleomycin, etoposide and cisplatin compared with bleomycin, etoposide and carboplatin in good-prognosis metastatic nonseminomatous germ cell cancer: a multiinstitutional Medical Research Council/EORTC trial. J Clin Oncol 1997; 15: 1844–52.

68. DeWit R, Stoter G, Kaye SB et al. Importance of bleomycin in combination chemotherapy for good-prognosis testicular nonseminoma: a randomized study of the EORTC Genitourinary Tract Cancer Cooperative Group. J Clin Oncol 1997; 15: 1837–43.

69. De Wit R, Stoter G, Sleijfer DT et al. Four cycles of BEP versus four cycles of VIP in patients with intermediate-prognosis metastatic testicular non-seminoma: a randomized study of the EORTC Genitourinary Tract Cancer Cooperative Group. Br J Cancer 1998; 78: 828–32.

70. Bokemeyer C, Kollmannsberger C, Meisner C et al. First-line high dose chemotherapy compared with standard-dose PEB/VIP chemotherapy in patients with advanced germ cell tumors: a multivariate and matched-pair analysis. J Clin Oncol 1999; 17: 3450–6.

71. Loehrer PJ, Gonin R, Nichols CR et al. Vinblastine plus ifosfamide plus cisplatin as initial salvage therapy in recurrent germ cell tumor. J Clin Oncol 1998; 16: 2500–4.

72. Miller KD, Loehrer PJ, Gonin R et al. Salvage chemotherapy with vinblastine, ifosfamide, and cisplatin in recurrent seminoma. J Clin Oncol 1997; 15: 1427–31.

73. Motzer RJ, Mazumdar M, Bajorin DF et al. High-dose carboplatin, etoposide and cyclophosphamide with autologous bone marrow transplantation in first-line therapy for patients with poor-risk germ cell tumors. J Clin Oncol 1997; 15: 2546–52.

74. Bamberg M, Shmidberger H, Meisner C et al. Radiotherapy for stage I, IIA/B testicular seminoma. Int J Cancer 1999; 83: 823–7.

75. Fossa SD, Horwich A, Russel JM et al. Optimal planning target volume for stage I testicular seminoma: a Medical Research Council randomized trial. J Clin Oncol 1999; 17: 1146–54.

76. Oliver RT, Mason MD, Mead GM et al. Radiotherapy versus single-agent carboplatin in adjuvant treatment of stage I seminoma: a randomised trial. Lancet 2005; 366: 293–300.

77. Warde P, Gospodarowicz MK, GoodmanPJ et al. Stage I testicular seminoma: results of adjuvant irradiation and surveillance. J Clin Oncol 1995; 13: 2255–62.

78. Aparicio J, Germa JR, Garcia del Muro X et al. Risk-adapted management for patients with clinical stage I seminoma: the Second Spanish Germ Cell Cancer Cooperative Group study. J Clin Oncol 2005; 23: 8717–23.

79. Schmidberger H, Bamberg M, Meisner C et al. Radiotherapy in stage IIA and IIB testicular seminoma with reduced portals: a prospective multicenter study. Int J Radiat Oncol Biol Phys 1997; 39: 321–6.

80. Krege S, Boergermann C, Baschek R et al. Single agent carboplatin for CS IIA/B testicular seminoma. A phase II study of the German Testicular Cancer Study Group. Ann Oncol 2006; 17: 276–80.

81. Oldenburg J, Alfsen GC, Lien HH et al. Postchemotherapy retroperitoneal surgery remains the necessary in patients with nonseminomatous testicular cancer and minimal residual tumor masses. J Clin Oncol 2003; 21: 3310–17.

82. Heidenreich A, Seger M, Schrader AJ, Hofmann R, Engelmann UH. Surgical considerations in residual tumor resection following inductive chemotherapy for advanced testicular cancer. Eur Urol 2004; (Suppl 3): 162–632.

83. Steyerberg EW, Keizer HJ, Fossa SD et al. Prediction of residual retroperitoneal mass histology after chemotherapy for metastatic nonseminomatous germ cell tumor: multivariate analysis of individual patient data from six study groups. J Clin Oncol 1995; 13: 1177–87.

84. Vergouwe Y, Steyerberg EW, de Wit R et al. External validation of a prediction rule for residual mass histology in testicular cancer: an evaluation for good prognosis patients. Br J Cancer 2003; 88: 843–7.

85. Albers P, Weissbach L, Krege S et al. German Testicular Cancer Study Group. Prediction of necrosis after chemotherapy of advanced germ cell tumors: results of a prospective multicenter trial of the German Testicular Cancer Study Group. J Urol 2004; 171(5): 1835–8.

86. Herr HW. Does necrosis on frozen section analysis of a mass after chemotherapy justify a limited retroperitoneal resection in patients with advanced testis cancer? Br J Urol 1997; 80: 653–7.

87. Baniel J, Foster RS, Gonin R, Bihrle R, Donohue JP. Complications of post-chemotherapy retroperitoneal lymph node dissection. J Urol 1995; 153: 976–9.

88. Fizazi K, Tjulandin S, Salvioni R et al. Viable malignant cells after primary chemotherapy for disseminated nonseminomatous germ cell tumors: prognostic factors and role of postsurgical chemotherapy – results from an international study. J Clin Oncol 2001; 19: 2647–57.

89. De Santis M, Becherer A, Bokemeyer C et al. 2-18Fluoro-deoxy-D-glucose positron emission tomography is a reliable predictor for viable tumor in postchemotherapy seminoma: an update of the prospective multicentric SEMPET trial. J Clin Oncol 2004; 22: 1034–9.

90. Becherer A, De Santis M, Karanikas G et al. FDG PET is superior to CT in the prediction of viable tumour in post-chemotherapy seminoma residuals. Eur J Radiol 2005; 54: 284–8.

91. Kondagunta GV, Bacik J, Donadio A et al. Combination of paclitaxel, ifosfamide and cisplatin is an effective second-line therapy for patients with relapsed testicular germ cell tumors. J Clin Oncol 2005; 23: 6549–55.

Sexual Dysfunction

CHAPTER 15

Treatment of erectile dysfunction in the elderly

Kok Bin Lim and Gerald B Brock

Introduction

The world's population is aging and expanding at an exponential rate. The human race entered the 19th century with a billion people, the 20th century with 1.6 billion, and today it exceeds 6 billion. The largest increase is predicted to occur in the aging population, those individuals over the age of 65 years. In 1950, less than 5% of the population was older than 65 years; by 2000, more than 400 million (7%) were over 65 years. This percentage is predicted to increase to 15% by 2050, swelling to over 1.5 million elderly. Life expectancy in the developed world over the same time period has increased from 47 years in 1900 to 80 by 2010.[1,2] This is attributed in part to developments in modern medicine and improved sanitation that occurred in the 20th century.

The prevalence of erectile dysfunction (ED) is related to aging as evidenced by the Massachusetts Male Aging Study (MMAS). Erectile dysfunction is defined as the persistent inability to attain and/or maintain a penile erection sufficient to complete a satisfactory sexual intercourse. In order to meet the definition of ED, it should cause distress to the patient or the couple. This is important because even though a significant proportion of elderly men would report some form of ED, only a minority seek treatment.

As the average life expectancy has increased, more elderly men are likely to come forward to ask for medical assistance, encouraged by the availability of oral therapy.

Epidemiology

The association between aging and male ED has been shown in several epidemiologic studies. In 1948, Kinsey et al first showed that sexual activity and erectile function declined with aging.[3] This study on 15 000 individuals between the ages of 10 and 80 years remains the largest population-based study on male sexual behavior. It describes an incidence of ED of 25% in 65-year-old men and 75% in men above 80. Likewise, the Baltimore Longitudinal Study of Aging reported that, by age 55 years, ED was a problem in 8% of healthy men and the prevalence increased to 25%, 55%, and 75% for ages 65, 75, and 80 respectively.[4]

The most contributive epidemiologic study to date is the Massachusetts Male Aging Study (MMAS), a community-based multidisciplinary survey of health and aging in men. In 1290 men whose ages ranged from 40 to 70 years, the mean probability of some degree of ED was 52%. Between the ages of 40 and 70 years, the probability of complete ED tripled from 5.1 to 15%, while the probability of moderate ED doubled from 17 to 34%. Within the same age range, the probability of minimal ED remained constant at 17%. While an estimated 60% of men were potent at age 40, this decreased to 33% at age 70 years. Whenever age was tested by multivariate linear regression or multivariate analysis of variance in conjunction with another predictor of ED, age invariably proved to be statistically significant at $P < 0.001$.[5]

Furthermore, coital activity also rapidly declined with age. The Duke Longitudinal Study found that 95% of men aged 46 to 50 years have intercourse at least once a week, but by the age of 66 to 71, only 28% report weekly coital activity.[6] The main reasons reported by men as to why they are not sexually active are the lack of a suitable partner, health, and medical problems.

Physiology of normal erectile function

Penile erection is a neurovascular phenomenon under psychogenic control. This psychogenic/neural control can be conceptualized into three main areas: local neural pathways, midbrain and spinal cord pathways, and higher brain centers.[7,8]

Local neural pathways

The local neural pathways incorporate both the genital and pelvic nerves and plexi. It can be divided into the autonomic (sympathetic and parasympathetic) and somatic (sensory and motor) systems. The cavernous nerves are mixed postganglionic parasympathetic and sympathetic neurons that supply the erectile tissue, thus controling the tone of the smooth muscles. The motor innervation is via the pudendal nerve that leads into the bulbocavernous and ischiocavernous muscles. Contraction of the latter muscles is important in the rigid erection phase as it constricts and compresses the corpora cavernosa, while rhythmic contraction of the bulbocavernous muscles is important for the expeling of semen during ejaculation. The afferent arc consists of sensory receptors in the penile skin that send sensory input via the dorsal nerve of the penis, connecting to the pudendal nerve and then the sacral spinal cord.

The spinal cord and midbrain

The lumbar spinal cord is the first level of reflex organization for coordination and generation of sexual responses. These spinal reflexes can be regulated by descending signals from the midbrain and higher centers. The spinal reflexes usually rest in an inhibited state; the efferent side is directed to non-sexual function, inducing flaccidity and lack of engorgement. Local sensory input and descending spinal signals can change this balance and activate a prosexual cascade of parasympathetic activity, reduced sympathetic output, and somatic muscular support.

Sensory information is conveyed cephalad through spinothalamic, spinoreticular, and vagal pathways. Various regions in the midbrain have been identified in the neural pathways of normal sexual function. The nucleus paragigantocellularis (NPG) receives ascending sensory input and has neurons that innervate the penis. It appears to have a role in orgasm but is not vital to erection. The most common neurotransmitter identified here is serotonin. The peri-aqueductal gray area has a large number of connections with hypothalamic sites involved in sexual response. One of these sites is the paraventricular nucleus (PVN), which has a major role in controlling genital response. It consists mainly of oxytocinergic and dopaminergic receptors. Its neurons send direct projections via the NPG onto neurons that innervate the penis. It also has direct projections to pelvic and autonomic efferents as well as being reciprocally connected to the medial pre-optic area (MPOA). The MPOA serves a vital role in sexual behavior and is potentially modulated by sex hormones (Figure 15.1).

Higher brain centers

The impact of imagination on human sexual behavior has been studied. In man, enhancing the central pro-erectile signals by enhanced imagination or by pharmacologic means improves erection. Studies with functional magnetic resonance imaging (MRI) have identified sexual imagery to be associated with activation in the dominant hemisphere, especially the occipital cortex, inferior frontal lobe, cingulate gyrus, corpus callosum, thalamus, caudate nucleus, globus pallidus, and inferior temporal lobe.

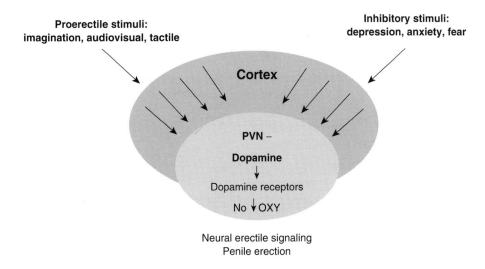

Figure 15.1

Smooth muscle

The tone of the smooth muscles determines the hemodynamic events that maintain the penis in the flaccid or rigid state. This in turn depends on the intracellular calcium levels.

Smooth muscle contraction

Contraction of the penile arteries and trabecular smooth muscles is mediated by α_1-adrenergic receptors that can be mediated by adrenergic nerve terminals or circulating catecholamines.[9] Activation of the α_1 receptors initially provokes the release of intracellular calcium from sarcoplasmic reticulum and subsequently extracellular calcium entry by opening the calcium channel on the smooth muscle cell membrane. This increase is transient and, when the intracellular calcium returns to basal levels, the calcium-sensitizing pathways take over. During this transient phase, the increased intracellular calcium activates the calcium–calmodulin-dependent myosin light chain kinase (MLCK) which phosphorylates myosin light chain.[10,11] This causes vasoconstriction

of the penile arteries and contraction of the trabecular smooth muscles which result in reduction of the arterial inflow and collapse of lacunar spaces. The contraction of the trabecular smooth muscles causes decompression of the draining venules from the cavernous bodies and promotes venous drainage from the lacunar spaces.[12,13] The main neurotransmitters involved are endothelin,[14] angiotensin II,[15] and constrictor prostanoids, $PGF_{2\alpha}$ and thromboxane A_2 (TXA_2).[16]

Smooth muscle relaxation

An initial stimulus starting from the supraspinal centers travels through the spinal cord and reaches the corpora cavernosa, ultimately traveling along the cavernous nerves. Terminal branches of the cavernous nerves release several neurotransmitters that are involved in initiating the erectile process. In addition, endothelial cells lining the walls of the cavernous sinusoids release active mediators, namely nitric oxide (NO), vasoactive intestinal polypeptide, acetylcholine, and a number of prostaglandins such as PGI_2 and PGE_1. In particular, NO activates guanylyl

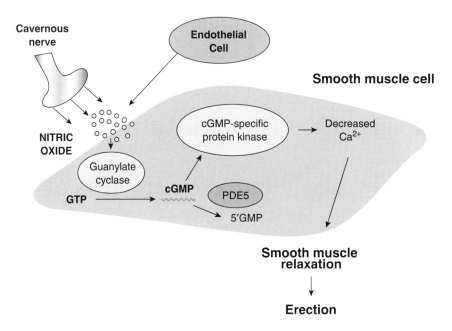

Figure 15.2

cyclase which converts cyclic guanosine triphosphate (cGTP) to cyclic guanosine monophosphate (cGMP), thus increasing intracellular cGMP levels. cGMP signals by three different ways: ion channels, phosphodiesterases, and protein kinases. Through these interactions, the cGMP induces loss of contractile tone by reducing intracellular calcium. This is achieved via hyperpolarization, closure of voltage-gated calcium channels, and sequestration of calcium by intracellular organelles.[17] This NO-induced increase in cGMP levels can be attenuated by phosphodiesterase V (PDE5) which metabolizes cGMP.[18] Ultimately, this leads to relaxation of the smooth muscle cells within the walls of the penile arteries and sinusoids.[19] The relaxation of the intracavernosal sinusoids leads to the corpora cavernosa filling with blood and the subsequent compression of the subtunical venous plexus against the inner surface of the tunica albuginea. This activates the veno-occlusive mechanism of the corpora cavernosa that traps blood within the corpora cavernosa, forming an isovolumetric reservoir. Any further arterial inflow

then leads to an increase in intracorporeal pressure and penile rigidity[20] (Figure 15.2).

When ejaculation and orgasm are achieved, norepinephrin is released by adrenergic fibers within the corpora cavernosa and smooth muscle contraction ensues with subsequent penile detumescence.[8]

Pathophysiology of erectile dysfunction in the aging male

With normal aging, there are changes in the physiology of the male erectile function. During arousal, the aging male presents a prolongation of the excitement phase with delayed erection, a lengthening of the plateau phase with a longer interval to ejaculation, and decreased penile rigidity. During orgasm, a shorter ejaculation event with an increased incidence of resolution without ejaculation is often observed. During postorgasm, the aging male has a more rapid detumescence and an increased refractory period.[21]

Abnormalities in erectile function have been characterized as neurogenic (failure to initiate), arteriogenic (failure to fill), and venogenic (failure to store).[22] However, the term venogenic ED should be viewed as mainly identifying the abnormalities in the corpus cavernosum anatomy and histology leading to the alteration of the cavernous veno-occlusive mechanism.[23] In addition, abnormalities of the sex hormones may significantly affect the quality of penile erections (endocrine-based ED). The process of aging may affect all pillars of the erectile process including nerves, arteries, veins, cavernous tissue, and hormones.

Effect of aging on smooth muscle function

The most prominent pathologic features of age-related histopathologic changes are fibrosis and smooth muscle atrophy. Studies with penile cavernosal tissue have shown that age-related fibrosis and smooth muscle atrophy produce an adverse effect on the mechanical properties of the penile erectile tissue and interfere with erection.

Using computerized image analysis, the percentage of smooth muscle cells was measured in patients of different age with normal erections. Less than 40 years old, the percentage was 46%; between 41 and 60 years, it was 40%; and over 60 years of age, it was 35%. This decrease in smooth muscle content may be responsible for the decline in erectile functions in older men. In addition, the rigidity of penile erection depends on the corporal veno-occlusive mechanism, which allows intracavernous pressure to increase during erection.[24]

Currently, age-related smooth muscle dysfunction is poorly understood. Atherosclerosis-induced arterial insufficiency is a common clinical problem in the elderly.[25] The abdominal aorta and its branches, especially the bifurcation of the iliac arteries, are involved earliest and most severely by atherosclerotic lesions.[26] Atherosclerosis of the aorto-iliac arterial bed can potentially compromise the blood supply of the lower genitourinary tract. Major risk factors for atherosclerosis such as hypertension, hypercholesterolemia, smoking, and diabetes

mellitus, have also been found to be associated with smooth muscle degeneration.[27]

Numerous studies have shown that atherosclerosis and tissue ischemia affect both arterial inflow and the veno-occlusive mechanism of the corpora cavernosa.[28] The severity of arterial occlusion has been correlated with the reduced proportion of smooth muscle in the corpus cavernosum. The reduction in smooth muscle content of the corpus cavernosum is associated with the impairment of cavernosal expandability and results in veno-occlusive dysfunction.[29] Hypoxia-induced overexpression of TGF-β_1 is believed to play a key role in the process of ischemia-induced damage.[30] Under normal conditions, TGF-β_1 maintains cell numbers by inhibiting cell proliferation and by controlling the mitogenic actions of platelet-derived growth factor (PDGF), a companion cytokine. TGF-β_1 also regulates the amount of extracellular matrix (ECM) by balancing new synthesis and deposition of ECM by degradation and removal with proteases. Under ischemic conditions, TGF-β_1 has been shown to be an essential mediator of tissue fibrosis. Overproduction of TGF-β_1 decreases the smooth muscle to connective tissue ratio by inducing the expression of collagen, fibronectin, and proteoglycans while inhibiting the growth of smooth muscle cells and the activity of collagenase.[31] In addition, TGF-β_1 gene expression is significantly increased in the older rat penile tissues as compared to the young rats.[32] It appears that the histologic alterations start distally in the very small penile arteries.[33] The patient develops a corporeal veno-occlusive dysfunction, whereas the cavernous arteries do not demonstrate any pathologic alteration at Doppler examination. Later, the pathophysiologic mechanism progresses and provokes severe arterial disease. At this stage, fibrosis of the corpora cavernosum becomes clinically evident.

Another important role of cavernosal oxygen tension appears to be regulation of prostanoid production in the corpus cavernosum. It has been shown that low oxygen tension decreases basal and acetylcholine-stimulated production of prostacyclin, PGI_2, TXA_2, $PGF2_\alpha$, and PGE_2 by inhibiting the activity of prostaglandin H synthase.[34] Decreased levels of PGE_1 also correlated with

211

increased expression of TGF-β_1 mRNA in human corpus cavernosum smooth muscle cells.[35] It is likely that the effect of low oxygen tension on prostanoid production also has a role in ischemia-induced cavernosal fibrosis.[36]

Bakircioglu et al investigated the effect of aging on trabecular smooth muscle content and caveolin-1 protein expression in rodent penile smooth muscle cells.[37] Caveolae are specialized plasma membrane invaginations on the surface of most cells. They are involved in transporting macromolecules across capillary endothelial cells by transcytosis, photocytosis, and signal transduction. Caveolae contain various signal transduction molecules including G protein, which is involved in regulating intracellular calcium homeostasis and the endothelial form of nitric oxide synthase. Caveolin is a family of integral membrane proteins associated with caveolae and trans-Golgi network derived vesicles. The suggested functions of caveolin-1 include cholesterol transport, caveolae formation, G protein subunit regulation, oncogenic transformation, insulin signaling, and endothelial nitric oxide synthase regulation. When both young and old rats were evaluated, immunostaining for caveolin-1 was noted in each group in the sarcolemma of smooth muscle cells and endothelium of trabecular sinusoids, but the staining pattern was less intense and the percentage of smooth muscle cells positive for caveolin-1 was reduced in the aged versus the young rats. In addition, young trabecular smooth muscle had more caveolae in the sarcolemma on electron microscopy and a higher expression of caveolin-1 protein on Western blot analysis, suggesting that a reduced expression of caveolin-1 may contribute to ED in aged rats.

Besides the histologic modification observed with penile ischemia, oxygen tension appears to be an important regulator of NO production. With reduced O_2 level, a reduction in smooth muscle cell relaxation has been observed.[38]

Hormonal changes in aging

With prolonged life expectancy, men can expect to live one-third of their lives with some form of hormone deficiency. Hormonal changes in the aging male are associated with changes in the body mass index, osteoporosis, and sleep and mood disorders.

Andropause is characterized by a gradual decline in serum total and bioavailable testosterone due to a decrease in testicular Leydig cell number and in their secretory capacity, as well as an age-related decrease in episodic and stimulated gonadotropin secretion.[39] Mean serum total testosterone levels decrease by 30% between ages 25 and 75 years, whereas mean serum free testosterone levels decrease by as much as 50% over the same period. This steeper decline in free testosterone levels is explained by an age-associated increase in sex hormone binding globulin.[40] With the decrease in androgens, luteinizing hormone (LH) and follicle stimulating hormone (FSH) increase transitionally.[41] The MMAS showed that, between the ages of 40 and 70 years, there was an annual decrease in the hormones, as shown in Table 15.1.[42]

Table 15.1 *Hormonal changes due to aging*

Testosterone	0.4%
Free testosterone	1.2%
Albumin bound testosterone	1%
Androstenedione	1.3%
Androstanediol	0.8%
Androstanediol – glucoronide	0.6%

Studies have also shown that levels of DHEA and DHEA-S decrease with age, so that by age 60 years, plasma levels for DHEA-S are one-third of those at ages 20 to 25. Our understanding of DHEA and DHEA-S has been limited because of a lack of DHEA-specific receptor, which is a prerequisite for the production of hormonal effects. Recent animal studies, however, revealed a putative DHEA-specific receptor on the plasma membrane of bovine aortic endothelial cells.[43] This receptor is coupled to the G family protein that promotes the production of endothelial nitric oxide synthase (eNOS). A further recent study by Williams et al showed evidence that supports the existence of a DHEA-specific receptor in human vascular smooth muscle cells (VSMCs).[44] VSMC proliferation contributes to remodeling of blood vessels and may be relevant with regard to sexual function which involves many vascular mechanisms.

DHEA is a neurosteroid, suggesting the possibility of specific effects on the nervous system. Neurosteroids are steroids persisting in the brain or nerves after castration and adrenalectomy, and hence are produced by neural synthesis from cholesterol. In vitro and in vivo effects on brain neurotransmission have been demonstrated in animal studies for DHEA.[45]

Overall, it can be seen that all fractions of biologically active gonadal and adrenal androgens decrease with age.

There are a variety of symptoms associated with decreasing androgen levels. Not all of these symptoms are directly related to a decrease in androgens but may be due to a concomitant decrease in the conversion product of androgens. It should be noted that each individual has his own threshold level of androgens; symptomatology generally occurs at the level of < 10 nmol testosterone, but in some men it may occur at < 12–15 nmol.

Finally, the third endocrine system of interest that gradually reduces its activity with aging is the growth hormone (GH)/insulin-like growth factor (IGF) axis. This reduction is associated with changes in lean muscle mass, bone density, hair distribution, and the pattern of obesity. GH administration reverses these alterations.[46] It has also been identified as an anti-apoptotic agent in a neuronal model. This has profound implications in the prevention of degradation of neurofibril proteins in Alzheimer's disease. Although the majority of evidence favors the use of androgens in the treatment of some of the manifestations of androgen deficiency in the aging male, recent studies indicate that elderly men respond to GH administration alone as well. In terms of sexual functioning, even though the literature is sparse regarding the role of GH, its administration does improve peripheral circulation and emotional status.[47]

Role of testosterone on penile erection

The possible regulatory roles for androgens in penile erection physiology have been most extensively studied in animals. A clear statement regarding androgen control in the erection physiology of humans is not currently possible based on existing evidence. In rats and rabbits, castration reduces trabecular smooth muscle content and increases connective tissue.[48] Androgen replacement prevents smooth muscle loss comparable to that observed in control animals.

Cavernosal androgen receptor activity in the rats varies widely with age, with maximal levels at puberty and markedly lower levels thereafter. This age-related reduction in the number of androgen receptors is androgen mediated and is irreversible.[49] This age-dependent decline in the androgen receptor coincides with and appears to be responsible for the cessation of penile growth.[50]

Androgens seem to stimulate and maintain the activity of the enzyme nitric oxide synthase (NOS). In adult rats, the decrease in NOS activity that followed castration was restored with androgen replacement, whereas no additional NOS activity was observed when intact animals were given additional androgens.[51] NADPH diaphorase staining decreases by more than half in cavernosal nerves after 10 days of castration but returns to near normal values following testosterone replacement.[52] There is decreased NOS activity in castrated compared to intact or testosterone replaced animals.[53] Measurement of NOS enzyme protein showed that, in castrated animals, there is less than half the quantity of NOS protein compared to testosterone replaced animals.[54]

In dogs, castration leads to a decline in the ratio of intracavernosal pressure to peak systolic pressure and there is also evidence of higher outflow rates in the castrated animals.[55] In rabbits, when strips of cavernosal tissue precontracted with α-adrenergic agonists were subjected to electrical field stimulation, there was a greater degree of relaxation in strips from castrated than intact animals.[56] The contraction in response to norepinephrine may also be hormonally dependent, with strips from intact rabbits showing a greater degree of contraction than tissues from castrated animals in response to the same concentration of agonist.[57] The relaxation in response to field stimulation was greater in castrated than in intact animals although relaxation in response to NO donor drugs was not different between the two groups, suggesting that basal NOS may be adequate to mediate the erectile response.[57]

In humans, several studies have reported that the episodes of nocturnal penile tumescence (NPT) and quality of spontaneous erections are diminished in hypogonadal men. Treatment with testosterone improves the quality of the erection and NPT frequency.[57] However, libido and visual erectile mechanisms may require smaller amounts of testosterone than normal blood levels. This explains why some hypogonadal men can have normal erections and NPT frequency.[58] In surgically castrated patients, levels of androgen adequate to maintain some degree of penile erection may be secreted by the adrenal cortex.[59]

Evidence from animal studies also demonstrated that normal androgen level is a prerequisite for a PDE-5 inhibitor to work appropriately. The same study showed that androgen deprivation, either by surgical or medical means, leads to fundamental structural alterations in the corpus cavernosum and results in failure of the veno-occlusive mechanisms.[60]

Other effects of testosterone

As testosterone decreases with advancing age, visceral fat and body mass index (BMI) increase. A large visceral fat depot is a strong predictor of a number of conditions, including diabetes mellitus, hypertension, cardiovascular disease, high triglyceride levels, and low high-density lipoprotein (HDL) cholesterol. Obesity is a multimorbid disease state that leads to insulin resistance, glucose intolerance, hyperglycemia, and type 2 diabetes mellitus (DM). Congestive heart failure is experienced at an increased frequency among this population as well. These associated comorbidities could also contribute to ED in aged men.[61,62]

Other contributory factors to erectile dysfunction

Comorbidities

When discussing age-related issues, it is often difficult to separate and to distinguish between the natural aging process, aging amplifiers, and an acute or chronic illness or intercurrent diseases. The aging male in particular has the risk of developing gender-specific urologic diseases such as prostate cancer, benign prostate hyperplasia, and incontinence disorders, which could contribute to ED either because of the disease per se or its therapy. Other diseases associated with an increased incidence due to aging are shown in Table 15.2. Many of these conditions can impact on sexual function. Furthermore, the drugs used to treat some of these conditions also have an effect on sexual function, for example thiazide diuretics, β-adrenergic antagonists, α_2-adrenoceptor agonists such as methyldopa, tricyclic antidepressants, and certain antipsychotic drugs.[63–65]

Table 15.2 *Diseases associated with aging*

Cardiovascular diseases
Malignancy
Degenerative diseases such as osteoporosis and arthritis
Metabolic diseases such as diabetes mellitus
Dementia such as Alzheimer's disease

Diabetes mellitus

Among all the endocrine causes of ED, diabetes mellitus (DM) occupies the most prominent position and it should be ruled out in all males with erectile insufficiency. The documentation of ED does not exclude other etiology of ED in diabetic patients. Organic factors are, however, most prominent in the causality of ED in the diabetic male and appear quite early in the course of the disease. The primary organic, pathophysiologic factors causing diabetic ED can be categorized as vascular, neurologic, and hypogonadism.

Vasculopathy

The vascular changes are quite prominent as shown by an observational study by Wang et al that looks at diabetic males with ED.[66] Duplex ultrasound examinations after intracorporeal injection of PGE_1 revealed 87.2% to have moderate and severe cavernous arterial insufficiency. This increased to 100% when hypertension or alcohol abuse were added risk factors to DM. In other studies, increased incidence of endothelial dysfunction was found as evidenced by reduced fibrinolysis, enhanced expression of endothelin 1, decreased prostacyclin release, increased adhesion molecule expression, and increased platelet adhesion.[67]

A major consequence of endothelial dysfunction is decreased production and/or action of NO. It has been documented that diabetic rats exhibit a marked decrease in penile NOS activity and a reduced nNOS content in penile tissue.[68]

Hyperglycemia in DM causes other metabolic changes that can affect penile physiology. Sobrevia and Mann, in an extensive review of the literature, noted that elevated blood sugar causes regional hemodynamic changes and endothelial-dependent relaxation is impaired. Protein kinase C is activated and oxygen free radicals are generated which inactivate NO and may cause further endothelial damage.[69]

Neuropathy

An observational study on patients with insulin-dependent diabetes mellitus (IDDM) revealed 60% had cardiac autonomic neuropathy, 68% had diabetic cystopathy, while 80% had signs of peripheral neuropathy. The surprising thing is that ED was the most common symptom and not postural hypotension.[70] Bemelmans et al, in a case-controlled study, looked at 27 impotent and 30 potent IDDM men as well as 102 impotent, non-diabetic men. Neurologic testing showed that 85% of the impotent diabetic men had some form of neuropathy versus 40% of the potent, diabetic men and 44% of impotent, non-diabetic men. They also found that poor diabetic control, as measured by the HbA_{1c} levels, correlated with increased sexual dysfunction.[71]

Hypogonadism

DM lowers testosterone level and hypogonadism can be another factor contributing to ED in this population. The MMAS longitudinal epidemiologic study on 1709 men, aged 40 to 70 years, looked at 1156 men 7 to 10 years later. They found that testosterone and SHBG levels were predictive of new cases of diabetics. The odds ratio for future diabetes is 1.58 for a decrease of 1 SD in free testosterone (4 ng/dl) and 1.89 for 1 SD decrease in

SHBG (16 nmol/l). This was consistent with prior cross-sectional data from this study.[72]

Prostate cancer

It should be noted that prostate cancer may be present in hypogonadal men and a rate of 29% has been reported in men aged 60 and over.[73] One of the presenting symptoms of prostate cancer is sudden onset of ED when the prostate cancer cells have invaded the cavernosal nerves. However, the main association of prostate cancer with ED is following definitive management of the disease by radiation or radical prostatectomy. The primary mechanism of ED after surgery is usually neurologic, but a contributory vascular cause has also been described.[74] The neurologic lesion occurs in either the pelvic plexus or cavernosal nerves. The incidence used to be in the vicinity of 100% but, with the advent of nerve-sparing procedures, maintenance of erectile capability varies from 30 to 65%, depending on the surgical technique, the pathologic staging, age of the patient, and level of pretreatment sexual functioning.[75]

Recovery of erectile function after radical pelvic surgery can be slow, over the course of 12–18 months. Early treatment (with self-administered intracavernosal injection of vasoactive agents) has been shown to improve the recovery of erectile function. It is believed that the pharmacologically induced erections prevent the structural tissue changes associated with prolonged ischemia, which in turn is due to infrequent or no erections during the nerve recovery process.[76]

Management of erectile dysfunction in the aging male

It is important to stress that many older men (and their partners) do experience sexual dysfunction but do not want (or seek) any form of treatment because they are not bothered by it themselves. This was recently confirmed in an epidemiologic study in the Netherlands where a representative sample of the city population ($n = 1215$, aged between 40 and 80) was interviewed about the prevalence of ED and its impact on quality of life. There was an age-related increase in the prevalence of ED that reached 37% in the 70–79-year age group and an age-related decrease in the proportion of men who were bothered by ED (73% in the 40–49-year age group to 46% in the 70–79-year age group).[77] This must be kept in mind when interviewing the aging male who has requested medical help for any possible reason. The readily available, easy to handle, and self-administered questionnaires designed to investigate the patient's sexual health have facilitated the evaluation of sexual concerns.[78]

The management of ED in the aged male is the same as any ailment; it would require a detailed history and physical examination assisted by some laboratory tests.

History should be focused on the type of sexual problem (i.e. ED vs premature ejaculation vs loss of libido) as patients sometimes get confused themselves. What is more important is that the clinician must identify the risk factors for ED which comprise serious medical conditions and lifestyle factors. This includes ischemic heart disease, hypertension, DM, perineal or pelvic trauma, dyslipidemia, depression, previous pelvic surgery, smoking, alcohol, and substance abuse. Most of these risk factors are more commonly found in the aging population and need to be investigated extensively. A psychosocial history is also important in order to obtain information on the couple's relationship (if one exists) and the partner's health. It is our experience that the partner would probably be in the menopausal phase of her life and could potentially suffer from some form of sexual dysfunction herself.

The physical examination should include both systemic review and a focus on the genitalia. The general assessment would include determining the height and weight for calculating the body mass index, verifying blood pressure, and identifying any peripheral vasculopathy and sensory loss. A digital rectal examination (DRE) of the prostate gland and rectum should always be performed in the aging male as they are at risk of developing prostate and rectal cancer.

Laboratory tests should be offered to all aging males presenting with ED. Serum glucose and lipids should be done. Prostate-specific antigen (PSA) testing is offered to those under 70 years of age with risk factors for prostate cancer as well as those with suspicious DRE. In addition, total testosterone and prolactin levels should be tested in patients who are PDE-5 inhibitor failures and those with symptoms of andropause. Other tests could be performed if indicated clinically.

Treatment options

There are two main types of treatment for ED, namely medical therapy and surgical therapy. Sandwiched in between, the option of sexual counseling and psychologic therapy should always be offered.

Medical therapy

Medical therapy is broadly classified into three main groups:

1. oral medication
2. local/topical therapy, e.g. intraurethral alprostadil and various topical agents
3. injections, e.g. intracavernosal PGE_1.

Oral therapy

The first line of therapy would include oral drug therapy, vacuum devices, and sex therapy. The latter is usually less frequently indicated as the proportion of aging patients with pure psychogenic ED is less than for their younger counterparts. The vacuum device is able to create a rigid erection in the majority of cases regardless of the patient's age. However, its use is troublesome and it is usually acceptable to patients with a stable relationship with their partners where the patient–partner's confidentiality is not a problem. The use of vacuum devices has been dramatically reduced since the advent of sildenafil and the other PDE-5 inhibitors.

There are two main classes of oral drugs available, either centrally acting or peripherally acting.

Peripherally acting agents – the PDE-5 inhibitors

Sildenafil has certainly revolutionized the therapeutic approach to ED in the aging male. A selective and competitive inhibitor of PDE-5, it has been shown to be an effective and well-tolerated oral agent for treating ED of broad-spectrum etiology.[79] Recently it has been joined by another two compounds, vardenafil and tadalafil.

As mentioned previously, the normal pathway for penile erection is initiated by sexual arousal which stimulates release of NO from nerve endings in the penis and vascular endothelial tissue. The NO in turn stimulates the guanylyl cyclase that increases the production of cGMP.[20] This leads to the activation of cGMP-dependent protein kinase and, after local phosphorylation of proteins, there is a reduction in intracellular calcium, leading to smooth muscle relaxation and accumulation of blood in the corpus cavernosum.[19] Therefore, cGMP is vital in the process of penile erection, which is constantly being degraded by the enzyme PDE-5.[18] This is where sildenafil comes into play, as an inhibitor of PDE-5; it reduces the degradation of cGMP and maintains a higher intracellular level of cGMP in both the corpus cavernosum and the vessels supplying it. This increases relaxation of the smooth muscle which dilates the corporeal sinusoids, resulting in increased blood flow and allowing an erection to occur.

The PDE-5 inhibitors do not increase the level of NO but potentiate its effect to facilitate an erection. Without sexual arousal, which triggers the nerve–NO pathway, these inhibitors are ineffective.

The most commonly experienced adverse events are headache, flushing, and dyspepsia, which occur in 10–15% of patients. Most of these adverse events are mild to moderate in nature. Visual disturbances may be experienced by a small number of patients receiving sildenafil (4%). These have been described as a transient and mild color tinge in vision or blurred vision.

Centrally acting agents – the dopamine agonists

Penile erections are initiated by central stimuli as discussed in previous chapters. These stimuli send inputs to the medial preoptic area (MPOA) and paraventricular nucleus (PVN). The PVN contains dopaminergic neurons which impinge on oxytocin-containing neurons. The PVN is the nucleus where apomorphine, the dopaminergic agonist, acts. From here, signals are transmitted to brainstem nuclei such as periaqueductal gray, raphe nuclei and then to the periphery of the erectile axis.[80]

Dopamine is one of the neurotransmitters involved in the initiation of erection.[81] Dopamine receptors are divided into two main families, the D1 and D2 like receptors. Apomorphine has a higher affinity for the D2 like receptors that are thought to be the main site for the induction of erection in the PVN.[82] Hence, apomorphine acts as a conditioner in the PVN, increasing the response to sexual stimuli, resulting in enhanced erections induced in the periphery. NO is required as a cofactor at the PVN in order to activate the oxytocinergic neurons. Hence, adequate sexual stimulation is needed to allow the erectogenic effect of apomorphine to work. Apomorphine is available in a sublingual form in some countries.

Others

Yohimbine is derived from the cortex of the *Coryanthe yohimbe* tree. Its main pharmacologic action is α_2-adrenoceptor antagonism. The α_2-adrenoceptors are located both centrally and peripherally. The site of action of yohimbine in humans is not well defined. It may have both peripheral and central actions. Central α_2-adrenoceptors are implicated in the regulation of sexual behavior.[83] Yohimbine has been demonstrated to increase sexual motivation in experienced male rats and induce sexual activity in sexually naïve or inactive rats.[84]

Peripherally, yohimbine acts antagonistically on postjunctional α_2-adrenoceptors that mediate contraction of the corpus cavernosum and helps facilitate penile erection. Recent data also indicate that yohimbine may mediate relaxation of the human and rabbit corpus cavernosum via release of NO from the endothelium.[85]

Local/topical therapy

Intraurethral suppositories may be used, for example MUSE, which contains alprostadil, a naturally occurring PGE_1, which relaxes corpus cavernosal

Table 15.3 *Comparison between the PDE–5 inhibitors*

	Tadalafil (Cialis)	Sildenafil (Viagra)	Vardenafil (Levitra)
Usual dose	10 mg	50 mg	10 mg
Onset	15–45 mins	20–60 mins	15–30 mins
Half-life	17.5 hours	1–2 hours	45 mins
Duration	24–36 hours	4 hours	4–5 hours
Affected by food	No	Yes	Yes
Metabolism	CYP3A4	CYP3A4 (major) CYP2C9 (minor)	CYP3A4 (major) CYP2C9 (minor)
Drug interactions	CYP3A4 inhibitors CYP2C9 inducers	CYP3A4 inhibitors CYP2C9 inducers	CYP3A4 inhibitors
Side-effects	Headache Dyspepsia Nasal congestion Flushing Back pain	Headache Flushing Dyspepsia Nasal congestion Visual disturbances	Headache Flushing Dyspepsia Nasal congestion Dizziness
Contraindications	Patients taking nitrates or alpha blockers Known hypersensitivity to PDE-5 inhibitors	Patients taking nitrates or alpha blockers Known hypersensitivity to PDE-5 inhibitors	Patients taking nitrates or alpha blockers Known hypersensitivity to PDE-5 inhibitors
Cautions	Heart disease Stroke Peptic ulcers Low blood pressure Liver impairment Renal impairment Prolonged erection (>4 hours) Bleeding disorders Blood cell problems Retinitis pigmentosa	Heart disease Stroke Peptic ulcers Low blood pressure Liver impairment Renal impairment Prolonged erection (>4 hours) Bleeding disorders Blood cell problems Retinitis pigmentosa	Heart disease Stroke Peptic ulcers Low blood pressure Liver impairment Renal impairment Prolonged erection (>4 hours) Bleeding disorders Blood cell problems Retinitis pigmentosa
Dosage forms	5, 10, 20 mg	25, 50, 100 mg	10, 20 mg

smooth muscle. Its action is discussed under the section on intracavernosal injection.

Topical therapy

Topical therapy for ED has been proposed as one of the means to circumvent some of the problems associated with intracavernosal injection and intraurethral suppository. It has an intrinsic appeal to patients as it could potentially avoid the systemic effects of oral therapy while being perceived as minimally invasive as it does not require any needles or intraurethral manipulations. Topical therapy may also be beneficial to patients unresponsive to systemic therapy or who are on medications that contraindicate such oral treatment (e.g. nitrates).

Currently, it remains under clinical trial and is not available for widespread use.

Intracavernosal injection

The use of alprostadil or other vasoactive drug mixtures is a reliable option for treating ED. The erectogenic effect is usually superior to that of PDE-5 inhibitors in terms of penile rigidity and onset of action.[86] Although some form of manual dexterity is required to handle the intracorporeal injection, new injecting devices are now available and make this treatment more readily accessible by the elderly.

PGE$_1$ Alprostadil or PGE$_1$ mediates relaxation of corpus cavernosum smooth muscle by increasing the intracellular concentration of cAMP via activation of EP prostaglandin receptors.[87] PGE$_1$ may also act by inhibiting the release of norepinephrine from sympathetic nerves[88] and suppressing angiotensin II secretion in the cavernosal tissues.[89]

Papaverine In vitro, papaverine induces relaxation of corpus cavernosum smooth muscle, cavernous sinusoids, penile arteries and penile veins, and attenuates contractions caused by stimulation of adrenergic nerves and exogenous norepinephrine.[90] In addition, in vivo studies in the rat model documented that intracavernosal injection of papaverine elicited a significant and prolonged increase in intracavernous pressure.[91]

Papaverine is also a non-specific phosphodiesterase inhibitor that causes an increase in intracellular cAMP and cGMP, leading to corporeal smooth muscle relaxation and penile erection. Papaverine may also regulate cavernosal smooth muscle tone via inhibition of voltage-dependent calcium channels independent of cAMP.[92]

Phentolamine Phentolamine is a non-selective α-adrenoceptor antagonist with similar affinity for α$_1$- and α$_2$-adrenoceptors. It induces the relaxation of corpus cavernosum erectile tissue by antagonism of the α$_1$- and α$_2$-adrenoceptors.[93] Furthermore, it delays detumescence, contributing to the maintenance of penile erection.

Combination therapy Phentolamine, papaverine, and PGE$_1$ are the vasoactive agents most commonly used in combination therapy to treat ED. Understandably, combination therapy is not only more efficacious, it is also associated with a reduction in the incidence of side-effects and cost per dose.

Surgical therapy

This option includes various penile implants and medical devices.

Penile implants

Penile implants are usually considered for patients who do not respond to other less invasive forms of therapy or for whom those therapies were contraindicated, such as patients on nitrates. There are various types of implants, ranging from inflatable to malleable, the selection of choice being guided by the surgeon according to the patient's body habitus and manual dexterity. A patient with a larger penis is best served by a three-piece inflatable. Those with limited manual dexterity or those having difficulty manipulating the hydraulic devices are encouraged to choose a semi-rigid rod.

The operation is usually performed under general or regional anesthesia. The complication rate is minimal if proper preoperative precautions and preparations are observed; potential complications are perforation of the corpora and urethra, migration of the prosthesis, infection, and mechanical failure. Generally, the patients' satisfaction with this procedure is about 90%, the highest among all available treatment modalities. The 5-year mechanical survival rate is reported to be about 90 to 95%.[94,95]

Vacuum constriction devices

Vacuum constriction devices (VCDs) cause rigidity by creating negative pressure suction and trapping the blood in the penis with an elastic band, disc, or O ring around the base of the penile shaft. Excessive negative pressure can cause bruising and hematoma and hence a vacuum pressure regulator is essential. The constriction can be maintained without risk for 30 minutes.[96,97]

Table 15.4 Types of testosterone replacement

Name	Example	Route	Dosage	Advantages	Disadvantages
Testosterone injection (e.g., testosterone enanthate, cypionate)	Andro-LA, testo-LA, depo-testosterone	IM	200–400 mg every 2–4 weeks	2–4-Week dosing, relatively low cost	Painful intramuscular injection, contraindicated in bleeding disorders, produces mood swings as testosterone levels fluctuate
Testosterone undecanoate				Longer duration, 8–12 weeks	
Sublingual and buccal lozenge		SL		Bypass first pass hepatic metabolism	Multiple daily dosing
17-α alkylated androgens (methyltestosterone, fluoxymesterone), testosterone undecanoate	Android-10, Virilon / Andriol	OR	10–50 mg per day in divided doses / 160–240 mg in 3–5 divided doses daily	Easily administered, suitable in bleeding disorders	Potentially hepatotoxic, frequent administration required, low and erratic bioavailability, GI intolerance / Less hepatotoxic, more expensive
Scrotal patch	Testoderm	TD	5–15 mg daily	Suitable in bleeding disorders, easily administered, mimics circadian rhythm of testosterone in normal men	Less scrotal irritation or discomfort, need shaving
Non-scrotal skin patch	Androderm		5 mg daily		Skin irritation, 10–20% discontinuation rate due to dermal intolerance
Testosterone cream, gel	Androgel	TD	5–10 mg daily	Less skin irritation, suitable in bleeding disorders, easily	Potential transfer of testosterone to female partner by skin contact

(Continued)

220

Table 15.4 Types of testosterone replacement

Name	Example	Route	Dosage	Advantages	Disadvantages
				administered, mimics circadian rhythm of testosterone in normal men	
Subdermal implant (testosterone pellet)		Depot	800 mg 6 monthly	Convenience	Invasive (requires minor office surgery), not suitable for older men who may need to terminate treatment rapidly, extrusions about 10%

The devices usually consist of a transparent plastic chamber, a manual or battery-operated vacuum, and elastic bands or other constriction devices. There are no absolute contraindications for this procedure, even for those patients with some form of coagulopathy or on anticoagulation.

The VCD causes penile rigidity sufficient for vaginal penetration in most men regardless of the cause of ED. The probability of achieving proper intercourse is as high as 80%. However, the dropout rate can be as high as 50% as well, with longer follow-up.[97,98] The complications encountered are usually minor, such as petechiae due to rupture of capillaries after use. Ecchymoses and hematoma are rare. Altered climax and impaired ejaculation have also been reported.

A word of caution regarding treatment of ED in the aging patient. It has been shown that most of these patients suffer from diffuse atherosclerotic disease that often affects the heart. Sexual activity should be viewed as any other form of physical activity, and the sudden commencement or increase in sexual activity due to the use of any effective erectogenic treatment should be evaluated by a clinician from a cardiovascular perspective in those individuals deemed to be at risk.

Role of hormone replacement

Androgen deficiency in men is increasingly recognized as an important health and quality of life issue. The goals of treatment include restoration of sexual functioning, libido, and sense of well-being. In addition, androgen replacement can prevent or delay osteoporosis and optimize bone density, maintain virilization, improve mental acuity, and restore normal hormone levels. Testosterone replacement therapy should maintain physiologic levels not only of serum testosterone but also of its metabolites, including dihydrotestosterone (DHT) and estradiol. Flexible dosing, convenient administration, infrequent application, and prolonged action are important features of an effective androgen replacement therapy.

However, the use of hormones in the elderly still remains controversial. Muscle weakness, anemia, lowered bone mass, and mood disturbances rapidly normalized in middle-aged hypogonadal men during testosterone replacement therapy. It is not known at this moment whether testosterone therapy in older men has similar beneficial effects and whether it can be done safely. On the specific activity of androgens on ED, reports suggest a marginal synergistic effect when testosterone is added to PDE-5 inhibitors in hypogonadal men who failed the latter as a single therapy, apparently mediated by an increased inflow in the cavernosal arteries.[99] These studies only involved small groups of patients who were followed for a limited period.[100] Only a prospective, double-blind, placebo-controlled study evaluating the effect of testosterone administration to aging hypogonadal men with ED could answer these questions.

Prior to any testosterone substitution or replacement therapy, an assessment for prostate cancer should be conducted through PSA measurement and DRE. As previously mentioned, prostate cancer can be present in hypogonadal men.[73] Whether testosterone also promotes the development of prostate cancer remains to be determined. Morales reported a meta-analysis of 13 evaluable studies of testosterone therapy and found no significant changes in PSA levels or prostate cancer detection rate, although the follow-up was not long.[101]

It is necessary to monitor men on testosterone therapy every 3 months during the first year and, if they are stable, at 1-year intervals thereafter. The dosage applied should be based on clinical improvement and not necessarily on the achievement of normal hormone levels. During testosterone therapy, lipid and cholesterol levels should be monitored, as well as liver and cardiovascular function. The latter is important as hematocrit can increase after 3 months of therapy.

Types of hormone replacement therapies

Current testosterone preparations for treating the aging male include oral testosterone undecanoate, injectable testosterone esters, transdermal testosterone patches, and subdermal testosterone implants, as well as testosterone gels.

Injectable

An imporved intramuscular injection with a longer half-life could reduce side-effects such as those due to the transient supraphysiologic levels experienced in the first few days after injection and the subnormal levels felt just prior to the next injection. Longer-acting injections (4–6 months) are probably not suitable for the elderly male. In cases of serious side-effects, a rapid withdrawal of testosterone replacement should be possible.

Oral

The maximal plasma concentration level is generally observed within 2–3 hours after ingestion, but after 6–8 hours the levels return to pretreatment levels. Hence replacements should be administered 2 or 3 times daily, always with a meal to improve absorption. The dose required should be determined on the basis of plasma levels and clinical effects.[102]

Transdermal

Transdermal scrotal and permeation-enhanced non-scrotal patches provide physiologic testosterone levels in hypogonadal men.[103] The peak levels are reached 2–4 hours after application and subsequently decrease to two-thirds of peak levels after 22–24 hours, mimicking the normal circadian variation. The non-scrotal patches cause local skin irritation although newer formulations have fewer such side-effects. The patches also have the advantage of enabling the therapy to the stopped immediately when necessary.

Gel

Various hydro-alcoholic testosterone gels have now become available. When administered, a variable percentage of the testosterone applied becomes bioavailable and, with daily applications, normal levels of testosterone can be reached and maintained.[104]

Anti-aging products and other hormone replacement therapies

DHEA

The use of DHEA remains controversial, with recent data showing a slight beneficial effect in women but not in men.[105] Self-administration of DHEA occurs on a massive scale as it is sold as a health product, but so far no side-effects have been reported. Currently, there is no convincing evidence about DHEA and its relations with ED, although recent data support the possibility of DHEA-specific receptors on vascular endothelial and smooth muscle cells, suggesting the likelihood of a vascular involvement of DHEA in ED.[106] However, it would require well-designed studies with specific end-points aimed at investigating the effects of deficiency of adrenal androgens and the results of replacement therapy in humans to resolve this issue of long-term effects of DHEA therapy.

Growth hormone

GH administration in aging patients at this point in time is not advisable due to its narrow dose limits and potential side-effects, which include flu-like symptoms, myalgia, arthralgia, carpal tunnel syndrome, edema, and impaired glucose tolerance. Contraindications to GH usage are type I DM, active or history of cancer, intracranial hemorrhage, diabetic retinopathy, and severe cardiac insufficiency.

Future treatment

Gene therapy

Despite the introduction of oral therapy, there is still room for improvement in the treatment of ED. First, there is a need for better treatment for moderate to severe ED. Second, the currently approved medical therapies require some form of planning prior to intercourse. Gene therapy represents a viable option in the future. Champion et al used adenoviral-mediated gene transfer of eNOS in aged rats which were subsequently submitted to cavernous nerve stimulation.[107] These authors demonstrated that the enhanced expression of eNOS employing an adenoviral vector significantly increased the erectile response to cavernosal nerve stimulation in the aged rats, similar to the response observed in young rats. The same authors also found a significant decrease in calcitonin gene related peptide (CGRP) in the penis of aged rats and subsequently performed an adenoviral-mediated gene transfer of prepro-CGRP. The aged rats showed a significant increase in cavernosal CGRP and cAMP levels 5 days after the gene transfer procedure, whereas cGMP levels remained unchanged. More importantly, a significant increase was seen in the erectile response to cavernosal nerve stimulation in the aged rat.[108]

Because neuropathy is a significant factor in many cases of organic ED, Bakirciogla et al explored the possibility of brain-derived neurotropic factor gene therapy to restore nerve-stimulated intracavernosal pressure (ICP) in a rat model with neurogenic impotence.[109] The results revealed that the treatment group had a significantly elevated nerve stimulated ICP response and this was correlated with a significant increase in the number of NOS positive nerve fibers observed. Another method is to use an angiogenic factor such as vascular endothelial derived growth factor (VEGF) as treatment for ED. Direct intracorporeal injection in a rat model of vascular insufficiency had restorative effects on nerve stimulated ICP response.[110]

Potassium channels provide an important mechanism for the regulation of corporeal smooth muscle cell tone and also represent a convergence point for mediating the effects of a wide array of neurotransmitters, neuromodulators, and hormones. Gene therapy employing this method has enabled the restoration of sufficient corporeal smooth muscle relaxation to result in normal penile erection.[111]

Finally, another approach is re-implantation of genetically modified cells into the corpus cavernosum. Wesells and Williams had established the feasibility of using autologous transplantation of endothelial cells into the corpus cavernosum of rats. The long-term viability and duration of this option are as yet unknown. Certainly, it opens up another therapeutic possibility.[112]

Conclusions

The weight of scientific evidence supports the statement that ED in the elderly male is generally multifactorial in origin. Treatment options should be individualized with all risks and benefits clearly defined for the patient and partner. Currently, we lack the ability to identify the underlying etiology of erectile difficulties in individual patients and thus direct therapy towards symptoms rather than reversal of the causative factors. With improved technologies and better understanding of the underlying molecular and genetic basis of erectile function, new therapeutic management is being devised. The role of hormone replacement therapy as well as anti-aging products in the aging male has yet to be fully defined. Clear statements concerning their use will be possible only after completion of large-scale, randomized, placebo-controlled studies.

References

1. Diczfalusy E. The aging male and developed countries in the 21st centuries. Aging Male 2002; 5(3): 139–46.
2. United Nations Department of Economic and Social Affairs. Population Division. World Population Prospects: The 2000 Revision. New York: United Nations.
3. Kinsey AC, Pomeroy WB, Martin CE. Sexual Behaviour in the Human Male. Philadelphia, PA: WB Saunders Co, 1948: 218–62.
4. Morley JE. Impotence. Am J Med 1986; 80(5): 897–905.
5. Feldman HA, Goldstein I, Hatzichristou D et al. Impotence and its medical and psychosocial correlates: results of the Massachusetts male aging study. J Urol 1994; 151: 54–61.
6. Pfeiffer E, Verwoerdt A, Wang HS. Sexual behaviour in aged men and women. Arch Gen Psy 1968; 19(6): 753–8.
7. McKenna KE. Some proposals regarding the organization of the central nervous system control of penile erection. Neurosci Biobehav Rev 2000; 24: 535–40.
8. Andersson KE, Wagner G. Physiology of penile erection. Physiol Rev 1995; 75: 191–236.
9. Saenz de Tejada I, Kim N, Lagan I et al. Regulation of adrenergic activity in penile corpus cavernosum. J Urol 1989; 142(4): 1117–21.
10. Himpens B, Missiaen L, Casteels R. Calcium homeostasis in vascular smooth muscle. J Vasc Res 1995; 32(4): 207–19.
11. Berridge MJ. Inositol triphosphate and calcium signalling. Nature 1993; 361: 315–25.
12. Hatzichristou DG, Saenz de Tejada I, Kupferman S et al. In vivo assessment of trabecular smooth muscle

tone, its application in pharmaco-cavernosometry and analysis of intracavernous pressure determinants. J Urol 1995; 153(4): 1126–35.

13. Fournier GR, Juenemann KP, Lue TF et al. Mechanisms of venous occlusion during canine penile erection: an anatomic demonstration. J Urol 1987; 137(1): 163–7.

14. Christ GJ, Lerner SE, Kim DC et al. Endothelin 1 as a putative modulator of erectile dysfunction: I. Characteristics of contraction of isolated corporal tissue strips. J Urol 1995; 153(6): 1998–2003.

15. Becker AJ, Uckert S, Stief CG et al. Possible role of bradykinin and angiotensin II in the regulation of penile erection and detumescence. Urol 2001; 57: 193–8.

16. Minhas S, Cartledge JJ, Eardley I et al. The interaction of nitric oxide and prostaglandins in the control of corporal smooth muscle tone: evidence for production of a cyclooxygenase derived endothelium contracting factor. BJU Int 2001; 87: 882–8.

17. Moncada S, Palmer RMJ, Higgs EA. Nitric oxide: physiology, pathophysiology and pharmacology. Pharmacol Rev 1991; 43: 109–42.

18. Kuthe A, Montorsi F, Andersson KE et al. Phosphodiesterase inhibitors for the treatment of erectile dysfunction. Curr Opin Investig Drugs 2002; 3: 1489–95.

19. Carvajal JA, Germain AM, Huidobro-Toro JP et al. Molecular mechanism of cGMP mediated smooth muscle relaxation. J Cell Physiol 2000; 184: 409–20.

20. Burnett AL, Lowenstein CJ, Bredt DS et al. Nitric oxide: a physiologic mediator of penile erection. Science 1992; 257: 401–3.

21. Davidson JM, Chen JJ, Crapo L et al. Hormonal changes and sexual functioning in aging men. J Clin Endocrinol Metab 1983; 57: 71–7.

22. Benet AE, Melman A. The epidemiology of erectile dysfunction. Urol Clin North Am 1995; 22: 699–709.

23. Saenz de Tejada I, Moroukian P, Tessier J et al. Trabecular smooth muscle modulates the capacitor function of the penis. Studies on a rabbit model. Am J Physiol 1991; 260: H1590–5.

24. Wespes E, Sattar AA, Golzarian J et al. Corporeal veno-occlusive dysfunction: predominantly intracavernous muscular pathology. J Urol 1997; 157: 1678–80.

25. Rose G. Epidemiology of atherosclerosis. BMJ 1991; 303: 1537–9.

26. Krane RJ, Goldstein I, Saenz de Tejada I. Impotence. NEJM 1989; 321: 1648–59.

27. Johnstone MT, Creager SJ, Scales KM et al. Impaired endothelium dependent vasodilation in patients with insulin dependent diabetes mellitus. Circulation 1993; 88: 2510–16.

28. Azadzoi KM, Siroky MB, Goldstein I. Study of etiologic relationship of arterial atherosclerosis to corporeal veno-occlusive dysfunction in the rabbit. J Urol 1996; 155: 1795–800.

29. Mulligan T, Katz PG. Why aged men become impotent. Arch Intern Med 1989; 149: 1365–6.

30. Nehra A, Gettman MT, Nugent M et al. Transforming growth factor beta-1 (TGF beta-1) is sufficient to induce fibrosis of rabbit corpus cavernosum in vivo. J Urol 1999; 162: 910–15.

31. Border WA, Noble NA. Transforming growth factor β in tissue fibrosis. NEJM 1994; 331: 1286–92.

32. Dahiya R, Chui R, Perinchery G et al. Differential gene expression of growth factors in young and old rat penile tissues is associated with erectile dysfunction. Int J Impot Res 1999; 11: 201–6.

33. Wespes E, Raviv G, Vanegas JP et al. Corporeal veno-occlusive dysfunction: a distal arterial pathology? J Urol 1998; 160: 2054–7.

34. Morisaki N, Kawano M, Koyama N. Effects of TGF-β1 on growth of aortic smooth muscle cells. Influences on interaction with growth factors, cell state, cell phenotype and cell cycle. Atherosclerosis 1991; 88: 227–34.

35. Moreland RB, Traish AM, McMillin MA et al. PGE1 suppresses the induction of collagen synthesis by TGF-β1 in human corpus cavernosum smooth muscle. J Urol 1995; 153: 826–34.

36. Daley JT, Brown ML, Watkins T et al. Prostanoid production in rabbit corpus cavernosum: I. Regulation by oxygen tension. J Urol 1996; 155: 1482–7.

37. Bakirciogla ME, Sievert KD, Nunes L et al. Decreased trabecular smooth muscle and caveolin-1 expression in the penile tissue of aged rats. J Urol 2001; 166: 734–8.

38. Kim N, Vardi Y, Padma-Nathan H et al. Oxygen tension regulates the nitric oxide pathway. Physiological role in penile erection. J Clin Invest 1993; 91: 437–42.

39. Bremner S, Vitiello MV, Prinz PN. Loss of circadian rhythmicity in blood testosterone levels with aging in normal men. J Clin Endocrinol Metab 1983; 56: 1278–81.

40. Vermeulen A, Kaufman JM, Giagulli VA. Influence of some biological indices on sex hormone binding globulin and androgen levels in aging or obese males. J Clin Endocrinol Metab 1996; 81: 1821–6.

41. Morley JE, Kaiser FE, Perry HM III et al. Longitudinal changes in testosterone, luteinising hormone and follicle stimulating hormone in healthy older men. Metabolism 1997; 46(4): 410–13.

42. Feldman HA, Longcope C, Derby CA. Age trends in the level of serum testosterone and other hormones in middle-aged men: longitudinal results

from the Massachusetts Male Aging Study. J Clin Endocrinol Metab 2002; 87: 589–98.

43. Liu D, Dillon JS. Dehydroepiandrosterone activates endothelial cell nitric-oxide synthase by a specific plasma membrane receptor couplet to Gai2,3. J Biol Chem 2002; 277: 21379–88.

44. Williams MR, Ling S, Dawood T et al. Dehydroepiandrosterone inhibits human vascular smooth muscle cell proliferation independent of ARs and ERs. J Clin Endocrinol Metab 2002; 87: 176–81.

45. Zwain IH, Yen SSC. Dehydroepiandrosterone (DHEA): biosynthesis and metabolism in the brain. Endocrinology 1999; 140(2): 880–7.

46. Munzer T, Harrnan M, Hees P et al. Effects of GH and/or sex steroid administration on abdominal subcutaneous and visceral fat in healthy aged and men. J Clin Endocrinol Metab 2001; 86: 3604–10.

47. Rudman D, Feller AG, Nagraj AS. Effects of human growth hormone in men over 60 years old. NEJM 1990; 323: 1–6.

48. Traish AM, Park K, Dhir V et al. Effects of castration and androgen replacement on erectile function in a rabbit model. Endocrinology 1999; 140: 1861–8.

49. Takane KK, George FW, Wilson JD. Androgen receptor of rat penis is down regulated by androgen. Am J Physiol 1990; 258: E46–50.

50. Takane KK, Wilson JD, McPhaul MJ. Decreased levels of the androgen receptor in the mature rat phallus are associated with decreased levels of androgen receptor messenger ribonucleic acid. Endocrinology 1991; 129: 1093–100.

51. Garban H et al. Restoration of normal adult penile erectile response in aged rats by long term treatment with androgens. Biol Reprod 1995; 53: 1365–75.

52. Zvara P, Sioufi R, Schipper H et al. Nitric oxide mediated erectile activity is a testosterone dependent event: a rat erection model. Int J Impot Res 1995; 7: 209–19.

53. Lugg J, Rajfer J, Gonzalez-Cadavid NF. Dihydrotestosterone is the active androgen in the maintenance of nitric oxide mediated penile erection in the rat. Endocrinology 1995; 136: 1495–501.

54. Chammes SL et al. The effect of androgen on nitric oxide synthase in the male reproductive tract of the rat. Fert Steril 1995; 63: 1101–7.

55. Muller SC, Hsieh JT, Lue TF et al. Castration and erection. An animal study. Eur Urol 1988; 15: 118–24.

56. Holmquist F, Persson K, Bodker A et al. Some pre- and post-junctional effects of castration in rabbit isolated corpus cavernosum and urethra. J Urol 1994; 152: 1011–16.

57. Carani C, Bancroft J, Granata A et al. Testosterone and erectile function, nocturnal penile tumescence and rigidity and erectile response to visual erotic stimuli in hypogonadal and eugonadal men. Psychoneuroendocrinology 1992; 17(6): 647–54.

58. Buena F, Swerdloff RS, Steiner BS et al. Sexual function does not change when serum testosterone levels are pharmacologically varied within normal male range. Fertil Steril 1993; 59: 1118–23.

59. Greenstein A, Plymate SR, Kartz PG. Visually stimulated erection in castrated men. J Urol 1995; 153: 650–2.

60. Traish AM, Munarriz R, O'Connell L et al. Effects of surgical or medical castration on erectile function in an animal model. J Androl 2003; 24: 381–7.

61. Kloner R, Padma Nathan H. Erectile dysfunction in patients with coronary artery diseases. Int J Impot Res 2005; 17(3): 209–15.

62. El Sakka AI, Morsy AM, Fagih BI et al. Coronary artery risk factors in patients with erectile dysfunction. J Urol 2004; 172(1): 251–4.

63. Barksdale JD, Gardner SF. The impact of first line anti-hypertensive drugs on erectile dysfunction. Pharmacotherapy 1999; 19: 573–81.

64. Chang SW, Fine R, Siegel D et al. The impact of diuretic therapy on reported sexual function. Arch Intern Med 1991; 151: 2402–8.

65. Mitchell JE, Popkin MK. Antipsychotic drug therapy and sexual dysfunction in men. Am J Psychiatry 1982; 139: 633–7.

66. Wang CJ, Shen SY, Wu CC et al. Penile blood flow study in diabetic impotence. Uro Int 1993; 50: 209–12.

67. De Angelis L, Marfella MA, Siniscalchi M et al. Erectile and endothelial dysfunction in type II diabetes: a possible link. Diabetologia 2001; 44(9): 1155–60.

68. Vernet D, Cai L, Garban H et al. Reduction of penile nitric oxide synthase in diabetic BB/WORdp (type I) and BBZ/WORdp (type II) rats with erectile dysfunction. Endocrinology 1995; 136: 5709–17.

69. Sobrevia L, Mann GE. Dysfunction of the endothelial nitric oxide signaling pathway in diabetes and hyperglycemia. Exp Physiol 1997; 82: 423–52.

70. Nijhawan S, Mathur A, Singh V et al. Autonomic and peripheral neuropathy in insulin dependent diabetics. J Assoc Phys India 1993; 41: 565–6.

71. Bemelmans BL, Meuleman EJ, Doesburg WH et al. Erectile dysfunction in diabetic men: the neurological factor revisited. J Urol 1994; 151: 884–9.

72. Stellato RK, Feldman HA, Hamdy O et al. Testosterone, sex hormone-binding globulin and the development of type II diabetes in middle aged men: prospective results from the Massachusetts male aging study. Diabetes care 2000; 23: 490–4.

73. Morgentaler A, Bruning CO, DeWolff WC. Occult prostate cancer in men with low serum testosterone. JAMA 1996; 276: 1904–6.

74. Lue TF. Impotence after radical pelvic surgery: physiology and management. Uro Int 1991; 46: 259–65.

75. Quinlan DM, Epstein JI, Carter BS et al. Sexual function following radical prostatectomy: influence of preservation of neurovascular bundles. J Urol 1991; 145: 998–1002.

76. Schwartz EJ, Wong P, Graydon RJ. Sildenafil preserves intracorporeal smooth muscle after radical retropubic prostatectomy. J Urol 2004; 171: 771–4.

77. Meuleman EJ, Donkers LH, Kiemeney B. Erectile dysfunction: prevalence and quality of life. The Boxmeer study. Aging Male 2000; 3(Suppl): 12.

78. Rosen RC, Riley A, Wagner G et al. The international index of erectile function (IIEF): a multidimensional scale for assessment of erectile dysfunction. Urology 1997; 49: 822–30.

79. Montorsi F, McDermott TED, Morgan R. Efficacy and safety of fixed dose oral Sildenafil in the treatment of erectile dysfunction of various etiologies. Urology 1999; 53: 1011–18.

80. Chen KK, Chan JY, Chang LS. Dopaminergic neurotransmission at the paraventricular nucleus of hypothalamus in central regulation of penile erection in the rat. J Urol 1999; 162: 237–42.

81. Melis MR, Succu S, Argiolas A et al. Dopamine agonists increase nitric oxide production in the paraventricular nucleus of the hypothalamus: correlation with penile erection. Eur J Neurosci 1996; 8: 2056–63.

82. Rampin O, Jerome N, Suaudeau C. Proerectile effects of apomorphine in mice. Life Sci 2003; 72: 2329–36.

83. Sala M, Braida D, Leone MP et al. Central effect of yohimbine on sexual behaviour in the rat. Physiol Behav 1990; 47(1): 165–73.

84. Clark JT, Smith ER, Davidson JM. Enhancement of sexual motivation in male rats by yohimbine. Science 1984; 225(4664): 847–9.

85. Filippi S, Luconi M, Granchi S et al. Endothelium dependency of yohimbine induced corpus cavernosum relaxation. Int J Impot Res 2002; 14(4): 295–307.

86. Shabsigh R, Padma-Nathan H, Gittleman M et al. Intracavernous alprostadil alphadex (Edex/Viridal) is effective and safe in patients with erectile dysfunction after failing sildenafil (Viagra). Urology 2000; 55: 477–80.

87. Lin JS, Lin YM, Jou YC et al. Role of cyclic adenosine monophosphate in prostaglandin E1 induced penile erection in rabbits. Eur Urol 1995; 28(3): 259–65.

88. Molderings GJ, van Ahlen H, Gothert M. Modulation of noradrenaline release in human corpus cavernosum by presynaptic prostaglandin receptors. Int J Impot Res 1992; 4: 19–25.

89. Kifor I, Williams GH, Vickers MA et al. Tissue angiotensin II as a modulator of erectile function, I. Angiotensin peptide content, secretion and effects in the corpus cavernosum. J Urol 1997; 157(5): 1920–5.

90. Kirkeby HJ, Forman A, Andersson KE. Comparison of the papaverine effects on isolated human penile circumflex veins and corpus cavernosum. Int J Impot Res 1990; 2: 49–54.

91. Rehman J, Chenven E, Brink PR et al. Diminished neurogenic but not pharmacologic induced intracavernosal pressure responses in the 3 month Streptozotocin (STZ) diabetic rat. Am J Physiol 1997; 272: H1960–71.

92. Iguchi M, Nakajima T, Hisada T et al. On the mechanism of papaverine inhibition of the voltage dependent calcium current in isolated smooth muscle cells from the guinea pig trachea. J Pharmacol Exp Ther 1992; 263(1): 194–200.

93. Traish A, Gupta S, Gallant C et al. Phentolamine mesylate relaxes penile corpus cavernosum tissue by adrenergic and non adrenergic mechanisms. Int J Impot Res 1998; 10(4): 215–23.

94. Deuk Choi Y, Jin Choi Y, Hwan Kim J et al. Mechanical reliability of the AMS 700 CMX inflatable penile prosthesis for the treatment of male erectile dysfunction. J Urol 2001; 165: 822–4.

95. Debocq F, Tefilli MV, Gheiler EL et al. Long term mechanical reliability of multicomponent inflatable penile prosthesis: comparison of device survival. Urology 1998; 52: 277–81.

96. Oakley N, Moore KT. Vacuum devices in erectile dysfunction: indications and efficacy. Br J Urol 1998; 82(5): 673–81.

97. Montague DK, Barada JH, Belker AM et al. Clinical guidelines panel on erectile dysfunction: summary report on the treatment of organic erectile dysfunction. The American Urological Association. J Urol 1996; 156(6): 2007–11.

98. Dutta TC, EID JF. Vacuum constriction devices for erectile dysfunction: a long term prospective study of patients with mild, moderate and severe dysfunction. Urology 1999; 54(5): 891–3.

99. Zhang XH, Morelli A, Luconi M et al. Testosterone regulates phosphodiesterase 5 expression and in vivo responsiveness to tadalafil in rat corpus cavernosum. Eur Urol 2005; 47(3): 409–16.

100. Shabsigh R, Kaufman JM, Steidle C et al. Randomized study of testosterone gel as adjunctive therapy to sildenafil in hypogonadal men with erectile dysfunction who do not respond to sildenafil alone. J Urol 2004; 172(2): 658–63.

101. Morales A. Androgen replacement therapy and prostate safety. Eur Urol 2002; 37: 1–4.

102. Morales A, Johnston B, Heaton JW et al. Oral androgens in the treatment of hypogonadal impotent men. J Urol 1994; 152: 1115–18.

103. Meikle AW, Mazer NA, Moellmer JF et al. Enhanced transdermal delivery across nonscrotal skin produces physiological concentrations of testosterone and its metabolites in hypogonadal men. J Clin Endocrinol Metab 1992; 74: 623–8.

104. Wang C, Berman N, Longstreth JA et al. Pharmacokinetics of transdermal testosterone gel in hypogonadal men: application of gel at one site versus four sites. A general clinical research centre study. J Clin Endocrinol Metab 2000; 85: 964–9.

105. Baulieu EE, Thomas G, Legrain S et al. DHEA, DHEA sulphate and aging: contribution of the DHEA age study to a sociobiomedical issue. Proc Natl Acad Sci USA 2000; 97: 4279–84.

106. Reiter WJ, Pycha A, Schatzl G et al. Dehydroepiandrosterone in the treatment of erectile dysfunction: a prospective, double-blind, randomized, placebo-controlled study. Urology 1999; 53: 590–4.

107. Champion HC, Bivalacqua TJ, Hyman AL et al. Gene transfer of endothelial nitric oxide synthase to the penis augments erectile responses in the aged rat. Proc Natl Acad Sci USA 1999; 96: 11648–52.

108. Bivalacqua TJ, Champion HC, Abdel-Mageed AB et al. Gene transfer of prepro-CGRP restores erectile function in the aged rat. Biol Reprod 2001; 65: 1371–7.

109. Bakirciolgla ME, Lin CS, Fan P et al. The effect of adeno-associated virus mediated brain derived neurotrophic factor in an animal model of neurogenic impotence. J Urol 2001; 165: 2103–9.

110. Lee MC, El-Sakka Al, Graziottin TM et al. The effect of vascular endothelial growth factor on a rat model of traumatic arteriogenic erectile dysfunction. J Urol 2002; 167: 761–7.

111. Christ GJ, Rehman J, Day N et al. Intracorporeal injection of hSlo cDNA in rats produces physiologically relevant alterations in penile function. Am J Heart Circ Physiol 1998; 275: H600–8.

112. Wessells H, Williams SK. Endothelial cell transplantation into the corpus cavernosum: moving towards cell-based gene therapy. J Urol 1999; 162: 2162–4.

CHAPTER 16

Assessment of the aging man with sexual dysfunction

Sidney Glina

Introduction

The increase in life expectancy over the past century has meant that individuals over the age of 65 years form an increasingly large proportion of our population. It is projected that by 2025 the population above 65 years of age will increase by 82%.[1] As sexual functioning declines with age, sexual dysfunction has become a main health concern.

Age is considered a major risk factor for various sexual disorders. Kinsey et al[2] made the first report in 1948 about sexual behavior in the human male. They studied 12 000 men and found an incidence of erectile dysfunction (ED) of 2% in men younger than 20 years and 25% in men aged 56 to 75 years. Also, probably the best known epidemiologic study on male sexual function, the Massachusetts Male Aging Study, showed that 52% of men in the Massachusetts area claimed some level of ED and the prevalence was also age-related.[3] Rosen et al[4] showed that ejaculatory disorders are strongly related to age. The aging male tends to have a significant decrease in sexual desire[5] and sexual activity is reported to decrease; 53% of older married couples at the age of 60 have sexual activities while only 24% of couples over the age of 76 have any sexual encounter.[6]

Although the incidence of sexual dysfunction increases in old age, this can be primarily related to the increased rate of health problems, rather than aging per se. A history of cardiopathy, diabetes, hypertension, neuropathy, or pelvic surgery/radiation increases the risk of ED. More than one associated condition increases the risk. In comparison with non-diabetic and non-hypertensive men, the odds ratio of ED was 1.4 for hypertensive men without diabetes, 4.6 for diabetic men without hypertension, and 8.1 for men with both diseases. Smoking is also an important risk factor.[7] It was reported that, in comparison with never smokers, the odds ratio of ED was 1.7 for current smokers and 1.6 for ex-smokers, and it increased with the duration of the habit.[8] These health factors are more prevalent in older people and hence it is perhaps not surprising to find an increase in biologically caused sexual problems in the elderly. Also many drugs, highly utilized by older adults, are related to sexual dysfunction. Antihypertensives such as thiazide diuretic and non-selective β-blockers, antidepressants, antipsychotic agents, and anti-androgens, among others, have been incriminated as a cause of sexual dysfunction.[9]

However the importance of psychosocial risk factors should not be dismissed. Psychologic conditions such as depression and psychosocial stresses (such as divorce, death of the spouse, lack of partners, loss of social status, loss of job, health-related family problems) are highly prevalent in older adults and contribute to sexual disorders.[10]

Assessment of a patient with erectile dysfunction

During the last two decades significant advances have been made in the understanding of male sexual dysfunction and ED can be caused by psychologic factors, arterial insufficiency, neurogenic disturbances, caverno-veno-occlusive dysfunction (CVOD), hormonal insufficiency, drugs, and Peyronie's disease.

In every disease the diagnostic work-up should be very detailed to find the correct etiology and to determine the best treatment. However, for ED, the exact cause frequently cannot be found or there is no 'best' treatment, but an effective way to restore a patient's sexual function. Principally after the development of an effective oral agent, the treatment of ED became simpler. Instead of an extensive diagnostic work-up, the physician should emphasize to the patient the therapeutic options, their effectiveness, and the adverse effects, and both of them, preferably with the agreement of the partner, must decide on the treatment. This is known as the goal-directed approach or patient-centered care.[11]

However, in every case a minimal work-up should be done. A detailed *anamnesis* is important to reveal the real problem. Is the erection impaired or has the patient a decrease in libido, premature ejaculation, or a difficult relationship with his partner? These are different conditions from ED and deserve different care, and many patients classify all of them as ED. Sexual inquiry is most often conducted by face-to-face interview, although self-reported questionnaires might help. These tools are simple and provide validated and cost-efficient identification of the problem.[11]

The goal of the *sexual history* is to evaluate the whole sexual function of the couple. When a patient complains of ED it is, for example, important to learn whether the erectile disorder happens in every intercourse or is partner-related, if it is difficult to initiate and/or to maintain the erection at masturbation or only during intercourse, and whether morning or nocturnal erection is rigid. The presence of a rigid and sustainable erection in any of these situations normally means that the organic aspects of erection function are normal. Basic topics for a sexual history are summarized in Table 16.1.

Following the sexual history a *medical history* should be taken and the objectives are to identify possible comorbid medical conditions and to assess the use of concomitant medications. Many underlying conditions such as diabetes, depression, cardiovascular disease, dislipidemia, hypogonadism, or past pelvic surgery can be severe risk factors for or the cause of ED. Furthermore, ED can be a marker of an underlying silent morbid condition such as diabetes or coronary artery disease.[12] In addition, the patient can be taking an ED-associated drug such as finasteride or an antihypertensive agent; withdrawing it or substituting it by another agent may solve the problem. The use of some medications such as the nitrates also constitutes a contraindication for the use of phosphodiesterase type 5 inhibitors.

A *psychosocial assessment* is fundamental to understanding the patient's ED. Multiple psychologic factors can contribute to or cause sexual dysfunction. Depression, loss of a partner, disease or death of a family member, professional and financial stress, and intracouple relationship distress should be identified during patient interview. An initial psychologic evaluation can be done by the urologist or general practitioner with some experience, but in some cases a referral to a psychologist or psychiatrist makes it easier and can increase the adherence to a planned psychotherapy.

In many cases the *differentiation between ED of physical and psychologic origin* can be done by history. Psychogenic ED usually has an acute onset, it is partner-related or can be situational; the patient usually presents some of the psychologic factors discussed above and he can refer normal erections in various circumstances as at masturbation or at night or morning. Organic ED has a gradual onset, patients generally refer to other comorbidities, and masturbation, nocturnal, or morning erections are rare and poor. It is important to consider that many times both psychologic and physical factors can be coexisting.

Although rarely identifying the cause of the ED, the *physical exam* of the patient can reveal conditions that determine different treatments: signs of hypogonadism, atropic testes, hepatomegaly, or penile fibrosis. Decreased testicular pain sensitivity

Table 16.1 *Basic topics for a sexual history (adapted from Rosen et al[11])*

Defining the problem:
1. Do you consider your sexual frequency satisfactory? (Libido disorder)
2. Do you feel sexually aroused frequently? (Libido disorder)
3. When you are sexually stimulated can you get and maintain a hard enough erection for a vaginal penetration? (Erection disorder)
4. Are you able to ejaculate when you have sexual activity? Is it too rapid? (Ejaculation disorder)

Erection domain:
1. Was the onset of your erectile dysfunction gradual or acute?
2. When did you have or try your last sexual intercourse?
3. Were your able to get an erection at that time?
4. Were your able to maintain the erection until your ejaculate?
5. What is the percentage of intercourses you have not been able to get or maintain the erection?
6. Do you have morning or nocturnal erections? How do you grade this erection according to rigidity (0–10)?
7. Do you have an erection at masturbation? How do you grade this erection according to rigidity (0–10)?
8. Have you noticed if the erection is better in any situation or with different partners (if you have more than one)?
9. Do you have any pain during erection?
10. Is there any curvature or bend in your penis?

can be the only signal of a diabetic autonomic neuropathy and the absence of a dorsal artery pulse can be the sign of a vascular disease. Also, this can be the unique opportunity for a digital rectal exam of the prostate.

In a patient with ED a *minimal laboratory check-up* is advisable to identify a possible cause of the sexual dysfunction as hypogonadism and to identify possible silent comorbidities. The check-up should include lipid profile, fasting glucose, testosterone, and PSA.[11]

In some situations for patients with primary ED, when there is a medico-legal dispute, or when patients want to know the etiology of their ED a *complementary work-up* should be added. There are various guidelines for this complementary evaluation[11] and I usually ask for a psychologic interview with a sexologist, the bioavailable or free testosterone level (plus prolactin, when there is a concomitant low libido), and an office pharmaco-induced erection test or an outpatient nocturnal penile tumescence (NPT) test with Rigiscan.

In this way it is possible to evaluate the various etiologies of ED: psychologic factors (anamnesis and psychologic interview), arterial insufficiency (patient should present a negative pharmaco-induced erection test, or abnormal NPT; must be confirmed by duplex ultrasound and arteriography if a vascular restoration is planned), neurogenic disturbances (history of possible neuropathies such as diabetes, alcohol abuse, medullar lesions, and an abnormal NPT), caverno-veno-occlusive dysfunction (negative pharmaco-induced erection test or abnormal NPT), hormonal insufficiency (low testosterone level), drug-induced ED (by medical history), and Peyronie's disease (anamnesis and physical exam).

Cavernosometry and cavernosography have a low value in the ED evaluation. First, they rely on a pharmaco-induced relaxation of the smooth muscle of the corpora cavernous and we still do have not an easy and reliable method to confirm it.[13] Thus, an abnormal cavernosometry can mean a caverno-venous-occlusive dysfunction (CVOD) or incomplete relaxation due to anxiety. Second, there is still no adequate test or a reliable normality criterion for the CVOD.[14] The diagnosis of CVOD can be made after a negative pharmaco-induced erection test, with self-stimulation or redosing of the vasoactive agents and a negative home test (autoinjection with vasoactive drugs at home and tentative sexual intercourse).

Other exams as neurologic testing are useful only in selected cases for a research protocol or medico-legal reasons.[11] However most neurologic exams (evoked potentials, peripheral electromyography, and latency time of dorsal nerve) check pathways other than the autonomic system that is responsible for the erection. Electromyography of the corpora cavernosa remains an experimental tool and needs to be studied further before it enters clinical practice.[11]

Where are the patients?

The main challenge sexual medicine experts face is the low treatment procurement by sexual dysfunction patients. Although ED is a very common medical condition very few patients receive treatment. Chew et al reported that only 11.6% of patients with ED had received treatment for this condition in the Perth, Australia area.[15]

Although ED can produce a negative impact on quality of life of patients and their partners,[16] it is difficult the patient to seek medical aid. In my practice patients take an average of 4 years to look for medical care for their sexual problems.

It is important to understand that ED is not a problem for every man. In a survey conducted in the UK around 20% of men claimed some sexual dysfunction,[17] although 23% of them considered that this dysfunction was not an important issue. However, 49% of men and 39% of women with sexual dysfunction wanted professional help for their sexual problems, and only 12% of these men and 6% of these women had received this help.

Patients are used to consulting their physicians because of other medical conditions such as diabetes, hypertension, and lower urinary tract symptoms, and do not complain about their sexual disorders.[18] Most of them are embarrassed to broach this subject with the doctor.[19] Cultural attitudes may contribute to the expectation that older people are, or ought to be, asexual.[20] Although sex roles have changed and

there has been more freedom of sexual expression since the 1960s, the stereotypes that older people are physically unattractive, uninterested in sex, and incapable of achieving sexual arousal are still widely held. Thus when they face a sexual problem they think that is 'normal' for old people.

ED is still also underdiagnosed because patients do not complain and physicians do not ask their patients about their sexual function. This is mainly because, in general, physicians are not prepared to deal with sexual medicine, ED is not seen as a medical condition, others do not feel comfortable with the subject, and ED is a time-consuming issue.

However, it is important for the physician to know that ED shares the same risk factors as any cardiovascular disease and can be considered as a marker of those diseases. In many cases the sexual dysfunction precedes a major cardiovascular event.[12] Furthermore, treatment of ED can improve the quality of life and the relationship of the couple[21] and it increases the adherence of the patient to the treatment of other major medical conditions.[22] In addition, there are tools such as the self-reported questionnaires, including the Sexual Health Inventory for Men (SHIM) among others, that reduce the time of ED diagnosis and facilitate patient–physician communication.[23] Lastly patients can be referred to experts if a physician is not comfortable treating sexual dysfunction.

Ejaculation disorders in the aging male

Ejaculation disorders in the aging male are much less studied than erectile dysfunction. Masters and Johnson[24] reported that, among other alterations in the sexual response of aging men, ejaculation time is longer compared to that of young adults, with longer periods of coitus. However in the clinical setting many aging adults complain of a decrease in the volume of ejaculate, delayed ejaculation, sometimes an inability to reach orgasm and ejaculation, and less frequently rapid or premature ejaculation.

In a survey of sexual function in men aged 50–80 years from five Asian countries Li et al found that ejaculation disorders were present in 68% of

Table 16.2 *Causes of delayed ejaculation, anejaculation and anorgasmia (MOD) in the aging male (adapted from McMahon et al[29])*

Psychogenic
Inhibited ejaculation (cultural, religious factors)

Anatomic causes
Prostate enlargement
Transurethral resection of prostate
Bladder neck incision
Diabetic autonomic neuropathy
Spinal cord injury
Radical prostatectomy
Open prostate surgery
Proctocolectomy
Bilateral sympathectomy
Abdominal aortic aneurismectomy
Para-aortic lymphadenectomy
Radiotherapy of prostate

Endocrine
Hypogonadism
Hypothyroidism

Drug-related
Tricyclic and serotonine-uptake inhibitors
Phenothiazine
Alpha-blockers
Alcohol abuse
Marijuana
Cocaine

respondents (52% reported bothersomeness) and pain on ejaculation was experienced by 19% of the men in the study (88% reported bothersomeness).[25]

Lue et al classified the delayed ejaculation, anejaculation, and retrograde ejaculation as male orgasmic dysfunction (MOD) and estimated that its prevalence is the same as for ED in the aging male.[26]

The etiology of MOD can be any medical disease, drug, or surgical procedure that interferes with either central control of ejaculation, the peripheral sympathetic nerve supply to the vas and bladder neck, the somatic afferent nerve supply to the pelvic floor, or the somatic afferent nerve supply to the penis.[25] Prostate or bladder neck surgery can lead to retrograde ejaculation or loss of orgasmic sensation in 80% and 35% of men,[27] respectively; both have been prevalent in men with lower urinary tract symptoms.[24] Also drugs as alpha-blockers and serotonin-uptake inhibitors, commonly used in aging males, can cause MOD. Causes of MOD are summarized in Table 16.2.

Low-volume ejaculate can be caused by prostate enlargement, diabetic autonomic neuropathy, or hypogonadism. Painful ejaculation may have psychologic or organic causes and the main cause is acute or chronic prostatitis.[28]

Lifelong premature or rapid ejaculation (PE) can go on affecting an older adult, but some men begin to refer PE because they are afraid to lose the erection (PE secondary to DE) or to low frequency of intercourse.[29]

Table 16.3 *Basic topics for sexual history taking in the aging male with ejaculation disorders (adapted from Rosen et al[11])*

1. Are you able to ejaculate when you have sex?
2. Are you able to ejaculate when you masturbate?
3. Do you ejaculate when you want to?
4. Do you ejaculate before your partner wants you to?
5. Are there situations where your ejaculation comes too quickly?
6. Is there any partner with whom you ejaculate too quickly?
7. Do you take too long to ejaculate?
8. Have you noticed a reduction in the volume of what you ejaculate?
9. Do you have difficulty reaching orgasm?
10. Is your orgasm satisfying?
11. Do you have pain when you ejaculate?
12. Have you seen blood in your semen?
13. If you have any problem with your ejaculation or orgasm, for how long has it been happening?

Assessment of the aging male with ejaculation disorders

As in other sexual dysfunctions, an aging male with any ejaculation disorder should be evaluated with a detailed *sexual history*. The main goal is to define the precise disorder and to learn whether it is situational, partner-related, lifelong, or acquired. The patient should be asked whether there is any problem with his erection and the frequency of intercourse. Details about his ejaculatory response, including the presence or absence of orgasm and the level of sexual satisfaction, or patient and partner distress, must be part of the history. Table 16.3 summarizes basic topics for sexual history taking of these patients.

A basic *medical history* should be obtained with special focus on the use of prescribed and recreational medications, because of the influence of some drugs on the ejaculatory response.

A *physical examination* might be relevant in cases of delayed ejaculation or anejaculation to establish the status of the testicles and epididymes, the presence of the vas deferens, and the sensation of the genitalia.[25]

Testosterone determination is probably the only *biochemical investigation* to be done in aging men with MOD to rule out possible hypogonadism. Bioavailable testosterone or the calculated free testosterone is the most reliable assay to establish the androgenic status

of the aging adult. Other laboratory-based evaluations, such as neurophysiologic studies, are not recommended for routine evaluation.[25]

Hypoactive sexual desire in aging men

Hypoactive sexual desire (HSD) is a condition that is characterized by the absence or decreased frequency of a man's desire for sexual activity. HSD is identified when it causes distress or dissatisfaction to the patient and/or the partner. It is not defined by the number of sexual encounters alone, because it is well known that in stable long-term relationships sexual frequency declines, although satisfaction may remain high. The Diagnostic and Statistical Manual of Mental Disorders, 4th edition (DSM IV), defines hypoactive sexual desire disorder as persistently or recurrently deficient (or absent) sexual fantasy and desire for sexual activity, leading to marked distress or interpersonal difficulty.[30]

Laumann et al, in an international survey of 13 618 men aged 40–80 years from 29 countries, reported a prevalence of lack of sexual interest from 12.5 to 28.0%, according to geographic area. The significant risk factors for low sexual desire were older age, depression, and poor health condition.[31]

Table 16.4 *Medical and psychologic factors associated with HSD[36]*

- Androgen deficiency
- Hyperprolactinemia
- Anger and anxiety
- Depression
- Relationship conflict
- Stroke
- Antidepressant therapy
- Epilepsy
- Post-traumatic stress syndrome
- Renal failure
- Coronary disease and heart failure
- Aging
- HIV
- Body-building and eating disorders

There are many theories about the physiology of sexual desire,[32] but it clearly depends on the balance of a normal hormonal environment and equilibrated psychosocial response.[33] The role of testosterone and perhaps of several other androgens appears to be necessary for the experience of sexual desire in its drive component. It appears that a minimum level of androgen is required for a man to be able to experience sexual desire.[34] HSD is considered the most common sexual pattern associated with depression,[35] and this is one of the major risk factors for HSD.[30]

HSD is a condition that can be a hidden cause of other sexual dysfunctions, mainly ED.[36] It is critical that the clinician identifies this condition; lack of success in the treatment of other disorders can be explained by the presence of an untreated HSD. Medical and psychologic factors associated with HSD are summarized in Table 16.4.[37]

Diagnosis of hypoactive sexual desire in the aging male

As in other sexual dysfunctions, patient history is the main tool for the diagnosis of HSD. Many patients complain about a secondary ED and the physician should be aware of the possibility that erection ability is impaired because of a lack of sexual desire. The diagnosis of HSD is not difficult if the clinician asks directly about desire, interest, or sexual activity.

It is important to differentiate whether the patient has a complete lack of sexual interest or whether there is a decrease in sexual desire related to a partner or situation. In the first case a major cause, such as hypogonadism, hyperprolactinemia, or depression, can be suspected. In the second case the patient will go on showing interest in other sexual activities, such as masturbation, and a relationship conflict can be suspected.

Basic topics for *sexual history taking* in men with HSD are listed in Table 16.5, modified from Rosen et al.[11]

A *medical history* is fundamental because there are underlying conditions or situations that can initiate HSD. It is not uncommon that a man who has undergone major heart surgery develops a secondary HSD because of a fear of death during sexual activities. *Depression* deserves special attention and it can be identified through the clinical interview; however, in many instances the use of screening tools can be useful. There are many scales that have been developed for depression detection. A short and useful tool, developed for the geriatric population, might be of help for the clinician unfamiliar with depression or with restricted time during the consultation, and this is shown in Table 16.6.[38] The

Table 16.5 *Basic topics for sexual history taking in men with HSD*

1. Do you still look forward to sex?
2. Do you still enjoy sexual activity?
3. Do you have sexual fantasies?
4. Do you have sexual dreams?
5. How frequently do you masturbate?
6. How easily sexually aroused (turned on) are you?
7. Do you read magazines or watch movies with erotic themes?
8. Do you find your partner sexually attractive?
9. Do you enjoy sexual activities with your partner?

Table 16.6 *Five-item version of the Geriatric Depression Scale*[37, 38]

1. Are you basically satisfied with your life?
2. Do you often get bored?
3. Do you often feel helpless?
4. Do you prefer to stay home rather than going out and doing new things?
5. Do you feel pretty worthless the way you are now?

Positive answers for depression screening are 'yes' to questions 2, 3, 4, and 5 and a 'no' to question 1.
A score of 0 to 1 positive answer suggests the patient is not depressed, a score of 2 or higher indicates possible depression.

briefness of the scale (only 5 items) and good psychometric properties make this a useful instrument for the detection of depression among older men.[39]

Physical examination can reveal secondary signs of hypogonadism and, rarely, a gynecomastia secondary to hyperprolactinemia.

Laboratory evaluation should include the measurement of serum testosterone, preferably bioavailable testosterone or calculated free testosterone, and prolactin. Additional laboratory tests (e.g. thyroid function, HIV tests) may be performed at the discretion of the physician, based on medical history and clinical suspicions.

Conclusions

The population is getting older and sexual dysfunction is a major health concern in the elderly. It is important that physicians are aware that patients do not complain easily about sexual dysfunction, despite its negative impact on a couple's quality of life. But they want to be asked about their sexual function. Furthermore, sexual dysfunction, mainly ED, can be a silent marker of underlying medical conditions. Thus, it is a duty of a physician to at least be concerned with those disorders. In general, history taking is the main tool for the diagnosis of a sexual dysfunction and it requires just time and interest to do it.

References

1. Lunenfeld B. Aging male. Aging Male 1998; 1: 1–7.
2. Kinsey AC, Pomeroy W, Martin CE. Age and sexual outlet. In: Kinsey AC, Pomeroy WB, Martin CE, eds. Sexual Behavior in the Human Male. Philadelphia, PA: WB Saunders, 1948: 218–62.
3. Feldman HA, Goldstein I, Hatzichristou DG et al. Impotence and its medical and psychosocial

correlates: results of the Massachusetts Male Aging Study. J Urol 1994; 151: 54–61.

4. Rosen R, Altwein J, Boyle P et al. Lower urinary tract symptoms and male sexual dysfunction: the multinational survey of the aging male (MSAM-7). Eur Urol 2003; 44: 637–49.

5. Schiavi RC, Schreiner-Engel P, Mandeli J. Healthy aging and male sexual function. Am J Psychiatry 1990; 147: 766–71.

6. Marsiglio W, Donnely D. Sexual relations in later life: a national study of married persons. J Gerontol 1991; 46: S338–44.

7. Polsky JY, Aronson KJ, Heaton JP et al. Smoking and other lifestyle factors in relation to erectile dysfunction. BJU Int 2005; 96: 1355–9.

8. Parazzini F, Menchini Fabris F, Bortolotti A et al. Frequency and determinants of erectile dysfunction in Italy. Eur Urol 2000; 31: 43–9.

9. Tejada IS, Ângulo J, Cellek S et al. Physiology of erectile function and pathophysiology of erectile dysfunction. In: Lue TF, Basson R, Rosen R et al, eds. Sexual Medicine. Paris: Health Publications, 2004: 287–344.

10. Cole MJ. Psychological Approach in Treatment. Edinburgh: Churchill Livingstone, 1993.

11. Rosen R, Hatzichristou DG, Broderick G et al. Clinical Evaluation and Symptom Scales: Sexual Dysfunction Assessment in Men. In: Lue TF, Basson R, Rosen R et al, eds. Sexual Medicine. Paris: Health Publications 2004: 173–220.

12. Ortiz J, Ortiz ST, Mônaco CG et al. Erectile dysfunction: a marker for myocardial perfusion impairment? Arq Bras Cardiol 2005; 85: 241–6.

13. Hatzichristou DG, Saenz de Tejada I, Kupferman S et al. In vivo assessment of trabecular smooth muscle tone, its application in pharmaco-cavernosometry and analysis of intracavernous pressure determinants. J Urol 1995; 153: 1126–34.

14. Glina S, Silva MFR, Puech-Leão P, Reis JMS et al. Veno-occlusive dysfunction of corpora cavernosa: comparison of diagnostic methods. Int J Impot Res 1995; 7: 1–10.

15. Chew KK, Earle CM, Stuckey BG et al. Erectile dysfunction in general medicine practice: prevalence and clinical correlates. Int J Impot Res 2000; 12: 41–5.

16. Althof SE. Quality of life and erectile dysfunction. Urology 2002; 59: 803–10.

17. Dunn KM, Croft PR, Hackett GI. Satisfaction in the sex life of a general population sample. J Sex Marital Ther 2000; 26: 141–51.

18. Hoesl CE, Woll EM, Burkart M et al. Erectile dysfunction is prevalent, bothersome and underdiagnosed in patients consulting urologists for benign syndrome. Eur Urol 2005; 47: 511–17.

19. Kuru AF, Sahin H, Akay AF et al. Erectile dysfunction rates and request for treatment in patients attending outpatient urology clinics and those accompanying them. Int Urol Nephrol 2004; 36: 223–6.

20. Deacon S, Minichiello V, Plummer D. Sexuality and older people: revisiting the assumptions. Educ Gerontol 1995; 21: 497–513.

21. Hultling C, Giuliano F, Quirk F et al. Quality of life in patients with spinal cord injury receiving Viagra (sildenafil citrate) for the treatment of erectile dysfunction. Spinal Cord 2000; 38: 363–70.

22. Nurnberg HG, Seidman SN, Gelenberg AJ et al. Depression, antidepressant therapies and erectile dysfunction: clinical trials of sildenafil citrate in treated and untreated patients with depression. Urology 2002; 60: 58–66.

23. Temeltas G, Gunduz MI, Ceylan Y et al. Is it necessary to use sexual health inventory for man routinely? Arch Androl 2005; 51: 207–12.

24. Masters WH, Johnson VE. Human Sexual Response. Boston, MA: Little, Brown, 1970.

25. Li MK, Garcia LA, Rosen R. Lower urinary tract symptoms and male sexual dysfunction in Asia: a survey of ageing men from five Asian countries. BJU Int 2005; 96: 1339–54.

26. Lue TF, Basson R, Giuliano F et al. Summary of the recommendations on sexual dysfunction in men. In Lue TF, Basson R, Rosen R et al, eds. Sexual Medicine. Paris: Health Publications, 2004: 605–28.

27. Yeni E, Unal D, Verit A et al. Minimal transurethral prostatectomy plus bladder neck incision versus standard transurethral prostatectomy in patients with benign prostatic hyperplasia: a randomized prospective study. Urol Int 2002; 69: 283–6.

28. Luzzi G. Male genital pain disorders. Sexual Relationship Ther 2003; 18: 225–35.

29. MacMahon CG, Abdo C, Incrocci L et al. Disorder of orgasm and ejaculation in men. In Lue TF, Basson R, Rosen R et al, Eds. Sexual Medicine. Paris: Health Publications, 2004: 409–68.

30. American Psychiatric Association. Diagnostic and Statistical Manual of Mental Disorders, 4th edn, text revision edn. Washington, DC: American Psychiatric Association, 2000.

31. Laumann EO, Nicolosi A, Glasser D et al. Int J Impot Res 2005; 17: 39–57.

32. Kaplan HS. The Sexual Desire Disorders: Dysfunctional Regulation of Sexual Motivation. New York: Brunner/Mazel, 1995.

33. Levine SB. The nature of sexual desire: a clinician's perspective. Arch Sexual Behav 2003; 32: 279–85.

34. Morales A, Buvat J, Gooren L et al. Endocrine aspects of men sexual dysfunction. In: Lue TF, Basson R, Rosen R et al, eds. Sexual Medicine, Paris. Health Publications, 2004: 345–82.

35. Althof SE, Leiblum SR, Chevert-Measson M et al. Psychological and interpersonal dimension of sexual function and dysfunction. In: Lue TF, Basson R,

Rosen, R et al, eds: Sexual Medicine, Paris. Health Publications, 2004: 73–116.

36. Corona G, Mannucci E, Petrone L et al. Psycho-biological correlates of hypoactive sexual desire in patients with erectile dysfunction. Int J Impot Res 2004; 16: 275–81.

37. Meuleman, EJ, Van Lankvled J. Hypoactive sexual desire disorder: an underestimated condition in men. BJU Int 2005; 95: 201–96.

38. Hoyl MT, Alessi CA, Harker JO et al. Development and testing of a five-items version of the Geriatric Depression Scale. J Am Geriatr Soc 1999; 47: 873–8.

39. Rinaldi P, Mecocci P, Benedetti C et al. Validation of the five-item Geriatric Depression Scale in elderly subjects in three different settings. J Am Geriatr Soc 2003; 51: 694–8.

Endocrine System

CHAPTER 17

Endocrinology of the aging male: an overview

John E Morley

Introduction

Multiple changes in the endocrine system occur with aging. In general, these appear to stem from an alteration in the pulse generator within cells which regulates the normal rhythmic secretion of hormones. The chaotic secretion of releasing hormones in the hypothalamus results in a diminished secretion of pituitary hormones.[1] In the pancreatic islets chaotic secretion of insulin plays a role in the development of the age-related insulin decline.[2] Aging is also associated with a decrease in receptor and/or post-receptor activity.[3] The combination of all these factors results in the aging male having the appearance of hormone deficiency. This has led many authorities to suggest that aging is due to an endocrine pause, with the corollary to this being that hormone replacement can result in the reversal of the aging process. This has led to the mythologic concepts of the andropause, adrenopause, somatopause, or menopause as the central drivers of aging. In turn, this has resulted in an anti-aging industry which sells the 'hormonal fountain of youth' as the magic pathway to rejuvenation.[4] However, it is more rational to accept that hormonal replacement is as likely to produce negative effects.

The major changes in circulating hormones that occur with aging are outlined in Table 17.1.

Endocrine disease and aging

The decline in hormone levels that occurs with aging puts older men at risk of developing endocrine deficiency disorders. Thus with aging there is an increased prevalence of hypothyroidism, hypogonadism, and diabetes mellitus. There is also an increased likelihood of older persons having polyglandular failure.

A typical presentations occur commonly in older persons. Apathetic thyrotoxicosis is the classic example of an unusual presentation in the older person. About 7% of older persons with thyrotoxicosis present with proximal myopathy, atrial fibrillation, depression, weight loss, and blepharptosis (hooded eyes). Persons with adrenocorticol insufficiency often present with weight loss, abdominal pain, and diarrhea or constipation. Pheochromocytoma can present with severe weight loss associated with worsening hypertension due to the catecholamine excess. Hypothyroidism presents insidiously with fatigue, cognitive problems, hypertension, and depression. Hyperparathyroidism can present with anorexia, weight loss, and cognitive impairment. Systemic mastocytosis patients may present with syncope, flushing, diarrhea, and gastroesophageal reflux disorder. Endocrine disorders need to be high on the differential diagnosis for all older persons presenting with weight loss, delirium, or dementia.

Table 17.1 *Hormones and aging*

Decreased	Unchanged	Increased
Growth hormone	Thyroxine	Norepinephrine
Insulin growth factor-I	Gastric inhibitory peptide	ACTH
Testosterone	Glucagon releasing peptide	Insulin
Estrogen (women)	Prolactin	Cholecystokinin
Dehydroepiandrosterone	TSH	Amylin
Pregnenolone	Epinephrine	Parathyroid hormone
25 (OH) Vitamin D	Ghrelin	FSH
Aldosterone	—	—
Triiodothyronine	—	—

With aging there is an increase in ectopic hormone production which parallels the increase in cancer. This applies particularly to ectopic ACTH production and the syndrome of inappropriate antidiuretic hormone from lung cancers; skin hemangiomas (endotheliomas) can result in overproduction of endothelin, resulting in hypertension.

The approach to hormone replacement changes with aging. Thus, the decrease in the rate of thyroid hormone plasma clearance leads to a need to reduce the replacement dose of L-thyroxine. If this is not done, then the older person can develop accelerated osteoporosis, atrial fibrillation, and weight loss. In persons with hypothyroidism who have angina or dyspnea, a slightly lower replacement dose may lead to amelioration of these symptoms.

Polypharmacy is common with aging and thus the effects of medications on hormones need to be considered. For example, phenytoin displaces thyroxine from its binding hormone and alters its rate of turnover, and rifomysin increases the thyroxine replacement dose needed. Coumadin and oral hypoglycemics interact to produce increased hypoglycemia and increased bleeding time. Lipid-lowering agents can increase the effectiveness of coumadin, resulting in an increased prothrombin time. High doses of vitamin A cause increased processing of pre-pro PTH to PTH, resulting in hypercalcemia. When older persons are on multiple medications, there is reduced compliance that can result in inadequate compliance, with older persons failing to take appropriate replacement doses.

Some endocrine disorders occur virtually exclusively in older persons. These include osteoporosis, late onset hypogonadism, and Paget's disease.

Insulin resistance syndrome

The prevalence of the insulin resistance syndrome increases with aging such that over 40% of persons over 60 years of age have the metabolic syndrome.[5] Males are slightly more likely to develop the metabolic syndrome than are females. The metabolic syndrome is classically related to the accumulation of visceral fat. The International Diabetes Foundation has defined the syndrome as requiring an increased waist circumference[6] (Table 17.2). The key features of the syndrome include hypertension, diabetes mellitus, increased uric acid, increased plasminogen activator inhibitor-I, hypertriglyceridemia, low HDL cholesterol, increased small dense LDL, myosteatosis, and non-alcoholic steatohepatitis. This syndrome is associated with increased myocardial infarction, stroke, frailty, disability, and mortality. Persons with the metabolic syndrome or diabetes mellitus have low testosterone levels and there is some evidence that low testosterone is associated with insulin resistance.[7] Older persons who receive GnRH agonists for prostate

Table 17.2 *International Diabetes Foundation: definition of the metabolic syndrome*

Central obesity: Waist circumference greater than 94 cm for Europids or 90 cm for Chinese men and 80 cm for women
Plus any 2 of the following:

- Triglycerides >1.7 mmol/l (150 mg/dl)
- Reduced HDL <1.03 mmol/l (40 mg/dl) in males or <1.29 mmol/l (50 mg/dl) in females
- Raised blood pressure >130 mmHg systolic and >85 mmHg diastolic
- Raised fasting blood glucose >5.6 nmol/l (100 mg/dl)

cancer have a very high incidence of diabetes mellitus.[8]

Three studies (the Da Qing, the Finnish Diabetes Prevention study, and the Diabetes Prevention Program) have all shown that lifestyle intervention with a heavy emphasis on exercise decreases the future incidence of diabetes.[9,10] Metformin was ineffective in persons over 60 years of age. The DREAM study has shown that thiazoliclinediones may prevent the occurrence of diabetes.[11]

Hormonal replacement and aging

A longitudinal study has shown that 25 (OH) vitamin D levels decline with aging.[12] Vitamin D replacement in older persons with low vitamin D levels prevents hip fracture, decreases falls, improves muscle strength, and decreases death.[13] Vitamin D levels should be measured in all older men and, if levels are below 30 mg/dl, vitamin D should be replaced until values are above this level.

There is little evidence to support growth hormone replacement in older men.[14] While it may increase muscle mass, it does not appear to improve strength. There is some evidence that in malnourished older persons growth hormone may produce weight gain and improve function.[15] Both animal and human studies suggest that low physiologic levels of growth hormone are more predictive of survival than are higher levels.

Ghrelin is produced in the fundus of the stomach. Ghrelin increases growth hormone, food intake, and memory. These effects are mediated through nitric oxide. The effects of aging on ghrelin are controversial.

Insulin growth factor-1 (IGF-1) levels decline with aging and decline further in malnourished older persons. IGF-1 administration increases muscle bulk but not strength and produces hypoglycemia. IGF-3 or mechanogrowth factor is produced in muscle in response to resistance exercise. Growth hormone can further increase these levels, but not in the absence of exercise. Mechanogrowth factor (MGF) increases muscle strength, predominantly by recruiting satellite cells.[16] Stem cell replacement with MGF reverses the muscle atrophy present in old rats.

Melatonin is produced in the pineal gland. Melatonin produces a small enhancement of sleep length and quality; it also has some antioxidant activity. The French 'red wine paradox' in which red wine drinkers appear to do better is thought to be due to riservatol in red wine. Riservatol produces its effects by activation of melatonin receptors.

Dehydroepiandrosterone (DHEA) levels decline markedly with aging. Despite extravagant claims for its efficaciousness for reversing the aging process, a year-long study using 50 mg of DHEA daily failed to show any effects on muscle mass or strength.[17]

There is much enthusiasm to replace testosterone in older men with late life hypogonadism or andropause.[18] Small studies suggest that testosterone replacement improves muscle mass, strength, libido, erectile dysfunction, visuospatial memory, and bone mineral density. Testosterone also increases the hematocrit. Long-term side-effects of testosterone therapy, especially on the prostate, are uncertain. Testosterone may also worsen sleep apnea. A recent study suggested low testosterone may be associated with increased mortality.[19] Low testosterone is also associated with increased atherosclerotic burden.[20] There is a need for a large, multi-center study to determine the true role of testosterone replacement in older men.

Conclusions

Over the last decade there have been major advances in our understanding of the interactions of hormones in aging in older men. These advances have created a Pandora's box of possible hormone replacements that may enhance the quality of life and/or promote longevity. Unfortunately, at present there are inadequate numbers of studies to allow clear recommendations on the utility of hormonal replacement in older men.

References

1. Veldhuis JD. Nature of altered pulsatile hormone release and neuroendocrine network signaling in human ageing: clinical studies of the somatotropic, gonadotropic, corticotropic and insulin axes. Novartis Found Symp 2000; 227: 163–85; discussion 185–9.

2. Meneilly GS, Veldhuis JD, Elahi D. Pulsatile insulin secretion in elderly patients with diabetes. Diabetes Res Clin Pract 2006; 73(2): 218–20.

3. Morley JE. Hormones and the aging process. J Am Geriatr Soc 2003; 51(7 Suppl): S333–7.

4. Morley JE. Is the hormonal fountain of youth drying up? J Gerontol A Biol Sci Med Sci 2004; 59(5): 458–60.

5. Morley JE. The metabolic syndrome and aging. J Gerontol A Biol Sci Med Sci 2004; 59(2): 178–83; discussion 184–92.

6. Alberti KG, Zimmet P, Shaw J. Metabolic syndrome – a new world-wide definition. A consensus statement from the International Diabetes Federation. Diabet Med 2006; 23(5): 469–80.

7. Kaplan SA, Meehan AG, Shah A. The age related decrease in testosterone is significantly exacerbated in obese men with the metabolic syndrome. What are the implications for the relatively high incidence of

8. Keating NL, O'Malley AJ, Smith MR. Diabetes and cardiovascular disease during androgen deprivation therapy for prostate cancer. J Clin Oncol 2006; 24(27): 4448–56.

9. Pan XR, Li GW, Hu YH et al. Effects of diet and exercise in prevention of NIDDM in people with impaired glucose tolerance. The DA Qing IGT and Diabetes Study. Diabetes Care 1997; 20(4): 527–44.

10. Crandall J, Schade D, Ma Y, Fujimoto WY, Barrett-Connor E, Fowler S, Dagogo-Jack S, Andres R. The influence of age on the effects of lifestyle modification and metformin in prevention of diabetes. J Gerontol A Biol Sci Med Sci 2006; 61: 1075–81.

11. DREAM (Diabetes Reduction Assessment with ramipril and rosiglitazone Medication) Trial Investigators; Gerstein HC, Yusuf S, Bosch J et al. Effect of rosiglitazone on the frequency of diabetes in patients with impaired glucose tolerance or impaired fasting glucose: a randomized controlled trial. Lancet 2006; 23: 368(9541): 1096–105.

12. Perry HM 3rd, Horowitz M, Morley JE, Patrick P, Vellas B, Baumgartner R, Garry PJ. Longitudinal changes in serum 25-hydroxyvitamin D in older people. Metabolism 1999; 48(8): 1028–32.

13. Venning G. Recent developments in vitamin D deficiency and muscle weakness among elderly people. BMJ 2005; 5; 330(7490): 524–6.

14. Kim MJ, Morley JE. The hormonal fountains of youth: myth or reality? J Endocrinol Invest 2005; 28(11 Suppl Proc): 5–14.

15. Chu LW, Lam KS, Tam SC, Hu WJ, Hui SL, Chiu A, Chiu KC, Ng P. A randomized controlled trial of low-dose recombinant human growth hormone in the treatment of malnourished elderly medical patients. J Clin Endocrinol Metab 2001; 86: 1913–20.

16. Goldspink G. Age-related muscle loss and progressive dysfunction in mechanosensitive growth factor signaling. Ann NY Acad Sci 2004; 1019: 294–8.

17. Percheron G, Hogrel JY, Denot-Ledunois S, Fayet G, Forette F, Baulieu EE, Fardeau M, Marini JF. Double-blind placebo-controlled trial. Arch Intern Med 2003; 24: 163(6): 720–7.

18. Haren MT, Kim MJ, Tariq SH, Wittert GA, Morley JE. Andropause: a quality-of-life issue in older males. Med Clin North Am 2006; 90(5): 1005–23.

19. Shores MM, Matsumoto AM, Sloan KL, Kivlahan DR. Low serum testosterone and mortality in male veterans. Arch Intern Med 2006; 166(15): 1660–5.

20. Svartberg J, von Muhlen D, Mathiesen E, Joakimsen O, Bonaa KH, Stensland-Bugge E. Low testosterone levels are associated with carotid atherosclerosis in men. J Intern Med 2006; 259(6): 576–82.

Chapter 18

Androgen deficiency and its management in elderly men

Louis JG Gooren and Bruno Lunenfeld

Introduction

Among the many processes of aging, endocrine changes are relatively easy to identify and quantify with the presently available methods for determining hormone levels, which are reliable and sensitive. The question has been raised whether there exists a counterpart to aging in women (unfortunately labeled as menopause) in the male. It has become clear that levels of testosterone do indeed show an age-related decline but the characteristics of this age-related decline of testosterone are so fundamentally different from the menopause that drawing parallels generates more confusion than clarity. In men testosterone production is affected in a slowly progressive way as part of the normal aging process. It will rarely be manifest in men under the age of 50 years and becomes usually only quantitatively significant in men over 60 years of age. This age-related decline of testosterone shows considerable interindividual variation. Some men in their eighties will still have normal testosterone levels. Unlike the menopause, the age-associated decline of testosterone does not present itself in an 'all or none' fashion. The majority of women are able to retrospectively identify their age of menopause. Men are unable to pinpoint the start of their decline of testosterone.

So, the age-related decline of testosterone calls for terminology not reminiscent of the female menopause. When scientific investigation started to produce evidence of an age-related decline of testosterone, terms such as male menopause, male climacteric, or andropause were introduced. For the reasons given above, they should not be used. (Partial) androgen decline in the aging male (ADAM or PADAM) is a much better description. The term late onset hypogonadism (LOH) is probably now the preferred term.[1] Some would rather use the term symptomatic LOH, indicating that there must be signs and symptoms of the age-related decline of testosterone to qualify as a clinical entity. While being an acceptable term, it is of note that the testosterone deficiency in LOH is usually less profound and less manifest than in other hypogonadal states, but it may be clinically significant and deserves the attention of the medical profession.

Increased longevity compels the medical profession, and the society at large, to foster effective medical approaches that prolong independent, and if possible enjoyable living as long as possible. There is evidence from longitudinal studies that one of the key elements in independent living is the capacity to carry out the so-called activities of daily living for which muscle strength and bone mineral density are pivotal. These two decline by 1–2% per year. Furthermore, aging is associated with increased visceral fat mass, insulin resistance, falls and fractures, decreased muscle mass and strength, and decreased physical and mental performance, all reminiscent of a state of androgen deficiency. There is ample evidence that these signs and symptoms in younger men can be reversed by testosterone replacement treatment. Whether comparable improvements can be achieved in elderly men, and whether this is safe, is now being studied.

The notion of an andropause or male menopause, or as it is termed now LOH, is not rarely viewed with some skepticism by the medical profession.[2] This is a concept that all too readily lends itself to opportunistic exploitation by anti-aging entrepreneurs, usually working outside the public health sector, who tout 'rejuvenation cures'. The history of this field, which includes names like Voronoff and Lespinasse and, surprisingly, even such reputable scientists as Brown-Sequard and Steinach, is not illustrious.[3] It is feared that those who peddle the indiscriminate use of androgens, growth hormone, melatonin, and adrenal androgens will perpetuate this quackery in the present time.[2] Only well-designed studies into the endocrinology of aging, with clear clinical objectives and proper terminology, can ensure that history does not repeat itself and that the baby is not thrown out with the bathwater.

Neuroendocrine mechanisms of aging

Most of the hormone deficiencies associated with aging are based on neuroendocrine mechanisms.[4] One of the best known examples of age-related decline of hormone is the menopause. Originally believed to result from 'exhaustion of the ovary', it is becoming clear that neuroendocrine mechanisms orchestrate the loss of reproductive capacity in women. Its sequels can be alleviated by the administration of estrogens, the end products of ovarian hormone production, though this clinical practice is now hotly debated.[5] The basis of the decline of testosterone is also largely, but not exclusively, explained by neuroendocrine mechanisms, all leading to a diminished stimulation of the pituitary to produce the stimulatory hormone of the peripheral endocrine gland. There are also testicular factors contributing to the decline of testosterone production with aging (for review see references 6 and 7). Healthy elderly men maintain high-frequency, but low-amplitude luteinizing hormone (LH) secretion

patterns. Further, there is evidence that, with the same circulating levels of testicular steroids, the feedback signal to the hypothalamus is stronger than in younger men, thus diminishing output of LH when testosterone levels decline.[7,8] The patterns of LH release are significantly more disorderly. These observations indicate that age reduces hypothalamic luteinizing hormone releasing hormone (LHRH) outflow (release and delivery) to the gonadotrope cells in the pituitary.[9]

Administration of human chorionic gonadotropin to elderly men produces a diminished response of testosterone compared to young men, particularly in obese men,[10,11] pointing to an impairment of testicular steroidogenesis.

As indicated above, among the many processes of aging, endocrine changes are relatively easy to identify and quantify with reliable, sensitive, and highly specific methods for determining hormone levels. It is not only the reproductive hormones that decline with aging. The production of the sleep-related pineal hormone melatonin declines with aging. Adrenal androgen levels start to decline in both sexes from the age of 30 years (adrenopause), becoming very low at and beyond age 80 years. The levels of the main adrenal hormone cortisol do not fall with aging. The question has arisen whether the imbalance between the catabolic cortisol and anabolic testosterone contributes to the sarcopenia of old age.[12] Growth hormone secretion also undergoes an age-related decline (somatopause). While insulin levels generally do not fall with aging, sensitivity to the biologic action of insulin decreases considerably with aging. Changes in calcium, water and electrolyte metabolism, and thyroid function all characterize aging. These changes often have clinical relevance. Hypothyroidism or hyperthyroidism may be associated with forms of senile dementia, a diagnosis that can often be overlooked. Asthenia and muscle weakness may find their cause in disturbances of the electrolytes or androgen and growth hormone physiology. Therefore, the relationship between aging and hormonal changes is a two-way street: aging affects the endocrine system but endocrine dysfunction may also mimic symptoms of the aging process in aging subjects.

The attraction of identifying hormonal factors in the aging process is that they lend themselves to relatively easy correction. Admittedly, it would be simple-minded to interpret all age-related changes of hormones as deficiencies awaiting correction.[13] There is still substantial research to be done to ascertain whether the replacement of age-related reductions in hormone production is meaningful and, even more so, whether it is safe. Hormones such as estrogens, androgens, and growth hormone are potential factors in the development and growth of tumors that occur in old age. This contribution will focus primarily on the age-related decline of testosterone, for which the term late onset hypogonadism (LOH) was recommended by the International Society for the Study of the Aging Male (ISSAM), the International Society of Andrology (ISA), and the European Association of Urology (EAU) to replace the previous terminology of andropause, androgen deficiency of the aging male (ADAM), and partial androgen deficiency of the aging male (PADAM).[14] It is a clinical and biochemical syndrome associated with advancing age and characterized by typical symptoms and a deficiency in serum testosterone levels. It may result in significant detriment in the quality of life and adversely affect the function of multiple organ systems.

Prevalence

Quantitative aspects of the decline of androgen levels in aging

Several studies document that androgen levels decline with aging (for review see reference 15). Longitudinal studies[16–18] have documented a statistical decline of plasma testosterone by approximately 30% in healthy men between the ages of 25 and 75 years. Since plasma levels of sex hormone-binding globulin (SHBG) increase with aging, plasma testosterone not bound to SHBG decreases even more, by about 50%, over that period. Studies in twins have shown that genetic factors account for 63% of the variability of plasma testosterone levels, and for 30% of the variability of SHBG levels.[19] Also systemic diseases, increasing with age, are a cause of declining plasma levels of testosterone.[20]

While it now has been shown, beyond doubt, that plasma testosterone, and in particular bioavailable and free testosterone, decline with aging, it remains uncertain what percentage of men becomes actually testosterone deficient with aging in the sense that they will suffer the clinical consequences from testosterone deficiency, and will potentially benefit from testosterone replacement. In a study of 300 healthy men between the ages of 20 and 100 years,[21] defining their reference range of total plasma testosterone between 11 and 40 nmol/l, one man was found with subnormal testosterone in the age group between 20 and 40 years, but more than 20% were above the age of 60 years; however 15% of men above the age of 80 years still had testosterone values above 20 nmol/l! It follows that only a certain proportion of men has lower-than-normal testosterone values in old age. There are several problems. For androgen deficiency it is difficult to rely on clinical symptoms, particularly in elderly men. In adult persons who have previously been eugonadal, symptoms of testosterone deficiency emerge only gradually and insidiously. So, only the physical signs of long-standing testosterone deficiency will be clinically recognized. Further, stringent criteria to diagnose testosterone deficiency have not been formulated, neither in the young nor in the elderly male population. In the elderly population testosterone deficiency is difficult to identify since symptoms of aging mimic symptoms of testosterone deficiency. It has not become clear whether, for aging men, other criteria for testosterone deficiency should be established than for younger men.

Testosterone has a number of physiologic functions in the male. In adulthood it is responsible for the maintenance of reproductive capacity and of secondary sex characteristics; it has positive effects on mood and libido, anabolic effects on bone and muscle, and it affects fat distribution and the cardiovascular system. Threshold plasma values of testosterone for each of these functions are becoming established. The studies of Bhasin et al[22] and of Kelleher et al,[23] analyzing the dose–response relationships between plasma testosterone and biologic effects, show that low-to-midnormal plasma levels of testosterone suffice for most biologic actions of testosterone. Another consideration is whether these threshold values change over the life-cycle. Theoretically, it is possible that in old age androgen levels suffice for some but not for all androgen-related functions. With regard to anabolic actions, elderly men are as responsive to testosterone as young men.[22] Male sexual functioning in (young) adulthood can be maintained with lower-than-normal values.[24,25] However, there are indications that the threshold required for behavioral effects of testosterone increases with aging,[26] recently confirmed in a laboratory setting indicating that libido and erectile function require higher testosterone levels in old age compared to younger men,[27] but also apparent from clinical observation[28] and suggested by a meta-analysis.[29]

Pathophysiology

Correlations between androgen levels and symptoms of male aging

Before addressing the impact of LOH on sexual functioning more specifically, some age-related physical and mental changes will be reviewed. These topics are reviewed more extensively elsewhere in this volume. Most non-endocrinologists associate the role of testosterone with sexual functioning only. Recent insights show convincingly that testosterone has a wide impact on male physical and mental functioning far beyond sexual functions only. Testosterone deficiency affects general health profoundly. This is of particular relevance since the quality of health is associated with sexual functioning.[30]

Body composition

Body composition is seriously affected by the aging process (for reviews see references 7 and 31–33). Aging is almost universally accompanied by an increase in abdominal fat mass and a decrease of muscle mass. Androgens have a substantial impact on muscle mass and on fat distribution, and therefore the relationship between these signs of aging and testosterone levels has been assessed.

Increase in fat mass

Several studies have convincingly documented an inverse correlation between abdominal fat mass and free testosterone levels and it appears independent of age. This finding has clinical relevance: the amount of visceral fat is highly significantly associated with an increased risk of cardiovascular disease, impaired glucose tolerance, and non-insulin dependent diabetes mellitus (the dysmetabolic syndrome, or just metabolic syndrome).[7,32,34–38] Whether the abdominal, and more specifically visceral obesity is the consequence of the low testosterone levels or vice versa, is not yet clear. It is clear, however, that visceral obesity leads to a decrease of testosterone levels, mainly via a decrease in SHBG levels.

Decline in muscle mass and strength

There is an impressive age-associated decline in muscle mass (12 kg between ages 20 and 70 years).[39–42] This loss of muscle mass is a major contributor to the age-associated decline in muscle strength and fatigue. Maximal muscle strength shows a correlation with muscle mass, independent of age. This is again related to the occurrence of falls, fractures, and the consequent limitations of independent living. The correlation between testosterone levels and muscle mass appears stronger than the correlation with muscle strength.

Bone mineral density

With aging there is an exponential increase in bone fracture rate,[7,31,43] which carries a clear association with the age-related decrease of bone mineral density (BMD). In view of the significance of sex steroids in the maintenance of BMD at all ages, the question whether the partial androgen deficiency in aging males plays an important role in the decrease of BMD is pertinent. A pivotal role of androgens in the decrease of BMD has, however, been difficult to establish. Not all scientific findings agree. Indeed, some studies find a significant, though weak, correlation between androgen levels and BMD at some but not all bone sites. Others are unable to establish a correlation. Some large-scale studies of several hundred elderly men have demonstrated that bone density in the radius, spine, and hip is correlated with levels of bioavailable testosterone.[43] Interestingly, the correlation with levels of bioavailable estradiol was much more prominent, probably pointing to the significance of estrogens in men, also in old age.[44]

Cardiovascular function

Premenopausal women suffer significantly less from cardiovascular disease than men, and traditionally it has been thought that the relationship between sex steroids and cardiovascular disease is predominantly determined by the relatively beneficial effects of estrogens and by the relatively detrimental effects of androgens on lipid profiles (for review see references 35, 37, and 38). Nevertheless, the vast majority of cross-sectional studies in men are not in agreement with this assumption; they show a positive correlation between free testosterone levels and HDL cholesterol, and a negative correlation with fibrinogen, plasminogen activator inhibitor-1, and insulin levels as well as with coronary heart disease,[45] but not with cardiovascular mortality.

Recent research shows the effects of sex steroids on biologic systems other than lipids. Fat distribution, endocrine/paracrine factors produced by the vascular wall (such as endothelins and nitric oxide), and blood platelets and coagulation must also be considered in the analysis of the relationship between sex steroids and cardiovascular disease.[46]

The above review articles emphasize the fact that short-term studies actually have shown a benefit to the cardiovascular system,[35,37] and that the therapeutic use of testosterone in men need not be restricted by concerns regarding cardiovascular side-effects.[38]

Cognitive performance

There is some evidence to suggest that testosterone may influence performance of cognitive tasks (for review see references 47–49), which is supported by the finding that testosterone administration to older men enhances performance on measures of spatial cognition. The correlation between testosterone levels and cognitive performance such as spatial ability or mathematic reasoning has been confirmed in Western and non-Western cohorts of healthy males.

Testosterone has also been associated with general mood elevating effects. Some studies have found associations between lowered testosterone levels and depressive symptoms. Depression is not rare in aging men and impairs their quality of life,[50] so the effects that declining levels of androgens may have on mood and on specific aspects of cognitive functioning in aging are well worth researching.

The impact of androgens on sexual functioning in elderly men

Aging is the most robust factor predicting erectile difficulties. It is obvious that aging *per se* is associated with a deterioration of the biologic functions mediating erectile function: hormonal, vascular, and neural processes. This is often aggravated by intercurrent disease in old age, such as diabetes mellitus and cardiovascular disease, and by the use of medical drugs. The following will address the role of testosterone, which, as indicated above, is only one of the elements which may explain sexual dysfunction with aging.

Erectile response in mammals is centrally and peripherally regulated by androgens. Severe hypogonadism in men usually results in loss of libido and potency. The insight into the more precise mechanisms of the action of androgens on sexual functions is of rather recent date. Studies in the 1980s showed that androgens particularly exert effects on libido and that sleep-related erections are androgen sensitive, but erections in response to erotic stimuli, somewhat surprisingly, are relatively androgen-independent.[51,52] Later studies modified this view somewhat, showing that penile responses to erotic stimuli with regard to the duration of response, maximal degree of rigidity, and speed of detumescence were related to circulating androgens.[53,54]

It was repeatedly shown in hypogonadal patients (with a wide age range) that sexual functions required androgen levels below or at the low end of reference values of testosterone.[22,24,25]

The above considerations – the relative androgen-independence of erections in response to erotic stimuli and the relatively low androgen levels required – were reasons to believe that testosterone was not a useful treatment for men with erectile difficulties whose testosterone levels were usually only marginally low.

An even more important element in the disregard of testosterone as a treatment option was the advent of intracorporeal smooth muscle relaxants (papaverine, prostaglandin E1), later superseded by the PDE-5 inhibitors, which when introduced in 1998 were hailed as the ultimate successful treatment of erectile dysfunction.

There are a number of recent developments which shed new light on testosterone treatment of erectile dysfunction in aging men:

1. The recent insight that, in contrast to the results obtained in younger men,[22,24,25] elderly men might require higher levels of testosterone for normal sexual functioning.[27,55] Actually, reviews of the literature on the effect of testosterone administration to elderly men on libido and erectile potency are quite encouraging.[29,56,57]

2. Several studies have now indicated that the administration of PDE-5 inhibitors is not always sufficient to restore erectile potency in men,[58-61] and that administration of testosterone improves the therapeutic response to PDE-5 inhibitors considerably.[59-61]

3. There is growing insight that testosterone has profound effects on tissues of the penis involved in the mechanism of erection and that testosterone deficiency impairs the anatomic and physiologic substrate of erectile capacity, reversible upon androgen replacement. These data come mainly from animal experimentation but a number of studies support their relevance for the human as well. There are androgen receptors in the corpus cavernosum.[62] Morelli et al[63] have shown that the synthesis of PDE-5 in the corpus cavernosum is upregulated by androgens. Aversa et al[59] demonstrated that the arterial inflow into the penis is improved by androgen administration. In a review paper[64] the authors, remarking that data on testosterone effects on the penis in the human are still limited, found it reasonable to extrapolate animal dependency on androgens for molecular activity in the penile tissue to the human.

The above provides compelling evidence for a re-examination of the merits of testosterone administration to aging men with erectile dysfunction. It has become clear that the beneficial effects of PDE-5 inhibitors are only optimally expressed in a eugonadal environment.[65] Obviously, the past and present experience[66-68] indicate that testosterone replacement alone may not suffice to restore erectile potency. Since erectile dysfunction is so strongly age-related, it is evident that, inherent in the process of aging, etiology is multifactorial, and combinations of drugs might be needed to restore it. It is a matter of clinical judgment what type of treatment should be tried first, PDE-5 inhibitors or testosterone, but it is important to remember that insufficient success of one type of treatment might require addition of the other.

Diagnosis

Screening

It is difficult to make a fair assessment of the infirmity associated with the aging process. Part of it will be due to 'natural aging' and part of it to emerging disease processes, which will be increasingly part of life with aging. 'Natural aging' and emerging diseases affect individual subjects to varying degrees. In addition, hormone deficiencies do not affect all men to the same degree. Clinical entities such as hypertension and diabetes mellitus range from mild to severe. Therefore it is useful to have tools that provide a 'grip' on signs and symptoms of aging. Such an instrument also facilitates assessment of the success of interventions in these populations.

The development of rate scales is a difficult venture. The validation of questionnaires is an arduous process. Translation into another language implies a new validation in that language to test whether questions are understood and interpreted linguistically and culturally in the same way as in the original language. The first rating scale was introduced by Morley and coworkers.[69,70] This scale tests whether certain symptoms are more likely to be present in aging men with declining levels of bioavailable testosterone. This rating scale has been subject to criticism.

A recently developed instrument is the Aging Males' Symptoms (AMS) rating scale.[72,73] This measures somatic, sexual, and psychologic aspects of an aging male's life. It was originally developed to measure response to reatment, rather than to diagnose symptoms of age-related decline of testosterone. Originally developed in the German language it has now been validated for English[72] (Appendix 1), and validations for other European languages are now available.[74,75] Validations in other languages and in other geographic areas are welcomed. Experience with the rating scale is not universally positive,[76] and some authors have argued that the problems encountered by aging men go well beyond symptoms attributable to androgen deficiency.[77]

Biochemical diagnosis

The laboratory reference values of testosterone and free testosterone show a wider range than those for most other hormones (for instance thyroid hormones), which makes it difficult to establish whether measured values of testosterone in patients are normal or abnormal. Is a patient whose plasma levels of testosterone fall from the upper to the lower range of normal testosterone levels (a drop of as much as 50%) testosterone deficient? Levels may well remain within the reference range but may be inappropriately low for that particular individual. In thyroid pathophysiology plasma TSH proves to be a better criterion of thyroid hyper/hypofunction than plasma T4 or T3, but it is uncertain whether plasma LH is a reliable indicator of male hypogonadism in the elderly man. With aging there are reductions in LH pulse frequency and amplitude. Several studies have found that LH levels are elevated in response to the decline in testosterone levels with aging, but less so than is observed in younger men with similarly decreased testosterone levels.[15] This may be due to a shift in the setpoint of the negative feedback of testosterone on the hypothalamic/solidus pituitary unit, resulting in an enhanced negative feedback action, which consequently leads to a relatively lower LH output in response to lowered circulating levels of testosterone. Another variable that might be significant in the assessment of androgen status in old age is plasma levels of SHBG. Its levels increase even with healthy aging, possibly due to a decrease in growth hormone production and an increase in the ratio of free estradiol over free testosterone.[15]

The above has outlined the many unresolved questions as to the verification of deficiencies in the biologic action of androgens in old age and what plasma testosterone levels conclusively represent androgen deficiency. Consequently, a pragmatic approach to this issue must be taken in order to let aging androgen-deficient men benefit from replacement therapy while the above theoretic but important questions are resolved by clinical investigations. The question has received serious attention in the past years.[1,78] Vermeulen[21] argues that there is no generally accepted cut-off value of plasma testosterone for defining androgen deficiency, and in the absence of convincing evidence for an altered androgen requirement in elderly men, he considers the normal range of free testosterone levels in young males also valid for elderly men. In his healthy male, non-obese, population aged 20–40 years ($n = 150$), the mean of log transformed early morning testosterone levels was 21.8 nmol/l (627 ng/dl); the mean minus 2 SD was 12.5 nmol/l (365 ng/dl) and minus 2.5 SD 11 nmol/l (319 ng/dl). For free testosterone, measured by equilibrium dialysis or calculated from testosterone and SHBG levels,[14] the mean was 0.5 nmol/l (14 ng/dl), minus 2 SD 0.26 nmol/l (7.4 ng/dl), and minus 2.5 SD 0.225 nmol/l or 6.5 ng/dl. If one takes as the lower normal limit and threshold of partial androgen deficiency a conservative value of 11 nmol/l for total testosterone and 0.225 nmol/l for free testosterone, which represent the lower 1% values for healthy young males, then it appears that more than 30% of men over 75 years old have subnormal free testosterone levels. It should be mentioned that direct free testosterone assays using a testosterone analog do not yield a reliable estimate of free testosterone.[79] The age-associated decline in free testosterone levels has both a testicular (decreased Leydig cell number) and central origin, the latter being characterized by a decrease in the orderliness and amplitude of LH pulses in elderly men. Hence, many elderly men have normal LH levels and an increase in LH levels is unlikely to be required for the diagnosis of hypogonadism in elderly men.

Another variable that might be significant in assessment of the androgen status in old age is plasma levels of SHBG. Vermeulen and coworkers[79] demonstrated that the free testosterone value calculated by the ratio total testosterone/SHBG (according to a second-degree equation following the mass action law) as determined by immunoassay appears to be a rapid, simple, and reliable indicator of bioavailable and free testosterone, comparable to testosterone values obtained by equilibrium dialysis. Some algorithms have been placed on the internet as so-called bioavailable testosterone calculators (www.issam.ch, www.get-back-on-track.com/en/tools/kalkulator.php, and www.him-link.com), making these algorithms readily available for distant users. It is redundant to measure/calculate bioavailable/free testosterone if plasma total testosterone appears to be in the truly hypogonadal (< 6 nmol/l)or in the truly eugonadal range (>15 nmol/l).[80] So, without much in the way of solid criteria for testosterone deficiency, determination of values of testosterone and SHBG might provide a reasonable index of the androgen status of an aging person.

To avoid a false diagnosis of hypogonadism, measurement of testosterone should preferably take place before 11 am in view of the diurnal rhythm of plasma testosterone, which is less marked in elderly men compared to young men, but is usually not absent. The consequences of lower-than-normal values of testosterone may have a great impact, such as testosterone replacement. If indeed plasma testosterone values/calculated bioavailable/free testosterone are so low that testosterone supplementation is considered, it may be worthwhile to repeat the measurement a couple of weeks later. The stress of a common cold and the like may temporarily depress testosterone secretion. Otherwise, serial measurements of testosterone in (elderly) men are fairly stable.[81,82] For the measurement of total testosterone commercial radioimmunoassays and non-radioactive immunoassays kits, as well as automated platform immunoassays that mostly use chemiluminescence detection, are widely available and provide fairly accurate measurements between 10 and 35 nmol/l. Below 10 nmol/l their accuracy is considerably less. However, reference values vary significantly from laboratory to laboratory, and from measurement method to method. Consequently, it is advisable that every laboratory establishes its own 'normal range' of testosterone in men.[83,84]

As already mentioned, in the absence of a reliable, clinically useful biologic parameter of androgen action, these laboratory criteria of hypogonadism of aging men are somewhat arbitrary but for the time being the best available to provide guidance. Algorithms have been developed to guide the clinician with regard to the interpretation of the results of laboratory measurements of testosterone and SHBG.

Different countries have different health economies with regard to reimbursement of laboratory measurements. In fact, measurement of SHBG is only helpful at the low end of reference values of testosterone. If values are clearly in the normal range additional measurement of SHBG is redundant. A value of total testosterone level below 6.5 nmol/l is sufficient proof of hypogonadism and a value above 13.0 nmol/l rules out hypogonadism in adult males. This strategy leads to significant time and cost savings.[80]

Treatment

Suitable testosterone preparations

If it turns out that some men benefit from androgen supplements, are there suitable testosterone preparations available to treat them? The androgen deficiency of the aging male is only partial and consequently only supplementation will be required. Preferably, administration of testosterone should leave their own residual testosterone production intact.

Parenteral testosterone preparations

Intramuscular preparations have been the mainstay of androgen replacement therapy since the 1950s. Injectable esters of testosterone have been available for the longest time and their effects are well recognized. They are inexpensive and safe but their use carries several major drawbacks even for young hypogonadal males. Plasma testosterone levels fluctuate strongly following administration. The most widely used pharmaceutic forms are the hydrophobic long chain testosterone esters in oily depot, enanthate, and the cypionate, given intramuscularly (im) at a dose of 200–250 mg/2 weeks. They yield transient supraphysiologic levels the first 2–3 days after injection, followed by a steady decline to subphysiologic levels just prior to the next injection.[85] These fluctuations in testosterone levels are experienced by some of the patients as unpleasant and accompanied by changes in energy, libido, and mood. The transient supraphysiologic levels might increase the frequency of side-effects, such as polycythemia.[7,86]

A new depot im injection containing 1000 mg of testosterone undecanoate (TU) in 4 ml of castor oil has recently become available. This is a new treatment modality for androgen supplementation or therapy. Several studies have documented its use in hypogonadal men.[87,88] In short, after two loading doses of 1000 mg TU at 0 and 6 weeks, repeated injections at 12-week intervals are sufficient to maintain testosterone levels in the reference range of eugonadal men. It has been argued that this preparation is less suitable for initiation of testosterone treatment of aging men.[89] It is thought that the long duration of action might constitute a problem in the event that a prostate malignancy is diagnosed. Experienced urologists, however, reason that the delay between diagnosing prostate cancer and its treatment is usually much longer than 12 weeks, without an adverse effect on the outcome.[85] In addition, current recommendations advocate initial follow-up at 3-month intervals for the first year, which fits very well in the schedule of TU injections. In the highly hypothetic situation that a tumor is discovered, further treatment would be discontinued and the use of an antiandrogen may be considered. So, certainly after the first uneventful year of androgen administration, it seems reasonable to administer long-acting testosterone preparations to elderly men.[89]

Oral testosterone undecanoate

Testosterone undecanoate is testosterone esterified in the 17β position with a long aliphatic side-chain, undecanoic acid, dissolved in oil and encapsulated in soft gelatin. TU is designed to deliver testosterone to the systemic circulation via the intestinal lymphatic route, thereby circumventing first-pass inactivation in the liver. Therefore it is free from liver toxicity and brings serum testosterone levels within physiologic range. The esterification of testosterone with undecanoate renders TU

sufficiently lipophilic to be incorporated in chylomicrons formed during the process of lipid digestion in the intestine. These chylomicrons are then transported via the intestinal lymphatic system. Of the 40 mg capsules, 63% (25 mg) is testosterone. After ingestion its route of absorption from the gastrointestinal tract is shifted from the portal vein to the thoracic duct.[90] For its adequate absorption from the gastro-intestinal tract it is essential that oral TU is taken with a meal that contains dietary fat 23 g lipids (for example: 2 cups of decaffeinated coffee, 2 rolls of bread, 2 slices of cheese, 2 slices of ham, 20 g jam, 20 g butter 460 kcal, or, 48 g carbohydrates and 14 g protein 1 cup of milk, 2 eggs).[91]

Without dietary fat the resorption and the resulting serum levels of testosterone are minimal.[91] Maximum serum levels are reached 2 to 6 hours after ingestion. To increase shelf-life the preparation has recently been reformulated and the oil in the capsule is now castor oil. Studies show that there is dose proportionality between serum testosterone levels and the dose range of 20–80 mg.[90] With a dose of 120–240 mg per day over 80% of hypogonadal men showed plasma testosterone levels in the normal range over 24 hours.[90]

On the basis of its flexible dosing, TU is also probably best suited to supplement the reduced, but still present, endogenous testicular testosterone production in the aging male with lower than normal, but not severely hypogonadal levels, of testosterone.[90] Long-term use has been proven to be safe, as demonstrated in a 10-year observation.[92]

Transbuccal testosterone administration

Transbuccal administration of testosterone provides a means of oral administration of testosterone. The resorption of testosterone through the oral mucosa avoids intestinal absorption and subsequent hepatic inactivation of testosterone. Two studies have assessed the efficacy of transbuccal administration of testosterone.[93,94] Both studies found that administration of 30 mg of testosterone formulated as a bioadhesive buccal tablet twice daily generated plasma testosterone and DHT levels in the normal range in hypogonadal men.[93,94] Gum irritation was noted in approximately 3% of men.

Transdermal delivery

Testosterone can be delivered to the circulation through the intact skin, both genital and non-genital.[90] The daily physiologic requirement of testosterone of 5–7 mg can be achieved by the trandermal route of delivery. Excipients are generally required to enhance absorption and improve bioavailability. Transdermal administration delivers testosterone at a controlled rate into the systemic circulation avoiding hepatic first pass and reproducing the diurnal rhythm of testosterone secretion, without the peak and trough levels observed with long-acting testosterone injections.

Transdermal patches

Scrotal patches were first designed to deliver testosterone through the scrotal skin, where the permeability is 5 times greater than for other skin sites. It required weekly scrotal shaving, and was difficult for some patients to apply and maintain in position for 24 hours. Transdermal scrotal testosterone administration is associated with high levels of DHT as a result of high concentrations of 5α-reductase in the scrotal skin.[90] The patch may be irritating and the use is not feasible if the scrotal surface is inadequate. To overcome these limitations, non-scrotal skin patches have been developed. These patches have a reservoir containing testosterone with a permeation-enhancing vehicle and gelling agents.[93] Improvements have been reported in sexual function, libido, energy level, and mood.[93]

The most common adverse effects are local skin reactions. Fifty percent of men participating in a clinical trial reported transient, mild to moderate erythema at some time during therapy. However, most of these reactions were associated with application of the patch over a bony prominence or on parts of the body that could have been subject to prolonged pressure during sleep or sitting.

Testosterone gel

Testosterone gel is also used for replacement therapy. The gel is hydro-alcoholic and between 5 and 10 g of 1% gel (10 mg testosterone per gram gel) are administered per day, amounting to between 50 and 100 mg testosterone in total.[90,95] The pharmacokinetics of testosterone gel has been extensively studied. Serum testosterone levels rose 2–3-fold 2 hours after application and rose further to 4–5-fold after 24 hours. Thereafter serum testosterone remained steadily in the upper range of normal and returned to baseline within 4 days after termination of the gel application. Mean DHT levels followed the same pattern as testosterone and were at or above the normal adult male range. Serum E_2 levels rose and followed the same pattern as testosterone. The application of the testosterone gel at either one site or four sites did not have a substantial impact on the pharmacokinetic profile.[96] Later studies showed that 9–14% of the testosterone administered is bioavailable. Steady-state testosterone levels are achieved 48–72 hours after the first application. Serum testosterone and free testosterone are similar on days 30, 90, and 180 after the start of administration. The formulation of the testosterone gel allows easy dose adjustments (50–75–100 mg testosterone gel).[97]

The clinical efficacy of transdermal testosterone gel on various androgen-dependent target organ systems has been very well documented.[96] The safety profile showed that PSA levels rose in proportion to the increase of testosterone levels but did not exceed normal values. Skin irritation was noted in 5.5% of patients in the study.[96,98] Remarkably, washing of the site of application 10 minutes after application of the gel did not affect pharmacokinetic profiles.[99] Transfer from one person to another was found to be insignificant. No increase in serum testosterone was found after intense rubbing of skins with persons whose endogenous testosterone levels had been suppressed.[99]

Recently, a new formulation of testosterone gel has been introduced,[100] and in view of its clinical success new formulations will follow.

Androgens and growth hormone

Signs associated with aging show a striking similarity with features observed in adults who are growth hormone (GH)-deficient, and therefore speculation has arisen that (some of the) features of aging must be ascribed to the age-related decline in GH, and can potentially be remedied with GH replacement (for review see references 101 and 102).

The interrelationship between sleep and the somatotropic axis is well documented. This relationship is relevant since most aging subjects experience a deterioration of their sleep. During aging, slow wave sleep and GH decline concurrently, raising the possibility that the age-related decline of GH is also a reflection of age-related alterations in sleep–wake patterns.[103]

Unlike the situation in androgen physiology it is much more difficult to establish who is GH-deficient in adulthood. The pulsatile nature of GH secretion and the large number of factors determining circulating levels of GH complicate the matter considerably in the sense that a single measurement of GH does not provide meaningful information. A single measurement of insulin-like growth factor-1 (IGF-1) is a reasonable first indicator of GH status. In subjects over the age of 40 years an IGF-1 value of 15 nmol/l or higher excludes a deficiency of GH. Further, treatment with GH is not without problems and still cannot be considered routine medical practice.

Both androgens and GH have potent anabolic effects and their decline may be related to the sarcopenia of old age. The expression of the biologic effects of each hormone depends on adequate circulating levels of the other. In androgen-deficient men, the manifestation of anabolic effects of GH administration is suboptimal, and vice versa.

Several studies have addressed the combined effects of androgens and GH and found that they were greater than the effect of either hormone alone.[104–108] Other studies have investigated the impact of androgens on GH physiology. The insight is still limited and not all studies are in agreement. One study did not find that the age-related decline of testosterone had any impact on GH output.[109] Others are more affirmative. One study argued that a certain threshold of androgens is a condition to ensure the GH-derived hepatic production of IGF-1 that mediates the majority of the biologic effects of GH.[110] Other systematic studies of the mechanism by which testosterone impacts on GH have found that high testosterone levels augment GH and IGF-1 production in the elderly male,[111] maybe by attenuating the feedback of IGF-1 and GH on their own production and thus generating a higher

output.[112] Further testosterone enhances GH secretion upon stimulation with GH-releasing peptide.[113]

So, while treatment of elderly men with GH is still a delicate issue which should be left to clinicians with extensive experience, improving the androgen milieu might be an option to optimize the effects of residual GH secretion in elderly subjects.

Risks of androgen therapy

Absolute contraindications

The absolute contraindication for testosterone therapy is the suspected or documented presence of prostate cancer or breast cancer. Although there is no evidence that testosterone or any other androgen initiates prostate cancer, it is generally accepted that testosterone therapy may accelerate an already existing prostate cancer.[1,89,114] Relative contraindications and cautions include severe congestive heart failure for concern of fluid retention and polycythemia, and severe sleep apnea.[1,89,114]

Relative risks
Benign prostatic hyperplasia
The development of benign prostatic hyperplasia occurs only in the presence of androgens; reduction in serum testosterone induced by chemical or surgical castration reduces prostate volume. It was reported that prostate volume, as determined by ultrasonography, increases significantly during testosterone therapy, mainly during the first 6 months, to a level equivalent to that of men without hypogonadism.[115,116] However, urine flow rates, postvoiding residual urine volumes, and prostate voiding symptoms did not change significantly in these studies. This apparent paradox is explained by the poor correlation between prostate volume and urinary symptoms. However, several follow-up studies[114,117] have not shown an exacerbation of voiding symptoms due to benign prostatic hyperplasia during testosterone therapy, and complications such as urinary retention have not occurred at higher rates than in controls receiving placebo. Clinicians should nevertheless be aware that individual men with hypogonadism may occasionally

have increased voiding symptoms with testosterone therapy.

Risk of developing a prostate carcinoma under androgen treatment

Several studies have found benefits (and risks!) of androgen replacement to aging men and there is a large degree of consensus that it is responsible medical practice to prescribe androgens to elderly men with proven clinical and biochemical hypogonadism. With regard to potential risks, most authors will agree that testosterone as such does not induce a malignant development of prostate cells.[118–121] More than 60 years of worldwide use of testosterone have failed to elicit a signal through case reporting or national adverse-event monitoring of an associated risk of developing a prostate carcinoma. Overall, studies, some placebo-controlled, using various testosterone formulations, over periods ranging from several months to 15 years, in men with a wide range of ages, have not revealed an increased risk of prostate cancer over the background prevalence,[118,120–129] which is estimated to lie around 0.55% per annum,[130] though a recent meta-analysis found that testosterone replacement in older men was associated with a significantly higher risk of detection of prostate events.[131]

The wary attitude the medical profession has always had towards the relationship between androgens and prostate cancer may loosen somewhat in view of some recent publications. There is now some evidence that men who harbor a precancerous lesion of the prostate (prostatic intraepithelial neoplasia or PIN), and who receive testosterone treatment, are not at higher risk of developing overt prostate cancer than controls without PIN.[132] Also men who have undergone radical prostatectomy because of cancer (and whose PSA levels remain undetectable) are now beginning to receive androgens, again without much of an adverse outcome.[133,134]

Most studies have found that there is no relation between circulating testosterone levels and the occurrence of prostate carcinomas,[118,120,135,136] but a recent report identified a relation with calculated free testosterone values.[137] There is, however, agreement that once malignant transformation has become established, androgens play a role in

stimulating malignant cell activity. Progression of the malignancy is initially likely to be slow because of the long doubling time until the latter stages of cancer when further genetic mutations occur and when cell death is outpaced by cell proliferation. However comforting this information may be, androgens are still prescribed to elderly men with a degree of trepidation that a prostate carcinoma not discovered with available diagnostic means might be stimulated by androgen treatment. And, in fact, if the population of aging men is large enough, prostate cancers will certainly become manifest for the simple reason that aging as such is the strongest predictor of the occurrence of prostate carcinomas. The attending physician may face legal procedures and the arguments pro treatment will be countered by dissenting opinions on the risks of androgen administration to elderly men. The latter may be less informed but might prevail. Therefore, it seems timely to address the, one could say, thorny issue of the occurrence of a prostate carcinoma in men receiving androgen treatment. What is the medical significance of such an occurrence? Prostate cancers do occur after testosterone administration to (elderly) men.[138–142] A recent study reported 20 cases of prostate cancer in men receiving testosterone in six urology practices[143] becoming manifest within months to a few years after initiation of testosterone administration. Unfortunately, the total number of testosterone-treated men in this setting was not reported, so it was not possible to determine what percentage of men was diagnosed with prostate cancer while receiving testosterone treatment. This could then have been set against the normal statistical occurrence of prostate carcinoma of men at that age. Interestingly, it appeared in this study that digital rectal examination (DRE) was more significant than PSA values in detecting these cancers.[143]

So, it is clear that some men will be diagnosed with prostate cancer in the course of their testosterone treatment. Will this patient have suffered a setback in his health and life expectancy and has the prescription of androgens to that man been a regrettable decision or even a mistake? If a long-acting testosterone preparation has been prescribed, is the patient even worse off? One way of approaching these questions is to consider the impact of delay in treatment on long-term cancer control and outcome of prostate cancer. One study[144] found possible indications that a delay of treatment negatively affected prostate cancer cure rates. The study found that results of PSA levels, Gleason score, and TNM stage at the time of diagnosis did affect biochemical disease-free survival rates. However, more recent studies contradict this notion.[145] It appeared that a delay of a few months of surgery did not adversely affect the recurrence-free survival rates following radical prostatectomy. Two other studies arrived at similar conclusions.[146,147] Delays of up to several months[146] or up to a year from diagnostic biopsy to radical prostactectomy do not impact on long-term biochemical cancer control rates. Several urologists feel that patients receiving testosterone replacement (for good reasons) and whose plasma testosterone levels are in the physiologic range, are in a similar situation to eugonadal men diagnosed with prostate cancer. Men receiving testosterone treatment are usually much more frequently medically examined compared to other men of similar age, therewith increasing the probability of early diagnosis of prostate cancer.

Several of the recommendations of testosterone administration to elderly men with LOH argue in favor of short-acting testosterone preparations.[1,14,89] The reasoning is that in case an intercurrent disease develops, such as prostate malignancy, the impact of the extra androgens provided by the administration of testosterone will be short-lived. Is this recommendation rational in view of the facts that (1) there is an early diagnosis in this group of men who supposedly are monitored, following the guidelines, with an absolute minimum of DRE + PSA determination once a year, and (2) delays between diagnostic biopsies and treatment of several months up to one year did not affect the recurrence rate as measured by PSA levels? The modern testosterone preparations generate physiologic testosterone levels for a maximum duration of 10–14 weeks. This span of time matches the delays that usually take place between diagnostic biopsy and actual treatment intervention. So, it would seem that the choice of preparation is not of great pathophysiologic relevance.

A further case in point that long-acting testosterone preparations are not detrimental to the patient diagnosed with prostate cancer might be that neoadjuvant androgen deprivation before surgical radical prostatectomy appears so far to have no clear benefits to the patient (for review see references 148–150).

Prostate surveillance under treatment with testosterone

Digital rectal examination combined with monitoring with PSA should lead to early diagnosis, and potential cure, of most prostate cancers emerging under testosterone therapy. Obviously, men eligible for androgen treatment with an abnormal PSA level and/or abnormal DRE should first undergo prostate biopsy. The standard recommendation is that DRE + PSA measurement should take place every 3–4 months in the first year of treatment, and subsequently every year, maybe every 2 years if there are no major changes.[1,14,114] There should be a low threshold for biopsy if the PSA level rises substantially or if there is a change on DRE, such as the development of a nodule, asymmetry, or areas of increased firmness. Conventionally, the cut-off for normal/abnormal values of PSA has been set at 4.0 ng/ml, but the rates of increase over time are more significant than absolute values. New guidelines have been developed. It appeared in follow-up studies of tens of thousands of men that the risk of having prostate cancer is also alarmingly high if PSA values range from 2 to 4 ng/ml, which implies that the commonly accepted cut-off value of PSA of 4 ng/ml as safe is no longer acceptable.[151,152] Meanwhile the majority of the prostate cancer experts agree that rather than the absolute value of PSA, its velocity during the observational period is of importance and that an increase in PSA of more than 0.5 ng/ml over 2 following years is an indication for a prostate biopsy and withdrawal from testosterone replacement therapy. The present recommendations are as follows: *Biopsy should be recommended if the PSA velocity exceeds 0.2–0.5 ng/ml/year in men with a total PSA level less than 2.5 ng/ml or if the PSA velocity is greater than 0.75 ng/ml/year and the total PSA is above 4 ng/ml.*[153]

Androgens and hematopoiesis

Young hypogonadal men have lower red blood cell counts and hematocrits than age-matched controls; the values in the former increase upon administration of androgens.[154] Healthy older men tend to have similar or slightly lower hematocrit values than young adult men.[154] Androgens stimulate erythropoiesis,[155] and in most studies a 2–5% increase of the haematocrit over baseline has been observed, but with 6–25% of subjects developing erythrocytosis with hematocrits over 50%[156] (for review see reference 7). Erythrocytosis may increase the risk of stroke and requires corrective measures such as temporary interruption or dose adaptation of testosterone administration and/or phlebotomy. There is evidence that the risk of erythrocytosis is related to the achieved levels of testosterone with the mode of testosterone administration.[7,86]

Two studies of elderly men receiving androgen administration have shown increases in hematocrit of up to 7%.[129,157] Androgen replacement therapy may result in polycythemia.[158,159] In some cases of polycythemia, phlebotomy or withholding androgen administration is required. There is very likely a relationship with (peak) levels of testosterone associated with the treatment modality. Parenteral testosterone injections with high peak levels of testosterone produced higher hematocrit values compared to oral and transdermal testosterone treatment modalities.[86] Studies with relatively new parenteral testosterone undecanoate, which generates plasma testosterone levels within the physiologic range, have not shown induction of erythrocytosis.[87,88,160]

Androgens and sleep apnea

Sleep apnea is a relatively uncommon but debilitating disorder occuring almost exclusively in men, particularly when they age. In men suffering from sleep apnea, low total and free testosterone levels have been found,[161,162] which may be secondary to their abdominal (visceral) obesity. Several androgen replacement studies provide evidence that androgen administration to hypogonadal men may induce or exacerbate sleep apnea in elderly men.[163–165] In a study by Matsumoto et al,[166] it was shown that androgen levels may play a role in the pathogenesis of obstructive sleep apnea and that this may be a complication of testosterone therapy, though the relevance of androgens for obstructive sleep apnoea could not be shown in a study wherein the pure anti-androgen flutamide was used and no improvement of sleep apnea was observed.[167] Since these apneic events and the ensuing oxygen desaturation may lead to cardiovascular complications it is pertinent to ask elderly men about this symptom and to measure and follow-up hematocrit values before and during androgen administration. Care must be exercised in men who are overweight, heavy smokers, or who have chronic obstructive airway disease.

Summary

It is now clear that a certain proportion of men will develop hypogonadism when they age. This diagnosis must be documented by the presence of clinical signs and symptoms and measurement of plasma testosterone levels. In these cases it is justified to provide treatment with androgens. Proper safeguards must be in place to secure safety of testosterone replacement at an advanced age.

References

1. Nieschlag E, Swerdloff R, Behre HM et al. Investigation, treatment and monitoring of late-onset hypogonadism in males. ISA, ISSAM, and EAU recommendations. Eur Urol 2005; 48: 1–4.
2. Handelsman DJ, Liu PY. Andropause: invention, prevention, rejuvenation. Trends Endocrinol Metab 2005; 16: 39–45.
3. Schultheiss D, Jonas U, Musitelli S. Some historical reflections on the ageing male. World J Urol 2002; 20: 40–4.
4. Smith RG, Betancourt L, Sun Y. Molecular endocrinology and physiology of the aging central nervous system. Endocr Rev 2005; 26: 203–50.
5. Harman SM, Naftolin F, Brinton EA, Judelson DR. Is the estrogen controversy over? Deconstructing

the Women's Health Initiative Study: a critical evaluation of the evidence. Ann NY Acad Sci 2005; 1052: 43–56.

6. Liu PY, Iranmanesh A, Nehra AX, Keenan DM, Veldhuis JD. Mechanisms of hypoandrogenemia in healthy aging men. Endocrinol Metab Clin North Am 2005; 34: 935–55, ix.

7. Kaufman JM, Vermeulen A. The decline of androgen levels in elderly men and its clinical and therapeutic implications. Endocr Rev 2005; 26: 833–76.

8. Veldhuis JD, Iranmanesh A. Short-term aromatase-enzyme blockade unmasks impaired feedback adaptations in luteinizing hormone and testosterone secretion in older men. J Clin Endocrinol Metab 2005; 90: 211–18.

9. Veldhuis JD, Iranmanesh A, Mulligan T. Age and testosterone feedback jointly control the dose-dependent actions of gonadotropin-releasing hormone in healthy men. J Clin Endocrinol Metab 2005; 90: 302–9.

10. Foresta C, Bordon P, Rossato M, Mioni R, Veldhuis JD. Specific linkages among luteinizing hormone, follicle-stimulating hormone, and testosterone release in the peripheral blood and human spermatic vein: evidence for both positive (feed-forward) and negative (feedback) within-axis regulation. J Clin Endocrinol Metab 1997; 82: 3040–6.

11. Isidori AM, Caprio M, Strollo F et al. Leptin and androgens in male obesity: evidence for leptin contribution to reduced androgen levels. J Clin Endocrinol Metab 1999; 84: 3673–80.

12. Crawford BA, Liu PY, Kean MT, Bleasel JF, Handelsman DJ. Randomized placebo-controlled trial of androgen effects on muscle and bone in men requiring long-term systemic glucocorticoid treatment. J Clin Endocrinol Metab 2003; 88: 3167–76.

13. Lamberts SW, Romijn JA, Wiersinga WM. The future endocrine patient. Reflections on the future of clinical endocrinology. Eur J Endocrinol 2003; 149: 169–75.

14. Nieschlag E, Swerdloff R, Behre HM et al. Investigation, treatment and monitoring of late-onset hypogonadism in males: ISA, ISSAM, and EAU recommendations. Int J Androl 2005; 28: 125–7.

15. Kaufman JM, Vermeulen A. The decline of androgen levels in elderly men and its clinical and therapeutic implications. Endocr Rev 2005.

16. Moffat SD, Zonderman AB, Metter EJ et al. Longitudinal assessment of serum free testosterone concentration predicts memory performance and cognitive status in elderly men. J Clin Endocrinol Metab 2002; 87: 5001–7.

17. Morley JE, Kaiser FE, Perry HM 3rd et al. Longitudinal changes in testosterone, luteinizing hormone, and follicle-stimulating hormone in healthy older men. Metabolism 1997; 46: 410–13.

18. Araujo AB, O'Donnell AB, Brambilla DJ et al. Prevalence and incidence of androgen deficiency in middle-aged and older men: estimates from the Massachusetts Male Aging Study. J Clin Endocrinol Metab 2004; 89: 5920–6.

19. Meikle AW, Bishop DT, Stringham JD, West DW. Quantitating genetic and nongenetic factors that determine plasma sex steroid variation in normal male twins. Metabolism 1986; 35: 1090–5.

20. Handelsman DJ. Testicular dysfunction in systemic disease. Endocrinol Metab Clin North Am 1994; 23: 839–56.

21. Vermeulen A. Androgen replacement therapy in the aging male – a critical evaluation. J Clin Endocrinol Metab 2001; 86: 2380–90.

22. Bhasin S, Woodhouse L, Casaburi R et al. Testosterone dose–response relationships in healthy young men. Am J Physiol Endocrinol Metab 2001; 281: E1172–81.

23. Kelleher S, Conway AJ, Handelsman DJ. Blood testosterone threshold for androgen deficiency symptoms. J Clin Endocrinol Metab 2004; 89: 3813–17.

24. Gooren LJ. Androgen levels and sex functions in testosterone-treated hypogonadal men. Arch Sex Behav 1987; 16: 463–73.

25. Buena F, Swerdloff RS, Steiner BS et al. Sexual function does not change when serum testosterone levels are pharmacologically varied within the normal male range. Fertil Steril 1993; 59: 1118–23.

26. Schiavi RC, Rehman J. Sexuality and aging. Urol Clin North Am 1995; 22: 711–26.

27. Gray PB, Singh AB, Woodhouse LJ et al. Dose-dependent effects of testosterone on sexual function, mood, and visuospatial cognition in older men. J Clin Endocrinol Metab 2005; 90: 3838–46.

28. Steidle C, Schwartz S, Jacoby K, Sebree T, Smith T, Bachand R. AA2500 testosterone gel normalizes androgen levels in aging males with improvements in body composition and sexual function. J Clin Endocrinol Metab 2003; 88: 2673–81.

29. Jain P, Rademaker AW, McVary KT. Testosterone supplementation for erectile dysfunction: results of a meta-analysis. J Urol 2000; 164: 371–5.

30. Lewis RW, Fugl-Meyer KS, Bosch R et al. Epidemiology/risk factors of sexual dysfunction. J Sex Med 2004; 1: 35–9.

31. Isidori AM, Giannetta E, Greco EA et al. Effects of testosterone on body composition, bone metabolism and serum lipid profile in middle-aged men: a meta-analysis. Clin Endocrinol (Oxf) 2005; 63: 280–93.

32. Makhsida N, Shah J, Yan G, Fisch H, Shabsigh R. Hypogonadism and metabolic syndrome: implications for testosterone therapy. J Urol 2005; 174: 827–34.

33. Moretti C, Frajese GV, Guccione L et al. Androgens and body composition in the aging male. J Endocrinol Invest 2005; 28: 56–64.

34. Kapoor D, Malkin CJ, Channer KS, Jones TH. Androgens, insulin resistance and vascular disease in men. Clin Endocrinol (Oxf) 2005; 63: 239–50.

35. Liu PY, Death AK, Handelsman DJ. Androgens and cardiovascular disease. Endocr Rev 2003; 24: 313–40.

36. Pitteloud N, Hardin M, Dwyer AA et al. Increasing insulin resistance is associated with a decrease in Leydig cell testosterone secretion in men. J Clin Endocrinol Metab 2005; 90: 2636–41.

37. Shabsigh R, Katz M, Yan G, Makhsida N. Cardiovascular issues in hypogonadism and testosterone therapy. Am J Cardiol 2005; 96: 67–72M.

38. Wu FC, von Eckardstein A. Androgens and coronary artery disease. Endocr Rev 2003; 24: 183–217.

39. Hughes VA, Frontera WR, Wood M et al. Longitudinal muscle strength changes in older adults: influence of muscle mass, physical activity, and health. J Gerontol A Biol Sci Med Sci 2001; 56: B209–17.

40. Hughes VA, Frontera WR, Roubenoff R, Evans WJ, Singh MA. Longitudinal changes in body composition in older men and women: role of body weight change and physical activity. Am J Clin Nutr 2002; 76: 473–81.

41. Frontera WR, Hughes VA, Fielding RA, Fiatarone MA, Evans WJ, Roubenoff R. Aging of skeletal muscle: a 12-yr longitudinal study. J Appl Physiol 2000; 88: 1321–6.

42. Bhasin S, Woodhouse L, Casaburi R et al. Older men are as responsive as young men to the anabolic effects of graded doses of testosterone on the skeletal muscle. J Clin Endocrinol Metab 2005; 90: 678–88.

43. Vanderschueren D, Vandenput L, Boonen S, Lindberg MK, Bouillon R, Ohlsson C. Androgens and bone. Endocr Rev 2004; 25: 389–425.

44. Seeman E. Estrogen, androgen, and the pathogenesis of bone fragility in women and men. Curr Osteoporos Rep 2004; 2: 90–6.

45. Crandall C, Palla S, Reboussin B et al. Cross-sectional association between markers of inflammation and serum sex steroid levels in the postmenopausal estrogen/progestin interventions trial. J Womens Health (Larchmt) 2006; 15: 14–23.

46. Nigam A, Bourassa MG, Fortier A, Guertin MC, Tardif JC. The metabolic syndrome and its components and the long-term risk of death in patients with coronary heart disease. Am Heart J 2006; 151: 514–21.

47. Lessov-Schlaggar CN, Reed T, Swan GE et al. Association of sex steroid hormones with brain morphology and cognition in healthy elderly men. Neurology 2005; 65: 1591–6.

48. Janowsky JS. The role of androgens in cognition and brain aging in men. Neuroscience 2006; 138: 1015–20.

49. Cherrier MM. Androgens and cognitive function. J Endocrinol Invest 2005; 28: 65–75.

50. Carnahan RM, Perry PJ. Depression in aging men: the role of testosterone. Drugs Aging 2004; 21: 361–76.

51. Bancroft J, Wu FC. Changes in erectile responsiveness during androgen replacement therapy. Arch Sex Behav 1983; 12: 59–66.

52. Bancroft J. Hormones and human sexual behavior. J Sex Marital Ther 1984; 10: 3–21.

53. Carani C, Granata AR, Bancroft J, Marrama P. The effects of testosterone replacement on nocturnal penile tumescence and rigidity and erectile response to visual erotic stimuli in hypogonadal men. Psychoneuroendocrinology 1995; 20: 743–53.

54. Granata AR, Rochira V, Lerchl A, Marrama P, Carani C. Relationship between sleep-related erections and testosterone levels in men. J Androl 1997; 18: 522–7.

55. Seftel AD, Mack RJ, Secrest AR, Smith TM. Restorative increases in serum testosterone levels are significantly correlated to improvements in sexual functioning. J Androl 2004; 25: 963–72.

56. Morley JE, Perry HM 3rd. Androgen treatment of male hypogonadism in older males. J Steroid Biochem Mol Biol 2003; 85: 367–73.

57. Gooren LJ, Saad F. Recent insights into androgen action on the anatomical and physiological substrate of penile erection. Asian J Androl 2006; 8: 3–9.

58. Park K, Ku JH, Kim SW, Paick JS. Risk factors in predicting a poor response to sildenafil citrate in elderly men with erectile dysfunction. BJU Int 2005; 95: 366–70.

59. Aversa A, Isidori AM, Spera G, Lenzi A, Fabbri A. Androgens improve cavernous vasodilation and response to sildenafil in patients with erectile dysfunction. Clin Endocrinol (Oxf) 2003; 58: 632–8.

60. Kalinchenko SY, Kozlov GI, Gontcharov NP, Katsiya GV. Oral testosterone undecanoate reverses erectile dysfunction associated with diabetes mellitus in patients failing on sildenafil citrate therapy alone. Aging Male 2003; 6: 94–9.

61. Shabsigh R. Testosterone therapy in erectile dysfunction. Aging Male 2004; 7: 312–18.

62. Schultheiss D, Badalyan R, Pilatz A et al. Androgen and estrogen receptors in the human corpus cavernosum penis: immunohistochemical and cell culture results. World J Urol 2003; 21: 320–4.

63. Morelli A, Filippi S, Mancina R et al. Androgens regulate phosphodiesterase type 5 expression and functional activity in corpora cavernosa. Endocrinology 2004; 145: 2253–63.

64. Lewis RW, Mills TM. Effect of androgens on penile tissue. Endocrine 2004; 23: 101–5.

65. Rochira V, Balestrieri A, Madeo B, Granata AR, Carani C. Sildenafil improves sleep-related erections in hypogonadal men: evidence from a randomized, placebo-controlled, crossover study of a synergic role for both testosterone and sildenafil on penile erections. J Androl 2006; 27: 165–75.

66. Mulhall JP, Valenzuela R, Aviv N, Parker M. Effect of testosterone supplementation on sexual function in hypogonadal men with erectile dysfunction. Urology 2004; 63: 348–52; discussion 352–3.

67. Guay AT, Jacobson J, Perez JB, Hodge MB, Velasquez E. Clomiphene increases free testosterone levels in men with both secondary hypogonadism and erectile dysfunction: who does and does not benefit? Int J Impot Res 2003; 15: 156–65.

68. Greenstein A, Mabjeesh NJ, Sofer M, Kaver I, Matzkin H, Chen J. Does sildenafil combined with testosterone gel improve erectile dysfunction in hypogonadal men in whom testosterone supplement therapy alone failed? J Urol 2005; 173: 530–2.

69. Morley JE, Perry HM 3rd, Kevorkian RT, Patrick P. Comparison of screening questionnaires for the diagnosis of hypogonadism. Maturitas 2006; 53: 424–9.

70. Morley JE, Charlton E, Patrick P et al. Validation of a screening questionnaire for androgen deficiency in aging males. Metabolism 2000; 49: 1239–42.

71. Tancredi A, Reginster JY, Schleich F et al. Interest of the androgen deficiency in aging males (ADAM) questionnaire for the identification of hypogonadism in elderly community-dwelling male volunteers. Eur J Endocrinol 2004; 151: 355–60.

72. Heinemann LA, Saad F, Zimmermann T et al. The Aging Males' Symptoms (AMS) scale: update and compilation of international versions. Health Qual Life Outcomes 2003; 1: 15.

73. Daig I, Heinemann LA, Kim S et al. The Aging Males' Symptoms (AMS) scale: review of its methodological characteristics. Health Qual Life Outcomes 2003; 1: 77.

74. Myon E, Martin N, Taieb C, Heinemann LA. Experiences with the French Aging Males' Symptoms (AMS) scale. Aging Male 2005; 8: 184–9.

75. Valenti G, Gontero P, Sacco M et al. Harmonized Italian version of the Aging Males' Symptoms scale. Aging Male 2005; 8: 180–3.

76. T'Sjoen G, Goemaere S, De Meyere M, Kaufman JM. Perception of males' aging symptoms, health and well-being in elderly community-dwelling men is not related to circulating androgen levels. Psychoneuroendocrinology 2004; 29: 201–14.

77. T'Sjoen G, Feyen E, De Kuyper P, Comhaire F, Kaufman JM. Self-referred patients in an aging male clinic: much more than androgen deficiency alone. Aging Male 2003; 6: 157–65.

78. Black AM, Day AG, Morales A. The reliability of clinical and biochemical assessment in symptomatic late-onset hypogonadism: can a case be made for a 3-month therapeutic trial? BJU Int 2004; 94: 1066–70.

79. Vermeulen A, Verdonck L, Kaufman JM. A critical evaluation of simple methods for the estimation of free testosterone in serum. J Clin Endocrinol Metab 1999; 84: 3666–72.

80. Gheorghiu I, Moshyk A, Lepage R, Ahnadi CE, Grant AM. When is bioavailable testosterone a redundant test in the diagnosis of hypogonadism in men? Clin Biochem 2005.

81. Vermeulen A, Verdonck G. Representativeness of a single point plasma testosterone level for the long term hormonal milieu in men. J Clin Endocrinol Metab 1992; 74: 939–42.

82. Tancredi A, Reginster JY, Luyckx F, Legros JJ. No major month to month variation in free testosterone levels in aging males. Minor impact on the biological diagnosis of 'andropause'. Psychoneuroendocrinology 2005; 30: 638–46.

83. Wang C, Catlin DH, Demers LM, Starcevic B, Swerdloff RS. Measurement of total serum testosterone in adult men: comparison of current laboratory methods versus liquid chromatography-tandem mass spectrometry. J Clin Endocrinol Metab 2004; 89: 534–43.

84. Matsumoto AM, Bremner WJ. Serum testosterone assays – accuracy matters. J Clin Endocrinol Metab 2004; 89: 520–4.

85. Schurmeyer T, Nieschlag E. Comparative pharmacokinetics of testosterone enanthate and testosterone cyclohexanecarboxylate as assessed by serum and salivary testosterone levels in normal men. Int J Androl 1984; 7: 181–7.

86. Jockenhovel F, Vogel E, Reinhardt W, Reinwein D. Effects of various modes of androgen substitution therapy on erythropoiesis. Eur J Med Res 1997; 2: 293–8.

87. Schubert M, Minnemann T, Hubler D et al. Intramuscular testosterone undecanoate: pharmacokinetic aspects of a novel testosterone formulation during long-term treatment of men with hypogonadism. J Clin Endocrinol Metab 2004; 89: 5429–34.

88. Harle L, Basaria S, Dobs AS. Nebido: a long-acting injectable testosterone for the treatment of male hypogonadism. Expert Opin Pharmacother 2005; 6: 1751–9.

89. Nieschlag E, Swerdloff R, Behre HM et al. Investigation, treatment and monitoring of late-onset hypogonadism in males. Aging Male 2005; 8: 56–8.

90. Gooren LJ, Bunck MC. Androgen replacement therapy: present and future. Drugs 2004; 64: 1861–91.

91. Bagchus WM, Hust R, Maris F, Schnabel PG, Houwing NS. Important effect of food on the bioavailability of oral testosterone undecanoate. Pharmacotherapy 2003; 23: 319–25.

92. Gooren LJ. A ten-year safety study of the oral androgen testosterone undecanoate. J Androl 1994; 15: 212–15.

93. Dobs AS, Matsumoto AM, Wang C, Kipnes MS. Short-term pharmacokinetic comparison of a novel testosterone buccal system and a testosterone gel in testosterone deficient men. Curr Med Res Opin 2004; 20: 729–38.

94. Wang C, Swerdloff R, Kipnes M et al. New testosterone buccal system (Striant) delivers physiological testosterone levels: pharmacokinetics study in hypogonadal men. J Clin Endocrinol Metab 2004; 89: 3821–9.

95. Ebert T, Jockenhovel F, Morales A, Shabsigh R. The current status of therapy for symptomatic late-onset hypogonadism with transdermal testosterone gel. Eur Urol 2005; 47: 137–46.

96. Wang C, Cunningham G, Dobs A et al. Long-term testosterone gel (AndroGel) treatment maintains beneficial effects on sexual function and mood, lean and fat mass, and bone mineral density in hypogonadal men. J Clin Endocrinol Metab 2004; 89: 2085–98.

97. Meikle AW, Matthias D, Hoffman AR. Transdermal testosterone gel: pharmacokinetics, efficacy of dosing and application site in hypogonadal men. BJU Int 2004; 93: 789–95.

98. Dobs AS, Meikle AW, Arver S et al. Pharmacokinetics, efficacy, and safety of a permeation-enhanced testosterone transdermal system in comparison with bi-weekly injections of testosterone enanthate for the treatment of hypogonadal men. J Clin Endocrinol Metab 1999; 84: 3469–78.

99. Rolf C, Knie U, Lemmnitz G, Nieschlag E. Interpersonal testosterone transfer after topical application of a newly developed testosterone gel preparation. Clin Endocrinol (Oxf) 2002; 56: 637–41.

100. McNicholas T, Ong T. Review of Testim gel. Expert Opin Pharmacother 2006; 7: 477–84.

101. Harman SM, Blackman MR. Use of growth hormone for prevention or treatment of effects of aging. J Gerontol A Biol Sci Med Sci 2004; 59: 652–8.

102. Toogood AA. The somatopause: an indication for growth hormone therapy? Treat Endocrinol 2004; 3: 201–9.

103. Obal F Jr, Krueger JM. GHRH and sleep. Sleep Med Rev 2004; 8: 367–77.

104. Harman SM, Blackman MR. The effects of growth hormone and sex steroid on lean body mass, fat mass, muscle strength, cardiovascular endurance and adverse events in healthy elderly women and men. Horm Res 2003; 60: 121–4.

105. Blackman MR, Sorkin JD, Munzer T et al. Growth hormone and sex steroid administration in healthy aged women and men: a randomized controlled trial. JAMA 2002; 288: 2282–92.

106. Huang X, Blackman MR, Herreman K et al. Effects of growth hormone and/or sex steroid administration on whole-body protein turnover in healthy aged women and men. Metabolism 2005; 54: 1162–7.

107. Gibney J, Wolthers T, Johannsson G, Umpleby AM, Ho KK. Growth hormone and testosterone interact positively to enhance protein and energy metabolism in hypopituitary men. Am J Physiol Endocrinol Metab 2005; 289: E266–71.

108. Giannoulis MG, Sonksen PH, Umpleby M et al. The effects of growth hormone and/or testosterone in healthy elderly men: a randomized controlled trial. J Clin Endocrinol Metab 2006; 91: 477–84.

109. Orrego JJ, Dimaraki E, Symons K, Barkan AL. Physiological testosterone replenishment in healthy elderly men does not normalize pituitary growth hormone output: evidence against the connection between senile hypogonadism and somatopause. J Clin Endocrinol Metab 2004; 89: 3255–60.

110. Jorgensen JO, Christensen JJ, Vestergaard E, Fisker S, Ovesen P, Christiansen JS. Sex steroids and the growth hormone/insulin-like growth factor-I axis in adults. Horm Res 2005; 64(2): 37–40.

111. Veldhuis JD, Keenan DM, Mielke K, Miles JM, Bowers CY. Testosterone supplementation in healthy older men drives GH and IGF-I secretion without potentiating peptidyl secretagogue efficacy. Eur J Endocrinol 2005; 153: 577–86.

112. Veldhuis JD, Anderson SM, Iranmanesh A, Bowers CY. Testosterone blunts feedback inhibition of growth hormone secretion by experimentally elevated insulin-like growth factor-I concentrations. J Clin Endocrinol Metab 2005; 90: 1613–17.

113. Veldhuis JD, Patrie JT, Brill KT et al. Contributions of gender and systemic estradiol and testosterone concentrations to maximal secretagogue drive of burst-like growth hormone secretion in healthy middle-aged and older adults. J Clin Endocrinol Metab 2004; 89: 6291–6.

114. Morales A. Testosterone treatment for the aging man: the controversy. Curr Urol Rep 2004; 5: 472–7.

115. Behre HM, Bohmeyer J, Nieschlag E. Prostate volume in testosterone-treated and untreated hypogonadal men in comparison to age-matched normal controls. Clin Endocrinol (Oxf) 1994; 40: 341–9.

116. Jin B, Conway AJ, Handelsman DJ. Effects of androgen deficiency and replacement on prostate zonal volumes. Clin Endocrinol (Oxf) 2001; 54: 437–45.

117. Schultheiss D, Machtens S, Jonas U. Testosterone therapy in the ageing male: what about the prostate? Andrologia 2004; 36: 355–65.

118. Carter HB, Pearson JD, Metter EJ et al. Longitudinal evaluation of serum androgen levels in men with and without prostate cancer. Prostate 1995; 27: 25–31.

119. Slater S, Oliver RT. Testosterone: its role in development of prostate cancer and potential risk from use as hormone replacement therapy. Drugs Aging 2000; 17: 431–9.

120. Heikkila R, Aho K, Heliovaara M et al. Serum testosterone and sex hormone-binding globulin concentrations and the risk of prostate carcinoma: a longitudinal study. Cancer 1999; 86: 312–15.

121. Hsing AW. Hormones and prostate cancer: what's next? Epidemiol Rev 2001; 23: 42–58.

122. Morgentaler A, Bruning CO 3rd, DeWolf WC. Occult prostate cancer in men with low serum testosterone levels. JAMA 1996; 276: 1904–6.

123. Thompson IM, Goodman PJ, Tangen CM et al. The influence of finasteride on the development of prostate cancer. N Engl J Med 2003; 349: 215–24.

124. Andriole G, Bostwick D, Brawley O et al. Chemoprevention of prostate cancer in men at high risk: rationale and design of the reduction by dutasteride of prostate cancer events (REDUCE) trial. J Urol 2004; 172: 1314–17.

125. Clark RV, Hermann DJ, Cunningham GR, Wilson TH, Morrill BB, Hobbs S. Marked suppression of dihydrotestosterone in men with benign prostatic hyperplasia by dutasteride, a dual 5alpha-reductase inhibitor. J Clin Endocrinol Metab 2004; 89: 2179–84.

126. Andriole GL, Roehrborn C, Schulman C, Slawin KM, Somerville M, Rittmaster RS. Effect of dutasteride on the detection of prostate cancer in men with benign prostatic hyperplasia. Urology 2004; 64: 537–41; discussion 542–3.

127. Giovannucci E, Stampfer MJ, Krithivas K et al. The CAG repeat within the androgen receptor gene and its relationship to prostate cancer. Proc Natl Acad Sci USA 1997; 94: 3320–3.

128. Chamberlain NL, Driver ED, Miesfeld RL. The length and location of CAG trinucleotide repeats in the androgen receptor N-terminal domain affect transactivation function. Nucleic Acids Res 1994; 22: 3181–6.

129. Tenover JS. Effects of testosterone supplementation in the aging male. J Clin Endocrinol Metab 1992; 75: 1092–8.

130. Makinen T, Tammela TL, Stenman UH et al. Second round results of the Finnish population-based prostate cancer screening trial. Clin Cancer Res 2004; 10: 2231–6.

131. Calof OM, Singh AB, Lee ML et al. Adverse events associated with testosterone replacement in middle-aged and older men: a meta-analysis of randomized, placebo-controlled trials. J Gerontol A Biol Sci Med Sci 2005; 60: 1451–7.

132. Rhoden EL, Morgentaler A. Testosterone replacement therapy in hypogonadal men at high risk for prostate cancer: results of 1 year of treatment in men with prostatic intraepithelial neoplasia. J Urol 2003; 170: 2348–51.

133. Kaufman JM, Graydon RJ. Androgen replacement after curative radical prostatectomy for prostate cancer in hypogonadal men. J Urol 2004; 172: 920–2.

134. Kaufman J. A rational approach to androgen therapy for hypogonadal men with prostate cancer. Int J Impot Res 2005.

135. Shaneyfelt T, Husein R, Bubley G, Mantzoros CS. Hormonal predictors of prostate cancer: a meta-analysis. J Clin Oncol 2000; 18: 847–53.

136. Stattin P, Lumme S, Tenkanen L et al. High levels of circulating testosterone are not associated with increased prostate cancer risk: a pooled prospective study. Int J Cancer 2004; 108: 418–24.

137. Parsons JK, Carter HB, Platz EA, Wright EJ, Landis P, Metter EJ. Serum testosterone and the risk of prostate cancer: potential implications for testosterone therapy. Cancer Epidemiol Biomarkers Prev 2005; 14: 2257–60.

138. Ebling DW, Ruffer J, Whittington R et al. Development of prostate cancer after pituitary dysfunction: a report of 8 patients. Urology 1997; 49: 564–8.

139. Loughlin KR, Richie JP. Prostate cancer after exogenous testosterone treatment for impotence. J Urol 1997; 157: 1845.

140. Curran MJ, Bihrle W 3rd. Dramatic rise in prostate-specific antigen after androgen replacement in a hypogonadal man with occult adenocarcinoma of the prostate. Urology 1999; 53: 423–4.

141. Rhoden EL, Morgentaler A. Risks of testosterone-replacement therapy and recommendations for monitoring. N Engl J Med 2004; 350: 482–92.

142. Sengupta S, Duncan HJ, Macgregor RJ, Russell JM. The development of prostate cancer despite late onset androgen deficiency. Int J Urol 2005; 12: 847–8.

143. Gaylis FD, Lin DW, Ignatoff JM, Amling CL, Tutrone RF, Cosgrove DJ. Prostate cancer in men using testosterone supplementation. J Urol 2005; 174: 534–8; discussion 538.

144. Nam RK, Jewett MA, Krahn MD et al. Delay in surgical therapy for clinically localized prostate cancer and biochemical recurrence after radical prostatectomy. Can J Urol 2003; 10: 1891–8.

145. Graefen M, Walz J, Chun KH, Schlomm T, Haese A, Huland H. Reasonable delay of surgical treatment in men with localized prostate cancer – impact on prognosis? Eur Urol 2005; 47: 756–60.

146. Khan MA, Mangold LA, Epstein JI, Boitnott JK, Walsh PC, Partin AW. Impact of surgical delay on long-term cancer control for clinically localized prostate cancer. J Urol 2004; 172: 1835–9.

147. Boorjian SA, Bianco FJ Jr, Scardino PT, Eastham JA. Does the time from biopsy to surgery affect biochemical recurrence after radical prostatectomy? BJU Int 2005; 96: 773–6.

148. Selli C, Milesi C. Neoadjuvant androgen deprivation before radical prostatectomy. A review. Minerva Urol Nefrol 2004; 56: 165–71.

149. Namiki S, Saito S, Tochigi T et al. Impact of hormonal therapy prior to radical prostatectomy on the recovery of quality of life. Int J Urol 2005; 12: 173–81.

150. Homma Y, Akaza H, Okada K et al. Radical prostatectomy and adjuvant endocrine therapy for prostate cancer with or without preoperative androgen deprivation: five-year results. Int J Urol 2004; 11: 295–303.

151. Thompson IM, Pauler DK, Goodman PJ et al. Prevalence of prostate cancer among men with a prostate-specific antigen level < or = 4.0 ng per milliliter. N Engl J Med 2004; 350: 2239–46.

152. Kundu SD, Grubb RL, Roehl KA, Antenor JA, Han M, Catalona WJ. Delays in cancer detection using 2 and 4-year screening intervals for prostate cancer screening with initial prostate specific antigen less than 2 ng/ml. J Urol 2005; 173: 1116–20.

153. Catalona WJ, Loeb S. The PSA era is not over for prostate cancer. Eur Urol 2005; 48: 541–5.

154. Shahidi NT. Androgens and erythropoiesis. N Engl J Med 1973; 289: 72–80.

155. Claustres M, Sultan C. Androgen and erythropoiesis: evidence for an androgen receptor in erythroblasts from human bone marrow cultures. Horm Res 1988; 29: 17–22.

156. Drinka PJ, Jochen AL, Cuisinier M, Bloom R, Rudman I, Rudman D. Polycythemia as a complication of testosterone replacement therapy in nursing home men with low testosterone levels. J Am Geriatr Soc 1995; 43: 899–901.

157. Morley JE, Perry HM 3rd, Kaiser FE et al. Effects of testosterone replacement therapy in old hypogonadal males: a preliminary study. J Am Geriatr Soc 1993; 41: 149–52.

158. Sih R, Morley JE, Kaiser FE, Perry HM 3rd, Patrick P, Ross C. Testosterone replacement in older hypogonadal men: a 12-month randomized controlled trial. J Clin Endocrinol Metab 1997; 82: 1661–7.

159. Hajjar RR, Kaiser FE, Morley JE. Outcomes of long-term testosterone replacement in older hypogonadal males: a retrospective analysis. J Clin Endocrinol Metab 1997; 82: 3793–6.

160. Nieschlag E, Buchter D, Von Eckardstein S, Abshagen K, Simoni M, Behre HM. Repeated intramuscular injections of testosterone undecanoate for substitution therapy in hypogonadal men. Clin Endocrinol (Oxf) 1999; 51: 757–63.

161. Santamaria JD, Prior JC, Fleetham JA. Reversible reproductive dysfunction in men with obstructive sleep apnoea. Clin Endocrinol (Oxf) 1988; 28: 461–70.

162. Grunstein RR, Handelsman DJ, Lawrence SJ et al. Neuroendocrine dysfunction in sleep apnea: reversal by continuous positive airways pressure therapy. J Clin Endocrinol Metab 1989; 68: 352–8.

163. Liu PY, Yee B, Wishart SM et al. The short-term effects of high-dose testosterone on sleep, breathing, and function in older men. J Clin Endocrinol Metab 2003; 88: 3605–13.

164. Schneider BK, Pickett CK, Zwillich CW et al. Influence of testosterone on breathing during sleep. J Appl Physiol 1986; 61: 618–23.

165. Sandblom RE, Matsumoto AM, Schoene RB et al. Obstructive sleep apnea syndrome induced by testosterone administration. N Engl J Med 1983; 308: 508–10.

166. Matsumoto AM, Sandblom RE, Schoene RB et al. Testosterone replacement in hypogonadal men: effects on obstructive sleep apnoea, respiratory drives, and sleep. Clin Endocrinol (Oxf) 1985; 22: 713–21.

167. Stewart DA, Grunstein RR, Berthon-Jones M, Handelsman DJ, Sullivan CE. Androgen blockade does not affect sleep-disordered breathing or chemosensitivity in men with obstructive sleep apnea. Am Rev Respir Dis 1992; 146: 1389–93.

CHAPTER 19

Growth hormone and aging in men

Marc R Blackman

Introduction

Aging in man is associated with a progressive loss of function, leading to decreased homeostasic capacity, initially in response to various stressors, and subsequently under baseline conditions. Both aging and growth hormone (GH) deficiency are associated with decreased skeletal muscle, bone mass, strength, increased total and intra-abdominal fat, dyslipidemia, glucose intolerance, reduced cardiac endurance and immunologic function, and altered quality of life.[1,2] Recent studies suggest that administration of recombinant GH to non-elderly GH-deficient men ameliorates or attenuates these abnormalities.[1,2] Because normal aging in men is associated with a decline in GH secretion and serum insulin-like growth factor I (IGF-I) levels,[1,2] it has been hypothesized that the above-noted alterations in body composition and function in older persons may be due in part to decrements in the function of the GH–IGF-I axis. To assess this possibility, the effects of different hormone replacement paradigms are being investigated in selected populations of elderly men. A major goal of this research effort is to assess whether tropic factors such as GH, GH-releasing hormone (GHRH), or other GH-releasing peptides or non-peptide mimetics can be used effectively, safely, ethically, and economically to prolong physical and functional independence, and to reduce morbidity and frailty in aged men.

Physiologic changes in the GH–IGF-I axis with aging

Age-related changes of spontaneous and stimulated GH release

GH is an important anabolic hormone that exerts stimulatory effects on protein synthesis and on lipolysis.[3] Pituitary GH release is regulated primarily by the interaction of the hypothalamic peptides GHRH, which stimulates,[4] and somatostatin, which inhibits,[5] GH production.

GH secretion is maximal during puberty, occurring mostly during the night, especially during deep (stages 3–4) slow wave sleep (SWS). Sleep–wake homeostasis is the primary contributor to the temporal organization of GH secretion, whereas the influence of circadian rhythmicity is much less important.[6] In young, healthy men, nearly 60–70% of GH release occurs during delta (stages 3–4) SWS.[6] The usual nocturnal sleep-onset GH secretory pulse results from a burst of hypothalamic GHRH release occurring contemporaneously with a diminished somatostatin tone, although the nocturnal GH surge can occur prior to sleep onset in both sexes. Young adult men given agents that increase SWS, such as γ-hydroxybutyrate, exhibit concomitant increases in nocturnal and 24-hour GH secretion,[7] suggesting that such drugs may be useful GH secretagogs.

Beginning in early to mid-adulthood, GH production decreases at a rate of about 14% per decade, primarily a result of a decrease in the amplitude of nocturnal GH pulses. By late adulthood, daily spontaneous GH secretion is decreased by 50–70% that exhibited in the third to fourth decades.[2] The acute secretory response of GH to pituitary stimulation with GHRH is reduced in healthy old versus young individuals. This reduced GH secretory response is thought to result from a decrease in the secretion or action of GHRH, and from a rise in somatostatinergic tone.[2]

Elderly people and GH-deficient younger adults have decreased delta sleep.[8,9] In a recent cross-sectional survey of 149 healthy men aged 16–83 years, the amount of deep SWS decreased by about 80% from young (16–25 years) to mid (36–50 years) adulthood, in temporal association with a nearly 75% reduction in spontaneous GH secretion. SWS, independent of age, was a major determinant of 24-hour and nocturnal GH release.[10]

GH binding proteins

Circulating GH binding protein (GHBP) levels decrease after the fifth to sixth decades in healthy men.[11] Whether the age-related decline in GHBP is a consequence of a decrease in peripheral GH receptors, the putative source of GHBPs, or a reduction in GH secretion with aging, and the possible physiologic significance of these alterations remain to be established.

IGF-I

Baseline serum levels of IGF-I are derived primarily from release of hepatic IGF-I, which tends to remain relatively constant throughout the day. IGF-I levels can be augmented directly, by the administration of GH or various GH secretagogs, and indirectly by physical activity and aerobic exercise.

Circulating IGF-I is more than 95% bound to one or more of six specific binding proteins (IGFBPs), of which IGFBP-3 is the predominant circulating binding protein.[12] The major role of the IGFBPs is to prolong the circulating half-life of IGF-I[13] and enhance or restrict the bioavailability of IGF-I to the target tissues.[12] Recent evidence suggests that the IGFBPs may have mitogenic and metabolic properties of their own.

In cross-sectional studies, levels of IGF-I in unextracted serum or plasma decreased with age in men, so that IGF-I levels were 30–50% lower in the seventh than the third decade.[14] A low serum IGF-I concentration (defined arbitrarily as a value below the lowest 2.5th centile of the comparison group) occurred in 85% of healthy elderly compared with young men and in 26% of chronically institutionalized compared with healthy elderly men.[15,16] Comorbid illness and aging exert independent and additive inhibitory effects on serum IGF-I levels. Using assay methods that reduce or eliminate IGFBPs, such as acid-ethanol extraction, cross-sectional studies have revealed steadily falling IGF-I levels, from a peak of nearly 500 mg/l in young adulthood to values averaging about 100 mg/l by age 80.[17]

Baseline serum IGF-I levels are directly related to spontaneous 24-hour GH secretion in young, but not older, adults.[17] This may reflect the confounding influences of diminished hepatic synthetic function and reserve, as well as other age-related variables that independently modify IGF-I, including abdominal obesity, hyperinsulinemia, hyperglycemia, aerobic capacity, changing levels of gonadal steroids, the menopause, and various disease states. Serum IGF-I is thus a less useful indicator of GH secretion in elderly persons than in younger adults. There is to date no consensus on the optimal clinical method of assessing age-related decrements in GH release.

Changes of IGF-binding proteins with age

Levels of IGFBP-3, the major plasma IGF-I binding protein, decrease with age in men.[18] In elderly persons, plasma levels of IGFBP-3 are positively correlated with levels of IGF-I, but only weakly related to spontaneous GH release.[18] Age-related alterations in the secretory physiology of the other IGFBPs remain to be elucidated.

GH, IGF-I, and the gonadal axis

Plasma levels of GH and IGF-I are influenced by endogenous and exogenous gonadal steroids. There is a significant positive relationship between endogenous estradiol levels and spontaneous GH release in healthy elderly men.[19] In older men, some investigators have reported that there are no significant correlations between serum testosterone levels and either GHRH-stimulated or spontaneous GH secretion.[19] More recently, however, significant positive correlations have been observed between serum testosterone levels and spontaneous and GHRH-stimulated GH secretion in elderly men who had age-related reductions in serum testosterone levels.[20–22] The above observations highlight the importance of considering the influence of the sex steroid milieu in studies of the effects of aging on endogenous GH secretion.

The influence of nutritive status on the somatotropic axis

GH release is suppressed during hyperglycemia[23] and chronic malnutrition, whereas hypoglycemia and acute fasting stimulate GH secretion.[24] The threshold for, and magnitude of, GH release appear to be similar in young and elderly adults.[25] GH release is decreased with obesity,[26] particularly with intra-abdominal adiposity.[27] There is a reduction in the frequency of GH secretory bursts and a significant shortening of the circulatory half-life of GH, both of which reduce integrated daily plasma GH concentrations.[27] By comparison with normal weight controls, obese men also have diminished GHRH-stimulated GH secretion,[26] which is partly reversible by exogenous administration of GHRH, arginine, and pyridostigmine, perhaps because of increased somatostatinergic tone.

Similarly, plasma IGF-I has been inversely correlated with adiposity and body mass index (BMI)[28] and, especially, with measures of intra-abdominal obesity.[29] This relationship is independent of age,[28] is partly reversible with weight loss, and may explain the association of low levels of IGF-I with cardiovascular risk factors such as hypertension, hyperlipidemia, hyperglycemia, and insulin resistance.[30]

Physical activity, exercise, and aerobic capacity

The acute GH response to aerobic or resistance exercise is reduced with age.[29,31] Basal and exercise-stimulated plasma IGF-I levels are higher in physically conditioned versus sedentary young men. Because of the general decline in physical activity with advancing age, a decrease in aerobic capacity ($VO_{2\,max}$) may contribute to diminished serum IGF-I levels in elderly persons. Although a positive correlation between $VO_{2\,max}$ and IGF-I levels has been reported in healthy men of various ages, this association may be less robust in elderly men.[32] A sustained program of moderate-intensity resistance exercise training in elderly persons for 1 year failed to increase IGF-I levels.[33] Several current investigations are underway to assess whether chronic aerobic or resistance exercise training elicits an increase in spontaneous GH release and/or IGF-I levels in healthy or frail elderly people.

The effects of age-related GH decline on physiologic outcomes

Both aging and GH deficiency in adults are associated with clinically significant decreases in lean body and muscle mass, skeletal muscle strength (sarcopenia),[34] and whole body and skeletal muscle protein synthesis. Aerobic capacity (exercise tolerance) also tends to be reduced. Similarly, bone density is diminished and calcium balance is negative. There are, in addition, increases in total and intra-abdominal fat accompanied by higher levels of total and low-density lipoprotein (LDL) cholesterol. Reduced strength, endurance, and lean mass may contribute to falls and frailty. Increased abdominal fat, particularly the visceral as opposed to subcutaneous component, is associated with an elevated 'bad' (LDL) cholesterol, increased insulin resistance, and greater cardiovascular disease risk (the so-called 'syndrome X'). Low bone mass (osteopenia) is associated with an increased risk of fractures, which are responsible in turn for serious morbidity and mortality in elderly men.[35,36] Administration of GH to GH-deficient non-elderly adults for 6–12 months improved muscle strength[37,38] and lean body mass,[39] decreased total and abdominal fat,[40] reduced total and LDL cholesterol[41] and serum leptin levels, and resulted in gain of bone mass after 18–24 months of treatment[42] and improved quality of life.[43] In GH-deficient adults, glucose tolerance and insulin sensitivity tend to worsen within the first few months of GH administration, and improve thereafter, concurrent with the reduction in total and intra-abdominal fat.

The effects of GH replacement In GH-deficient elderly persons

Various metabolic outcomes have been assessed in short-term GH intervention studies conducted in older persons. Treatment of elderly patients with human GH for 2 weeks increased fat oxidation,[44] and decreased total and LDL cholesterol, with an early transient rise in very low-density lipoprotein (VLDL) and triglycerides and no change in high-density lipoprotein (HDL).[45] Both healthy[46,47] and unhealthy[48,49] older adults treated with GH for periods between 2 weeks,[44] 4 weeks,[50] and 6 months[46] exhibit dose-dependent increases in nitrogen, phosphate, and sodium balance, IGF-I, mid-arm circumference, and/or body weight. An increase in *de novo* protein synthesis was demonstrated after GH administration in postsurgical[44,49] but not healthy[51] older individuals.

Administration of GH for periods up to 6 months leads to substantial, predictable changes in body composition. A landmark study[52] demonstrated that administration of recombinant human GH (rhGH) to healthy men >60 years old could produce highly significant increases in lean body mass and reductions in total body fat over a 6-month period. However, subsequent trials have failed to demonstrate significant improvements in strength or bone mass in men or women treated with rhGH for up to 12 months.[46,53,54]

Administration of recombinant human IGF-I

The effects of IGF-I administration have been assessed in healthy non-obese and obese postmenopausal women, but, to date, have not been reported in elderly men. In older women, short-term (e.g. 4 weeks) administration of high doses of IGF-I improved anabolism and body composition, in association with significant side-effects, whereas low-dose IGF-I promoted lesser, but beneficial, changes in body composition with fewer side-effects.[50,55,56] In contrast, long-term (12 months) administration of IGF-I in low doses did not significantly alter body composition, bone density, or indices of psychologic function in older women, suggesting that any benefit from monotherapy with IGF-I may be transient in this population group.[57] Whether similar results would be obtained in selected populations of aged men remains to be determined.

GH secretagogs

Several GH-releasing peptides and related non-peptide GH secretagogs have been synthesized which exert potent stimulatory effects on pulsatile GH release. These novel GH secretagogs exert anti-somatostatinergic functional effects mediated via an endogenous GH secretagog receptor,[58] which, along with a naturally occurring ligand for this GH secretagog receptor,[59] has recently been identified. The physiologic role(s) of both synthetic and naturally occurring GH secretagogs, and their contribution to the age-related decline in GH production, remain to be elucidated.[60–63]

Adverse effects of GH therapy

Several categories of adverse effects are relatively common during treatment of non-elderly adults with GH, whereas others are as yet unproved but of potential concern.[64] The former group includes effects related to salt and water retention (edema, hypertension, headache, papilledema, pseudotumor cerebri), to arthralgias and carpal tunnel syndrome, and to metabolic dysfunction, whereas the latter group relates to possible stimulation of benign or malignant tissue growth. Short-term administration of GH elicited supraphysiologic increases in IGF-I in some older individuals, along with hyperinsulinemia, impaired glucose tolerance, decreased daily sodium excretion, and edema.[47] However, in other studies in which elderly men were treated for up to 6 months with low doses of GH, either no adverse effects[48] or modest increases in mean systolic blood pressure and fasting plasma glucose concentrations within the normal range[52] were noted. The adverse effects of GH on salt and water retention appear to be dose-dependent, and are more often evident with supraphysiologic increases in circulating IGF-I levels.[65] However, even low-dose regimens of GH administration are non-physiologic, and serum GH profiles after parenteral administration of GH differ substantially from the normal, diurnal pattern of pulsatile GH secretion. Although there is no definitive evidence that administration of GH enhances risk for *de novo* carcinogenesis in either GH-deficient children or young adults,[1,64] it is uncertain whether GH replacement in elderly persons with age-related decrements in GH secretion enhances the risk for *de novo* mutagenesis, or of promotion or propagation of pre-existent malignant diseases.

Conclusions

There is a physiologic, age-related decline in spontaneous (nocturnal) GH release and IGF-I levels which begins in the third decade and continues into advanced old age, so that GH and IGF-I measurements in the elderly are often indistinguishable from those in younger adults with pathologic GH deficiency. This physiologic decline in GH and IGF-I, like pathologic GH deficiency in non-elderly adults, is associated with adverse changes in body composition such as diminished muscle and bone mass and increased intra-abdominal fat, with their attendant increased risks of muscle weakness, osteoporosis, obesity, diabetes mellitus, dyslipidemia, and cardiovascular disease.

Whether the decline of somatotropic function with age represents a treatable hormone deficiency state with associated adverse outcomes (e.g. muscle weakness, osteoporosis, etc.), or an age-appropriate adaptive response protecting frail older persons from increased susceptibility to homeostatic disturbances, is the focus of much current research. Recent studies suggest that administration of GH to elderly people for periods up to 6 months can reverse or attenuate some of these changes in body composition and metabolic function, but whether these effects lead to improvements in physiologic and functional status, and the quality and duration of life, remains to be established. Whether the possible clinical improvements after GH administration will be outweighed by undesirable side-effects, and whether they would be sufficient to justify the economic costs, also deserve further inquiry, as does the potential use of the newer, orally active GH-releasing peptides and related non-peptide secretagogs. Finally, the decision to treat otherwise healthy older people with GH or GH secretagogs will inevitably evoke certain ethical considerations, including a re-examination of the distinction between physiologic aging and disease, and a redefinition of what constitutes normative and successful aging.

References

1. Corpas E, Harman SM, Blackman MR. Human growth hormone and human aging. Endocr Rev 1993; 14: 20–39.
2. O'Connor KO, Stevens TE, Blackman MR. GH and aging. In: Juul A, Jorgenson JOL, eds. Growth Hormone in Adults. Cambridge, UK: Cambridge University Press, 1996: 323–66.
3. Rudman D. Growth hormone, body composition and aging. J Am Geriatr Soc 1985; 33: 800–7.
4. Cronin MJ, Thorner MO. Basic studies with growth hormone-releasing factor. In: DeGroot LJ, ed. Endocrinology, Vol. 1. Philadelphia, PA: WB Saunders, 1989: 183–91.
5. Reichlin S. Somatostatin. N Engl J Med 1983; 309: 1495–501.
6. van Cauter E, Plat L, Copinschi G. Interrelations between sleep and somatotropic axis. Sleep 1998; 21: 553–66.
7. Van Cauter E, Plat L, Scharf MB et al. Simultaneous stimulation of slow-wave sleep and growth hormone secretion by gamma-hydroxybutyrate in normal young men. J Clin Invest 1997; 100: 745–53.
8. Prinz PN, Weitzman ED, Cunningham GR, Karacan I. Plasma growth hormone during sleep in young and aged men. J Gerontol 1983; 38: 519–24.
9. Astrom C, Lindholm J. Growth hormone deficient young adults have decreased deep sleep. Neuroendocrinology 1990; 51: 82–4.
10. van Cauter E, Leproult R, Plat L. Differential rates of aging of slow wave sleep and REM sleep in normal men: impact on growth hormone and cortisol levels. JAMA 2000; 284: 861–8.
11. Hattori N, Kurahachi H, Ikekubo K et al. Effects of sex and age on serum GH binding protein levels in

normal adults. Clin Endocrinol (Oxf) 1991; 35: 295–7.

12. Ooi GT. Insulin-like growth factor-binding proteins (IGFBPs): more than just 1,2,3. Mol Cell Endocrinol 1990; 71: C39–43.

13. Guler HP, Zapf J, Schmid C, Froesch ER. Insulin-like growth factors I and II in healthy man. Estimations of half-lives and production rates. Acta Endocrinol (Copenh) 1989; 121: 753–8.

14. Clemmons DR, Van Wyk JJ. Factors controlling blood concentration of somatomedin C. Clin Endocrinol Metab 1984; 13: 113–43.

15. Rudman D, Nagraj HS, Mattson D, Erve RR, Rudman IW. Hyposomatomedinemia in the nursing home patient. J Am Geriatr Soc 1986; 34: 427–30.

16. Abbassi AA, Drinka PJ, Mattson DE, Rudman D. Low circulating levels of insulin-like growth factors and testosterone in chronically institutionalized elderly men. J Am Geriatr Soc 1993; 41: 975–82.

17. Florini JR, Prinz PN, Vitirello MV, Hintz RL. Somatomedin-C levels in healthy young and old men. Relationships to peak and 24-hour integrated levels of growth hormone. J Gerontol 1985; 40: 2–7.

18. Corpas E, Harman SM, Blackman MR. Serum IGF-binding protein-3 is related to IGF-I, but not to spontaneous GH release, in healthy old men. Horm Metab Res 1992; 24: 543–5.

19. Ho KY, Evans WS, Blizzard RM et al. Effects of sex and age on 24-hour profile of growth hormone secretion in men: importance of endogenous estradiol concentrations. J Clin Endocrinol Metab 1987; 64: 51–8.

20. Corpas E, Harman SM, Piñeyro MA et al. GHRH 1–29 twice daily reverses the decreased GH and IGF-I levels in old men. J Clin Endocrinol Metab 1992; 75: 530–5.

21. Iranmanesh A, Lizarralde G, Veldhuis JD. Age and relative adiposity are specific negative determinants of the frequency and amplitude of growth hormone (GH) secretory bursts and the half-life of endogenous GH in healthy men. J Clin Endocrinol Metab 1991; 73: 1081–8.

22. Blackman MR, Christmas C, Münzer T et al. Influence of testosterone on the GH–IGF-I axis in healthy elderly men. In: Veldhuis JD, Giustina A, eds. Sex–Steroid Interactions with Growth Hormone. New York: Springer-Verlag, 1999: 44–53.

23. Press M, Tamborlane WV, Thorner MO et al. Pituitary responses to growth hormone releasing factor in diabetes: failure of glucose-mediated suppression. Diabetes 1984; 33: 804–6.

24. Ho KY, Veldhuis J, Johnson ML et al. Fasting enhances growth hormone secretion and amplifies the complex rhythms of growth hormone secretion in man. J Clin Invest 1988; 81: 968–75.

25. Meneilly GS, Cheung E, Tuokko H. Altered responses to hypoglycemia of healthy elderly people. J Clin Endocrinol Metab 1994; 78: 1341–8.

26. Williams T, Berelowitz M, Jaffe SN et al. Impaired growth hormone (GH) responses to GH-releasing factor (GRF) in obesity: a pituitary defect reversed with weight reduction. N Engl J Med 1984; 311: 1403–7.

27. Iranmanesh A, Lizarralde G, Veldhuis JD. Age and relative adiposity are specific negative determinants of the frequency and amplitude of growth hormone (GH) secretory bursts and the half-life of endogenous GH in healthy men. J Clin Endocrinol Metab 1991; 73: 1081–8.

28. Copeland KC, Colletti RB, Devlin JD, McAuliffe TL. The relationship between insulin-like growth factor-1, adiposity and aging. Metabolism 1990; 39: 584–7.

29. Hagberg JM, Seals DR, Yerg JE et al. Metabolic responses to exercise in young and old athletes and sedentary men. J Appl Physiol 1988; 65: 900–8.

30. Rasmussen MH, Frystyk J, Andersen T et al. The impact of obesity, fat distribution and energy restriction on insulin-like growth factor-1 (IGF-1), IGF-binding protein-3, insulin and growth hormone. Metabolism 1994; 43: 315–19.

31. Craig BW, Brown R, Everhart J. Effects of progressive resistance training on growth hormone and testosterone levels in young and elderly subjects. Mech Ageing Dev 1989; 49: 159–69.

32. Poehlman ET, Copeland KC. Influence of physical activity on insulin-like growth factor in healthy younger and older men. J Clin Endocrinol Metab 1990; 71: 1468–73.

33. Pyka G, Taaffe DR, Marcus R. Effect of a sustained program of resistance training on the acute growth hormone response to resistance exercise in older adults. Horm Metab Res 1994; 26: 330–3.

34. Cuneo RC, Salomon F, Wiles CM, Sönksen PH. Skeletal muscle performance in adults with growth hormone deficiency. Horm Metab Res 1990; 33(Suppl 4): 55–60.

35. Jackson HA, Kleerkoper M. Osteoporosis in men: diagnosis, pathophysiology, and prevention. Medicine 1990; 69: 137–52.

36. Nguyen TV, Eisman JA, Kelly PJ, Sambrook PN. Risk factors for osteoporotic fractures in elderly men. Am J Epidemiol 1996; 144: 255–63.

37. Cuneo R, Salomon F, Wiles CM et al. Growth hormone treatment in growth hormone-deficient adults. II. Effects on exercise performance. J Appl Physiol 1991; 70: 695–700.

38. Johannsson G, Grimby G, Sunnerhagen KS, Bengtsson B-A. Two years of growth hormone (GH) treatment increase isometric and isokinetic muscle strength in GH-deficient adults. J Clin Endocrinol Metab 1997; 82: 2877–84.

39. Amato G, Carella C, Fazio S et al. Body composition, bone metabolism, and heart structure and function in growth hormone (GH) deficient adults before and after GH replacement therapy at low doses. J Clin Endocrinol Metab 1993; 77: 1671–6.

40. Gertner JM. Effects of growth hormone on body fat distribution in adults. Horm Res 1993; 40: 10–15.

41. Cuneo RC, Salomon F, Watts GF et al. Growth hormone treatment improves serum lipids and lipoproteins in adults with growth hormone deficiency. Metabolism 1993; 42: 1519–23.

42. Johannsson G, Rosen T, Bosaeus I et al. Two years of growth hormone (GH) treatment increases bone mineral content and density in hypopituitary patients with adult-onset GH deficiency. J Clin Endocrinol Metab 1996; 81: 2865–73.

43. Burman P, Broman JE, Hettat J et al. Quality of life in adults with growth hormone (GH) deficiency: response to treatment with recombinant human GH in a placebo-controlled 21-month trial. J Clin Endocrinol Metab 1995; 80: 3585–90.

44. Ponting GA, Halliday D, Teale JD, Sim AJW. Postoperative positive nitrogen balance with intravenous hyponutrition on growth hormone. Lancet 1988; 2: 438–9.

45. Oscarsson J, Ottosson M, Wiklund O et al. Low dose continuously infused growth hormone results in increased lipoprotein A and decreased low density lipoprotein cholesterol concentrations in middle aged men. Clin Endocrinol (Oxf) 1994; 41: 109–16.

46. Holloway L, Butterfield G, Hintz R et al. Effects of recombinant human growth hormone on metabolic indices, body composition, and bone turnover in healthy elderly women. J Clin Endocrinol Metab 1994; 79: 470–9.

47. Marcus R, Butterfield G, Holloway L et al. Effects of short term administration of recombinant human growth hormone to elderly people. J Clin Endocrinol Metab 1990; 70: 519–27.

48. Kaiser FE, Silver AJ, Morley JE. The effect of recombinant human growth hormone on malnourished older individuals. J Am Geriatr Soc 1991; 39: 235–40.

49. Binnerts A, Wilson JHP, Lamberts SWJ. The effects of human growth hormone administration in elderly adults with recent weight loss. J Clin Endocrinol Metab 1988; 67: 1312–16.

50. Thompson J, Butterfield GE, Marcus R et al. The effects of recombinant human insulin-like growth factor-I and growth hormone on body composition in elderly women. J Clin Endocrinol Metab 1995; 80: 1845–52.

51. Zachwieja JJ, Bier DM, Yarasheski KE. Growth hormone administration in older adults: effects on albumin synthesis. Am J Physiol 1994; 266: E840–4.

52. Rudman D, Feller AG, Nagraj HS et al. Effect of human growth hormone in men over 60 years old. N Engl J Med 1990; 323: 1–6.

53. Papadakis M, Grady D, Black D et al. Growth hormone replacement in healthy older men improves body composition but not functional ability. Ann Intern Med 1996; 124: 708–16.

54. Taafe DR, Pruitt L, Reim J et al. Effect of recombinant human growth hormone on the muscle strength response to resistance exercise in elderly men. J Clin Endocrinol Metab 1994; 79: 1361–6.

55. Butterfield GE, Thompson J, Rennie MJ et al. Effect of rhGH and rhIGF-I treatment on protein utilization in elderly women. Am J Physiol 1997; 272: E94–9.

56. Thompson J, Butterfield GE, Gylfadottir UK et al. Effects of human growth hormone, insulin-like growth factor-I, and diet and exercise on body composition of obese postmenopausal women. J Clin Endocrinol Metab 1998; 83: 1477–84.

57. Friedlander AI, Butterfield GE, Moynihan S et al. One year of insulin-like growth factor-I treatment does not affect bone density, body composition, or psychological measures in postmenopausal women. J Clin Endocrinol Metab 2001; 86: 1496–503.

58. Howard AD, Feighner SD, Cully DF et al. A receptor in pituitary and hypothalamus that functions in growth hormone release. Science 1996; 273: 974–7.

59. Kojima M, Hosoda H, Date Y et al. Ghrelin is a growth-hormone-releasing acylated peptide from stomach. Nature (London) 1999; 402: 656–60.

60. Copinschi G, Leproult R, Van Onderbergen A et al. Prolonged oral treatment with MK-677, a novel growth hormone secretagogue, improves sleep quality in man. Neuroendocrinology 1997; 66: 278–86.

61. Fuh VL, Bach MA. Growth hormone secretagogues: mechanisms of action and use in aging. Growth Horm IGF Res 1998; 8: 13–20.

62. Murphy MG, Bach MA, Plotkin D et al. Oral administration of the growth hormone secretagogue MK-677, markers of bone turnover in healthy and functionally impaired elderly adults. The MK-677 Study Group. J Bone Miner Res 1999; 14: 1182–8.

63. Murphy MG, Weiss S, McClung M et al. Effects of alendronate and MK-677 (a growth hormone secretagogue), individually and in combination, on markers of bone turnover and bone mineral density in postmenopausal osteoporotic women. J Clin Endocrinol Metab 2001; 86: 1116–25.

64. Consensus: critical evaluation of the safety of recombinant human growth hormone administration: statement from the Growth Hormone Research Society. J Clin Endocrinol Metab 2001; 86: 1868–70.

65. Cohn L, Feller AG, Draper MW et al. Carpal tunnel syndrome and gynecomastia during growth hormone treatment of elderly men with low circulating IGF-1 concentrations. Clin Endocrinol (Oxf) 1993; 39: 417–25.

CHAPTER 20

The thyroid

Mary H Samuels and Jerome M Hershman

Serum thyroid hormone and thyrotropin concentrations in the elderly

Thyroid function has been extensively studied in the elderly. Early studies reported significant alterations in thyroid hormone and thyrotropin (TSH) levels, as well as blunted TSH responses to exogenous thyrotropin-releasing hormone (TRH) in older subjects. However, more recent studies revealed that most of these alterations are due to the effects of illness and medications on thyroid hormone levels. Acute or chronic non-thyroidal illness decreases serum tri-iodothyronine (T_3) levels, and more severe illness also decreases serum thyroxine (T_4) levels. Serum TSH levels are usually normal, but decrease as the illness becomes more severe, and TSH responses to TRH are blunted. During recovery from acute illness, serum TSH and T_4 rise in parallel, and TSH may temporarily exceed the normal range. Glucocorticoids and dopamine reduce TSH levels, and amiodarone and propranolol block conversion of T_4 to T_3, thus elevating serum T_4 and lowering T_3 levels. For these reasons, interpretation of thyroid function tests in the elderly must include an assessment of possible effects of non-thyroidal illness or medications.[1]

In healthy elderly subjects, T_4 production decreases by approximately 25%, but serum T_4 levels are unchanged, due to reductions in T_4 clearance. T_3 production and degradation decrease by approximately 30%, and serum T_3 levels may be slightly lower compared to young subjects while remaining in the normal range.[2] One study reported decreased 24-hour mean serum TSH levels in healthy elderly men, suggesting that 24-hour TSH secretion may be decreased in the elderly.[3]

Hypothyroidism

Prevalence

The prevalence of overt hypothyroidism in the elderly ranges between 0.6 and 3%, depending on the population studied. In most studies, the prevalence is lower among men than among women, because of the increased rate of autoimmune hypothyroidism in women.[4] Subclinical (or mild) hypothyroidism, defined as an elevated serum TSH and normal serum free T_4 concentration, occurs with increasing frequency as subjects age, and is present in approximately 8–15% of the elderly population. Subclinical hypothyroidism is also more common in women (range 7–21% for women vs 2–15% for men).[5–7] Elderly subjects with subclinical hypothyroidism have at least a 2–3% annualized rate of progression to overt hypothyroidism. This rate increases to 4–5% per year if antithyroid antibodies are present.[8] The strongest predictor of progression from subclinical to overt hypothyroidism is the TSH level; baseline TSH levels of less than 10 mU/l associated with low incidence rates of overt hypothyroidism.[9]

Clinical features

It is a common impression that the typical clinical features of hypothyroidism are less pronounced in the elderly. However, one study that addressed this question systematically found that most symptoms and signs of hypothyroidism were present to similar degrees in young and old hypothyroid patients.[10] Specifically, fatigue, weakness, mental status changes, depression, hoarseness, dry skin, decreased heart rate, and slowed deep tendon reflexes were equally common in both age groups. However, elderly patients had fewer complaints of weight gain, cold intolerance, paresthesias, and muscle cramps. Thus, it appears that the major difficulty in diagnosing hypothyroidism in the elderly is not the lack of symptoms, but rather their non-specific nature. Clinical findings of hypothyroidism in the elderly are often attributed to medical illnesses, medication use, depression, or the aging process.

Causes

Most hypothyroidism in the elderly is due to autoimmune (Hashimoto's) thyroiditis, which explains the increased prevalence among elderly women, compared with men.[6,11] There is an age-dependent increase in the prevalence of antithyroid antibodies; 16% of older women and 9% of older men have antithyroid peroxidase antibodies. Between 40 and 70% of older subjects with elevated TSH levels have antithyroid antibodies, although only a minority of older subjects with antithyroid antibodies have elevated TSH levels. Euthyroid subjects with high levels of antithyroid peroxidase antibody have increased rates of development of subclinical and eventually overt hypothyroidism.

Apart from Hashimoto's thyroiditis, other causes of hypothyroidism in the elderly include thyroid surgery or radiation therapy to the neck, radioiodine treatment of Graves' disease, recovery from subacute or silent thyroiditis, and under-replacement of thyroxine in subjects with known hypothyroidism. In addition, drugs such as lithium, iodine-containing compounds (for example, radiocontrast agents or amiodarone), and interferon-alpha can cause hypothyroidism. The issue of hypothyroidism due to iodinated radiocontrast agents or amiodarone is particularly important in the elderly, since older patients are more likely to receive these agents. TSH levels should be monitored routinely in subjects receiving amiodarone, or in subjects with suggestive symptoms within 6 months of radiocontrast administration.

Treatment

Overt hypothyroidism in an elderly patient should be treated with synthetic levothyroxine, rather than other thyroid hormone preparations such as desiccated thyroid extract or combinations of L-thyroxine and L-tri-iodothyronine. The latter preparations contain unacceptably high levels of tri-iodothyronine, which can precipitate or exacerbate cardiac conditions. A meta-analysis showed that there is no additional benefit when tri-iodothyronine is used together with L-thyroxine.[12] The goal of treatment is attainment of a normal serum TSH level. The replacement dose of L-thyroxine in the elderly is lower than replacement doses used in young subjects, since the elderly have decreased metabolism of thyroxine.[11] It is usually prudent to begin with a low starting does of L-thyroxine (25 μg per day or less), especially in a patient with long-standing hypothyroidism and/or known cardiac disease. The dose is gradually increased every 4–8 weeks until the TSH is normalized. A number of medications commonly taken by elderly patients can interfere with L-thyroxine absorption, including iron and calcium supplements, and care must be taken to separate these medications from thyroid hormone doses. In addition, elderly patients with impaired gastric acid secretion due to atropic gastritis or proton pump inhibitors may require increased L-thyroxine doses.[13] In rare cases, the development of angina precludes the use of full replacement doses of thyroxine. In these cases, it is appropriate to consider surgical therapy or angioplasty while the patient is still hypothyroid,[14] followed by attempts to achieve euthyroidism once the angina is well controlled.

It is unclear whether all elderly patients with subclinical hypothyroidism should be treated. Such treatment would prevent progression to overt hypothyroidism and treat the subtle tissue effects of mild hypothyroidism, including neurocognitive symptoms, cardiovascular effects, and hyperlipidemia. In support of this, recent epidemiologic studies report associations between subclinical hypothyroidism and prevalent or incident cardiovascular disease or overall mortality,[15,16] although there are negative studies as well.[17,18] L-Thyroxine therapy of subclinical hypothyroidism improves surrogate markers of cardiovascular disease, including lipid profiles, endothelial function, and carotid intimal thickness. However, there are no intervention studies that measure cardiovascular or all-cause mortality endpoints. Based on a synthesis of the available data, there is general agreement that elevation of serum TSH above 10 mU/l is an indication for treatment with levothyroxine.[19] In contrast, asymptomatic mild elevations of TSH may be best left untreated, at least in the oldest old patients.[17,20] Patients with suggestive symptoms, abnormal cardiac function, or hyperlipidemia may benefit most from therapy for subclinical hypothyroidism, but this has not been rigorously tested.

Hyperthyroidism

Prevalence

Hyperthyroidism occurs in 0.2–2% of the elderly population, with somewhat higher rates in elderly women compared with elderly men.[5,6,21] Subclinical hyperthyroidism, defined as a suppressed serum level of TSH with normal free thyroid hormone concentrations, occurs in about 2% of elderly subjects,[2,21] with a variable progression to overt hyperthyroidism.[21,22]

Clinical features

Elderly hyperthyroid patients do not manifest the same degree of adrenergic symptoms and signs as younger hyperthyroid subjects.[23,24] Older patients have decreased rates of fatigue, weakness, nervousness, sweating, heat intolerance, hyperphagia, diarrhea, tremor, tachycardia, and hyperactive reflexes, compared with young patients with hyperthyroidism. Instead, older patients tend to present with confusion, anorexia, and atrial fibrillation. This phenomenon has been termed 'apathetic hyperthyroidism' in the elderly. Such patients can be mistakenly diagnosed with cancer, heart disease, dementia, or gastrointestinal illness rather than hyperthyroidism, leading to extensive and unnecessary testing.

Causes

The causes of hyperthyroidism in the elderly are similar to the causes of hyperthyroidism in young subjects, and include Graves' disease, toxic multinodular goiter, toxic adenoma, subacute or silent thyroiditis, or over-replacement with thyroid hormone preparations.[8,25] Graves' disease is less common in the elderly, while toxic multinodular goiter is more common. In addition, the development of hyperthyroidism in an elderly patient sometimes occurs after administration of amiodarone or an iodine-containing radiocontrast agent.

Risks

There are two specific risks associated with hyperthyroidism that are particularly important in older patients. First, overt hyperthyroidism has marked effects on the cardiovascular system, including enhanced myocardial contractility, accelerated heart rate, increased cardiac output, and peripheral vasodilatation. This may lead to increased myocardial oxygen demand, cardiac hypertrophy, or angina in older patients. In addition, the risk of atrial fibrillation is increased by overt or subclinical hyperthyroidism, especially in older subjects.[18,26] Results from the Framingham Study showed that 28% of subjects with subclinical hyperthyroidism developed atrial fibrillation over 10 years, compared with 11% of age-matched euthyroid subjects.[16] Second, hyperthyroidism leads to excess bone resorption and the development of osteoporosis, especially in postmenopausal women.[27] It may also contribute to osteoporosis in elderly men.

Treatment

The treatment of hyperthyroidism in the elderly depends on the cause of the disease, severity of the hyperthyroidism, and condition of the patient. Graves' disease is treated by radioactive iodine-131 or thionamide therapy. Toxic multinodular goiters and toxic adenomas are treated with radioactive iodine (at higher doses than those used to treat Graves' disease) or surgery, with the choice depending on the patient's suitability for surgery and the presence of any worrisome nodules that would warrant excision.

The decision whether to treat subclinical hyperthyroidism is difficult, since treatment options are complicated and carry some risks, and since the overall risk of subclinical hyperthyroidism has not been well quantified. A T_3 level should initially be obtained to rule out T_3 toxicosis. One should decide whether to treat subclinical hyperthyroidism based on the presence of symptoms (remembering that hyperthyroidism may be masked in elderly patients), risks for osteoporosis, and risks for atrial fibrillation or other cardiac events. In some cases, it may be prudent to initiate a trial of antithyroid drug therapy. This affords the physician and the patient a chance to see whether symptoms and other parameters improve with treatment of the subclinical hyperthyroidism. Because subjects with serum TSH less than 0.1 mU/l have a high incidence of atrial fibrillation,[18,26] the etiology should be determined and treatment should be given to these patients.

Thyroid nodules

Prevalence

Thyroid nodules, either solitary or multiple, increase in frequency with aging. The frequency of detection of nodules by ultrasonography varied from 13 to 67% in different studies.[28] The prevalence of thyroid nodules is somewhat higher in women than in men. Thyroid nodules in asymptomatic individuals ('incidentalomas') have been identified frequently by ultrasonography, which is much more sensitive than palpation. In one study the prevalence of incidentalomas was 67% by high-resolution ultrasonography and only 21% by neck palpation.[29] A large autopsy series showed that 50% of the population with no known history of thyroid disease had discrete nodules, and in 35% the nodules were greater than 2 cm in diameter.[30]

Clinical evaluation

Evaluation of the thyroid nodule focuses on the detection of malignancy. Although thyroid nodules are more frequent in women, the likelihood of malignancy is somewhat higher in men. Radiation exposure during childhood predisposes to thyroid nodules and thyroid carcinoma, but the latency period probably does not exceed 50 years, so that the chance of radiation-induced thyroid cancer from childhood exposure is low in the elderly. A family history of thyroid cancer suggests familial medullary thyroid cancer as a component of multiple endocrine neoplasia (MEN) type 2 or familial papillary cancer. Multinodular goiter is also prevalent in many families.

Most thyroid nodules are asymptomatic. Hemorrhage into a thyroid nodule or cyst may cause rapid enlargement and pain. Rapid growth of a nodule over a period of several weeks is suspicious of malignancy. Persistent hoarseness may result from recurrent laryngeal paralysis by cancer or a large multinodular goiter.

On physical examination, a firm fixed nodule is more likely to be malignant, but many differentiated carcinomas have a normal consistency. Lymphadenopathy suggests malignancy. The distinction between a solitary nodule and multinodular goiter by neck palpation is limited. In approximately 50% of cases of a clinically solitary nodule on palpation, the lesion was subsequently found to be a dominant nodule in a multinodular goiter on histologic examination.[31] The relative risk of cancer in solitary versus multinodular thyroid glands is controversial. Many studies have reported lower rates of thyroid carcinoma in palpable multinodular glands (5–13%), compared with the solitary nodules (9–25%), but other studies have found similar incidences of cancer in solitary nodules and in multinodular glands.

Diagnostic tests

A low serum TSH concentration suggests the presence of either an autonomously functioning adenoma, or a toxic multinodular goiter. Elevated antiperoxidase and antithyroglobulin antibody titers indicate lymphocytic thyroiditis, which may present as a nodule. The serum thyroglobulin level is not a useful test to distinguish benign from malignant nodules, because it is increased with any goitrous process.

In the past, radionuclide scanning of nodular thyroid glands was recommended as part of the standard evaluation. This is not a cost-effective approach, since almost all nodules in euthyroid patients are non-functioning. Therefore, the current evaluation of a suspected thyroid nodule or multinodular goiter starts with a serum TSH level. If the patient has a suppressed TSH level, a radionuclide scan is appropriate, but otherwise the patient should proceed directly to an ultrasound and fine needle aspiration biopsy, based on criteria detailed below.

Thyroid 'incidentalomas' are found by ultrasound of the neck, computed tomography, magnetic resonance imaging, and even positron emission tomography scans performed for other indications. Thyroid nodules as small as 2 mm can be detected very effectively with current high-resolution ultrasonography using a 12-MHz to 16-MHz probe. Nodules as small as 5 mm can be biopsied by fine-needle aspiration (FNA) biopsy.

Thyroid ultrasound scanning discriminates cystic from solid lesions. It has proved useful to differentiate thyroid from non-thyroid neck masses and to localize nodules deep within the gland that are not palpable. Cystic nodules constitute 10–20% of all thyroid nodules, and a significant fraction may harbor papillary carcinomas.[32] Ultrasonography is now used routinely to guide FNA biopsy.

Fine-needle aspiration biopsy provides reliable information and is the most effective method of diagnosing the cause of the nodule. Utilization of FNA biopsy has dramatically reduced the need for surgery to diagnose benign thyroid nodules. In a large series of patients who had FNA biopsy of the thyroid, benign cytology was found in 69% (mainly colloid goiter), malignant cytology in 3.5% and suspicious cytology in 10%.[33] The suspicious category is often called 'follicular lesion,' and makes up about 20 to 30% of the nodules in current series. This could represent a follicular adenoma, hyperplastic nodule in a colloid goiter, follicular cancer, or a follicular variant of papillary carcinoma. Only one-tenth to one-quarter of follicular lesions that are surgically removed are cancers. The diagnosis of follicular lesion is responsible for nearly one-half of thyroid operations on nodules. In patients with nodules that are follicular lesions, a radioiodine scan may be helpful. 'Hot' or functional nodules are rarely malignant.

Because of the high frequency of thyroid nodules and the impracticality of biopsying all of the detectable nodules, the Society of Radiologists in Ultrasound issued a consensus statement about the indications for biopsy of thyroid nodules.[34] The statement pointed out that none of the sonographic criteria that are suspicious for malignancy are sufficiently sensitive to be strong indications for biopsy without considering the size of the nodule. It recommends biopsy of nodules as small as 1 cm if there are microcalcifications because they probably represent psammoma bodies of papillary carcinoma. Other criteria for FNA biopsy include solid nodules larger than 1.5 cm, mixed solid and cystic nodules larger than 2 cm, or substantial growth of a nodule since the prior examination. The other sonographic criteria suggesting malignancy, namely hypoechogenicity, irregular margins, and increased vascularity within the nodule, were regarded as not sufficiently sensitive or specific to be strong indicators for biopsy.

Management

Treatment of the thyroid nodule depends on the functional state of the nodule and the cytologic diagnosis of the FNA biopsy. The hyperfunctioning 'hot' nodule is treated with radioiodine ablation or surgery. The vast majority of thyroid nodules are benign and can be managed medically. Medical management with thyroid hormone suppressive therapy is based on the assumption that growth of the nodule is TSH dependent. Spontaneous regression of thyroid nodules may occur. L-Thyroxine suppressive therapy is useful for nodules that do not decrease in size over several months of initial observation, but is contraindicated in elderly men with cardiac disease, and should be used with caution in elderly patients in general. In a randomized, double-blind, placebo-controlled trial of T_4 treatment of solitary thyroid nodules for 18 months, 27% of those given L-thyroxine had a volume reduction > 50% and 27% had a volume reduction of 20–50%, compared with only 17% and 14%, respectively, in the placebo group.[35] The therapy should reduce the serum TSH to the lower limit of the normal range in order to avoid the complications of subclinical thyrotoxicosis noted above. Generally, patients are followed by ultrasound or palpation at intervals of 4 to 6 months.

If the cytologic diagnosis indicates malignancy or is strongly suspicious for malignancy, the nodule should be removed surgically.

Thyroid cancer

Thyroid cancer accounts for 2.2% of all cancers in the USA, and mortality from thyroid cancer is less than 0.3% of all cancer deaths. Thyroid cancer is classified into five major types: papillary, follicular, medullary, anaplastic, and thyroid lymphoma.

Papillary carcinoma is the most common type of thyroid cancer and accounts for 80% of all thyroid cancers. Although its prognosis is generally favorable, it is more aggressive in the elderly.[36] Surgery, either near-total or total thyroidectomy, is the initial treatment of choice for papillary carcinoma. Radioiodine therapy is used as an adjunct to surgery to treat patients with residual or recurrent papillary cancer in the neck.[37] The prophylactic use of radioactive iodine ablation after surgery reduces the mortality rate and increases survival; it is generally given to any older person with papillary cancer.

Recent data show that there is a 2.4-fold increase in thyroid cancer during the past three decades. Analysis of these data indicates that the increased incidence is entirely due to more papillary thyroid cancers, primarily those smaller than 2 cm.[38] An Italian study of 243 papillary thyroid microcarcinomas, defined as smaller than 10 mm, found that none of those smaller than 8 mm had distant metastases during follow-up for a median of 5.1 years.[39] None of the patients had cancer-related mortality. A study of 211 Japanese patients with papillary microcarcinomas, diagnosed by FNA biopsy and not resected, showed that tumors smaller than 7 mm tended not to enlarge or spread to lymph nodes over a 4-year period of follow-up by ultrasound.[40]

Thyroid hormone in a suppressive dose is prescribed after thyroidectomy to reduce recurrence. TSH stimulates growth of thyroid tumors that contain TSH receptors. The dose of L-thyroxine should be adjusted to keep the TSH suppressed to subnormal levels without causing clinical thyrotoxicosis. L-Thyroxine doses may need to be more conservative in elderly patients with thyroid cancer who have cardiac disease or atrial fibrillation.

Follicular thyroid carcinoma accounts for about 10% of all thyroid cancers in the USA and occurs more frequently in the elderly. Hurthle cell carcinoma, a variant of follicular thyroid carcinoma, carries a poorer prognosis. Tumor recurrence in distant sites is more frequently seen with follicular than with papillary carcinoma, and occurs with higher prevalence in highly invasive tumors. Treatment includes total thyroidectomy, and iodine-131 therapy to ablate residual tumor. Radioiodine is the principal treatment of metastatic tumors. If the tumor does not concentrate the isotope, external radiation may be effective. As with papillary carcinoma, thyroxine therapy should be given to suppress serum TSH levels to the subnormal range.

In patients with differentiated thyroid cancer, either papillary or follicular, who have been treated by thyroidectomy and radioiodine ablation, the serum thyroglobulin is a sensitive marker for recurrence of the thyroid cancer and has replaced routine radioiodine scans in follow-up of these patients.[41] Measurement of thyroglobulin under TSH stimulation, endogenous or exogenous, is more sensitive than suppressed thyroglobulin.[42]

Medullary carcinoma accounts for 2–4% of thyroid cancers and is derived from the calcitonin-secreting cells or parafollicular cells. Elevated serum calcitonin levels establish the diagnosis and correlate with tumor mass. About 20–30% are familial tumors and are associated with other endocrine neoplasias (MEN 2A or 2B). The recognition of point mutations in RET proto-oncogene on chromosome 10 has enhanced the ability to detect these neoplasms at an early and potentially curable stage in suspected family members. Approximately 70–80% of medullary carcinoma is sporadic and diagnosed later in life, mostly after age 50 years.[43] The preferred treatment consists of total thyroidectomy and a modified radical neck dissection on the side of the tumor and the central compartment.

Anaplastic thyroid carcinoma is the most aggressive and lethal cancer. It accounts for 2% of thyroid cancer. In 28–70% of patients, there is a previous differentiated thyroid carcinoma.[44] The peak occurrence is in the seventh decade; nearly all patients are 60 years or older. It presents with a rapidly growing thyroid mass. Treatment includes surgery followed by external radiation and chemotherapy, but only a small percentage survive more than 1 year.

Thyroid lymphoma accounts for about 1% of thyroid malignancies and is almost always accompanied by chronic lymphocytic thyroiditis. The patients are usually over 60 years of age, and there is a female preponderance. This tumor nearly always arises from B-cell lymphocytes. It presents as a rapidly enlarging thyroid mass in a patient with Hashimoto's disease. FNA biopsy may suggest the diagnosis, but definitive diagnosis usually requires an open biopsy. Surgical removal of the lymphoma by total thyroidectomy is unwise. Treatment with external radiation and four to six courses of chemotherapy usually produces a permanent remission.[45]

References

1. Langton JE, Brent GA. Nonthyroidal illness syndrome: evaluation of thyroid function in sick patients. Endocrinol Metab Clin North Am 2002; 31: 159–72.
2. Hershman JM, Pekary AE, Berg L et al. Serum thyrotropin and thyroid hormone levels in elderly and middle-aged euthyroid persons. J Am Geriatr Soc 1993; 41: 823–8.
3. Barreca T, Franceschini R, Messina V et al. 24-Hour thyroid-stimulating hormone secretory pattern in elderly men. Gerontology 1985; 31: 119–23.
4. Sawin CT, Castelli WP, Hershman JM et al. The aging thyroid. Thyroid deficiency in the Framingham Study. Arch Intern Med 1985; 145: 1386–8.
5. Livingston EH, Hershman JM, Sawin CT, Yoshikawa TT. Prevalence of thyroid disease and abnormal thyroid tests in older hospitalized and ambulatory persons. J Am Geriatr Soc 1987; 35: 109–14.
6. Tunbridge WMG, Evered DC, Hall R et al. The spectrum of thyroid disease in a community: the Whickham survey. Clin Endocrinol 1977; 7: 481–93.
7. Canaris GJ, Manowitz MR, Mayor G, Ridgway EC. The Colorado thryoid disease prevalence study. Arch Intern Med 2000; 160: 526–34.
8. Vanderpump MPJ, Tunbridge WMG, French JM et al. The incidence of thyroid disorders in the community: a twenty-year follow-up of the Whickham survey. Clin Endocrinol 1995; 43: 55–68.
9. Diez JJ, Iglesias P. Spontaneous subclinical hypothyroidism in patients older than 55 years: an analysis of natural course and risk factors for the development of overt thyroid failure. J Clin Endocrinol Metab 2004; 89: 4890–7.
10. Doucet J, Trivalle C, Chassagne PH et al. Does age play a role in the clinical presentation of hypothyroidism? J Am Geriatr Soc 1994; 42: 984–6.
11. Sawin CT, Bigos ST, Land S, Bacharach P. The aging thyroid. Relationship between elevated serum thyrotropin level and thyroid antibodies in elderly patients. Am J Med 1985; 79: 591–4.
12. Grozinsky-Glasberg S, Fraser A, Nahshoni E et al. Thyroxine–triiodothyronine combination therapy versus thyroxine monotherapy for clinical hypothyroidism: meta-analysis of randomized controlled trials. J Clin Endocrinol Metab 2006; 91: 2592–9.
13. Centanni M, Gargano L, Canettieri G et al. Thyroxine in goiter, Helicobacter pylori infection, and chronic gastritis. N Engl J Med 2006; 354: 1787–95.
14. Ladenson PW, Levin AA, Ridgway EC, Daniels GH. Complications of surgery in hypothyroid patients. Am J Med 1984; 77: 261–6.
15. Imaizumi M, Akahoshi M, Ichimaru S et al. Risk for ischemic heart disease and all-cause mortality in subclinical hypothyroidism. J Clin Endocrinol Metab 2004; 89: 3365–70.
16. Walsh JP, Bremner AP, Bulsara MK et al. Subclinical thyroid dysfunction as a risk factor for cardiovascular disease. Arch Intern Med 2005; 165: 2467–72.
17. Gussekloo J, van Exel E, de Craen AJ et al. Thyroid status, disability and cognitive function, and survival in old age. JAMA 2004; 292: 2591–9.
18. Cappola AR, Fried LP. Arnold AM et al. Thyroid status, cardiovascular risk, and mortality in older adults. JAMA 2006; 295: 1033–41.
19. Surks MI, Ortiz E, Daniels GH et al. Subclinical thyroid disease: scientific review and guidelines for diagnosis and management. JAMA 2004; 291: 228–38.
20. Cooper DS. Thyroid disease in the oldest old. JAMA 2004; 292: 2651–4.
21. Sawin CT, Geller A, Kaplan MM et al. Low serum thyrotropin (thyroid stimulating hormone) in older persons without hyperthyroidism. Arch Intern Med 1991; 151: 165–8.
22. Stott DJ, McLellan AR, Finlayson J et al. Elderly patients with suppressed serum TSH but normal free thyroid hormone levels usually have mild thyroid overactivity and are at increased risk of developing overt hyperthyroidism. Q J Med 1991; 285: 77–84.
23. Davis PJ, Davis FB. Hyperthyroidism in patients over the age of 60 years. Clinical features in 85 patients. Medicine 1974; 53: 161–79.
24. Tibaldi JM, Barzel US, Albin J, Surks M. Thyrotoxicosis in the very old. Am J Med 1986; 81: 619–22.
25. Charkes ND. The many causes of subclinical hyperthyroidism. Thyroid 1996; 6: 391–6.
26. Sawin CT, Geller A, Wolf PA et al. Low serum thyrotropin concentrations as a risk factor for atrial fibrillation in older persons. N Engl J Med 1994; 331: 1249–52.
27. Lee MS, Kim SY, Lee MC et al. Negative correlation between the change in bone mineral density and serum osteocalcin in patients with hyperthyroidism. J Clin Endocrinol Metab 1990; 70: 766–70.

28. Tan GH, Gharib H. Thyroid incidentalomas: management approaches to nonpalpable nodules discovered incidentally on thyroid imaging. Ann Intern Med 1997; 126: 226–31.

29. Ezzat S, Sarti DA, Cain DR, Braunstein GD. Thyroid incidentalomas. Prevalence by palpation and ultrasonography. Arch Intern Med 1994; 154: 1838–40.

30. Mortensen JD, Woolner LB, Bennett WA. Gross and microscopic findings in clinically normal thyroid glands. J Clin Endocrinol Metab 1955; 15: 1270–6.

31. Wheeler MH. Investigation of the solitary thyroid nodule. Clin Endocrinol 1996; 44: 245–7.

32. Mazzaferri EL. Management of a solitary thyroid nodule. N Engl J Med 1993; 328: 553–9.

33. Gharib H, Goellner JR. Fine needle aspiration biopsy of the thyroid: an appraisal. Ann Intern Med 1993; 118: 282–9.

34. Frates MC, Benson CB, Charboneau JW et al. Management of thyroid nodules detected at US: Society of Radiologists in Ultrasound consensus conference statement. Radiology 2005; 237: 794–800.

35. Wemeau JL, Caron P, Schvartz C et al. Effects of thyroid-stimulating hormone suppression with levothyroxine in reducing the volume of solitary thyroid nodules and improving extranodular nonpalpable changes: a randomized, double-blind, placebo-controlled trial by the French Thyroid Research Group. J Clin Endocrinol Metab 2002; 87: 4928–34.

36. Vini J, Hyer SL, Marshall J, A'Hern R, Harmer C. Long-term results in elderly patients with differentiated thyroid carcinoma. Cancer 2003; 97: 2736–42.

37. Dulgeroff AJ, Hershman JM. Medical therapy for differentiated thyroid carcinoma. Endocr Rev 1994; 15: 500–15.

38. Davies L, Welch HG. Increasing incidence of thyroid cancer in the United States, 1973–2002. JAMA 2006; 295: 2164–7.

39. Roti E, Rossi R, Trasforini G et al. Clinical and histological characteristics of papillary thyroid microcarcinoma: results of a retrospective study in 243 patients. J Clin Endocrinol Metab 2006; 91: 2171–8.

40. Ito Y, Tomada C, Uronon T et al. Papillary microcarcinoma of the thyroid: how should it be treated? World J Surg 2004; 28: 1115–21.

41. Cooper DS, Doherty GM, Haugen BR et al. Management guidelines for patients with thyroid nodules and differentiated thyroid cancer. Thyroid 2006; 16: 109–42.

42. Pacini F, Molinaro E, Lippi F et al. Prediction of disease status by recombinant human TSH-stimulated serum Tg in the postsurgical follow-up of differentiated thyroid carcinoma. J Clin Endocrinol Metab 2001; 86: 5686–90.

43. Sizemore GW. Medullary carcinoma of the thyroid gland. Semin Oncol 1987; 14: 306–14.

44. Ain K. Anaplastic thyroid cancer. Thyroid 1998; 8: 715–26.

45. Matsuzuka F, Miyauchi A, Katayama S et al. Clinical aspects of primary thyroid lymphoma: diagnosis and treatment based on our experience of 119 cases. Thyroid 1993; 3: 93–9.

Aging and Body Composition

CHAPTER 21

Aging, testosterone, and body composition

Alex Vermeulen

Introduction

Normal aging in males is associated with important changes in body composition, characterized by a decline in fat-free mass, organ mass, and total body water, as well as by an increase in fat mass. These changes have important clinical implications: the decrease in muscle mass induces a decrease in muscle strength, with as a corollary decreased statural stability with increased tendency to fall, which, together with the age-associated osteoporosis leads to an increase in bone fracture rate, whereas the increase in abdominal fat induces insulin resistance with impaired glucose tolerance, leading eventually to diabetes mellitus, atherogenic lipid profile atherosclerosis, and an increased risk of cardiovascular disease.

Aging is accompanied by important changes in the endocrine system: a decrease in Leydig cell function and growth hormone (GH) secretion, decreased adrenal androgen secretion, and decreased melatonin secretion. As androgens as well as GH are known to increase lean body and muscle mass, whereas hypogonadism and GH deficiency are accompanied by an increased fat mass, it is tempting to postulate a causal relationship between the altered endocrine function and the age-associated changes in body composition.

Many factors, however, influence body composition and age-associated changes in lifestyle and energy balance, and a decrease in physical activity, contribute to the age-associated changes in body composition. Moreover, some of the endocrine changes observed in elderly males may be the consequence rather the cause of changes in body composition: abdominal obesity, for example, induces a decrease in GH levels as well as a decrease in hepatic sex hormone-binding globulin (SHBG) synthesis, with as a consequence a decrease in total and free testosterone levels, which can be normalized by weight loss.[1,2]

Hence, age-associated changes in body composition are determined by a complex interplay of hormonal and non-hormonal factors and it remains difficult to unravel the possible cause and effect relationships between changes in hormone levels and changes in body composition in the aging male.

Changes in body composition with age

Although symptoms of aging have a multifactorial origin, in view of the similarity of aging symptoms and the symptoms of androgen deficiency in young adults, it is generally believed that the age-associated decrease in androgen levels may play an important role in this symptomatology. It should be realized, however, that the androgen deficiency in aging males is only partial, showing moreover an important interindividual variability, that the decline in androgen levels is slow, and that aging is accompanied by a decline in almost all physiologic functions. Hence, strong correlations of symptoms with androgen levels can hardly be expected and a causal role of the latter in the clinical symptomatology will be difficult to establish.

Aging is accompanied by an *increase in fat mass*, especially abdominal visceral fat. In a study of community-dwelling, healthy men it was found that fat mass increased from 22.3% of body weight in 61 middle-aged men (mean age 42 years) to 29.4% in 271 healthy elderly men (mean age 76 years); the body mass index (BMI) was similar in both groups, but lean body mass was 20% lower in the elderly. The ratio of visceral over subcutaneous abdominal fat increased highly significantly ($P < 001$) with age from a ratio of 0.33 at age 30 to a ratio of 1.33 at age 60 years[3] Seidell et al[4,5] reported that, in a healthy population, age correlates with abdominal fat independently of BMI, whereas subcutaneous fat increases with the degree of obesity.

Fat mass is strongly negatively associated with (free) testosterone levels[3,6] and this is independent of age, the negative correlation with fat mass being almost exclusively determined by abdominal fat.[3] As, however, adiposity is a negative determinant of serum testosterone,[3] it is not evident whether the decrease in plasma testosterone is causal to the age-associated increase of (abdominal) fat. Nevertheless, some studies show that low testosterone levels predict visceral obesity, as well as the development of the metabolic syndrome and diabetes 7–10 years later[7,8] Laaksonen et al[8] reported that subjects with testosterone levels in the lowest third, after correction for BMI, were 1.7 times more likely to develop the metabolic syndrome. Similarly, Ho et al,[9] in the Rancho Bernardo study, following 294 elderly men over a period of 8 years, observed that low total testosterone levels, but not biotestosterone levels, corrected for BMI and systolic blood pressure, predicted diabetes mellitus (odds ratio 2.7; 95% confidence limits: 1.1–6.6).

However, as well as androgens, other hormonal and non-hormonal factors codetermine the age-associated changes in body fat. The decrease in GH and IGF-1 levels with age play an important role in the age-associated changes in body composition with an increase in body fat, and GH treatment may

be more effective than testosterone supplementation in reducing abdominal fat mass (see Chapter 22 by Sattler). Androgens (and estrogens), on the other hand amplify endogenous GH secretion,[10] which illustrates again the complexity of the mechanisms governing the age-associated changes in body composition. Nevertheless, the negative correlation of testosterone levels with abdominal fat persists after correction for serum GH and IGF-1 levels.[3]

With a rare exception,[11] most studies, moreover, show that testosterone supplementation in elderly men induces a modest decrease of 1–2% in fat mass.[12–17] Page et al[16] reported an even more significant decrease in fat mass of 6.3%. Hence it may be concluded that the decline in testosterone levels is coresponsible for the age-associated increase in abdominal fat.

The increase in visceral fat has important metabolic consequences: elevated free fatty acids, triglycerides, cholesterol, hyperinsulinism with impaired glucose tolerance, decreased HDL cholesterol levels and hypertension (metabolic syndrome), resulting ultimately in increased frequency of cardiovascular incidents and reduced life expectancy. Fasting insulin levels are highly significantly correlated with the abdominal/gluteal fat ratio,[3] in accordance with the generally accepted view that abdominal (visceral) fat is the major determinant of insulin resistance. Moreover, it has been observed that low testosterone levels by themselves adversely affect insulin sensitivity and the lipoprotein profile, hence contributing directly to the development of impaired glucose tolerance and the metabolic syndrome.[7]

Testosterone deficiency in young males leads to a *decrease in lean body mass and muscle strength*.[18] Bross et al[19] reported an age-associated decrease in muscle mass by as much as 35–40% in males between the ages of 20 and 80 years. The decrease in muscle mass is characterized by a decrease in the number of muscle fibers, especially type II fibers,[20] and a decline in muscle strength.

However, although exogenous androgen administration has myotrophic effects, increasing protein synthesis, increasing muscle fiber cross-sectional area, and reducing muscle degradation,[14,21,22] the correlation between endogenous (free) testosterone levels and muscle mass is less clear. Many authors[3,6,23] found no association of testosterone levels with lean body mass in a large group of community-dwelling elderly men and, in the Baltimore longitudinal study of aging, Roy et al[23] did not find any, age-corrected, correlation in men aged 20 to 90 years. Other authors, however,[6,24,25] did find an association of free testosterone levels and muscle mass, but not always with muscle strength.[24] Hence the evidence that the age-associated decline in testosterone levels is causal for the decrease in muscle mass with age is not consistent.

Androgen supplementation in elderly men causes a moderate increase in lean body mass,[10,16] but the effects on muscle strength are controversial, some authors reporting negative,[12,15,17] others[14,16,26,27] positive effects (see Chapter 23 by Sheffield-Moore).

Aging is accompanied by a progressive *bone loss*, leading to osteoporosis and an exponential increase in the incidence of fractures of hip and spine.[28,29] However, although hypogonadism in young men is accompanied by accelerated bone loss, the role of partial androgen deficiency of elderly males is still unsettled. Whereas several authors[30–33] found a significant correlation between prevalent bone mineral density (BMD) and plasma (free) testosterone levels, others[34,35] did not find any correlation. Cross-sectional studies consistently showed, however, a positive association of prevalent BMD with free or bioavailable plasma estradiol levels,[6,32,35–39] which to a large extent have a direct or indirect (via peripheral aromatization of testosterone) testicular origin and also decrease with age. Nevertheless, there is strong evidence that testosterone itself also plays a direct role in the development and maintenance of BMD, as shown by the effects of selective androgen receptor blockade on BMD in men with prostate cancer,[40] and the subnormal BMD in patients with complete androgen insensitivity, notwithstanding high estrogen levels.[41]

As to the effects of androgen substitution on BMD in elderly males, they seem to be most pronounced in patients with low basal testosterone levels,[12,17] although other authors observed that the effects were positively correlated with the magnitude of the increase in testosterone levels but not with basal levels.[42]

Unexpectedly, studying the effects of dehydro-epiandrosterone (DHEA) supplementation (50 mg/day for 1 year) on body composition and bone mineral density in 30 men over 60 years of age, with low basal dehydroepiandrosterone sulfate (DHEAS) levels, Jankowski et al[43] observed a tendency to an increase in hip BMD, without significant changes in fat or fat-free mass. These finding require confirmation by additional studies.

Conclusions

In conclusion, aging in males is accompanied by an individually variable decrease in (free) testosterone levels, a moderate decrease in free estradiol levels, and a dramatic decrease in DHEAS levels. Available data strongly suggest that, besides other hormonal (GH) and non-hormonal factors, this decrease in free testosterone and estradiol plays a contributory role in the decrease in muscle mass and BMD as well as in the age-associated increase in (abdominal) fat mass. Whereas the decrease in muscle mass and BMD plays a role in the increased tendency to falls and bone fracture rate, with its consequent invalidity, and increased morbidity and even mortality, the increase in abdominal fat mass has important metabolic consequences, reaching from hyperlipidemia, over the metabolic syndrome, to diabetes mellitus and cardiovascular disease.

References

1. Vermeulen A, Kaufman JM, Giagulli VA. Influence of some biological indices on sex-hormone-binding-globulin and androgen levels in ageing and obese males. J Clin Endocrinol Metabol 1996; 81: 1821–6.

2. Pritchard J, Despres JP, Gagnon J et al. Plasma adrenal, gonadal and conjugated steroids before and after long-term exercise induced negative energy balance in identical twins. Metabolism 1999; 48: 1120–7.

3. Vermeulen A, Goemaere S, Kaufman JM. Sex hormones, body composition and aging. Aging Male 1999; 2: 8–16.

4. Seidell JC, Björntorp P, Sjöström L, Kvist H, Sannerstedt R. Visceral fat accumulation in men is positively associated with insulin, glucose and

C-peptide levels and negatively with testosterone. Metab Clin Exp 1990; 39: 897–901.

5. Seidell JC, Oosterlee A, Duerenberg P, Hautvast JGAJ, Ruys JHGJ. Abdominal fat depots measured with computed tomography: effects of degree of obesity, sex and age. Eur J Clin Nutr 1988; 42: 805–13.

6. Van den Beld AW, de Jong FH, Grobbee DE, Pols HA, Lamberts SW. Measures of bio-available testosterone and estradiol and their relationships with muscle strength, bone density and body composition in elderly men. J Clin Endocrinol Metab 2000; 85: 3276–82.

7. Stellato RK, Feldman HA, Hamdy O, Horton ES, McKinlay JB. Testosterone, sex-hormone-binding globulin and the development of type 2 diabetes mellitus in middle-aged men. Diabetes Care 2000; 23: 490–4.

8. Laaksonen DE, Niskanen R, Purnonen K et al. Testosterone and sex-hormone-binding-globulin predict the metabolic syndrome and diabetes in middle aged men. Diabetes Care 2004; 27: 1036–41.

9. Oh JY, Barrett-Connor E, Wedick NM, Wingard DL. Endogenous sex hormones and the development of type 2 diabetes in older men and women; the Rancho Bernardo study. Diabetes Care 2002; 25: 55–60.

10. Ho KY, Weissberger AJ. Secretory patterns of growth hormone according to age and sex. Horm Res 1990; 33(Suppl 4): 7–11.

11. Sih R, Morley JE, Kaiser FE et al. Testosterone replacement in older men: a 12 month randomized controlled trial. J Clin Endocrinol Metab 1997; 82: 1661–7.

12. Kenny AM, Prestwood KM, Gruman CA, Marcello KM, Raisz LG. Effects of trandermal testosterone on bone and muscle in older men with low bio-available testosterone levels. J Gerontol A Biol Sci Med Sci 2001; 56: M266–72.

13. Blackman MB, Sorkin JD, Munzer T et al. Growth hormone and sex steroid administration on healthy aged women and men. A randomized controlled trial. JAMA 2002; 288: 2282–9.

14. Ferrando AA, Sheffield-Moore M, Yeckel CW et al. Testosterone administration to older men improves muscle function: molecular and physiological mechanisms. Am J Physiol Endocrinol Metab 2002; 282: E601–7.

15. Wittert GA, Chapman IM, Haren MT et al. Oral testosterone supplementation increases muscle mass and decreases fat mass in healthy elderly men with low normal gonadal status. J Gerontol A Bio Sci Med Sci 2003; 58: 618–25.

16. Page ST, Amory JK, Dubois-Bowman FD et al. Exogenous testosterone alone or with finasteride increases physical performance, grip strength and lean body mass in older men with low serum testosterone. J Clin Endocrinol Metab 2005; 90: 1502–10.

17. Snyder PJ, Peachey H, Hannoush P et al. Effect of testosterone treatment on bone mineral density in men over 65 years of age. J Clin Endocrinol Metab 1999; 84: 1966–72.

18. Mauras N, Hayes V, Welch S et al. Testosterone deficiency in young men: marked alterations in whole body protein kinetics, strength and adiposity. J Clin Endocrinol Metab 1998; 83: 1886–92.

19. Bross R, Javanbakht M, Bhasin S. Anabolic interventions for aging associated sarcopenia. J Clin Endocrinol Metab 1999; 84: 3420–30.

20. Larsson L. Histochemical characteristics of human skeletal muscle during aging. Acta Physiol Scand 1983; 117: 469–71.

21. Frontera WR, Hughes V, Fielding RA et al. Ageing of skeletal muscle: a 12 year longitudinal study. J Appl Physiol 2000; 88: 1321–6.

22. Sinha-Hikim I, Cornford M, Gaytan H, Lee ML, Bhasin S. Effects of testosterone supplementation on skeletal muscle fiber hypertrophy and satellite cells in community-dwelling older men. J Clin Endocrinol Metab 2006; 91: 3024–33.

23. Roy TA, Blackman LR, Harman SM et al. Interrelationships of serum testosterone and free testosterone index with FFM and strength in aging men. Am J Physiol Endocrinol Metab 2002; 283: E284–94.

24. Szulc P, Munoz F, Claustrat B et al. Bio-available estradiol may be an important determinant of osteoporosis in men: the MINOS study. J Clin Endocrinol Metab 2001; 86: 192–9.

25. Abbasi AA, Drinka PJ, Mattson DE, Rudman D. Low circulating levels of insulin-like growth factors and testosterone in chronically institutionalized elderly men. J Am Geriatr Soc 1993; 41: 975–82.

26. Sheffield-Moore M, Yeckel C, Gilkison C et al. Testosterone administration improves muscle function: molecular and physiological mechanisms. Am J Physiol Endocrinol Metab 2002; 282: E601–7.

27. Snyder PJ, Peachey H, Hannoush P et al. Effect of testosterone treatment on body composition and muscle strength in men over 65 years of age. J Clin Endocrinol Metab 1999; 84: 2647–53.

28. Oden A, Dawson A, Dere W et al. Lifetime risk of hip fractures is underestimated. Osteoporos Int 1998; 8: 599–603.

29. Cooper C, Campion G, Melton LJ. Hip fractures in the elderly: a worldwide projection. Osteoporos Int 1992; 2: 285–9.

30. Murphy S, Khaw KT, Cassidy Y, Compston JE. Sex hormones and bone mineral density in elderly men. Bone Miner 1993; 20: 133–40.

31. Kenny AM, Gallagher JC, Prestwood KM, Gruman CA, Raisz LG. Bone density, bone turnover and hormone levels in men over 75. J Gerontol A Biol Sci Med Sci 1998; 53: M419–25.

32. Greendale GA, Edelstein S, Barrett-Connor E. Endogenous sex steroids and bone mineral density in older women and men: the Rancho Bernardo study. J Bone Miner Res 1997; 12: 1833–43.

33. Jackson JA, Riggs MW, Spiekerman AM. Testosterone deficiency as risk factor for hip fractures in men: a case control study. Am J Med Sci 1992.

34. Goderie-Plomp HW, Van der Klift M, de Ronde W et al. Endogenous sex hormones, sex hormone-binding globulin and the risk of incident vertebral fractures in elderly men and women: the Rotterdam Study. J Clin Endocrinol Metab 2004; 89: 3261–9.

35. Gennari L, Merlotti D, Martini G et al. Longitudinal association between sex hormone levels, bone loss, and bone turnover in elderly men. J Clin Endocrinol Metab 2003; 88: 5327–33.

36. Khosla S, Melton LJ, Atkinson EJ, O'Fallon WM. Relationship of serum steroid levels to longitudinal changes in bone density in young versus elderly men. J Clin Endocrinol Metab 2001; 86: 3555–61.

37. Amin S, Zhang YQ, Sawin DT et al. Association of hypogonadism and estradiol levels with bone mineral density in elderly men from the Framingham study. Ann Intern Med 2000; 133: 951–63.

38. Szulc P, Claustrat B, Marchand F, Delmas PD. Increased risk of falls and increased bone resorption in elderly men with partial androgen deficiency: the MINOS study. J Clin Endocrinol Metab 2003; 88: 5240–7.

39. Goemaere S, Van Pottelbergh I, Zmierczak H et al. Inverse association between bone turnover rate and bone mineral density in community-dwelling men > 70 years of age: no major role of sex steroid status. Bone 2001; 29: 286–91.

40. Diamond T, Campbell J, Bryant C, Lynch W. The effect of combined androgen blockade on bone turnover and bone mineral densities in men treated for prostate carcinoma: longitudinal evaluation and response to intermittent etidronate therapy. Cancer 1998; 83: 1561–6.

41. Sobel V, Schwarz B, Yuan-Shan Zhu, Cordero JJ, Imperato-McGinley J. Bone mineral density in the complete androgen insensitivity and 5α-reductase deficiency syndromes. J Clin Endocrinol Metab 2006; 91: 3017–23.

42. Amory JK, Watts NB, Easley KA et al. Exogenous testosterone or testosterone with finasteride increase bone mineral density in older men with low serum testosterone. J Clin Endocrinol Metab 2004; 89: 503–10.

43. Jankowski, C, Gozansky WS, Schwarz RS et al. Effects of dehydroepiandrosterone replacement therapy on bone mineral density in older adults: a randomized controlled trial. J Clin Endocrinol Metab 2006; 91: 2986–93.

CHAPTER 22

Growth hormone and body composition in the aging male

Fred Sattler

Introduction

Growth hormone (GH) is a 191 amino acid, single-chain peptide synthesized in the somatotropic cells of the anterior pituitary gland and is often referred to as the 'master anabolic hormone.' Its biologic activity is mediated through signal transduction of a ubiquitous GH-specific transmembrane receptor. Additional effects are mediated through insulin-like growth factor 1 (IGF-1; known as the 'second message' of GH) that is synthesized largely in the liver and most other tissues. During the human aging process, daily secretion and integrated plasma concentrations of GH decrease as do IGF-1 levels.

Aging is also associated with a number of complications including loss of muscle mass (sarcopenia), increase in total and trunk fat, loss of bone mineral density, and the occurrence of metabolic derangements including dyslipidemia and insulin resistance that relate to these changes in body composition and predispose men to adverse health effects including impaired physical function, frailty, bone fractures, hypertension, and complications of atherosclerosis. Whether these undesirable effects are merely normal physiologic adaptations to aging or are in part due to the decline in GH production and secretion is uncertain. Regardless, there has been increasing interest in the potential for therapy with GH as the possible 'fountain of youth' to increase muscle mass, strength, and vigor. Hence, the relationship of GH to changes in body

composition and function during aging and evidence supporting replacement therapy with GH are the focus of this chapter. Care will be taken to consider and contrast the basis and principles of GH replacement therapy for older relatively healthy persons versus treatment of adult patients with overt hypothalamic–pituitary disease that is often associated with multiple hormone deficiencies.

Growth hormone physiology

A complex neuroendocrine network controls the mass of GH secreted per burst from the anterior pituitary. The integrated secretion of GH each day is diurnal with variable frequency and an amplitude of pulsatile release that is greatest 1 to 2 hours after subjects fall asleep. Smaller pulses occur during the day but are generally below the level of detection for most conventional assays. Hypothalamic peptidyl agonists and antagonists regulate the mass of GH secreted per burst from the pituitary gland. Facilitative signals include GH-releasing hormone (GHRH) and possibly ghrelin and GH-releasing peptides (GHRPs), whereas GH secretion is inhibited by somatostatin. Evidence suggests that decreased GH secretory-burst mass in normal aging is related to diminished GHRH or ghrelin/GHRPs, or somatostatin excess.[1,2]

A number of physiologic factors also affect the integrated GH secretion, including level of sleep, exercise and physical activity, stress hormones, body composition, nutritional status, and metabolic signals. For example, fasting, malnutrition, severe inflammation, and obesity have profound inhibitory effects on GH production. Obesity is common in older men and is associated with diminished spontaneous and stimulated GH secretion along with enhanced metabolic clearance of the hormone. These effects are possibly due to increased hypothalamic somatostatinergic tone, GHRH hyporeactivity, hyperinsulinism, or elevated free fatty acids.

Once secreted, 40–50% of the serum GH is bound to GH-binding protein (GHBP, a circulating extracellular domain of the GH receptor), which retards clearance of the hormone. Although GHBP levels are relatively constant until about 60 years of age, levels of GHBP decline thereafter up to the 10th decade of life. Supplemental androgen therapy upregulates GHBP.

Insulin like growth factor 1

IGF-1 is a proinsulin peptide, synthesized by most tissues, that mediates primarily mitogenic and proliferative actions that overlap a number of the biologic activities of GH (Table 22.1). IGF-1 binds to a discrete (type 1 IGF-1) receptor that differs from the insulin receptor to produce both cytokine-like paracrine and autocrine effects, but it also circulates and functions as a systemic hormone. The liver appears to be the primary source of systemic IGF-1, which mediates some of the systemic effects of GH (i.e., second message of GH). Blood levels of IGF-1 indirectly reflect the mass of secreted GH and serve to inhibit hypothalamic–pituitary secretion of GH. During negative caloric balance or catabolism, IGF-1 synthesis decreases and GH secretion increases, producing a state of GH resistance due to the reduction in GH effects mediated through IGF-1.

Because of the ubiquity of IGF-1 synthesis and widespread distribution of IGF-1 and GH receptors, it is difficult to clearly differentiate which of the biologic activities of GH are directly regulated and which are mediated through the IGF-1 system. Regardless, in determining IGF-1 levels, consideration must be given to caloric balance, stress, underlying disease, and factors that affect synthesis of IGF-1 by the liver and other tissues. Finally,

testosterone supplementation to high physiologic levels may increase IGF-1 secretion by the liver,[3] which could provide an additional anabolic stimulus.

Deficiencies of GH and IGF-1 with aging

The declines in GH production and secretion, GHBP, and IGF-1 levels that occur with aging are often referred to as the 'somatopause' and are the basis for speculation that these anabolic hormones are related to the body composition, metabolic, and functional changes that occur with aging. Indeed, after puberty, GH levels decrease exponentially with aging.[4] In particular, GH production has been reported to decline by 14% per decade[5] and may decline by up to 50% every 7 years in men, beginning in adulthood.[2] Elderly men may produce as little as 50 μg/day compared with pubertal boys who produce 1.0–1.5 mg/day.[6] In a study in men greater than 60 years of age, 35% were GH-deficient,[7] and GH secretion for healthy adults in their seventies was less than 50% of that in 20-year-olds.[8] Similarly, serum IGF-1 levels continue to decline through the 8th and 9th decades of life.[9] Eighty-five percent of healthy 59–98-year-old men had low serum IGF-1 levels below the 2.5th percentile of younger men.[10]

Diminished GH secretion in adults has been associated with a number of body composition, metabolic, and functional changes (Table 22.2). This constellation of symptoms, signs, and measurements has been largely determined from persons with hypopituitarism and multiple hormone deficiencies due to tumors, injury, or radiation to the hypothalamus or pituitary glands. However, there is some evidence that similar findings occur in older persons without a history or evidence of these CNS abnormalities, but with isolated low GH secretion during provocative testing.[11,12] Regardless, the constellation of findings is similar to those expected with hypogonadism or aging, making it difficult to assess their relationship to GH deficiency per se in older persons. Replacement doses of GH may appreciably ameliorate or even correct many of these abnormalities (as will be described below), especially in persons with hypopituitarism, supporting

Table 22.1 *Biologic effects of growth hormone and IGF-1*

Growth hormone	IGF-1	Both hormones
Amino acid transport into muscle	DNA and RNA synthesis	Insulin antagonism
Total body protein synthesis	Muscle hypertrophy	Islet cell synthesis
Lipolysis	Renal PO_4 and Na retention	Nitrogen retention
Fat oxidation	Linear bone growth	Somatic growth
IGF-1 production	Chondrocyte expansion	Erythropoiesis
IGFBP-3[a] and ALS[b] production	SO_4 incorporation into cartilage	Immune enhancement
Somatostatin secretion		

[a], IGF binding protein-3; [b], Acid labile subunit, which is part of the ternary complex of IGFBP-3 and IGF-1 that is the primary carrier of IGF-1 in the blood stream.

the supposition but not establishing with certainty that GH deficiency was causally related since these patients also had other hormonal abnormalities that may not have been optimally corrected.

Clinical evidence of GH deficiency due to aging

Loss of lean tissue and skeletal muscle strength

In some men, loss of muscle mass, maximal voluntary strength, and physical function occurs with aging[5] despite normal testosterone levels, suggesting that other anabolic mediators (e.g. GH and IGF-1) may be impaired and contributing to these undesirable effects. Declines in both GH and IGF-1 have been associated with progressive loss of total lean tissue from the 2nd to 7th decades.[9,10,13] In 121 men of 65–97 years of age, IGF-1 levels were highly correlated with muscle mass in one study.[14]

The importance of GH in regulating body composition and physical function is inferred from GH-treatment studies. In adult-onset GH deficiency from pituitary disease, treatment with GH increased lean tissue by 2 to 5.5 kg,[15] presumably through the known effects of GH to increase nitrogen retention and protein synthesis while decreasing protein oxidation.[16–18] Increases in cross-sectional area of muscle suggest that part of the increase in lean body mass (LBM) during treatment with GH involves

skeletal muscle.[19–21] Maximal voluntary quadriceps force and torque were not increased with short-term therapy up to 6 months in some studies,[20,22,23] suggesting that beneficial effects demonstrable by imaging may merely relate to hydration effects that would be measured as increases in appendicular LBM. However, increases in strength were demonstrable after 6–36 months of treatment in other studies of patients with pituitary diseases,[19,21,24,25] suggesting that there had been accretion of functional myofibrillar proteins. Regardless, it is unclear whether declines in GH secretion or IGF-1 levels during aging are responsible for losses in muscle mass and strength and whether replacing either hormone will consistently benefit body composition or physical strength and function during the normal aging process.

Bone mineral density is decreased and the risk of bone fractures is increased in patients with hypopituitarism.[26] Treatment with GH improves bone mineralization but it is not clear whether treatment reduces the risk of fractures.[27,28]

Accumulation of central adipose mass and metabolic complications

GH is also an important regulator of adiposity. In adults with GH deficiency due to pituitary disease fat mass is increased,[29] and it has been shown by CT and MRI that the fat accumulates centrally within the abdominal cavity.[30,31] In these patients, GH replacement therapy results in a reduction in fat

Table 22.2 Manifestations of adult growth hormone deficiency

Body composition

Decreased lean body mass
Decreased skeletal and myocardial muscle mass
Increased total and trunk adiposity
Decreased bone mineral density and osteoporosis
Dry thin skin, wrinkles

Metabolism

Decreased total body protein synthesis
Decreased lipolysis and fat oxidation
Hyperinsulinism related to obesity
Increased total and LDL cholesterol
Elevations of serum fibrinogen
Elevations of systemic plasminogen activator inhibitor 1

Function

Elevated blood pressure
Impaired cardiac function (left ventricular wall thinning, decreased stroke volume, and cardiac output)
Decreased maximum voluntary muscle strength
Anemia and diminished oxygen-carrying capacity
Decreased aerobic exercise capacity
Decreased vitality and energy
Decreased quality of life (e.g. depression, isolation)
Increased cardiovascular mortality

mass of 4–6 kg.[15] Anthropometric measurements and CT and MRI imaging indicate that reductions occur primarily in the abdominal region[29] and involve the visceral fat.[30,31]

In this population, increased adipose tissue is often associated with elevations of total serum cholesterol, LDL-C, and apolipoprotein B, fasting triglycerides and with insulin resistance and hypertension, whereas HDL cholesterol is decreased.[15] This metabolic profile may be associated with accelerated atherosclerosis and premature death due to cardiovascular disease.[32–35] Importantly, carotid artery ultrasonography has demonstrated increased intima media thickening (IMT) in these patients.[36] The commonly accepted mechanism for these metabolic changes involves the liberation of free fatty acids, which can be oxidized by peripheral tissues or taken up by the liver where they are re-esterified to triglycerides.[37–39] Treatment with GH in these patients

invariably reduces this atherogenic lipid profile.[15] Of importance, arterial IMT, a morphologic surrogate of coronary atherosclerosis, has been negatively correlated with IGF-1 levels and was significantly reduced as early as 3 months after initiation of GH treatment in subjects with adult onset GH deficiency.[40,41] Finally, treatment with GH for 6 months has decreased C-reactive protein and pulse wave velocity,[42] providing further evidence for the potential of GH treatment to reduce cardiovascular risks.

Controversial issues related to the GH deficiency syndrome

Interpretation of a body of data provides conflicting evidence as to whether manifestations attributable to GH deficiency are truly due to diminished secretion of this hormone during aging. First, many of the studies describing the constellation of findings thought to be due to GH deficiency involved patients with pathologic pituitary disease. A number of these reports were published prior to specific hormone assays or provocative testing procedures necessary to diagnose specific hormone deficiencies. Second, suboptimal therapy for other concomitant hormone deficiencies may have complicated assessment of GH deficiency in these patients. For example, overtreatment with cortisol may lead to increases in central obesity and insulin resistance. Undertreatment with thyroid hormone may be associated with obesity and elevation of LDL-C, whereas overtreatment may result in worsening osteopenia. Undertreatment with androgens may perpetuate the ongoing deficiency or even loss of lean tissue, muscle mass, and voluntary strength while sustaining central obesity. Third, a number of reports described increased mortality due to GH deficiency,[32,34,35] one of the most compelling reasons to justify GH replacement therapy. However, not all studies described excess atherosclerotic disease and a number of patients in these reports had received cranial radiation, which could adversely affect cerebral vasculature predisposing such individuals to unfavorable outcomes. Finally, there are few data describing a GH deficiency syndrome in relatively healthy older patients without other hormone deficiencies but who have low GH secretion during provocative testing. Whether the global benefits of GH treatment for patients with pituitary disease can be extrapolated to older relatively healthy adults has been a lingering question for years.

Diagnosis of GH deficiency associated with aging

Dynamic tests of GH secretion

Because of the pulsatile nature of GH secretion, single blood tests are not useful to diagnose GH deficiency. For research purposes, 24-hour or overnight sampling at least every 20 minutes and preferably every 10–15 minutes followed by deconvolusion analysis is the most definitive way to assess hypothalamic–pituitary function of the GHRH–GH system, but this is highly cumbersome and not appropriate for routine clinical management. There are several standard methods that utilize dynamic tests to identify clinical conditions associated with impaired GH secretions (Table 22.3). The insulin tolerance test (ITT) is recommended by the Growth Hormone Research Society[43] and is considered by many as the gold standard. However, the test has potential risks related to the necessity to induce hypoglycemia, namely at least a 50% drop in blood sugar from baseline or glucose level < 40 mg/dl. Thus, the ITT must be monitored closely, making this a resource-intensive test, and it is contraindicated in patients with a history of ischemic heart disease or seizures.

Several other stimulatory tests including GHRH, GHRPs, arginine, L-dopa, clonidine, somatostatin rebound, or vigorous aerobic exercise are alternative approaches used by clinicians. Although GHRP-2 bolus injection appears to be the most potent of the individual provocative tests,[44] bolus injection of GHRH followed by arginine infusion for 30 minutes appears to be a useful, reproducible, age-independent alternative to the ITT with a sensitivity and specificity of 90–95%, similar to the ITT. However, protocols (e.g. timing and intervals for blood collection and GH cut-off points with newer second and third generation GH assays) have not been well standardized.[45]

Obesity, hypothyroidism, or hypercortisolism blunt the response to GHRH stimulation, whereas malnutrition, catabolic conditions, and inflammation may be associated with elevated GH responses. For example, the evoked response to GHRH plus arginine was negatively affected by obesity as assessed by BMI.[46] These caveats should be considered when evaluating the results of any of the dynamic tests.

IGF-1 and IGFBP levels

Serum or plasma IGF-1 levels decline with age.[47] Because systemic IGF-1 levels and its major carrier protein IGFBP-3 are highly GH dependent, and serum or plasma IGF-1 or IGFBP-3 levels fluctuate very little over 24 hours, measurement of IGF-1 or IGFBP-3 is sometimes used to screen for GH deficiency. In patients with a history of or findings consistent with pituitary disease, IGF-1 levels less

Table 22.3 *Dynamic tests of growth hormone secretory capacity*

Stimulatory tests	Dosage and route of administration
Insulin tolerance test	0.05–0.15 U/kg intravenous (iv) bolus
Glucagon	1 mg intramuscularly or subcutaneously
GHRH[a]	1.0 μg/kg iv bolus
GHRP-2[b] (heralexin)	1.0 μg/kg iv bolus
GHRH + GHRP	Variable
Arginine	0.5 g/kg or 30 g infused iv over 30 minutes
L-Dopa	500 mg orally
Arginine + GHRH	GHRH iv bolus followed by a 30 minute infusion of arginine
Arginine + L-dopa	L-Dopa given orally followed by a 30 minute infusion of arginine
Clonidine	250 μg orally

[a], Growth hormone releasing hormone; [b], Growth hormone releasing peptide-2.

than 77.2 or 84 μg/l[45,48] were associated with a high predictive probability of GH deficiency. However, IGF-1 levels are affected by nutritional status and inflammation as well as age and may be normal in up to 30–40% of hypopituitary patients, especially men greater than 60 years of age.[47] Thus, measurement of these peptides should probably be used for diagnosis only in conjunction with dynamic tests of GH secretion.

Effects of GH treatment in aging men without pathologic pituitary disease

During the normal aging process there is a decline in muscle strength and functional performance, which is associated with poor medical outcome and impaired quality of life. The potential for treatment with GH has largely been extrapolated from a number of prospective and placebo-controlled studies that have demonstrated benefits of recombinant human GH (rhHG) when administered for at least 6 months in adults with primarily pituitary disease.[20,29,30,49–55] Increases in lean tissue ranged from 1.1 to 5.5 kg or up to 7%, with decreases in adipose tissue of 1.5 to 5.7 kg or up to 10% of total body fat. Effects on metabolic and functional markers were more variable but it was clear that rhGH treatment improved body composition (fat-free mass and adipose tissue) in these studies. However, the numbers of subjects studied were relatively small and reports of treatment greater than 6 months are more limited.[52,53] Further, the number of studies involving relatively healthy older patients without pathologic pituitary disease is even more limited and will be reviewed in the remainder of this section.

Effects of GH treatment on lean tissue, strength, and physical performance

In older relatively healthy men, GH deficiency is not as profound as in men with pituitary disease.[56] Thus, it is not surprising that there are only a limited number of controlled studies involving GH treatment for this population (Tables 22.4 and 22.5). In these studies, subjects generally had low IGF-1 levels, a putative marker of GH deficiency. During treatment, increases in IGF-1 were of similar magnitude to increases in younger persons given GH, indicating that systemic responsiveness to GH treatment was preserved and that the low levels of IGF-1 were likely due to GH deficiency.

In the first study of 21 men 61–81 years old, subjects were assigned to treatment with 0.03 mg/kg biosynthetic GH three times weekly or no treatment for 6 months. Study therapy with rhGH resulted in a significant 8.8% increase in LBM by ^{40}K analysis.[7,72] Changes in strength and function

Table 22.4 *Effects of growth hormone therapy on lean tissue, bone, and strength in older men*

Study	Age (years)	n	Dose (mg/kg/week)	Length of Rx	Effects on LBM (total and regional)	Effects on strength, power, and aerobics	Effects on bone
Rudman[a,7,72]	61–81	21	0.09	12 months	↑ 8.8%	NR[b]	↑ 1.6% lumbar spine BMD[c]
Welle[a18]	62–74	10	0.09	3 months	↑ 3.3 ± 0.7 kg (total LBM)[d] ↑ 3.3 ± 1.1 kg (muscle)	↑ 14 ± 5% knee torque[e]	NR
Marcus[71]	>60	6	0.21–0.84	7 days	↓ urinary nitrogen	N/A[f] after just 7 Rx days	↑ bone remodeling
Papadakis[a58]	70–85	52	0.09	6 months	↑ 4.3%	NC[g] in handgrip, knee torque, VO$_2$max[h]	↑ 0.9% in total BMC[i]
Blackman[a59]	71 ± 1.7	74	0.09	6 months	↑ 3.1 kg	NC in 1-RM strength ↑ 8.3% in VO$_2$max	↑ osteocalcin, pro-collagen peptide
Lange[a,f60,61]	74 ± 1.0	31	0.05	3 months	↑ 2.46 ± 0.51 NC in leg CSA[k]	NC in isokinetic quad strength or leg power	NC in BMC
Hennessey[a,j 62]	71 ± 1.3	31	0.015	6 months	↑ type I/II fibers	↑ 21.3% in knee extension	NR
Taaffe[a,j 23,63]	65–82	18	0.14	10 weeks	↑ 1.4 kg (3.3%)	NC in 10 strength exercise	NR
Yarasheski[a,j 64]	67 ± 1	23	0.09–0.17	16 weeks	↑ 4.8 ± 0.6 kg	NC in 9 strength exercise	NR

a, Controlled study; sample size includes placebo and no treatment; b, not reported; c, bone mineral density; d, lean body mass; e, both knee extension and flexion; f, not available; g, non-significant change, $P > 0.05$; h, maximum consumption of oxygen in one minute; i, bone mineral content; j, with resistance exercise, see text; k, cross-sectional area.

Table 22.5 *Effects of growth hormone therapy on adipose tissue, and metabolic and functional markers in older men*

Study[a]	Length	Adipose tissue	Insulin sensitivity	Lipids	Cognitive	Quality of life
Rudman[7,72]	12 months	↓ 14.4%	Hyperglycemia in 3	NR[b]	NR	NR
Marcus[71]	7 days	NR	Impaired OGTT[c]	↓ cholesterol at all doses of GH	NR	NR
Papadakis[58]	6 months	↓ 13.1%	NR	NR	↑ trails B; NC[d] in MMS[f]/ DDS[g]	NC in GDS[e]
Blackman[59,70]	6 months	↓ 3.2 kg ↓ 14% (abdomen) ↓ 21 cm² in VAT	↓ glucose tolerance in 7; diabetes in 2	NR	NR	NR
Lange[60]	3 months	↓ 2.27 ± 0.54 kg	NR	NR	NR	NR
Taaffe[23]	10 weeks	↓ 0.8 kg (12.3%)	NR	NR	NR	NR
Yarasheski[64]	16 weeks	↓ 2.6 ± 0.8 kg	NR	NR	NR	NR
Johannssong[h,25]	9 months	↓ 9.2 ± 2.4% ↓ 18 ± 7.6% VAT	NC in GDR,[i] fasting insulin, or glucose	↓ cholesterol (0.7 mmol/l) ↓ triglycerides (0.31 mmol/l)	NR	NR

a, number of subjects and doses are listed in Table 22.4; b, not reported; c, oral glucose tolerance test (OGTT) in 5 subjects receiving 0.12 mg/kg/day but OGTT was normal in subject receiving lower doses; d, non-significant change, $P > 0.05$; e, Geriatric Depression Scale; f, Mini Mental Status test; g, Digital Symbol Substitution test; h, subjects aged 48–66 years; i, glucose disposal rate at 9 months.

were not assessed. In a second study involving 10 men 62–74 years of age, rhGH therapy (0.03 mg/kg 3 times weekly) for 6 months produced significant increases in total LBM of 3.3 ± 0.7 kg using ^{40}K counting and muscle mass of 3.3 ± 1.1 kg by urinary creatinine excretion, with a $14 \pm 5\%$ increase in isokinetic thigh strength.[18] In a third study of 52 healthy 70–85-year-old men, rhGH (0.03 mg/kg 3 times weekly) significantly increased LBM by 4.3% by DEXA scanning and ultrasonography, but there was no change in handgrip strength, isokinetic knee torque, or VO$_2$max (maximum consumption of oxygen in one minute) testing after 3 months compared with controls.[58] In a fourth study, 74 healthy men 73 ± 1.3 years old were randomized to receive rhGH at 0.03 mg/kg thrice weekly with or without testosterone supplementation or placebo for 26 weeks.[59] Those receiving GH alone experienced a significant 3.1 kg increase in LBM by DEXA. There was no change in 1-repetition maximum (1-RM) voluntary strength of the quadriceps but VO$_2$max significantly increased by 8.3%.

In a fifth study utilizing a factorial design with or without resistance training (RT), 31 healthy 74 ± 1-year-old men randomized to rhGH (final average dose of about 7.2 ± 0.8 μg/kg/day) or placebo, treatment with GH alone for 12 weeks increased fat-free mass by 2.5 ± 0.5 kg, but there were no significant changes in isokinetic quadriceps strength, leg power, or muscle fiber cross-sectional area (CSA).[60] However, the myosin heavy chain 2X isoform increased significantly, suggesting that GH may have rejuvenated the effects of IGF-1 on skeletal muscle, as suggested by increased local expression of IGF-1Ea (exon a, spliced variant) and mechano growth factor (IGF-1Ec) mRNA in these subjects.[61] Finally, in a similarly designed study involving 31 men aged 71 ± 1.3 years, treatment with GH alone significantly increased CSA area of both type I and II muscle fibers of the vastus lateralis after 3 months in seven older subjects who received only GH.[62] Although knee extension 1-RM strength increased non-significantly by 23.1% with GH alone ($P = 0.098$) versus a non-significant decline of 16.2% with placebo ($P = 0.096$), the effect of GH on strength by multivariate analysis was highly significant.

Interaction of GH treatment with resistance exercise

Several studies provide further information about the potential of GH treatment in older men to augment strength and function (Table 22.4). In 18 men 65–82 years of age with low IGF-1 levels and who had previously completed 14 weeks of progressive resistance training (PRT), addition of rhGH (0.02 mg/kg/day) for 10 weeks did not increase type I or II muscle fiber CSA or strength compared to placebo during continued PRT, although fat-free mass increased and fat mass decreased significantly by DEXA scanning for those receiving GH.[23,63] The authors concluded that deficits in GH with aging cannot explain the threshold or plateau effects of PRT in older persons who experience initial benefits with this form of exercise. In a second study of 23 sedentary 67 ± 1-year-old men with low serum IGF-1 levels assigned to concurrent PRT and randomized to rhGH (12.5–24 μg/kg/day) or placebo for 16 weeks, total fat-free mass increased more with GH, but increments in vastus lateralis protein synthesis rates, urinary creatinine excretion, and training-specific isotonic and isokinetic strength were similar in both groups.[64] Results of these two studies are similar to the factorial designed study by Hennessey et al which showed no benefits of the addition of GH to RT.[62] In these studies, PRT may have provided a maximal stimulus for muscle hypertrophy, as demonstrated in an animal model,[65] or the populations studied were too small to demonstrate small but important enhancements with GH. In addition, testosterone levels were not reported and thus some study participants may have had suboptimal testosterone status, thereby limiting the effects of GH treatment, as will be discussed later.

These data provide limited but compelling evidence that treatment with rhGH augments LBM, but limited evidence that treatment benefits skeletal muscle protein synthesis. Moreover, the studies provide limited support that the changes in body composition are associated with meaningful increases in muscle strength or power, aerobic endurance, or physical function after short periods of treatment.

Interpreting the results of GH treatment on lean tissue and physical function

Several caveats must be considered when interpreting these studies. First, much of the increase in LBM with GH treatment may have been visceral and not somatic or may have even represented fluid accumulation which is measured as lean tissue by a number of imaging procedures. The study by Welle et al[18] was the only investigation to show significant improvements in strength (knee flexion and extension torque), which suggests that there was in fact accretion of myofibrillar contractile proteins. Second, these were relatively healthy ambulatory subjects with limited evidence of frailty or physical impairment. It is possible that the effects of therapy might be different if treatment was evaluated in a more physically impaired population. Third, the treatment regimens may have confounded results related to the common use of an albeit convenient every other day dosing schedule. Data and experience suggest that adverse events are dose related. It is uncertain whether more physiologic strategies using lower doses given on a daily basis each evening would have been more tolerable. Finally, the treatment duration was relatively short in these studies (generally 6 months or less) and it is possible that more prolonged therapy, for example, of 1 to 2 years, may have produced different results with benefits including augmented strength and physical function.

Effects of GH treatment on bone

In studies of men with adult-onset GH deficiency, there is a biphasic response to therapy with increases in biochemical markers of bone remodeling generally occurring during the first 6 months of therapy with little or no effect on bone mineral density (BMD), whereas treatment for 12–18 months or longer is often associated with enhancement of bone mineral content (BMC) and BMD with little or minimal change in markers of bone turnover.[15,53,66,67] As shown in Table 22.4, there was evidence in three of the studies in aging men that rhGH increased BMD or BMC, with increases in markers of bone remodeling in a fourth study.[68] Regardless, in these subjects and in the conglomerate of adults with GH deficiency due to pituitary disease, there is no evidence that treatment with rhGH decreases risks for fractures[28] and there are probably more cost-efficient ways to treat osteopenia and osteoporosis in older men such as with bisphosphonates.

Effects of GH treatment on body fat and measures of metabolism

As indicated earlier, GH status appears to be important in regulating adiposity. Indeed, IGF-1 levels are inversely related to percent total body fat and visceral adipose tissue (VAT).[6,69] Further, in adults with GH deficiency due to pituitary disease, fat mass is increased,[29] and by CT and MRI the fat accumulates centrally within the abdominal cavity.[30,31] In these patients, GH replacement therapy results in reductions in fat mass of 4–6 kg.[15] Anthropometric measurements and CT and MRI imaging indicate that reductions occur primarily in the abdominal region[29] and involve reductions in visceral fat.[30,31]

The potential for treatment of obesity in adults without pituitary disease is supported by a placebo-controlled study of 30 relatively healthy men 48–66 years old with abdominal obesity and low serum IGF-1 levels[25] (Table 22.5). In that report, treatment with GH ($9.5\,\mu g/kg/day$) for 9 months resulted in significant reductions in total body adipose tissue, abdominal subcutaneous adipose tissue (SAT), and VAT of $9.2 \pm 2.4\%$, $6.1 \pm 3.2\%$, and $18.1 \pm 7.6\%$, respectively, by ^{40}K counting and CT imaging. These changes were associated with significant reductions in total cholesterol (0.7 mmol/l), fasting triglycerides (0.31 mmol/l), fibrinogen, and diastolic blood pressure, but fasting glucose, insulin levels, and systolic blood pressure were unchanged. The glucose disposal rate (GDR) during a hyperinsulinemic euglycemic clamp decreased modestly after 6 weeks of GH treatment but was identical to the GDR in the placebo group at 9 months.

The studies involving only men more than 60 years of age and without pituitary disease also reported significant decreases in total and abdominal fat (Table 22.5). The decreases in fat ranged from 0.8–3.2 kg or 12.3–14.4% of total body fat. One of the studies reported significant decreases in both abdominal SAT ($-27\ cm^2$) and VAT ($-21 cm^2$).[70] Such improvements in central adiposity are expected to be of importance, since increased abdominal VAT, and possibly SAT, is an important component of the metabolic syndrome and therefore predisposes older persons to increased risk for atherosclerotic complications and diabetes. In further support of these observations, IMT of the carotid artery, an early morphologic change associated with atherosclerosis, has been negatively correlated with IGF-1 levels but was significantly reduced as early as 3 months after initiation of GH treatment, albeit in adults with GH deficiency due to hypopituitarism.[40,41]

Interpreting the results of GH treatment on body fat and metabolism

Whether reductions in body fat during GH therapy in older, relatively healthy persons will actually translate into reduced risk factors for cardiovascular complications is uncertain. In none of the treatment studies of older persons without pituitary disease were changes in lipids or fibrinolysis reported, except in the short 7-day treatment study involving only six men[71] and except for the one trial that also included middle-aged men as well as some older subjects[25] (Table 22.5). Despite improvements in central obesity in these studies, the adverse effect warranting special attention was the occurrence of impaired glucose tolerance (IGT) and overt diabetes, which were reported in three of the studies of GH in older adults (Table 22.5).[57,59,71] This observation is consistent with reports of early IGT in patients with pituitary disease treated with GH.

Potential for adverse events

In the studies of older men without overt pituitary disease, there were appreciable treatment-associated side-effects including edema, myalgias and joint pain, carpal tunnel syndrome, headaches, gynecomastia, and the occurrence of IGT and even diabetes.[57–60,71,72] In a number of cases these adverse events were treatment limiting. Fluid retention is probably the most common adverse event during treatment with GH and is associated with increased plasma renin activity. Isotopic studies suggest that

fluid retention is out of proportion to the hydration effects due to the intracellular accretion of protein[64] and therefore reflects accumulation of extracellular water.

Impaired glucose tolerance and diabetes[7,59,71,73] are in part due to the tendency of GH to cause hyperinsulinism, and the impaired ability of insulin to suppress hepatic glucose output or to facilitate peripheral glucose disposal.[74,75] However, the beneficial effects of GH on reducing total and abdominal fat and increasing lean tissue and possibly skeletal muscle mass later in the course of therapy may result in restoration of insulin sensitivity to levels similar to those prior to treatment.[25,73,76]

In studies of GH treatment for adults, the number and severity of adverse events have been related to increased levels of IGF-1 during GH treatment,[57,58,77–80] and evidence suggests that dose and older age are important factors in determining tolerability of this therapy.[81–83] Symptoms and findings generally regress and often disappear completely after several weeks when the dose is reduced, treatment is terminated, or even during continued treatment. However, it is not clear whether lower doses will have the same benefits on body composition that have been clearly demonstrable in older men (Tables 22.4 and 22.5).

Need for additional scientific direction

Potential to improve muscle mass and strength

If GH supplementation is to be of value in treatment of the somatopause, therapy would need to augment the loss of muscle that occurs with aging (sarcopenia) and ameliorate or prevent frailty by increasing skeletal muscle strength. In this regard, evidence indicates that hypertrophy of skeletal muscle (by imaging and muscle fiber analysis) and enhancement of contractile fiber protein synthesis are possible in the elderly with anabolic stimuli.[84,85] In fact, increases in skeletal muscle mass and protein synthesis with resistance training are comparable to those achieved in young men.[86,87] These increases in muscle mass, contractile myofibrillar proteins, and adaptations may be associated with augmentation in maximal voluntary strength.[85,88,89] However, there is only limited evidence that treatment with GH increases voluntary skeletal muscle strength or function in older, relatively healthy men.

Understanding the relationship of low testosterone and low GH secretion

Relatively low testosterone and IGF-1 compared to youthful levels may each occur in up to 80% of elderly persons and may be associated with sarcopenia.[10] In the New Mexico Aging Process study, levels of testosterone and IGF-1 along with physical inactivity were the strongest predictors of muscle loss.[90] Yet, the interaction of testosterone and the GH axes in regulating muscle mass, strength, and physical function has not been extensively studied in the elderly, despite some evidence that testosterone levels and spontaneous GHRH-stimulated GH secretion are related in older men. Available data suggest that testosterone is the primary regulator of net muscle protein and potential for hypertrophy. In experimentally induced hypogonadism (mean testosterone of $30\,\eta g/dl$), significant decline in muscle IGF-1 mRNA and increase in muscle IGFBP-4 (an inhibitor of myofibrillar protein synthesis) occurred after 10 weeks, but there was no decrease in either mean or peak serum GH and IGF-1 levels, or GH production rates.[91] Whereas testosterone treatment of elderly men augments muscle protein synthesis, muscle mass, and strength and is associated with increased IGF-1 mRNA and decreased IGFBP-4 in muscle.[92]

These observations suggest that the effects of androgens on myocytes may be independent of systemic levels of GH or IGF-1. However, at higher doses to achieve systemic levels in the upper physiologic range (similar to youthful levels), testosterone is a potent stimulus for hepatic production of IGF-1[3,93] and augments 24-hour basal, pulsatile, and entropic GH production.[93] Thus, there may be systemic interactions between these hormonal axes, which may occur at lower levels of testosterone in the elderly whose tissues appear more sensitive to the actions of testosterone.[94]

The effects of modulating systemic levels of GH or IGF-1 in regulating muscle physiology have been less thoroughly evaluated. It is known that upregulation of autocrine or paracrine expression and secretion of IGF-1 is associated with increased myofibrillar protein and DNA synthesis. Local production of IGF-1 stimulates satellite nuclei to proliferate, differentiate, and to fuse with myofibers to maintain or re-establish the myonucleus to myofiber size ratios of the enlarged muscle fibers.[95] The potential of systemic levels of GH or IGF-1 to affect local changes in muscle is suggested by forearm infusions of GH or IGF-1, which increase local muscle protein synthesis.[96–98] Moreover, in hypogonadism induced by GnRH antagonism, treatment with rhGH significantly increased skeletal muscle androgen receptors and IGF-1 while decreasing IGFBP-4, indicating that systemic therapy with GH has the potential to upregulate muscle protein synthesis.[99] Finally, GH treatment was reported to increase myosin heavy chains in skeletal muscle.[100] Thus, increasing systemic GH may enhance the local effects of IGF-1 in skeletal muscle and may augment the effects of androgens by increasing androgen receptors in muscle cells.

When levels of testosterone and GH are both augmented, anabolic effects may be amplified. In androgen- and GH-deficient boys, therapy with both hormones resulted in a synergistic response in body composition and linear growth.[101,102] In elderly subjects, fixed doses of rhGH plus testosterone produced greater increases in LBM than either alone.[59] However, the optimal levels of these hormones acting in concert to increase muscle mass and achieve functional benefits in the elderly are unknown. Moreover, testosterone and GH may regulate different types of muscle adaptations. Androgens significantly increase muscle force and power by increasing type II fibers, which are necessary for activities such as stair climbing and rising from a chair, whereas therapy with GH up to 6 months appears to have little effect on muscle strength, but VO$_2$max may be significantly increased,[19,59] suggesting that type I fibers are primarily increased. Treatment with GH also increases the anaerobic ventilatory threshold[19] and results in a lower O$_2$ consumption at the same aerobic power output,[103] which may allow daily tasks to be done with less physiologic fatigue. Thus, the effects of GH and testosterone on muscle appear different and may be complementary.

It is possible that for GH treatment to enhance skeletal muscle mass and function in older men, low testosterone levels may have to be normalized to the physiologic range or youthful levels. Indeed, in healthy aged men with relatively low IGF-1 and testosterone levels, treatment with GH enhanced total body protein synthesis.[104] Testosterone supplementation enhanced the effects of GH but per se did not enhance protein synthesis. Whereas, in experimentally induced clinically severe hypogonadism, treatment with GH maintained protein synthesis rates, fat oxidation, and fat-free mass similar to the pretreatment eugonadal state and produced marked increases in IGF-1 and androgen receptor mRNA concentrations in skeletal muscle.[105] The latter study suggests that GH positively influences body composition in the absence of the anabolic effects of testosterone. Additional studies will be necessary to further elucidate the individual importance and interaction of these two anabolic hormones in maintaining or augmenting myofibrillar muscle protein synthesis during the aging process.

Determining the effects of GH treatment on cardiovascular risk factors during aging

Data provided in this chapter suggest that treatment of otherwise healthy older men will significantly decrease total body, abdominal, and even visceral fat. However, there are few data to indicate whether, in fact, these benefits translate into improved blood pressure, atherogenic lipid profiles, insulin sensitivity, fibrinolysis, left ventricular mass, or cardiac function in older men with abdominal obesity and components of the metabolic syndrome, as has been demonstrated in adult patients with pituitary disease.[106–109] In addition, the potential for deleterious effects, even if short term, on insulin sensitivity is worrisome. Regardless, in the context of cost–benefit considerations, demonstration that GH supplementation improves multiple components of the metabolic syndrome or survival as well as body composition would provide compelling evidence in favor of providing this therapy during the aging process for older individuals with diminishing GH secretion. The adage that more studies are needed couldn't be more relevant.

References

1. Veldhuis JD, Iranmanesh A, Weltman A. Elements in the pathophysiology of diminished growth hormone (GH) secretion in aging humans. Endocrine 1997; 7(1): 41–8.
2. Giustina A, Veldhuis JD. Pathophysiology of the neuroregulation of growth hormone secretion in experimental animals and the human. Endocr Rev 1998; 19(6): 717–97.
3. Hobbs CJ, Plymate SR, Rosen CJ, Adler RA. Testosterone administration increases insulin-like growth factor-I levels in normal men. J Clin Endocrinol Metab 1993; 77(3): 776–9.
4. Rudman D, Kutner MH, Rogers CM et al. Impaired growth hormone secretion in the adult population: relation to age and adiposity. J Clin Invest 1981; 67(5): 1361–9.
5. Iranmanesh A, Lizarralde G, Veldhuis JD. Age and relative adiposity are specific negative determinants of the frequency and amplitude of growth hormone (GH) secretory bursts and the half-life of endogenous GH in healthy men. J Clin Endocrinol Metab 1991; 73(5): 1081–8.
6. Veldhuis JD, Liem AY, South S et al. Differential impact of age, sex steroid hormones, and obesity on basal versus pulsatile growth hormone secretion in men as assessed in an ultrasensitive chemiluminescence assay. J Clin Endocrinol Metab 1995; 80(11): 3209–22.
7. Rudman D, Feller AG, Nagraj HS et al. Effects of human growth hormone in men over 60 years old [see comments]. N Engl J Med 1990; 323(1): 1–6.
8. Harris TB, Kiel D, Roubenoff R et al. Association of insulin-like growth factor-I with body composition, weight history, and past health behaviors in the very old: the Framingham Heart Study. J Am Geriatr Soc 1997; 45(2): 133–9.
9. Roubenoff R, Kehayias JJ. The meaning and measurement of lean body mass. Nutr Rev 1991; 49(6): 163–75.
10. Abbasi AA, Drinka PJ, Mattson DE, Rudman D. Low circulating levels of insulin-like growth factors and testosterone in chronically institutionalized elderly men. J Am Geriatr Soc 1993; 41(9): 975–82.
11. Corpas E, Harman SM, Blackman MR. Human growth hormone and human aging. Endocr Rev 1993; 14(1): 20–39.
12. Cuneo RC, Salomon F, McGauley GA, Sonksen PH. The growth hormone deficiency syndrome in adults. Clin Endocrinol (Oxf) 1992; 37(5): 387–97.

13. Watkins JC, Roubenoff R, Rosenberg IH. Body Composition: Measure and Screening of Change with Age. Boston, MA: Foundation for Nutritional Advancement, 1992.

14. Baumgartner RN, Waters DL, Gallagher D, Morley JE, Garry PJ. Predictors of skeletal muscle mass in elderly men and women. Mech Ageing Dev 1999; 107(2): 123–36.

15. Carroll PV, Christ ER, Bengtsson BA et al. Growth hormone deficiency in adulthood and the effects of growth hormone replacement: a review. Growth Hormone Research Society Scientific Committee. J Clin Endocrinol Metab 1998; 83(2): 382–95.

16. Russell-Jones DL, Weissberger AJ, Bowes SB et al. The effects of growth hormone on protein metabolism in adult growth hormone deficient patients. Clin Endocrinol (Oxf) 1993; 38(4): 427–31.

17. Brill KT, Weltman AL, Gentili A et al. Single and combined effects of growth hormone and testosterone administration on measures of body composition, physical performance, mood, sexual function, bone turnover, and muscle gene expression in healthy older men. J Clin Endocrinol Metab 2002; 87(12): 5649–57.

18. Welle S, Thornton C, Statt M, McHenry B. Growth hormone increases muscle mass and strength but does not rejuvenate myofibrillar protein synthesis in healthy subjects over 60 years old. J Clin Endocrinol Metab 1996; 81(9): 3239–43.

19. Cuneo RC, Salomon F, Wiles CM, Hesp R, Sonksen PH. Growth hormone treatment in growth hormone-deficient adults. I. Effects on muscle mass and strength. J Appl Physiol 1991; 70(2): 688–94.

20. Whitehead HM, Boreham C, McIlrath EM et al. Growth hormone treatment of adults with growth hormone deficiency: results of a 13-month placebo controlled cross-over study. Clin Endocrinol (Oxf) 1992; 36(1): 45–52.

21. Jorgensen JO, Thuesen L, Muller J et al. Three years of growth hormone treatment in growth hormone-deficient adults: near normalization of body composition and physical performance. Eur J Endocrinol 1994; 130(3): 224–8.

22. Jorgensen JO, Pedersen SA, Thuesen L et al. Beneficial effects of growth hormone treatment in GH-deficient adults. Lancet 1989; 1(8649): 1221–5.

23. Taaffe DR, Pruitt L, Reim J et al. Effect of recombinant human growth hormone on the muscle strength response to resistance exercise in elderly men. J Clin Endocrinol Metab 1994; 79(5): 1361–6.

24. Jorgensen JO, Pedersen SA, Thuesen L et al. Long-term growth hormone treatment in growth hormone deficient adults. Acta Endocrinol (Copenh) 1991; 125(5): 449–53.

25. Johannsson G, Marin P, Lonn L et al. Growth hormone treatment of abdominally obese men reduces abdominal fat mass, improves glucose and lipoprotein metabolism, and reduces diastolic blood pressure. J Clin Endocrinol Metab 1997; 82(3): 727–34.

26. Wuster C, Abs R, Bengtsson BA et al. The influence of growth hormone deficiency, growth hormone replacement therapy, and other aspects of hypopituitarism on fracture rate and bone mineral density. J Bone Miner Res 2001; 16(2): 398–405.

27. Clanget C, Seck T, Hinke V et al. Effects of 6 years of growth hormone (GH) treatment on bone mineral density in GH-deficient adults. Clin Endocrinol (Oxf) 2001; 55(1): 93–9.

28. Johansson AG. Gender difference in growth hormone response in adults. J Endocrinol Invest 1999; 22(5 Suppl): 58–60.

29. Salomon F, Cuneo RC, Hesp R, Sonksen PH. The effects of treatment with recombinant human growth hormone on body composition and metabolism in adults with growth hormone deficiency. N Engl J Med 1989; 321(26): 1797–803.

30. Bengtsson BA, Eden S, Lonn L et al. Treatment of adults with growth hormone (GH) deficiency with recombinant human GH. J Clin Endocrinol Metab 1993; 76(2): 309–17.

31. Snel YE, Doerga ME, Brummer RM, Zelissen PM, Koppeschaar HP. Magnetic resonance imaging-assessed adipose tissue and serum lipid and insulin concentrations in growth hormone-deficient adults. Effect of growth hormone replacement. Arterioscler Thromb Vasc Biol 1995; 15(10): 1543–8.

32. Rosen T, Bengtsson BA. Premature mortality due to cardiovascular disease in hypopituitarism. Lancet 1990; 336(8710): 285–8.

33. Bulow B, Hagmar L, Mikoczy Z, Nordstrom CH, Erfurth EM. Increased cerebrovascular mortality in patients with hypopituitarism. Clin Endocrinol (Oxf) 1997; 46(1): 75–81.

34. Bates AS, Van't Hoff W, Jones PJ, Clayton RN. The effect of hypopituitarism on life expectancy. J Clin Endocrinol Metab 1996; 81(3): 1169–72.

35. Tomlinson JW, Holden N, Hills RK et al. Association between premature mortality and hypopituitarism. West Midlands Prospective Hypopituitary Study Group. Lancet 2001; 357(9254): 425–31.

36. Markussis V, Beshyah SA, Fisher C, Sharp P, Nicolaides AN, Johnston DG. Detection of premature atherosclerosis by high-resolution ultrasonography in symptom-free hypopituitary adults. Lancet 1992; 340(8829): 1188–92.

37. Hussain MA, Schmitz O, Mengel A et al. Comparison of the effects of growth hormone and insulin-like growth factor I on substrate oxidation and on insulin sensitivity in growth hormone-deficient humans. J Clin Invest 1994; 94(3): 1126–33.

38. Angelin B, Rudling M. Growth hormone and hepatic lipoprotein metabolism. Curr Opin Lipidol 1994; 5(3): 160–5.

39. Laursen T, Jorgensen JO, Jakobsen G, Hansen BL, Christiansen JS. Continuous infusion versus daily injections of growth hormone (GH) for 4 weeks in GH-deficient patients. J Clin Endocrinol Metab 1995; 80(8): 2410–18.

40. Pfeifer M, Verhovec R, Zizek B et al. Growth hormone (GH) treatment reverses early atherosclerotic changes in GH-deficient adults. J Clin Endocrinol Metab 1999; 84(2): 453–7.

41. Colao A, Di Somma C, Rota F et al. Short-term effects of growth hormone (GH) treatment or deprivation on cardiovascular risk parameters and intima-media thickness at carotid arteries in patients with severe GH deficiency. J Clin Endocrinol Metab 2005; 90(4): 2056–62.

42. McCallum RW, Sainsbury CA, Spiers A et al. Growth hormone replacement reduces C-reactive protein and large-artery stiffness but does not alter endothelial function in patients with adult growth hormone deficiency. Clin Endocrinol (Oxf) 2005; 62(4): 473–9.

43. Consensus guidelines for the diagnosis and treatment of adults with growth hormone deficiency: summary statement of the Growth Hormone Research Society Workshop on Adult Growth Hormone Deficiency. J Clin Endocrinol Metab 1998; 83(2): 379–81.

44. Veldhuis JD, Patrie JT, Brill KT et al. Contributions of gender and systemic estradiol and testosterone concentrations to maximal secretagogue drive of burst-like growth hormone secretion in healthy middle-aged and older adults. J Clin Endocrinol Metab 2004; 89(12): 6291–6.

45. Hartman ML, Crowe BJ, Biller BM et al. Which patients do not require a GH stimulation test for the diagnosis of adult GH deficiency? J Clin Endocrinol Metab 2002; 87(2): 477–85.

46. Bonert VS, Elashoff JD, Barnett P, Melmed S. Body mass index determines evoked growth hormone (GH) responsiveness in normal healthy male subjects: diagnostic caveat for adult GH deficiency. J Clin Endocrinol Metab 2004; 89(7): 3397–401.

47. Hilding A, Hall K, Wivall-Helleryd IL et al. Serum levels of insulin-like growth factor I in 152 patients with growth hormone deficiency, aged 19–82 years, in relation to those in healthy subjects. J Clin Endocrinol Metab 1999; 84(6): 2013–19.

48. Biller BM, Samuels MH, Zagar A et al. Sensitivity and specificity of six tests for the diagnosis of adult GH deficiency. J Clin Endocrinol Metab 2002; 87(5): 2067–79.

49. Cuneo RC, Salomon F, Watts GF, Hesp R, Sonksen PH. Growth hormone treatment improves serum lipids and lipoproteins in adults with growth hormone deficiency. Metabolism 1993; 42(12): 1519–23.

50. Beshyah SA, Sharp PS, Gelding SV, Halliday D, Johnston DG. Whole-body leucine turnover in adults on conventional treatment for hypopituitarism. Acta Endocrinol (Copenh) 1993; 129(2): 158–64.

51. Eden S, Wiklund O, Oscarsson J, Rosen T, Bengtsson BA. Growth hormone treatment of growth hormone-deficient adults results in a marked increase in Lp(a) and HDL cholesterol concentrations. Arterioscler Thromb 1993; 13(2): 296–301.

52. Hansen TB, Vahl N, Jorgensen JO, Christiansen JS, Hagen C. Whole body and regional soft tissue changes in growth hormone deficient adults after one year of growth hormone treatment: a double-blind, randomized, placebo-controlled study. Clin Endocrinol (Oxf) 1995; 43(6): 689–96.

53. Baum HB, Biller BM, Finkelstein JS et al. Effects of physiologic growth hormone therapy on bone density and body composition in patients with adult-onset growth hormone deficiency. A randomized, placebo-controlled trial. Ann Intern Med 1996; 125(11): 883–90.

54. Johannsson G, Grimby G, Sunnerhagen KS, Bengtsson BA. Two years of growth hormone (GH) treatment increase isometric and isokinetic muscle strength in GH-deficient adults [see comments]. J Clin Endocrinol Metab 1997; 82(9): 2877–84.

55. Attanasio AF, Bates PC, Ho KK et al. Human growth hormone replacement in adult hypopituitary patients: long-term effects on body composition and lipid status – 3-year results from the HypoCCS Database. J Clin Endocrinol Metab 2002; 87(4): 1600–6.

56. Toogood AA, O'Neill PA, Shalet SM. Beyond the somatopause: growth hormone deficiency in adults over the age of 60 years. J Clin Endocrinol Metab 1996; 81(2): 460–5.

57. Cohn L, Feller AG, Draper MW, Rudman IW, Rudman D. Carpal tunnel syndrome and gynaecomastia during growth hormone treatment of elderly men with low circulating IGF-I concentrations. Clin Endocrinol (Oxf) 1993; 39(4): 417–25.

58. Papadakis MA, Grady D, Black D et al. Growth hormone replacement in healthy older men improves body composition but not functional ability [see comments]. Ann Intern Med 1996; 124(8): 708–16.

59. Blackman MR, Sorkin JD, Munzer T et al. Growth hormone and sex steroid administration in healthy aged women and men: a randomized controlled trial. JAMA 2002; 288(18): 2282–92.

60. Lange KH, Andersen JL, Beyer N et al. GH administration changes myosin heavy chain isoforms in skeletal muscle but does not augment muscle strength or hypertrophy, either alone or combined with resistance exercise training in healthy elderly men. J Clin Endocrinol Metab 2002; 87(2): 513–23.

303

61. Hameed M, Lange KH, Andersen JL et al. The effect of recombinant human growth hormone and resistance training on IGF-I mRNA expression in the muscles of elderly men. J Physiol 2004; 555(Pt 1): 231–40.

62. Hennessey JV, Chromiak JA, DellaVentura S et al. Growth hormone administration and exercise effects on muscle fiber type and diameter in moderately frail older people. J Am Geriatr Soc 2001; 49(7): 852–8.

63. Taaffe DR, Jin IH, Vu TH, Hoffman AR, Marcus R. Lack of effect of recombinant human growth hormone (GH) on muscle morphology and GH-insulin-like growth factor expression in resistance-trained elderly men. J Clin Endocrinol Metab 1996; 81(1): 421–5.

64. Yarasheski KE, Zachwieja JJ, Campbell JA, Bier DM. Effect of growth hormone and resistance exercise on muscle growth and strength in older men. Am J Physiol 1995; 268(2 Pt 1): E268–76.

65. Goldberg AL, Goodman HM. Relationship between growth hormone and muscular work in determining muscle size. J Physiol (Lond) 1969; 200(3): 655–66.

66. Ohlsson C, Bengtsson BA, Isaksson OG, Andreassen TT, Slootweg MC. Growth hormone and bone. Endocr Rev 1998; 19(1): 55–79.

67. Hansen TB, Brixen K, Vahl N et al. Effects of 12 months of growth hormone (GH) treatment on calciotropic hormones, calcium homeostasis, and bone metabolism in adults with acquired GH deficiency: a double blind, randomized, placebo-controlled study. J Clin Endocrinol Metab 1996; 81(9): 3352–9.

68. Christmas C, O'Connor KG, Harman SM et al. Growth hormone and sex steroid effects on bone metabolism and bone mineral density in healthy aged women and men. J Gerontol A Biol Sci Med Sci 2002; 57(1): M12–18.

69. Marin P, Kvist H, Lindstedt G, Sjostrom L, Bjorntorp P. Low concentrations of insulin-like growth factor-I in abdominal obesity. Int J Obes Relat Metab Disord 1993; 17(2): 83–9.

70. Munzer T, Harman SM, Hees P et al. Effects of GH and/or sex steroid administration on abdominal subcutaneous and visceral fat in healthy aged women and men. J Clin Endocrinol Metab 2001; 86(8): 3604–10.

71. Marcus R, Butterfield G, Holloway L et al. Effects of short term administration of recombinant human growth hormone to elderly people. J Clin Endocrinol Metab 1990; 70(2): 519–27.

72. Rudman D, Feller AG, Cohn L et al. Effects of human growth hormone on body composition in elderly men. Horm Res 1991; 36(Suppl 1): 73–81.

73. Rosenfalck AM, Fisker S, Hilsted J et al. The effect of the deterioration of insulin sensitivity on beta-cell function in growth-hormone-deficient adults following 4-month growth hormone replacement therapy. Growth Horm IGF Res 1999; 9(2): 96–105.

74. Jorgensen JO, Moller J, Alberti KG et al. Marked effects of sustained low growth hormone (GH) levels on day-to-day fuel metabolism: studies in GH-deficient patients and healthy untreated subjects. J Clin Endocrinol Metab 1993; 77(6): 1589–96.

75. Ho KK, O'Sullivan AJ, Hoffman DM. Metabolic actions of growth hormone in man. Endocr J 1996; 43 (Suppl): S57–63.

76. Johnston DG, Al-Shoumer KA, Chrisoulidou A et al. Long-term effects of growth hormone therapy on intermediary metabolism and insulin sensitivity in hypopituitary adults. J Endocrinol Invest 1999; 22(5 Suppl): 37–40.

77. Holmes SJ, Shalet SM. Factors influencing the desire for long-term growth hormone replacement in adults. Clin Endocrinol (Oxf) 1995; 43(2): 151–7.

78. Thompson JL, Butterfield GE, Marcus R et al. The effects of recombinant human insulin-like growth factor-I and growth hormone on body composition in elderly women. J Clin Endocrinol Metab 1995; 80(6): 1845–52.

79. Holloway L, Butterfield G, Hintz RL, Gesundheit N, Marcus R. Effects of recombinant human growth hormone on metabolic indices, body composition, and bone turnover in healthy elderly women. J Clin Endocrinol Metab 1994; 79(2): 470–9.

80. Chipman JJ, Attanasio AF, Birkett MA et al. The safety profile of GH replacement therapy in adults. Clin Endocrinol (Oxf) 1997; 46(4): 473–81.

81. Kehely A, Bates PC, Frewer P et al. Short-term safety and efficacy of human GH replacement therapy in 595 adults with GH deficiency: a comparison of two dosage algorithms. J Clin Endocrinol Metab 2002; 87(5): 1974–9.

82. Yuen K, Ong K, Husbands S et al. The effects of short-term administration of two low doses versus the standard GH replacement dose on insulin sensitivity and fasting glucose levels in young healthy adults. J Clin Endocrinol Metab 2002; 87(5): 1989–95.

83. Gillberg P, Bramnert M, Thoren M, Werner S, Johannsson G. Commencing growth hormone replacement in adults with a fixed low dose. Effects on serum lipoproteins, glucose metabolism, body composition, and cardiovascular function. Growth Horm IGF Res 2001; 11(5): 273–81.

84. Frontera WR, Meredith CN, O'Reilly KP, Knuttgen HG, Evans WJ. Strength conditioning in older men: skeletal muscle hypertrophy and improved function. J Appl Physiol 1988; 64(3): 1038–44.

85. Singh MA, Ding W, Manfredi TJ et al. Insulin-like growth factor I in skeletal muscle after weight-lifting exercise in frail elders Am J Physiol 1999; 277(1 Pt 1): E135–43.

86. Luthi JM, Howald H, Claassen H et al. Structural changes in skeletal muscle tissue with heavy-resistance exercise. Int J Sports Med 1986; 7(3): 123–7.

87. Hasten DL, Pak-Loduca J, Obert KA, Yarasheski KE. Resistance exercise acutely increases MHC and

mixed muscle protein synthesis rates in 78–84 and 23–32 yr olds. Am J Physiol Endocrinol Metab 2000; 278(4): E620–6.

88. Moritani T, deVries HA. Potential for gross muscle hypertrophy in older men. J Gerontol 1980; 35(5): 672–82.

89. Larsson L. Physical training effects on muscle morphology in sedentary males at different ages. Med Sci Sports Exerc 1982; 14(3): 203–6.

90. Baumgartner RN, Waters DL, Gallagher D, Morley JE, Garry PJ. Predictors of skeletal muscle mass in elderly men and women. Mech Ageing Dev 1999; 107(2): 123–36.

91. Mauras N, Hayes V, Welch S et al. Testosterone deficiency in young men: marked alterations in whole body protein kinetics, strength, and adiposity. J Clin Endocrinol Metab 1998; 83(6): 1886–92.

92. Urban RJ, Bodenburg YH, Gilkison C et al. Testosterone administration to elderly men increases skeletal muscle strength and protein synthesis. Am J Physiol Endocrinol Metab 1995; 269: E820–6.

93. Gentili A, Mulligan T, Godschalk M et al. Unequal impact of short-term testosterone repletion on the somatotropic axis of young and older men. J Clin Endocrinol Metab 2002; 87(2): 825–34.

94. Winters SJ, Sherins RJ, Troen P. The gonadotropin-suppressive activity of androgen is increased in elderly men. Metabolism 1984; 33(11): 1052–9.

95. Adams GR. Role of insulin-like growth factor in the regulation of skeletal muscle adaptation to increased loading. In: Hollooszy JO, ed. Exercise and Sport Medicine Reviews, Baltimore, Philadelphia, Hong Kong, London, Munich, Sydney, Tokyo: Williams and Wilkins, 1998; 28: 31–60.

96. Fryburg DA, Gelfand RA, Barrett EJ. Growth hormone acutely stimulates forearm muscle protein synthesis in normal humans. Am J Physiol 1991; 260(3 Pt 1): E499–504.

97. Fryburg DA. Insulin-like growth factor I exerts growth hormone- and insulin-like actions on human muscle protein metabolism. Am J Physiol 1994; 267(2 Pt 1): E331–6.

98. Fryburg DA, Jahn LA, Hill SA, Oliveras DM, Barrett EJ. Insulin and insulin-like growth factor-I enhance human skeletal muscle protein anabolism during hyperaminoacidemia by different mechanisms. J Clin Invest 1995; 96(4): 1722–9.

99. Hayes VY, Urban RJ, Jiang J et al. Recombinant human growth hormone and recombinant human insulin-like growth factor I diminish the catabolic effects of hypogonadism in man: metabolic and

100. Fong Y, Rosenbaum M, Tracey KJ et al. Recombinant growth hormone enhances muscle myosin heavy-chain mRNA accumulation and amino acid accrual in humans. Proc Natl Acad Sci USA 1989; 86(9): 3371–4.

101. Van der Werff ten Bosch JJ, Bot A. Growth hormone and androgen effects in the third decade. Acta Endocrinol Suppl 1986; 279: 29–34.

102. Pertzelan A, Blum I, Grunebaum M, Laron Z. The combined effect of growth hormone and methandrostenolone on the linear growth of patients with multiple pituitary hormone deficiencies. Clin Endocrinol (Oxf) 1977; 6(4): 271–6.

103. Irving BA, Patrie JT, Anderson SM et al. The effects of time following acute growth hormone administration on metabolic and power output measures during acute exercise. J Clin Endocrinol Metab 2004; 89(9): 4298–305.

104. Huang X, Blackman MR, Herreman K et al. Effects of growth hormone and/or sex steroid administration on whole-body protein turnover in healthy aged women and men. Metabolism 2005; 54(9): 1162–7.

105. Hayes VY, Urban RJ, Jiang J et al. Recombinant human growth hormone and recombinant human insulin-like growth factor I diminish the catabolic effects of hypogonadism in man: metabolic and molecular effects. J Clin Endocrinol Metab 2001; 86(5): 2211–19.

106. Colao A, di Somma C, Pivonello R et al. The cardiovascular risk of adult GH deficiency (GHD) improved after GH replacement and worsened in untreated GHD: a 12-month prospective study. J Clin Endocrinol Metab 2002; 87(3): 1088–93.

107. Maison P, Chanson P. Cardiac effects of growth hormone in adults with growth hormone deficiency: a meta-analysis. Circulation 2003; 108(21): 2648–52.

108. Colao A, Di Somma C, Cuocolo A et al. Does a gender-related effect of growth hormone (GH) replacement exist on cardiovascular risk factors, cardiac morphology, and performance and atherosclerosis? Results of a two-year open, prospective study in young adult men and women with severe GH deficiency. J Clin Endocrinol Metab 2005; 90(9): 5146–55.

109. Maison P, Griffin S, Nicoue-Beglah M et al. Impact of growth hormone (GH) treatment on cardiovascular risk factors in GH-deficient adults: a meta-analysis of blinded, randomized, placebo-controlled trials. J Clin Endocrinol Metab 2004; 89(5): 2192–9.

CHAPTER 23

Androgens and lean body mass in the aging male

Melinda Sheffield-Moore, Shanon Casperson, and Randall J Urban

Introduction

Considerable public interest and scientific effort has been directed towards the study of the aging male, with particular attention being focused on whether androgens can assist in the maintenance of lean body mass and strength with age. It is well established that with advancing age men undergo a gradual but inevitable decline in gonadal function, often resulting in undiagnosed hypogonadism. A few of the associated symptoms of age-related male hypogonadism or andropause are loss of lean body mass, increased adiposity, and decline in muscle strength and function. It is therefore not surprising that age-related sarcopenia poses a major health concern in old age and is identified worldwide as a significant public-health problem.[1,2]

Of primary concern is the progressive reduction in lean muscle mass and strength that occurs with aging. While the mechanisms for the decline are only just beginning to be explained,[3] the resulting loss of contractile tissue and functional capacity contributes to the increase prevalence of lower-extremity weakness and bone resorption, thus increasing fall-related disability (i.e. bone fracture) in the aging male.[4,5] Indeed, the ability to counteract progressive losses in skeletal muscle mass and strength in older men has considerable implications. By attenuating or even preventing these losses, older individuals will have an improved quality of life, prolonged independent living, and a significantly reduced dependence on structured health-care. Apart from the obvious pitfalls of age-related sarcopenia, there are also metabolic consequences to be considered. These may include a depressed basal metabolic rate, hypothalamic disruption of thermoregulation, glucose intolerance, altered lipid metabolism, and enhanced osteoporosis. Thus, as the population of older men grows the need to develop therapies to counteract losses in skeletal muscle mass and strength associated with aging takes on added significance.

Recent evidence suggests that, in controlled pharmacologic dosing and replacement therapies, androgens are clinically beneficial to various patient populations suffering from muscle wasting.[4] In particular, hypogonadal men benefit from testosterone therapy via enhanced skeletal muscle mass, increased bone density, and increased protein synthesis.[5] Moreover, changes in body composition, both increases in lean body mass and decreases in fat mass, are strongly correlated to dosage and type of drug being administered.[6–9] This chapter discusses the effects of androgens on skeletal muscle mass, strength, protein synthesis, and molecular markers of muscle in aging men.

Androgens and andropause

The maintenance of skeletal muscle mass and function in the aging male is complicated by the decline in androgens associated with a syndrome termed andropause. In contrast to the menopause in women, the andropause does not occur in all men, and its presentation and pathophysiology may vary.[10,11] Decreased potency and libido, increased fatigability, decreased muscle strength and mass, osteopenia and osteoporosis, increased adipose tissue, and depressed mood are clinical features that define andropause.[10–12] Other symptoms of andropause include prostatic gland hypertrophy and signs of feminization, for example gynecomastia.[12] Moreover, a significant reduction in serum testosterone concentrations is a core physiologic event in those affected by andropause, with the lowest androgen levels seen in men who are aged 70 years and older. While there is no definitive age of onset of andropause, serum testosterone concentrations decrease as men age,[13–16] and significant endogenous reductions in testosterone can occur as early as the fifth decade.[13] As a man ages, sex hormone-binding globulin (SHBG) concentration increases,[17] and although serum total testosterone concentrations are influenced by SHBG, serum free testosterone concentrations also decrease in healthy aging men.[14,15] Moreover, bioavailable testosterone declines with aging[18] while dihydrotestosterone (DHT) concentrations remain unchanged.[19] Unfortunately, as yet, we do not know the full health impact of these age-related hormonal changes in older men.

It is well accepted that serum testosterone concentrations decline with age; however, the association between lower serum testosterone levels and sarcopenia is less clear. The hypothesized relationship is that age-related reductions in serum testosterone prevent the maintenance of lean muscle mass, which in turn leads to muscle weakness, increased risk for falls, and diminished performance of daily living skills. For example, we know that when eugonadal young men are made hypogonadal with a gonadotropin-releasing hormone analog, lean body mass and muscle strength are lost.[20] Considering that 85% of healthy older men (ages 60–98) have serum testosterone concentrations below 480 ng/dl,[21] based upon a normal range of 480–1270 ng/dl in healthy 20–30-year-old males, the potential exists for significant numbers of men

to be affected by sarcopenia. In fact, chronically institutionalized or rehabilitating older men have been shown to have lower serum testosterone concentrations[22,23] compared to their healthy counterparts[22] indicating that the severity of loss of muscle function correlates with serum testosterone concentration. Thus, a definite link has been established between lower serum testosterone concentrations and reduced skeletal muscle function in older men. However, sarcopenia occurs in both men and women with aging, so testosterone is not the only factor implicated in muscle loss. Nevertheless, androgens are possible therapeutic alternatives to slow age-associated sarcopenia.

Androgens and muscle protein synthesis

During the last few years the scientific community has established that exogenous administration of androgens induces myotropic effects in the skeletal muscle of eugonadal males. Both testosterone and its synthetic analog oxandrolone were proven capable of inducing myotropic effects in the skeletal muscle of postabsorptive young[6,8,24,27] and older men.[6,8,25–27] In older men, long-term testosterone administration has an anabolic effect by reducing muscle protein degradation in the fasted state.[28] However, in young men after 5 days of androgen administration there was an increase in the rate of protein synthesis (i.e. fractional synthetic rate of muscle protein).[29] Overall, these findings have provided the physiologic and molecular evidence that androgens deserve attention in the clinical arena, as a pharmacologic intervention against losses in the lean body mass associated with age.

While natural androgens such as testosterone clearly stimulate muscle protein synthesis in young and prevent muscle breakdown in the old, they also process androgenic or virilizing effects in humans. Skeletal muscle, bone, and kidneys all show protein-building effects as a result of the androgen-induced positive nitrogen balance. However, the possible side-effects of androgen-replacement therapy limit the clinical use of these androgens to specific patient populations such as hypogonadal men because of these safety considerations. Efforts are being made to find alternative anabolic agents that can be used in women and children as well as men.

We recently demonstrated that a 14-day administration of oxandrolone in moderate doses stimulates muscle protein anabolism in older women.[30] Interestingly, our data suggest that the mechanism by which this is accomplished differs from those previously studied in men. Specifically, our data show that skeletal muscle of older women is anabolically responsive to an androgen and may be capable of achieving similar benefits of longer-term androgen supplementation as demonstrated in their older male counterparts. However, further research is needed in women to better understand the intracellular mechanisms stimulating muscle protein anabolism and the timeframe needed for protein accretion to occur. If the optimal dose and timing of androgen can be determined in older men and women that give a maximal anabolic response with minimal side-effects, the expectation is that androgens could be very beneficial in modulating age-related sarcopenia.

Androgens and muscle strength

As men age and lose lean body mass and circulating levels of serum testosterone, physical strength is compromised. Evidence from a 12-year longitudinal study of aging skeletal muscle indicates that the quantitative loss in muscle cross-sectional area is a major contributor to the decline in muscle strength seen with aging.[31] In fact, a correlation has been shown between circulating levels of testosterone and strength improvement in older adults involved in a resistance training program.[6] In particular, maximal strength correlates with muscle mass regardless of age, but decreases with age to a greater extent than does muscle mass. Thus, the expectation of increasing muscle strength by increasing lean body mass via the administration of therapeutic doses of androgen alone is intriguing.

The primary goal of hormone replacement therapy using androgens in the older male is to maintain strength and function of the appendicular muscles. A few studies have accomplished this by

administering therapeutic doses of androgens in hypogonadal men.[3,6,25,32] However, others have been unable to demonstrate increases in muscle strength with testosterone administration alone.[33,34] Still others have demonstrated that while testosterone administration alone improves strength and power, it does not change specific tension. Hence this leads to the conclusion that resistance exercise contributes to contractile property changes of skeletal muscle which are not obtained by testosterone administration alone.[6] In the absence of definitive findings, it is reasonable to consider that a combination of hormone replacement therapy, physical activity (i.e. resistance training), and nutritional intervention will result in optimal increases in muscle strength. However, the equally important variables of power, fatigability, and activities of daily living must not be overlooked when considering intervention programs, whether it be androgen therapy alone or in combination with exercise and nutrition. To date there is a lack of evidence relating testosterone administration and improvements in physical function. However, studies have shown that there is no relationship between fatigability and testosterone dose.[6,32] Clearly, more work is required in the aging male to determine the extent to which androgen replacement therapy positively affects measures of strength, power, and fatigability.

Molecular aspects of androgen action

The specific mechanism responsible for the increase in muscle mass and strength during androgen administration is not known. We do know that androgens induce their specific response via the androgen receptor (AR), which in turn regulates the transcription of androgen-responsive target genes. While an accumulation of DNA is therefore essential for muscle growth, we do not know the exact mechanisms of androgen-induced DNA accretion in skeletal muscle. A study in eugonadal young men and in cultured muscle satellite cells has shown that androgens increase muscle mass in part by acting on several cell types to regulate the differentiation of mesenchymal precursor cells in the skeletal muscle, although satellite cells and myonuclei are the predominant sites of AR expression.[35] Stimulation of satellite cell replication can also be caused by increases in the insulin-like growth factor-1 (IGF-1) gene. In one study, muscle hypertrophy stimulated by IGF-1 was caused by an increase in both myosin heavy chain content and the mean number of nuclei per myotube.[36] These new data support our previous finding that the increase in muscle protein synthesis that occurs with testosterone administration is mediated by increasing intramuscular concentrations of IGF-1. We found that in healthy older men, testosterone given for 1 month increased IGF-1 mRNA concentrations in muscle while also decreasing mRNA concentrations of the inhibitory IGF binding protein-4.[37]

Myostatin (also designated growth differentiation factor 8) is a member of the transforming growth factor-β (TGF-β) superfamily that is a potent regulator of muscle growth. Serum myostatin-immunoreactive protein concentrations are increased in 60–92-year-old men and women with muscle wasting from sarcopenia of aging.[38] Concentrations of mRNA encoding myostatin are decreased in skeletal muscle of young and older men and women after heavy-resistance exercise.[39] However, expression of mRNA encoding myostatin in skeletal muscle of older men is not different from that of younger men,[40] and low-dose growth hormone (GH) and testosterone administration in older men does not alter this expression.[41] Two studies, one showing that myostatin regulates muscle mass throughout the lifespan,[42] and the other showing that myostatin deficiency in a mouse with muscular dystrophy improved muscle function,[43] give great promise to the possibility of using myostatin antagonists. However, future studies should investigate myostatin expression at different doses of androgen and at crucial time points of androgen administration.

Conclusions

While advances in medicine have enabled older persons to live longer, often their quality of life is less than optimal. This is in part due to the alterations in body composition associated with the aging process. Although there is sufficient evidence to believe that androgen therapy is clinically warranted in older men afflicted with symptoms of sarcopenia, we are far from understanding the timing or mechanisms of age-associated sarcopenia. Moreover, we have not yet quieted the debate of the appropriate androgen regimen to be administered to aging males to prevent age-associated sarcopenia. The present review clearly demonstrates the need for additional cross-sectional and longitudinal studies examining the timing, dosing, and molecular mechanisms responsible for slowing progressive sarcopenia in the aging male.

References

1. Dutta C, Hadley EC. The significance of sarcopenia in old age. J Gerontol 1995; 50A: 1–4.
2. Schwartz RS. Trophic factor supplementation: effect on the age-associated changes in body composition. J Gerontol 1995; 50A: 151–6.
3. Greenland LJS, Nair KS. Sarcopenia – consequences, mechanisms, and potential therapies. Mech Ageing Develop 2003; 124: 287–99.
4. Evens WJ. Functional and metabolic consequences of sarcopenia. J Nutr 1997; 127: 998–1003S.
5. Szulc P, Claustrat B, Marchand F, Delmas PD. Increased risk of falls and increased bone resorption in elderly men with partial androgen deficiency: the MINOS study. J Clin Endocrinol Metab 2003; 88(11): 5240–7.
6. Herbst K, Bhasin S. Testosterone action on skeletal muscle. Curr Opin Clin Nutr Metab Care 2004; 7: 271–7.
7. Kong A, Edmonds P. Testosterone therapy in HIV wasting syndrome: systematic review and meta-analysis. Lancet Infect Dis 2002; 2: 692–9.
8. Bhasin S, Woodhouse L, Storer TW. Androgen effects on body composition. Growth Horm IGF Res 2003; 13(Suppl A): S63–71.
9. Woodhouse L, Gupta N, Bhasin M et al. Dose-dependent effects of testosterone on regional adipose distribution in healthy young men. J Clin Endocrin Metab 2004; 89: 718–26.
10. Mastrogiacomo I, Feghali G, Foresta C, Ruzza G. Andropause: incidence and pathogenesis. Arch Androl 1982; 9: 293–6.
11. Vermeulen A. The male climacterium. Am Med 1993; 25: 531–4.
12. Urban RJ, Veldhuis VJ. Hypothalamopituitary concomitants of ageing. In: Sowers JR, Felicetta JV, eds.

The Endocrinology of Aging. New York: Raven Press, 1988: 41–74.

13. Moroa EV, Verkhratsky NS. Hypophysealgonadal system during male aging. Arch Gerontol Geriatr 1985; 4: 13–19.

14. Nankin HR, Caulkins JH. Decreased bioavailable testosterone in aging normal and impotent men. J Clin Endocrinol Metab 1986; 63: 1418–20.

15. Tenover JS, Matsumoto AM, Plymate SR, Bremner WJ. The effects of aging in normal men on bioavailable testosterone and luteinizing hormone secretion: response to clomiphene citrate. J Clin Endocrinol Metab 1987; 65: 1118–25.

16. Vermeulen A. Clinical review 24: androgens in the aging male. J Clin Endocrinol Metab 1991; 73: 221–4.

17. Purifoy FE, Koopmans LH, Mayes DM. Age differences in serum androgen levels in normal adult males. Hum Biol 1981; 57: 71.

18. Morley JE, Kaiser FE, Perry HM III et al. Longitudinal changes in testosterone, lutenizing hormone, and follicle-stimulating hormone in healthy older men. Metabolism 1997; 46: 410–13.

19. Gary A, Feldman HA, McKinley JB, Longcope C. Age, disease and changing sex hormone levels in middle-aged men: results of the Massachusetts Male Aging Study. J Clin Endocrinol Metab 1991; 73: 1016–25.

20. Mauras N, Hayes V, Welch S et al. Testosterone deficiency in young men: marked alterations in whole body protein kinetics, strength, and adiposity. J Clin Endocrinol Metab 1998; 83: 1886–92.

21. Rudman D, Shetty KR. Unanswered questions concerning the treatment of hyposomatotropism and hypogonadism in elderly men. J Am Geriatr Soc 1994; 42: 522–7.

22. Abbasi AA, Drinka PJ, Mattson DE, Rudman D. Low circulating levels of insulin-like growth factors and testosterone in chronically institutionalized elderly men. J Am Geriatr Soc 1993; 41: 975–82.

23. Kasasih Jb, Abbasi AA, Rudman D. Serum insulin-like growth factor-I and serum testosterone status of elderly in an inpatient rehabilitation unit. Am J Med Sci 1996; 311: 169–73.

24. Ferrando AA, Sheffield-Moore M, Yeckel CW et al. Testosterone administration to older men improves muscle function: molecular and physiological mechanisms. Am J Physiol Endocrinol Metab 2002; 282: E601–7.

25. Schroeder ET, Zheng L, Yarasheski KE et al. Treatment with oxadrolone and the durability of effects in older men. J Appl Physiol 2004; 96: 1055–62.

26. Page ST, Amory JK, Bowman FD et al. Exogenous testosterone alone or with finasteride increases physical performance, grip strength and lean body mass in older men with low serum testosterone. J Clin Endocrinol Metab 2005; 90(3): 1502–10.

27. Schroeder ET, Terk M, Satller F. Androgen therapy improves muscle mass and strength but not muscle quality: results from two studies. Am J Physiol Endocrinol Metab 2003; 285: E16–24.

28. Ferrando A, Sheffield-Moore M, Paddon-Jones D, Wolfe R, Urban R. Differential anabolic effects of testosterone and amino acid feeding in older men. J Clin Endocrinol Metab 2003; 88(1): 358–62.

29. Sheffield-Moore M, Urban R, Wolfe S et al. Short term oxandrolone administration stimulates net muscle protein synthesis in young men. J Clin Endocrinol Metab 1999; 84: 2705–11.

30. Sheffield-Moore M, Paddon-Jones D, Casperson SL et al. Androgen therapy induces muscle protein anabolism in older women J Clin Endocrinol Metab 2006; 91(10): 3844–9.

31. Frontera WR, Hughes VA, Fielding RA et al. Ageing of skeletal muscle: a 12 year longitudinal study. J Appl Physiol 2000; 88: 1321–6.

32. Storer TW, Magliano L, Woodhouse L et al. Testosterone dose-dependently increases maximal voluntary strength and leg power, but does not affect fatigability or specific tension. J Clin Endocrinol Metab 2003; 88: 1478–85.

33. Snyder PJ, Peachey HM III, Kiaser FE et al. Effects of testosterone replacement therapy in old hypogonadal males: a preliminary study. J Am Geriatr Soc 1993; 41: 149–52.

34. Tenover JS. Effects of testosterone supplementation in the aging male. J Clin Endocrinol Metab 1992; 75: 1092–8.

35. Sinha-Hikim I, Taylor W, Nestor F et al. Androgen receptor in human skeletal muscle and cultured muscle satellite cells: up-regulation by androgen treatment. J Clin Endocrinol Metab 2004; 89(10): 5245–55.

36. Jacquemin V, Furling D, Bigot A, Butler-Browne G, Mouly V. IGF-1 induces human myotube hypertrophy by increasing cell recruitment. Exp Cell Res 2004; 299(1): 148–58.

37. Ferrando A, Sheffield-Moore M, Yeckel C et al. Testosterone administration to older men improves muscle function: molecular and physiological mechanisms. Am J Physiol Endocrinol Metab 2002; 282: E601–7.

38. Yarasheski KE, Bhasin S, Sinha-Hikim I, Pak-Loduca J, Gonzakz-Cadavid NF. Serum myostatin-immunoreactive protein is increased in 60–92 year old women and men with muscle wasting. J Nutr Health Aging 2002; 6: 343–8.

39. Roth SM, Martel GS, Farrell RE et al. Myostatin gene expression is reduced in humans with heavy-resistance strength training: a brief communication. Exp Biol Med 2003; 228: 706–9.

40. Welle S, Bhatt K, Shah B, Thornton C. Insulin-like growth factor-1 and myostatin mRNA expression in muscle: comparison between 62–77 and 21–31 yr old men. Exp Gerontol 2002; 37: 833–9.

41. Marcell TJ, Harman SM, Urban RJ et al. Comparison of GH, IGF-I, and testosterone with mRNA of receptors and myostatin in skeletal muscle in older men. Am J Physiol 2001; 281: E1159–64.

42. Grobet L, Pirottin D, Farnir F et al. Modulating skeletal muscle mass by postnatal, muscle-specific inactivation of the myostatin gene. Genesis 2003; 35: 227–38.

43. Bogdanovich S, Krag TO, Barton ER et al. Functional improvement of dystrophic muscle by myostatin blockade. Nature 2002; 420: 418–21.

CHAPTER 24

Visceral obesity, androgens, and the risks of cardiovascular disease

Louis JG Gooren

Introduction

For a long time adipose tissue was considered an inactive reserve depot of fat. It is now increasingly recognized that adipose tissue itself is active tissue, directly and actively involved in the control of body weight and energy balance via secretion of a large number of molecules with regulatory potential (adipokines), such as leptin, adiponectin, resistin, interleukin-6 (IL-6), tumor necrosis factor (TNF), and plasminogen activator inhibitor-1 (PAI-1). The identification of these secretory factors has increased insight into how an excess of body fat is related to metabolic disturbances, diabetes mellitus, and cardiovascular disease, an association that was earlier only understood in epidemiologic terms.[1,2]

Moreover, the production by the liver of C-reactive protein (CRP), an acute phase inflammatory protein, and fibrinogen, of which the levels are elevated in subjects with increased risk of cardiovascular disease, is triggered by various pro-inflammatory cytokines derived from numerous sources, such as macrophages, monocytes, and the adipose tissue. Several large population studies indicate that biomarkers of inflammation predict an increased risk for cardiovascular disease and that several aspects of cardiovascular disease can be viewed as having aspects of an inflammatory process.[3–6]

Adipose tissue is metabolically regulated by several genetic, hormonal, and nutritional factors.[7]

The primary metabolic function of the adipocyte or fat cell, the smallest functional unit of the adipose tissue, is to store fat in the form of triglycerides when the energy intake is in excess, and to release free fatty acids as energy supply in times of starvation. The amount of triglycerides in adipose tissue is a reflection of the balance between energy intake and energy expenditure over time. Several physiologic mechanisms regulate the amount of body fat in order to maintain a rather constant energy storage. It is reasonable to believe that the highly efficient and precisely regulated mechanism to conserve energy in the form of adipose tissue has, primarily, evolved to ensure an adequate supply of energy in times of scarcity of food, necessary for individual survival and for the energy demands that pregnancy and lactation put on women. In modern times this evolutionary adaptive mechanism may overshoot its usefulness and may no longer be favorable for survival in today's Western world, rather the contrary! Obesity carries a large number of health risks and shortens life expectancy. The current wide availability of highly palatable, calorically dense foods and the sedentary lifestyle promote weight gain. Obesity is a condition that is characterized by an excess storage of triglycerides in adipose tissue. Its development probably involves a very complex interaction between genetic, environmental, and developmental factors.[8–10]

The clinical relevance of visceral obesity

It is now commonly accepted that a preferential accumulation of fat in the abdominal region is associated with an increased risk of non-insulin-dependent diabetes mellitus (NIDDM) and cardiovascular disease, not only in obese subjects but even in non-obese subjects.[11] A large number of cross-sectional studies have established a relationship between abdominal obesity and cardiovascular risk factors such as hypertension, dyslipidemia (elevated levels of cholesterol, triglycerides, and low-density lipoproteins and low levels of high-density lipoproteins), and impaired glucose tolerance with hyperinsulinemia, a cluster known as the 'insulin resistance syndrome' or 'metabolic syndrome'.[12–14] The term metabolic syndrome is now preferred. Meanwhile two definitions of the syndrome have been proposed, which largely overlap but take a different approach. The definition of the National Cholesterol Education program tries to define risks for cardiovascular disease while the definition adopted by the WHO assigns greater value to the metabolic derangements and requires the measurement of insulin.[15] In the adult population, between 15 and 25% are suffering from the metabolic syndrome, depending on the prevalence of obesity in that society. It is increasingly recognized that geographic factors must be taken into consideration in the definition of the metabolic syndrome.[16,17]

The explanation of the association between abdominal obesity and the insulin resistance syndrome is still hypothetic, but the identification of the secretory products of the fat cell (adipokines) and their pathophysiologic significance have added to our understanding.[2,5] The visceral fat depot has three characteristics that distinguish it from the subcutaneous fat stores: (1) it has a high metabolic activity with a high turnover of triglycerides producing large amounts of free fatty acids (FFAs) and adipokines, (2) it drains on the portal vein which drains directly into the liver (the hypothesis states that the liver is unable to handle this high flow of FFAs and adipokines leading to a disturbance in glucose and lipid metabolism), and (3) high levels of FFAs and of adipokines may reduce insulin

clearance leading to hyperinsulinemia, may further enhance hepatic gluconeogenesis, and may reduce glucose uptake by the muscles, resulting in peripheral insulin resistance. Poor fibrinolysis and low-grade inflammation are components of the metabolic syndrome and add to the cardiovascular risks.

While this cluster of risk factors is now well documented, the causal relationships between the single components of the cluster are still uncertain but are beginning to be understood. Hyperinsulinemia, either primary or secondary to obesity, and the accompanying insulin resistance are the characteristic elements of the metabolic syndrome and are probably responsible for the glucose intolerance, dyslipidemia, and elevated blood pressure through cause and effect relationships. Hyperinsulinemia and insulin resistance are causally related to hypertension through direct effects on the vascular tone, stimulation of the adrenergic system, and inhibition of natriuresis. Both environmental factors (physical exercise and eating patterns) and genetic factors play a role in visceral obesity and insulin resistance (for review see reference 18). In the treatment of the metabolic syndrome changes of lifestyle (exercise and eating patterns) should take priority over pharmacotherapy, which can improve remaining cardiovascular risk markers.[10]

Adipokines

The fat cell has traditionally been viewed as a rather passive element in the regulation of reserve energy stores, with its main role to serve as the site of triglyceride storage in times of caloric excess, and of release of free fatty acids in times of increased energy needs. However, several decades ago the theory developed that the fat cell might play a more active role and actually senses excessive energy storage, and, in response, provides a signal that leads to restriction of food intake and induced energy expenditure, thus keeping body weight and fat mass within certain limits. As indicated above, in recent years it was demonstrated that the fat cell functions as an endocrine cell, producing and secreting molecules with regulatory potential such as IL-6, TNF,

PAI-1, leptin, adiponectin, and resistin.[19–22] One of the first discovered hormonal signals of the fat cell was leptin, which represents an important step in a better understanding of obesity.[23] The largest proportion of leptin is produced by the fat cells; the subcutaneous fat cells probably produce more leptin than the visceral fat cells. So, the leptin signal to decrease food intake coming from visceral fat may be weaker than the signal originating from subcutaneous fat. Leptin may be involved in reproductive physiology as well. It is well known that severe weight loss in women is associated with amenorrhea and that puberty in girls develops only when they have attained a certain critical body mass. Leptin is in all likelihood the signal provided by the adipose tissue to the central nervous system to initiate the release of gonadotropin-releasing hormones, and to discontinue its release when fat mass falls below a critical value, as is the case in anorexia nervosa or in women who exercise excessively (athletes).[24]

There are sex differences in leptin. Circulating leptin levels in women are considerably higher than in men. This may be explained partially by the fact that women store their excess fat predominantly subcutaneously in the gluteofemoral region and men more in the abdominal/visceral area, the latter localization producing less leptin. Also sex steroids affect leptin levels, with an increase produced by estrogens and a suppressive effect exerted by androgens. Puberty in boys is associated with an initial rise in leptin levels (probably as a result of aromatization of rising levels of testosterone to estradiol) followed by a decline when their androgen levels increase in the further course of puberty. Androgen replacement in hypogonadal men lowers leptin levels, maybe also as a result of the decrease in subcutaneous fat, but also as a result of the direct suppressive effect on androgens on its production.

Leptin may be a factor in the association between adiposity and decreased testosterone levels. In men there appears to be a correlation between body mass index and fat mass on the one hand and leptin levels on the other. Leptin receptors are present on the Leydig cell and inhibit the testosterone generated by administration of human chorionic gonadotropin.[25] This may be a model for a less effective stimulation of testosterone production by luteinizing hormone when circulating leptin levels are high, as is the case in obesity. Another study found a correlation between adiposity, insulin, and leptin on the one hand which correlated negatively with testosterone levels.[26] More studies have found that insulin is an important determinant of leptin levels. Feeding and overfeeding increase insulin levels which leads, in turn, to an increase in leptin, and vice versa.[27]

The main target of leptin is the central nervous system. By modulating neurotransmitters in the hypothalamus it increases energy expenditure and inhibits appetite and weight gain. Leptin may enhance hepatic fatty acid oxidation. Leptin influences neuropeptides affecting appetite and anorexia. The question has arisen whether obesity is an abnormality of leptin physiology. Indeed, both animals and humans with abnormalities of the gene involved in the production of leptin are very obese. In animals this can be partially corrected by the administration of exogenous recombinant leptin. Most obese subjects with the metabolic syndrome have high circulating levels of leptin.[28] These high levels may be interpreted as a state of leptin insensitivity, explaining why the physiologic responses to leptin (reduced food intake and increased physical activity) fail to take place. It may be a deficient transport of leptin into the brain,[29] or deficient receptor or postreceptor mechanisms of leptin making its action less efficient.

Will the administration of exogenous leptin ever become a tool in the hopeless task of weight reduction? The first studies have been carried out and indeed hold promise (for review see reference 30). In the studies where leptin was administered to human subjects visceral fat decreased earlier in the course of weight loss than subcutaneous fat, which is promising in view of the relation of visceral fat to cardiovascular disease and diabetes mellitus. It is not yet clear which subjects are particularly eligible for leptin administration; results of leptin administration on adiposity varied strongly between subjects. The long-term efficacy and safety of recombinant leptin have not been studied. Treatment with leptin sensitizers and analogs may be easier to administer and more potent than the subcutaneous administration of recombinant leptin.[31] A strong correlation between low levels of adiponectin and increased insulin resistance has been established in animal experimentation and humans.[32,33]

Patients with diabetes, patients with the metabolic syndrome, and obese subjects have lower levels of adiponectin than controls.[34,35] Adiponectin improves insulin resistance in vivo. Circulating adiponectin levels correlate negatively with insulin and PAI-1, and positively with insulin sensitivity and HDL-C.[36] There are sex differences in circulating adiponectin levels. Men have lower adiponectin levels than women. This sex difference becomes manifest in puberty and can be related to rising plasma levels of testosterone in puberty.[37] The role of androgens is further supported by the effects of testosterone administration to hypogonadal men.[38]

Resistin, another adipocyte-derived cytokine, impairs glucose tolerance.[39,40] Resistin levels are increased in obesity and downregulated by thiazolidenedones. Its role awaits further delineation.

IL-6 is an important adipocyte signaling molecule, released from predominantly visceral but also subcutaneous fat upon sympathetic nervous system activation (such as with stress). Approximately 25–30% of circulating IL-6 is derived from adipose tissue.[41] The venous drainage of IL-6 via the portal vein to the liver enhances CRP and fibrinogen production. Together with the high concentration of free fatty acids originating from visceral fat, IL-6 mediates a number of the effects of visceral fat on the metabolic syndrome.

IL-10 is a potent anti-inflammatory cytokine. IL-10 levels are low in the metabolic syndrome.[42] TNF is another pro-inflammatory cytokine secreted by monocytes/macrophages, endothelial cells, and to a large extent by adipocytes. TNF levels are strongly correlated with body mass index. Weight loss reduces levels of TNF. Levels of TNF are important regulators of insulin sensitivity.[43]

Sex differences in fat distribution

Adult men and women differ in their fat distribution; the regional distribution of body fat is a characteristic of masculinity and femininity. In premenopausal women a larger proportion of fat is stored in peripheral fat depots such as breasts, hips, and thighs. Men tend to deposit excess fat in the abdominal regions (both subcutaneous and intra-abdominal or visceral fat depots) and generally have a larger visceral fat depot than (premenopausal) women. As regional localization of body fat is considered a secondary sex characteristic, it is likely that sex steroids are involved in the male and female patterns of fat deposition. This view is strengthened by the observation that variations in sex steroid levels in different phases of (reproductive) life parallel regional differences in fat storage and fat mobilization. Until puberty boys and girls do not differ very much in the amount of body fat and its regional distribution, although girls may have somewhat more body fat than boys. From puberty on differences become manifest. The ovarian production of estrogens and progesterone induces an increase in total body fat as well as selective fat deposition in the breast and gluteofemoral region. Pubertal boys show a strong increase in fat-free mass while the amount of total body fat does not change very much. Adolescent boys lose subcutaneous fat but accumulate fat in the abdominal region, which in most boys is not very visible in that stage of development but clearly demonstrable with imaging techniques.[44] The sex-steroid-induced regional distribution is not an all-or-none mechanism; it is a preferential accumulation of excess fat. Obese men and women still show their sex-specific fat accumulation but store their fat also in the 'fat depots of the other sex.'

It is not only the fat distribution that differs between the sexes from puberty on, the dynamics of fat cell size and fat metabolism are also different. The amount of fat in a certain depot is dependent on the number and size of the fat cells. Fat cells in the gluteal and femoral region are larger than in the abdominal region. The activity of lipoprotein lipase, the enzyme response for accumulation of triglycerides in the fat cell, is higher in the gluteofemoral region than in the abdominal area. Conversely, lipolysis is regulated by hormone-sensitive lipase, which in turn is regulated by several hormones and by the sympathetic nervous system. Catecholamines stimulate lipolysis via the β-adrenergic receptor while α_2-adrenoreceptors inhibit lipolysis. Hormones affect the catecholamine receptors. Testosterone stimulates the β-adrenergic receptor while estrogens/progesterone favor α_2-adrenoreceptors. Insulin stimulates fat accumulation.

It is not an unreasonable speculation that the sex-steroid-dependent fat distribution serves (or maybe better has served!) the different roles of men and women in reproduction. The visceral fat depot has a high metabolic activity which a high turnover of triglycerides with sets rather acutely large amounts of free fatty acids (FFAs). The visceral fat depot drains on the portal vein, which drains its blood in the liver providing FFAs as fuel for quick and high degrees of physical activity. So the reserve energy supplies of men can be mobilized fast and are readily available to fuel metabolism. Women's fat stores lend themselves less to rapid mobilization. Pregnancy and lactation are situations that release energy from female stores at the buttocks and thighs, but do so at a slow pace. Again, these sex differences are not absolute but a matter of predominance.

As indicated above, a large number of studies have documented that visceral obesity is associated with low plasma total testosterone levels.[45–48] Part of the explanation for the low total testosterone levels might be the lower plasma levels of sex hormone-binding globulin (SHBG) encountered in obese men; these men are often hyperinsulinemic which, again, might be part of the explanation for the low-ered levels of SHBG.[49] Normally, an increase in SHBG levels is observed in aging men, in all like-lihood due to a decrease in growth hormone and IGF-I levels with aging.[39] Studies have found that low total and free testosterone levels are associated with coronary artery disease in men and into low levels of plasma total testosterone with cardiovascular risk factors in healthy men,[50] and that these are not independent variables.[51,52] From another study it appeared that rather than age per se, it is the value of plasma testosterone that is related to features of the metabolic syndrome.[52] A prospective study found that men with low testosterone and low SHBG levels are more likely to develop insulin resistance and subsequent diabetes mellitus type II.[53] It could be established that sleep apnea and daytime sleepiness are much more related to visceral obesity than to general obesity and their occurrence was related to plasma insulin and leptin levels.[54] Inflammatory cytokines released from adipose tissue produce fatigue and sleepiness in these men.

Relationships between sex steroids and fat distribution in adulthood and aging

While the evidence that pubertal sex steroids induce a sex-specific fat distribution with preferential abdominal/visceral fat accumulation in males and preferential gluteofemoral fat accumulation in females is quite solid, later in life a number of paradoxes occur in the relationship between sex steroids and fat distribution.

Acquired adult-onset hypogonadism in men is associated with a higher amount of subcutaneous fat than in eugonadal men, but the amount of visceral fat appears to be not less than in a comparison group of eugonadal men.[55] So, apparently while androgens induce visceral fat accumulation, once fat has been stored in the visceral depot it does not need continued androgen stimulation as opposed to maintenance of bone and muscle mass, which were lower in the men with adult onset hypogonadism than in eugonadal controls.[49] Induction of androgen deficiency in healthy men by administration of an LHRH agonist leads to an increase in fat mass.[56] Correlation studies in large groups of subjects have shown that visceral fat increases with aging. There is an inverse correlation between the amount of visceral fat and plasma insulin on the one hand and levels of testosterone and SHBG on the other. Therefore, the effects of overfeeding and starvation on sex steroid levels are interesting. In an experiment, 12 pairs of identical twins were overfed for 120 days, resulting in an average weight gain of 8 kg. The excess fat was accumulated both subcutaneously and abdominally/viscerally, with a clear preference for the latter localization. Plasma testosterone levels did not decline but SHBG levels declined. Even though plasma testosterone did not decline there was a significant negative correlation between changes in visceral fat and in plasma testosterone. In other words: a gain in visceral fat led to a decrease in plasma testosterone. A further correlation that appeared was between fasting insulin and changes in abdominal fat and in testosterone.[57] The latter is interesting in view of the fact that plasma levels of insulin are negatively correlated with SHBG.[58,59] In vitro studies have shown that insulin inhibits hepatic production of SHBG. Lower SHBG levels lead to a fall in total plasma testosterone since this leads to an increase in free testosterone in the first instance and subsequently to a higher metabolic breakdown of testosterone. It could be shown that a higher degree of visceral obesity was correlated with lower SHBG levels and with higher levels of 3α-diol-G, a metabolite of testosterone, indicating that a lowering of SHBG induces testosterone metabolism. Plasma insulin was positively associated with 3α-diol-G.[58]

Conversely, weight loss produced an increase in testosterone itself[58,59] and/or an increase in SHBG.[60,61] The study of Pritchard et al[57] found that the rise in testosterone levels correlated inversely with loss of abdominal fat and with plasma insulin. Collectively, these studies suggest that a high degree of visceral adiposity is associated with high insulin levels and low SHBG levels and low total plasma testosterone, and with an increase in metabolites of testosterone, and vice versa.

Correlation studies cannot unravel the cause and effect relationships between the correlates, whether low testosterone induces visceral fat deposition or whether a large visceral fat depot leads to low testosterone levels. Prospective studies have confirmed that lower endogenous androgens predict central adiposity in men,[62] and that these low testosterone levels are significantly inversely associated with levels of blood pressure, fasting plasma glucose and triglyceride, body mass index, and HDL cholesterol.[63] A study in Japanese–American men found that low testosterone levels predicted an increase in visceral fat 7.5 years later.[64] Unfortunately, SHBG levels were not measured but baseline testosterone levels were significantly correlated with fasting C-peptide and fasting insulin levels while adjustment for baseline visceral fat diminished the association between baseline testosterone and plasma insulin, evidencing a role of the amount of visceral fat in their interrelationship. The amount of visceral fat at baseline also predicted an increase in visceral fat over the follow-up period of 7.5 years. The latter is important since in all follow-up studies the hypotestosteronemia associated with visceral obesity may already have been presented when the subjects were initially included in the study. It does not come as a surprise that subjects with a degree of visceral obesity at a younger age show an increase thereof in their later life, as was the case in the study of Tsai et al.[64] A 5-year follow-up study of Swedish men indicated that elevated plasma cortisol and low testosterone were prospectively associated with an increased incidence of cardiovascular-related events and diabetes mellitus type 2.[65] A cautionary note is that middle-aged and elderly men with risk factors for cardiovascular disease usually have lower plasma testosterone levels than healthy men, and these epidemiologic findings may be self-serving in their predictions. The already existing excess of visceral fat in the men in the study may have been the mechanism of low testosterone in these men.

It is of note that, with aging, plasma testosterone levels also show a decline independently of the amount of visceral fat.

Elevated androgen levels in women increase the amount of visceral fat in women, women with the polycystic ovarian syndrome being the classic example.[12] In the medical literature, this is often presented as a paradox in the sense that high levels of androgens in women and low levels of androgens in men are associated with visceral obesity. The paradox is partially semantic: high testosterone levels in women (for instance 3–5 nmol/l) mean (very) low androgens in men. So the use of the terms high and low testosterone must be related to the sex. A further element is the relation to age. Women with the polycystic ovarian syndrome are relatively young (of reproductive age) when they come to the attention of the medical profession while the relationship between visceral obesity and low androgen levels in men is typically an epidemiologic finding in elderly men. Apparently, similar to the situation in androgen-naïve teenage boys, androgens in women with polycystic ovarian syndrome are capable of visceral fat accumulation when these women are exposed to androgens postpubertally when their polycystic ovaries start to produce androgens.

In postmenopausal women there is a larger degree of (male type) upper body fat accumulation in comparison to the former gluteofemoral fat storage. Following menopause, androgen levels drop considerably in women. So, obviously premenopausal estrogen/progesterone levels are required to maintain a premenopausal female type of fat distribution, also evidenced by the fact that postmenopausal hormone replacement (partially) restores the premenopausal fat distribution.[66]

Increasing testosterone and the effects on adipose tissue

It is a widely held belief that androgens have an atherogenic effect and thus lead to cardiovascular disease. Two review papers have examined this relationship and conclude that it is not tenable to regard testosterone as a culprit in the etiology of cardiovascular disease.[67,68] It rather appears that lower-than-normal testosterone levels in men are associated with cardiovascular risk factors of which visceral obesity, with its association with cardiovascular risk factors, might be the intermediate. Visceral adiposity is associated with low testosterone levels in cross-sectional studies, and from this type of study the cause and effect relationship is not immediately evident. Does visceral adiposity induce low levels of testosterone, or do low levels of testosterone induce visceral adiposity? Some prospective studies argue that low testosterone predicts visceral adiposity.[62–65] Several studies have examined the effects of testosterone administration on adipose tissue in men. Some have found a decrease in fat mass with testosterone replacement therapy,[69–72] while others found no change.[73,74] But longer-term studies of testosterone supplementation of older men have consistently demonstrated a decrease in fat mass.[75–79] In one study wherein young men were made testosterone deficient with an LHRH agonist, testosterone deficiency was associated with gains in subcutaneous, intermuscular, and intra-abdominal fat. Graded restoration of plasma testosterone with exogenous testosterone led to a dose-dependent reduction in adipose tissue with no quantitative differences between trunk and peripheral non-trunk fat mass.[80]

Testosterone inhibits the expression of the activity of lipoprotein lipase, the main enzymatic regulator of triglyceride uptake in the fat cell, preferentially in abdominal fat and less so in femoral fat, and, maybe, mobilizes lipids from the visceral fat depot. A study of testosterone administration restoring testosterone levels to midnormal values with a duration of 8–9 months found a decrease in the visceral fat mass, a decrease in fasting glucose and lipid levels, and an improvement in insulin sensitivity; in addition, a decrease in diastolic blood pressure was observed.[81] More studies are needed to examine whether raising testosterone levels in viscerally obese men will lead to a reduction in visceral fat and an improvement in the cardiovascular and diabetogenic risk factors associated with it. One study could not confirm this,[82] but others found more promising results.[83,84]

Estrogens and the metabolic syndrome

Estrogens in men, which are largely a product of peripheral aromatization of androgens, are receiving increasing attention. Traditionally conceptualized as 'female hormones', estrogens appear to have unexpected but important effects on the male reproductive/metabolic system.[85,86]

The discovery of one man with deficient estrogen action (on the basis of a receptor mutation) and four others with deficient estrogen synthesis, and further studies in knockout mouse models suggest strongly that in the virtual absence of estrogen action, symptoms of the metabolic syndrome develop. For example, atherosclerosis at an early age, insulin resistance, visceral obesity, and a high-risk lipid profile were present, and improved upon administration of estrogens to the men with deficient estrogen synthesis.[85,86] It would seem that a low-to-absent estrogen action in men is a factor in the metabolic syndrome. In support of a role of estrogens is the increased risk of cardiovascular disease in men with a variation in the estrogen receptor alpha gene.[43] The circulating testosterone levels in these men were rather high than low and symptoms deteriorated upon administration of testosterone. So, this observation distinguishes these cases from the men studied in population studies which predict an increased cardiovascular risk in men with low testosterone levels,[62–64] and improvement upon testosterone administration.[65–67] The men in the studies which found that low testosterone levels predict an increased cardiovascular risk[62–67] certainly did not have low plasma estradiol levels. Plasma estradiol levels in men show no tendency to decline with aging.[85] So, a number of paradoxes are presented here for which presently no plausible explanation exists. Speculatively, it might be that the protective effects that androgens seem to have on the occurrence of the metabolic syndrome are only manifest in an endocrine milieu where there is a normal degree of biologic action of estrogens,[87] potentially through interaction of estrogens with androgen receptors.[88]

The epidemic of obesity and what to do about it?

Obesity is reaching epidemic proportions in the developed but also the developing world. Sixty-three percent of men and 55% of women are overweight in the United States. Twenty-two percent are grossly overweight with a body mass index (body weight in kg divided by the square of the height in m) over $30 \, kg/m^2$. The prevalence of obesity has doubled in the past decade (for review see reference 89). The consequences are serious. Approximately 80% of obese adults have at least one and 40% have two or more associated diseases such as diabetes, hypertension, cardiovascular disease, gallbladder disease, cancers, and last but not least diseases of the locomotor system such as arthrosis. In the USA 300 000 people die more or less directly from the consequences of obesity and the costs for the national health-care budget amount to 10%, making it not only a personal medical problem but also a public health problem. The frequency of overweight is maximal between the ages of 50 and 60 years and shows subsequently a tendency to decline slowly. Most people over 75 years are no longer very obese. Genetics are significant. Studies in identical twins show that 60–70% of overweight can be ascribed to genetic factors and 30–40% to environmental influences. If both parents are obese,

approximately 80% of the children will be overweight and with one obese parent the likelihood is 40%. If neither parent is obese the likelihood is less than 10%.

Body mass index provides a better index than body weight itself to describe the degree of obesity. There is now solid evidence that fat distribution (a large visceral fat depot) is a strong predictor of cardiovascular disease and of the development of diabetes mellitus type II. Visceral fat is quantitatively most reliably assessed with computerized tomography or magnetic resonance imaging, which is too costly to become a method of mass screening and probably redundant in assessing an individual case. A number of studies document that surrogate measures provide a reasonable indication of the amount of visceral fat accumulation. A waist to hip ratio >0.95, waist circumference of more than 101 cm, and sagittal diameter >23 cm (measured with the patient supine) are all indications of visceral obesity. These patterns of body fat distribution are also linked to a negative biochemical cardiovascular risk profile.[90] So, it is possible with simple means to determine overweight and fat distribution patterns. The above values have typically been obtained in a Caucasian population. However, in Chinese subjects as well the waist to hip ratio provides additional information on cardiovascular risk,[91] but different criteria apply for Asians.[92] In Asians a BMI of 23–25 is overweight and >25 obesity, and a waist circumference >90 cm means abdominal obesity.

The pathophysiology of obesity is poorly understood. That obesity is a discrepancy between food intake on the one hand and energy expenditure on the other is simple, but what physiologic mechanisms are involved, and how these could be influenced to redress obesity, are much more difficult questions. The central nervous systems coordinates the checks and balances with the arcuate and paraventricular nuclei in the hypothalamus as key players. Afferent vagal and sympathetic stimuli and hormonal messages such as insulin, leptin, cholecystokinin, and glucocorticoid modulate in the hypothalamus the neuropeptides involved in appetite and satiety. Efferent signals to the sympathetic and parasympathetic nervous system and to the thyroid regulate food intake and energy expenditure.[93]

Recent identification of novel appetite-regulating hormones has revealed the complex interactions of humoral factors in the regulation of feeding behavior in mammals. One of these hormones, ghrelin, a natural ligand of the orphan receptor GHS-R, purified from the stomach, is able to stimulate growth hormone release from pituitary cells. Ghrelin stimulates appetite by acting on the hypothalamic arcuate nucleus, the region known to control food intake. As an orexigenic peptide, ghrelin is therefore an endogenous regulator of feeding behavior from the peripheral tissues to the central nervous system.[94] It is reasonable to assume that part of the success of surgical procedures in the treatment of morbid obesity is based on the reduction of ghrelin from the stomach.[95,96] This information has not led to powerful tools for intervention.

A number of hormonal diseases are associated with increased fat accumulation (hypothyroidism, hypercortisolism) but they are rarely the explanation for overweight. Obesity associated with endocrine disease has rather characteristic physical features and can be recognized relatively easily by a trained eye. Measurement of thyroid hormone and cortisol are, therefore, rarely useful in the diagnostic work-up of obesity.

Treatment is far from simple. Diet treatment is only marginally successful. In a review of 21 study populations with 3030 subjects, of whom 70% of subjects could be followed for 3–14 years, the mean initial weight loss was 4–28 kg, but 0–49% (median 15%) successfully maintained the initial weight loss of at least 9–11 kg.[97] It is even more difficult, after an initial success, to maintain a reduced weight in the long term.[97] It is evident that the combination of reduced caloric intake and increase in energy expenditure will lead to a reduction in weight, though the sad thing is that, being on a weight-reducing diet, the body develops counter regulations as if the weight loss was undesired and to be counterbalanced, slowing the loss of weight. The addition of drugs to a weight-reducing diet has a limited degree of success,[98] and it is difficult, even with drugs, to achieve a weight reduction of more than 5–6%. In a recent review fluoxetine induced a weight reduction of 5.8 kg after 52 weeks, with considerable side-effects, such as tremor, sweating, and somnolence. Orlistat led to a reduction of 2.6 kg at 26 weeks, but with gastro-intestinal complaints. Sibutramine induced a weight loss of 4.5 kg at 26 weeks but was associated with palpitations.[99] Metformin, a drug used in the treatment of type 2 diabetes, may reduce appetite and caloric intake. New drugs are being developed.[100] Surgical procedures, such as gastric banding, gastric bypass, biliopancreatic diversion, or duodenal switch, are increasing successful, though there are considerable risks.[101–103]

It has to be admitted that the fight against obesity is largely unsuccessful and probably cannot be won in the setting of clinical therapeutic medicine, but must come from health education teaching sensible eating and encouraging greater physically activity, starting early in life.[104,105] Eating patterns are very resistant to change.

Lack of success in the battle against obesity leads to frustration on the side of the patient and the physician who, not having powerful tools, tells the patients that s/he lacks willpower and must take his/her responsibility.

References

1. Devaraj S, Rosenson RS, Jialal I. Metabolic syndrome: an appraisal of the pro-inflammatory and procoagulant status. Endocrinol Metab Clin North Am 2004; 33: 431–53.
2. Nigro J, Osman N, Dart AM et al. Insulin resistance and atherosclerosis. Endocr Rev 2006; 27: 242–59.
3. Ross R. Atherosclerosis is an inflammatory disease. Am Heart J 1999; 138: S419–20.
4. Libby P. Inflammation in atherosclerosis. Nature 2002; 420: 868–74.
5. Haffner SM. The metabolic syndrome: inflammation, diabetes mellitus, and cardiovascular disease. Am J Cardiol 2006; 97: 3–11A.
6. Juge-Aubry CE, Henrichot E, Meier CA. Adipose tissue: a regulator of inflammation. Best Pract Res Clin Endocrinol Metab 2005; 19: 547–66.
7. Schwartz MW, Seeley RJ. The new biology of body weight regulation. J Am Diet Assoc 1997; 97: 54–8.
8. Natali A, Ferrannini E. Hypertension, insulin resistance, and the metabolic syndrome. Endocrinol Metab Clin North Am 2004; 33: 417–29.
9. Grundy SM. Metabolic syndrome: part II. Endocrinol Metab Clin North Am 2004; 33: xi–xiii.

10. Stone NJ, Saxon D. Approach to treatment of the patient with metabolic syndrome: lifestyle therapy. Am J Cardiol 2005; 96(4A): 15–21E.

11. Kannel WB, Cupples LA, Ramaswami R et al. Regional obesity and risk of cardiovascular disease; the Framingham Study. J Clin Epidemiol 1991; 44: 183–90.

12. Bjorntorp P. Abdominal obesity and the metabolic syndrome. Ann Med 1992; 24: 465–8.

13. Despres JP, Marette A. Relation of components of insulin resistance syndrome to coronary disease risk. Curr Opin Lipidol 1994; 5: 274–89.

14. Assmann G, Nofer JR, Schulte H. Cardiovascular risk assessment in metabolic syndrome: view from PROCAM. Endocrinol Metab Clin North Am 2004; 33: 377–92.

15. Lakka HM, Laaksonen DE, Lakka TA et al. The metabolic syndrome and total and cardiovascular disease mortality in middle-aged men. JAMA 2002; 288: 2709–16.

16. Seclen S, Villena A, Gonzalez-Villalpando C et al. Geographic variations of the International Diabetes Federation and the National Cholesterol Education Program–Adult Treatment Panel III definitions of the metabolic syndrome in nondiabetic subjects. Diabetes Care 2006; 29: 685–91.

17. Shiwaku K, Anuurad E, Enkhmaa B et al. Predictive values of anthropometric measurements for multiple metabolic disorders in Asian populations. Diabetes Res Clin Pract 2005; 69: 52–62.

18. Natali A, Ferrannini E. Hypertension, insulin resistance, and the metabolic syndrome. Endocrinol Metab Clin North Am 2004; 33: 417–29.

19. Trayhurn P, Wood IS. Adipokines: inflammation and the pleiotropic role of white adipose tissue. Br J Nutr 2004; 92: 347–55.

20. Hutley L, Prins JB. Fat as an endocrine organ: relationship to the metabolic syndrome. Am J Med Sci 2005; 330: 280–9.

21. Yu YH, Ginsberg HN. Adipocyte signaling and lipid homeostasis: sequelae of insulin-resistant adipose tissue. Circ Res 2005; 96: 1042–52.

22. Kershaw EE, Flier JS. Adipose tissue as an endocrine organ. J Clin Endocrinol Metab 2004; 89: 2548–56.

23. Koerner A, Kratzsch J, Kiess W. Adipocytokines: leptin – the classical, resistin – the controversial, adiponectin – the promising, and more to come. Best Pract Res Clin Endocrinol Metab 2005; 19: 525–46.

24. Woods SC, Benoit SC, Clegg DJ et al. Regulation of energy homeostasis by peripheral signals. Best Pract Res Clin Endocrinol Metab 2004; 18: 497–515.

25. Isidori AM, Caprio M, Strollo F et al. Leptin and androgens in male obesity: evidence for leptin contribution to reduced androgen levels. J Clin Endocrinol Metab 1999; 84: 3673–80.

26. Van Den Saffele JK, Goemaere S, De Bacquer D et al. Serum leptin levels in healthy ageing men: are decreased serum testosterone and increased adiposity in elderly men the consequence of leptin deficiency? Clin Endocrinol (Oxf) 1999; 51: 81–8.

27. Doucet E, St Pierre S, Almeras N et al. Fasting insulin levels influence plasma leptin levels independently from the contribution of adiposity: evidence from both a cross-sectional and an intervention study. J Clin Endocrinol Metab 2000; 85: 4231–7.

28. Ford ES. Factor analysis and defining the metabolic syndrome. Ethn Dis 2003; 13: 429–37.

29. Mantzoros CS. The role of leptin in human obesity and disease: a review of current evidence. Ann Intern Med 1999; 130: 671–80.

30. Flier JS. Obesity wars: molecular progress confronts an expanding epidemic. Cell 2004; 116: 337–50.

31. Kobayashi K. Adipokines: therapeutic targets for metabolic syndrome. Curr Drug Targets 2005; 6: 525–9.

32. Chandran M, Phillips SA, Ciaraldi T et al. Adiponectin: more than just another fat cell hormone? Diabetes Care 2003; 26: 2442–50.

33. Do D, Alvarez J, Chiquette E, Chilton R. The good fat hormone: adiponectin and cardiovascular disease. Curr Atheroscler Rep 2006; 8: 94–9.

34. Kondo H, Shimomura I, Matsukawa Y et al. Association of adiponectin mutation with type 2 diabetes: a candidate gene for the insulin resistance syndrome. Diabetes 2002; 51: 2325–8.

35. Weyer C, Funahashi T, Tanaka S et al. Hypoadiponectinemia in obesity and type 2 diabetes: close association with insulin resistance and hyperinsulinemia. J Clin Endocrinol Metab 2001; 86: 1930–5.

36. Pellme F, Smith U, Funahashi T et al. Circulating adiponectin levels are reduced in nonobese but insulin-resistant first-degree relatives of type 2 diabetic patients. Diabetes 2003; 52: 1182–6.

37. Bottner A, Kratzsch J, Muller G et al. Gender differences of adiponectin levels develop during the progression of puberty and are related to serum androgen levels. J Clin Endocrinol Metab 2004; 89: 4053–61.

38. Lanfranco F, Zitzmann M, Simoni M, Nieschlag E. Serum adiponectin levels in hypogonadal males: influence of testosterone replacement therapy. Clin Endocrinol (Oxf) 2004; 60: 500–7.

39. Steppan CM, Lazar MA. Resistin and obesity-associated insulin resistance. Trends Endocrinol Metab 2002; 13: 18–23.

40. Rea R, Donnelly R. Resistin: an adipocyte-derived hormone. Has it a role in diabetes and obesity? Diabetes Obes Metab 2004; 6: 163–70.

41. Vozarova B, Weyer C, Hanson K et al. Circulating interleukin-6 in relation to adiposity, insulin action, and insulin secretion. Obes Res 2001; 9: 414–17.

42. Esposito K, Pontillo A, Giugliano F et al. Association of low interleukin-10 levels with the metabolic syndrome in obese women. J Clin Endocrinol Metab 2003; 88: 1055–8.

43. Arner P. The adipocyte in insulin resistance: key molecules and the impact of the thiazolidinediones. Trends Endocrinol Metab 2003; 14: 137–45.

44. Roemmich JN, Clark PA, Mai V et al. Alterations in growth and body composition during puberty: III. Influence of maturation, gender, body composition, fat distribution, aerobic fitness, and energy expenditure on nocturnal growth hormone release. J Clin Endocrinol Metab 1998; 83: 1440–7.

45. Seidell JC, Bjorntorp P, Sjostrom L et al. Visceral fat accumulation in men is positively associated with insulin, glucose, and C-peptide levels, but negatively with testosterone levels. Metabolism 1990; 39: 897–901.

46. Khaw KT, Barrett-Connor E. Lower endogenous androgens predict central adiposity in men. Ann Epidemiol 1992; 2: 675–82.

47. Despres JP, Couillard C, Gagnon J et al. Race, visceral adipose tissue, plasma lipids, and lipoprotein lipase activity in men and women: the Health, Risk Factors, Exercise Training, and Genetics (HERITAGE) family study. Arterioscler Thromb Vasc Biol 2000; 20: 1932–8.

48. Prud'homme D, Bouchard C, Tremblay A et al. Relationships between endogenous steroid hormone, sex hormone-binding globulin and lipoprotein levels in men: contribution of visceral obesity, insulin levels and other metabolic variables. Atherosclerosis 1997; 133: 235–44.

49. Kaufman JM, Vermeulen A. Declining gonadal function in elderly men. Baillières Clin Endocrinol Metab 1997; 11: 289–309.

50. Simon D, Charles MA, Nahoul K et al. Association between plasma total testosterone and cardiovascular risk factors in healthy adult men: the Telecom Study. J Clin Endocrinol Metab 1997; 82: 682–5.

51. Pitteloud N, Mootha VK, Dwyer AA et al. Relationship between testosterone levels, insulin sensitivity, and mitochondrial function in men. Diabetes Care 2005; 28: 1636–42.

52. Blouin K, Despres JP, Couillard C et al. Contribution of age and declining androgen levels to features of the metabolic syndrome in men. Metabolism 2005; 54: 1034–40.

53. Stellato RK, Feldman HA, Hamdy O et al. Testosterone, sex hormone-binding globulin, and the development of type 2 diabetes in middle-aged men: prospective results from the Massachusetts male aging study. Diabetes Care 2000; 23: 490–4.

54. Vgontzas AN, Papanicolaou DA, Bixler EO et al. Sleep apnea and daytime sleepiness and fatigue: relation to visceral obesity, insulin resistance, and hypercytokinemia. J Clin Endocrinol Metab 2000; 85: 1151–8.

55. Katznelson L, Rosenthal DI, Rosol MS et al. Using quantitative CT to assess adipose distribution in adult men with acquired hypogonadism. Am J Roentgenol 1998; 170: 423–7.

56. Mauras N, Hayes V, Welch S et al. Testosterone deficiency in young men: marked alterations in whole body protein kinetics, strength, and adiposity. J Clin Endocrinol Metab 1998; 83: 1886–92.

57. Pritchard J, Despres JP, Gagnon J et al. Plasma adrenal, gonadal, and conjugated steroids before and after long-term overfeeding in identical twins. J Clin Endocrinol Metab 1998; 83: 3277–84.

58. Tchernof A, Labrie F, Belanger A et al. Androstane-3alpha,17beta-diol glucuronide as a steroid correlate of visceral obesity in men. J Clin Endocrinol Metab 1997; 82: 1528–34.

59. Vermeulen A, Kaufman JM, Giagulli VA. Influence of some biological indexes on sex hormone-binding globulin and androgen levels in aging or obese males. J Clin Endocrinol Metab 1996; 81: 1821–6.

60. Wang C, Catlin DH, Starcevic B et al. Low fat high fiber diet decreased serum and urine androgens. J Clin Endocrinol Metab 2005; 90: 3550–9.

61. Leenen R, van der KK, Seidell JC et al. Visceral fat accumulation in relation to sex hormones in obese men and women undergoing weight loss therapy. J Clin Endocrinol Metab 1994; 78: 1515–20.

62. Khaw KT, Barrett-Connor E. Lower endogenous androgens predict central adiposity in men. Ann Epidemiol 1992; 2: 675–82.

63. Zmuda JM, Cauley JA, Kriska A et al. Longitudinal relation between endogenous testosterone and cardiovascular disease risk factors in middle-aged men. A 13-year follow-up of former Multiple Risk Factor Intervention Trial participants. Am J Epidemiol 1997; 146: 609–17.

64. Tsai EC, Boyko EJ, Leonetti DL et al. Low serum testosterone level as a predictor of increased visceral fat in Japanese-American men. Int J Obes Relat Metab Disord 2000; 24: 485–91.

65. Rosmond R, Wallerius S, Wanger P et al. A 5-year follow-up study of disease incidence in men with an abnormal hormone pattern. J Intern Med 2003; 254: 386–90.

66. Tchernof A, Poehlman ET. Effects of the menopause transition on body fatness and body fat distribution. Obes Res 1998; 6: 246–54.

67. Wu FC, von Eckardstein A. Androgens and coronary artery disease. Endocr Rev 2003; 24: 183–217.

68. Liu PY, Death AK, Handelsman DJ. Androgens and cardiovascular disease. Endocr Rev 2003; 24: 313–40.

69. Brodsky IG, Balagopal P, Nair KS. Effects of testosterone replacement on muscle mass and muscle protein synthesis in hypogonadal men – a clinical research center study. J Clin Endocrinol Metab 1996; 81: 3469–75.

70. Katznelson L, Rosenthal DI, Rosol MS et al. Using quantitative CT to assess adipose distribution in adult men with acquired hypogonadism. Am J Roentgenol 1998; 170: 423–7.

71. Snyder PJ, Peachey H, Berlin JA et al. Effects of testosterone replacement in hypogonadal men. J Clin Endocrinol Metab 2000; 85: 2670–7.

72. Dobs AS, Bachorik PS, Arver S et al. Interrelationships among lipoprotein levels, sex hormones, anthropometric parameters, and age in hypogonadal men treated for 1 year with a permeation-enhanced testosterone transdermal system. J Clin Endocrinol Metab 2001; 86: 1026–33.

73. Bhasin S, Storer TW, Berman N et al. Testosterone replacement increases fat-free mass and muscle size in hypogonadal men. J Clin Endocrinol Metab 1997; 82: 407–13.

74. Wang C, Eyre DR, Clark R et al. Sublingual testosterone replacement improves muscle mass and strength, decreases bone resorption, and increases bone formation markers in hypogonadal men – a clinical research center study. J Clin Endocrinol Metab 1996; 81: 3654–62.

75. Rebuffe-Scrive M, Marin P, Bjorntorp P. Effect of testosterone on abdominal adipose tissue in men. Int J Obes 1991; 15: 791–5.

76. Snyder PJ, Peachey H, Hannoush P et al. Effect of testosterone treatment on body composition and muscle strength in men over 65 years of age. J Clin Endocrinol Metab 1999; 84: 2647–53.

77. Rolf C, von Eckardstein S, Koken U. Testosterone substitution of hypogonadal men prevents the age-dependent increases in body mass index, body fat and leptin seen in healthy ageing men: results of a cross-sectional study. Eur J Endocrinol 2002; 146: 505–11.

78. Marin P, Oden B, Bjorntorp P. Assimilation and mobilization of triglycerides in subcutaneous abdominal and femoral adipose tissue in vivo in men: effects of androgens. J Clin Endocrinol Metab 1995; 80: 239–43.

79. Marin P, Arver S. Androgens and abdominal obesity. Baillières Clin Endocrinol Metab 1998; 12: 441–51.

80. Woodhouse LJ, Gupta N, Bhasin M et al. Dose-dependent effects of testosterone on regional adipose tissue distribution in healthy young men. J Clin Endocrinol Metab 2004; 89: 718–26.

81. Marin P, Oden B, Bjorntorp P. Assimilation and mobilization of triglycerides in subcutaneous abdominal and femoral adipose tissue in vivo in men: effects of androgens. J Clin Endocrinol Metab 1995; 80: 239–43.

82. Turner L, Conway AJ, Jimenez M et al. Do reproductive hormones modify insulin sensitivity and metabolism in older men? A randomized, placebo-controlled clinical trial of recombinant human chorionic gonadotropin. Eur J Endocrinol 2003; 148(1): 55–66.

83. Shabsigh R, Katz M, Yan G, Makhsida N. Cardiovascular issues in hypogonadism and testosterone therapy. Am J Cardiol 2005 26; 96(12B): 67–72M.

84. Kapoor D, Malkin CJ, Channer KS et al. Androgens, insulin resistance and vascular disease in men. Clin Endocrinol (Oxf) 2005; 63: 239–50.

85. Vermeulen A, Kaufman JM, Goemaere S et al. Estradiol in elderly men. Aging Male 2002; 5: 98–102.

86. Rochira V, Granata AR, Madeo B et al. Estrogens in males: what have we learned in the last 10 years? Asian J Androl 2005; 7: 3–20.

87. Phillips GB. Is atherosclerotic cardiovascular disease an endocrinological disorder? The estrogen–androgen paradox. J Clin Endocrinol Metab 2005; 90: 2708–11.

88. Panet-Raymond V, Gottlieb B, Beitel LK et al. Interactions between androgen and estrogen receptors and the effects on their transactivational properties. Mol Cell Endocrinol 2000; 167: 139–50.

89. Must A, Spadano J, Coakley EH et al. The disease burden associated with overweight and obesity. JAMA 1999; 282: 1523–9.

90. Zhu S, Heymsfield SB, Toyoshima H et al. Race-ethnicity-specific waist circumference cutoffs for identifying cardiovascular disease risk factors. Am J Clin Nutr 2005; 81: 409–15.

91. Wildman RP, Gu D, Reynolds K et al. Are waist circumference and body mass index independently associated with cardiovascular disease risk in Chinese adults? Am J Clin Nutr 2005; 82: 1195–202.

92. Misra A, Wasir JS, Vikram NK. Waist circumference criteria for the diagnosis of abdominal obesity are not applicable uniformly to all populations and ethnic groups. Nutrition 2005; 21: 969–76.

93. Toni R, Malaguti A, Castorina S et al. New paradigms in neuroendocrinology: relationships between obesity, systemic inflammation and the neuroendocrine system. J Endocrinol Invest 2004; 27: 182–6.

94. Korbonits M, Grossman AB. Ghrelin: update on a novel hormonal system. Eur J Endocrinol 2004; 151(Suppl 1): S67–70.
95. Williams DL, Cummings DE. Regulation of ghrelin in physiologic and pathophysiologic states. J Nutr 2005; 135: 1320–5.
96. Leonetti F, Silecchia G, Iacobellis G et al. Different plasma ghrelin levels after laparoscopic gastric bypass and adjustable gastric banding in morbid obese subjects. J Clin Endocrinol Metab 2003; 88: 4227–31.
97. Ayyad C, Andersen T. Long-term efficacy of dietary treatment of obesity: a systematic review of studies published between 1931 and 1999. Obes Rev 2000; 1: 113–19.
98. Mathys M. Pharmacologic agents for the treatment of obesity. Clin Geriatr Med 2005; 21: 735–46, vii.
99. Norris SL, Zhang X, Avenell A et al. Efficacy of pharmacotherapy for weight loss in adults with type 2 diabetes mellitus: a meta-analysis. Arch Intern Med 2004; 164: 1395–404.
100. Bailey CJ. Drugs on the horizon for diabesity. Curr Diab Rep 2005; 5: 353–9.
101. Buchwald H, Avidor Y, Braunwald E et al. Bariatric surgery: a systematic review and meta-analysis. JAMA 2004; 292: 1724–37.
102. Fernandez AZ Jr, Demaria EJ, Tichansky DS et al. Multivariate analysis of risk factors for death following gastric bypass for treatment of morbid obesity. Ann Surg 2004; 239: 698–702.
103. Crookes PF. Surgical treatment of morbid obesity. Annu Rev Med 2006; 57: 243–64.
104. Stone NJ. Focus on lifestyle change and the metabolic syndrome. Endocrinol Metab Clin North Am 2004; 33: 493–508.
105. Hogan M. Physical and cognitive activity and exercise for older adults: a review. Int J Aging Hum Dev 2005; 60: 95–126.

Nutrition, Digestion and Metabolism

CHAPTER 25

Nutrition in older men

David R Thomas

Introduction

The effect of nutritional intake on men's health can be divided into three dimensions. First, food is essential to life. Good health is dependent on an adequate intake of energy and protein, and dietary sources of essential vitamins and minerals. Absence of essential nutrients can lead to primary disease (malnutrition syndromes). Second, nutritional intake has been associated with the risk of developing future disease. Good nutritional health has been linked to the prevention of premature mortality (lengthening lifespan) and to prevention of the development of chronic conditions (burden of disease). Finally, disease itself impacts nutritional health. A variety of diseases affect both nutritional intake (anorexia) and nutritional status (cachexia).

Morbidity and mortality differ between genders. Life expectancy at birth for men is 74.5 years, while life expectancy for women is 79.9 years. Over the lifespan, women outlive men by an average of 5.4 years. The top 10 causes of death in men, accounting for about 80% of deaths, are shown in Table 25.1. More than half of the deaths in men result from cardiovascular disease and cancer, both of which have been linked to nutrition.

The accumulation of chronic diseases leads to a 'burden of illness' and impacts health-related quality of life. There are gender-specific differences in the prevalence of chronic conditions in older

Table 25.1 *Top 10 causes of mortality in men: United States 2002*

Rank	Cause	Percentage of male deaths
1	Heart disease	28.4
2	Cancer	24.1
3	Unintentional injuries	5.8
4	Stroke	5.2
5	Chronic obstructive pulmonary disease	5.1
6	Diabetes	2.8
7	Influenza and pneumonia	2.4
8	Suicide	2.1
9	Kidney disease	1.6
10	Chronic liver disease and cirrhosis	1.5
Total		79

Table 25.2 *Prevalence of selected chronic conditions by age greater than 65 years and sex: United States 2001–2002*

Condition	Male	Female
More common in men		
All types heart disease	37.2	27.1
Coronary heart disease	27.1	17
Stroke	9.9	8.2
Any cancer	24.7	17.9
Prostate cancer	9	—
Skin cancer	8.2	4.8
Colorectal cancer	3.1	1.9
Melanoma	1.7	0.6
Lung cancer	1.2	0.5
Diabetes	17.6	13.8
Ulcer	15.3	12
Emphysema	6.6	3.8
More common in women		
Hypertension	47.2	52.2
Arthritic symptoms	30.6	31.8
Sinusitis	11	16.4
Kidney disease	3.2	12.0
Asthma	7.2	9.1
Hay fever	5.8	7.1
Chronic bronchitis	5.3	6.8
Liver disease	1.2	3.4

persons over the age of 65 years, as shown in Table 25.2. Heart disease and cancer account for almost two-thirds of prevalent conditions in older men, but less than half of prevalent conditions in older women. All but one of these prevalent conditions – stroke – have a higher mortality in men than in women. Prevention of these disorders by nutritional intervention has the potential to greatly impact the health status of older men.

A variety of gender-related differences may explain this disproportionate difference in mortality and morbidity. Body fat distribution differs between men and women, with men more likely to accumulate abdominal fat (apple-shaped obesity) and women more likely to accumulate fat around the hips (pear-shaped obesity). The apple-shaped obesity is associated with an increased risk of heart disease, diabetes, cancer, and stroke. Sex hormone differences may explain the fat distribution differences among genders.

Men are more likely to smoke, drink alcohol, use illicit drugs, and behave aggressively compared to women. Risk-taking behaviors certainly account for some of these differences. Aggressive behavior may explain an increased risk of mortality from accidents, suicide, and homicide. Nevertheless, the major contributors to morbidity and mortality in men are cardiovascular disease and cancer – conditions that have been related to nutritional risk factors.

The effect of age on nutrition

The daily volume of foods and beverages declines as a function of age. Total energy intake decreases substantially with age, by 1000 to 1200 kcal in men in the seventh decade. Older adults tend to consume less energy-dense sweets and fast foods, and consume more energy-dilute grains, vegetables, and fruits. Men exhibit a greater decrease in food intake, over the lifespan, than do women.[1] The cumulative effect of decreases in food intake and the anorexia of aging places older men at risk for nutritional deficiencies.[2,3] Lower food intake among the elderly has been associated with lower intakes of calcium, iron, zinc, B vitamins, and vitamin E. This low-energy intake or low-nutrient density of the diet may increase the risk of diet-related illnesses. Fifty percent of older adults have a vitamin and mineral intake less than the RDA, while 10–30% have subnormal levels of vitamins and minerals.[4]

Physiologic changes associated with age, including slower gastric emptying, altered hormonal responses, decreased basal metabolic rate, and altered taste and smell, may also contribute to lowered energy intake. Other factors such as marital status, income, education, socioeconomic status, diet-related attitudes and beliefs, and convenience likely play a role as well.[5]

Testosterone levels decline with aging and in the presence of co-existing disease can reach very low levels.[6,7] Notably, low testosterone levels are associated with elevated circulating leptin levels, an anorectic and lipolytic hormone produced by adipocytes. These changes probably account for age- and disease-related anorexia, weight loss, and cachexia in some hypogonadal men.[8,9]

The effect of nutrition on prevention of disease

A large body of epidemiologic evidence suggests that eating a diet rich in sources of vitamins and other nutrients has a protective effect on development of disease. Table 25.3 summarizes examples of the epidemiologic associations of nutrients with specific disease states. The data from randomized, controlled trials show (with a few exceptions) that supplementation with vitamin supplements does not have much effect on disease states. Table 25.4 summarizes examples of randomized, controlled trials and meta-analytic reviews for nutrients and specific diseases.

Cardiovascular disease

Cereal fiber consumption late in life is associated with a 21% lower risk of cardiovascular disease,

comparing the highest quintile of intake with the lowest quintile after adjustment for age, sex, education, diabetes, ever smoking, pack-years of smoking, daily physical activity, exercise intensity, alcohol intake, and fruit and vegetable fiber consumption. Neither fruit nor vegetable fiber intake were associated with development of cardiovascular disease. Higher cereal fiber intake was also associated with a lower risk of total stroke and ischemic stroke when analyzed separately. Dark breads such as wheat, rye, or pumpernickel were associated with a 24% lower risk of developing cardiovascular disease, compared to other sources.[10]

In one of the largest epidemiologic observations, 71 910 female participants in the Nurses' Health study and 37 725 male participants in the Health Professionals' Follow-up Study who were free of major chronic disease were followed for incidence of cardiovascular disease, cancer, or death. Total fruit and vegetable intake was inversely associated with risk of cardiovascular disease but not with overall cancer incidence. The benefit occurred in persons who had five or more daily servings. Of the food groups analyzed, green leafy vegetable intake showed the strongest inverse association with major chronic disease and cardiovascular disease. For an increment of one serving per day of green leafy vegetables, relative risks were 0.95 (95% CI: 0.92–0.99) for major chronic disease and 0.89 (95% CI: 0.83–0.96) for cardiovascular disease.[11] These findings suggest that high consumption of fruits and vegetables results in a small reduction in risk of cardiovascular disease. There was no association found between fruit and vegetable intake (either total or of any particular group) and overall cancer incidence. For men and women combined, persons in the highest quintile of total fruit and vegetable consumption did not have a lower risk for major chronic disease compared to those in the lowest quintile.

A number of specific diets have been proposed to decrease the incidence of cardiovascular disease. The Mediterranean diet is characterized by a high intake of vegetables, legumes, fruits, and cereals (in the past largely unrefined); a moderate to high intake of fish; a low intake of saturated lipids but high intake of unsaturated lipids, particularly olive

Table 25.3 *Observational studies on vitamin intake and health*

Study	Subjects	Outcome	Measure	Results
Robinson et al[87]	750 patients vs 800 controls	Coronary artery disease	Homocysteine concentrations >80th percentile	Increased risk
Robinson et al[87]	750 patients vs 800 controls	Coronary artery disease	Vitamin B6 < 20th percentile	Increased risk
Muntwyler et al[20]	83 639 male US physicians with no history of CVD or cancer	Cardiovascular disease or cardiovascular mortality	Self-reported use of vitamins E, C, or multivitamins	No association
Cancer Prevention Study[88]	26 593 male smokers, aged 50–69 years	Cerebral infarction	Dietary intake of beta carotene	0.77 (0.61–0.99)
Cancer Prevention Study[88]	26 593 male smokers, aged 50–69 years	Cerebral infarction	Lycopene, lutein, zeaxanthin, vitamin C, flavonols, flavones, vitamin E	No association
Tabak et al[33]	Finland (n = 1248), Italy (n = 1386), and the Netherlands (n = 691) middle-aged men	Pulmonary function	Higher intake of fruits, vegetables	Higher forced vital capacity
Tabak et al[33]	Finland (n = 1248), Italy (n = 1386), and the Netherlands (n = 691) middle-aged men	Pulmonary function	Higher intake of vitamin C, beta-carotene	No association
Tabak et al[33]	Finland (n = 1248), Italy (n = 1386), and the Netherlands (n = 691) middle-aged men	Pulmonary function	Higher intake of vitamin E	No association
Hung et al[4]	71 910 women participants in the Nurses' Health study and 37 725 men in the Health Professionals Follow-up Study, free of major chronic disease, 14-year follow-up	Cardiovascular disease or cancer	Total fruit and vegetable intake	Chronic disease = 0.95 (0.89–1.01); cardiovascular disease = 0.88 (0.81–0.95); cancer = 1.00 (0.95–1.05)

Table 25.4 *Randomized, controlled studies on vitamin intake and health*

Study	Subjects	Outcome	Intervention	Results
MRC/BHF Heart Protection Study[77]	20 536 subjects followed 5 years	All-cause, vascular or non-vascular mortality, or major coronary events, stroke, revascularization, and cancer	Vitamin E 600 mg/d, vitamin C 250 mg/d, and beta-carotene 20 mg/d vs placebo	No difference
The Beta-Carotene and Retinol Efficacy Trial[78]	18 314 subjects, 45–74 years, at high risk, followed 4 years	Lung cancer	Beta-carotene and retinyl palmitate vs placebo	28% higher incidence and 17% higher total mortality in the supplemented group
The SU.VI.MAX Study[79]	13 017 persons, age 45–60, followed 7.5 years	Cardiovascular disease or cardiovascular mortality	120 mg ascorbic acid, 30 mg vitamin E, 6 mg beta-carotene, 100 µg selenium, 20 mg zinc vs placebo	No association
HOPE trial[80]	3994 persons > 55 years with CVC or DBM, followed 7 years	Cardiovascular events and cancer	Vitamin E 400 IU/d vs placebo	No difference in cancer incidence, cancer mortality, cardiovascular events; higher risk of CHF and hospitalization for CHF
Meta-analysis of 7 trials[89]	4119 persons	Age-related macular degeneration, progression to advanced disease	Antioxidant vitamin and zinc	0.72, CI 0.52–0.98
Meta-analysis of 7 trials[89]	4119 persons	Age-related macular degeneration, prevention	Vitamin E, beta-carotene, or both	No benefit
Girodon et al[90]	725 institutionalized elderly subjects > 65 years,	Antibody titers, respiratory infections, urinary tract	Trace elements (zinc and selenium sulfide) or vitamins (beta-carotene,	Antibody titers after influenza vaccine higher in groups receiving

Table 25.4 *(Continued)*

Study	Subjects	Outcome	Intervention	Results
	followed 2 years	infections, survival rate	ascorbic acid, and vitamin E) vs placebo	trace elements alone or with vitamins, but the vitamin group had significantly lower antibody titers; no effect on infections or survival
Chandra et al[91]	96 institutionalized subjects	Infection, antibiotics	Vitamin A 400 units, beta-carotene 16 mg; thiamine 2.2 mg; riboflavin 1.5 mg; niacin 16 mg; vitamin B6 3.0 mg; folate 400 µg; vitamin B12 4.0 µg; vitamin C 80 mg; vitamin D 4 µg; vitamin E 440 mg; iron 16 mg; zinc 14 mg; copper 1.4 mg; selenium 20 µg; iodine 0.2 mg; calcium 200 mg; and magnesium 100 mg vs placebo (calcium, 200 µg, and magnesium, 100 mg)	23 vs 48 fewer infection-related illness days; 18 vs 32 fewer days taking antibiotics
Meta-analysis[81]	135 967 participants in 19 clinical trials	All-cause mortality	Vitamin E, all doses	Higher mortality
Meta-analysis[82]	135 967 participants in 19 clinical trials	Alzheimer's dementia	Vitamin E 2000 IU/d	Longer duration to institutionalization, higher mortality

oil; a low to moderate intake of dairy products, mostly cheese and yogurt; a low intake of meat; and a modest intake of ethanol, mostly as wine. The effect of the Mediterranean diet was first thought to be due to lowering of cholesterol levels, but emphasis has recently shifted from the low content of saturated lipids toward its high content of olive oil and

a vague constellation of other characteristics. In epidemiologic studies, respondents rated their adherence to a typical Mediterranean diet on a scale of 1 to 10. Sixty-three percent of subjects had poor to average compliance with the diet (score 1 to 4), and no effect on mortality was seen. A 43% decrease in mortality was seen in those who had better than average adherence to the diet and a 75% reduction in mortality was seen in those with very good adherence to the diet.[12] Two randomized controlled trials have demonstrated that a Mediterranean diet high in alpha-linolenic acids in patients who have had a myocardial infarction,[13] or a Mediterranean diet modified with whole grains, fruits, vegetables, and nuts in patients with diagnosed cardiovascular disease, can reduce cardiovascular mortality.[14]

The effect of the Mediterranean diet extended to persons over the age of 60 years, who had no coronary heart disease, stroke, or cancer at baseline. However, the effect size was smaller, averaging a 7% decrease in mortality for each 2-step increment of diet compliance score. Moreover, the effect was not homogeneous across all geographic areas, with Greece showing the most effect size and no effect seen in the Netherlands or in Germany.[15]

Other epidemiologic data suggest a clear association between elevated homocysteine levels and higher risk of stroke and cardiovascular disease. Folate levels, which are dependent on homocysteine levels, are predictive of cardiovascular risk. The risk of stroke is also higher for persons who consume fewer fruits and vegetables.

Taken together, the association between homocysteine levels and vascular disease is strong. An association has been shown for carotid disease (5 studies), coronary disease (2 studies), peripheral vascular disease (1 study), and aortic atherosclerotic disease (1 study). An increased risk of cardiovascular disease and high levels of homocysteine levels has been shown in 10 of 13 case-control studies and 1 cohort study. A decreased risk for cardiovascular disease has been observed with high levels of folate (3 of 5 prospective and 1 of 2 retrospective studies) and vitamin B6 (2 of 2 prospective and 2 of 2 retrospective studies), but not with high levels of vitamin B12 (1 prospective and 2 retrospective studies).[16] Whether or not decreasing homocysteine levels by dietary or pharmacologic interventions will reduce cardiovascular mortality is not known.

Randomized, controlled trials of specific supplements have failed to demonstrate a consistent or significant effect of any single vitamin or combination of nutrients on incidence of or death from cardiovascular disease.[17] Vitamin E plus vitamin C plus beta-carotene showed no difference in all-cause, vascular, or non-vascular mortality, or secondary measures including major coronary events, stroke, revascularization, and cancer compared to placebo.[18] There is some concern that these vitamins may blunt the protective HDL2 cholesterol response to HDL cholesterol-targeted therapy.[19]

Other studies have not supported a link between supplemental vitamins and disease. The self-reported intake of vitamins E, C, or multivitamins was not associated with a decreased incidence of cardiovascular disease or cardiovascular mortality after adjusting for known cardiovascular risk factors in a large observational study of male physicians.[20]

Lung cancer

Four placebo-controlled trials have not shown a benefit of beta-carotene, alone or in combination with alpha-tocopherol or retinol, or alpha-tocopherol alone on the development of lung cancer. For people with risk factors for lung cancer, no reduction in lung cancer incidence or mortality was found in those taking vitamins alone compared with placebo. For people with no known risk factors of lung cancer, none of the vitamins or their combinations appeared to have any effect. In fact, in combination with retinol, a statistically significant increase in risk of lung cancer incidence was found compared to placebo.[21]

Colon cancer

A diet that is low in fat and high in fiber, fruits, and vegetables does not appear to reduce the risk of recurrence of colorectal adenomas. In 2079 men and women aged 35 years or older who had one or more confirmed colorectal adenomas, randomly assigned a low fat (20% of total calories), high fiber (18 g of dietary fiber per 1000 kcal) diet containing 3.5 servings per 100 kcal of fruits and vegetables (3.5 servings per 1000 kcal), the rate of recurrence of large adenomas and advanced adenomas did not differ significantly from the group assigned to their usual diet.[22]

Prostate cancer

Six hundred and eighty-nine men who were randomized to intensive counseling to consume a diet low in fat and high in fiber, fruits, and vegetables were compared to 661 men who were given a standard brochure on a healthy diet. Measurement of prostate-specific antigen at baseline and annually for 4 years showed no differences between groups.[23]

Bladder cancer

Micronutrient intake, including lutein, zeaxanthin, anhydrolutein, alpha-cryptoxanthin, beta-cryptoxanthin, lycopene, dihydrolycopene, alpha-carotene, beta-carotene, total carotenoids, retinol, alpha-tocopherol, beta-tocopherol, gamma-tocopherol, delta-tocopherol, and total tocopherols, were examined in men who developed bladder cancer after 20 years of surveillence and compared to age-matched controls. There were statistically significant inverse linear trends in risk for alpha-carotene, beta-carotene, lutein plus zeaxanthin, beta-cryptoxanthin, and total carotenoids. However, after adjustment for pack-years of cigarette smoking none of the inverse trends remained significant.[24]

Diabetes

In a study of 3042 subjects randomly enrolled using the 2001 Census data, who had no clinical evidence of cardiovascular disease, 33% of the men and 13% of the women fulfilled the NCEP ATP III criteria for the metabolic syndrome. In this group who met the criteria for the metabolic syndrome, 58% of men and 72% of women were sedentary.[25]

Glycemic control is central to improving outcome in diabetes.[26] Weight loss has been strongly associated with an improvement in glycemic control.[27] Dietary advice has been a cornerstone of the treatment of diabetes. A number of interventions have been reviewed in a formal meta-analysis.[28] Eighteen trials were identified. Dietary approaches in this review included low-fat/high-carbohydrate diets, high-fat/low-carbohydrate diets, low-calorie (1000 kcal per day) and very-low-calorie (500 kcal per day) diets, and modified fat diets. Two trials compared the American Diabetes Association exchange diet with a standard reduced fat diet and five studies assessed low-fat diets versus moderate-fat or low-carbohydrate diets. Two studies assessed the effects of a very-low-calorie diet versus a low-calorie diet. Six studies compared dietary advice

with dietary advice plus exercise and three other studies assessed dietary advice versus dietary advice plus behavioral approaches. No high-quality data were found on the efficacy of the dietary treatment of type 2 diabetes. Exercise, however, improved glycolysated hemoglobin at 6 and 12 months in people with type 2 diabetes.

Few data exist for or against the use of low-carbohydrate diets, particularly among participants older than age 50 years, for use longer than 90 days, or for diets of 20 g/day or less of carbohydrates. Weight loss in diabetics using low-carbohydrate diets was principally associated with decreased caloric intake and increased diet duration, but not with reduced carbohydrate content.[29]

Low intakes of vitamin C[30] and zinc[31] have been epidemiologically associated with a higher prevalence of diabetes. In other trials of diabetic individuals, no associations were observed between glycolysate hemoglobin and intake of vitamin C, or intake of vitamin E or beta-carotene.[32]

Pulmonary disease

Lung function studies illustrate the sometimes confusing data from epidemiologic surveys. Forced expiratory volume was associated with intake of vitamin E in Finland, but only with dietary intake of fruit in Italy, and only with beta-carotene intake in the Netherlands. However, in all three countries, men with above-average intakes of both fruit and vegetables had a higher forced expiratory volume than those with a low intake of both foods. However, after adjustment for energy intake, the association of all three antioxidants disappeared.[33] Differences across populations, even over relatively small distances, confound these studies. Six controlled trials on supplementation of vitamin C in persons with asthma showed no appreciable benefit on asthma outcome.[34]

Osteoporosis

Osteoporosis, a metabolic bone disease characterized by low bone mass, microarchitectural deterioration of bone tissue, and increased susceptibility to fracture, is now recognized to be a disease of both men and women. By bone mineral density standards, the prevalence of osteoporosis is approximately 2 million men in the United States. The age-related decline in bone mineral density in men seems to result from a decline in the levels of bioavailable estrogen. Alternatively, genetic polymorphisms may predispose men to a weakened, osteoporotic phenotype.[35] The treatment of osteoporosis in men, including bisphosphonates, calcium, and intermittent parathyroid hormone, is similar to that in women.

Vitamin and mineral nutrition

Evidence of epidemiologic associations of vitamins and disease states has been found for nine vitamins. Inadequate folate status is associated with neural tube defects and some cancers. Folate and vitamins B6 and B12 are required for homocysteine metabolism and are associated with coronary heart disease risk. Vitamin E and lycopene may decrease the risk of prostate cancer. Vitamin D is associated with decreased occurrence of fractures when taken with calcium.[36] Zinc, beta-carotene, and vitamin E appear to slow the progression of macular degeneration, but do not reduce the incidence.

In observational studies (case-control or cohort design), people with a high intake of antioxidant vitamins by regular diet or as food supplements generally have a lower risk of myocardial infarction and stroke than people who are low consumers of antioxidant vitamins. The association in observation studies has been shown for carotene and ascorbic acid, as well as tocopherol. The use of various dietary supplements, including vitamins, to prevent or delay disease or aging rests for the most part on epidemiologic associations. It does appear from these data that a diet rich in vitamins is associated with a tendency to improved health.

However, the results from controlled trials are dismal. In randomized controlled trials, antioxidant vitamins as food supplements have no beneficial effects in the primary prevention of myocardial infarction and stroke. Thus, the apparent beneficial results of a high intake of antioxidant vitamins reported in observational studies have not been confirmed in large randomized trials.[37]

Baseline intake of carotenes and vitamin C, or vitamin E in supplemental or dietary (non-supplemental)

form, or in both forms, was not related to a decreased risk of dementia of the Alzheimer's type after 4 years of follow-up.[38]

The discrepancy between different types of studies is probably explained by the fact that dietary composition and supplement use is a component in a cluster of healthy behavior. An alternative hypothesis is that there are as yet unknown essential organic compounds in certain foods.

Much of the enthusiasm for the use of vitamin or mineral supplements to prevent disease or increase longevity results from the belief that supplementation is harmless. However, serious adverse events have been reported. Toxicity may result from excessive doses of vitamin A during early pregnancy and from other fat-soluble vitamins taken in high doses. There is increasing concern from randomized, controlled trials that beta-carotene and vitamin E may be associated with a higher mortality risk.

The most prudent approach is to recommend a daily intake of fruits and vegetables as a likely source of essential nutrients. Failing compliance with a natural source of essential nutrients, and in populations at high risk of vitamin deficiency, vitamin supplements should be encouraged. Vitamin supplements should be used as replacement doses guided by the recommended daily allowances, and super-therapeutic doses should be avoided.

The effect of nutrition on disease

Obesity is associated with greater morbidity and poorer health-related quality of life than smoking, problem alcohol drinking, or poverty,[39] and has been argued to be the number one health problem in the United States. In general population studies, the relationship between mortality and body mass index (BMI) has been reported as a J-shaped or a U-shaped curve.[40] Excess risk of death has been observed at both extremes of high and low weight. This relationship is clear in the young and middle-aged population, but becomes more controversial in the older population (see Table 25.5).

Data from the Framingham Heart Study[84] demonstrate an increased mortality risk for both men and women at the highest extremes of BMI,

Table 25.5 *Association of mortality and high body weight*

Study	Characteristic	Relative risk	95% CI
Cancer Prevention Study I[92]	30–44-year-old men	1.10	1.04–1.16
	65–74-year-old men	1.03	1.02–1.05
	30–44-year-old women	1.08	1.05–1.11
	65–74-year-old women	1.02	1.02–1.03
Cancer Prevention Study II[93]	65–74-year-old men, BMI 26.5–27.9	1.1	1.0–1.3
	> 75-year-old men, BMI 26.5–27.9	1.1	0.97–1.2
	65–74-year-old women, BMI 26.5–27.9	1.04	0.9–1.2
	> 75 year-old women BMI 26.5–27.9	1.07	1.0–1.2
	65–74-year-old men, BMI 30–31.9	1.4	1.2–1.7
	> 75 year-old men, BMI 30–31.9	1.2	1.0–1.3
	65–74-year-old women, BMI 30–31.9	1.3	1.2–1.5
	> 75-year-old women BMI 30–31.9	1.3	1.2–1.4
Nurses' Health Study[94]	BMI 29–31.9 vs BMI 19	2.1	
	BMI > 32 vs BMI 19	2.2	
Framingham Heart Study[84]	BMI > 70th percentile	2.0	
EPESE[85]	BMI highest quintile vs middle quintile		
	Men	1.33	1.13–1.57
	Women	1.31	1.12–1.53
Cardiovascular Health Study[47]	BMI > 20	None	
NHANES I[86]	BMI > 30 vs BMI 22 to 30	None	
Community study[83]	BMI > 27	None	

NHANES, National Health and Nutrition Examination Survey Epidemiological Follow-Up Study; EPESE, Established Populations for Epidemiologic Studies of the Elderly.

even when accounting for potential effects of excess weight on serum cholesterol level, blood glucose level, and systolic blood pressure. At the upper extreme, risk of death was 2-fold higher over the entire follow-up period for persons with BMI above the 70th percentile at both 55 and 65 years of age.

Data from Established Populations for Epidemiologic Studies of the Elderly (EPESE)[85] demonstrate that mortality risk was approximately 40% higher for persons in the heaviest quintile of BMI at age 50 compared with persons in the middle quintile. In the Cardiovasular Health Study (CHS) data, a BMI greater than 32 in men was associated with an age-adjusted 18% increase in mortality.[47] Conversely, a BMI greater than 34 in women was associated with only an 8% increase in mortality.

Greater BMI was associated with higher mortality in men and women up to 75 years of age in the Cancer Prevention Study I.[41] However, the magnitude of the risk associated with greater BMI diminishes with age. For example, for mortality from cardiovascular disease, the relative risk associated with an increment of 1 in the BMI was 10% for 30–44-year-old and 3% for 65–74-year-old men.

A body mass index of 25 to 30 was not associated with excess mortality using the National Health and Nutrition Examination Survey (NHANES) data compared to the normal weight category of 18.5 to less than 25.[86] Excess mortality began only at a BMI of greater than 30. These findings are consistent with the increases in life expectancy in the United States and the declining mortality rates from ischemic heart disease.[42]

Paradoxically, although the prevalence of obesity in the United States has increased dramatically in recent decades, the major risk factors for cardiovascular disease except diabetes have decreased over time across all body mass index groups. Compared with obese persons in 1960–62, obese persons in 1999–2000 had a 21% lower prevalence of high cholesterol level, an 18% lower prevalence of high blood pressure, and a 12% lower smoking prevalence. The lower prevalence of risk factors was associated with an increase in lipid-lowering and antihypertensive medication use, particularly among obese persons. Although the prevalence of diabetes was stable within BMI groups, other cardiovascular disease risk factors declined considerably over time.[43]

A BMI of greater than $27 \, kg/m^2$ has not been significantly related to risk of mortality.[44,45] In older patients, only a slight elevation in mortality rates occurred at a BMI of greater than $35 \, kg/m^2$.[46,47] Overall, the data suggest that a BMI >27 kg/m^2 does not convey the same degree of increased mortality risk in older adults.[48] Current standards have defined overweight for all ages as a BMI of 27.8 or more for men and 27.3 or more for women.[49] Andres et al have has suggested that a BMI of 24 to 30 is the desirable range for people aged 60 to 69.[50] Although there is increased mortality at extremes of body weight, these data would seem to support using higher desirable weights for older adults.

Only limited data support the notion that intentional weight loss reduces total mortality. However, mortality is only a small part of the substantial burden of disease caused by obesity-related conditions such as hypertension,[51,52] diabetes mellitus,[53,54] coronary artery disease,[55–58] degenerative arthritis,[59] and cancers of the breast,[60,61] uterus,[62] and colon.[63] Short-term reductions in caloric intake (dieting) have favorable effects on blood pressure, cholesterol, and metabolic rate. These benefits require at least a 20% reduction in caloric intake.[64]

Weight loss has been shown to reduce disease-specific risks such as hypertension and type 2 diabetes.[65] However, it should be noted that overweight/

obesity-related comorbidities, particularly those associated with the insulin resistance syndrome (e.g., hypertension, dyslipidemias, and hyperinsulinemia) can be improved rather independently of weight loss.[66,67] Blood pressure can be lowered in the absence of weight loss by dietary changes.[68] The effect on blood pressure by non-pharmacologic interventions can be maintained for 3–5 years despite significant increases in body weight.[69] Other trials in coronary artery disease have shown prevention effects to be independent of weight loss.[70] The data suggest that improvement in comorbid conditions can be improved with lifestyle changes, but that the effect is independent of whether weight loss occurs.

The effect of disease on nutrition

Body weight increases with age in women, at least until their seventies. However, in men body weight tends to decline after age 70, in part due to hormonal effects and sarcopenia.[71]

Cachexia is a major cause of weight loss and increased mortality, affecting an estimated 5 million persons in the United States. Clinically, cachexia manifests with excessive weight loss in the setting of ongoing disease, usually with a disproportionate muscle wasting. Although numerous diseases are associated with cachexia, the underlying pathophysiologic mechanisms are unclear.[72] Cachexia is frequently a complication of disease states, including congestive cardiomyopathy, end-stage renal disease, chronic obstructive pulmonary disease, acquired immunodeficiency syndrome, rheumatoid arthritis, and cancer.[73]

Cytokines associated with disease states directly result in feeding suppression and lower intake of nutrients. Interleukin-1 beta and tumor necrosis factor act on the glucose-sensitive neurons in the ventromedial hypothalamic nucleus (a 'satiety' site) and the lateral hypothalamic area (a 'hunger' site).[74] The data suggest that cytokine levels are commonly associated with disease conditions characterized by cachexia, and may play a role in appetite suppression, mortality, and weight loss.

When observational data for persons with the lowest and highest BMI have been adjusted for

Table 25.6 *Association of weight loss and mortality*

Study	Characteristics	Factors	Relative risk	95% CI
NHANESI[86]	BMI 22–26, who lost > 10% of maximum lifetime weight within the 10 years before the study	Men Women	2.1 3.6	
EPESE[85]	Lost 10% or more of body weight between age 50 and follow-up	Men Women	1.69 1.62	1.45–1.97 1.38–1.90
CHS[47]	Involuntary weight loss of 10 lb or more in the year before baseline	Men (% mortality) Women (% mortality)	33.0% 16.2%	
Community Study[83]	288 frail elders 78 ± 8 years, home support services; followed 3–5 years	Weight loss at baseline Male gender Age at baseline	1.76 2.71 1.40	1.15–2.71 1.73–4.24 1.06–1.86

NHANES, National Health and Nutrition Examination Survey Epidemiological Follow-Up Study; EPESE, Established Populations for Epidemiologic Studies of the Elderly; CHS, Cardiovascular Health Study.

weight loss, weight loss rather than current BMI becomes the salient factor (Table 25.6). The presence of pre-existing illness may confound the association between weight loss and death, either because of earlier deaths from non-cardiovascular disease or because weight loss serves as a marker for more severe cardiovascular disease. In the NHANES I dataset, risk of mortality was higher for both men and women who lost 10% or more of their maximum lifetime weight within the 10 years before the study, even when controlling for current weight. The effect of pre-existing illness was adjusted for by excluding deaths within the first 5 and first 8 years of the study. This adjustment weakened the association between weight loss and increased risk for death from non-cardiovascular disease in women. There was a strong association between weight loss and increased risk for death from cardiovascular disease among men and women even with a maximum BMI between 26 and 29 (relative risks of up to 2.1 and 3.6, respectively).[75]

In the EPESE, persons who lost 10% or more of body weight between age 50 and old age had a 60%

increased risk of mortality compared with persons of stable weight. Exclusion of participants who lost 10% or more of their weight and adjustment for health status eliminated the higher risk of death associated with low weight. This inverse association of weight and mortality in old age appears to reflect illness-related weight loss from heavier weight in middle age.

In the CHS, the age-adjusted death rate for people who reported an unintended loss of 10 lb or more in the year before evaluation (16.2% for women and 33.0% for men) was much higher than the death rate for those who lost weight through diet or exercise (5% in women and 16.4% in men), or who maintained or gained weight (9.5% in women and 14% in men). People who had lost 10% or more of their body weight since age 50 also exhibited a relatively higher death rate (15.9% in women and 30.3% in men). The relationship between BMI and mortality disappeared after excluding those who lost weight since age 50. Weight loss between baseline and age 50 was a critical risk factor for higher mortality, rather than being overweight.

From the NHANES I data, an increased risk in women with a lower BMI occurred only among those who had lost more than 8.5% of their reported lifetime maximum weight. Women who had lost weight had a higher risk than women with a low BMI. In fact, women with a low BMI, but whose weight remained stable, had the lowest risk of mortality. Thus, the effect of weight loss on mortality is more profound than current weight, even when accounting for factors associated with weight loss and increased mortality risk.[76]

Summary and clinical relevance

Epidemiologic data suggest that nutrition affects future health. Older men in particular are prone to diseases which have been linked to nutrition. A healthy diet, defined as higher consumption of fruits and vegetables, a reduction in fat intake, and adequate vitamin D, has been associated with a lower prevalence of cardiovascular disease and reduction in fractures. Unfortunately, supplementation of specific nutrients has not been as successful in disease prevention. Finally, the presence of disease itself impacts nutritional health, leading to anorexia and cachexia syndromes. Optimizing nutritional intake may be associated with a reduction in prevalence and burden of disease in older men.

References

1. Morley JE. Anorexia of aging – physiologic and pathologic. Am J Clin Nutr 1997; 66: 760–73.
2. Morley JE, Thomas DR. Anorexia and aging: pathophysiology. Nutrition 1999; 15: 499–503.
3. Thomas DR. Distinguishing starvation from cachexia. Geriatr Clin North Am 2002; 18: 883–92.
4. Wakimoto P, Block G. Dietary intake, dietary patterns, and changes with age: an epidemiological perspective. J Gerontol Series A Biol Sci Med Sci 2001; 56: 65–80.
5. Drewnowski A, Shultz JM. Impact of aging on eating behaviors, food choices, nutrition, and health status. J Nutr Health Aging 2001; 5: 75–9.
6. Morley JE, Kaiser FE, Perry HM et al. Longitudinal changes in testosterone, luteinizing hormone, and follicle-stimulating hormone in healthy older men. Metab Clin Exper 1997; 46: 410–13.
7. Bhasin S. Testosterone supplementation for aging-associated sarcopenia. J Gerontol Med Sci 2003; 58A: 1002–8.
8. Baumgartner RN, Waters DL, Gallagher D, Morley JE, Garry PJ. Predictors of skeletal muscle mass in elderly men and women. Mech Ageing Devel 1999; 107: 123–36.
9. Wittert GA, Chapman IM, Haren MT, Mackintosh S, Coates P, Morley JE. Oral testosterone supplementation increases muscle and decreases fat mass in healthy elderly males with low-normal gonadal status. J Georntol Med Sci 2003; 58A: 618–25.
10. Mozaffarian D, Kumanyika SK, Lemaitre RN et al. Cereal, fruit, and vegetable fiber intake and the risk of cardiovascular disease in elderly individuals. JAMA 2003; 289(13): 1659–66.
11. Hung HC, Joshipura KJ, Jiang R et al. Fruit and vegetable intake and risk of major chronic disease. J Natl Cancer Inst 2004; 96: 1577–84.
12. Trichopoulou A, Bamia C, Trichopoulos D. Mediterranean diet and survival among patients with coronary heart disease in Greece. Arch Intern Med 2005; 165(8): 929–35.
13. de Lorgeril M, Renaud S, Mamelle N et al. Mediterranean alpha-linolenic acid-rich diet in secondary prevention of coronary heart disease. Lancet 1994; 343: 1454–9.
14. Singh RB, Dubnov G, Niaz MA et al. Effect of an Indo-Mediterranean diet on progression of coronary artery disease in high risk patients (Indo-Mediterranean Diet Heart Study): a randomised single-blind trial. Lancet 2002; 360: 1455–61.
15. Trichopoulou A, Orfanos P, Norat T et al. Modified Mediterranean diet and survival: EPIC-elderly prospective cohort study. BMJ 2005; 330(7498): 991.
16. Anonymous. Review: high levels of homocysteine are associated with an increased risk for cardiovascular disease. ACP J Club 2000; 132: 73.
17. Morris CD, Carson S. Routine vitamin supplementation to prevent cardiovascular disease: a summary of the evidence for the US Preventive Services Task Force. Ann Intern Med 2003; 139: 56–70.
18. Antioxidant vitamins did not reduce death, vascular events, or cancer in high-risk patients. ACP Journal Club 2003; 138: 3.
19. Brown BG, Cheung MC, Lee AC, Zhao XQ, Chait A. Antioxidant vitamins and lipid therapy – end of a long romance? Arterioscler Thromb Vasc Biol 2002; 22: 1535–46.
20. Muntwyler J, Hennekens CH, Manson JE, Buring JE, Gaziano JM. Vitamin supplement use in a low-risk population of US male physicians and subsequent cardiovascular mortality. Arch Intern Med 2002; 162: 1472–6.

21. Caraballoso M, Sacristan M, Serra C, Bonfill X. Drugs for preventing lung cancer in healthy people. Cochrane Database System Rev 2003; 3.

22. Schatzkin A, Lanza E, Corle D et al. Lack of effect of a low-fat, high-fiber diet on the recurrence of colorectal adenomas. Polyp Prevention Trial Study Group. N Engl J Med 2000; 342(16): 1149–55.

23. Shike M, Latkany L, Riedel E et al. and the Polyp Prevention Trial Study Group. Lack of effect of a low-fat, high-fruit, -vegetable, and -fiber diet on serum prostate-specific antigen of men without prostate cancer: results from a randomized trial. Am Soc Clin Oncol 2002; 20(17): 3592–8.

24. Nomura AMY, Lee J, Stemmermann GN, Franke AA. Serum vitamins and the subsequent risk of bladder cancer. J Urol 2003; 170(4 Part 1): 1146–50.

25. Pitsavos C, Panagiotakos DB, Chrysohoou C, Kavouras S, Stefanadis C. The associations between physical activity, inflammation, and coagulation markers, in people with metabolic syndrome: the ATTICA study. Eur J Cardiovasc Prevent Rehab 2005; 12(2): 151–8.

26. Turner RC, Millns H, Neil HA et al. Risk factors for coronary artery disease in non-insulin dependent diabetes mellitus: United Kingdom Prospective Diabetes Study (UKPDS: 23). BMJ 1998; 316(7134): 823–8.

27. Grylls WK, McKenzie JE, Horwath CC, Mann JI. Lifestyle factors associated with glycaemic control and body mass index in older adults with diabetes. Eur J Clin Nutr 2003; 57(11): 1386–93.

28. Moore H, Summerbell C, Hooper L et al. Dietary advice for treatment of type 2 diabetes mellitus in adults. Cochrane Database System Rev 2005; 4.

29. Bravata DM, Sanders L, Huang J et al. Efficacy and safety of low-carbohydrate diets: a systematic review. JAMA 2003; 289(14): 1837–50.

30. Sargeant LA, Wareham NJ, Bingham S et al. Vitamin C and hyperglycemia in the European Prospective Investigation into Cancer – Norfolk (EPIC-Norfolk) study: a population-based study. Diabetes Care 2000; 23(6): 726–32.

31. Singh RB, Niaz MA, Rastogi SS et al. Current zinc intake and risk of diabetes and coronary artery disease and factors associated with insulin resistance in rural and urban populations of North India. J Am Coll Nutr 1998; 17(6): 564–70.

32. Shoff SM, Mares-Perlman JA, Cruickshanks KJ et al. Glycosylated hemoglobin concentrations and vitamin E, vitamin C, and beta-carotene intake in diabetic and nondiabetic older adults. Am J Clin Nutr 1993; 58(3): 412–16.

33. Tabak C, Smit HA, Rasanen L et al. Dietary factors and pulmonary function: a cross sectional study in middle aged men from three European countries. Thorax 1999; 54: 1021–6.

34. Ram FSF, Rowe BH, Kaur B. Vitamin C supplementation for asthma. Cochrane Database System Rev 2003; 3.

35. Stock H, Schneider A, Strauss E. Osteoporosis: a disease in men. Clin Orthopaed Rel Res 2004; (425): 143–51.

36. Fairfield KM, Fletcher RH. Vitamins for chronic disease prevention in adults – scientific review. JAMA 2002; 287(23): 3116–26.

37. Asplund K. Antioxidant vitamins in the prevention of cardiovascular disease: a systematic review. J Intern Med 2002; 251: 372–92.

38. Luchsinger JA, Tang MX, Shea S, Mayeux R. Antioxidant vitamin intake and risk of Alzheimer disease. Arch Neurol 2003; 60: 203–8.

39. Sturm R, Wells KB. Does obesity contribute as much to morbidity as poverty or smoking? Pub Health 2001; 115: 229–235.

40. Weindruch R, Sohal RS. Caloric intake and aging. N Engl J Med 1997; 337: 986–94.

41. Stevens J, Cai J, Pamuk ER et al. The effect of age on the association between body-mass index and mortality. N Engl J Med 1998; 338: 1–7.

42. Flegal KM, Graubard BI, Williamson DF, Gail MH. Excess deaths associated with underweight, overweight, and obesity. JAMA 2005; 293(15): 1861–7.

43. Gregg EW, Cheng YJ, Cadwell BL et al. Secular trends in cardiovascular disease risk factors according to body mass index in US adults. JAMA 2005; 293(15): 1868–74.

44. Landi F, Zuccala G, Gambassi G et al. Body mass index and mortality among older people living in the community. J Am Geriatr Soc 1999; 47: 1072–6.

45. Dorn JM, Schisterman EF, Winkelstein W, Trevisan M. Body mass index and mortality in a general population sample of men and women. Am J Epidemiol 1997; 146: 919–31.

46. Landi F, Onder G, Gambassi G et al. Body mass index and mortality among hospitalized patients. Arch Intern Med 2000; 160: 2641–4.

47. Diehr P, Bild DE, Harris TB et al. Body mass index and mortality in nonsmoking older adults: the Cardiovascular Health Study. Am J Public Health 1998; 88: 623–9.

48. Thomas DR, Morley JE. Obesity after menopause. Infertil Reprod Med Clin North Am 2001; 12: 605–23.

49. Kuczmarski RJ, Flegal KM, Campbell SM, Johnson CL. Increasing prevalence of overweight among US adults: the National Health and Nutrition Examination Surveys, 1960 to 1991. JAMA 1994; 272: 205–11.

50. Andres R, Elahi D, Tobin JD et al. Impact of age on weight goals. Ann Intern Med 1985; 103: 1030–3.

51. Stamler R, Stamler J, Riedlinger WF, Algera G, Roberts RH. Weight and blood pressure. Findings in hypertension screening of 1 million Americans. JAMA 1978; 240: 1607–10.

52. Reeder BA, Senthilselvan A, Despres JP et al. The association of cardiovascular disease risk factors with abdominal obesity in Canada. CMAJ 1997; 157: S39–45.

53. Colditz GA, Willet WC, Rotnizky A, Manson J. Weight gain as a risk factor for clinical diabetes mellitus in women. Ann Intern Med 1995; 122: 481–6.

54. Manson JE, Nathan DM, Krolewski AS et al. A prospective study of exercise and incidence of diabetes among U.S. male physicians. JAMA 1992; 268: 63–7.

55. Willett WC, Manson JE, Stampfer MD et al. Weight, weight change and coronary heart disease in women. Risk within the 'normal' weight range. JAMA 1995; 273: 461–5.

56. Hubert HB, Fienleib M, McNamara PM et al. Obesity as an independent risk factor for cardiovascular disease: a 26-year follow-up of participants in the Framingham Heart Study. Circulation 1983; 67: 968–77.

57. Rabkin SW, Mathewson FAL, Hsu PH. Relation of body weight to development of ischemic heart disease in a cohort of young North American men after a 26 year observation period: the Manitoba Study. Am J Cardiol 1977; 39: 452–8.

58. Harris TB, Launer LJ, Madans J, Feldman JJ. Cohort study of effects of being overweight and change in weight on risk of coronary heart disease in old age. BMJ 1997; 314: 1791–4.

59. Sahyoun NR, Hochberg MC, Helmick CG, Harris T, Pamuk ER. Body mass index, weight change, and incidence of self-reported physician-diagnosed arthritis among women. Am J Pub Health 1999; 89: 391–4.

60. Paffenberger RS Jr, Kampert JB, Chang HG. Characteristics that predict risk of breast cancer before and after menopause. Am J Epidemiol 1980; 112: 258–68.

61. Lubin F, Ruder AM, Wax Y et al. Overweight and changes in weight throughout life in breast cancer etiology. A case-control study. Am J Epidemiol 1985; 122: 579–88.

62. Kelsey JL, LiVolsi VA, Holford TR et al. A case-control study of cancer of the endometrium. Am J Epidemiol 1982; 116: 333–42.

63. Phillips RL, Snowdown DA. Dietary relationships with fatal colorectal cancer among Seventh Day Adventists. J Natl Cancer Inst 1985; 74: 307–17.

64. Velthuis-te Wierik EJ, van den Berg H, Schaafsma G, Hendriks HF, Brouwer A. Energy restrictions, a useful intervention to retard human ageing? Results of a feasibility study. Eur J Clin Nutr 1994; 48: 138–48.

65. Diabetes Prevention Program Research Group. Reduction in the incidence of type 2 diabetes with lifestyle intervention or metformin. N Engl J Med 2002; 346: 393–403.

66. de Lorgeril M, Renaud S, Mamelle N et al. Mediterranean alpha-linolenic acid-rich diet in secondary prevention of coronary heart disease. Lancet 1994; 343: 1454–9.

67. Weintraub MS, Rosen Y, Otto R, Eisenberg S, Breslow SL. Physical exercise conditioning in the absence of weight loss reduces fasting and postprandial triglyceride-rich lipoprotein levels. Circulation 1989; 79: 1007–14.

68. Appel LJ, Moore TJ, Obarzanek E et al. A clinical trial of the effects of dietary patterns on blood pressure. DASH Collaborative Research Group. N Engl J Med 1997; 336: 1117–24.

69. Leserman J, Stuart EM, Mamish ME et al. Nonpharmacologic intervention for hypertension: long-term follow-up. J Cardiopulm Rehabil 1989; 9: 316–24.

70. Gaesser GA. Thinness and weight loss: beneficial or detrimental to longevity? Sci Sports Exercise 1999; 31: 1118–28.

71. Thomas DR, Morley JE. Obesity after menopause. Infertil Reprod Med Clin North Am 2001; 7.

72. Morley JE, Thomas DR, Wilson MM. Cachexia: Pathophysiology. AM J Clin Nutr 2006; 83: 735–43.

73. Thomas DR. Distinguishing starvation from cachexia. Geriatr Clin North Am 2002; 18: 883–92.

74. Espat NJ, Moldawer LL, Copeland EM 3rd. Cytokine-mediated alterations in host metabolism prevent nutritional repletion in cachectic cancer patients. J Surg Oncol 1995; 58: 77–82.

75. Pamuk ER, Williamson DF, Serdula MK, Madans J, Byers TE. Weight loss and subsequent death in a cohort of U.S. adults. Ann Intern Med 1993; 119: 744–8.

76. Rumpel C, Harris TB, Madans J. Modification of the relationship between the Quetelet Index and mortality by weight-loss history among older women. Ann Epidemiol 1993; 3: 448–50.

77. Heart Protection Study Collaborative Group. MRC/BHF Heart Protection Study of antioxidant vitamin supplementation in 20,536 high-risk individuals: a randomised placebo-controlled trial. Lancet 2002; 360: 23–33.

78. Omenn GS, Goodman GE, Thornquist MD et al. Effects of a combination of beta carotene and vitamin A on lung cancer and cardiovascular disease. N Engl J Med 1996; 334(18): 1150–5.

79. Hercberg S, Galan P, Preziosi P et al. The SU.VI.MAX Study: a randomized, placebo-controlled trial of the health effects of antioxidant vitamins and minerals. Arch Intern Med 2004; 164: 2335.

80. Lonn E, Bosch J, Yusuf S et al, HOPE and HOPE-TOO Trial Investigators. Effects of long-term vitamin E supplementation on cardiovascular events and cancer: a randomized controlled trial. JAMA 2005; 293(11): 1338–47.

81. Miller ER 3rd, Pastor-Barriuso R, Dalal D et al. Meta-analysis: high-dosage vitamin E supplementation may increase all-cause mortality. Ann Intern Med 2005; 142: 37–46.

82. Miller ER 3rd, Pastor-Barriuso R, Dalal D et al. Meta-analysis: high-dosage vitamin E supplementation may increase all-cause mortality. Ann Intern Med 2005; 142: 37–46.

83. Landi F, Zuccala G, Gambassi G et al. Body mass index and mortality among older people living in the community. J Am Geriatr Soc 1999; 47: 1072–6.

84. Harris T, Cook EF, Garrison R et al. Body mass index and mortality among nonsmoking older persons: the Framingham study. JAMA 1988; 259: 1520–4.

85. Losonczy KG, Harris TB, Cornoni-Huntley J et al. Does weight loss from middle aged to old age explain the inverse weight mortality relation in old age? Am J Epidemiol 1995; 141: 312–21.

86. Cornoni-Huntley JC, Harris TB, Everett DF et al. An overview of body weight of older persons, including the impact on mortality. The National Health and Nutrition Examination Survey I-Epidemiologic Follow-Up Study. J Clin Epidemiol 1991; 44: 743–53.

87. Robinson K, Arheart K, Refsum H et al. Low circulating folate and vitamin B6 concentrations: risk factors for stroke, peripheral vascular disease, and coronary artery disease. European COMAC Group. Circulation 1998; 97(5): 437–43.

88. Leppala JM, Virtamo J, Fogelholm R et al. Controlled trial of alpha-tocopherol and beta-carotene supplements on stroke incidence and mortality in male smokers. Arterioscl Thromb Vasc Biol 2000; 20(1): 230–5.

89. Evans JR. Meta-analysis of seven trials: Antioxidant vitamin and mineral supplements for slowing the progression of age-related macular degeneration. Cochrane Eyes and Vision Group. Cochrane Database Syst Rev 2006; 4.

90. Giroden F, Galan P, Monget AL et al. Impact of trace elements and vitamin supplementation on immunity and infections in institutionalized elderly patients: a randomized controlled trial. MIN. VIT. AOX. geriatric network. Arch Intern Med 1999; 159(7): 748–54.

91. Chandra RK. Effect of vitamin and trace-element supplementation on immune responses and infection in elderly subjects. Lancet 1992; 340(8828): 1124–7.

92. Stevens J, Cai J, Pamuk ER et al. Cancer Prev I The effect of age on the Association between Body-Mass Index and Mortality Cancer Prev I. N Engl J Med 1998; 338: 1–7.

93. Calle EE, Thum MJ, Petrelli JM, Rodriguez C, Heath CW. Body-mass index and mortality in a prospective cohort of U.S. adults. Cancer Prev II. N Engl J Med 1999; 341: 1097–105.

94. Manson JE, Willet WC, Stampfer MJ et al. Body weight and mortality among women. N Engl J Med 1995; 333(11): 677–85.

CHAPTER 26

Obesity in middle-aged men

Richard YT Chen and Gary A Wittert

Prevalence of obesity in middle-aged men

Obesity, which is the long-term outcome of energy intake in excess of energy expenditure, is emerging as a worldwide epidemic. Although childhood obesity is now increasingly common, epidemiologic studies indicate that the onset of obesity in most men tends to occur in young adulthood, and progresses through middle and old age. While there is no proper definition for 'middle age', it is arbitrarily characterized by most studies as the age group of 40–65 years. The United States National Health and Nutrition Surveys of 1988–94 (NHANES III) reported an obesity prevalence of 19.9% amongst men, based on a body mass index (BMI) of 30.0 or greater.[1] Although the prevalence of overweight (BMI ≥ 25.0) Japanese men aged 15 years or older was much lower at 1.6% in 1993, recent data indicate the prevalence has risen to 32% in 2001 amongst those aged 40–49 years.[2]

Age-related changes in body composition

Body weight increases until approximately the age of 60–65 years, and decreases in over 60% of the population thereafter. Muscle mass peaks between the third and fourth decades, followed by a decline of about 1.2 kg per decade in men. Muscle mass and strength decrease by approximately 15% and 30%, respectively, between the second and seventh decades.[3] Factors which may be responsible for, or are at least associated with these changes, include decreased physical activity, inadequate nutrition, vascular disease, increased activity of the cytokines interleukin-1 (IL-1), interleukin-6 (IL-6), and tumor necrosis factor alpha (TNF-α), and decreased levels of the anabolic hormones testosterone, dehydroepiandrosterone (DHEA), growth hormone (GH), and insulin-like growth factor-1 (IGF-1).[4] Fat mass also increases with age and tends to be redistributed viscerally around the abdomen,[3,5] although current data suggest that age-related visceral adiposity affects women more than men.[6]

Mechanisms of weight gain

Energy expenditure

Energy expenditure decreases by around 165 kcal/decade in men, primarily due to changes in voluntary physical activity and, to a lesser extent, a reduction in resting metabolic rate (RMR).[7] In a population-based cohort of 33 466 men aged 45–79 years in central Sweden, total daily physical activity was found to decrease by approximately 4% by age 50 as compared to age 15. Physical activity was 2.6% lower in obese men compared to those with normal weight. Men with self-rated poor health had 11.3% lower levels of physical activity than those reporting very good health.[8,9] The progressive decline in RMR is explained by both a loss of fat-free mass and a decrease in physical activity.[10]

Energy intake

Food intake is regulated by a complex system involving orexigenic (appetite-stimulating) and anorexigenic (appetite-inhibiting) hormones that link hypothalamic satiety centers with gastrointestinal function and energy stores. After BMI adjustment, the plasma levels of acylated (but not desacyl) ghrelin, which is the active form of ghrelin, were higher in female subjects than those in males.[11] Ghrelin production and release is increased by fasting and low protein diets, and inhibited by somatostatin, growth hormone, and high fat diets, and has been shown to activate neuropeptide Y (NPY) and agouti-related peptide (AgRP) neurons in the hypothalamus.[12] NPY and AgRP, which are capable of orexigenic stimulation themselves while simultaneously antagonizing anorexigenic melanocortin pathways, increase appetite, gastric motility, and triglyceride stores in adipocytes, but reduce energy expenditure, resulting in net body weight gain.[12] Conversely, the actions of NPY and AgRP are inhibited by the anorexigenic stimulus of leptin, produced from adipose tissue, especially after a meal. Leptin levels are lower in men, compared to women, and this does not appear to change with age.[13] Other gastrointestinal peptides, such as cholecystokinin (CCK), glucagon-like peptide-1 (GLP-1), pancreatic polypeptide (PP), and peptide YY (PYY) 3–36, act in synergy with leptin to reduce gastric emptying, resulting in increased gastric distension, which has been identified as a satiety signal to inhibit food intake.[12] Ghrelin and leptin are, thus, complementary, but antagonistic, in their actions on hypothalamic satiety and gastrointestinal functions.

Obesity in humans is characterized by low ghrelin levels; weight loss leads to an increase in ghrelin levels, indicating that ghrelin plays an important role in the long-term maintenance of body weight despite its low levels.[14] The sustained suppression of ghrelin levels in patients who have lost weight through gastric bypass surgery further supports this view.[15] The lack of ghrelin suppression after a meal in obese persons may also result in persistent food intake.[16] The higher circulating levels of free (bioactive) leptin in obese persons suggest the presence of leptin resistance, as they do not result in reduced caloric intake.[13] Energy intake decreases with advancing age, but probably to a lesser extent than energy expenditure.[10] In a cross-sectional study of 15 266 healthy men aged 55–79 years, total energy and energy from fat, but not from other nutrients, increased linearly with increasing BMI, which increased by 0.53 and 0.14 kg/m² for every 500 kcal of fat and total energy consumed, respectively.[17]

Overall mortality

There is a large body of evidence showing that higher BMI values are associated with higher mortality in middle-aged men. In a prospective 14-year survey of 457 785 men,[18] the lowest rate of death from all causes was found at a BMI between 23.5 and 24.9, and relative risk was not significantly elevated for BMI values between 22.0 and 26.4. Mortality increased with increasing BMI thereafter for all categories of causes of death, even in healthy non-smoking subjects. Particularly in men, a high BMI was highly predictive of death from cardiovascular disease, with a relative risk of 2.90.[18] Similarly, a 10-year follow-up showed that, amongst 39 756 men aged < 65 years, overall and cardiovascular mortality rose linearly with increasing BMI, the relative risk for overall mortality being 1.97 for BMI ≥ 30.0.[19] Obesity-related mortality appears to be influenced by differences in ethnicity and gender. Amongst Caucasian subjects aged 30–64 years, women had comparatively lower mortality risks than men for BMI > 28.0.[18] The same study found that, amongst subjects in the highest BMI category, Afro-American men had a lower mortality risk compared with Caucasian men. On the other hand, a 7-year study of more than 10 000 Japanese subjects aged 40–69 years reported a higher mortality risk in overweight women compared with men, where a higher mortality risk was not evident.[2] Deaths from cardiovascular disease and cancers predominated.[18,20]

Disease-specific risks

Metabolic syndrome, type 2 diabetes mellitus, and cardiovascular disease

The metabolic syndrome is a cluster of abnormalities – glucose intolerance, hyperinsulinemia, obesity, hypertension, and dyslipidemia – that is associated with insulin resistance, and an increased risk of development of type 2 diabetes mellitus (T2DM) and cardiovascular disease.[21] Data from the NHANES III survey revealed that the prevalence of the metabolic syndrome (defined using the National Cholesterol Education Program clinical criteria[21]) rises with age, being < 10%, 20%, and 45% in men aged 20–29 years, 40–49 years, and 60–69 years, respectively.[22] In parallel, data from the Framingham Study show that the incidence of T2DM rises exponentially from the age of 20–30 years onwards.[23] The metabolic syndrome itself is associated with increased cardiovascular mortality, indicating that atherogenic macrovascular changes begin before the onset of overt T2DM.[24]

Male gender and age over 44 years have been reported to be associated with higher risk of incident T2DM.[25] A prospective study involving 7735 British men aged 40–59 years showed that the risk of cardiovascular mortality, fatal and non-fatal myocardial infarctions, and new-onset T2DM rose progressively from a BMI > 24.0.[26] Another Finnish study of 1209 men aged 42–60 years, who were healthy at baseline, reported that cardiovascular mortality, after adjusting for smoking and LDL cholesterol levels, was 2.9–4.2 times greater in men with the metabolic syndrome compared with those without.[27] A similar study of 1336 middle-aged Lithuanian subjects showed that cardiovascular disease risk was 1.8 times higher in men aged 45–64 years with the metabolic syndrome compared to those without.[28]

Obesity, particularly central visceral adiposity, plays an important role in the progression from metabolic syndrome to the onset of T2DM by promoting insulin resistance and hyperinsulinemia. In support of this is a study involving 575 middle-aged Japanese men showing that a high visceral fat area correlated strongly with impaired glucose tolerance and the development of metabolic syndrome.[29] A prospective relationship between abdominal adiposity and the risk of T2DM was also found among 1972 male participants in the Department of Veterans Affairs Normative Aging Study cohort.[30] Insulin secretion decreases with age even after adjusting for differences in adiposity, fat distribution,

and physical activity.[31] Hepatic uptake of elevated free fatty acid release through the breakdown of triglycerides (TGs) by insulin-resistant adipocytes leads to increased hepatic production of TGs, atherogenic small dense low-density lipoprotein (LDL), and reduced high-density lipoprotein (HDL) levels. Prolonged lipotoxicity may impair β-cell function, induce further insulin resistance, and impair glucose tolerance.[32] C-reactive protein (CRP) levels rise proportionately with increasing number of components of the metabolic syndrome,[33] and endothelial inflammatory processes induced by sustained dyslipidemia ultimately result in atherosclerosis.[34] New-onset atrial fibrillation and atrial flutter have also been associated with obesity in middle-aged men.[35] Higher levels of plasma renin activity, angiotension-converting enzyme, and aldosterone found in centrally obese subjects are believed to perpetuate hypertension.[36]

Cancers

A prospective study involving 900 000 subjects (average age 57 years) found that men with BMI ≥ 40.0 had a higher age-adjusted mortality risk of 52% from cancers, whereas there was no evidence of increased risk among the leanest subjects.[20] Interestingly, women in the same BMI category had an even greater mortality risk of 62%. Gastrointestinal cancers, particularly involving the liver, pancreas, stomach, and colon, predominate. The relative risk of cancer appeared to rise exponentially with increasing BMI. The positive association between obesity and mortality from cancers is consistent with animal studies showing that tumor incidence and tumor growth may be reduced through dietary restriction.[37] It has been suggested that non-alcoholic steatohepatitis leading to cryptogenic cirrhosis may account for the increased incidence of hepatocellular carcinoma in obese persons.[38] Generally, however, the biologic mechanisms linking obesity and cancer mortality are still poorly understood; moreover, it is unclear to what extent obesity affects cancer treatment and outcome.[39]

Pulmonary function

Obstructive sleep apnea (OSA), with its attendant risks of the development of hypertension, stroke, and myocardial infarction, is a well-known complication of obesity. It has been suggested that abdominal obesity may weaken respiratory muscle dynamics, causing negative pressure to develop during inspiration and resulting in upper airway collapse and the development of OSA over time.[40] Reduction in baroreceptor sensitivity (BRS), leading to elevated sympathetic activity, is thought to play an important role in the development of hypertension that affects about 40% of OSA sufferers.[41]

OSA has been shown to correlate positively with a reduction in the pulsatile secretion of luteinizing hormone, resulting in some degree of androgen deficiency, in obese middle-aged men.[42] Basal levels of IGF-1 are markedly lower in obese men with OSA, and there is evidence that OSA results in impairment of growth hormone secretion and sensitivity.[43] OSA may contribute to the development of insulin resistance, independently of BMI, and elevated plasma leptin levels are thought to be a marker of OSA, as they are reduced with continuous positive airway pressure (CPAP) therapy.[41]

Relative androgen deficiency

Plasma total testosterone levels are significantly lower in men with visceral obesity compared to their lean counterparts, independently of age.[44,45] The cause and effect relationship between relative androgen deficiency and obesity is controversial. Conventionally, the former had been thought to predispose towards the development of metabolic syndrome and T2DM,[46-48] and the relative androgen deficiency that results from visceral adiposity may have an adverse effect on metabolic status per se.[49] Obesity, insulin resistance, and glucose homeostasis have been reported to improve with testosterone therapy in middle-aged men.[50,51] Further supporting evidence arises from the fact that although sustained weight loss in centrally obese men led to higher serum testosterone levels, no relationship was seen between changes in androgen levels and insulin sensitivity.[52] However, a cross-sectional study of 400 men aged 40–80 years showed that higher levels of serum testosterone were associated with better insulin sensitivity and a reduced risk of the metabolic syndrome, independently of insulin

levels and body composition.[53] Testosterone replacement is effective in reducing fat mass, by inducing lipolysis, and increasing muscle mass and strength by increasing muscle protein synthesis and growth through greater expression of IGF-1.[54] Plasma testosterone levels in men are also inversely associated with circulating leptin concentrations, even after adjusting for fat mass,[55] and testosterone therapy reduces leptin levels.[56]

Dementia

Obese men (BMI ≥ 30.0) were reported to have a 30% increased risk of developing dementia in a 27-year longitudinal study involving 10 276 subjects aged 40–45 years at baseline, although the outcome was not statistically significant after adjusting for mid-life and late-life comorbidities.[57] Obese women were twice as likely to have dementia compared to those of normal weight. As elevated levels of CRP are associated with increased adiposity[58] and dementia,[59] there are postulations that obesity-related inflammatory processes may be responsible for neuronal degradation, cerebral atrophy, and consequent cognitive decline.[60]

Stroke

A 23-year study of 9151 middle-aged men, who were free of cardiovascular disease at baseline, reported that truncal obesity carried a higher relative risk of up to 1.5 for stroke mortality even after adjusting for systolic blood pressure, BMI, cigarette smoking, and socioeconomic status.[61] In a Swedish cohort of 7402 healthy men aged 47–55 years who were followed up over 28 years, a high BMI was associated with an increased risk of total, ischemic and unspecified strokes, but not hemorrhagic stroke.[62]

Other comorbidities

Gastroesophageal reflux is commonly associated with obesity, although it has been reported that esophageal motility is not different from lean controls.[63] Accelerated osteoarthritis of weight-bearing joints, depression, low self-esteem, and body-image disturbance are other well-known associations of obesity.[64]

Table 26.1 *Classification of weight by BMI*

BMI (kg/m²)	WHO (2000) Classification	NHLBI (1998) Terminology	WPRO (2000) BMI (kg/m²)	WPRO (2000) Classification
<18.5	Underweight	Underweight	<18.5	Underweight
18.5–24.9	Normal range	Normal range	18.5–22.9	Normal range
25.0–29.9	Pre-obese	Overweight	23.0–24.9	Overweight at risk
30.0–34.9	Obese I	Obese I	25.0–29.9	Obese I
35.0–39.9	Obese II	Obese II	≥30.0	Obese II
≥40.0	Obese III	Obese III		

WHO (2000): World Health Organization. Obesity. Preventing and Managing the Global Endemic. WHO Technical Report Series no 894. Geneva: WHO, 2000.
NHLBI (1998): The Obesity Task Force of the National Heart, Lung and Blood Institute. Clinical Guidelines on the Identification, Evaluation, and Treatment of Overweight and Obesity in Adults – The Evidence Report. Obes Res 1998; 6: 51–209S.
WPRO (2000): Steering Committee. The Asia-Pacific perspective: redefining obesity and its treatment. Melbourne: International Diabetes Institute, 2000.

Assessment of obesity

Assessment should include quantifying and categorizing the individual's obesity status, detection of any existing obesity-related comorbidities, and understanding his current behavioral pattern pertaining to energy balance.

Anthropometric assessment

While precise methods of assessing body composition utilizing dual energy X-ray absorptiometry (DEXA) or bioelectrical impedance analysis (BIA) are available, measurement of BMI, calculated as weight (in kilograms) divided by the square of height (in meters), has conventionally been used as a clinical screening tool to identify overweight and obese subjects. The BMI provides an estimate of body fat and has been shown, in longitudinal population studies, to be positively correlated with increased morbidity and mortality.[64,65] In recognition of the fact that the prevalence of overweight and obesity are generally lower in Asian populations, lower BMI cutoffs have been adopted for the Asia-Pacific region since 2000 by the International Obesity Task Force in collaboration with the World Health Organization Western Pacific Regional Office (Table 26.1).[66] However, the BMI does not distinguish between lean or fat tissue, which may lead to erroneous conclusions. As it is the increased amount of abdominal visceral fat mass that is particularly linked to higher risk of obesity-related disease states and mortality, waist circumference measurement (made at the end of normal expiration at the level of the iliac crest) is a more appropriate indicator of abdominal adiposity, especially in older men.[67,68] A high waist circumference (defined as ≥102 cm) in non-smoking men may be a better predictor of all-cause mortality than high BMI.[68] Moreover, population studies have shown that a large waist circumference is associated with increased cardiovascular risk independently of BMI.[64] In a large prospective study involving Japanese subjects aged 40–69 years, men had a lower proportion of body fat, as well as a lower mortality risk, compared to women for the same value of BMI.[2]

Risk assessment

In addition to anthropometric data, a detailed medical history to elicit symptoms, or the presence of established disease, concerning coronary disease, cerebrovascular disease, T2DM, and OSA should be

Table 26.2 *Age-specific energy balance equations for men aged 30–60 years (World Health Organization)*

Activity level	Activity factor
Light	1.55
Moderate	1.78
Heavy	2.10

Resting energy expenditure (REE)
per day = (11.3 × W) + (16 × H) + 901 kcal
Estimated total energy expenditure
total energy expenditure (TEE) = REE × activity
factor. 500–1000 kcal per day is subtracted from
the TEE to achieve energy deficit of
3500–7000 kcal per week.
W, weight in kilograms; H, height in meters.
Source: http://www.fao.org/DOCREP/003/AA040E/AA
040E00.HTM.

obtained. Metabolic status, paying particular attention to glucose tolerance, lipid profile, and hyperuricemia, should be evaluated. Liver function should be assessed for the presence of steatohepatitis. Disease conditions that may contribute towards obesity, such as Cushing's syndrome and hypothyroidism, must be excluded. The impact of obesity on the individual's social function should also be addressed.

Dietary assessment

An attempt should be made to fully understand the patient's food preferences and portions. A 3–7-day food journal (including weekends) documenting dietary patterns and behaviors, or a food frequency questionnaire, is useful and may reveal an underlying psychiatric binge-eating disorder. Age- and gender specific energy equations – which estimate energy intake against energy expenditure – are helpful in targeting net negative energy balance so as to initiate gradual weight loss and achieve desired body weight (Table 26.2).

Assessment of energy expenditure

Physical activity patterns may also be assessed through an activity journal or questionnaire.

Barriers to exercise, such as osteoarthritis, existing cardiopulmonary disease, and lack of time, confidence, or social support, should be noted.

Treatment of obesity

The objectives are to attain weight loss and maintain desired weight, and to treat existing obesity-related disorders. A successful weight-loss program requires an individualized multidisciplinary approach involving the patient's regular physician, endocrinologist, dietitian, nutritionist, exercise consultant, and, in some cases, the general surgeon.

Lifestyle modification

Although, hypertension, dyslipidemia, and glucose intolerance can be ameliorated independently of weight loss, the ability to modify behavioral factors and optimize cardiovascular risk factors is associated with the maintenance of good health. Beginning a moderately vigorous sports activity, quitting cigarette smoking, maintaining normal blood pressure, and avoiding obesity were separately associated with lower rates of death from all causes and from coronary heart disease among middle-aged and older men.[69]

Promoting energy deficit

Net negative energy balance, with the aim of achieving some degree of weight loss, is best attained through a combination of reduced energy intake in conjunction with increased energy expenditure. Realistic targets should be set. An initial goal of a minimum of 7–10% weight loss is preferable rather than targeting the ideal BMI at once, which may not be attainable.[70] A rate of weight loss of about 0.5–1.0 kg/week, which translates into a calorie deficit of 3500–7000 kcal/week, is recommended.[71] A 10 kg reduction in weight may result in a systolic blood pressure reduction of 5–20 mmHg.[72] In a 20-year prospective study, weight loss was associated with a lower risk of incident T2DM in middle-aged men, although it did not produce any significant cardiovascular benefit except in those with BMI ≥ 27.5.[73] However, for overweight individuals in good health, there is no evidence to show that mortality rates are reduced with weight loss.[74]

Low-energy diets of 1000–1500 kcal/day may require multivitamin and mineral supplementation, particularly vitamins B6, B12, and folic acid to restrict serum homocysteine levels. A folic acid intake of 800 μg/day has been reported to reduce coronary disease and stroke by 16% and 24%, respectively.[75] Diets reduced in (particularly refined) carbohydrate, and low in saturated fat, with increased protein and high in fiber (10–25 g/day) may particularly benefit individuals with metabolic syndrome or T2DM.[70] Substitution of monounsaturated fat for carbohydrate reduces postprandial glycemia and hypertriglyceridemia.[76] A meta-analysis revealed that dietary sodium restriction had a minimal effect on blood pressure reduction.[77]

Regular exercise is the best predictor of successful weight maintenance. An increase in physical activity leads to improved insulin sensitivity and glucose tolerance, with a corresponding reduction in all-cause and cardiovascular mortality.[74] Aerobic training is better than resistive training in raising the resting metabolic rate in middle-aged men.[78] Improvements in fitness have been shown to attenuate age-related increases in adiposity. People who exercise regularly appear to accumulate less adipose tissue in the upper and central body regions as they get older, potentially reducing the risk for the metabolic disorders associated with upper body obesity.[79]

Pharmacotherapy

Pharmacotherapy is primarily aimed at initiating weight loss, weight loss maintenance, and risk reduction. The current evidence for long-term efficacy is limited to sibutramine (2 years) and orlistat (4 years), with 46% and 16% of subjects, respectively, achieving ≥10% reduction of initial body weight.[80] The addition of orlistat results in further weight loss, reduces waist circumference and insulin resistance, and improves β-cell function and dyslipidemia in obese diabetic subjects who are already on metformin.[81] Sibutramine produces similar improvements in metabolic profile.[82] Both sibutramine and orlistat, in conjunction with cognitive behavioral therapy, have been reported to promote weight loss in obese subjects with binge eating disorder.[83,84] In the XENDOS study, orlistat has been reported to reduce the rate of incident T2DM in middle-aged obese subjects with impaired glucose tolerance.[25] However, 12 months of treatment with orlistat failed to influence the predicted 10-year cardiovascular disease risk in middle-aged obese subjects with one or more cardiovascular risk factors.[85] Administration of leptin in humans led to some degree of weight loss in obese individuals.[86]

Surgery

Bariatric surgery produces sustained, long-term weight loss. Most of the current literature on the effects of bariatric surgery involves more women than men, but there is no evidence supporting any gender differences in outcome. It is thought that the suppression of plasma ghrelin levels after Roux-en-Y gastric bypass (RYGBP) is responsible for the maintenance of postsurgical weight loss.[87] By contrast, plasma ghrelin levels are seen to rise 1 year after restrictive surgery, which may explain the superiority of bypass surgery in maintaining weight loss compared with restrictive surgery.[88] RYGBP surgery has been reported to reduce insulin resistance (measured using a homeostasis model) 6 days after surgery, even before any appreciable weight loss has occurred, implying a possible role of gastrointestinal humoral mechanisms in maintaining insulin resistance.[89] Fat mass before biliopancreatic diversion (BPD) surgery was found to be the strongest predictor of weight loss 2 years after BPD while, conversely, age and the presence of T2DM were strong negative predictors.[90] Middle-aged, morbidly obese individuals who underwent bariatric surgery had a lower incidence of T2DM and hypertriglyceridemia at 10 years, as well as a more favorable metabolic profile, compared with controls, although no difference was noted in hypertension incidence.[91]

References

1. Flegal KM, Carroll MD, Juczmarski RJ, Johnson CL. Overweight and obesity in the United States: prevalence and trends, 1960–1994. Int J Obes Relat Metab Disord 1998; 22: 39–47.
2. Hayashi R, Iwasaki M, Otani T et al. Body mass index and mortality in a middle-aged Japanese cohort. J Epidemiol 2005; 15: 70–7.

3. Hughes VA, Frontera WR, Roubenoff R, Evans WJ, Singh MA. Longitudinal changes in body composition in older men and women: role of body weight change and physical activity. Am J Clin Nutr 2002; 76: 473–81.

4. Morley JE, Baumgartner RN, Roubenoff R, Mayer J, Nair KS. Sarcopenia. J Lab Clin Med 2001; 137: 231–43.

5. Beaufrere B, Morio B. Fat and protein redistribution with aging: metabolic considerations. Eur J Clin Nutr 2000; 54: S48–53.

6. Perissinotto E, Pisent C, Sergi G, Grigoletto F. Anthropometric measurements in the elderly: age and gender differences. Br J Nutr 2002; 87: 177–86.

7. Elia M. Obesity in the elderly. Obes Res 2001; 9: S244–8.

8. Norman A, Bellocco R, Vaida F, Wolk A. Total physical activity in relation to age, body mass, health and other factors in a cohort of Swedish men. Int J Obes Relat Metab Disord 2002; 26: 670–5.

9. Norman A, Bellocco R, Vaida F, Wolk A. Age and temporal trends of total physical activity in Swedish men. Med Sci Sports Exerc 2003; 35: 617–22.

10. Poehlman ET. Energy expenditure and requirements in aging humans. J Nutr 1992; 122: 2057–65.

11. Akamizu T, Shinomiya T, Irako T, Fukunaga M, Nakai Y, Kangawa K. Separate measurement of plasma levels of acylated and desacyl ghrelin in healthy subjects using a new direct ELISA assay. J Clin Endocrinol Metab 2005; 90: 6–9.

12. Inui A, Asakawa A, Bowers CY et al. Ghrelin, appetite, and gastric motility: the emerging role of the stomach as an endocrine organ. FASEB J 2004; 18: 439–56.

13. Mann DR, Johnson AOK, Gimpel T, Castracane VD. Changes in circulating leptin, leptin receptor, and gonadal hormones from infancy until advanced age in humans. J Clin Endocrinol Metab 2003; 88: 3339–45.

14. Hansen TK, Dall R, Hosoda H et al. Weight loss increases circulating levels of ghrelin in human obesity. Clin Endocrinol 2002; 56: 203–6.

15. Hasler WL. The stomach and weight reduction: the role of ghrelin. Gastroenterology 2003; 124: 575–7.

16. English PJ, Ghatei MA, Malik IA, Bloom SR, Wilding JP. Food fails to suppress ghrelin levels in obese humans. J Clin Endocrinol Metab 2002; 87: 2984–7.

17. Satia-Abouta J, Patterson RE, Schiller RN, Kristal AR. Energy from fat is associated with obesity in U.S. men: results from the Prostate Cancer Prevention Trial. Prev Med 2002; 34: 493–501.

18. Calle EE, Thun MJ, Petrelli JM, Rodriguez C, Heath CWJ. Body-mass index and mortality in a prospective cohort of US adults. N Engl J Med 1999; 341: 1097–105.

19. Baik I, Ascherio A, Rimm EB et al. Adiposity and mortality in men. Am J Epidemiol 2000; 152: 264–71.

20. Calle EE, Rodriguez C, Walker-Thurmond K, Thun MJ. Overweight, obesity, and mortality from cancer in a prospectively studied cohort of US adults. N Engl J Med 2003; 348: 1625–30.

21. Expert Panel on Detection, Evaluation, And Treatment of High Blood Cholesterol In Adults (Adult Treatment Panel III), Executive Summary of The Third Report of The National Cholesterol Education Program (NCEP) JAMA 2001; 285: 2486–97.

22. Ford ES, Giles WH, Dietz WH. Prevalence of the metabolic syndrome among US adults: findings from the Third National Health and Nutrition Examination Survey. JAMA 2002; 287: 356–9.

23. Wilson PW, Anderson KM, Kannel WB. Epidemiology of diabetes in the elderly. The Framingham Study. Am J Med 1986; 80: 3–9.

24. Haffner SM, Stern MP, Hazuda HP, Mitchell BD, Patterson JK. Cardiovascular risk factors in confirmed prediabetic individuals. Does the clock for coronary heart disease start clicking before the onset of clinical diabetes? JAMA 1990; 263: 2893–8.

25. Torgerson JS, Hauptman J, Boldrin MN, Sjostrom L. XENical in the prevention of diabetes in obese subjects (XENDOS) study: a randomized study of orlistat as an adjunct to lifestyle changes for the prevention of type 2 diabetes in obese patients. Diabetes Care 2004; 27: 155–61.

26. Shaper AG, Wannamethee SG, Walker M. Body weight: implications for the prevention of coronary heart disease, stroke, and diabetes mellitus in a cohort of middle-aged men. BMJ 1997; 314: 1311.

27. Lakka H-M, Laaksonen DE, Lakka TA et al. The metabolic syndrome and total and cardiovascular disease mortality in middle-aged men. JAMA 2002; 288: 2709–16.

28. Cerniauskiene LR, Reklaitiene R, Luksiene DI et al. Association of metabolic syndrome with ischaemic heart disease among middle-aged Kaunas population. Medicina (Kaunas) 2005; 41: 435–41.

29. Mori Y, Hoshino K, Yokota K, Yokose T, Tajima N. Increased visceral fat and impaired glucose tolerance predict the increased risk of metabolic syndrome in Japanese middle-aged men. Exp Clin Endocrinol Diabetes 2005; 113: 334–9.

30. Cassano PA, Rosner B, Vokonas PS, Weiss ST. Obesity and body fat distribution in relation to the incidence of non-insulin-dependent diabetes mellitus. A prospective cohort study of men in the normative aging study. Am J Epidemiol 1992; 136: 1474–86.

31. Muller DC, Elahi D, Tobin JD, Andres R. The effect of age on insulin resistance and secretion: a review. Semin Nephrol 1996; 16: 289–98.

32. McGarry JD, Dobbins RL. Fatty acids, lipotoxicity and insulin secretion. Diabetologia 1999; 42: 128–38.

33. Festa A, D'Agostino RJ, Howard G, Mykkanen L, Tracy RP, Haffner SM. Chronic subclinical inflammation as part of the insulin resistance syndrome: the Insulin Resistance Atherosclerosis Study (IRAS). Circulation 2000; 102: 42–7.

34. Quinones MJ, Nicholas SB, Lyon CJ. Insulin resistance and the endothelium. Curr Diab Rep 2005; 5: 246–53.

35. Frost L, Hune LJ, Vestergaard P. Overweight and obesity as risk factors for atrial fibrillation or flutter: the Danish Diet, Cancer, and Health Study. Am J Med 2005; 118: 489–95.

36. Ruano M, Silvestre V, Castro R et al. Morbid obesity, hypertensive disease and the renin–angiotensin–aldosterone axis. Obes Surg 2005; 15: 670–6.

37. Dunn SE, Kari FW, French J et al. Dietary restriction reduces insulin-like growth factor I levels, which modulates apoptosis, cell proliferation, and tumour progression in p53-deficient mice. Cancer Res 1997; 57: 4667–72.

38. Qian Y, Fan JG. Obesity, fatty liver and liver cancer. Hepatobiliary Pancreat Dis Int 2005; 4: 173–7.

39. Adami H-O, Trichopoulos D. Obesity and mortality from cancer. N Engl J Med 2003; 348: 1623–4.

40. Shinohara E, Kihara S, Yamashita S et al. Visceral fat accumulation as an important risk factor for obstructive sleep apnoea syndrome in obese subjects. J Intern Med 1997; 241: 11–18.

41. Coughlin S, Calverley P, Wilding J. Sleep disordered breathing – a new component of syndrome x? Obes Rev 2001; 2: 267–74.

42. Luboshitzky R, Lavie L, Shen-Orr Z, Herer P. Altered luteinizing hormone and testosterone secretion in middle-aged obese men with obstructive sleep apmoea. Obes Res 2005; 13: 780–6.

43. Gianotti L, Pivetti S, Lanfranco F et al. Concomitant impairment of growth hormone secretion and peripheral sensitivity in obese patients with obstructive sleep apnea syndrome. J Clin Endocrinol Metab 2002; 87: 5052–7.

44. Seidell JC, Bjorntorp P, Sjostrom L, Kvist H, Sannerstedt R. Visceral fat accumulation in men is positively associated with insulin, glucose, and C-peptide levels, but negatively with testosterone levels. Metabolism 1990; 39: 897–901.

45. Vermeulen A, Goemaere S, Kaufman JM. Testosterone, body composition and aging. J Clin Invest 1999; 22: 110–16.

46. Laaksonen DE, Niskanen L, Punnonen K et al. Sex hormones, inflammation and the metabolic syndrome: a population-based study. Eur J Endocrinol 2003; 149: 601–8.

47. Stellato RK, Feldman HA, Hamdy O, Horton ES, McKinlay JB. Testosterone, sex hormone-binding globulin, and the development of type 2 diabetes in middle-aged men: prospective results from the Massachusetts Male Aging Study. Diabetes Care 2000; 23: 490–4.

48. Haffner SM, Shaten J, Stern MP, Smith GD, Kuller L. Low levels of sex hormone-binding globulin and testosterone predict the development of non-insulin dependent diabetes mellitus in men: MRFIT Research Group Multiple Risk Factor Intervention Trial. Am J Epidemiol 1996; 143: 889–97.

49. Phillips GB, Jing TY, Heymsfield SB. Relationships in men of sex hormones, insulin, adiposity, and risk factors for myocardial infarction. Metabolism 2003; 52: 784–90.

50. Marin P, Holmang S, Jonsson L et al. The effects of testosterone treatment on body composition and metabolism in middle-aged obese men. Int J Obes Relat Metab Disord 1992; 16: 991–7.

51. Boyanov MA, Boneva Z, Christov VG. Testosterone supplementation in men with type 2 diabetes, visceral obesity and partial androgen deficiency. Aging Male 2003; 6: 1–7.

52. Niskanen L, Laaksonen DE, Punnonen K et al. Changes in sex hormone-binding globulin and testosterone during weight loss and weight maintenance in abdominally obese men with the metabolic syndrome. Diabetes Obes Metab 2004; 6: 208–15.

53. Muller M, Grobbee DE, den Tonkelaar I, Lamberts SWJ, van der Schouw YT. Endogenous sex hormones and metabolic syndrome in aging men. J Clin Endocrinol Metab 2005; 90: 2618–23.

54. Mudali S, Dobs AS. Effects of testosterone on body composition of the ageing male. Mech Ageing Dev 2004; 125: 297–304.

55. Luukka V, Personen U, Huhtaniemi I. Inverse correlation between serum testosterone and leptin in men. J Clin Endocrinol Metab 1998; 81: 4433.

56. Hislop MS, Rantanjee BD, Soule SG, Marais AD. Effects of anabolic-androgenic steroid use or gonadal testosterone suppression on serum leptin concentration in men. Eur J Endocrinol 1999; 141: 40–6.

57. Whitmer RA, D Gunderson EP, Barrett-Connor E, Quesenberry Jr CP, Yaffe K. Obesity in middle age and future risk of dementia: a 27 year longitudinal population based study. BMJ 2005; 330: 1360.

58. Das UN. Is obesity an inflammatory condition? Nutrition 2001; 17: 953–66.

59. Schmidt R, Schmidt H, Curb JD et al. Early inflammation and dementia: a 25-year follow-up of the Honolulu-Asia aging study. Ann Neurol 2002; 52: 168–74.

60. Yaffe K, Kanaya A, Lindquist K et al. The metabolic syndrome, inflammation, and risk of cognitive decline. JAMA 2004; 292: 2237–42.

61. Tanne D, Medalie JH, Goldbourt U. Body fat distribution and long-term risk of stroke mortality. Stroke 2005; 36: 1021–5.

62. Jood K, Jern C, Wilhelmsen L, Rosengren A. Body mass index in mid-life is associated with a first stroke

in men: a prospective population study over 28 years. Stroke 2004; 35: 2764–9.

63. Di Francesco V, Baggio E, Mastromauro M et al. Obesity and gastro-esophageal acid reflux: physiopathological mechanisms and role of gastric bariatric surgery. Obes Surg 2004; 14: 1095–102.

64. Kushner RF, Blatner DJ. Risk assessment of the overweight and obese patient. J Am Diet Assoc 2005; 105: S53–62.

65. McTigue KM, Harris R, Hemphill B et al. Screening and interventions for obesity in adults: summary of the evidence for the US Preventive Services Task Force. Ann Intern Med 2003; 139: 933–49.

66. Steering Committee. The Asia-Pacific perspective: redefining obesity and its treatment. Melbourne: International Diabetes Institute, 2000.

67. Baumgartner RN, Heymsfield SB, Roche AF. Human body composition and the epidemiology of chronic disease. Obes Res 1995; 3: 73–95.

68. Seidell JC, Visscher TL. Body weight and weight change and their health implications for the elderly. Eur J Clin Nutr 2000; 54: S33–9.

69. Paffenbarger RS Jr, Hyde RT, Wing AL et al. The association of changes in physical-activity level and other lifestyle characteristics with mortality among men. N Engl J Med 1993; 328: 538–45.

70. Plodkowski RA, Krenkel J Combined treatment for obesity and the metabolic syndrome. J Am Diet Assoc 2005; 105: S124–30.

71. National Institutes of Health Clinical Guidelines on the Identification, Evaluation, and Treatment of Overweight and Obesity in Adults – The Evidence Report. Obes Res 1998; 6 (Suppl 2): 51–209.

72. Chobanian AV, Bakris GL, Black HR et al. The Seventh Report of the Joint National Committee on Prevention, Detection, Evaluation, and Treatment of High Blood Pressure: the JNC 7 report. JAMA 2003; 289: 2560–72.

73. Wannamethee SG, Shaper AG, Walker M. Overweight and obesity and weight change in middle aged men: impact on cardiovascular disease and diabetes. J Epidemiol Community Health 2005; 59: 134–9.

74. Gaesser GA. Thinness and weight loss: beneficial or detrimental to longevity? Med Sci Sports Exerc 1999; 31: 1118–28.

75. Wald DS, Law M, Morris JK. Homocysteine and cardiovascular disease: evidence on causality from a meta-analysis. BMJ 2002; 325: 1202.

76. Franz MJ, Bantle JP, Beebe CA et al. Evidence-based nutrition principles and recommendations for the treatment and prevention of diabetes and related complications. Diabetes Care 2003; 26 (Suppl 1): S51–61.

77. Jurgens G, Graudal NA. Effects of low sodium diet versus high sodium diet on blood pressure, renin, aldosterone, catecholamines, cholesterols, and

triglyceride. Cochrane Database Syst Rev: 2004; CD004022.

78. Toth MJ, Gardner AW, Poehlman ET. Training status, resting metabolic rate, and cardiovascular disease risk in middle-aged men. Metabolism 1995; 44: 340–7.

79. Kohrt WM, Malley MT, Dalsky GP, Holloszy JO. Body composition of healthy sedentary and trained, young and older men and women. Med Sci Sports Exerc 1992; 24: 832–7.

80. Ioannides-Demos LL, Proietto J, McNeil JJ. Pharmacotherapy for obesity. Drugs 2005; 65: 1391–418.

81. Berne C. A randomized study of orlistat in combination with a weight management programme in obese patients with Type 2 diabetes treated with metformin. Diabet Med 2005; 22: 612–18.

82. Filippatos TD, Kiortsis DN, Liberopoulos EN, Mikhailidis DP, Elisaf MS. A review of the metabolic effects of sibutramine. Curr Med Res Opin 2005; 21: 457–68.

83. Grilo CM, Masheb RM, Salant SL. Cognitive behavioral therapy guided self-help and orlistat for the treatment of binge eating disorder: a randomized, double-blind, placebo-controlled trial. Biol Psychiatry 2005; 57: 1193–201.

84. Milano W, Petrella C, Casella A et al. Use of sibutramine, an inhibitor of the reuptake of serotonin and noradrenaline, in the treatment of binge eating disorder: a placebo-controlled study. Adv Ther 2005; 22: 25–31.

85. Swinburn BA, Carey D, Hills AP et al. Effect of orlistat on cardiovascular disease risk in obese adults. Diabetes Obes Metab 2005; 7: 254–62.

86. Heymsfield SB, Greenberg AS, Fujioka K et al. Recombinant leptin for weight loss in obese and lean adults: a randomized, controlled, dose-escalation trial. JAMA 1999; 282: 1568–75.

87. Cummings DE, Weigle DS, Frayo RS et al. Plasma ghrelin levels after diet-induced weight loss or gastric bypass surgery. N Engl J Med 2002; 346: 1623–30.

88. Nijhuis J, van Dielen FM, Buurman WA, Greve JW. Ghrelin, leptin and insulin levels after restrictive surgery: a 2-year follow-up study. Obes Surg 2004; 14: 783–7.

89. Wickremesekera K, Miller G, Naotunne TD, Knowles G, Stubbs RS. Loss of insulin resistance after Roux-en-Y gastric bypass surgery: a time course study. Obes Surg 2005; 15: 474–81.

90. Valera-Mora ME, Simeoni B, Gagliardi L et al. Predictors of weight loss and reversal of comorbidities in malabsorptive bariatric surgery. Am J Clin Nutr 2005; 81: 1292–7.

91. Sjostrom L, Lindroos AK, Peltonen M et al. Lifestyle, diabetes, and cardiovascular risk factors 10 years after bariatric surgery. N Engl J Med 2004; 351: 2683–93.

CHAPTER 27

Diabetes in the elderly male: nutritional aspects

John E Morley

We have to lament that our mode of cure is so contrary to the inclinations of the sick. Though perfectly aware of the efficacy of the [diet] regimen, and the impropriety of deviations, yet they commonly trespass, concealing what they feel as a transgression on themselves. They express a regret that a medicine could not be discovered however nauseous or distasteful, which would suppress the necessity of any restriction of diet.

John Rollo, 1798

Introduction

Over half of all diabetics in the United States are over 60 years of age. Diabetes occurs more commonly in males than in females (Figure 27.1). In men aged 65 to 74 years, 21% have diabetes with 43% of them being undiagnosed. In the older old (75 years of age or older), 24% of men have diabetes with a quarter of them being undiagnosed. Approximately, two-thirds of older diabetics are being treated, but only 16% have adequate control. In nursing homes approximately 30% of patients have diabetes mellitus. Most older persons with diabetes mellitus are now living in the developing world.

Diabetes accelerates the aging process. At the cellular level, hyperglycemia decreases the DNA unwinding rate, increases collagen cross-linking, decreases $Na^+K^+ATPase$ activity, and increases capillary basement membrane thickening.[1] Clinically,

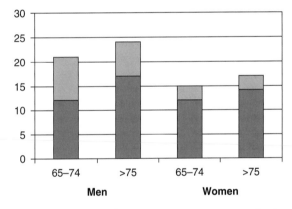

Figure 27.1 *Diabetes occurs more commonly in males than in females.*

diabetics are more likely to have cataracts and other visual disturbances, increased atherosclerosis, decreased cognition, increased dysphoria, injurious falls, and a decline in functional status compared to age-matched controls.

Pathogenesis of diabetes in older persons

With aging there is a decrease in both insulin-mediated glucose disposal and non-insulin-mediated glucose utilization.[2] In addition, many older persons have a decrease in glucose-induced insulin release.

355

Table 27.1 *Comparison of diabetes mellitus in young, middle-aged, and old males*

	Type 1	Type 1½	Type 2
Age	**Young**	**Old**	**Middle-aged**
Body habitus	Thin	Thin with visceral adiposity	Obese
Insulin levels	Very low	Low	High
Insulin-mediated glucose disposal	Normal	Mild decrease	Markedly decreased
Non-insulin-mediated glucose disposal	Normal	Decreased	Normal
Fasting hepatic glucose output	Increased	Normal	Increased
Therapeutic agent of choice	Insulin	Thiazolidinedione	Metformin

Obesity is associated with a decline in the production of gastrointestinal incretins, viz glucagon-like peptide-1 and gastric inhibitory peptide, which leads to reduced insulin levels. In younger type 2 diabetics, fasting hepatic glucose output is increased, whereas this is much less common in older persons. In addition, it is now recognized that unlike in middle aged type 2 diabetics, older diabetics are often not obese.

With aging, a number of mitochondrial abnormalities tend to accumulate. This leads to a reduction in mitochondrial flux and, therefore, a reduction in the utilization of intracellular lipid.[3] Thus, triglycerides and free fatty acids accumulate within the cell leading to autophosphorylation of insulin receptor substrate that leads to reduced activation of the glucose transporter (GLUT) when insulin activates its receptor.

Because of these differences in diabetes between middle-aged and older diabetics, we have suggested that older diabetics have a type 1½ diabetes, i.e., their diabetes is intermediate between types 1 and 2 (Table 27.1).[4]

The metabolic syndrome

The Dutchman, Nicholaes Tulp, was the first to describe the hypertriglyceridemia syndrome. GB Morgagni (1682–1771) described a syndrome of visceral obesity, hypertension, hyperuricemia, atheroma, and sleep apnea. In 1977, Haller named this the metabolic syndrome, and in 1991 Ferrannini called it the insulin resistance syndrome. The criteria for the metabolic syndrome are shown in Table 27.2. Like diabetes, the metabolic syndrome increases with age, reaching nearly 44% of the population aged 60 to 69 years. It is also slightly more common in men than in women.

The metabolic syndrome can be considered the 'couch potato' syndrome. It occurs in persons with a genetic predisposition who overeat and do not exercise and, thus, develop predominantly visceral obesity. Visceral obesity is associated with the increased production of tumor necrosis factor alpha, interleukin-6, and leptin, and a decline in adiponectin, leading to insulin resistance and hyperinsulinemia. The components of the metabolic syndrome include diabetes mellitus, hypertension, hyperuricemia, coagulation abnormalities, lipid abnormalities, myosteatosis (fatty infiltration into muscle), and non-alcoholic steatohepatitis (Figure 27.2). This leads to a 2- to 4-fold increase in the risk of developing myocardial infarction and cerebrovascular accidents. In a person with hypertension, having the other components of metabolic syndrome doubles their cardiovascular risk, and increases the risk of chronic renal disease and microalbuminuria.

The major lipid abnormality of the metabolic syndrome is hypertriglyceridemia. The increased levels of triglycerides lead to a reduction in high-density lipoprotein (HDL) (including HDL-2

Table 27.2 *Criteria for the metabolic syndrome*

Criteria	NCEP ATP III[26]	1999 WHO[27]
Insulin resistance	—	Essential
Fasting glucose (mmol/l)	> 6.1	> 6.1
2-hour glucose (mmol/l)	—	> 7.8
Blood pressure (mm/Hg)	> 130/85	> 140/80
Triglycerides (mmol/l)	> 1.0	> 0.9
HDL (mmol/l)		
males	< 1.0	< 0.9
females	< 1.3	< 1
Body mass index	—	> 30
Waist to hip ratio		
males	—	> 0.9
females	—	> 0.85
Waist circumference		
males	> 102 (Asian 90)	—
females	> 88 (Asian 80)	—
Microalbuminuria (mg/g creatinine)	—	> 30

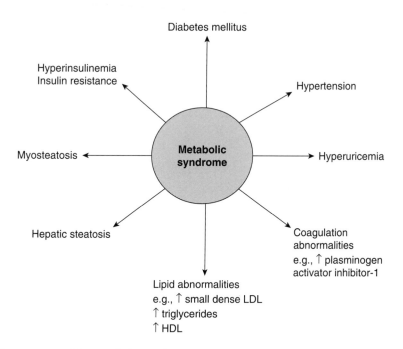

Figure 27.2 *Components of the metabolic syndrome.*

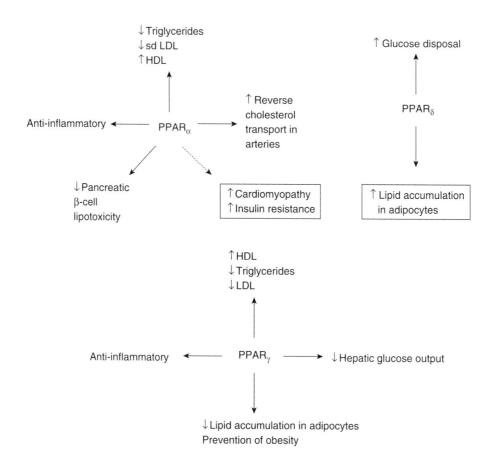

Figure 27.3 *Effects of the PPARs that may be involved in the metabolic syndrome.* ↑, *= increase;* ↓, *= decrease; boxed effects are negative; sd, = small dense.*

particles with the loss of apolipoprotein-A1) and an increase in small dense low-density lipoprotein (LDL) particles. Small dense LDL is highly atherogenic, being retained preferentially by the arterial wall and being readily oxidized. Cholesterol ester transfer protein exchanges very-low-density lipoprotein (VLDL) triglycerides for LDL cholesterol. The hydrolysis of triglyceride-rich LDL leads to the formation of small dense LDL particles. The cardiovascular risk in persons with small dense LDL particles is 3-fold higher than in those with large fluffy LDL particles. Triglyceride elevation appears to be less of a risk factor in men than in women.

There is increasing evidence that the nuclear receptor family of peroxisome proliferator activated receptors (PPARs) are important cellular mediators of the metabolic syndrome (Figure 27.3). PPARα agonists (e.g., gemfibrozil or fenofibrate) decrease triglycerides and small dense LDL and increase HDL, are anti-inflammatory (decrease CRP, cytokines, and cell adhesion molecules), increase reverse cholesterol transport in atherosclerosis, and decrease β-cell lipotoxicity in the pancreatic islets. However, in muscle and heart they have negative effects, increasing insulin resistance in muscle and producing a cardiomyopathy. PPARδ agonists (e.g., thiazolidinediones) increase glucose disposal and have an anabolic role to increase cellular incorporation of lipids. A PPARδ resistance syndrome has been reported that consists of insulin resistance, hypertension, dyslipidemia, diabetes mellitus, hepatic steatosis, and partial lipodystrophy. A common genetic variant of PPARδ (Pro 12 Ala) results in type 2 diabetes associated with an increase in body mass index. PPARδ activation leads to decreased hepatic glucose output, increased HDL cholesterol, decreased serum triglycerides, reduced adipose tissue, increased muscle endurance capacity, and anti-inflammatory effects in macrophages.

Centenarians tend to have high levels of large fluffy LDL. In older males treatment should be targeted at lowering small dense LDL and not total LDL or cholesterol. Further understanding of PPAR metabolism should lead to appropriate drugs to move this area forward.

Reasons for maintenance of euglycemia in diabetics

Maintenance of diabetic control is important for many reasons:[5]

- Prevention of hyperglycemic comas
- Prevention of retinopathy, neuropathy, and nephropathy
- Prevention of glucose toxicity
  - accelerated aging
  - trace mineral loss in urine
  - infection
  - dehydration
  - incontinence/nocturia
  - excess pain
  - cognitive decline.

Diabetes and functional status

Multiple studies have shown that diabetes mellitus is associated with a decline in functional status in older persons.[6,7] Diabetes leads to diabetics reading less, gardening less, using the telephone less, writing letters less, and going out socially less.[8] Diabetics are more likely to have injurious falls than non-diabetics.[6]

Diabetes and the stomach

Hyperglycemia is associated with delayed stomach emptying.[9] This is associated with worse gastrointestinal symptoms such as heartburn, nausea, dysphagia, diarrhea, constipation, fecal incontinence, and postprandial fullness. Changes in the rate of stomach emptying also alter the ability to adequately control diabetes. Elevated glucose levels 2 hours following a meal are more closely associated with cardiovascular disease than are fasting glucose levels.[10]

Both older persons and persons with diabetes may have marked falls in blood pressure following a meal.[11] This is due to glucose and is produced by release of the vasodilatory peptide, calcitonin gene related peptide.[12] This effect is more common in the morning and is variable. It is associated with falls, syncope, stroke, myocardial infarction, and death.

Diabetics have increased gut wall permeability.[13] This leads to translocation of bacteria into the lymphatic and portal systems. These bacteria release lipopolysaccharides which activate monocytes to produce tumor necrosis factor alpha and interleukin-6. This excess of cytokines results in sarcopenia and immune dysfunction. Our studies have suggested that the prebiotic oligofructosaccharides attenuate production of mRNA for both interleukin-6 and tumor necrosis factor.

Diet and diabetes

It is now well recognized that therapeutic diabetic diets have little effect on glycemic control in older diabetics.[14,15] These should no longer be used at all in institutional settings. As older persons who lose weight, particularly men, have poor outcomes, weight loss needs to be avoided.[16]

However, as shown in Figure 27.4, avoidance of extremely high postprandial levels of glucose and triglycerides and delayed return to baseline levels can be remarkably toxic to tissues, especially arteries. Smoothing of the postprandial curves can be done by enriching the diet either in fiber or unsaturated fatty acids.[17] Administration of omega-3 fatty acids not only lowers triglyceride

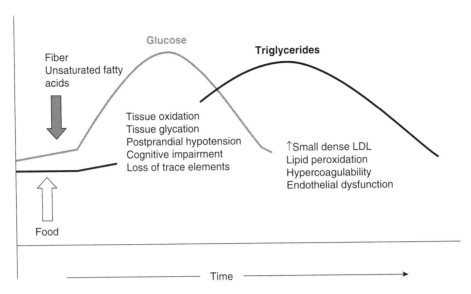

Figure 27.4 *Effect of food on glucose and triglycerides and their effects on tissues and function in diabetics. Fiber and unsaturated fatty acids modulate the glycemic and triglyceride curves and accelerate the return to basal levels.*

levels in diabetics, but also decreases lipid peroxidation and increases glutathione peroxidase.[18] Fish oils also increase learning and memory, which is often impaired in diabetics.

Zinc and diabetes

Diabetics lose zinc in the urine and have poor zinc absorption.[19,20] About 9% of diabetics are zinc deficient. Zinc deficiency leads to immune dysfunction, e.g., decreased phytohemagglutin. T-cell proliferation and zinc serum thymic factor increased lipid peroxidation, decreased antioxidant activity, decreased wound healing, decreased testosterone, and decreased insulin growth factor-1.

Vitamin D, diabetes, and frailty

With aging there is a decline in vitamin D levels.[21] In men with type 2 diabetes there is a marked increase in hip fractures.[22] Hypovitaminosis D is common in medical patients with diabetes.[23] Vitamin D supplementation with calcium improves strength and performance in older persons with low vitamin D levels.[24]

Other nutritional issues[25]

- Low magnesium is common in diabetes and may be related to increased systolic hypertension.
- The role of chromium remains unclear in age-related hyperglycemia.
- High copper levels may accelerate atherosclerosis.
- Vitamin B12 deficiency is common in diabetics and leads to increased homocysteine. This is related to increased atherosclerosis, cognitive decline, and hip fracture.
- High doses of vitamin C and E can interfere with the glucose oxidation reaction used to measure blood glucose levels.

Conclusions

As so aptly pointed out by Aretaeus of Cappadocia, 'diabetes mellitus is a mysterious disease … where the flesh and limbs melt into the urine.' The dietary management of older persons with diabetes requires their diets being tailored to the needs of the person with, in most cases, weight maintenance being the goal. Hypertriglyceridemia, the main cause of small dense LDL, requires attention in older persons with diabetes or insulin resistance. Unsaturated fatty acids may be important in this setting. Zinc replacement should be considered in diabetics with either vascular or pressure ulcers. Postprandial hyperglycemia needs to be limited wherever possible. Older diabetics need to receive calcium and vitamin D to prevent hip fracture. The need for magnesium and vitamin B12 should be regularly monitored in older diabetics. Finally, malnutrition is common in hospitalized and institutionalized older diabetics. They often will require increased calories to reach this goal.

References

1. Hartnell JM, Morley JE, Mooradian AD. Reduction of alkali-induced white blood cell DNA unwinding rate: a potential biomarker of aging. J Gerontol 1989; 44: B125–30.
2. Meneilly GS, Tessier D. Diabetes in elderly adults. J Gerontol Med Sci 2001; 56: M5–13.
3. Petersen KF, Befroy D, Dufour S et al. Mitochondrial dysfunction in the elderly: possible role in insulin resistance. Science 2003; 300: 1140–2.
4. Morley JE. Diabetes mellitus: a major disease of older persons. J Gerontol Med Sci 2000; 55: M255–6.
5. Morley JE, Perry HM 3rd. The management of diabetes mellitus in older individuals. Drugs 1991; 41: 548–65.
6. Rodriquez-Saldana J, Morley JE, Reynoso MT et al. Diabetes mellitus in a subgroup of older Mexicans: prevalence, association with cardiovascular risk factors, functional and cognitive impairment, and mortality. J Am Geriatr Soc 2002; 50: 111–16.
7. Miller Dk, Lui LY, Perry HM 3rd, Kaiser FE, Morley JE. Reported and measured physical functioning in older inner-city diabetic African Americans. J Gerontol Med Sci 1999; 54A: M230–6.
8. Sinclair AJ. Diabetes in the elderly: a perspective from the United Kingdom. Clin Geriatr Med 1999; 15: 225–37.
9. Rayner CK, Horowitz M. Gastrointestinal motility and glycemic control in diabetes: the chicken and the egg revisited? J Clin Invest 2006; 116: 299–302.
10. Leiter LA, Ceriello A, Davidson JA et al. International Prandial Glucose Regulation Study Group. Clin Ther 2005; 27(Suppl B): S42–56.
11. Morley JE. Editorial: postprandial hypotension – the ultimate Big Mac attack. J Gerontol Med Sci 2001; 56A: M741–3.
12. Edwards BJ, Perry HM 3rd, Kaiser FE et al. Relationship of age and calcitonin gene-related peptide to postprandial hypotension. Mech Ageing Development 1996; 87: 61–73.
13. Mooradian AD, Morley JE, Levine AS, Prigge WF, Gebhard RL. Abnormal intestinal permeability to sugars in diabetes mellitus. Diabetologia 1986; 29: 221–4.
14. Coulston AM, Mandelbaum D, Reaven GM. Dietary management of nursing home residents with non-insulin-dependent diabetes mellitus. Am J Clin Nutr 1990; 51: 67–71.
15. Tariq SH, Karcic E, Thomas DR et al. The use of a no-concentrated-sweets diet in the management of type 2 diabetes in nursing homes. J Am Dietetic Assoc 2001; 101: 1463–6.
16. Wilson MM, Morley JE. Invited review: aging and energy balance. J Appl Physiol 2003; 95: 1728–36.
17. Gerhard GT, Ahman A, Meeuws K et al. Effects of a low-fat diet compared with those of a high-monounsaturated fat diet on body weight, plasma lipids and lipoproteins, and glycemic control in type 2 diabetes. Am J Clin Nutr 2004; 80: 668–73.
18. Neff LM. Evidence-based dietary recommendations for patients with type 2 diabetes mellitus. Nutr Clin Care 2003; 6: 51–61.
19. Niewoehner CB, Allen JI, Boosalis M, Levine AS, Morley JE. Role of zinc supplementation in type II diabetes mellitus. Am J Med 1986; 81: 63–8.
20. Kinlaw WB, Levine AS, Morley JE, Silvis SE, McClain CJ. Abnormal zinc metabolism in type II diabetes mellitus. Am J Med 1983; 75: 273–7.
21. Perry HM 3rd, Horowitz M, Morley JE et al. Longitudinal changes in serum 25-hydroxyvitamin D in older people. Metabolism 1999; 48: 1028–32.
22. Holmberg AH, Johnell O, Nilsson PM et al. Risk factors for hip fractures in a middle-aged population: a study of 33 000 men and women. Osteoporos Int 2005; 16: 2185–94.
23. Chiu KC, Chu A, Go VL, Saad MF. Hypovitaminosis D is associated with insulin resistance and beta cell dysfunction. Am J Clin Nutr 2004; 59: 820–5.
24. Bischoff-Ferrari HA, Orav EJ, Dawson-Hughes B. Effect of cholecalciferol plus calcium on falling in ambulatory older men and women: a 3-year randomized controlled trial. Arch Intern Med 2006; 166: 424–30.
25. Mooradian AD, Morley JE. Micronutrient status in diabetes mellitus. Am J Clin Nutr 1987; 45: 877–95.
26. National Institute of Health. Third Report of the Nation Cholesterol Education Program Expert Panel on Detection, Evaluation, and Treatment of High Blood Cholesterol in Adults (Adult Treatment Panel III). Bethesda, MD: National Institutes of Health; NIH Publication 2001: 01–3670.
27. Hanley AJ, Wagenknecht LE, D, Agostino RB, Zinman B, Haffer SM. Identification of subjects with insulin resistance and beta-cell dysfunction using alternative definitions of the metabolic syndrome. Diabetes. 2003; 52: 2740–47.

CHAPTER 28

Lipids through the ages

Margaret-Mary G Wilson

There are no such things as applied sciences, only applications of science.
Louis Pasteur
French biologist & bacteriologist (1822–1895)[1]

Introduction

Discovery of the low-density lipoprotein (LDL) receptors by Brown and Goldstein in 1976 facilitated aggressive research into the clinical implications and therapeutic modulation of lipid disorders.[2] Several decades later, knowledge of basic physiologic concepts of lipoprotein metabolism remains critical to fully understanding the management of dyslipidemias.

Dyslipidemia describes abnormal lipid metabolism resulting in quantitative or qualitative changes in lipoprotein particles that increase the risk of coronary heart disease. Physiologically significant changes include decreased concentration of high-density lipoprotein (HDL) cholesterol, hypertriglyceridemia, elevated concentration of LDL, and/or increased density of LDL particles. Several mechanisms have been implicated in the etiology of dyslipidemias. Genetic theories such as mutations of dominantly expressed genes encoding receptors, enzymes, or proteins involved in lipoprotein metabolism have been implicated in familial hyperlipidemia. However, dyslipidemia is more likely to result from a polygenic manifestation of environmental influences on genetic make-up.[3–5]

Clinical implications of dyslipidemias in older adults are manifest in the pathogenesis of atherosclerotic vascular disease. Extensive data link the treatment of dyslipidemias with a reduction in the incidence of coronary artery disease and cerebrovascular disease. Dietary and lifestyle changes are generally considered the first-line therapy for the management of dyslipidemias. Failure to reach target goals generally justifies institution of lipid-lowering agents. Available data from a meta-analysis of randomized trials indicate that statins, the most commonly used lipid-lowering medications, reduce the risk of coronary heart disease by 31% and all-cause mortality by 21% regardless of age and gender.[6] Similar studies support the use of statins in the secondary prevention of cerebrovascular events.[7]

Cholesterol, diet, and atherogenesis

Although the precise role of dietary modulation in atherogenesis is not fully understood, limitations of dietary restriction as an effective lipid-lowering strategy are becoming increasingly evident as alternative theories of atherogenesis evolve. Nonetheless, the effect of diet on vascular reactivity, lipid metabolism kinetics, and antioxidant potential continues to prompt aggressive research into the development of therapeutic modalities targeting atherosclerosis.

Data from human studies indicate that elevated atherogenic lipoproteins, regardless of the mechanism of increase, are a major prerequisite for disease. Evidence also supports a pivotal role for the

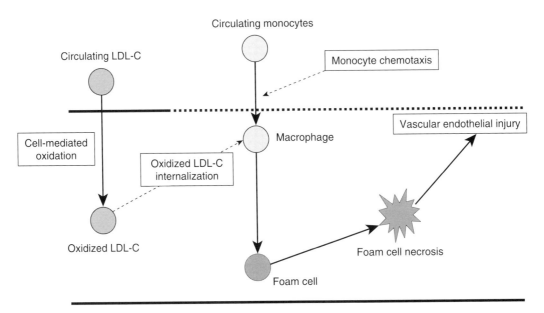

Figure 28.1 *Vascular endothelium and atherogenic inflammation.*

endothelium, as an inflammatory mediator, and positions oxidatively modified LDL as a major player in monocyte recruitment and foam cell formation (Figure 28.1).[8]

Animal models provide convincing evidence that diet is implicated in the atherogenic response to vascular injury. Following ingestion of a high fat and high cholesterol diet, apolipoprotein E (apoE)-deficient mice accumulate lipoprotein particles within the vascular intima. Consequently, monocytes migrate into the intima and transform into foam cells that rapidly result in the formation of fatty streaks and fibrous plaques, markers of advanced atherosclerosis.[9] Animal studies show that consumption of oxidized cholesterol produces increased aortic wall cholesterol concentration and accelerated development of atherosclerotic lesions. When rabbits were fed oxidized fatty acids or oxidized cholesterol, the fatty streak lesions in the aorta were increased by 100%. Moreover, dietary oxidized cholesterol significantly increased aortic lesions in apoE- and LDL receptor-deficient mice.[10] Furthermore, consumption of cholesterol-rich processed foods modulates absorption kinetics and tissue uptake of chylomicrons by delaying plasma clearance.[11] These

findings explain the increased frequency of coronary atherosclerosis in immigrant Indian populations with a relatively high consumption of ghee, a butter product rich in cholesterol oxides.[12] Similarly, a Western diet rich in oxidized fats would increase the risk of arterial atherosclerosis.

Oxidized LDL particles are implicated in the inflammatory phase of atherogenesis. Suggested pathogenetic mechanisms include liberation of growth factors, such as macrophage colony stimulating factor, inhibition of endothelial nitrous oxide synthase, and preferential binding of monocytes over neutrophils.[13] Dietary factors may also influence atherogenesis by modulating the burden of intracellular oxidative metabolic stress. ApoE-deficient mice on a lipid-poor diet exhibit comparatively low vascular lipid hydroperoxide content and reduced reactive molecular oxygen generation.[14] Dietary intervention has been shown to enhance atherosclerotic disease regression and improve clinical outcome. Data from a systematic review by Hooper and others show that reduction of dietary fat intake can result in an overall decrease in serum cholesterol by 11%. In the same study

Table 28.1 *Statin therapy and hyperlipidemia: primary prevention trials*

Trials	Significant risk reduction
West of Scotland Coronary Prevention Study Group (WOSCOPS)[46] Air Force/Texas Coronary Atherosclerosis Prevention Study (AFCAPS/TexCAPS)[48] Anglo-Scandinavian Cardiac outcomes trial – Lipid Lowering Arm (ASCOT-LLA)[49] Collaborative Atorvastatin Diabetes study (CARDS)[70]	Non-fatal MI + cardiac deaths: 40% All-cause mortality: 28% 1st acute coronary event + sudden cardiac death: 37% Non-fatal + fatal MI: 36% Non-fatal + fatal stroke: 27% Acute coronary events: 35% Stroke: 47%

cardiovascular morbidity and mortality was reduced by 16% and 9%, respectively.[15] Similar data from a meta-analysis of 19 randomized controlled trials showed a reduction ranging from 8.5% at 3 months to 5.5% at 12 months following modification of dietary lipid consumption.[16] Benefits of dietary modulation in lowering serum lipids are also evident from data derived from studies examining the efficacy of Step I and II dietary recommendations from the United States National Cholesterol Education Program in lowering serum lipid levels.[17]

Dietary macronutrient interactions may play a role in atherogenesis by altering the metabolic balance of oxidation damage and defense. The latter theory has been proffered as a likely explanation for the cardioprotective effect of the 'Mediterranean diet', which encourages increased consumption of mono- and unsaturated fatty acids, particularly linolenic acid, by increasing the ratio of plant foods to animal products in the diet.[18–22] Several factors may explain the cardioprotective effect of the Mediterranean diets, including the relatively high concentration of flavinoids. Flavinoids are among the most potent antioxidants.[23] In addition, quercetin, a specific flavinoid present in large quantities in most Mediterranean plant foods, is a potent inhibitor of free radical damage and platelet aggregation. Guercetin also facilitates regeneration of oxidized tocopherol.[24]

The National Cholesterol Education Program (NCEP) Adult Treatment Panel III (ATP III) recommends lifestyle changes in diet and physical activity in the management of hyperlipidemia. Nevertheless, despite several studies indicating the efficacy of non-pharmacologic measures, dyslipidemia is most commonly treated with drug therapy.[25,26]

Lipid-lowering pharmacologic therapy

Statins are generally considered the ideal drug choice for the management of hyperlipidemias. These agents exert their lipid-lowering effect by inhibiting the action of the enzyme 3-hydroxy-3-methylglutaryl coenzyme A (HMG-CoA) reductase, thereby blocking hepatic synthesis of cholesterol. Several primary and secondary prevention trials support a beneficial role for statin therapy in coronary artery disease (Tables 28.1 and 28.2). One of the earliest studies to indicate a positive benefit from statin therapy was the Scandinavian Simvastatin Survival Study (4S), which showed survival benefit from lipid-lowering therapy in hyperlipidemic patients with proven coronary artery disease (CAD). Simvastatin therapy was also associated with a significant reduction in the incidence of non-fatal cardiac events and revascularization procedures.[27]

Results from both the Cholesterol and Recurrent Events (CARE) trial and the Long-term Intervention with Pravastatin in Ischemic Disease (LIPID) trial demonstrated positive benefit from pravastatin. In the CARE trial patients with CAD who did not have very high lipid levels (LDL < 240) exhibited a significant reduction in fatal and non-fatal cardiac events,

Table 28.2 *Statin therapy and hyperlipidemia: secondary prevention trials*

Trials	Significant risk reduction
Scandinavian Simvastatin Survival Study (4S)[27]	All-cause mortality: 30% Coronary mortality: 42% Revascularization: 37%
Cholesterol and Recurrent Events (CARE) trial[28]	Fatal or non-fatal MI: 24% CABG: 26% Angioplasty: 23% Stroke: 31%
Long-term Intervention with Pravastatin in Ischemic disease (LIPID)[29]	Cardiac death: 24% All-cause mortality: 22%
Heart Protection Study (HPS)[32]	All-cause mortality: 13% Cardiac events, strokes, revascularization: 25%
Veterans' Affairs High-Density Lipoprotein Cholesterol Intervention Trial (VA-HIT)[33]	CAD, non-fatal MI, stroke: 24% Coronary event: 22%
Myocardial Ischemia Reduction with Aggressive Cholesterol Lowering (MIRACL)[36]	All-cause mortality, non-fatal MI, resuscitated cardiac arrest, recurrent ischemia requiring hospitalization: 16%

strokes, and revascularization procedures following pravastatin therapy.[28,29] Data also indicated that patients with lipid levels well within normal also benefited from statin therapy.[30] In the LIPID trial pravastatin therapy was associated with a 24% reduction in cardiac death and a 22% reduction in all-cause mortality. Thus, both the CARE and LIPID trials lent credence to the efficacy of statin therapy in patients with CAD and normal cholesterol levels.[29,31]

In the Heart Protection Study (HPS), patients at high risk of a coronary event benefited from simvastatin 40 mg daily, regardless of LDL level, over a 5-year period. All-cause mortality was reduced by 13% and there was a 25% reduction in cardiac events, strokes, and revascularization procedures over a 5-year period.[32] The Veterans' Affairs High-Density Lipoprotein Cholesterol Intervention Trial (VA-HIT) examined the effect of raising HDL cholesterol levels in patients with average LDL and triglyceride levels using gemfibrozil. Although benefit from gemfibrozil therapy was not evident until after 2 years of treatment, there was a significant reduction in the incidence of strokes, transient ischemic attacks, and carotid endarterectomies.[33] Further analyses revealed specific benefit in men with CAD who had diabetes. This cohort exhibited a 32% reduction in cardiac events and a 41% reduction in cardiac deaths.[34] Gemfibrozil therapy had a negligible effect on LDL levels in the VA-HIT study. It has been suggested that the combined use of statin and gemfibrozil may achieve the optimal lipid profile, however the increased risk of statin-induced myopathy with this combination outweighs any conceivable benefit.

Benefits of early and aggressive lipid lowering in patients with acute coronary syndrome were specifically addressed in the Myocardial Ischemia Reduction with Aggressive Cholesterol Lowering (MIRACL) trial. This study showed that initiation of atorvastatin (80 mg/day) therapy 24–96 hours after an acute coronary syndrome reduced the incidence of cardiac arrest with resuscitation, non-fatal myocardial infarction, non-fatal stroke, and recurrent symptomatic myocardial ischemic events requiring emergency hospitalization. Atorvastatin therapy in the MIRACL trial did not reduce the risk of coronary artery bypass surgery or revascularization procedures. Notably, in the MIR-ACL trial there was no lower limit to the LDL level acceptable for inclusion in the trial and the mean LDL level for subjects on atorvastatin therapy was 72 mg/dl.[35,36] Initiation of statin therapy immediately after an acute coronary syndrome (ACS) is also supported by data from two other randomized controlled trials, the Pravastatin Turkish Trial, and the Lipid-Coronary Artery Disease (L-CAD) study. Additionally, Pitt and others in the Aggressive Lipid-Lowering Therapy Compared with Angioplasty in Stable Coronary Artery Disease (AVERT) trial concluded that, in low-risk patients with stable coronary artery disease, aggressive lipid-lowering therapy may be as effective as angioplasty and usual care in reducing the incidence of coronary ischemic events. In contrast to the aforementioned studies, data from the Fluvastatin on Risk Diminishing After Acute Myocardial Infarction (FLORIDA) study failed to show any clinical benefit.[37,38]

Head-to-head trials examining the comparative efficacy of statins, such as the Reversal of Atherosclerosis with Aggressive Lipid Lowering (REVERSAL), the Pravastatin or Atorvastatin Evaluation and Infection Therapy trial (PROVE-IT), and the Treating to New Targets (TNT) trial, all demonstrated positive cardiovascular benefit from high-dose statin therapy in subjects with coronary artery disease.[39] In addition, the Reversal of Atherosclerosis with Aggressive Lipid Lowering (REVERSAL) trial examined regression of coronary atherosclerosis, demonstrating a reduction in plaque volume with atorvastatin therapy.[40–43] Notably the TNT trial was the first study specifically designed to examine goals of therapy. Results of this study showed that subjects who attained a therapeutic LDL target of 75 mg/dl had significantly greater reductions in strokes, non-fatal cardiac events, and cardiac deaths.[44,45]

The West of Scotland Coronary Prevention Study (WOSCOPS) was the first study to examine the effect of statins as primary prevention. Pravastatin administered over a 6-month period to middle-aged men (45–64 years) with hyperlipidemia (mean LDL levels 192 mg/dl), but without a history of CAD, resulted in a 40% risk reduction in non-fatal myocardial infarction or cardiac deaths, and a 28% reduction

in all-cause mortality.[46] Findings of the Air Force/Texas Coronary Atherosclerosis Prevention Study (AFCAPS/TexCAPS) extended the benefits of statins as primary prevention to patients with even lower LDL cholesterol levels (mean 150 mg/dl). Following 5 years of statin therapy, there was a significant reduction in the incidence of fatal and non-fatal acute coronary syndromes as well as sudden cardiac death.[47,48] Similar findings were observed in the Anglo-Scandinavian Cardiac Outcomes Trial – Lipid Lowering Arm (ASCOT-LLA), where hypertensive patients with multiple risk factors for CAD, regardless of lipid levels, demonstrated a significant reduction in non-fatal and fatal MI and strokes within 12 months of atorvastatin therapy.[49,50]

Approach to hyperlipidemia in the aging adult

Based on results of the aforementioned studies, recommendations of the Expert Panel on Detection, Evaluation and Treatment of High Blood Cholesterol in Adults were incorporated into the revised National Cholesterol and Education Program guidelines. Proponents of the revisions favor a lower threshold for the initiation of statin therapy and a therapeutic goal for serum LDL levels of < 70 mg/dl in high-risk adult patients.[51]

Clinical applicability of statin therapy in the geriatric patient population is less clear as subjects over the age of 75 years are poorly represented in the majority of these studies. Thus the assumption that hypercholesterolemia has equally sinister implications in older adults is based mainly on data extrapolated from younger subjects. In the Heart Protection Study (HPS), a comparable reduction in the incidence of adverse cardiac and vascular events was achieved in younger subjects and subjects over 65 years.[32] However, few patients over the age of 80 years were included in the study, thus the clinical implications of the findings in the HPS cannot be extended to octogenarians or beyond. Positive benefits were observed following statin therapy in the pravastatin in elderly individuals at risk of vascular disease (PROSPER) trial. Older subjects aged between 70 and 82 years with pre-existing vascular disease or an elevated risk of vascular disease exhibited a reduction in fatal and non-fatal cardiac events. However, there were no demonstrable effects on stroke-related events or all-cause mortality.[52] Further analysis of data from the PROSPER study failed to show any benefit from the use of pravastatin as primary prevention. Positive data relating to the clinical efficacy of statin therapy as primary prevention in octogenarians and older adults are lacking.

Previous data from the Framingham study suggest that the positive correlation between total serum cholesterol and all-cause mortality levels off in the seventh decade of life. Thereafter, past the age of 80 years, a negative correlation emerges.[53,54] Data from older subjects in the Established Population for the Epidemiologic Study of the Elderly (EPESE) trial and the Cardiovascular Health Study failed to show a positive association between hyperlipidemia and adverse cardiac events, cardiac mortality, or all-cause mortality. Indeed, paradoxically, patients with lower cholesterol levels had lower survival rates.[55] In the EPESE trial there was no association between hypercholesterolemia or low HDL cholesterol and all-cause mortality, cardiac deaths, or hospitalization for acute coronary syndrome in subjects older than 70 years.[56,57]

In contrast, several studies have shown that hypocholesterolemia in older adults is associated with increased all-cause mortality in older nursing home residents and hospitalized older adults.[58–61] Similar data have been obtained even in high-functioning community-dwelling elders in whom it has been shown that low cholesterol levels are associated with an increased risk of premature death and functional decline.[62] Reasons for the association between low cholesterol levels and increased mortality in older subjects are unknown. One plausible hypothesis is that hypocholesterolemia may be associated with a corresponding depletion of antioxidant derivatives such as squalene and ubiquinone (CoQ10).[63] Thus, even if lipid-lowering therapy reduces cardiovascular events in older adults, any survival benefit derived from such treatment may be countered by the deleterious effects of hypocholesterolemia on noncardiac endpoints in older patients. Thus in spite of the fairly common practice of prescribing statin therapy to older adults perceived to be at risk, there is

limited evidence that treatment of hypercholesterolemia in octogenarians and nonagenarians will reduce morbidity or mortality.

Polypharmacy and age-related changes in pharmacokinetics and pharmacodynamics place older adults at increased risk of adverse effects and unwanted drug interactions. In 2001, cerivastatin was withdrawn by the Food and Drug Administration (FDA) due to reported episodes of myositis and fatal rhabdomyolysis occurring particularly in older patients.[64] Subsequently, in 2004, the FDA issued another public health alert advising caution in the prescription of rosuvastatin due to several reports of rhabdomyolysis and nephrotoxicity associated with use of this agent in older patients.[65,66]

Animal studies have shown carcinogenic effects associated with statin therapy at serum drug concentrations achieved in routine clinical practice.[67] Studies in human subjects also show a trend toward an increased risk of cancer in older adults treated with statins. Some workers have hypothesized that induction of HMG-CoA reductase and subsequent mevalonate synthesis in extrahepatic tissues may promote the growth of mevalonate-dependent cancers, such as breast cancer.[68] Nevertheless, available clinical studies provide little evidence to support objective clinical concerns about an increased cancer risk associated with statin use in the elderly. Analysis of data from the WOSCOPS, CARE, CARD, and LIPID trials did not reveal any difference in the incidence of fatal and non-fatal cancers between pravastatin and placebo groups.[69,70] Similarly, in the HPS and 4S study the trend toward an increase in non-melanoma skin cancer in women treated with simvastatin was not statistically significant.[27]

Currently, there are few studies in octogenarians and beyond that demonstrate convincing clinical benefit from the use of statins as lipid-lowering agents. Likewise, although low cholesterol levels are associated with increased mortality in older adults, there is little evidence to support a direct causal link. Thus, health-care providers should factor age into the decision to initiate statin therapy. In older adults, expected clinical benefits of treating hyperlipidemia such as longevity should be carefully weighed against complications such as adverse drug reactions, polypharmacy, and increased health-care costs. These complications may notably compromise quality of life and functional status and increase the risk of frailty in the affected elder.

References

1. Pasteur L, Chamberland, Roux. Summary report of the experiments conducted at Pouilly-le-Fort, near Melun, on the anthrax vaccination, 1881. Yale J Biol Med 2002; 75(1): 59–62.
2. Raju TN. The Nobel chronicles. 1985: Joseph Leonard Goldstein (b 1940), Michael Stuart Brown (b 1941). Lancet 2000; 355(9201): 416.
3. Austin MA, Hutter CM, Zimmern RL, Humphries SE. Genetic causes of monogenic heterozygous familial hypercholesterolemia: a HuGE prevalence review. Am J Epidemiol 2004; 160(5): 407–20.
4. Shoulders CC, Jones EL, Naoumova RP. Genetics of familial combined hyperlipidemia and risk of coronary heart disease. Hum Mol Genet 2004; 13(1): R149–60.
5. Greco K, Bayan M. Heart stopper genes: would you recognize a high risk patient? Online J Issues Nurs 2000; 5(3): 4.
6. LaRosa JC, He J, Vupputuri S. Effect of statins on risk of coronary disease: a meta-analysis of randomized controlled trials. JAMA 1999; 282(24): 2340–6.
7. Crouse JR III, Byington RP, Hoen HM, Furberg CD. Reductase inhibitor monotherapy and stroke prevention. Arch Intern Med 1997; 157(12): 1305–10.
8. Gimbrone MA Jr, Topper JN, Nagel T, Anderson KR, Garcia-Cardena G. Endothelial dysfunction, hemodynamic forces, and atherogenesis. Ann NY Acad Sci 2000; 902: 230–9.
9. Tamminen M, Mottino G, Qiao JH, Breslow JL, Frank JS. Ultrastructure of early lipid accumulation in ApoE-deficient mice. Arterioscler Thromb Vasc Biol 1999; 19(4): 847–53.
10. Staprans I, Pan XM, Rapp JH, Feingold KR. The role of dietary oxidized cholesterol and oxidized fatty acids in the development of atherosclerosis. Mol Nutr Food Res 2005; 49(11): 1075–82.
11. Rong JX, Shen L, Chang YH et al. Cholesterol oxidation products induce vascular foam cell lesion formation in hypercholesterolemic New Zealand white rabbits. Arterioscler Thromb Vasc Biol 1999; 19(9): 2179–88.
12. Jacobson MS. Cholesterol oxides in Indian ghee: possible cause of unexplained high risk of atherosclerosis in Indian immigrant populations. Lancet 1987; 2(8560): 656–8.
13. Lusis AJ. Atherosclerosis. Nature 2000; 407(6801): 233–41.
14. Guo Z, Mitchell-Raymundo F, Yang H et al. Dietary restriction reduces atherosclerosis and oxidative stress in the aorta of apolipoprotein E-deficient mice. Mech Ageing Dev 2002; 123(8): 1121–31.
15. Hooper L, Summerbell CD, Higgins JP et al. Dietary fat intake and prevention of cardiovascular disease: systematic review. BMJ 2001; 322(7289): 757–63.
16. Tang JL, Armitage JM, Lancaster T et al. Systematic review of dietary intervention trials to lower blood total cholesterol in free-living subjects. BMJ 1998; 316(7139): 1213–20.
17. Yu-Poth S, Zhao G, Etherton T et al. Effects of the National Cholesterol Education Program's Step I and Step II dietary intervention programs on cardiovascular disease risk factors: a meta-analysis. Am J Clin Nutr 1999; 69(4): 632–46.
18. Menotti A, Keys A, Aravanis C et al. Seven Countries Study. First 20-year mortality data in 12 cohorts of six countries. Ann Med 1989; 21(3): 175–9.
19. de LM, Salen P, Martin JL et al. Wine drinking and risks of cardiovascular complications after recent acute myocardial infarction. Circulation 2002; 106(12): 1465–9.
20. de LM, Salen P, Martin JL et al. Mediterranean diet, traditional risk factors, and the rate of cardiovascular complications after myocardial infarction: final report of the Lyon Diet Heart Study. Circulation 1999; 99(6): 779–85.
21. Trichopoulou A, Vasilopoulou E, Georga K. Macro- and micronutrients in a traditional Greek menu. Forum Nutr 2005; (57): 135–46.
22. Trichopoulou A, Vasilopoulou E. Mediterranean diet and longevity. Br J Nutr 2000; 84(2): S205–9.
23. Hale SL, Kloner RA. Effects of resveratrol, a flavinoid found in red wine, on infarct size in an experimental model of ischemia/reperfusion. J Stud Alcohol 2001; 62(6): 730–5.
24. Chen JW, Zhu ZQ, Hu TX, Zhu DY. Structure–activity relationship of natural flavonoids in hydroxyl radical-scavenging effects. Acta Pharmacol Sin 2002; 23(7): 667–72.
25. Cheng C, Graziani C, Diamond JJ. Cholesterol-lowering effect of the Food for Heart Nutrition Education Program. J Am Diet Assoc 2004; 104(12): 1868–72.
26. Pathak UN, Gurubacharya DL. Non-pharmacological therapy of hyperlipidaemia. Nepal Med Coll J 2003; 5(2): 109–12.
27. Stalenhoef AF. Scandinavian simvastatin study (4S). Lancet 1994; 344(8939–8940): 1766–7.
28. Bonner G. [Care study. Secondary prevention after myocardial infarct in moderately elevated total cholesterol.] Fortschr Med 1997; 115(17): 57–8.
29. Higashikata T. [Clinical trials on protective efficacy of statins for cardiovascular events due to hyperlipidemia

(J-LIT, 4S, CARE, LIPID etc).] Nippon Rinsho 2004; 62(3): 628–36.

30. Pfeffer MA, Sacks FM, Moye LA et al. Influence of baseline lipids on effectiveness of pravastatin in the CARE Trial. Cholesterol And Recurrent Events. J Am Coll Cardiol 1999; 33(1): 125–30.

31. Keech A, Colquhoun D, Best J et al. Secondary prevention of cardiovascular events with long-term pravastatin in patients with diabetes or impaired fasting glucose: results from the LIPID trial. Diabetes Care 2003; 26(10): 2713–21.

32. MRC/BHF Heart Protection Study of cholesterol lowering with simvastatin in 20,536 high-risk individuals: a randomised placebo-controlled trial. Lancet 2002; 360(9326): 7–22.

33. Robins SJ, Collins D, Wittes JT et al. Relation of gemfibrozil treatment and lipid levels with major coronary events: VA-HIT: a randomized controlled trial. JAMA 2001; 285(12): 1585–91.

34. Robins SJ, Rubins HB, Faas FH et al. Insulin resistance and cardiovascular events with low HDL cholesterol: the Veterans Affairs HDL Intervention Trial (VA-HIT). Diabetes Care 2003; 26(5): 1513–7.

35. Schwartz GG, Oliver MF, Ezekowitz MD et al. Rationale and design of the Myocardial Ischemia Reduction with Aggressive Cholesterol Lowering (MIRACL) study that evaluates atorvastatin in unstable angina pectoris and in non-Q-wave acute myocardial infarction. Am J Cardiol 1998; 81(5): 578–81.

36. Schwartz GG, Olsson AG, Ezekowitz MD et al. Effects of atorvastatin on early recurrent ischemic events in acute coronary syndromes: the MIRACL study: a randomized controlled trial. JAMA 2001; 285(13): 1711–8.

37. Wright RS, Murphy JG, Bybee KA, Kopecky SL, LaBlanche JM. Statin lipid-lowering therapy for acute myocardial infarction and unstable angina: efficacy and mechanism of benefit. Mayo Clin Proc 2002; 77(10): 1085–92.

38. Pitt B, Waters D, Brown WV et al. Aggressive lipid-lowering therapy compared with angioplasty in stable coronary artery disease. Atorvastatin versus Revascularization Treatment Investigators. N Engl J Med 1999; 341(2): 70–6.

39. Nissen SE, Tuzcu EM, Schoenhagen P et al. Effect of intensive compared with moderate lipid-lowering therapy on progression of coronary atherosclerosis: a randomized controlled trial. JAMA 2004; 291(9): 1071–80.

40. Nissen SE, Tuzcu EM, Schoenhagen P et al. Effect of intensive compared with moderate lipid-lowering therapy on progression of coronary atherosclerosis: a randomized controlled trial. JAMA 2004; 291(9): 1071–80.

41. Cannon CP, Braunwald E, McCabe CH et al. Intensive versus moderate lipid lowering with statins after acute coronary syndromes. N Engl J Med 2004; 350(15): 1495–504.

42. LaRosa JC, Grundy SM, Waters DD et al. Intensive lipid lowering with atorvastatin in patients with stable coronary disease. N Engl J Med 2005; 352(14): 1425–35.

43. Waters DD, Guyton JR, Herrington DM et al. Treating to New Targets (TNT) Study: does lowering low-density lipoprotein cholesterol levels below currently recommended guidelines yield incremental clinical benefit? Am J Cardiol 2004; 93(2): 154–8.

44. LaRosa JC, Grundy SM, Waters DD et al. Intensive lipid lowering with atorvastatin in patients with stable coronary disease. N Engl J Med 2005; 352(14): 1425–35.

45. Waters DD, Guyton JR, Herrington DM et al. Treating to New Targets (TNT) Study: does lowering low-density lipoprotein cholesterol levels below currently recommended guidelines yield incremental clinical benefit? Am J Cardiol 2004; 93(2): 154–8.

46. West of Scotland Coronary Prevention Study: implications for clinical practice. The WOSCOPS Study Group. Eur Heart J 1996; 17(2): 163–4.

47. Brown AS. Primary prevention of coronary heart disease: implications of the Air Force/Texas coronary atherosclerosis prevention study (AFCAPS/TexCAPS). Curr Cardiol Rep 2000; 2(5): 439–44.

48. Downs JR, Clearfield M, Weis S et al. Primary prevention of acute coronary events with lovastatin in men and women with average cholesterol levels: results of AFCAPS/TexCAPS. Air Force/Texas Coronary Atherosclerosis Prevention Study. JAMA 1998; 279(20): 1615–22.

49. Sever PS, Poulter NR, Dahlof B et al. Reduction in cardiovascular events with atorvastatin in 2,532 patients with type 2 diabetes: Anglo-Scandinavian Cardiac Outcomes Trial – Lipid-Lowering Arm (ASCOT-LLA). Diabetes Care 2005; 28(5): 1151–7.

50. Osende JI, Ruiz-Ortega M, Blanco-Colio LM, Egido J. Statins to prevent cardiovascular events in hypertensive patients. The ASCOT-LLA study. Nephrol Dial Transplant 2004; 19(3): 528–31.

51. Aronow WS. Should the NCEP III guidelines be changed in elderly and younger persons at high risk for cardiovascular events? J Gerontol A Biol Sci Med Sci 2005; 60(5): 591–2.

52. Shepherd J, Blauw GJ, Murphy MB et al. Pravastatin in elderly individuals at risk of vascular disease (PROSPER): a randomised controlled trial. Lancet 2002; 360(9346): 1623–30.

53. Kronmal RA, Cain KC, Ye Z, Omenn GS. Total serum cholesterol levels and mortality risk as a function of age. A report based on the Framingham data. Arch Intern Med 1993; 153(9): 1065–73.

54. Manolio TA, Cushman M, Gottdiener JS et al. Predictors of falling cholesterol levels in older adults:

the Cardiovascular Health Study. Ann Epidemiol 2004; 14(5): 325–31.

55. Krumholz HM, Vaccarino V, Mendes de Leon CF, Seeman TE, Berkman LF. Cholesterol and coronary heart disease mortality in elderly patients. JAMA 1996; 275(2): 110–1.

56. Krumholz HM, Seeman TE, Merrill SS et al. Lack of association between cholesterol and coronary heart disease mortality and morbidity and all-cause mortality in persons older than 70 years. JAMA 1994; 272(17): 1335–40.

57. Fried LP, Kronmal RA, Newman AB et al. Risk factors for 5-year mortality in older adults: the Cardiovascular Health Study. JAMA 1998; 279(8): 585–92.

58. Rudman D, Mattson DE, Nagraj HS et al. Antecedents of death in the men of a Veterans Administration nursing home. J Am Geriatr Soc 1987; 35(6): 496–502.

59. Rudman D, Mattson DE, Nagraj HS et al. Prognostic significance of serum cholesterol in nursing home men. J Parenter Enteral Nutr 1988; 12(2): 155–8.

60. Noel MA, Smith TK, Ettinger WH. Characteristics and outcomes of hospitalized older patients who develop hypocholesterolemia. J Am Geriatr Soc 1991; 39(5): 455–61.

61. Forette B, Tortrat D, Wolmark Y. Cholesterol as risk factor for mortality in elderly women. Lancet 1989; 1(8643): 868–70.

62. Reuben DB, Ix JH, Greendale GA, Seeman TE. The predictive value of combined hypoalbuminemia and hypocholesterolemia in high functioning community-dwelling older persons: MacArthur Studies of Successful Aging. J Am Geriatr Soc 1999; 47(4): 402–6.

63. Smith TJ. Squalene: potential chemopreventive agent. Expert Opin Invest Drugs 2000; 9(8): 1841–8.

64. Griffin JP. The withdrawal of Baycol (cerivastatin). Adverse Drug React Toxicol Rev 2001; 20(4): 177–80.

65. Wooltorton E. Rosuvastatin (Crestor) and rhabdomyolysis. CMAJ 2004; 171(2): 129.

66. Wolfe SM. Dangers of rosuvastatin identified before and after FDA approval. Lancet 2004; 363(9427): 2189–90.

67. Newman TB, Hulley SB. Carcinogenicity of lipid-lowering drugs. JAMA 1996; 275(1): 55–60.

68. Duncan RE, El-Sohemy A, Archer MC. Statins and cancer development. Cancer Epidemiol Biomarkers Prev 2005; 14(8): 1897–8.

69. Pfeffer MA, Keech A, Sacks FM et al. Safety and tolerability of pravastatin in long-term clinical trials: prospective Pravastatin Pooling (PPP) Project. Circulation 2002; 105(20): 2341–6.

70. Colhoun HM, Betteridge DJ, Durrington PN et al. Primary prevention of cardiovascular disease with atorvastatin in type 2 diabetes in the Collaborative Atorvastatin Diabetes Study (CARDS): multicentre randomised placebo-controlled trial. Lancet 2004; 364(9435): 685–96.

CHAPTER 29

Insulin resistance syndrome in older people

Angela Marie Abbatecola and Giuseppe Paolisso

Introduction

The insulin resistance syndrome (IRS), otherwise known as the metabolic syndrome (MS) or syndrome X, is made up of a constellation of cardiovascular and metabolic risk factors, all of which have been shown to be associated with cardiovascular disease (CVD)[1] as well as all-cause death.[2,3] Such factors have been mainly identified as: glucometabolic abnormalities (type 2 diabetes (DM2)), impaired glucose tolerance, or impaired fasting glucose), insulin resistance (IR), visceral obesity, dyslipidemia, hypertension, and altered blood coagulation. The central building stone of the IRS is a more generalized metabolic disorder known as insulin resistance, to which all individual components are linked. In fact, IR has been considered the unifying hypothesis for describing the pathophysiology of the IRS. In the next part of this chapter, we will focus our discussion on the link between age-related IR and the individual components of the IRS.

The exact components of the definition of the IRS vary according to those suggested by the World Health Organization (WHO),[4] the National Cholesterol Education Program's Adult Treatment Panel (NCEP:ATP III),[5] the European Group for the Study of Insulin Resistance (EGIR),[6] and the International Diabetes Federation (IDF).[7] Even though all four panels have agreed that the essential components of the syndrome are altered glucose metabolism, increased abdominal fat measures, and altered blood pressure and lipid profiles, they vary according to details among those components (Table 29.1). One important difference that needs to be highlighted is that the EGIR and the ATP III definitions of the IRS do not necessarily include diabetic individuals. The EGIR and ATP III definition specifically allow a more epidemiologic approach to defining the syndrome, especially when large numbers are available. It is widely known that in non-diabetic persons, a negative correlation exists between fasting insulin and insulin sensitivity, thus IR individuals could be defined as the 25% of the population with the highest IR or the highest fasting insulin concentrations. Indeed, fasting hyperinsulinemia is considered a surrogate of IR in many studies. Considering that there is no simple way to measure IR in diabetic persons and the gold standard for such measurement as seen by the WHO definition of the IRS is the clamp technique, the definitions provided by the EGIR, as well as the ATP III, would allow for a more simple approach on large-scale studies in non-diabetic individuals. In April 2005 a consensus report for the IRS was formulated according to the IDF definition. Interestingly, the criteria provided by IDF take into consideration both diabetic and non-diabetic individuals in a more simple approach (see Table 29.1).

Table 29.1 *Characteristics of the criteria for the MS according to WHO, NCEP-ATP III, EGIR, and IDF*

WHO

IFG/IGT, DM2, or IR (hyperinsulinemic, euglycemic clamp technique in the lowest 25%) + 2 or more of the following:
- BMI > 30 or WHR > 0.9 (men) or > 0.85 (women)
- Triglycerides ≥ 1.7 mmol/l or HDL < 0.9 (men) or < 1.0 (women)
- Blood pressure > 140/90 mmHg
- Microalbuminuria: urinary albumin excretion rate > 20 µg/min

EGIR

IR or fasting hyperinsulinemia (highest 25%) in non-diabetic individuals + 2 or more of the following:
- Waist circumference ≥ 94 cm (men) or ≥ 80 cm (women)
- Triglycerides ≥ 2.0 mmol/l or HDL < 1.0
- Blood pressure: ≥ 140/90 mmHg and/or medication
- Fasting hyperglycemia: FPG ≥ 6.1 mmol/l

ATP III

Three or more of the following risk factors:
- Waist circumference ≥ 102 cm (men) or ≥ 88 cm (women)
- Triglycerides ≥ 150 mg/dl
- HDL < 49 mg/dl (men) or < 50 mg/dl (women)
- Blood pressure: ≥ 130/85 mmHg
- FPG ≥ 6.1 mmol/l

IDF

- Triglycerides ≥ 150 mg/dl or specific treatment for such lipid abnormality
- HDL < 40 mg/dl (men) or < 50 mg/dl (women) or specific treatment for such lipid abnormality
- Blood pressure: ≥ 130/85 mmHg

Epidemiology

Considering that the world's older population has been growing for centuries, such a group of individuals is more likely to be exposed to a higher risk of developing chronic-degenerative diseases in old age and in particular the IRS. In fact, the Third National Health and Nutrition Survey (NHANES III) investigated the prevalence of the IRS in 8814 men and women 20 years of age and older.[8] These authors found that the prevalence of the IRS increased from 6.7% among participants aged 20–29 years to 43.5% and 42.0% for those age 60–69 years and 70 years and above, respectively.

Indeed, a striking increase in the number of older persons with the IRS has also taken place worldwide. Such an increase has also been associated with an inevitable global epidemic of both obesity and type 2 diabetes.[9] The rise in obesity and sedentary lifestyle in older persons, especially in the United States and Europe, has also been shown to play a significant role in the IRS.

Due to the great variability in the frequency of the syndrome among different populations, because of the differing frequencies of the abnormalities as well as the differing methodologies of measurement, the EGIR compared the frequency of the IRS taking into account the WHO (excluding DM2) and

EGIR criteria.[10] This group compared the frequency of the IRS in eight European countries over a large population sample (7276 men and 9363 women). From their study the IRS was more frequent in men than in women. According to WHO standards the frequency of IRS ranged from 8 to 20% in men less than 40 years of age, from 7 to 36% in men aged between 40 and 55 years, and from 17 to 47% in men over the age of 55 years. The same standards applied to women showed a frequency of IRS ranging from 3 to 8% in women less than 40 years of age, from 5 to 22% in women aged 40 to 55 years, and from 14 to 39% in women over the age of 55 years. The individual components and their frequency in men and women are reported in Figure 29.1.

Insulin resistance in older persons

As previously highlighted, the key player in the IRS is IR and, due to the fact that the aging process is significantly associated with an increase in IR per se, older persons with IRS need to be recognized as a delicate group of individuals with an increased risk of developing DM2 and CVD.

The aging process is associated with impaired glucose handling, mainly due to a decline in insulin action.[11–13] There is strong evidence that increased resistance to insulin action is one of the main components of diminished homeostatic glucose regulation in older persons. Insulin-mediated glucose uptake, measured by the glucose clamp technique, was demonstrated to progressively decline with aging.[14] The unifying hypothesis described by Barbieri et al,[15] explaining the relationship between IR and age, encompasses four main pathways, namely:

1. anthropometric changes (increase in fat mass with a parallel decline in fat free mass);
2. environmental changes (diet habits and reduced physical activity);
3. neurohormonal variations which may have an opposite effect of that of insulin at skeletal muscle and adipose levels;
4. a rise in oxidative stress.

Therefore, any one of the individual components of the IRS may have a greater clinical significance when found in older persons. Indeed, the management of IRS in older persons will lead clinicians to adopt precise measures. However, this approach has not been completely translated into clinical practice and many geriatricians claim that the administration of any available medical treatment is still conditioned to a previous diagnosis of specific disease. Therefore, only new clinical trials aimed at treating IRS components in older persons will need to focus on significant differences when treating older, middle-aged, and younger persons with IRS.

Insulin resistance and dyslipidemia

Increased plasma triglycerides, small dense low-density lipoprotein (LDL) cholesterol levels, and reduced high-density lipoprotein (HDL) cholesterol levels constitute the atherogenic dyslipidemia of IRS. In particular, IR is associated with:

1. hypertriglyceridemia and a subsequent increase in very low density lipoproteins (VLDLs);
2. small and dense LDLs;
3. lower HDL levels.

Visceral fat seems to have a major role and, indeed, the quantity of visceral fat tissue (as measured by computerized tomography (CT)), waist circumference, and IR are all significantly linked to one another.[16,17] Visceral fat tissue and IR are known to be at the basis of increased hepatic production of triglycerides and VLDL as well as reduced intravascular breakdown of VLDL and chylomicrons. In physiologic conditions, insulin inhibits lipolysis and promotes lipogenesis. By promoting the flow of intermediates through glycolysis, insulin promotes the formation of α-glycerol phosfate and fatty acids necessary for triglyceride formation. Insulin then stimulates fatty acid synthase, thus leading to increased fatty acid synthesis. At the same time, in the adipose tissue cell, insulin inhibits the breakdown of triglycerides by inhibiting the activity of a hormone-sensitive lipase, an enzyme necessary for triglyceride breakdown. This enzyme is also found

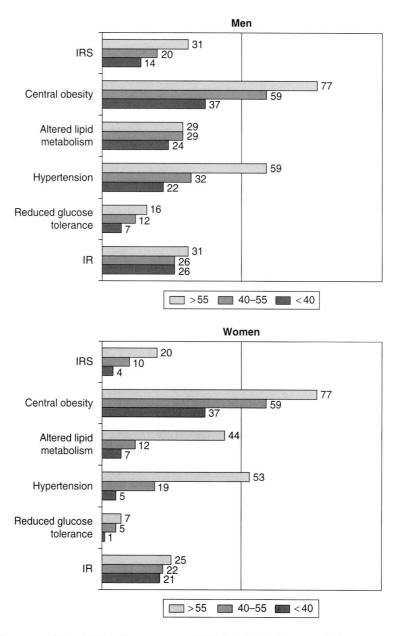

Figure 29.1 *Frequency (%) of IRS and components (WHO definition) in non-diabetic men and women.*

on the luminal surface of the endothelium of capillaries in both adipose tissue and skeletal muscle tissue. However, on the endothelium level, insulin increases the activity of the lipoprotein lipase, which, in turn, increases the breakdown of triglycerides in VLDLs as well as chylomicrons, thus playing an important role in the uptake of free fatty acids (FFAs) from the bloodstream to adipose tissue.

As a result, lipoproteins synthesized in the liver are taken up by adipose tissue and FFAs are ultimately stored as triglycerides. During an IR state, insulin action on adipose tissue is no longer effective in repressing the activity of such a lipoprotein lipase, thus a consequent rise in FFA plasma concentrations takes place.[18] On the vascular level, the reduced activity of the lipoprotein lipase results in a slower catabolism of chylomicrons and VLDLs and is clinically expressed as hypertriglyceridemia. Such triglycerides will be secreted by the liver as VLDL in circulation, thus creating a vicious cycle. Fasting hypertriglyceridemia has been identified as an independent risk factor for ischemic heart disease (IHD).[19] In particular, these authors reported that triglyceride-rich lipoproteins have different atherogenic potential. In addition to the direct atherogenic effect of triglyceride-rich lipoproteins, high triglyceride levels appear to be a marker of a series of other potentially atherogenic and prothrombotic changes (see below).

The second observation seen in the atherogenic profile during IR is the presence of small, dense, and highly atherosclerotic LDLs. The exact mechanism involved in the formation of small and dense LDL is not completely understood, however the hepatic lipase (HL), an enzyme found on the endoluminal surface of hepatic sinusoids, seems to have an important role on lipoprotein size and density formation. The HL specifically acts by hydrolyzing phospholipids and triglycerides found in HDLs and intermediate density lipoproteins (IDLs), but is also known to hydrolyze phospholipids and triglycerides in LDLs. In particular, it has been demonstrated that the more active the HL, the greater the release of phospholipids and triglycerides, thus resulting in the formation of smaller and more dense LDLs.[20] Considering that IR is associated with a significantly greater activity of the HL, this alteration may explain why a greater concentration of smaller and denser LDLs is found in such IR individuals. Furthermore, LDLs in the bloodstream of insulin-resistant persons have higher concentrations of triglycerides due to the cholesterol ester transfer protein (CETP), an enzyme that transfers triglycerides from VLDLs to LDLs,[21] thus forming the perfect substrate for highly active HL (no longer

insulin inhibited) and the formation of smaller and more dense LDLs. Small dense LDLs might be more atherogenic than normal dense LDLs due to the fact that they:

1. are more toxic to the endothelium
2. have a greater capability of crossing the endothelial membrane
3. have an increased susceptibility to oxidation and
4. are more selective to bound to scavenger receptors on monocyte-derived macrophages.[22]

The third altered lipid profile observed during IRS is the occurrence of lower HDL concentrations. As far as HDLs are concerned, they are smaller and more dense during an IR state and their size is inversely correlated with their triglyceride content, a phenomenon due to an increased catabolism of HDL itself.[23] The higher concentration of triglycerides in HDL is due to increased activity of CETP, an enzyme that also transfers triglycerides from VLDLs to HDLs.[21] Consequently, increased liver lipase activity (no longer effectively inhibited by insulin) results in a smaller core volume of HDL and thus the formation of smaller and more dense HDLs. During this phase, apoA-I normally present on the surface of HDL detaches and may be detected by its significantly higher urinary concentration.[24] These above alterations are particularly active during an IR state. Therefore, all three altered lipid profiles (hypertriglyceridemia, smaller and denser LDLs, and lower HDL concentrations) constitute the so-called atherogenic lipoprotein profile.[25] In fact, drugs known to improve IR by targeting each altered lipid profile of these components may reduce the risk of vascular events (see ahead).

Insulin resistance and obesity

A further component of the IRS is obesity and, in particular, the presence of extensive visceral fat tissue. Many studies have shown that increased visceral fat is a risk factor for age-related diseases such as hypertension, DM2, CVD, and reduced cognitive functioning.[26–29] It is well known that aging is associated with a decrease in lean body mass (especially muscle tissue) and a parallel rise in fat mass.[30] There is a slow, progressive redistribution of fat as intra-abdominal fat tends to increase and subcutaneous fat on the limbs tends to decrease. Data have repeatedly demonstrated that intra-abdominal fat is a major clinical parameter associated with IR. Although the mechanisms for the link between IR and intra-abdominal fat accumulation have not been fully elucidated, it has been suggested that a high lipolytic response of visceral adipose tissue to catecholamine exposes the liver to high FFA concentrations, which are known to play a role in IR (see above).

Increased adipose tissue present in overweight and obese individuals is no longer considered an inert bystander, but an active endocrine organ capable of regulating whole-body metabolism and other vital functions related to inflammation and immune responses.[31–33] These actions are mediated by a number of molecules that are secreted by adipocytes and act in an autocrine, paracrine, or endocrine fashion. Among those identified to date are leptin, adipsin, resistin, and adiponectin, which are believed to adapt metabolic fluxes to the amount of stored energy.[31] Therefore, understanding the regulation and expression of such adipokines in older individuals with different body fat density and distribution may indicate a new target for preventive measures, especially when considering cardiovascular functioning. The dysregulation of the adipokine network has been implicated in the etiology of IR and other components of the IRS, such as glucose intolerance, obesity, dyslipidemia, and hypertension.[34] In addition, there is a growing list of adipokines involved in the control of pro-inflammatory markers (tumor necrosis factor alfa (TNF-α), interleukin 6 (IL-6), IL-1β, IL-8, IL-10, transforming growth factor-β, nerve growth factor) and of the acute-phase response (plasminogen activator inhibitor-1, haptoglobin, serum amyloid A).[35,36] The production of these proteins by adipose tissue is increased in obesity, and raised circulating levels of several acute-phase proteins as well as inflammatory cytokines have led to the view that obesity, characterized by a chronic low-grade inflammatory state, is linked to IR and the IRS.

An increase in fat tissue, especially in the abdominal area, has also been associated with an increase in plasma levels of diverse pro-inflammatory cytokines. In particular, the increase in pro-inflammatory cytokines or adipokines including IL-6, resistin, TNF-α, and C-reactive protein (CRP) reflect overproduction by the expanded adipose tissue. This production supports evidence that monocyte-derived macrophages reside in adipose tissue and are at least in part the source of cytokine production locally and in the systemic circulation. The magnitude of such a vicious cycle remains unknown.

In recent years, much attention has been given to an anti-inflammatory adipokine, adiponectin, and it has also been shown to be involved in the modulation of IR.[37] In addition, adiponectin has demonstrated anti-atherogeneic effects.[38] In fact, in animal models of obesity, adiponectin has been shown to improve hyperglycemia and hyperinsulinemia without inducing weight gain or even inducing weight loss in some studies.[34,37,39] Furthermore, adiponectin modulates endothelial function and has an inhibitory effect on vascular smooth muscle cell proliferation.[40] Adiponectin also preferentially accumulates in the injured vascular walls where its ability to suppress macrophage-to-foam cell transformation need to be understood.[41] Some studies have shown that low concentrations of adiponectin are linked to myocardial infarction,[42] and to the progression of subclinical coronary heart disease.[43]

Previous works have demonstrated that the aging process itself is also associated with a dysregulation of the inflammatory response.[44–46] Such dysregulation is defined by the presence of high plasma concentrations of pro-inflammatory cytokines such as TNF-α, IL-6, and acute phase reactive proteins in older persons.[44,47] A growing body of evidence has also shown that TNF-α, IL-6, and CRP contribute to age-related IR.[45,47] In particular, diverse pro-inflammatory cytokine concentrations have been linked to aging, IR, and the IRS. These cytokines are probably important in controlling for the degree of IR since it has been shown that their serum concentrations are significantly higher in obese humans.

Insulin resistance and arterial hypertension

Arterial hypertension, another component of IRS, clusters with many metabolic diseases such as obesity, DM2, atherosclerosis, and dyslipidemic states. About 50 years ago, the association between IR and arterial hypertension was already documented.[48] Later on, numerous studies investigated the association in detail. In fact, one study specifically demonstrated that a strong association existed between hypertension, hyperinsulinemia, and reduced glucose tolerance in a large population of patients (n = 2475).[49] Another study evaluated the ability of hyperinsulinemia (as a surrogate measure of IR) to predict the development of coronary heart disease (CHD) and hypertension[50] in a healthy population. These authors found that 25% of the population with the highest insulin response (postglucose challenge) had a significantly higher increase in the incidence of hypertension (2-fold) or CHD (3-fold). Furthermore, these results were found independently of differences in age, gender, or body mass index (BMI). Indeed, these results indicate the importance of insulin resistance and/or hyperinsulinemia on vascular disease development over a 15-year time frame.

The mechanisms responsible for the relationship between IR and hypertension are multifactorial.[51] Firstly, it is important to note that insulin is a vasodilator when given intravenously to normal weight subjects,[52] and has a vasoconstrictor effect in IR aged and DM2 patients.[53] It is widely known that insulin is capable of stimulating the production of nitric oxide, thus resulting in increased blood flow, especially in skeletal muscle. Due to the fact that a common pathway exists between the insulin-dependent release of nitric oxide and the metabolic actions of insulin, any altered activity of such a pathway would result in both decreased vasodilation and reduced glucose skeletal muscle uptake. In fact, these alterations would explain the presence of increased peripheral blood flow, especially in skeletal muscle tissue, following an inadequate release of insulin-dependent nitric oxide release. Secondly, insulin has a direct effect on cardiac muscle tissue[54] by increasing cardiac output and rate through the activity of the sympathetic nervous system (SNS).[55] During an IR state, the SNS becomes hyperactive with subsequent peripheral vasoconstriction, increased heart rate, and hypertension. Thirdly, it is widely known that insulin has an antinatriuretic effect by the activation of the renin–angiotensin–aldosterone system.[56] Studies have also shown a significant and inverse relationship between IR and sodium diet restriction in both normal and high blood pressure patients.[57] Therefore, increased volume after renal sodium retention would contribute to a state of arterial volume-dependent hypertension. Lastly, another possible explanation between IR and hypertension may also be linked to a derangement of cations. The ATPase Na^+/K^+ pump is insulin sensitive and thus during IR a significant increase in intracellular sodium (Na^+) accompanies a consequent increase in intracellular calcium (Ca^{2+}).

Insulin resistance and hypercoagulability

During the IRS an alteration in the hemostatic system occurs and results in a potentially 'prothrombotic state' with severe vascular complications. Three main components of the hemostatic system are activated during an array of vascular tissue injury and include blood platelets, endothelial cells, and plasma coagulation factors. During an IR state, such reliability becomes less effective showing that insulin is intrinsically involved in the correct operation of such a system. Therefore, any alteration in the insulin-signaling pathway has been shown to result in amplified platelet activation and increased coagulation cascade activity accompanied by a parallel reduction in fibrinolysis.

Platelet activation

Insulin receptors are normally present on the surface of blood platelets and, when insulin binds to such receptors, the insulin signaling pathway is activated. Studies have shown that insulin is capable of reducing platelet response to adenosine diphosphate (ADP), thrombin, epinephrine, platelet-activating factor, as well as angiotensin II.[58,59] Furthermore, the activation of the insulin signaling pathway also results in lower platelet concentrations of calcium. Therefore, normal insulin action has an inhibitory/regulatory action on platelet aggregation. In an IR state such equilibrium is lost and a persistent prothrombic condition occurs with an increased risk for vascular obstruction.

Increased coagulation cascade activity

Increased levels of fibrinogen have been associated with IR. Fibrinogen is not only of fundamental importance in thrombin activity regulation, but also has a predictive value for future cardiovascular events.[60] In this context, it is important to underline that pro-inflammatory cytokine production from adipose tissue is known to markedly influence a hypercoagulable state by increasing hepatic fibrinogen production, as well as causing endothelial dysfunction towards a hypercoagulable condition. During IR there is a simultaneous increase in tissue factor (TF) and factor VII of the coagulation cascade, and this significantly enhances the activation of the coagulation cascade.

Abnormal fibrinolysis

Reduced fibrinolysis is a well-documented finding of the IRS and, in particular, IR is known to play a pivotal role. Normally, fibrinolysis is tightly controlled by the equilibrium between tissue plasminogen-activator (t-PA) and plasminogen activator inhibitor-1 (PAI-1). Persons with the IRS have increased PAI-1 levels which will inhibit t-PA, thus resulting in lower plasmin formation. PAI-1 levels have been shown to significantly increase during chronic inflammation and increased FFA levels. This may be explained by IR due to the fact that IR is associated with enhanced lipolysis and higher FFA concentrations (see above). These FFAs then catalyze the induction of the PAI-1 gene expression and PAI-1 production. Furthermore, the increased pro-inflammatory state found in such individuals is tightly related to IR.

Potential components of the IRS in the elderly

Oxidative stress

Recently, researchers have focused on the progressive changes that occur in the DNA structure and the potential consequences of such mutations. In particular, it has been suggested that excess and unopposed oxidative stress is the main cause of increasing mitochondrial DNA (mtDNA) mutations with aging and IRS. Accordingly, oxidative stress is characterized by an uncontrolled production of free radicals, derived from oxygen and produced by splitting a covalent bond into atoms or molecules with an unpaired electron, thereby forming highly reactive oxygen species (ROS). In normal physiologic conditions, the intramitochondrial environment is characterized by a substantial equilibrium between the production of ROS and the activity of antioxidant mechanisms, such as glutathione peroxidase (GSH-Px) and superoxide dismutase (SOD). However, when the endogenous production of ROS substantially increases with a parallel decrease in antioxidant agents, tissue damage due to such oxidative stress occurs. Studies suggest that the degree of unopposed oxidative stress is also predictive of mortality. In particular, the production of free radicals in the heart, kidney, and liver is inversely proportional to the maximum lifespan,[61] and the rate of mitochrondrial oxygen radical generation is negatively associated with animal longevity. In animal models, caloric restriction also decreases mitochondrial oxygen radical production and oxidative damage to mtDNA, decreasing the rate of aging, and some epidemiologic studies have suggested that dietary antioxidants may have a significant impact on age-related disease states.[62,63] The benefits from supplemental antioxidants remain unproven in clinical trials.

Oxidative stress also adversely impacts other vulnerable targets including lipid and protein components of membranes. Free radicals then facilitate lipid oxidation and a consequent reduction in trans-membrane transportation. This mechanism of uncontrolled oxidative stress (already active in older persons) becomes extremely active during the IRS and the link between IR and endothelial dysfunction may explain, in part, the increased risk for cardiovascular disease associated with IRS.

The mechanisms by which IR leads to endothelial dysfunction are certainly multiple and complex. All major abnormalities of the IRS, such as hyperglycemia, hypertension, dyslipidemia, and altered coagulation, are also directly linked to endothelial dysfunction. However, in regard to the link between IR and oxidative stress, it is important to underline recent observations. As previously mentioned, insulin has a direct vasodilatory effect mediated through stimulation of nitric oxide production in endothelial cells.[64] During an IR state the ability to stimulate nitric oxide becomes limited and at the same time an increase in ROS, such as superoxide, occurs. Pro-inflammatory cytokines, such as TNF-α and IL-6, work synergistically with ROS toward creating endothelial disarray and, thus, an increased risk for the development of vascular disease. Therefore, one may speculate that individuals who exhibit the IRS may have an abnormality in nitric oxide production by endothelial cells, and at the same time a constant stimulation of proatherogenic changes in the vasculature in response to IR.

Homocysteine

Homocysteine, a sulfur-containing amino acid formed during the metabolism of methionine, has emerged as a novel independent biomarker for the development of atherosclerotic disease in coronary, cerebral, and peripheral vascular beds. In fact, there is an increased risk for cardiovascular disease in those with elevated fasting plasma total homocysteine levels. One study showed that those individuals with hyperinsulinemia (considered a marker of IR) had significantly higher homocysteine levels than those with normal insulin levels. Plasma levels of insulin seem to influence homocysteine metabolism, possibly through the effects on glomerular filtration or by influencing the activity of key enzymes in homocysteine metabolism. The authors of this study also underlined that persons with two or more IRS phenotypes had significantly higher homocysteine levels compared to those with one or no IRS phenotype.[65] Interestingly, elevated homocysteine levels increase the risk for CVD in type 2 diabetes patients to a greater extent than among non-diabetic subjects.[66] In a large community-based population of non-diabetic individuals a modest association was found between IR and elevated homocysteine levels.[65] These authors found that the co-occurrence of specific features of IRS, especially hypertension and central obesity, was associated with more marked elevations in homocysteine levels.

The involvement of homocysteine as a contributory factor to vascular damage still remains controversial. However, the presence of high plasma levels of homocysteine may play an important role and these are capable of promoting oxidative damage to the endothelium of vascular cells through auto-oxidation, and the formation of homocysteine mixed disulfides and ROS.[67] In particular, oxidation of two homocysteine molecules results in the formation of oxidized disulfide, two protons and two electrons, while promoting the formation of ROS. Activation of ROS is only one of the many damaging effects of homocysteine, since it may act alone as well as in concert with other multiple injurious stimuli to damage endothelial cell function. The combined effect of hypercoagulability and IR strengthens the processes of oxidation, glycation, or homocysteinylation of LDLs necessary for the transformation in atherogenic particles. There are multiple metabolic toxicities associated with IRS, and in particular IR, which are also associated with the production of ROS, thus creating multiple injurious stimuli and a higher risk for accelerated atherosclerosis.

Cognitive functioning

The aging process is associated with significant decline in cognitive functioning. Indeed, many studies have tried to discover the mechanisms involved with cognitive decline in vulnerable older persons. Many of the same risk factors associated with CVD have also been recognized with a higher risk for developing compromised cognitive functioning. The risk of cognitive impairment, especially in older persons with IRS, needs to be recognized by physicians, due to the fact that its association with lower functional status in older persons opens new public health concerns. The IRS and its individual components have also been associated with increased risk of developing cognitive impairment and decline over 4 years in high-functioning older persons even after adjusting for comorbidities.[68] In particular, such decline was steeper in those who had high serum levels of inflammatory markers.

Age-related IR has been shown to be independently associated with reduced cognitive functioning in older non-diabetic persons.[69] To this regard, it is now well documented that insulin is a fundamental neuromodulator, contributing to neurobiologic processes in particular, energy homeostasis, and cognition. Interestingly, insulin and insulin receptors are selectively expressed in the brain.[70] Initially the majority of glucose transporters in the brain were considered insulin-insensitive; however, it has been recently shown that a significant element of brain glucose uptake is insulin sensitive and is essential for correct cognitive functioning.[71] Thus, an age-related reduction in glucose uptake due to altered insulin signaling can lead to a deficiency in energetic substrate that cannot be compensated by other metabolic pathways.[72,73] Interestingly, a significant increase in peripheral IR develops as individuals age, raising the possibility that a reduced efficiency of the metabolic pathway responsible for energy production is one of the mechanisms of cognitive decline in older persons.[74,75]

Collectively, these findings suggest that insulin contributes to normal cognitive functioning, and that insulin abnormalities exacerbate cognitive impairment, such as those associated with Alzheimer's disease. It is noteworthy that endothelial damage and vascular disease combined with IR are also responsible for an age-related decline in cognitive function even in the absence of dementia. Furthermore, any factors capable of lowering or increasing the risk of endothelial damage and/or affecting insulin action may have a role in cognitive function and cerebrovascular disease.

Muscle functioning

In older persons, poor muscle strength and poor physical performance often coexist. Midlife handgrip muscle strength has been recognized as an important factor that predicts old age functional ability.[76] Observational studies have consistently shown that chronic conditions such as coronary heart disease, diabetes, and pulmonary obstructive disease are associated with lower muscle strength.[76,77]

It is also widely known that insulin plays a pivotal role for muscle contraction by increasing glucose uptake and promoting intracellular glucose metabolism, thus it is plausible that age-related IR may be a determinant of reduced muscle functioning as seen clinically by lower muscle strength. One cross-sectional study showed that a significant association between IR and muscle strength exists in older non-diabetic persons independently of multiple confounders.[78]

In particular, insulin may also be an important determinant on muscle function since glucose uptake is necessary for adequate muscle contraction. Another important role played by insulin is its ability to repress whole body proteolysis, thus shifting total body metabolism towards an anabolic state. Therefore, it is plausible that an age-related IR may be a determinant of poor muscle strength in older persons with IRS. Furthermore, a reduction in insulin peripheral activity may reduce the muscle tissue anabolic rate leading to a relative catabolic state and, in turn, contributing to the impairment in muscle functioning. Indeed, insulin is known to play a pivotal role in muscle functioning by increasing glucose uptake and promoting intracellular glucose metabolism.

Therapeutic perspectives: no pills, one pill, or polypills?

Metabolic risk factors of the IRS include atherogenic dyslipidemia, hypertension, IR, prothrombotic state, and the proinflammatory state. Due to the fact that IR is the pivotal key player in the IRS, drug intervention should be aimed at improving insulin sensitivity, either directly through the use of drugs known to improve insulin sensitivity or indirectly through the use of drugs known to improve metabolic alterations associated with IR (Figure 29.2).

All of the risk factors linked to IR need to be treated in order to reduce the severity of IRS. The American Diabetes Association (ADA)[79] and the National Cholesterol Education Program (NCEP) have adopted guidelines for the complications related to IRS.[5] The cornerstones of IRS treatment are the management of weight and making certain that appropriate physical exercise is performed. In fact, education and training should be considered fundamental due to the fact that environmental influences such as improper nutrition and physical inactivity are considered root causes of IRS. Interventions in IRS with physical activity have

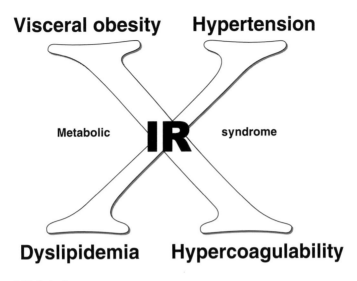

Figure 29.2 *IRS and IR-linked components.*

shown that regular and sustained physical activity will improve all risk factors of the IRS.[80,81] In regard to weight management, there is a general consensus that persons with IRS have to lower their intake of saturated fats, reduce consumption of simples sugars, and increase intake of fruits, vegetables, and whole grains.[82] Recommendations for carbohydrate and unsaturated fat intake remain controversial,[83] however it has been seen that low-fat diets promote weight reduction[84] and higher monosaturated fat intake reduces postprandial glycemia, reduces plasma triglyceride levels, and raises HDL concentrations.[83] Even though modifications in diet and exercise need to be adopted in the first-line approach for treating IRS, the use of pharmaceuticals is almost always necessary.

Thiazolidinediones (TZD or glitazones) are a new class of oral antidiabetic drugs which exert their insulin-sensitizing action by stimulation of the nuclear transcription factor peroxisome proliferator-activated receptor gamma (PPAR-γ). At present, pioglitazone and rosiglitazone are available for clinical use. Different activation levels of PPAR-γ and of cofactors determine the binding of PPAR-γ to distinct target genes, which in turn regulates their transcriptional activity. It is important to

recall that PPARs are members of the superfamily of nuclear hormone receptors which are transcription factors transmitting signals that originate from lipid-soluble factors to the genome. Nuclear receptors then bind to DNA at specific sites or response elements, which when linked able the receptor complex, which in turn can activate or repress the expression of a target gene. Three different PPAR genes have been identified, α, γ, and δ,[85] and are involved in distinct expression patterns which suggest their important functional differences. TZDs dramatically upgrade insulin sensitivity through the PPAR-γ and are then capable of lowering blood glucose levels through more active glucose transporters and by stimulating the insulin-signaling pathway.

Studies have also underlined that PPAR-γ agonists are capable of improving altered lipid metabolism associated with IR. PPAR-γ is highly expressed in adipose tissue, where it triggers adipocyte differentiation and also induces genes critical for adipogenesis. Adipose tissue serves as a major site of oxidized LDL (oxLDL) detoxification, thus removing it from the bloodstream and potentially inhibiting the formation of atherosclerotic lesions. Increasing clinical evidence also shows that rosiglitazone treatment significantly improves factors

383

associated with CVD, including endothelial activity, inflammatory processes, and dyslipidemia.[86,87] Moreover, one study comparing the effects of lipid metabolism of rosiglitazone and pioglitazone during an IR state demonstrated that both drugs were associated with lower FFA levels; however, only the pioglitazone-treated group was associated with significantly lower triglyceride levels.[88] Only future clinical trials in older persons in an IR state will be able to clarify whether significant protective factors from the use of TZDs are substantial.

TZDs are also capable of reducing oxLDLs in both lean and obese diabetic animals.[89] In particular, TZDs upregulated oxidized LDL receptor 1 (OLR1) in adipocytes by facilitating the exchange of coactivators for corepressors on the OLR1 gene in cultured mouse adipocytes. TZDs markedly stimulated the uptake of oxLDL into adipocytes, which required OLR1. Increased OLR1 expression, resulting from TZD treatment, significantly increased adipocyte cholesterol content and enhanced FA uptake. While the physiologic role of adipose tissue in cholesterol and oxLDL metabolism is still unknown, the induction of OLR1 may be a potential means through which PPAR-γ ligands may regulate lipid metabolism and insulin sensitivity in adipocytes.[89] Some caution should be used when treating older persons with PPAR-γ agonists due to the fact that these agents may cause water retention and altered hepatic detoxifying activity, thus magnifying a potential condition of cardiac failure and an inadequate removal of toxic compounds due to inappropriate liver metabolism.

PPAR-α agonists or fibrates are used to treat dyslipidemia, particularly in the case of high triglycerides and low HDL cholesterol. Fibrates (gemfibrozil, bezafibrate, fenofibrate) are another class of lipid-lowering drugs known to be generally effective on lowering elevated plasma triglycerides and cholesterol. There is a lack of controlled clinical trials with fibrates compared to statins, especially in older persons. However, the use of fibrates has been shown to have protective effects against further vascular events in survivors of myocardial infarction.[90] The more pronounced effect of fibrates is a decrease in plasma triglyceride-rich lipoproteins after linking to PPAR-α. PPAR-α is especially expressed in kidney, heart, and muscle tissue (all known to metabolize large concentrations of fatty acids). Fibrates are ligands for PPAR-α.[91]

The main mechanisms of action of fibrates are thus linked to the activation of key genes involved in lipid metabolism. The hypotriglyceridemic action of fibrates involves the combination effect of HL and apoC-III expression. HL is induced at the transcriptional level mediated by PPAR, while apoC-III is repressed. As a consequence, a reduced secretion of VLDL particles, together with enhanced catabolism of triglyceride-rich particles, thus explains such action. Secondly, fibrates are also known to increase hepatic uptake of FFAs, increase the removal of LDL particles, and stimulate the production of HDL and its major constituents, apoA-I and apoA-II.

Hypertriglyceridemia in association with an IR state is considered the main target for the use of fibrates in the IRS. In fact, in those persons undergoing therapy with fenofibrate, a 50% decrease in triglycerides and a simultaneous 10–30% increase in basal HDL were observed.[92] Fenofibrate was also found to be more effective in reducing plasma concentrations of oxidized LDLs and, in CVD high-risk individuals, the impact of accelerating chylomicron and VLDL catabolism underlines the ability of fibrates to act on postprandial lipid metabolism.[92] Only large clinical studies will confirm their effectiveness in reducing coronary events and total mortality in older high-risk individuals.

A very recent new drug named rimonabant, a selective cannabinoid-1 (CB1) blocker, decreases food intake and weight and increases adiponectin and insulin sensitivity. Drug interventions with rimonabant, such as the RIO-Europe study, addressed the effects of such therapy on weight loss, altered glucose metabolism, and dyslipidemia.[93] These authors found that at the 1-year follow-up, patients undergoing treatment with 20 mg of rimonabant had significant reductions in body weight and waist circumference. There was also a significant improvement in lipid and glucose parameters. There was a significant increase in HDL levels and a decrease in triglycerides as well as a significant reduction in IR as measured by the homeostasis model assessment index (HOMA).

The risk for CV events is significantly increased during an IR state and, due to the fact that enhanced lipid metabolism may ameliorate an IR state, lipid-lowering agents such as statins may have an important role. It is widely known that statins or 3-hydroxy-3-methylglutaryl-coenzyme A reductase inhibitors reduce the risk of CVD by reducing all apoB-containing lipoproteins and VLDL production. Statins are effective, both in primary and secondary prevention of CHD, in middle-aged and older (< 65 years) men and women, in both diabetics and non-diabetics with CHD.[94,95] Statins used in secondary prevention of CHD significantly reduce the risk of stroke. They also reduce daily attacks of myocardial ischemia. Statins have been shown to reduce LDLs by 20–50% and triglycerides by 10–40%, and to increase HDLs by 5–12%. In fact, ATP III of the National Cholesterol Education Program issued evidence-based guidelines for major clinical trials with statin therapy. According to the ATP III algorithm, persons are categorized into three risk categories:

1. established CVD and CVD risk equivalents
2. multiple (two or more risk factors)
3. zero to one risk factor.

CVD risks include non-coronary forms of atherosclerotic disease, diabetes, and multiple (two or more) CVD risk factors with a 10-year risk for CVD > 20%. Therefore, all persons with CVD or CVD risk equivalents may be considered high risk.

Therapy in high-risk CVD patients

The goal for LDL-lowering therapy is to achieve LDL levels less than 100 mg/dl in high-risk patients. Therefore, in persons with LDL levels < 100 mg/dl no further LDL-lowering therapy is recommended, while in high-risk patients with LDL levels ≥100 mg/dl, diet therapy should be initiated. When baseline LDL is ≥130 mg/dl, an LDL-lowering drug should be started simultaneously with diet therapy. In the presence of high triglycerides or low HDL, consideration may be given to using a fibrate.

Therapy in moderate-risk CVD patients

Moderate-risk persons have two or more risk factors and a 10-year risk between 10 and 20%. The recommendation in this case is to obtain LDL < 130 mg/dl. When LDL is 100–129 mg/dl at baseline or on lifestyle therapy, an initiation of an LDL-lowering drug to achieve LDL < 100 mg/dl is a therapeutic option.

When LDL-lowering drug treatment is initiated in high-risk or moderate-risk patients, it is advised that the goal of such therapy is to achieve at least a 30 to 40% reduction in LDL levels.

How do statins improve IR? Studies have reported that statins also have a beneficial impact on the chemical properties of lipoproteins by reducing oxidized LDLs, as well as small and dense VLDLs, all commonly observed during an IR state.[96] In particular, small doses of atorvastatin (10 mg) have been shown to reduce VLDLs and IDLs as well as apoB postprandial concentrations in persons with normal lipid profiles.[97] Furthermore, in patients with altered lipid profiles and altered glucose metabolism (reduced glucose tolerance or type 2 diabetes), treatment with atorvastatin reduced IR, as seen by the HOMA index,[98] and reduced small, dense atherogenic LDLs.[99] Simvastatin, rosuvastatin, and fluvastatin have also been shown to reduce oxLDLs, thus generalizing the so-called 'class effect' of statins. It has been hypothesized that a reduction in hepatic lipase activity during such therapy may be at the basis of such a phenomenon.

In regard to arterial hypertension and IR, mild elevations in blood pressure can often be controlled by lifestyle changes, including reduced sodium intake and weight loss. However, if hypertension persists despite such changes, antihypertensive drug treatment is usually required. It is widely known that the benefits demonstrated from reducing arterial hypertension lower the risk for CVD.[100] It also has been suggested that the use of angiotensin-converting enzyme (ACE) inhibitors or angiotensin receptor blockers are better first-line therapy for IRS patients.[101] The prothrombotic state characterized by high concentrations of fibrinogen, PAI-1, and increased platelet aggregation may be treated when necessary with low-dose aspirin or other antiplatelet drugs.[102] Indeed, such drugs are universally recommended in patients with established CVD. Their effectiveness in older persons with IRS in the absence of CVD has still not been verified through clinical trials. However, their use has been considered a prophylactic therapeutic option when the risk for CVD is high.[103]

Conclusions

IR is considered the root of the IRS and age-related IR will further derange metabolic changes normally occurring in older persons. The percentage of aged subjects in the populations of industrialized countries is dramatically increasing, thus predisposing more persons to development of the IRS. If one accepts that each single component of IRS is significantly linked to IR, physicians will need to focus on correcting IR in order to improve each metabolic component.

References

1. Hu G, Qiao Q, Tuomilehto J et al. DECODE Study Group. Prevalence of the metabolic syndrome and its relation to all-cause and cardiovascular mortality in nondiabetic European men and women. Arch Intern Med 2004 164(10): 1066–76.
2. Isomaa B, Almgren P, Tuomi T et al. Cardiovascular morbidity and mortality associated with the metabolic syndrome. Diabetes Care 2001; 24(4): 683–9.
3. Lakka HM, Laaksonen DE, Lakka TA et al. The metabolic syndrome and total and cardiovascular disease mortality in middle-aged men. JAMA 2002; 288(21): 2709–16.
4. Alberti KG, Zimmet PZ. Definition, diagnosis, and classification of diabetes mellitus and its complications. Part 1: diagnosis and classification of diabetes mellitus provisional report of a WHO consultation. Diabet Med 1998: 15: 539–53.
5. Executive Summary of the Third Report of the National Cholesterol Education Program (NCEP) Expert Panel on Detection, Evaluation, and Treatment of High Blood Cholesterol in Adults (Adult Treatment Panel III). JAMA 2001; 285: 2486–97.
6. Balkau B, Charles MA. Comment on the provisional report from the WHO consultation. European Group for the Study of Insulin Resistance (EGIR). Diabet Med 1999; 16: 442–3.
7. Holt RI. International Diabetes Federation redefines the metabolic syndrome. Diabetes Obes Metab 2005; 7(5): 618–20.
8. Ford ES, Giles WH, Dietz WH. Prevalence of the metabolic syndrome among US adults: findings from the third National Health and Nutrition Examination Survey. JAMA 2002 16; 287(3): 356–9.
9. Zimmet P, Alberti KG, Shaw J. Global and societal implications of the diabetes epidemic. Nature 2001; 414(6865): 782–7.
10. Balkau B, Charles MA, Drivsholm T et al. European Group For The Study Of Insulin Resistance (EGIR). Frequency of the WHO metabolic syndrome in European cohorts, and an alternative definition of an insulin resistance syndrome. Diabetes Metab 2002; 28(5): 364–76.
11. Fink RI, Kolterman OG, Griffin J, Olefsky JM. Mechanisms of insulin resistance in aging. J Clin Invest 1983: 71(6): 1523–35.
12. Rowe JW, Minaker KL, Pallotta JA, Flier JS. Characterization of the insulin resistance of aging. J Clin Invest 1983: 71(6): 1581–7.
13. Gumbiner B, Thorburn AW, Ditzler TM, Bulacan F, Henry RR. Role of impaired intracellular glucose metabolism in the insulin resistance of aging. Metabolism 1992: 41(10): 1115–21.
14. Ferrannini E, Vichi S, Beck-Nielsen H et al. Insulin action and age. European Group for the Study of Insulin Resistance (EGIR). Diabetes 1996: 45(7): 947–53.
15. Barbieri M, Rizzo MR, Manzella D, Paolisso G. Age-related insulin resistance: is it an obligatory finding? The lesson from healthy centenarians. Diabetes Metab Res Rev 2001; 17(1): 19–26.
16. Banerji MA, Chaiken RL, Gordon D, Kral JG, Lebovitz HE. Does intra-abdominal adipose tissue in black men determine whether NIDDM is insulin-resistant or insulin-sensitive? Diabetes 1995; 44(2): 141–6.
17. Fujimoto WY, Abbate SL, Kahn SE, Hokanson JE, Brunzell JD. The visceral adiposity syndrome in Japanese-American men. Obes Res 1994; 2: 364–71.
18. Laws A, Hoen HM, Selby JV et al. Differences in insulin suppression of free fatty acid levels by gender and glucose tolerance status. Relation to plasma triglyceride and apolipoprotein B concentrations. Insulin Resistance Atherosclerosis Study (IRAS) Investigators. Arterioscler Thromb Vasc Biol 1997; 17(1): 64–71.
19. Jeppesen J, Hein HO, Suadicani P, Gyntelberg F. Triglyceride concentration and ischemic heart disease: an eight-year follow-up in the Copenhagen Male Study. Circulation 1998; 97(11): 1029–36.
20. Zambon A, Austin MA, Brown BG, Hokanson JE, Brunzell JD. Effect of hepatic lipase on LDL in normal men and those with coronary artery disease. Arterioscler Thromb 1993; 13(2): 147–53.
21. Morton RE, Zilversmit DB. Purification and characterization of lipid transfer protein(s) from human lipoprotein-deficient plasma. J Lipid Res 1982; 23(7): 1058–67.

22. Krauss RM. Dense low density lipoproteins and coronary artery disease. Am J Cardiol 1995; 75(6): 53–7B.

23. Rashid S, Uffelman KD, Lewis GF. The mechanism of HDL lowering in hypertriglyceridemic, insulin-resistant states. J Diabetes Compl 2002; 16(1): 24–8.

24. Clay MA, Newnham HH, Barter PJ. Hepatic lipase promotes a loss of apolipoprotein A-I from triglyceride-enriched human high density lipoproteins during incubation in vitro. Arterioscler Thromb 1991; 11(2): 415–22.

25. Austin MA, King MC, Vranizan KM, Krauss RM. Atherogenic lipoprotein phenotype. A proposed genetic marker for coronary heart disease risk. Circulation 1990; 82(2): 495–506.

26. Pierson RN Jr. Body composition in aging: a biological perspective. Curr Opin Clin Nutr Metab Care 2003; 6(1): 15–20.

27. Kannel WB, Cupples LA, Ramaswami R et al. Regional obesity and risk of cardiovascular disease; the Framingham Study. J Clin Epidemiol 1991; 44(2): 183–90.

28. Harris TB, Launer LJ, Madans J, Feldman JJ. Cohort study of effect of being overweight and change in weight on risk of coronary heart disease in old age. BMJ 1997; 314(7097): 1791–4.

29. Elias MF, Elias PK, Sullivan LM, Wolf PA, D'Agostino RB. Lower cognitive function in the presence of obesity and hypertension: the Framingham heart study. Int J Obes Relat Metab Disord 2003; 27(2): 260–8.

30. Chumlea WC, Garry PJ, Hunt WC, Rhyne RL. Distributions of serial changes in stature and weight in a healthy elderly population. Hum Biol 1988; 60(6): 917–25.

31. Ahima RS, Flier JS. Adipose tissue as an endocrine organ. Trends Endocrinol Metab 2000; 11: 327–32.

32. Rajala MW, Scherer PE. Minireview: the adipocyte – at the crossroads of energy homeostasis, inflammation, and atherosclerosis. Endocrinology 2003; 144(9): 3765–73.

33. Lyon CJ, Law RE, Hsueh WA. Minireview: adiposity, inflammation, and atherogenesis. Endocrinology 2003; 144(6): 2195–200.

34. Fasshauer M, Paschke R. Regulation of adipocytokines and insulin resistance. Diabetologia 2003; 46(12): 1594–603.

35. Trayhurn P, Wood IS. Adipokines: inflammation and the pleiotropic role of white adipose tissue. Br J Nutr 2004; 92(3): 347–55.

36. Yudkin JS, Stehouwer CD, Emeis JJ, Coppack SW. C-reactive protein in healthy subjects: associations with obesity, insulin resistance, and endothelial dysfunction: a potential role for cytokines originating from adipose tissue? Arterioscler Thromb Vasc Biol 1999; 19: 972–8.

37. Chandran M, Phillips SA, Ciaraldi T, Henry RR. Adiponectin: more than just another fat cell hormone? Diabetes Care 2003; 26(8): 2442–50.

38. Cnop M, Havel PJ, Utzschneider KM et al. Relationship of adiponectin to body fat distribution, insulin sensitivity and plasma lipoproteins: evidence for independent roles of age and sex. Diabetologia 2003; 46(4): 459–69.

39. Salmenniemi U, Ruotsalainen E, Pihlajamaki J et al. Multiple abnormalities in glucose and energy metabolism and coordinated changes in levels of adiponectin, cytokines, and adhesion molecules in subjects with metabolic syndrome. Circulation 2004; 110(25): 3842–8.

40. Ouchi N, Kihara S, Arita Y et al. Novel modulator for endothelial adhesion molecules: adipocyte-derived plasma protein adiponectin. Circulation 1999; 100: 2473–6.

41. Okamoto Y, Arita Y, Nishida M. An adipocyte-derived plasma protein, adiponectin, adheres to injured vascular walls. Horm Metab Res 2000; 32: 47–50.

42. Pischon T, Girman CJ, Hotamisligil GS et al. Plasma adiponectin levels and risk of myocardial infarction in men. JAMA 2004; 291(14): 1730–7.

43. Maahs DM, Ogden LG, Kinney GL et al. Low plasma adiponectin levels predict progression of coronary artery calcification. Circulation 2005; 111(6): 747–53.

44. Paolisso G, Rizzo MR, Mazziotti G et al. Advancing age and insulin resistance: role of plasma tumor necrosis factor-alpha. Am J Physiol 1998; 275(2 Pt 1): E294–9.

45. Abbatecola AM, Ferrucci L, Grella R et al. Diverse effect of inflammatory markers on insulin resistance and insulin-resistance syndrome in the elderly. J Am Geriatr Soc 2004; 52(3): 399–404.

46. Franceschi C, Bonafe M, Valensin S et al. Inflammaging. An evolutionary perspective on immunosenescence. Ann NY Acad Sci 2000; 908: 244–54.

47. Hak AE, Pols HAP, Stehouwer CDA et al. Markers of inflammation and cellular adhesion molecules in relation to insulin resistance in nondiabetic elderly: the Rotterdam study. J Clin Endocrinol Metab 2001; 86: 4398–405.

48. Welborn TA, Breckenridge A, Rubinstein AH, Dollery CT, Fraser TR. Serum-insulin in essential hypertension and in peripheral vascular disease. Lancet 1966; 1(7451): 1336–7.

49. Modan M, Halkin H, Almog S et al. Hyperinsulinemia. A link between hypertension obesity and glucose intolerance. J Clin Invest 1985; 75(3): 809–17.

50. Zavaroni I, Bonini L, Gasparini P et al. Hyperinsulinemia in a normal population as a predictor of non-insulin-dependent diabetes mellitus,

hypertension, and coronary heart disease: the Barilla factory revisited. Metabolism 1999; 48(8): 989–94.

51. Ferrannini E, Buzzigoli G, Bonadonna R et al. Insulin resistance in essential hypertension. N Engl J Med 1987; 317(6): 350–7.

52. Steinberg HO, Brechtel G, Johnson A, Fineberg N, Baron AD. Insulin-mediated skeletal muscle vasodilation is nitric oxide dependent. A novel action of insulin to increase nitric oxide release. J Clin Invest 1994; 94(3): 1172–9.

53. Steinberg HO, Chaker H, Leaming R et al. Obesity/insulin resistance is associated with endothelial dysfunction. Implications for the syndrome of insulin resistance. J Clin Invest 1996; 97(11): 2601–10.

54. ter Maaten JC, Voorburg A, de Vries PM et al. Relationship between insulin's haemodynamic effects and insulin-mediated glucose uptake. Eur J Clin Invest 1998; 28(4): 279–84.

55. Grassi G, Seravalle G, Cattaneo BM et al. Sympathetic activation in obese normotensive subjects. Hypertension 1995; 25(4 Pt 1): 560–3.

56. DeFronzo RA, Cooke CR, Andres R, Faloona GR, Davis PJ. The effect of insulin on renal handling of sodium, potassium, calcium, and phosphate in man. J Clin Invest 1975; 55(4): 845–55.

57. Zavaroni I, Coruzzi P, Bonini L et al. Association between salt sensitivity and insulin concentrations in patients with hypertension. Am J Hypertens 1995; 8(8): 855–8.

58. Trovati M, Anfossi G. Insulin, insulin resistance and platelet function: similarities with insulin effects on cultured vascular smooth muscle cells. Diabetologia 1998; 41(6): 609–22.

59. Trovati M, Mularoni EM, Burzacca S et al. Impaired insulin-induced platelet antiaggregating effect in obesity and in obese NIDDM patients. Diabetes 1995; 44(11): 1318–22.

60. Anand SS, Yi Q, Gerstein H et al. Relationship of metabolic syndrome and fibrinolytic dysfunction to cardiovascular disease. Circulation 2003; 108(4): 420–5.

61. Sohal RS, Svensson I, Sohal BH, Brunk UT. Superoxide anion radical production in different animal species. Mech Ageing Dev 1989; 49(2): 129–35.

62. Gilgun-Sherki Y, Melamed E, Offen D. Antioxidant treatment in Alzheimer's disease: current state. J Mol Neurosci 2003; 21(1): 1–12.

63. Paolini M, Sapone A, Canistro D, Chieco P, Valgimigli L. Antioxidant vitamins for prevention of cardiovascular disease. Lancet 2003; 362(9387): 920.

64. Kuboki K, Jiang ZY, Takahara N et al. Regulation of endothelial constitutive nitric oxide synthase gene expression in endothelial cells and in vivo: a specific vascular action of insulin. Circulation 2000; 101(6): 676–81.

65. Meigs JB, Jacques PF, Selhub J et al. Fasting plasma homocysteine levels in the insulin resistance syndrome: the Framingham offspring study. Diabetes Care 2001; 24(8): 1403–10.

66. Hoogeveen EK, Kostense PJ, Beks PJ et al. Hyperhomocysteinemia is associated with an increased risk of cardiovascular disease, especially in non-insulin-dependent diabetes mellitus: a population-based study. Arterioscler Thromb Vasc Biol 1998; 18(1): 133–8.

67. Jakubowski H, Zhang L, Bardeguez A, Aviv A. Homocysteine thiolactone and protein homocysteinylation in human endothelial cells: implications for atherosclerosis. Circ Res 2000; 87(1): 45–51.

68. Yaffe K, Kanaya A, Lindquist K et al. The metabolic syndrome, inflammation, and risk of cognitive decline. JAMA 2004; 292: 2237–42.

69. Abbatecola AM, Paolisso G, Lamponi M et al. Insulin resistance and executive dysfunction in older persons. J Am Geriatr Soc 2004; 52(10): 1713–18.

70. Kyriaki G. Brain insulin: regulation, mechanisms of action and functions. Cell Mol Neurobiol 2003; 23: 1–25.

71. McEwen BS, Reagan LP. Glucose transporter expression in the central nervous system: relationship to synaptic function. Eur J Pharmacol 2004; 490: 13–24.

72. Messier C, Awad N, Gagnon M. The relationships between atherosclerosis, heart disease, type 2 diabetes and dementia. Neurol Res 2004; 26(5): 567–72.

73. Craft S, Dagogo-Jack SE, Wiethop BV et al. Effects of hyperglycemia on memory and hormone levels in dementia of the Alzheimer type: a longitudinal study. Behav Neurosci 1993; 107: 926–40.

74. Kalmijn S, Feskens EJM, Launer LJ, Stijnen T, Kromhout D. Glucose intolerance, hyperinsulinemia and cognitive function in a general population of elderly men. Diabetologia 1995; 38: 1096–102.

75. Kuhl DE, Metter EJ, Riege WH, Hawkins RA. The effects of normal aging on patterns of cerebral glucose utilization. Ann Neurol 1984; 15: S133–7.

76. Rantanen T, Guralnik JM, Foley D et al. Midlife hand grip strength as a predictor of old age disability. JAMA 1999; 281(6): 558–60.

77. Kallman DA, Plato CC, Tobin JD. The role of muscle loss in the age-related decline of grip strength: cross-sectional and longitudinal perspectives. J Gerontol 1990: 45(3): M82–8.

78. Abbatecola AM, Ferrucci L, Ceda GP et al. Insulin resistance and muscle strength in older persons. J Gerontol A Biol Sci Med Sci 2005; 60(10): 1278–82.

79. Franz MJ, Bantle JP, Beebe CA et al. Evidence-based nutrition principles and recommendations for the treatment and prevention of diabetes and related complications. Diabetes Care 2002; 25(1): 148–98.

80. Cook S, Weitzman M, Auinger P, Nguyen M, Dietz WH. Prevalence of a metabolic syndrome phenotype in adolescents: findings from the third National Health and Nutrition Examination Survey, 1988–1994. Arch Pediatr Adolesc Med 2003; 157(8): 821–7.

81. Lakka TA, Laaksonen DE, Lakka HM et al. Sedentary lifestyle, poor cardiorespiratory fitness, and the metabolic syndrome. Med Sci Sports Exerc 2003; 35(8): 1279–86.

82. National Cholesterol Education Program (NCEP) Expert Panel on Detection, Evaluation, and Treatment of High Blood Cholesterol in Adults (Adult Treatment Panel III). Third Report of the National Cholesterol Education Program (NCEP) Expert Panel on Detection, Evaluation, and Treatment of High Blood Cholesterol in Adults (Adult Treatment Panel III) final report. Circulation 2002; 106(25): 3143–421.

83. Grundy SM, Abate N, Chandalia M. Diet composition and the metabolic syndrome: what is the optimal fat intake? Am J Med 2002; 113 (Suppl 9B): 25–9S.

84. Klein S, Sheard NF, Pi-Sunyer X et al. Weight management through lifestyle modification for the prevention and management of type 2 diabetes: rationale and strategies. A statement of the American Diabetes Association, the North American Association for the Study of Obesity, and the American Society for Clinical Nutrition Am J Clin Nutr 2004; 80(2): 257–63.

85. Schoonjans K, Staels B, Auwerx J. Role of the peroxisome proliferator-activated receptor (PPAR) in mediating the effects of fibrates and fatty acids on gene expression. J Lipid Res 1996; 37(5): 907–25.

86. Gilling L, Suwattee P, DeSouza C, Asnani S, Fonseca V. Effects of the thiazolidinediones on cardiovascular risk factors. Am J Cardiovasc Drugs 2002; 2(3): 149–56.

87. Sidhu JS, Cowan D, Kaski JC. The effects of rosiglitazone, a peroxisome proliferator-activated receptor-gamma agonist, on markers of endothelial cell activation, C-reactive protein, and fibrinogen levels in non-diabetic coronary artery disease patients. J Am Coll Cardiol 2003; 42(10): 1757–63.

88. Buse JB, Tan MH, Prince MJ, Erickson PP. The effects of oral anti-hyperglycaemic medications on serum lipid profiles in patients with type 2 diabetes. Diabetes Obes Metab 2004; 6(2): 133–56.

89. Chui PC, Guan HP, Lehrke M, Lazar MA. PPARgamma regulates adipocyte cholesterol metabolism via oxidized LDL receptor 1. J Clin Invest 2005; 115(8): 2244–56.

90. Ericsson CG, Hamsten A, Nilsson J et al. Angiographic assessment of effects of bezafibrate on progression of coronary artery disease in young male postinfarction patients. Lancet 1996; 347(9005): 849–53.

91. Forman BM, Chen J, Evans RM. Hypolipidemic drugs, polyunsaturated fatty acids, and eicosanoids are ligands for peroxisome proliferator-activated receptors alpha and delta. Proc Natl Acad Sci USA 1997; 94(9): 4312–17.

92. Guerin M, Bruckert E, Dolphin PJ, Turpin G, Chapman MJ. Fenofibrate reduces plasma cholesteryl ester transfer from HDL to VLDL and normalizes the atherogenic, dense LDL profile in combined hyperlipidemia. Arterioscler Thromb Vasc Biol 1996; 16(6): 763–72.

93. Van Gaal LF, Rissanen A, Scheen A, Ziegler O, Rossner S. Effect of rimonabant on weight reduction and cardiovascular risk. Lancet 2005; 366(9483): 369–70.

94. Miettinen TA, Pyorala K, Olsson AG et al. Cholesterol-lowering therapy in women and elderly patients with myocardial infarction or angina pectoris: findings from the Scandinavian Simvastatin Survival Study (4S). Circulation 1997; 96(12): 4211–18.

95. Colquhoun D, Keech A, Hunt D et al. LIPID Study Investigators. Effects of pravastatin on coronary events in 2073 patients with low levels of both low-density lipoprotein cholesterol and high-density lipoprotein cholesterol: results from the LIPID study. Eur Heart J 2004; 25(9): 771–7.

96. Stein DT, Devaraj S, Balis D, Adams-Huet B, Jialal I. Effect of statin therapy on remnant lipoprotein cholesterol levels in patients with combined hyperlipidemia. Arterioscler Thromb Vasc Biol 2001; 21(12): 2026–31.

97. Parhofer KG, Barrett PH, Schwandt P. Atorvastatin improves postprandial lipoprotein metabolism in normolipidemic subjects. J Clin Endocrinol Metab 2000; 85(11): 4224–30.

98. Paolisso G, Barbagallo M, Petrella G et al. Effects of simvastatin and atorvastatin administration on insulin resistance and respiratory quotient in aged dyslipidemic non-insulin dependent diabetic patients. Atherosclerosis 2000; 150(1): 121–7.

99. Pontrelli L, Parris W, Adeli K, Cheung RC. Atorvastatin treatment beneficially alters the lipoprotein profile and increases low-density lipoprotein particle diameter in patients with combined dyslipidemia and impaired fasting glucose/type 2 diabetes. Metabolism 2002; 51(3): 334–42.

100. Chobanian AV, Bakris GL, Black HR et al. Seventh report of the Joint National Committee on

Prevention, Detection, Evaluation, and Treatment of High Blood Pressure. Hypertension 2003; 42(6): 1206–52.

101. Julius S, Kjeldsen SE, Brunner H et al. VALUE trial: long-term blood pressure trends in 13,449 patients with hypertension and high cardiovascular risk. Am J Hypertens 2003; 16(7): 544–8.

102. Colwell JA. Antiplatelet agents for the prevention of cardiovascular disease in diabetes mellitus. Am J Cardiovasc Drugs 2004; 4(2): 87–106.

103. Pearson TA, Blair SN, Daniels SR et al. AHA Guidelines for Primary Prevention of Cardiovascular Disease and Stroke: 2002 Update: Consensus Panel Guide to Comprehensive Risk Reduction for Adult Patients Without Coronary or Other Atherosclerotic Vascular Diseases. American Heart Association Science Advisory and Coordinating Committee. Circulation 2002; 106(3): 388–91.

CHAPTER 30

Free radicals and vitamins

Seema Joshi

Introduction

Aging is a generalized physiologic process that progressively decreases the ability of an organism to adapt to environmental change and increases its vulnerability to disease and death. Aging results in a diminution of reserves of most physiologic systems. It affects cells and the systems made up of them, as well as tissue components. Aging is a characteristic of all higher organisms. The diversity of age-related impairments has led many gerontologists to conclude that no general mechanism is likely to underlie these changes. Therefore, numerous theories have been advanced to explain the phenomenon of aging.

Theories on aging have tried to explain the variation in lifespan among cohort genetic strains and species and the loss of homeostasis during the latter part of life. These theories have also tried to identify factors responsible for lifespan extension and have tried to demonstrate how variation of senescent factors can manipulate the rate of aging. The theories on aging can be divided into two major categories. The first category attributes the process of aging to 'genetically programmed processes.' In this category aging is thought to be a consequence of purposeful events, governed by an internal clock or pacemaker. In the second category aging is attributed to the 'accumulation of damage to critical cellular or tissue constituents.' This theory envisions aging as the cumulative result of damage to tissues occurring over time, resulting in a progressive functional decline.[1-4]

Free radical theory

The 'free radical theory' of aging was first proposed in the 1950s. Harman suggested that the free radical theory provided an explanation for the inverse relationship between the average lifespan of mammalian species and their basal metabolic rate, clustering of degenerative diseases toward the terminal part of the lifespan, beneficial effects of caloric restriction on lifespan, and an increase in autoimmune manifestations with age.[5] Over the past three decades a great deal of evidence has been obtained in support of the free radical theory of aging. According to this theory, free radical reactions with biomolecules, such as proteins and lipid membranes, are responsible for the functional deterioration related to aging (Figure 30.1). Lipid peroxidation, protein oxidation, and oxidation of DNA occurring as a result of free radical damage have been found to increase with age. Also, caloric restriction has consistently been shown to reduce the levels of free radical damage in tissues of rodents. It has been seen that conditions that reduce oxidative stress and free radical damage tend to increase maximal lifespan. Studies with *Drosiphila melanogaster* show that flies overexpressing both superoxide dismutase and catalase have less free radical damage and longer lifespans.[4,6-10]

Production of free radicals

Free radicals are low molecular weight molecules with at least one unpaired electron. However,

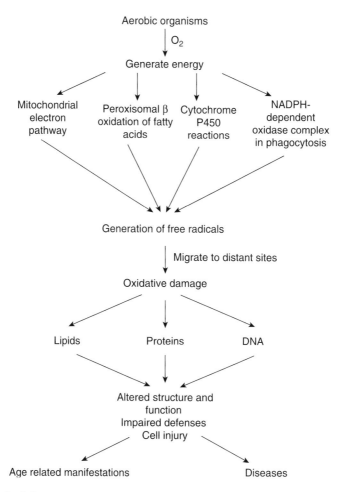

Figure 30.1 *Free radical theory.*

reactive oxygen species (ROS) refers to a number of chemically reactive molecules derived from oxygen which include superoxide ($O_2^{\cdot-}$), hydroxyl radical (HO·), hydrogen peroxide (H_2O_2), and hypochlorous acid (HOCl).[11-13] Aerobic organisms use oxygen to generate energy. In its ground state oxygen has little reactivity. Oxygen accepts electrons from other radicals one at a time. During mitochondrial respiration, a coordinated four-electron reduction of oxygen results in formation of water. However, the mitochondrial electron transport chain is not perfect; one and two electron transfers to oxygen result

in the generation of superoxide and hydrogen peroxide, these in turn are catalyzed by transition metals like iron and copper to form highly reactive hydroxyl radicals.[14,15]

Free radicals are generated during mitochondrial electron transport, peroxisomal β-oxidation of fatty acids, cytochrome P450 reactions, and by phagocytic cells. Mitochondria are a major source of toxic oxidants in cells. Mitochondria lack endogenous antioxidant mechanisms and depend on glutathione to remove hydrogen peroxide. They are thus potential targets for free radical induced

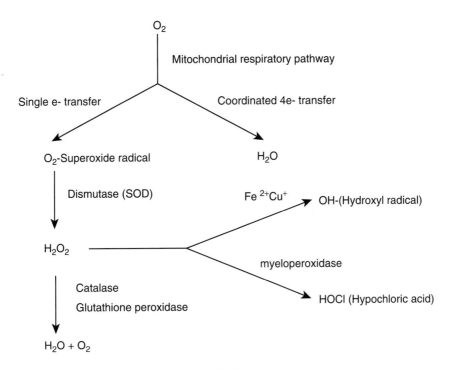

Figure 30.2 *Production and Metabolism of Free Radicals*

Mechanism of free radical induced damage

injury.[14,16,17] Free radicals formed as a result of partial reduction of oxygen leak from the mitochondria. They attack various cell components, form the toxic ROS that migrate to distant sites and damage biomolecules by modifying proteins, lipids, and nucleic acids. This in turn is thought to result in the development or enhancement of age-related manifestations.[5,18,19] Figure 30.2 illustrates the formation and metabolism of free radicals.

Free radicals lead to tissue injury by oxidative modification of proteins, lipids, and DNA. Oxidative damage of the lipid molecules occurs in three steps: initiation, propagation, and termination. Polyunsaturated fatty acids (PUFAs) create electron-rich hydrogens at CH_2 that are vulnerable

to react with the hydroxyl radical (OH·) and other free radicals. There occurs a radical-mediated extraction of a hydrogen atom from the methylene carbon. This step of the reaction with free radicals is called initiation. Subsequent molecular rearrangement and interaction with oxygen may result in the formation of a peroxyl radical that may propagate oxidative damage, attacking the hydrogens from other PUFAs. These propagation chain reactions are terminated by the cleavage of peroxyl radicals. Peroxidized lipids may disintegrate into cytotoxic and mutagenic compounds. Plasma lipid peroxides may represent the lipid peroxidation status of tissues. Some studies report an increase in the levels of plasma lipid peroxides with aging. A decrease in PUFA content in the system may be another method of determining lipid peroxidation, because PUFAs are the primary substrates of lipid peroxidation.[4,20–25]

Proteins, unlike lipids, are not as reactive; however, metal binding sites in proteins are highly susceptible to

Table 30.1 Antioxidant defense system

Enzymes:

Involved in the metabolism of free radicals

- superoxide dismutase (SOD)
- superoxide reductase (SOR)
- catalase
- glutathione peroxidase (GPx)

Involved in the repair of oxidative damage

- phospholipase A2
- glycosylases
- proteinases

Antioxidant molecules: scavengers of reactive oxygen species

- vitamin C
- vitamin E
- carotenoids
- ubiquinones
- lipoic acid

oxidative damage, resulting in irreversible modification. Oxidative damage occurs as a result of backbone or side chain modification of peptides. Backbone modification results in the formation of peroxyl radicals. This causes protein cross-linking or peptide-bond cleavage. However, side-chain modifications result in the loss of catalytic or structural function of the affected proteins which may have deleterious effects on cellular and organ functions. Propagating radicals as in lipid peroxidation may be involved in protein oxidation. There are several markers of protein oxidation, these include protein carbonyl derivatives, protein fragments, advanced glycation end products, and oxidized amino acid side chains.[26-29]

Antioxidant defense system

Cells and tissues possess antioxidant defense mechanisms against free radical induced damage. Damage from oxidative stress occurs when the production of free radicals exceeds the cell's capacity to protect itself. Cellular protective mechanisms that prevent free radical induced cell damage include:[4,14]

- scavenging free radicals,
- binding catalytic metal ions used for the formation of reactive oxygen species
- upregulating endogenous antioxidant defenses.

The antioxidant defense system includes antioxidant and oxidant repair enzymes, and antioxidant molecules (Table 30.1). The antioxidant enzyme system includes dismutases (SOD), superoxide reductases (SOR), catalase, and glutathione peroxidases (GPx). SOD catalyzes the dismutation of $O_2\cdot^-$ to H_2O_2. Catalase and glutathione peroxidases convert H_2O_2 to H_2O. Enzymes such as phospholipase A2, glycosylases, and proteinases are involved in the repair of oxidative damage. Phospholipase A2 cleaves lipid peroxides from phospholipids, reducing the impact of injury to biomembranes. Glycosylases are responsible for recognition and excision of oxidized bases from DNA. Similarly, proteinases degrade oxidized proteins.[4,14,15,30-33] Antioxidant molecules include vitamins C and E, lipoic acid, flavinoids, carotenoids, and ubiquinones. These molecules may act as ROS scavengers.[4,14]

Several aging interventional studies support the free radical theory of aging. Since free radicals and oxidative stress are considered important factors in the biology of aging, it is thought that modulation of oxidative stress may slow the aging process. Dietary components with antioxidant activity have received particular attention. It is suggested that they may have a potential role in modulating oxidative stress associated with aging and chronic conditions. Vitamin C, vitamin E, and beta-carotene are referred to as antioxidant vitamins. Epidemiologic evidence suggests that eating a diet rich in sources of vitamins has a protective effect on development of disease. However, this strong association of dietary intake of vitamins and disease in epidemiologic studies has not been shown in randomized clinical trials.[34,35]

Antioxidant vitamins

The process of aging is associated with increased pathogenesis. Several investigators have used exogenous antioxidants to slow the process of aging caused by oxidative damage from free radical reactions. Various natural and synthetic substances have been tested for their efficacy in disease prevention and life extension. Vitamins A, E, and C, also known as antioxidant vitamins, have been long proposed to prevent disease.[36–38]

Vitamin A and beta-carotene

Vitamin A refers to preformed retinol and the carotenoids that are converted to retinol. Vitamin A is found in animal products, including organ meats, fish, egg yolks, and fortified milk. Other natural sources include yellow, orange, and red plant compounds, such as carrots and green leafy vegetables. The current RDI for vitamin A is 1500 µg/l (5000 IU). It has been observed that the dietary intake of vitamin A decreases with age, however, hypovitaminosis A is uncommon even in the very old. Major dietary carotenoids are beta-carotene and lycophene. Carotenoids cannot be synthesized by the body and their supplies are dependent upon dietary intake. They are potent antioxidants and exert their antioxidant properties by scavenging free radicals.[35,39–41] Vitamin A has a number of biologic actions. It is essential for the prevention of xerophthalmia and phototransduction. Cellular differentiation and integrity are also dependent upon vitamin A.[42,43]

Role of dietary vitamin A supplementation in disease prevention

Coronary heart disease   Clinical trials generally have failed to demonstrate a beneficial effect of antioxidant supplements on cardiovascular morbidity and mortality. Vitamin A and beta-carotene supplements have shown no benefit for primary or secondary prevention of coronary heart disease (CHD) in randomized trials and have been associated with potential harm.[44,45] In the Physicians' Health Study, 2 years of supplementation with beta-carotene produced neither benefit nor harm in terms of the incidence of malignant neoplasms, cardiovascular disease, or death from all causes.[46] Another study suggested that the combination of beta-carotene and vitamin A had no benefit and that it may have an adverse effect on the incidence of lung cancer and on the risk of death from lung cancer, cardiovascular disease, and any cause in smokers and workers exposed to asbestos.[47] In the Women's Health Study and Alpha Tocopherol Beta Carotene (ATBC) cancer prevention study, supplementation with beta-carotene had no effect on cardiovascular disease.[48,49]

Cancer   The protective effects of dietary vitamin A against cancer seen in observational studies most likely represent the effect of beta-carotene. There exists discordance between data from epidemiologic studies of dietary vitamin A on possible cancer chemoprevention and that obtained from randomized controlled trials.

The risk of lung cancer among male smokers or asbestos workers receiving beta-carotene supplements was shown to be significantly increased in two large, randomized, placebo-controlled trials. An increase in the incidence and mortality of prostate cancer among subjects randomized to receive beta-carotene supplements was seen in the

ATBC cancer prevention study. This excess risk appeared to resolve over time once supplements were stopped.[47,50,51]

There have been several observational studies of vitamin A intake and breast cancer; the results of these studies have yielded varying results. In a study by Kushi et al, no association between dietary vitamin A and breast cancer was observed.[52] Another study suggested that a high intake of total carotenoids and docosahexaenoic acid may reduce the risk of breast cancer in women.[53] Data from the Nurses' Health Study suggest that premenopausal women, particularly those with a positive family history, have significant reductions in breast cancer risk with increasing dietary intake of alpha-carotene, beta-carotene, lutein/zeaxanthin, and total vitamin A.[54,55]

Beta-carotene supplements did not show a reduction in colorectal adenoma risk in the Polyp Prevention Study Group.[56]

Other conditions

Evidence obtained from observational studies reveals that high doses of vitamin A may be a risk factor for osteopenia and fractures.[57–59] Studies evaluating the effect of beta-carotene supplements on the risk of cataract formation showed no overall effect; however, there seemed to be a decreased risk among current smokers.[60]

At the present time, supplementation with vitamin A and beta-carotene is not recommended. Based upon current clinical data, vitamin A and beta-carotene lack clinical efficacy with respect to cancer prevention and may have adverse effects on the incidence of lung cancer and on the risk of death from lung cancer and cardiovascular disease.

Vitamin E

Vitamin E or tocopherol possesses potent antioxidant properties. It acts as a free radical scavenger and prevents lipid peroxidation. Alpha-tocopherol is the biologically active form of vitamin E. It prevents the oxidation of polyunsaturated fatty acids (PUFAs), a major structural component of cell membranes. Vitamin E is found in nuts, vegetable oils, whole grains, egg yolks, and green leafy vegetables. The predominant form in the human diet is gamma tocopherol; however, over-the-counter preparations of vitamin E contain alpha-tocopherol.[35,61]

Vitamin E deficiency is seen in conditions resulting from fat malabsorption. Deficiency may manifest as gait disturbance occurring as a result of neuronal degeneration. Neuronal degeneration leads to spinocerebellar ataxia, decreased deep tendon reflexes or areflexia, peripheral neuropathy, and posterior column destruction with impairment of proprioception and vibratory sense. It can cause a degenerative myopathy, ocular impairment, and brown bowel syndrome, a result of lipofuscin deposition and a reduction of red blood cell lifespan.[42,62,63]

Oxidation of low density lipoprotein (LDL) appears to be important in mediating the atherogenicity of LDL. Alpha-tocopherol reduces LDL susceptibility to oxidation.[64,65]

Role of dietary vitamin E supplementation in disease prevention

Coronary heart disease
Observational studies have supported the role of vitamin E in the prevention of CHD. Several studies have found a lower risk of CHD and death from CHD following supplementation with vitamin E.[66–68] Randomized controlled trials have not supported these observations and have found no benefits of vitamin E supplements in both primary and secondary prevention of CHD. The ATBC study showed no significant effect on the incidence of myocardial infarction and cardiac death.[44,49,69]

In one of a series of reports issued by the ATBC study the risk of fatal CHD increased in the groups that received either beta-carotene or the combination of alpha-tocopherol and beta-carotene; there was a non-significant trend of increased deaths in the alpha-tocopherol group.[70] In the HOPE trial, daily supplementation with vitamin E had no effect on progression of carotid intimal-medial thickness.[71] The HOPE-TOO trial (ongoing outcomes, a 2.5-year extension of the trial) showed that vitamin E at 400 IU was associated with an increase in heart failure.[72] In the Women's Angiographic Vitamin and Estrogen (WAVE) study, neither HRT nor antioxidant vitamin supplements provided cardiovascular benefit to postmenopausal women with coronary disease. Instead, a potential for harm was suggested with each treatment.[73] The GISSI prevention trial, the Cambridge Heart Antioxidant Study (CHAOS), and the Heart Protection Study showed no effect on cardiovascular mortality.[74–76]

Stroke   In the ATBC study, daily supplementation with vitamin E had no overall effect on stroke risk. However, a subgroup analysis suggested that vitamin E may increase the risk for subarachnoid hemorrhage and decrease the risk for ischemic stroke, particularly in men with hypertension.[77] The Health Professionals Follow-up Study showed no association between supplemental vitamin E and stroke risk.[78]

Cancer   Several studies have tried to examine the role of vitamin E in cancer prevention. Observational data from the Health Professionals Follow-up Study showed no association between vitamin E supplement use and all prostate cancers. However, it showed a decrease in risk of metastatic or fatal prostate cancer among smokers who consumed at least 100 IU of supplemental vitamin E daily.[79] The ATBC cancer prevention study observed a 32% decrease in prostate cancer incidence and a 41% decrease in prostate cancer mortality among men receiving alpha-tocopherol compared with placebo.[46] In a second report from the ATBC study a significant reduction in lung cancer risk was associated with higher serum vitamin E levels. The reduction in risk was greatest among men younger than age 60 years and among patients with fewer years of cumulative smoking exposure.[80]

Alzheimer's disease   Observational studies have suggested that increased dietary intake of vitamin E may have a protective effect against the development of Alzheimer's disease. In a longitudinal cohort study, supplementation with both vitamins E and C protected against the development of vascular dementia and improved cognitive function late in life.[81–83] A randomized trial of selegiline, vitamin E, both, or placebo among patients with Alzheimer's disease showed that both selegiline and vitamin E were independently associated with significant reductions in several outcomes, including functional decline.[84]

Immunity   There have been several studies reporting that vitamin E supplementation improves the immune response. However, randomized, placebo-controlled studies have found no reduction in the incidence of respiratory infections in institutionalized or non-institutionalized elderly patients receiving daily vitamin E supplements.[85–89]

All-cause mortality   A meta-analysis of vitamin E supplementation that did not stratify trials by dose of vitamin E found no significant effect of supplementation on all-cause mortality.[44] However, a recent meta-analysis that examined the dose–response relationship between vitamin E and overall mortality in a total of 19 randomized clinical trials found that vitamin E supplementation with a dose ≥400 IU/day was associated with a significantly increased risk of all-cause mortality.[90]

Current evidence for vitamin E supplementation is inconclusive. Data at present suggest that high-dose vitamin E (≥400 IU/day) increases all-cause mortality. Also, individuals taking anticoagulants should be particularly advised against high doses of vitamin E because of the synergistic action of vitamin E with these drugs.

Vitamin C

Vitamin C, also known as ascorbic acid, is a water-soluble vitamin. Deficiency of vitamin C can be seen in the frail elderly and is caused by insufficient dietary intake. The bioavailability of vitamin C is inversely related to the amount ingested as well as its form. Aging does not affect its absorption. Natural sources of vitamin C include citrus fruits, raw leafy vegetables, strawberries, melons, tomatoes, broccoli, and peppers. The vitamin C content of various foods depends upon the season of the year, the transport time to the store, the shelf time before purchase, the form of storage, and the method of cooking. It is heat labile and boiling can cause a 50 to 80% loss.[35,39,91]

Table 30.2 *Conclusions for antioxidant supplement use for disease-specific states[a]*

	CHD[b] 1°		2°	Heart failure	Stroke	Cancer	Dementia	Cataracts	All-cause mortality
Vitamin A	NB[c]		NB	—	—	↑ Lung cancer among smokers ↑ Prostate cancer risk and mortality	—	↓ Cataract formation among smokers	↑
Vitamin E	NB		NB[d]	↑ risk	NB[e]	↓ Prostate cancer incidence and mortality ↓ Lung cancer risk	Inconclusive[f]	—	↑
Vitamin C	Inconclusive[g]		NB	—	NB[h]	—	—	↓ Risk of cataract requiring extraction	—

[a] Based on current scientific evidence.
[b] Coronary heart disease.
[c] No benefit.
[d] Benefits seen in individuals with CRF on hemodialysis.
[e] Subgroup analysis revealed ↑ risk of subarachnoid hemorrhage and ↓ risk of ischemic stroke in individuals with hypertension.
[f] Observational studies and 1 RCT show a slowing of disease progression.
[g] Data from observational studies.
[h] Improvement in common carotid artery intima-media thickness; implications are unclear.

Vitamin C has antioxidant properties and reduces harmful free radicals; it is a reversible biologic reductant. It provides reducing equivalents for a number of biochemical reactions involving iron and copper. It therefore functions as a cofactor, enzyme complement, cosubstrate, or a strong antioxidant in a variety of reactions and metabolic processes.[39,92–95]

Vitamin C is involved in collagen and norepinephrine synthesis. Vitamin C is essential for the conversion of iron from the ferric (+3) to the ferrous (+2). This is important for the conversion of methemoglobin to hemoglobin and for the absorption of iron from the duodenum. Vitamin C has a role in prostaglandin and prostacyclin metabolism. It may be capable of attenuating the inflammatory response or even sepsis syndrome. Deficiency primarily affects the musculoskeletal and hematopoietic systems and results in scurvy. Scurvy can develop if the intake of vitamin C is less than 10 mg per day for 3 to 6 months.[63,96,97]

Role of dietary vitamin C supplementation in disease prevention

Coronary heart disease There has been conflicting evidence from epidemiologic studies for the role of vitamin C in the primary prevention of CHD. Several observational studies have shown a lower mortality rate in individuals consuming vitamin C supplements. The National Health and Nutrition Examination survey found that the relation of the standardized mortality ratio (SMR) for all causes of death to increasing vitamin C intake is strongly inverse for males and weakly inverse for females. The survey reported a 34% lower standardized mortality rate among individuals consuming 50 mg or more of vitamin C per day.[98] In the EPIC-Norfolk prospective study a 20 μmol/l rise in plasma ascorbic acid concentration, equivalent to about 50 g per day increase in fruit and vegetable intake, was associated with about a 20% reduction in risk of all-cause mortality ($P < 0.0001$), independent of age, systolic blood pressure, blood cholesterol, cigarette smoking habit, diabetes, and supplement use.[99] In a study by Gale et al, vitamin C concentration, whether measured by dietary intake or plasma concentration of ascorbic acid, was strongly related to subsequent risk of death from stroke but not from CHD.[100] A large, randomized trial of vitamin C for secondary prevention of CHD found no benefit of supplementation.[76]

Stroke A 20-year follow-up study of a cohort of elderly people found mortality from stroke to be highest in those with the lowest vitamin C status.[100] The Health Professionals Follow-up Study showed no association between supplemental vitamin C and stroke risk.[78] In the Antioxidant Supplementation in Atherosclerosis Prevention (ASAP) study, supplementation with a combination of vitamin E and slow-release vitamin C slowed down the atherosclerotic progression in hypercholesterolemic persons. In both sexes combined, the average annual increase in the mean common carotid artery intima-media thickness was 0.014 mm in the unsupplemented and 0.010 mm in the supplemented group.[101]

Cancer Some observational studies show an inverse relation of ascorbic acid to cancer mortality in men but not in women.[98,99] There currently exists very little evidence supporting the role of vitamin C in the prevention of cancer.

Other conditions There have been some reports of excessive use of vitamin C as a risk factor for calcium oxalate nephrolithiasis. However, a prospective epidemiologic study demonstrated that consumption of high doses of vitamin C lowered the relative risk of calcium oxalate stones compared to 250 mg or less of vitamin C per day.[102] Observational data suggest that micronutrients with antioxidant capabilities may retard the development of age-related cataract. In a prospective study, the risk of cataract was 45% lower among women who used vitamin C supplements for 10 or more years (relative risk 0.55 (0.32 to 0.96)).[103] However, in a randomized controlled study the use of a high-dose formulation of vitamin C, vitamin E, and beta-carotene in a relatively well-nourished older adult cohort had no apparent effect on the 7-year risk of development or progression of age-related lens opacities or visual acuity loss.[104]

Conclusions

Epidemiologic and population studies suggest beneficial effects of antioxidant vitamins such as vitamin E, vitamin C, and beta-carotene on cardiovascular disease (CVD) and malignancies. However, a preponderance of clinical trials has failed to demonstrate a beneficial effect of antioxidant supplements on CVD morbidity and mortality. Table 30.2 summarizes the conclusions for vitamin supplements based on the current scientific evidence available. A recent meta-analysis of studies of vitamin E supplementation for prevention of heart disease found no benefit and even an increase in all-cause mortality at dosages above 400 IU per day. Also, beta-carotene supplement use has not shown clinical efficacy and has been associated with an increased risk of lung and prostate cancer. Based on currently available data, the use of antioxidant vitamin supplements for the prevention and treatment of CVD and malignancies is not justified.

References

1. Katz MS, Gerety, MB. Internal Medicine, Stein, 5th edn. Chapter 373 Gerontology and Geriatric Medicine, Mosby.
2. Geriatric Medicine: An Evidence Based Approach, 4th edn. Molecular and Biologic Factors in Aging – Charles Mobbs, New York: Springer-Verlag, 2003.
3. Ganong WF. Review of Medical Physiology, 22nd edn. McGraw-Hill, 2005.
4. Poon HF, Calabrese V, Scapagnini G, Butterfield DA. Free radicals and brain aging. Clin Geriatr Med 2004; 20(2): 329–59.
5. Harman D. Free radical theory of aging. Mutat Res 1992; 275: 257–66.
6. Armbrecht HJ, Coe RM. The Theories of Aging. The Science of Geriatrics, Vol 1, New York: Springer, 2000.
7. Harman D. Prolongation of life: role of free radical reactions in aging. J Am Geriatr Soc 1969; 17(8): 721–35.
8. Sohal RS, Weindruch R. Oxidative stress, caloric restriction and aging. Science 1996; 273: 59–63.
9. Rao G, Xia E, Nadakavukaren MJ, Richardson A. Effect of dietary restriction on the age dependent changes in the expression of antioxidant enzymes in rat liver. J Nutr 1990; 120: 102–9.
10. Yu BP. Aging and oxidative stress: modulation by dietary restriction. Free Rad Biol Med 1996; 5: 651–68.
11. Nordberg J, Arner ES. Reactive oxygen species, antioxidants, and the mammalian thioredoxin system. Free Radic Biol Med 2001; 31(11): 1287–312.
12. Fridovich I. Fundamental aspects of reactive oxygen species, or what's the matter with oxygen? Ann NY Acad Sci 1999; 893: 13–18.
13. Halliwell B. Antioxidants in human health and disease. Annu Rev Nutr 1996; 16: 33–50.
14. Blumberg JB. Free radical theory of aging. The Science of Geriatrics, Vol 1. New York: Springer, 2000.
15. Turrens JF. Mitochondrial formation of reactive oxygen species. J Physiol 2003; 552(2): 335–4.
16. Fernandez-Checa JC et al. Oxidative stress: role of mitochondria and protection by glutathione. Biofactors 1998; 8(1–2): 7–11.
17. Sastre J, Pallardo FV, Vina J. The role of mitochondrial oxidative stress in aging. Free Radic Biol Med 2003; 35(1): 1–8.
18. Calabrese V, Bates TE, Stella AM. NO synthase and NO-dependent signal pathways in brain aging and neurodegenerative disorders: the role of oxidant/antioxidant balance. Neurochem Res 2000; 25(9–10): 1315–41.
19. Ventura B et al. Control of oxidative phosphorylation by Complex I in rat liver mitochondria: implications for aging. Biochim Biophys Acta 2002; 1553(3): 249–60.
20. Frankel EN. Chemistry of free radical and singlet oxidation of lipids. Progr Lipid Res 1984; 23(4): 197–221.
21. Halliwell B, Gutteridge JM. Biologically relevant metal ion-dependent hydroxyl radical generation. An update. FEBS Lett 1992; 307(1): 108–12.
22. Halliwel B, Chirico S. Lipid peroxidation: its mechanism, measurement and significance. Am J Clin Nutr 1993; 57: 715–25S.
23. Esterbauer H, Ramos P. Chemistry and pathophysiology of oxidation of LDL. Rev Physiol Biochem Pharmacol 1995; 127: 31–64.
24. Esterbauer H, Schaur RJ, Zollner H. Chemistry and biochemistry of 4-hydroxynonenal, malonaldehyde and related aldehydes. Free Radic Biol Med 1991; 11(1): 81–128.
25. Giusto NM et al. Age-associated changes in central nervous system glycerolipid composition and metabolism. Neurochem Res 2002; 27(11): 1513–23.
26. Dean RT, Fu S, Stocker R, Davies MJ. Biochemistry and pathology of radical mediated protein oxidation. Biochem J 1997; 324: 1–18.
27. Berlett BS, Stadman ER. Protein oxidation in aging, disease and oxidative stress. J Biol Chem 1997; 272: 20313–16.
28. Butterfield DA, Stadtman ER. Protein oxidation processes in aging brain. Adv Cell Aging Gerontol 1997; 2: 161–91.
29. Levine RL, Stadtman ER. Oxidative modification of proteins during aging. Exp Gerontol 2001; 36(9): 1495–502.
30. Bohr VA, Anson RM. DNA damage, mutation, and fine structure DNA repair in aging. Mutat Res 1995; 338: 25–34.
31. Holmes GE, Bernstein C, Bernstein H. Oxidative and other DNA damages as the basis of aging: a review. Mutat Res 1992; 275: 305–15.
32. Pacifici RE, Davies KJ. Protein, lipid and DNA repair systems in oxidative stress: the free radical theory of aging revisited. Gerontology 1991; 37: 166–80.
33. Stadtman ER. Role of oxidized amino acids in protein breakdown and stability. Methods Enzymol 1995; 258: 379–93.
34. McCall MR, Frei B. Can antioxidant vitamins materially reduce oxidative damage in humans? Free Radic Biol Med 1999; 26: 1034–53.
35. Thomas DR. Vitamins in health and aging. Clin Geriatr Med 2004; 20(2): 259–74.
36. Yu BP. Cellular defenses against damage from reactive oxygen species. Physiol Revs 1994; 74: 139–62.

37. Meydani M, Evans WJ, Handelman G et al. Protective effect of vitamin E on exercise induced oxidative damage in young and older adults. Am J Physiol 1993; 264: R992–8.

38. Yu BP, Kang CM, Han JS, Dong Soo K. Can antioxidant supplement slow the aging process? Biofactors 1998; 7(1/2): 93–9.

39. Larry JE. Vitamin Nutrition in the Elderly, Geriatric Nutrition: A Comprehensive Review, 2nd edn. New York: Raven Press, 1995.

40. Ross AC. Vitamin A and retinoids. In: Shils M, Olson J, Shike M, eds. Modern Nutrition in Health and Disease. Philadelphia, PA: Lippincott, 2000: 305.

41. Harrison EH. Enzymes catalyzing the hydrolysis of retinyl esters. Biochem Biophys Acta 1993; 1170: 99.

42. Pazirandeh S, Burns DL. Overview of fat soluble vitamins. UpToDate 2005 (version 13.1).

43. Jacobs P, Wood L. Vitamin A. Disease-A-Month, Vol 49, No 11. Mosby, Inc, 2003.

44. Vivekananthan DP, Penn MS, Sapp SK et al. Use of antioxidant vitamins for the prevention of cardiovascular disease: meta-analysis of randomised trials. Lancet 2003; 361: 2017.

45. http: //circ.ahajournals.org/cgi/content/full/110/5/637.

46. Hennekens CH, Buring JE, Manson JE et al. Lack of effect of long-term supplementation with beta carotene on the incidence of malignant neoplasms and cardiovascular disease. N Engl J Med 1996; 334(18): 1145–9.

47. Omenn GS, Goodman GE, Thornquist MD et al. Effects of a combination of beta carotene and vitamin A on lung cancer and cardiovascular disease. N Engl J Med 1996; 334(18): 1150–5.

48. Lee IM, Cook NR, Manson JE, Buring JE, Hennekens CH. Beta-carotene supplementation and incidence of cancer and cardiovascular disease: the Women's Health Study. J Natl Cancer Inst 1999; 91(24): 2102–6.

49. Virtamo J, Rapola JM, Ripatti S et al. Effect of vitamin E and beta carotene on the incidence of primary non-fatal myocardial infarction and fatal coronary heart disease. Arch Intern Med 1998; 158(6): 668–75.

50. The Alpha-Tocopherol, Beta Carotene Cancer Prevention Study Group. The effect of vitamin E and beta-carotene on the incidence of lung cancer and other cancers in male smokers. N Engl J Med 1994; 330: 1029.

51. Virtamo J, Pietinen P, Huttunen JK et al. Incidence of cancer and mortality following alpha-tocopherol and beta-carotene supplementation: a postintervention follow-up. JAMA 2003; 290: 476.

52. Kushi LH, Fee RM, Sellers TA et al. Intake of vitamins A, C, and E and postmenopausal breast cancer. Am J Epidemiol 1996; 144: 165.

53. Nkondjock A. Intake of specific carotenoids and essential fatty acids and breast cancer risk in Montreal, Canada. Am J Clin Nutr 2004; 79(5): 857–64.

54. Hunter DJ, Manson JE, Colditz GA et al. A prospective study of intake of vitamins C, E, and A and the risk of breast cancer. N Engl J Med 1993; 329: 234.

55. Zhang S, Hunter DJ, Forman MR et al. Dietary carotenoids and vitamins A, C, and E and risk of breast cancer. J Natl Cancer Inst 1999; 91: 547.

56. Greenberg ER, Baron JA, Tosteson TD et al. A clinical trial of antioxidant vitamins to prevent colorectal adenoma. Polyp Prevention Study Group. N Engl J Med 1994; 331: 141.

57. Melhus H, Michaelsson K, Kindmark A et al. Excessive intake of vitamin A is associated with reduced bone mineral density and increased risk for hip fracture. Ann Intern Med 1998; 129: 770.

58. Feskanich D, Singh V, Willett WC, Colditz GA. Vitamin A intake and hip fractures among postmenopausal women. JAMA 2002; 287: 47.

59. Michaelsson K, Lithell H, Vessby B, Melhus H. Serum retinol levels and the risk of fracture. N Engl J Med 2003; 348: 287.

60. Christen WG, Manson JE, Glynn RJ et al. A randomized trial of beta carotene and age-related cataract in US physicians. Arch Ophthalmol 2003; 121: 372.

61. Massey PB. Dietary supplements. Med Clin North Am 2002; 86(1): 127–47.

62. Perrig WJ, Perrig P, Stahelin HB. The relation between antioxidants and memory performance in the old and very old. J Am Geriatr Soc 1997; 45: 718–24.

63. Johnson KA. Vitamin nutrition in the older adult. Clin Geriatr Med 2002; 18(4): 773–99.

64. Reaven PD, Khouw A, Beltz WF, Parthasarathy S, Witztum JL. Effect of dietary antioxidant combinations in humans. Protection of LDL by vitamin E but not by beta-carotene. Arterioscler Thromb 1993; 13(4): 590–600.

65. Dieber-Rotheneder M, Puhl H, Waeg G, Striegl G, Esterbauer H. Effect of oral supplementation with D-alpha-tocopherol on the vitamin E content of human low density lipoproteins and resistance to oxidation. J Lipid Res 1991; 32(8): 1325–32.

66. Stampfer MJ, Hennekens CH, Manson JE et al. Vitamin E consumption and the risk of coronary disease in women. N Engl J Med 1993; 328(20): 1444–9.

67. Rimm EB, Stampfer MJ, Ascherio A et al. Vitamin E consumption and the risk of coronary heart disease in men. N Engl J Med 1993; 328(20): 1450–6.

68. Kushi LH, Folsom AR, Prineas RJ et al. Dietary antioxidant vitamins and death from coronary heart disease in postmenopausal women. N Engl J Med 1996; 334(18): 1156–62.

69. de Gaetano G. Low-dose aspirin and vitamin E in people at cardiovascular risk: a randomised trial in

general practice. Collaborative Group of the Primary Prevention Project. Lancet 2001; 357(9250): 89–95.

70. Rapola JM, Virtamo J, Ripatti S et al. Randomised trial of alpha-tocopherol and beta-carotene supplements on incidence of major coronary events in men with previous myocardial infraction. Lancet 1997; 349(9067): 1715–20.

71. Yusuf S, Dagenais G, Pogue J, Bosch J, Sleight P. Vitamin E supplementation and cardiovascular events in high-risk patients. The Heart Outcomes Prevention Evaluation Study Investigators. N Engl J Med 2000; 342(3): 154–60.

72. Lonn E, Bosch J, Yusuf S, Pogue J et al. Effects of long-term vitamin E supplementation on cardiovascular events and cancer. JAMA 2005; 293(11): 1338–47.

73. Waters DD, Alderman EL, Hsia J et al. Effects of hormone replacement therapy and antioxidant vitamin supplements on coronary atherosclerosis in postmenopausal women: a randomized controlled trial. JAMA 2002; 288(19): 2432–40.

74. Dietary supplementation with n-3 polyunsaturated fatty acids and vitamin E after myocardial infarction: results of the GISSI-Prevenzione trial. Gruppo Italiano per lo Studio della Sopravvivenza nell'Infarto miocardico. Lancet 1999; 354: 447.

75. Stephens NG, Parsons A, Scofield PM et al. Randomized controlled trial of vitamin E in patients with coronary disease: Cambridge Heart Antioxidant Study (CHAOS). Lancet 1996; 347: 781.

76. MRC/BHF Heart Protection Study of antioxidant vitamin supplementation in 20536 high-risk individuals: a randomised placebo-controlled trial. Lancet 2002; 360: 23.

77. Leppala JM, Virtamo J, Fogelholm R et al. Vitamin E and beta carotene supplementaion in high risk for stroke. Arch Neurol 2000; 57: 1503.

78. Ascherio A, Rimm EB, Hernan MA et al. Relation of consumption of vitamin E, vitamin C, and carotenoids to risk for stroke among men in the United States. Ann Intern Med 1999; 130: 963.

79. Chan JM, Stampfer MJ, Ma J et al. Supplemental vitamin E intake and prostate cancer risk in a large cohort of men in the United States. Cancer Epidemiol Biomarkers Prev 1999; 8: 893.

80. Woodson K, Tangrea JA, Barrett MJ et al. Serum alpha-tocopherol and subsequent risk of lung cancer among male smokers. J Natl Cancer Inst 1999; 91: 1738.

81. Masaki KH, Losonczy KG, Izmirlian G et al. Association of vitamin E and C supplement use with cognitive function and dementia in elderly men. Neurology 2000; 54: 1265.

82. Morris MC, Evans DA, Bienias JL et al. Dietary intake of antioxidant nutrients and the risk of incident Alzheimer disease in a biracial community study. JAMA 2002; 287: 3230.

83. Engelhart MJ, Geerlings MI, Ruitenberg A et al. Dietary intake of antioxidants and risk of Alzheimer disease. JAMA 2002; 287: 3223.

84. Sano M, Ernesto C, Thomas RG et al. A controlled trial of selegiline, alpha-tocopherol, or both as treatment for Alzheimer's disease. The Alzheimer's Disease Cooperative Study. N Engl J Med 1997; 336: 1216.

85. Meydani SN, Meydani M, Blumberg JB et al. Vitamin E supplementation and in vivo immune response in healthy elderly subjects. A randomized controlled trial. JAMA 1997; 277: 1380.

86. Serafini M. Dietary vitamin E and T cell-mediated function in the elderly: effectiveness and mechanism of action. Int J Dev Neurosci 2000; 18: 401.

87. Girodon F, Galan P, Monget AL et al. Impact of trace elements and vitamin supplementation on immunity and infections in institutionalized elderly patients: a randomized controlled trial. MIN. VIT. AOX. geriatric network. Arch Intern Med 1999; 159: 748.

88. Meydani SN, Leka LS, Fine BC et al. Vitamin E and respiratory tract infections in elderly nursing home residents: a randomized controlled trial. JAMA 2004; 292: 828.

89. Graat JM, Schouten EG, Kok FJ. Effect of daily vitamin E and multivitamin-mineral supplementation on acute respiratory tract infections in elderly persons: a randomized controlled trial. JAMA 2002; 288: 715.

90. Miller ER 3rd, Pastor-Barriuso R, Dalal D et al. Meta-analysis: high-dosage vitamin E supplementation may increase all-cause mortality. Ann Intern Med 2005; 142: 37.

91. Johnson KA. Vitamin nutrition in the older adult. Clin Geriatr Med 2002; 18(4): 773–99.

92. Jacob R. Vitamin C. In: Shils M, Olson J, Shike M, Ross AC, eds. Modern Nutrition in Health and Disease. Philadelphia, PA: Lippincott, 2000: 467.

93. Schorah CJ. The transport of vitamin C and effects of disease. Proc Nutr Soc 1992; 51: 189.

94. Kallner A, Hornig D, Pellikka R. Formation of carbon dioxide from ascorbate in man. Am J Clin Nutr 1985; 41: 609.

95. Garry PJ, Vanderjagt DJ, Hunt WC. Ascorbic acid intakes and plasma levels in healthy elderly. Ann NY Acad Sci 1987; 498: 90–9.

96. Willett WC, Stampfer MJ. What vitamins should I take, Doctor? N Engl J Med 2001; 345: 1819–24.

97. Levine M, Rumsey SC, Daruwala R et al. Criteria and recommendations for vitamin C intake. JAMA 1999; 281: 1415–23.

98. Enstrom JE, Comstock GW, Salkeld RM et al. Vitamin C intake and mortality among a sample of the United States population. Epidemiology 1992; 3: 194.

99. Khaw KT, Bingham S, Welch A et al. Relation between plasma ascorbic acid and mortality in men and women in EPIC-Norfolk prospective study: a prospective population study. European Prospective

Investigation into Cancer and Nutrition. Lancet 2001; 357: 657.

100. Gale CR, Martyn CN, Winter PD, Cooper C. Vitamin C and risk of death from stroke and coronary heart disease in cohort of elderly people. BMJ 1995; 310: 1563.

101. Salonen RM, Nyyssonen K, Kaikkonen J et al. Six-year effect of combined vitamin C and E supplementation on atherosclerotic progression: the Antioxidant Supplementation in Atherosclerosis Prevention (ASAP) Study. Circulation 2003; 107: 947.

102. Urivetzky et al. Ascorbic acid overdosing: a risk factor for calcium oxalate nephrolithiasis. J Urol 1992; 147: 1215.

103. Hankinson SE, Stampfer MJ, Seddon JM et al. Nutrient intake and cataract extraction in women: a prospective study. BMJ 1992; 305: 335.

104. A randomized, placebo-controlled, clinical trial of high-dose supplementation with vitamins C and E and beta carotene for age-related cataract and vision loss: AREDS report no. 9. Arch Ophthalmol 2001; 119: 1439.

CHAPTER 31

Resistance exercise

Charles P Lambert

Introduction

Sarcopenia is the age-related decline in skeletal muscle mass. Sarcopenia leads to decreased muscle strength, which in turn can lead to functional disability. Using the classification of moderate sarcopenia, which is a muscle mass that is between 1 and 2 standard deviations lower than the mean for young men (age 18–39 years) Janssen et al[1] reported that 45% of older men (≥ 60 years) fell into this category. Seven per cent of older men were classified as severely sarcopenic, which is 2 or more standard deviations below the mean for young men. Older men who were classified as moderately sarcopenic had problems stooping, crouching, or kneeling and had a decreased ability to perform the tandem stand test. Those men classified as severely sarcopenic, in addition to having the problems of those individuals who were moderately sarcopenic, also had a reduced ability to stand up from a chair.

The effect of sarcopenia on health-care costs is due to its relationship to physical disability. Janssen et al[2] calculated that the direct health-care cost due to sarcopenia in the US in 2000 was $18.5 billion ($7.7 billion for women and $10.8 billion for men). This totaled approximately 1.5% of the total health-care costs in the US. These investigators also calculated that a reduction of sarcopenia by 10% would have saved $1.1 billion in the year 2000.[2]

One intervention that has been shown to reduce muscle mass and strength losses is resistance training, also called strength training. Androgen (testosterone or anabolic steroid) administration is another means to increase muscle mass and strength in older individuals. However, in contrast to resistance exercise training there is no neurologic effect of androgen replacement. Increased motor-unit recruitment and increased motor-unit firing rates, as well as other adaptations within the nervous system, are responsible for the majority of the increases in strength early (during the first several weeks) in a resistance exercise training program.

Resistance exercise results in an increase in muscle size

Resistance training in the elderly results in muscle hypertrophy. In an early study, Fiatarone et al[3] reported that resistance training for 8 weeks (3 days/week, 3 sets/workout, 8 repetitions/set, and 80% of 1 repetition maximum (RM)) resulted in a 10.9% increase in quadriceps muscle size. The mean age of the individuals in that study was 90.2 years. In another early study, Frontera et al[4] reported that 12 weeks of resistance training similar to that performed by Fiatarone et al[3] resulted in a 9.3% increase in quadriceps muscle size. The individuals in that study were between the ages of 60 and 72. Hakkinen et al[5] reported an 8.5% increase in the cross-sectional area of the quadriceps femoris as a result of a 10-week progressive resistance training program in older men (mean age 60.8 years). Thus, from these studies one can expect about a 10% increase in muscle size with a typical 12-week progressive resistance training program. Since the loss in muscle mass in an elderly individual would appear to be greater than 10%, as the rate of loss is typically around 0.5–1.0% per year after the age of about 40,[6] longer resistance training studies appear to be warranted to determine whether the muscle mass loss of elderly individuals could be completely reversed.

Resistance exercise improves physical function

Seyennes et al[7] reported that 10 weeks of resistance training at 80% of 1 RM, 3 times/week in individuals with a mean age of 81.5 years resulted in a 55% increase in strength, 27.6% improvement in chair rising time, a 19.2% improvement in stair climbing power, and a 27.5% improvement in the 6-minute walk distance. Vincent et al[8] reported that 6 months of training similar to that of Seyennes et al[7] resulted in a 27.6% increase in leg press strength, a 14.6% improvement in leg extension strength, and a 5.8% improvement in stair climbing time. Sullivan et al[9] examined the effects of progressive resistance exercise (10 weeks, 80% of 1 RM, 3 times/week, 3 sets of 8) on strength and function in very frail elderly individuals. They found a 74% increase in leg press strength while the maximum safe gait speed increased in 53% of the individuals and the sit to stand maneuver times improved in 79% of the cases. Fiatarone et al[10] reported that 10 weeks of typical progressive resistance exercise in individuals with a mean age of 87.1 years increased strength by 113%. Additionally, gait velocity was improved by 11.8% and stair climbing power was improved by 28.4%.

Thus, based on these studies and others, progressive resistance exercise is effective in improving strength and measures of physical function in the elderly. Of note is that the increase in muscle mass or hypertrophy is typically less then the increase in measures of physical function. In addition to the increase in muscle mass observed as a result of progressive resistance training or androgen administration, progressive resistance training provides the added benefit of an improvement in neural components of strength, which are composed of improved motor unit recruitment and motor unit firing rates as well as a reduction in antagonist muscle co-activation.

Neural adaptations responsible for improvements in muscle strength

Increased motor-unit recruitment and faster motor-unit firing rates are adaptations that are typically called the neural component of improvements in muscle strength. Motor-unit recruitment and motor-unit firing rates are collectively referred to as muscle activation. It appears that the ability to activate an agonist muscle is maximal for most muscle groups in the elderly when using isometric contractions and a supramaximal electrical stimulus to assess muscle activation (for review see reference 11). However, linear equations relating muscle activation to maximal voluntary contractions have been used in the past. Stackhouse et al[12] have reported that the utilization of curvilinear equations may be more appropriate and have reported that the muscle activation deficits in older people relative to young may be about 11% rather than 2–4%. Thus, the use of curvilinear equations suggests that there may be room for improvement in muscle activation in older people as a result of resistance training. This room for improvement appears to be very small in light of the large improvements in muscle strength and small increases in muscle hypertrophy in the elderly as a result of resistance training.

There are a few possible explanations, in addition to agonist muscle activation, for the increase in strength:

1. There has been shown to be about a 12.5% reduction in muscle co-activation of antagonist muscle groups in ~70-year-old men with 6 months' resistance exercise training plus explosive exercise. Thus, a reduction in muscle co-activation may play a role.
2. Almost all of the studies of muscle activation have been performed with isometric exercise. There may be greater deficits in muscle activation in the elderly with dynamic exercise than isometric exercise (isometric exercise is the way muscle activation is usually assessed).

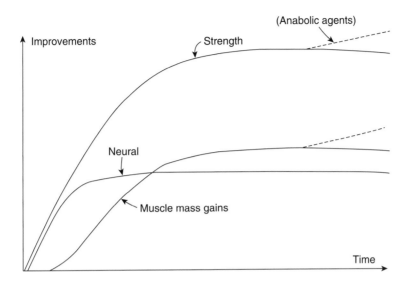

Figure 31.1 *Time course of resistance training induced adaptations (adapted from Sale[88]).*

3. It has been suggested[13] that there may be training-induced inhibition of Golgi tendon organs. The Golgi tendon organs act to stop the contraction in the direction of intended movement if the load becomes too heavy. Thus a load that used to be perceived as too heavy by the Golgi tendon organs before training may no longer be perceived that way after training and this results in the ability to move heavier loads.

Figure 31.1 depicts a theoretic model for the time course of the increases in strength, muscle mass, and neurologic adaptations for an individual involved in resistance training. An estimate for the intersection of the lines depicting neural and muscle mass gains is ~16–24 weeks.

Comparison of resistance exercise to testosterone replacement

Skeletal muscle protein synthesis in the elderly

Testosterone replacement in older men has been shown to increase muscle protein synthesis, strength, and muscle hypertrophy. However, there are side-effects associated with testosterone replacement, such as a large increase in the hematocrit which may reach dangerous levels, as well as the potential for stimulation of prostate cancer. Resistance exercise training has no known side-effects and most studies show that it is as efficacious or more efficacious for increasing muscle strength than testosterone administration (compare Tables 31.2 and 31.3, later).

Table 31.1 compares the mixed muscle protein synthesis response to a typical dose of testosterone administration and to one acute resistance exercise bout in the elderly. As can be seen from these studies, the mixed muscle protein synthetic response to an acute resistance training session is at least as much and may be greater than the response to testosterone replacement. Few studies have compared testostosterone replacement to resistance training in the same study. Recently, Sullivan et al[18] performed a study in very frail individuals with a 2 × 2 design, with the independent variables being exercise intensity (20% of 1 RM vs 80% of 1 RM) and testosterone administration (!00 mg of testosterone/week vs placebo). They found a significant resistance exercise effect on muscle strength but no significant effect of testosterone on muscle strength. In contrast, they found

Table 31.1 *Mixed skeletal muscle protein synthetic response to resistance training and testosterone administration in the elderly*

Acute resistance training studies	Testosterone replacement studies
Hasten et al:[14] 182% increase	Urban et al:[15] 80% increase
Sheffield-Moore el al:[16] 58% increase	Brodsky et al:[17] 42% increase

that testosterone significantly improved mid-thigh cross-sectional muscle area but resistance exercise did not. In contrast, Casaburi et al[19] reported similar increases in strength between resistance exercise vs testosterone replacement groups, but similar to the study of Sullivan et al,[18] they found that testosterone replacement alone increased lean body mass but resistance training alone did not. Casaburi et al[19] studied COPD patients with low testosterone levels (≤ 320 ng/dl).

Comparison of resistance exercise induced muscle protein synthesis to that of aerobic exercise

Sheffield-Moore et al[20] conducted a study evaluating the effects of an endurance exercise bout in older and younger men. The exercise duration was 45 minutes and the exercise intensity was ~40% of VO2 peak (moderate walking on a treadmill). They found the increase in muscle protein synthesis was 0.0363%/hour in the young men and 0.0830%/hour in the older men. This is similar to the increase as a result of resistance exercise: 0.030%/hour for the younger men and appears to be greater than that for resistance training in older men (0.044%/hour). Both the resistance exercise study and the aerobic exercise study were performed in the postabsorptive state. Thus, it appears that postexercise mixed muscle protein synthesis in the postabsorptive state does not explain the much greater increase in muscle mass accumulation that occurs for individuals who engage in resistance exercise training when compared to that for individuals engaged in aerobic exercise training.

Skeletal muscle strength gains: comparison of testosterone replacement and resistance exercise training

We have examined 13 studies of testosterone administration to the elderly in which the duration of administration ranged from 4 weeks to 3 years.[15,19,21–31] In addition, the administration method was intramuscular injection for 8 out of the 13 studies with the other administration methods being sublingual,[29] a transdermal gel application,[28,30] and a scrotal patch.[26] It was reported in two of the studies that there was no significant increase in strength.[26,27] The greatest increase in strength was ~110% (grip strength[24]) with the range of the other studies being a 7.5% decrease to a 63% increase[24] in strength. In addition, in the study with the greatest increase (~110%) there was a ~4% improvement in a timed physical performance test, whereas there was a 5.6% decrease in the timed physical performance test for the placebo group over 3 years. The mean increase in strength for the cited testosterone studies (Table 31.2) was 22.7%.

From 16 resistance training studies with most having a duration of 12 weeks and all of them having a frequency of 3 ×/week, the mean strength improvement was 57.4% with a range of 15.6–134.0% (Table 31.2). Based on these studies it would appear that the strength improvements induced by resistance exercise training in older adults are of much greater magnitude (possibly 2-fold greater) than the improvements induced by testosterone administration to older adults. This is important as it is strength, which is a combination of the amount of muscle mass available *and* neurologic factors, that dictates function as opposed to only muscle mass alone. Resistance training induces both neurologic and muscle mass accumulation whereas testosterone administration only results in gains in muscle mass. Further, it is strength (and/or power) that translates into improvements in the ability to perform functional activities not muscle mass per se. Of note also is that these greater changes in strength with resistance training occur after only 12 weeks, while the changes elicited by testosterone administration may take much longer (Tables 31.2 and 31.3).

Table 31.2 *Increases in strength with testosterone administration*

Study	Age (years)	Dose of testosterone	Mode of administration	Duration of administration	% Increase in strength
Snyder et al[26]	>65	6 mg/day	Scrotal patch	36 months	−7.5
Young et al[31]	30.2	200 mg/week	IM injection	6 months	9.1
Wang et al[29]	19–60 (all hypogonadal, total testosterone <250 ng/dl)	5 mg 3 × daily	Sublingual	6 months	6.3
Wang et al[30]	19–68 (all had a total testosterone of ≤300 ng/dl)	50 and 100 mg testosterone/ day	Transdermal testosterone gel	3 months	~8
Sih et al[25]	66 (bioavailable testosterone < 60 ng/dl)	200 mg/2 weeks	IM injection	12 months	63
Bhasin et al[21]	19–47 (hypogonadal)	100 mg/week	IM injection	3 months	Bench press + 22% Squat + 44%
Page et al[24]	71 (hypogonadal; total testosterone less than 350 ng/dl)	200 mg/2 weeks	IM injection	36 months	~110 grip strength
Urban et al[15]	67 (total testosterone ≤480 ng/dl)	100 mg/week	IM injection	4 months	~25
Morley et al[23]	77.6 (bioavailable testosterone < 70 ng/dl)	200 mg/2 weeks	IM injection	3 months	~13
Tenover[27]	66.7 (low total testosterone ≤400 ng/dl)	100 mg/week	IM injection	3 months	No change in grip strength
Wang et al[28]	19–68 (hypogonadal: ≤300 ng/dl)	5, 7.5, or 10 g AndroGel	Transdermal gel	36 months	Bench press: ~11.5 Leg press: ~18.8

(Continued)

Table 31.2 *(Continued)*

Study	Age (years)	Dose of testosterone	Mode of administration	Duration of administration	% Increase in strength
Kenny et al[22]	76 (low bioavailable testosterone)	5 mg/day	Transdermal patch	12 months	38
Casaburi et al[19]	~67 (chronic obstructive pulmonary disease patients; low testosterone: <320 ng/dl)	100 mg/week	IM injection	2.5 months	~17

Power vs strength in relation to physical function

The relationship between strength and performance on tests of physical function such as stair climbing, the ability to rise from a chair, and gait speed has been firmly established in the literature. Recently, investigators have been addressing the effect of power on performance of tests of physical function when compared to the effects of strength on these tests. Power is a combination of strength (aka force) and how fast that strength is applied, or in other words, the ability to apply strength quickly. Bean et al[45] examined the effects of leg power vs leg strength on measures of physical function and found that leg power explained more of the variation in physical function than did leg strength. Thus, it may be important to apply resistance training models that enhance muscle power over muscle strength. How exactly to do this awaits scientific inquiry.

High-force low-repetition training programs to induce improvements in muscle strength and power

Over the last two decades having older individuals resistance train at 80% of 1 RM for 3 sets of 8 repetitions has been the predominant way that resistance training programs have been administered. However,

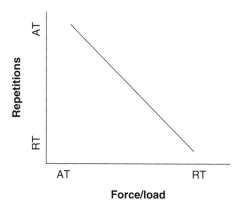

Figure 31.2 *Theoretic model of Specific Adaptations to Imposed Demands (SAID principle). AT, aerobic training; RT, resistance training.*

because of the exercise training principle known as the SAID principle – Specific Adaptations to Imposed Demands – it would follow that if a person wanted to improve the 1 RM he/she would have to train with a weight that is closer to the 1 RM than a weight he or she could perform 8 repetitions with. Figure 31.2 depicts a summary of the SAID principle.

Powerlifters and weightlifters have known this for years but to our knowledge very low repetition training with very high loads to increase strength has not been examined thoroughly in scientific studies and has not been applied to the elderly.

Table 31.3 *Increases in strength with resistance training*

Study	Gender	Mean age (years)	Duration (weeks)	Training % of 1 RM	% Increase in strength
Brown et al[32]	Men	60–70	12	70–90	48
Trappe et al[33]	Women	74	12	80	56
Trappe et al[34]	Men	74	12	80	50
Campbell et al[35]	8 men; 4 women	56–80	12	80	55.2
Harridge et al[36]	8 men; 3 women	85–97	12	80	134
Yarasheski et al[37]	8 women; 4 men	76–92	12	65–100	24.7
Griewe et al[38]	4 men; 4 women	82	12	85–90 of initial 1 RM	23.5
Frontera et al[4]	12 men	60–72	12	80	107.4
Casaburi et al[19]	12 men	~67; chronic obstructive pulmonary disease patients; low testosterone: <320 ng/dl	10	80	~17
Hakkinen et al[39]	10 men	61	10	8–10 RM, 3–5 RM, 15 RM	15.6
Moritani and deVries[40]	5 men	69.6	8	66% 1 RM	22.3
Balagopal et al[41]	?	71	12	80% 1 RM	37.4
Hagerman et al[42]		63.7	16	85–90% 1 RM	68.7
Jubrias et al[43]		69.2	24	60–70% 1 RM for 4 weeks, 70–85% 1 RM for remainder	64
Flynn et al[44]	Women	67–84	10	80% 1 RM	82
Fiatarone et al[10]	37 women; 63 men	87.1	10	80	113

Evidence suggesting that this kind of training leads to greater increases in strength than moderate load intermediate repetition training comes from a manuscript by Campos et al[46] (Table 31.4), in which resistance exercise in young individuals was performed at the 3–5 RM, the 9–11 RM, or the 20–28 RM for 8 weeks. The absolute and relative strength gains in the leg press and squat exercises were significantly greater for the group exercising at the 3–5 RM than for the other groups.

Resistance exercise and health-related variables

Resistance exercise and insulin sensitivity in individuals with impaired glucose tolerance and non-insulin-dependent diabetes mellitus

Data from the National Health and Nutrition Examination Survey suggest that approximately 8%

of the population of the United States have non-insulin-dependent diabetes mellitus.[47] There are many complications that result from this disease, not the least of which is coronary artery disease. Weight loss and aerobic exercise training have been commonly used to treat this disease and its precursor, impaired glucose tolerance. Resistance exercise, however, has received comparatively less attention, likely due to its low energy expenditure when compared with aerobic exercise of equal duration.

Early research by Yki-Jarvinen and Koivisto[48] suggested that, all things being equal, the greater the amount of muscle mass one has, the greater the glucose disposal rate. Thus, because one of the major adaptations of resistance exercise is an increase in muscle mass, it would follow that resistance exercise would be efficacious in improving insulin sensitivity. Miller et al[49] reported that glucose disposal expressed *relative to fat-free mass* during a hyperinsulinemic–euglycemic clamp was improved by 24% in men aged 50–65 years who had normal glucose tolerance. In addition, fasting plasma insulin levels and levels during an oral glucose tolerance test were lower after training. Thus an increase in muscle mass, or in this case fat-free mass, does not explain the improvement in glucose disposal as a result of a resistance training regimen.

Ryan et al[50] examined the effects of 24 weeks of progressive resistance training on insulin sensitivity in 18 men and women between the ages of 65 and 74 of whom had impaired glucose tolerance. Glucose utilization expressed relative to the concentration of insulin (M/I) tended to be improved (increased 10%, $P = 0.06$) as a result of the resistance exercise intervention.

Recently, Ibanez et al[51] reported that a high-intensity progressive resistance training regimen performed twice weekly for 16 weeks in older men (mean age 66.6 years) with type 2 diabetes resulted in a 46.3% improvement in insulin sensitivity as assessed using Bergman's minimal model procedure.

At least two studies have examined the effects of high-intensity resistance training on glycemic control in older individuals with type 2 diabetes. Castaneda et al[52] examined a 16-week high-intensity resistance training program in Latino men and women and found a 12.6% drop in glycosylated hemoglobin

concentrations and that 22 out of the 31 individuals in the resistance training group had a reduction of their intake of diabetes-related drugs. These positive changes were accomplished without a reduction in body weight. Ishii et al[53] examined the effects of resistance training (4–6 weeks, 5 ×/ week) on insulin sensitivity in non-insulin-dependent diabetics utilizing the hyperinsulinemic–euglycemic clamp technique. They performed this technique 2 days after the last bout of exercise to eliminate the effects of the last exercise bout. Much of the resistance exercise performed in that investigation was performed at 40–50% of 1 RM, with less than one minute of recovery between sets. Thus, the exercise performed in that investigation was at a lower intensity and with reduced recovery periods compared to traditionally performed progressive resistance training. Interestingly, in that investigation they found a 48% improvement in the glucose disposal rate when this rate was *normalized to lean body mass*. Thus, resistance training in this investigation improved insulin sensitivity via a mechanism other than an increase in lean body mass.

Comparison of resistance and aerobic exercise training on insulin sensitivity

In a very well controlled study in which body weight was maintained stable, Hughes et al[54] reported an 11% increase in glucose disposal in response to a euglycemic–hyperinsulinemic clamp as a result of 12 weeks of aerobic exercise training in older individuals with impaired glucose tolerance. Exercise was performed for 55 minutes/day and 4 days/week. This increase in glucose disposal appears to be similar to or less than in studies of resistance training. Thus, based on limited data it appears that resistance training and aerobic training result in similar improvements in glucose disposal. Clearly, more studies directly comparing these exercise modes are warranted.

Effects of resistance exercise training on blood lipids

An important area of consideration is whether resistance exercise favorably affects blood lipids in men. It appears that resistance exercise as typically performed to increase muscle strength and hypertrophy

Table 31.4 *Study design and results from Campos et al[46]*

Group	Number of repetitions/set	Rest period between sets	Number of sets	Statistical outcome with regard to strength (1 RM)	Statistical outcome with regard to muscular endurance (to fatigue at 60% of 1 RM)
Low repetition	3–5 at 3–5 RM	3 minutes	4	Significantly greater ($P \leq 0.05$) improvement than all other groups with regard to LP and S but not LE	
Intermediate repetition	9–11 at 9–11 RM	2 minutes	3	Significantly greater than control	
High repetition	20–28 at 20–28 RM	1 minute	2	Significantly greater than control	Significantly greater improvement than all groups for LP, S, and LE

LP, leg press; S, squat; LE, leg extension.

does not beneficially alter resting blood lipid concentrations in well controlled studies.[55,56]

The postprandial triglyceride concentration (lipemia) is more predictive of coronary artery disease risk than fasting triglyceride concentrations.[57] Additionally, in predicting the absence or presence of coronary artery disease in 61 male subjects with severe CAD and 40 control subjects, Patsch et al[57] reported that a single time point measurement of triglycerides 6 or 8 after a meal was accurate 68% of the time.

Petitt et al[58] reported that in 21–40-year-old men and women a resistance exercise bout of 10 exercises (3 × 10 repetitions at the 10 RM for each exercise), reduced the area under the triglyceride curve after a fat tolerance meal 16 hours after exercise by 16% compared to a control group, and by 18% compared to an aerobic exercise group. The resistance exercise also reduced baseline triglycerides by ~20%

16 hours after the resistance exercise bout compared to the two other groups. Thus, resistance exercise appears to lower this important risk factor related to coronary artery disease in young men and women. Future research should be aimed at determining whether there is a similar effect in older men and women.

Comparison of aerobic exercise training and resistance exercise training on blood lipids

Aerobic exercise training has been shown to reduce total cholesterol, total triglyceride, low-density lipoprotein (LDL) cholesterol, and the total cholesterol to high-density lipoprotein (HDL) ratio while increasing the HDL cholesterol.[59] Additionally, Kraus et al[60] reported that aerobic exercise has a beneficial effect on blood lipids in overweight men and women and they found that those who exercised the most (20 miles of jogging per week) incurred the greatest benefit. Thus, based on these data and those of Kokkinos et al,[55,56] it appears that aerobic exercise training is superior to resistance exercise training with regard to positive blood lipid alterations. However, based on the study described in the previous section, Petitt et al,[58] the postprandial triglyceride concentration is improved to a greater extent by resistance training than aerobic exercise training.

Resistance exercise and inflammatory cytokines

Aging is associated with an increase in inflammatory cytokines which may lead to chronic maladies such as the loss of skeletal muscle mass (sarcopenia), atherosclerosis, and cognitive impairment.[61] Further, an elevation in inflammatory cytokines is observed in many other chronic disease states. The loss of muscle mass induced by elevated inflammatory cytokines such as TNFα and IL-6 in the elderly may lead to physical disability.[62] TNFα has been shown to cause skeletal muscle protein degradation directly.[63] Recently, there has been interest in the effects of exercise on inflammatory cytokine concentrations in blood and in skeletal muscle. Gielen et al[64] reported that 6 months of aerobic exercise (cycling) reduced vastus lateralis TNFα by 37%, IL-6 by 42%, and IL-1β by 48%. In a very thorough investigation, Greiwe et al[38] reported that TNFα was markedly elevated in the skeletal muscle of elderly frail individuals and that 3 months of resistance exercise training 3 times per week decreased skeletal muscle TNFα protein expression by 34%, while TNFα mRNA was decreased by 46% in the frail elderly individuals. Further, Bruunsgaard et al[65] reported that the concentration of soluble TNF receptor-1 in plasma, a very good indicator of chronic plasma TNFα concentrations, prior to resistance exercise training, was inversely related to the improvement in strength in nursing home residents. This information taken together suggests that resistance exercise training as well as aerobic exercise training can reduce inflammatory cytokine production in muscle, which would presumably reduce muscle protein degradation, and that a pretraining elevation in inflammatory markers may attenuate the attainment of strength gains in nursing home residents.

Lipopolysaccharide (LPS) acts to stimulate cytokine production from monocytes. Exercise training acts to reduce LPS-stimulated cytokine production from monocytes. Toll-like receptors (TLRs) are present on the monocyte surface and act to bind LPS and initiate the cascade of events that lead to inflammatory cytokine production.

In a series of studies from Dr Michael Flynn's laboratory the role of exercise training status on TLR expression has been examined. He and his co-investigators hypothesized that the reduced inflammatory cytokine production in the trained state could be due to downregulation of TLRs on the monocyte. In a cross-sectional study, these investigators found a significant 190% reduction in TLR-4 in resistance-trained older women (aged 65–85) compared to women who did not resistance train.[66] In a subsequent study, these individuals found that, like their previous study, TLR-4 was downregulated in trained vs untrained women. However, they found no effect of acute resistance exercise on cell surface TLR-4 expression. Recently these investigators found that older women who were previously untrained and then were exercise trained had a reduction in TLR-4 in response to 12 weeks of resistance and aerobic exercise training.[67] Taken together, it appears that resistance training acts to downregulate the expression of TLR-4, which partly dictates inflammatory cytokine production from the monocyte.

Resistance exercise, muscle mass, and resting energy expenditure

It is clear that aging results in a reduction in muscle mass which is typically ~0.5–1.0% per year after the age of ~40.[11] It is also clear from a seminal study by Tzankoff and Norris[68] that the decline in muscle mass is mirrored by a decline in the resting metabolic rate. These investigators reported that muscle mass, as measured by 24-hour creatinine excretion, declined with increasing age after 45 years and that the relationship between oxygen consumption and muscle mass was very strong ($r = 0.644$). Bosy-Westphal et al[69] reported a Pearson correlation coefficient of 0.75 between fat-free mass measured by dual X-ray absorptiometry and resting metabolic rate over a wide range of body compositions. Thus, although fat-free mass contains bone, skin, blood, and organs, in addition to muscle, it may be an excellent surrogate to estimate muscle in relation to resting energy expenditure.

One obvious result of the loss of muscle mass and reduced resting energy expenditure with aging is a positive energy balance and deposition of fat. This would not be a beneficial adaptation. It is clear that acute exercise such as a resistance exercise bout can increase resting energy expenditure afterwards. In addition, theoretically the addition of muscle mass as a result of resistance exercise training should result in an increase in resting energy expenditure. In a well-designed study to address this question, Campbell et al[35] reported that 12 weeks of resistance training in men and women aged 56–80 resulted in a 1.4 kg increase in fat-free mass and a 6.8% increase in energy expenditure equivalent to an extra 4.6 kcal/hour, 110.4 kcal/day, 772.8 kcal/week, 40 186 kcal/yr, which, given 3500 kcal is 1 pound of fat, is equivalent to the expenditure of 11.5 lb of fat/year, which is not a trivial amount. Thus, it appears that a practically significant increase in resting energy expenditure can be achieved by older individuals undertaking a resistance exercise training protocol. Additionally, during the period of resistance exercise training there was a 2.2% drop in the body fat level. Thus, resistance exercise, predominantly through the addition of muscle mass, appears to be an excellent way to expend energy (calories).

Comparison of resistance exercise induced increase in resting metabolic rate to that of aerobic exercise

The results of most studies indicate no effect of aerobic exercise training on resting metabolic rate (RMR).[70–74] However, Sullo et al[75] reported that there is an increase in RMR with an increase in aerobic power in master athletes. Because aerobic exercise does not increase fat-free mass there appears to be no reason to believe that aerobic exercise would increase resting metabolic rate. Thus, it would appear that resistance training is a more appropriate form of training to increase resting energy expenditure.

Resistance exercise and bone density

The prevalence of osteoporosis in elderly men is ~3–6% based on data from the National Health and Nutrition Examination Survey (NHANES III).[76] Because of the high loads placed on bone, resistance training has been evaluated as a method for increasing bone density. Yarasheski et al[77] reported that 16 weeks of progressive resistance training (2 ×/week; 75–90% 1 RM; 5–10 repetitions/set) in 64–75-year-old men which involved all major muscle groups on Nautilus exercise machines resulted in a statistically significant increase in bone density at Ward's triangle (proximal femur). However, they did not find differences in whole body, lumbar spine, femoral neck, or greater trochanter bone densities. Compared to other investigations utilizing resistance training, the investigation of Yarasheski et al[77] would be considered to be using high-intensity resistance training.

Maddalozzo and Snow[78] had middle-aged men (mean age 54.6 years) perform 24 weeks (3×/week) of high-intensity (periodized: weeks 1–6: 70% 1 RM; weeks 7–10: 80% of 1 RM, weeks 10–12: 90+% of 1 RM; they performed this routine twice during the 24-week program) or moderate intensity (40–60% of 1 RM) resistance exercise. The moderate-intensity program was performed on machines while in the seated position while the high-intensity group used a functional standing free-weight program which incorporated physiologically taxing exercises such as free-weight deadlifts and squats. The high-intensity, but not the low-intensity, resistance exercise increased lumbar spine bone mineral density while the greater trochanter bone density was significantly increased as a result of both moderate- and high-intensity resistance training. No significant beneficial effect was observed at the femoral neck, total hip, or whole body.

Vincent and Braith[79] trained older (mean age 67.7 years) individuals 3 ×/week for 24 weeks using machines. Subjects in the low-intensity group trained at 50% of 1 RM while subjects in the high-intensity group trained at 80% of 1 RM. A significant improvement in the femoral neck was observed for the high-intensity group but no differences were observed for total body, anteroposterior spine, lateral spine, or Ward's triangle for low- or high-intensity groups.

Although these investigations report differential results it can be concluded that high-intensity resistance training (at least ~80% of 1 RM) would appear to be more beneficial at improving bone mineral density when compared to moderate-intensity resistance exercise. Future studies should incorporate very high-intensity resistance training (~90% of 1 RM) to determine the effects on bone mineral density as well as the effects on muscle strength.

Comparison of resistance exercise induced increase in bone density to that of aerobic exercise

At this time it is unclear whether bone mineral density in men is more positively affected by resistance exercise training or aerobic exercise training. However, non-weight-bearing aerobic activities such as swimming likely will not have a beneficial effect on bone density. There is a need for more research on this topic.

Resistance exercise and spontaneous physical activity

Fiatarone et al[10] examined the effects of resistance exercise with and without nutritional supplementation (360 kcal liquid; 60% carbohydrate, 23% fat, and 17% protein) on strength, physical function, and spontaneous physical activity in men and women with a mean age of 87.1 years. These investigators found a 113% improvement in strength and significant improvements in gait velocity and stair climbing power. Furthermore, these individuals showed a significant ~35% increase in spontaneous physical activity when exercise and exercise + supplement groups were combined compared to the supplement alone group + the control group. Thus, at least in this population of very old men and women, resistance training, likely through an increase in strength, can increase the amount of activity performed throughout the day. This is a very important additional benefit of resistance exercise training.

Resistance exercise and resting blood pressure and comparison with aerobic exercise

High blood pressure is a significant risk for developing cardiovascular disease. Because some individuals engage in resistance exercise as their sole source of structured physical activity, it would be important to know what effect if any resistance exercise has on blood pressure. In a recent meta-analysis Cornelissen and Fagard[80] examined the effect of dynamic resistance exercise on blood pressure. From 12 studies that did not differentiate between studies performed in hypertensives or normotensives and which were of varying durations (6–26 weeks), these investigators found that there was a −3.2 mmHg change in systolic and a −3.5 mmHg change in diastolic blood pressure following dynamic resistance exercise training. In a 2002 meta-analysis, Whelton et al[81] reported that systolic blood pressure was reduced by 3.84 mmHg and diastolic blood pressure by 2.58 mmHg as a result of aerobic exercise training. Thus, individuals should not abstain from resistance training because they assume there is no impact of resistance training on health-related variables such as blood pressure. Although the meta-analysis of Cornelissen and Fagard[80] involved only a small number of studies, the magnitude of the decrease in blood pressure for resistance training was similar to the magnitude of the reduction seen in aerobic training studies.[81] Thus, resistance and aerobic exercise training appear to be of similar value in reducing resting blood pressure.

Utility of resistance exercise during diet-induced weight loss

Resistance exercise training during weight loss induced by energy restriction typically results in maintenance of lean body mass,[82,83] while aerobic exercise training during diet-induced weight loss does not.[83] This is important as lean body mass is very metabolically active and thus combusts a large amount of energy. In contrast, aerobic exercise is better for inducing a caloric deficit for weight loss than resistance exercise training since aerobic exercise training burns more energy than resistance exercise of equal duration. As it would appear to maximize fat loss and maintain lean body mass, a combination of aerobic and resistance exercise training should be undertaken during diet-induced weight loss.

Role of resistance exercise in the treatment of osteoarthritis

Osteoarthritis is a joint disorder in which inflammation is the cause.[84] This inflammation leads to the

Table 31.5 *Summary of beneficial effects of resistance training and aerobic training on health-related variables*

Insulin sensitivity	Blood lipids	Muscle mass	Muscle strength	Resting metabolic rate	Bone density	Resting blood pressure
RT = AT	RT < AT	RT>>>>AT	RT>>>>AT	RT > AT	RT = AT	RT = AT

RT, resistance training; AT, aerobic training.

breakdown and loss of cartilage within the joint. Osteoarthritis affects ~20.7 million adults in the United States and is the most common type of arthritis.[85] Penninx et al[86] reported that the cumulative incidence of disability in activities of daily living in individuals with knee osteoarthritis was 52.5% in the control group, 37.8% in a resistance exercise group, and 36.4% during 18 months of resistance training, aerobic training, or a control intervention. Thus, both resistance training and aerobic training appear to be effective in reducing the number of people who become disabled as a result of knee osteoarthritis.

In a similar 18-month study, Ettinger et al[87] reported moderate improvements in pain, disability, and physical performance measures as a result of either resistance exercise or aerobic exercise when compared to a health education group. Thus, based on these data it appears that either resistance or aerobic exercise should be utilized to reduce the probability of an impairment in activities of daily living and/or to improve pain and physical performance measures in individuals with knee osteoarthritis.

Summary

The reduction in muscle mass with increasing age termed sarcopenia is very costly. Resistance exercise training appears to be far superior to androgen administration with regard to improving strength in older individuals. This is important as strength and not muscle mass is the primary determinant of physical function. With regard to improving muscular strength with resistance training, intensity is the major factor. The exercise intensity should be at least and probably more than 80% of the 1 RM to maximally improve muscle strength. Resistance training appears to be equally effective as aerobic exercise training with regard to improving insulin sensitivity and resting blood pressure, and increasing bone density (Table 31.5). Resistance training is superior to aerobic training with regard to improving muscle mass, muscle strength, and resting metabolic rate. Aerobic training appears to be more advantageous for improving most blood lipid measurements except for postprandial lipemia, for which resistance training appears to be more beneficial. Resistance training appears to be superior for maintaining muscle mass when compared to aerobic exercise during diet-induced weight loss, although aerobic exercise training appears to be more beneficial for creating an energy deficit than resistance exercise. For the aging male, resistance exercise training is an essential activity for improving many health-related variables. Resistance training should be undertaken by all men and the addition of aerobic exercise training will likely lead to additional improvements in many health-related variables.

References

1. Janssen I, Heymsfield SB, Ross R. Low relative skeletal muscle mass (sarcopenia) in older persons is associated with functional impairment and physical disability. J Am Geriatr Soc 2002; 50: 889–96.
2. Janssen I, Shepard DS, Katzmarzyk PT et al. The healthcare costs of sarcopenia in the United States. J Am Geriatr Soc 2004; 52: 80–5.

3. Fiatarone MA, Marks EC, Ryan ND et al. High-intensity strength training in nonagenarians. Effects on skeletal muscle. JAMA 1990; 263: 3029–34.

4. Frontera WR, Meredith CN, O'Reilly KP et al. Strength conditioning in older men: skeletal muscle hypertrophy and improved function. J Appl Physiol 1988; 64: 1038–44.

5. Hakkinen K, Newton RU, Gordon SE et al. Changes in muscle morphology, electromyographic activity, and force production characteristics during progressive strength training in young and older men. J Gerontol A Biol Sci Med Sci 1998; 53: B415–23.

6. Lambert C.P.a.E.W.J. Effects of aging and resistance exercise on determinants of muscle strength. J Am Aging Assoc 2002; 25: 73–8.

7. Seynnes O, Fiatarone Singh MA, Hue O et al. Physiological and functional responses to low-moderate versus high-intensity progressive resistance training in frail elders. J Gerontol A Biol Sci Med Sci 2004; 59: 503–9.

8. Vincent KR, Braith RW, Feldman RA et al. Resistance exercise and physical performance in adults aged 60 to 83. J Am Geriatr Soc 2002; 50: 1100–7.

9. Sullivan DH, Wall PT, Bariola JR et al. Progressive resistance muscle strength training of hospitalized frail elderly. Am J Phys Med Rehabil 2001; 80: 503–9.

10. Fiatarone MA, O'Neill EF, Ryan ND et al. Exercise training and nutritional supplementation for physical frailty in very elderly people. N Engl J Med 1994; 330: 1769–75.

11. Lambert CP, and Evans WJ. Adaptations to aerobic and resistance exercise in the elderly. Rev Endocr Metab Disord 2005; 6: 137–43.

12. Stackhouse SK, Stevens JE, Johnson CD et al. Predictability of maximum voluntary isometric knee extension force from submaximal contractions in older adults. Muscle Nerve 2003; 27: 40–5.

13. Brooks GA White FT, TP. Exercise Physiology: Human Bioenergetics and Its Applications. Mountain View: Mayfield Publishing Company, 1996.

14. Hasten DL, Pak-Loduca J, Obert KA et al. Resistance exercise acutely increases MHC and mixed muscle protein synthesis rates in 78–84 and 23–32 yr olds. Am J Physiol Endocrinol Metab 2000; 278: E620–6.

15. Urban RJ, Bodenburg YH, Gilkison C et al. Testosterone administration to elderly men increases skeletal muscle strength and protein synthesis. Am J Physiol 1995; 269: E820–6.

16. Sheffield-Moore M, Paddon-Jones D, Sanford AP et al. Mixed muscle and hepatic derived plasma protein metabolism is differentially regulated in older and younger men following resistance exercise. Am J Physiol Endocrinol Metab 2005; 288: E922–9.

17. Brodsky IG, Balagopal P, and Nair KS. Effects of testosterone replacement on muscle mass and muscle protein synthesis in hypogonadal men – a clinical research center study. J Clin Endocrinol Metab 1996; 81: 3469–75.

18. Sullivan DH, Roberson PK, Johnson LE et al. Effects of muscle strength training and testosterone on strength, muscle mass, and function in the frail elderly. Med Sci Sports and Exerc, in Press.

19. Casaburi R, Bhasin S, Cosentino L et al. Effects of testosterone and resistance training in men with chronic obstructive pulmonary disease. Am J Respir Crit Care Med 2004; 170: 870–8.

20. Sheffield-Moore M, Yeckel CW, Volpi E et al. Postexercise protein metabolism in older and younger men following moderate-intensity aerobic exercise. Am J Physiol Endocrinol Metab 2004; 287: E513–22.

21. Bhasin S, Storer TW, Berman N et al. Testosterone replacement increases fat-free mass and muscle size in hypogonadal men. J Clin Endocrinol Metab 1997; 82: 407–13.

22. Kenny AM, Prestwood KM, Gruman CA et al. Effects of transdermal testosterone on bone and muscle in older men with low bioavailable testosterone levels. J Gerontol A Biol Sci Med Sci 2001; 56: M266–72.

23. Morley JE, Perry HM 3rd, Kaiser FE et al. Effects of testosterone replacement therapy in old hypogonadal males: a preliminary study. J Am Geriatr Soc 1993; 41: 149–52.

24. Page ST, Amory JK, Bowman FD et al. Exogenous testosterone (T) alone or with finasteride increases physical performance, grip strength, and lean body mass in older men with low serum T. J Clin Endocrinol Metab 2005; 90: 1502–10.

25. Sih R, Morley JE, Kaiser FE et al. Testosterone replacement in older hypogonadal men: a 12-month randomized controlled trial. J Clin Endocrinol Metab 1997; 82: 1661–7.

26. Snyder PJ, Peachey H, Hannoush P et al. Effect of testosterone treatment on body composition and muscle strength in men over 65 years of age. J Clin Endocrinol Metab 1999; 84: 2647–53.

27. Tenover JS. Effects of testosterone supplementation in the aging male. J Clin Endocrinol Metab 1992; 75: 1092–8.

28. Wang C, Cunningham G, Dobs A et al. Long-term testosterone gel (AndroGel) treatment maintains beneficial effects on sexual function and mood, lean and fat mass, and bone mineral density in hypogonadal men. J Clin Endocrinol Metab 2004; 89: 2085–98.

29. Wang C, Eyre DR, Clark R et al. Sublingual testosterone replacement improves muscle mass and strength, decreases bone resorption, and increases

bone formation markers in hypogonadal men – a clinical research center study. J Clin Endocrinol Metab 1996; 81: 3654–62.

30. Wang C, Swedloff RS, Iranmanesh A et al. Transdermal testosterone gel improves sexual function, mood, muscle strength, and body composition parameters in hypogonadal men. Testosterone Gel Study Group. J Clin Endocrinol Metab 2000; 85: 2839–53.

31. Young NR, Baker HW, Liu G et al. Body composition and muscle strength in healthy men receiving testosterone enanthate for contraception. J Clin Endocrinol Metab 1993; 77: 1028–32.

32. Brown AB, McCartney N, Sale DG. Positive adaptations to weight-lifting training in the elderly. J Appl Physiol 1990; 69: 1725–33.

33. Trappe S, Godard M, Gallagher P et al. Resistance training improves single muscle fiber contractile function in older women. Am J Physiol Cell Physiol 2001; 281: C398–406.

34. Trappe S, Williamson D, Godard M et al. Effect of resistance training on single muscle fiber contractile function in older men. J Appl Physiol 2000; 89: 143–52.

35. Campbell WW, Crim MC, Young VR et al. Increased energy requirements and changes in body composition with resistance training in older adults. Am J Clin Nutr 1994; 60: 167–75.

36. Harridge SD, Kryger A, Stensgaard A. Knee extensor strength, activation, and size in very elderly people following strength training. Muscle Nerve 1999; 22: 831–9.

37. Yarasheski KE, Pak-Loduca J, Hasten DL et al. Resistance exercise training increases mixed muscle protein synthesis rate in frail women and men >/=76 yr old. Am J Physiol 1999; 277: E118–25.

38. Greiwe JS, Cheng B, Rubin DC et al. Resistance exercise decreases skeletal muscle tumor necrosis factor alpha in frail elderly humans. FASEB J 2001; 15: 475–82.

39. Hakkinen K, Kraemer WJ, Newton RU et al. Changes in electromyographic activity, muscle fibre and force production characteristics during heavy resistance/power strength training in middle-aged and older men and women. Acta Physiol Scand 2001; 171: 51–62.

40. Moritani T, deVries HA. Potential for gross muscle hypertrophy in older men. J Gerontol 1980; 35: 672–82.

41. Balagopal P, Schimke JC, Ades P et al. Age effect on transcript levels and synthesis rate of muscle MHC and response to resistance exercise. Am J Physiol Endocrinol Metab 2001; 280: E203–8.

42. Hagerman FC, Walsh SJ, Staron RS et al. Effects of high-intensity resistance training on untrained older men. I. Strength, cardiovascular, and metabolic responses. J Gerontol A Biol Sci Med Sci 2000; 55: B336–46.

43. Jubrias SA, Esselman PC, Price LB et al. Large energetic adaptations of elderly muscle to resistance and endurance training. J Appl Physiol 2001; 90: 1663–70.

44. Flynn MG, Fahlman M, Braun WA et al. Effects of resistance training on selected indexes of immune function in elderly women. J Appl Physiol 1999; 86: 1905–13.

45. Bean JF, Kiely DK, Herman S et al. The relationship between leg power and physical performance in mobility-limited older people. J Am Geriatr Soc 2002; 50: 461–7.

46. Campos GE, Luecke TJ, Wendeln HK et al. Muscular adaptations in response to three different resistance-training regimens: specificity of repetition maximum training zones. Eur J Appl Physiol 2002; 88: 50–60.

47. Harris MI, Flegal KM, Cowie CC et al. Prevalence of diabetes, impaired fasting glucose, and impaired glucose tolerance in U.S. adults. The Third National Health and Nutrition Examination Survey, 1988–1994. Diabetes Care 1998; 21: 518–24.

48. Yki-Jarvinen H, Koivisto VA. Effects of body composition on insulin sensitivity. Diabetes 1983; 32: 965–9.

49. Miller JP, Pratley RE, Goldberg AP et al. Strength training increases insulin action in healthy 50- to 65-yr-old men. J Appl Physiol 1994; 77: 1122–7.

50. Ryan AS, Hurlbut DE, Lott ME et al. Insulin action after resistive training in insulin resistant older men and women. J Am Geriatr Soc 2001; 49: 247–53.

51. Ibanez J, Izquierdo M, Arguelles I et al. Twice-weekly progressive resistance training decreases abdominal fat and improves insulin sensitivity in older men with type 2 diabetes. Diabetes Care 2005; 28: 662–7.

52. Castaneda C, Layne JE, Munoz-Orians L et al. A randomized controlled trial of resistance exercise training to improve glycemic control in older adults with type 2 diabetes. Diabetes Care 2002; 25: 2335–41.

53. Ishii T, Yamakita T, Sato T et al. Resistance training improves insulin sensitivity in NIDDM subjects without altering maximal oxygen uptake. Diabetes Care 1998; 21: 1353–5.

54. Hughes VA, Fiatarone MA, Fielding RA et al. Exercise increases muscle GLUT-4 levels and insulin action in subjects with impaired glucose tolerance. Am J Physiol 1993; 264: E855–62.

55. Kokkinos PF, Hurley BF, Smutok MA et al. Strength training does not improve lipoprotein-lipid profiles in men at risk for CHD. Med Sci Sports Exerc 1991; 23: 1134–9.

56. Kokkinos PF, Hurley BF, Vaccaro P et al. Effects of low- and high-repetition resistive training on lipoprotein-lipid profiles. Med Sci Sports Exerc 1998; 20: 50–4.

57. Patsch JR, Miesenbock G, Hopferwieser T et al. Relation of triglyceride metabolism and coronary artery disease. Studies in the postprandial state. Arterioscler Thromb 1992; 12: 1336–45.

58. Petit DS, Arngrimsson SA, Cureton KJ. Effect of resistance exercise on postprandial lipemia. J Appl Physiol 2003; 94: 694–700.

59. Tran ZV, Weltman A, Glass GV et al. The effects of exercise on blood lipids and lipoproteins: a meta-analysis of studies. Med Sci Sports Exerc 1983; 15: 393–402.

60. Kraus WE, Houmard JA, Duscha BD et al. Effects of the amount and intensity of exercise on plasma lipoproteins. N Engl J Med 2002; 347: 1483–92.

61. Krabbe KS, Pedersen M, Bruunsgaard H. Inflammatory mediators in the elderly. Exp Gerontol 2004; 39: 687–99.

62. Penninx BW, Kritchevsky SB, Newman AB et al. Inflammatory markers and incident mobility limitation in the elderly. J Am Geriatr Soc 2004; 52: 1105–13.

63. Li YP, and Reid MB. Effect of tumor necrosis factor-alpha on skeletal muscle metabolism. Curr Opin Rheumatol 2001; 13: 483–7.

64. Gielen S, Adams V, Mobius-Winkler S et al. Anti-inflammatory effects of exercise training in the skeletal muscle of patients with chronic heart failure. J Am Coll Cardiol 2003; 42: 861–8.

65. Bruunsgaard H, Bjerregaard E, Schroll M et al. Muscle strength after resistance training is inversely correlated with baseline levels of soluble tumor necrosis factor receptors in the oldest old. J Am Geriatr Soc 2004; 52: 237–41.

66. Flynn MG, McFarlin BK, Phillips MD et al. Toll-like receptor 4 and CD14 mRNA expression are lower in resistive exercise-trained elderly women. J Appl Physiol 2003; 95: 1833–42.

67. Stewart LK, Flynn MG, Campbell WW et al. Influence of exercise training and age on CD14+ cell-surface expression of toll-like receptor 2 and 4. Brain Behav Immun 2005; 19: 389–97.

68. Tzankoff SP, and Norris AH. Effect of muscle mass decrease on age-related BMR changes. J Appl Physiol 1977; 43: 1001–6.

69. Bosy-Westphal A, Eichhorn C, Kutzner D et al. The age-related decline in resting energy expenditure in humans is due to the loss of fat-free mass and to alterations in its metabolically active components. J Nutr 2003; 133: 2356–62.

70. Broeder CE, Burrhus KA, Svanevik LS et al. The effects of aerobic fitness on resting metabolic rate. Am J Clin Nutr 1992; 55: 795–801.

71. Davis JR, Tagliaferro AR, Kertzer R et al. Variations of dietary-induced thermogenesis and body fatness with aerobic capacity. Eur J Appl Physiol Occup Physiol 1983; 50: 319–29.

72. Gilbert JA, Misner JE, Boileau RA et al. Lower thermic effect of a meal post-exercise in aerobically trained and resistance-trained subjects. Med Sci Sports Exerc 1991; 23: 825–30.

73. LeBlanc J, Mercier P, Samson P. Diet-induced thermogenesis with relation to training state in female subjects. Can J Physiol Pharmacol 1984; 62: 334–7.

74. Schulz LO, Nyomba BL, Alger S et al. Effect of endurance training on sedentary energy expenditure measured in a respiratory chamber. Am J Physiol 1991; 260: E257–61.

75. Sullo A, Cardinale P, Brizzi G et al. Resting metabolic rate and post-prandial thermogenesis by level of aerobic power in older athletes. Clin Exp Pharmacol Physiol 2004; 31: 202–6.

76. Looker AC, Orwoll ES, Johnston CC Jr et al. Prevalence of low femoral bone density in older U.S. adults from NHANES III. J Bone Miner Res 1997; 12: 1761–8.

77. Yarasheski KE, Campbell JA, Kohrt WM. Effect of resistance exercise and growth hormone on bone density in older men. Clin Endocrinol (Oxf) 1997; 47: 223–9.

78. Maddalozzo GF, Snow CM. High intensity resistance training: effects on bone in older men and women. Calcif Tissue Int 2000; 66: 399–404.

79. Vincent KR, Braith RW. Resistance exercise and bone turnover in elderly men and women. Med Sci Sports Exerc 2002; 34: 17–23.

80. Cornelissen VA, Fagard RH. Effect of resistance training on resting blood pressure: a meta-analysis of randomized controlled trials. J Hypertens 2005; 23: 251–9.

81. Whelton SP, Chin A, Xin X et al. Effect of aerobic exercise on blood pressure: a meta-analysis of randomized, controlled trials. Ann Intern Med 2002; 136: 493–503.

82. Ballor DL, Katch VL, Becque MD et al. Resistance weight training during caloric restriction enhances lean body weight maintenance. Am J Clin Nutr 1988; 47: 19–25.

83. Bryner RW, Ullrich IH, Sauers J et al. Effects of resistance vs. aerobic training combined with an 800 calorie liquid diet on lean body mass and resting metabolic rate. J Am Coll Nutr 1999; 18: 115–21.

84. www.medterms.com.

85. www.Cureresearch.com.

86. Penninx BW, Messier SP, Rejeski WJ et al. Physical exercise and the prevention of disability in activities of daily living in older persons with osteoarthritis. Arch Intern Med 2001; 161: 2309–16.

87. Ettinger WH Jr, Burns R, Messier SP et al. A randomized trial comparing aerobic exercise and resistance exercise with a health education program in older adults with knee osteoarthritis. The Fitness Arthritis and Seniors Trial (FAST). JAMA 1997; 277: 25–31.

88. Sale DG. Neural adaptation to resistance training. Med Sci Sports Exerc 1988; 20: S135–45.

CHAPTER 32

Constipation and diarrhea

Syed H Tariq

Introduction

Both constipation and diarrhea are commonly seen in the elderly population. The epidemiology, causes, evaluation and treatment of constipation and diarrhea are described in detail.

Constipation

Constipation is a frequent concern in older adults and accounts for an increase in the use of the health-care system and a substantial proportion of health-care dollars spent on over-the-counter medications.[1-3] Almost half of all patients more than 65 years of age report constipation or the regular use of laxatives.[4] Chronic constipation can lead to fecal impaction, incontinence, and delirium, which necessitate hospitalization and severe curtailment of normal activities of daily living.[5-8]

Definition
Constipation is defined by patients as difficulty with defecation and complaints of hard stools or straining.

Physicians, on the other hand, describe constipation as less than three bowel movements per week. Constipation may be primary, if there is no obvious reason, or, secondary, resulting from altered bowel function because of metabolic abnormalities, medications, mechanical factors causing obstruction, or insufficient diet. Chronic constipation indicates that the symptoms have been present for more than 3 months. If chronic constipation is not responsive to the usual treatments, it requires further investigation for evidence of slow transit constipation, also known as pelvic outlet dysfunction. Although constipation can be part of irritable bowel syndrome (IBS), a new onset of IBS occurs less frequently in elders than in younger patients. The Rome criteria define constipation as outlined in Table 32.1, a consensus definition used by experts for the primary purpose of use in clinical trials.

Epidemiology
The prevalence of self-reported constipation, physician visits, and laxative use increases with aging, while the prevalence of stool frequency does not

---

Table 32.1 *Rome criteria for functional constipation*

Two or more of the following should be present for at least 12 weeks out of the preceding 12 months:

- Straining in more than 25% of defecations
- Lumpy or hard stools in more than 25% of defecations
- Sensation of incomplete evacuation in more than 25% of defecations
- Less than three defecations per week
- Manual evacuation or assistance to facilitate defecation 25% of the time

change with age.[4,9] Harari et al[4] reported a 10-fold increase in self-reported constipation in men from 0.6 to 6.3% from age 40 to 80 years, and an approximately 3-fold increase in women from 4 to 11%. They reported laxative use in about 30% of both elderly men and women without any significant decrease in bowel frequency. There is some evidence suggesting that lack of fiber, inactivity, and lack of fluid may contribute to constipation in otherwise healthy older people.[10,11] Women reported fewer bowel movements than did men and non-whites, and people of lower socioeconomic class also reported fewer bowel movements.[12]

In frail elders, up to 45% reported constipation as a health issue. The prevalence of constipation is higher in nursing home residents, a finding not well explained by the increased use of laxatives,[13] but it could be explained by a higher use of medications and other comorbidities.

The elderly perceive constipation as the presence of hard stools and straining, which correlates with self-reported constipation in this population.[14] Population-based studies reported constipation at 40% in community-dwelling older adults over the age of 64 years. The common risk factor for developing constipation in this population was the use of medication; i.e. non-steroidal anti-inflammatory drugs.[15]

In one study 20 to 30% of community-dwelling older adults used laxatives on at least a weekly basis. In nursing homes, it was reported that 59% of the residents used laxative at least on an intermittent basis.[16]

Economic impact and quality of life

Older adults treat constipation with over-the-counter products; thus, the economic impact of laxative use is likely considerably higher. At present there are no studies in the US addressing the economic aspect of laxative use. One study in the UK estimated the annual cost to the National Health Service for prescription laxatives at £43 million.[17]

The presence of chronic constipation impacts functioning in daily life and older adults affected by it rate their health lower than people without any gastrointestinal symptoms.[18] Health-related quality of life is reduced in patients with chronic constipation.[19]

The presence of constipation has been hypothesized to increase urinary tract symptoms, with treatment of constipation resulting in reduced urinary frequency, urgency, and dysuria.[20] Constipation is also associated with fecal incontinence, fecal impaction, and stercoral ulceration.[21,22] Effective strategies are needed for reducing the burden of illness and cost associated with constipation.

Causes of constipation

There are a number of causes of constipation in older adults as outlined in Table 32.2. The most common ones are medications and co-existent medical conditions. The reduced intake of dietary fiber is associated with constipation. In some studies, a high-fiber diet has been shown to be associated with lower laxative use;[23] however, other studies show no beneficial effect from fiber.[2] Dehydration and low calorie intake have been considered important risk factors for constipation in older adults; however it is not authenticated in studies.[1,5,24] Although immobility and reduced fluid and fiber intake are often implicated in the development of constipation, there is little evidence to support these myths. Reduced liquid intake does not appear to cause constipation,[25] likewise increased physical activity does not reverse constipation.[26] Reduced calorie intake[27] and increased psychologic distress[25] correlate well with constipation in the elderly, although the mechanism of the latter remains unknown.

Evaluation of constipation

History

The evaluation of constipation begins with a good understanding of the patient's perspective on their altered bowel function and the onset of constipation. In acute or subacute onset it is important to exclude structural lesions such as neoplasia or volvulus. The presence of weight loss along with rectal bleeding and/or iron deficiency anemia also requires examination of the colon to exclude cancer. Rectal pain, especially with defecation, suggests an anal disorder. The need for manual disimpaction, fecal urgency, and fecal or urinary incontinence are all important predictors of neurologic damage. Clear documentation of laxative use, its frequency,

Table 32.2 *Causes of constipation*

A. Medications

    a. Antidepressants (SSRIs and TCAs)
    b. Antipsychotics
    c. Antihistamines
    d. Anti-Parkinson's drugs
    e. Antacids (especially aluminum or calcium)
    f. Calcium supplements and calcium channel blockers
    g. Diuretics
    h. Iron
    i. Non-steroidal anti-inflammatory drugs
    j. Opiates
    k. Sucralfate

B. Metabolic

    a. Amyloidosis
    b. Chronic kidney disease
    c. Diabetes
    d. Electrolyte imbalance ($\downarrow$ calcium and magnesium)
    e. Hyperparathyroidism
    f. Hypothyroidism
    g. Scleroderma

C. Mechanical

    a. Anal stenosis
    b. Colonic neoplasia
    c. Strictures (intrinsic or extrinsic)

D. Neuropsychiatric

    a. Autonomic neuropathy
    b. Cerebrovascular accident
    c. Dementia
    d. Depression
    e. Parkinson's disease
    f. Multiple sclerosis

E. Other

    a. Decreased intake of calories, fiber, fluid
    b. Fever
    c. Immobility
    d. Poor access to toilet
    e. Weakness

efficacy, and duration of use, provides crucial historical data. Review of all medications currently used is important to determine whether any of them are contributing to constipation.

Physical examination

A careful general physical examination is required to explore evidence for a possible systemic disorder, excluding fecal impaction and assessing of anorectal

Table 32.3 *Agents used in the treatment of constipation*

Agent	Usual dosage
Fiber	
oat bran	1–6 tablespoons in divided dosages mixed with food
psyllium	1–2 tablespoons po 1–4 times/day
methylcellulose	1 heaped tablespoon (2 g) po 1–3 times/day
Osmotic laxatives	
lactulose	15–60 ml po in divided doses
sorbitol 70% solution	15–150 ml po in divided doses
magnesium citrate	120–300 ml po in divided doses daily
magnesium hydroxide	15–60 ml po at bedtime
polyethylene glycol	17 g po daily
Stimulant laxatives	
senna	8.6–17.2 g po daily
castor oil	15–60 ml po times one
bisacodyl	10–30 ml po daily
Enemas	
tap water	500–1000 ml up to twice weekly
sodium biphosphate	1 or 2 enemas weekly
oil retention	4.5 oz as needed up to 1 to 2 times weekly

function. Examination of the abdomen for masses and evidence of altered muscle tone and stool-filled bowel loops is an integral part of general examination. Inspection and digital rectal examination of the anal sphincter at rest, with squeezing, and with straining, are important in determining sphincter integrity, perineal descent, rectal masses, and prolapse.

Diagnostic tests

In the evaluation of constipation the following laboratory tests are often recommended: complete blood count, serum chemistry including electrolytes, kidney function, magnesium, calcium, and sensitive thyroid-stimulating hormone. Fecal occult blood testing and screening sigmoidoscopy/colonoscopy for neoplasm of the colon are indicated if not performed previously. Patients who are not responsive to medications or who have severe constipation need referral to a specialist (a gastroenterologist with expertise in manometry). Additional tests include colon transit measurement, colonic manometry, anorectal manometry, balloon expulsion testing, and defecography. Of patients undergoing extensive exhaustive investigations, the cause of constipation is determined in only about 50%.[28]

Treatment

Educating the patient and correcting any misconceptions regarding constipation is the initial step in the management of constipation. Discontinuation of laxatives, especially stimulants, is absolutely necessary if clinical constipation is not present. Fiber is generally a safe, inexpensive, first-line approach, which improves stool consistency and accelerates colon transit time.[29] An increase in fluid intake might be helpful in dehydrated patients, but may rarely improve symptoms of constipation in the chronically constipated.[11] Similarly, an increase in physical activity is also recommended without any clear evidence.[11,12] Agents used in the treatment of constipation are listed in Table 32.3.

Studies with psyllium generally show an improvement in stool form and frequency.[29,30] There is no role for stool softeners in the treatment of chronic constipation and they are not superior to psyllium.[31–33] Osmotic laxatives include polyethylene glycol (PEG), lactulose, sorbitol, magnesium salts, and saline salts. Saline and magnesium salts should not be used in renal, liver, and heart failure patients. There are no studies in older adults directly assessing PEG, but in younger adults, when compared to lactulose, it showed efficacy, safety, and fewer side-effects over a 6-month period.[34] Lactulose improved stool frequency, reduced the need for enemas, and reduced fecal impaction over a 12-week period.[35] A randomized controlled trial of lactulose and sorbitol in older adults found no difference in laxative effect and no strong preference of one laxative over the other by the study subjects.[36] Abdominal symptoms were similar between the two groups except for greater complaints of nausea in the lactulose group. The cost of sorbitol is generally lower and makes it a preferred agent for many patients.

Stimulant laxatives, when used in recommended doses, are unlikely to harm the colon. However, stimulant laxatives do result in electrolyte imbalance or abdominal pain in some patients.[37] An observational study using senna-containing concentrate as part of a program that included stool softener and increased fiber resulted in improved bowel evacuation and prevention of fecal impaction in nursing home residents.[38]

The role of enema in the treatment of constipation is limited to acute situations. Any enema must be used with caution owing to the risk of colonic perforation.[39] Soap enemas should not be used. Small-volume tap water enemas may be helpful in emptying the rectum; large-volume enemas can also be used, but can result in hyponatremia. Enemas containing phosphate are described to cause hyperphosphatemia, especially in renal insufficiency patients.

Prokinetic agents stimulate propulsion along with the gastrointestinal tract. Tegaserod, a 5HT4 agonist, improves the symptoms of constipation in adults.[40] There are no reported data for individuals over the age of 65 years. The use of neostigmine, an acetylecholinesterase inhibitor, is reserved for hospitalized patients with acute colonic pseudo-obstruction.[41]

Amitiza is the first selective chloride channel activator approved for therapeutic use and has been shown to offer effective relief of chronic idiopathic constipation in adults. Two double-blind, placebo-controlled studies showed that approximately 60% of patients who used amitiza experienced a spontaneous bowel movement within the first 24 hours.[58,59] Additionally, amitiza was shown to decrease abdominal bloating, abdominal discomfort, and constipation severity when administered over a 6–12-month treatment period. Amitiza works by increasing fluid secretion and motility in the intestine, and thereby increasing the passage of the stool and alleviating symptoms associated with chronic idiopathic constipation.

Refractory constipation may be treated with agents such as misoprostol and colchicine. Misoprostol is a prostaglandin agonist which stimulates intestinal secretion and transit time, but causes abdominal pain and cramping.[42] Colchicine can as used as it causes acute diarrhea, but it frequently causes abdominal pain which limits its use. Biofeedback can also be used in the treatment of dyssynergic defecation and slow transit time.[43] Patients with refractory constipation and slow transit time may benefit from subtotal colectomy and ileorectostomy,[44] but this is rarely required as most patients respond to laxatives.[45] Surgical therapy is most successful in patients without upper gut motility disorders or significant psychologic symptoms.[46]

Diarrhea

The average stool output for men is 100 g per day. Objectively, diarrhea is defined as a stool weight greater than 200 g in 24 hours. Clinically, diarrhea is a change in stools, usually defined as three or more loose or watery stools or more bloody stools in 24 hours.[47] Some of the associated symptoms include urgency, cramping, bloating, and incontinence.

Epidemiology

The true incidence of diarrhea in the elderly is not known, although diarrheal diseases are the second

Table 32.4 *Causes of diarrhea in the elderly*

Acute
Drugs
Diet
Infections
    bacterial
    viral
Protozoal
Ischemia

Chronic
Osmotic diarrhea
Secretory diarrhea
Malabsorption syndrome
Motility disorder
Inflammatory condition
Chronic infection
    bacterial
    parasitic
    protozoal
    viral

most common cause of death in the world.[48,49] Acute diarrhea causes considerable global morbidity and is a common presenting symptom in general practice in the US.[50] Infection is the most common cause of acute diarrhea, and is related to environmental conditions such as contaminated food and water supplies, inadequate sewage disposal, closed living and working conditions, and globalization of food products.[51]

The elderly are predisposed to infectious diarrhea, because of hypochlorhydria and achlorhydria, luminal stasis, or decreased mucosal immune function. Nursing home outbreaks of *Escherichia coli* (*E. coli*) O157:H7 infections have been documented with three times the morbidity and mortality compared to younger persons. The high mortality rates (16 to 35%) occur largely because the elderly are less capable of replenishing their losses and tolerating the intravascular hypovolemia associated with dehydration.[52]

Classification
Diarrhea is classified on the basis of duration and its causes are summarized in Table 32.4:

- acute – less than 2 weeks' duration
- chronic – more than 4 weeks' duration.

Acute diarrhea
Acute diarrhea is usually self-limiting and is acute in nature. The major causes are infection, recent drug change, and food intolerance. Sudden onset of bloody diarrhea could be caused by acute diverticulitis, inflammatory bowel disease, or ischemia, which could be the result of acute thrombosis or colitis.[53–55]

Bacterial causes of acute diarrhea can be a result of preformed exotoxin production (*Staphylococcus aureus*, *Bacillus cereus*, or *Clostridium perfringens*), enterotoxin production (enterotoxigenic *E. coli*, *Vibrio cholerae*), cytotoxin production (enterohemorrhagic *E. coli* O157:H5, *E. coli*, *Clostridium difficle*, or *Vibrio* parhemolytics), or invasion of the mucosa (shigella, salmonella, *Campylobacter jejuni*, enteroinvasive *E. coli*, *Yersinia enterocolitica*, *Chlamydia neisseria*, gonorrheae and *Listeria monocytogenes*).

Viral diarrhea may be inflammatory (cytomegalovirus) or non-inflammatory (norovirus and rotavirus). Norwalk virus is present throughout the year, while rotavirus is seen in the cooler months. The route of transmission is fecal–oral and it has caused epidemics in nursing homes.

Similarly, protozoal infections are also inflammatory (*Entamoeba histolytica*) or non-inflammatory (*Giardia lambia*, cryptosporidium, and cyclospora).

Chronic diarrhea
Chronic diarrhea can be divided into seven different categories.[56,57]

Osmotic diarrhea is characterized by a decrease in stool volume with fasting and an increased stool osmotic gap. Osmotic diarrhea is caused by lactase deficiency, laxative abuse, and malabsorption syndromes.

Deficiency of lactase, which is a disaccharidase, is common and should be considered in all patients with chronic diarrhea, especially after an episode of viral gastroenteritis, medical illness, or gastrointestinal surgery. Sorbitol is commonly used as a sweetener in gums, candies, and some medications and may cause diarrhea in some patients, especially in diabetics or in those who are trying to lose weight.

Factitious diarrhea is usually caused by the ingestion of magnesium- or phosphate-containing compounds (laxatives, antacids), though this is less likely to be seen in the elderly population. The fat substitute olestra is also believed to cause diarrhea and cramps in occasional patients.

Secretory diarrhea is caused by agents that trigger intestinal epithelial cells to secrete water and electrolytes into the intestinal lumen. Secretory diarrhea is usually of large volume (greater than 1 liter/day), and there is no change with fasting and a normal osmotic gap. Secretory diarrhea may be mediated by hormones (VIPoma, carcinoid tumors, and medullary carcinoma of the thyroid), villous adenoma, bile salt malabsorption (ileal resection, Crohn's ileitis, and postcholecystectomy), medications, and laxative abuse.

A *malabsorption syndrome* is characterized by weight loss and fecal fat greater than 10 g/24 hours. The common causes are bacterial overgrowth (motility disorders, e.g. diabetes, vagotomy, scleroderma, fistulas, small intestinal diverticula), small bowel mucosal disorders (celiac sprue, tropical sprue, Whipple's disease, eosinophilic gastroenteritis, small bowel resection, short bowel syndrome, Crohn's disease), pancreatic disease (chronic pancreatitis), lymphatic obstruction (lymphoma, carcinoid), infections (tuberculosis, *Mycobacterium avium* intracellulare (MAI), Kaposi's sarcoma, sarcoidosis, and retroperitoneal fibrosis.

Motility disorder is seen in systemic diseases (scleroderma, diabetes mellitus, hypertension), irritable bowel disease, and postsurgical cases (vagotomy, partial gastrectomy, and blind loop with bacterial overgrowth).

Inflammatory conditions are characterized by fever, hematochezia, and abdominal pain. The inflammatory conditions responsible for chronic diarrhea are ulcerative colitis, Crohn's disease, microscopic colitis, radiation enteritis, and malignancies of the gut.

The causes of *chronic infection* may be parasitic (*Giardia lambia*, *Entamoeba histolytica*), AIDS-related, viral (cytomegalovirus), bacterial (*Clostridium difficile*, *Mycobacterium avium* complex), or protozoal (Microsporida, Cryptosporidium, *Isospora belli*).

Factitious diarrhea is seen in 15% of patients caused by surreptitious laxative abuse or dilution of stool.

Diagnosis

Evaluation is indicated for patients with moderate or severe illness when clinical symptoms suggest bacterial infection, or when there is bloody diarrhea, acute diarrhea lasting longer than 8 hours, or larger-volume diarrhea (≥ 6 stools/24 hours).

In the initial evaluation it is important to determine whether the patient's problem is a result of fecal impaction, fecal incontinence, and/or actual diarrhea. Knowing the characteristics of the diarrhea would help in the differential diagnosis. History and physical examination provide clues to the etiology and determine the severity of the diarrhea: fever, signs of dehydration (orthostatic hypotension), delirium, and the presence of abdominal pain. Peritoneal signs may be present in infection with *C. difficile* or enterohemorrhagic *E. coli*.

Symptoms of food poisoning usually develop within 6 to 12 hours of ingestion of the toxin, and it takes about 12 to 48 hours after ingestion of *Salmonella* or *Campylobacter*. Blood in the stool is usually suggestive of inflammation or ulceration, infections (*Shigella*, *E. histolytica*, or enteroinvasive *E. coli*), and recent use of antibiotics could be associated with *C. difficile*. The presence of vascular disease, abdominal bruit, and/or painless bleeding suggests colonic ischemia. The initial work-up includes complete blood count, electrolytes, and renal and hepatic functions. Stools should be tested for blood, fecal leucocytes, qualitative fat, and, in patients with suspected *C. difficile*, electrolytes to calculate the osmotic gap to differentiate osmotic (a gap of >125) from secretory diarrhea (a gap of <50).

Stool cultures are indicated in patients with severe diarrhea and fever, bloody stools, fecal leukocytes, or prolonged illness (>14 days). Stool samples should be obtained for testing of ova and parasites in patients who travel extensively or live in an endemic area (three fresh samples are required for a 90% sensitivity). Qualitative 72-hour fecal fat collection is important when the cause of diarrhea remains obscure, fecal fat >9.5 g/100 g of stool is suggestive of biliary steatorrhea or pancreatic insufficiency.

Flexible sigmoidoscopy may be indicated in some cases to evaluate for pseudomembranes or ischemia. Specialized testing may be indicated in certain cases, for example, if one suspects hormone-secreting tumors, serum gastrin or vasoactive intestinal peptides, calcitonin and urine collection for 5-hydroxyindoleacetic acid, metanephrine, or histamine may be helpful. In lactase deficiency, the stool pH is usually 4 to 6 with an associated increase in short-chain fatty acids. Then a lactose-hydrogen breath test is indicated. In cases of surreptitious laxative abuse, a problem more common in elderly women, measurement of magnesium, sulfate, and phosphate in stool water is important.

A plain film of the abdomen may show pancreatic calcification, and a small-bowel follow-through examination may show ileal disease (Crohn's disease) or thickening of the mucosa in cases of lymphoma. Colonoscopy provides direct visualization of the colonic mucosa and is the procedure of choice for diagnosing inflammatory bowel disease, colorectal tumors, and radiation proctitis. Biopsy samples obtained from the colonic mucosa can be examined for the possibility of microscopic colitis. Upper gastrointestinal endoscopy may be needed to perform a biopsy (in case of celiac disease or Whipple's disease) or an aspirate of the small bowel (bacterial overgrowth). Serum tests of antigliadin immunoglobulin (IgA and IgG) antibodies and antiendomysial IgA antibodies are helpful in the diagnosis and treatment of patients with celiac sprue.

Treatment

The first priority for the management of diarrhea is to replace fluids and electrolytes. Patient who can tolerate oral fluids should receive oral rehydration solutions. In the elderly, the classic signs of dehydration that are seen in young adults are unreliable, such as skin turgor or dry mucosa. Rather, orthostatic hypotension and laboratory parameters such as hypernatremia, hyperosmolarity, increased ratio of BUN/Cr > 20, and prerenal azotemia are more reliable. Elderly persons with fluid loss require close monitoring and possible hospitalization. Food poisoning is usually self-limited, usually of brief symptomatic duration, and is treated using fluid support.

Empiric antibiotic treatment is indicated for patients with fever, evidence of toxicity, bloody stools, or traveler's diarrhea, and the usual drugs used in the treatment include ciprofloxacin 500 mg bid × 5 days, norfloxacin 400 mg bid × 5 days, and trimethoprim/sulfamethoxazole ds × 5 days. Although treatment can begin immediately, it is helpful to obtain a stool sample for bacterial culture first.

If toxin-producing or invasive bacteria are not suspected, then antidiarrheal drugs can be used. Empiric treatment can minimize diarrheal symptoms when the diagnostic evaluation is in progress. Soluble fiber adds form to the stool. Synthetic opioids such as loperamide and diphenoxylate are excellent first-line drugs. Loperamide is generally preferred, because the usual formulation of diphenoxylate incorporates atropine, which can cause significant adverse effects in elderly persons. When the diarrhea cannot be controlled with these drugs, stronger opioids are recommended. A somatostatin analog is a second-line drug for the treatment of chronic idiopathic diarrhea because of its need for injection and increased adverse effects. When bile acid diarrhea is suspected, cholestyramine may be tried.

Treatment of microscopic colitis consists of removing the offending agent when it is identified and the use of antidiarrheal drugs. Clinical improvement is reported with 5-aminosalicylate drugs. Corticosteroids are generally avoided.

Summary

Constipation and diarrhea are commonly seen in the older adult. It is important to recognize and treat these conditions to avoid complications. Untreated constipation can result in abdominal pain, fecal impaction, and even perforation.

References

1. Harari D, Gurwitz JH, Minaker JL. Constipation in the elderly. J Am Geriatr Soc 1993; 41: 1130–40.
2. Lederle FA. Epidemiology of constipation in elderly patients. Drugs utilization and cost-containment strategies. Drugs Ageing 1995; 6: 465–9.

3. Romero Y, Evans JM, Fleming, KC et al. Symposium on geriatrics – part VII: Constipation and fecal incontinence in the elderly population. Mayo Clin Proc 1996; 71: 81–92.

4. Harari D, Gurwitz JH, Avorn J et al. Bowel habit in relation to age and gender: findings from the National Health Interview survey and clinical implications. Arch Intern Med 1996; 156: 315–20.

5. Prather CM, Ortiz-Camacho CP. Evaluation and treatment of constipation and fecal impaction in adults. Mayo Clin Proc 1998; 73: 881–7.

6. Read NW, Abouzeky L, Read MD et al. Anorectal function in elderly patients with fecal impaction. Gastroenterology 1985; 89: 959–66.

7. Read NW, Celik AF, Katsinelos P. Constipation and incontinence in the elderly. J Clin Gastroenterol 1995; 20: 61–70.

8. Tariq SH, Morley ME, Prather CM. Health issues in the elderly: fecal incontinence: importance, clinical evaluation and treatment. Am J Med 2003; 115(3): 217–27.

9. Everhart JE, Go VL, Johannes RS et al. A longitudinal survey of self-reported bowel habits in the United States. Dig Dis Sci 1989; 34: 1153–62.

10. Annells M, Koch T. Constipation and the preached trio: diet, fluid intake, exercise. Int J Nurs Studies 2003; 40: 843–52.

11. Muller-Lissner SA, Kamm MA, Scarpignato C, Wald A. Myths and misconceptions about chronic constipation. Am J Gastroenterol 2005; 100: 232–42.

12. Higgins PD, Johanson JF. Epidemiology of constipation in North America: a systematic review. Am J Gastroenterol 2004; 99: 750–9.

13. Van Dijk KN, de Vries CS, van den Berg PB et al. Constipation as an adverse effect of drug use in nursing home patients: an overestimated risk. Br J Clin Pharmacol 1998; 46: 255–61.

14. Harari D, Gurwitz JH, Avorn J, Bohn R, Minaker KL. How do older persons define constipation? Implications for therapeutic management. J Gen Intern Med 1997; 12: 63–6.

15. Talley NJ, Fleming KC, Evans JM et al. Constipation in an elderly community: a study of prevalence and potential risk factors. Am J Gastroenterol 1996; 91: 19–25.

16. Lamy PP, Krug BH. Review of laxative utilization in a skilled nursing facility. J Am Geriatr Soc 1978; 26: 544–9.

17. Petticrew M, Watt I, Sheldon T. Systematic review of the effectiveness of laxatives in the elderly. Health Technology Assessment (Winchester, England) 1997; 1: i–iv, 1–52.

18. O'Keefe EA, Talley NJ, Zinsmeister AR, Jacobsen SJ. Bowel disorders impair functional status and quality of life in the elderly: a population-based study. J Gerontol Series A Biol Sci Med Sci 1995; 50: M184–9.

19. Glia A, Lindbergh G. Quality of life in patients with different types of functional constipation. Scand J Gastroenterol 1997; 32: 1083–9.

20. Charach G, Greenstien A, Rabinovich P. Alleviating constipation in the elderly improves lower urinary tract symptoms. Gerontology 2001; 47: 72–6.

21. Lynch AC, Dobbs BR, Keating J, Frizelle FA. The prevalence of fecal incontinence and constipation in a general New Zealand population: a postal survey. NZ Med J 2001; 114: 474–7.

22. Maull Ki, Kinning WK, Kay S. Stercoral ulceration. Am Surgeon 1982; 48: 20–4.

23. Hull C, Greco RS, Brooks DL. Alleviation of constipation in the elderly by dietary fiber supplementation. J Am Geriatr Soc 1980; 28: 400–14.

24. Wrenn K. Fecal impaction. N Engl J Med 1989; 321: 658–62.

25. Whitehead WE, Drinkwater D, Cheskin LJ, Heller BR, Schuster MM. Constipation in the elderly living at home. Definition, prevalence, and relationship to lifestyle and health status. J Am Geriatr Soc 1989; 37: 423–9.

26. Meshkinpour H, Selod S, Movahedi H et al. Effects of regular exercise in management of chronic idiopathic constipation. Dig Dis Sci 1998; 43: 2379–83.

27. Towers AL, Burgio KL, Locher JL. Constipation in the elderly: influence of dietary, psychological, and physiological factors. J Am Geriatr Soc 1994; 78: 701–6.

28. Halverson AL, Orkin BA. Which physiologic tests are useful in patients with constipation? Dis Colon Rectum 1998; 41: 735–9.

29. Badiali D, Corazziari E, Habib FI et al. Effect of wheat bran in treatment of chronic nonorganic constipation. A double-blind controlled trial. Dig Dis Sci 1995; 40: 349–56.

30. Cheskin LJ, Kamal N, Crowell MD, Schuster MM, Whitehead WE. Mechanisms of constipation in older persons and effects of fiber compared with placebo. J Am Geriatr Soc 1995; 43(6): 666–9.

31. Castle SC, Cantrell M, Israel DS, Samuelson MJ. Constipation prevention: empiric use of stool softeners questions. Geriatrics 1991; 46: 84–6.

32. McRorie JW, Daggy BP, Morel JG et al. Psyllium is superior to docusate sodium for treatment of chronic constipation. Aliment Pharmacol Therapeut 1998; 12: 491–7.

33. Ashraf W, Park F, Lof J, Quigley EM. Effects of psyllium therapy on stool characteristics, colon transit and anorectal function in chronic idiopathic constipation. Randomized controlled trial. Aliment Pharmacol Therapeut 1995; 9: 639–47.

34. Corazziari E, Badiali D, Bazzocchi G et al. Long term efficacy, safety, and tolerability of low daily doses of isosmotic polyethylene glycol electrolyte balanced solution (PMF-100) in the treatment of functional chronic constipation. Gut 2000; 46: 522–6.

35. Sanders JF. Lactulose syrup assessed in a double-blind study of elderly constipated patients. J Am Geriatr Soc 1978; 26: 236–9.

36. Lederle FA, Busch DL, Mattox KM, West MJ, Aske DM. Cost-effective treatment of constipation in the elderly: a randomized double-blind comparison of sorbitol and lactulose. Am J Med 1990; 89: 597–601.

37. Xing JH, Soffer EE. Adverse effects of laxatives. Dis Colon Rectum 2001; 44: 1201–9.

38. Maddi VI. Regulation of bowel function by a laxative/stool softener preparation in aged nursing home patients. J Am Geriatr Soc 1979; 27: 464–8.

39. Paran H, Butnaru G, Neufeld D, Magen A, Freund U. Enema-induced perforation of the rectum in chronically constipated patients. Dis Colon Rectum 1999; 42: 1609–12.

40. Johanson JF, Wald A, Tougas G et al. Effect of tegaserod in chronic constipation: a randomized, double-blind, controlled trial. Clin Gastroenterol Hepatol 2004; 2: 796–805.

41. Ponec RJ, Saunders MD, Kimmey MB. Neostigmine for the treatment of acute colonic pseudo-obstruction. N Engl J Med 1999; 341: 137–41.

42. Roarty TP, Weber F, Soykan I, McCallum RW. Misoprostol in the treatment of chronic refractory constipation: results of a long-term open label trial. Aliment Pharmacol Therapeut 1997; 11: 1059–66.

43. Enck P. Biofeedback training in disordered defecation. A critical review. Digest Dis Sci 1993; 38: 1953–60.

44. Nyam DC, Pemberton JH, Ilstrup DM, Rath DM. Long-term results of surgery for chronic constipation. Dis Colon Rectum 1997; 40: 273–9.

45. Rex DK, Lappas JC, Goulet RC, Madura JA. Selection of constipated patients as subtotal colectomy candidates. J Clin Gastroenterol 1992; 15: 212–17.

46. Redmond JM, Smith GW, Barofsky I et al. Physiological tests to predict long-term outcome of total abdominal colectomy for intractable constipation. Am J Gastroenterol 1995; 90: 748–53.

47. DuPont HL. Guidelines on acute infectious diarrhea in adults. The Practice Parameters Committee of the American College of Gastroenterology. Am J Gastroenterol 1997; 92: 1962–75.

48. Bern C, Martines J, de Zoysa I, Glass RI. The magnitude of the global problem of diarrhoeal disease: a ten-year update. Bull WHO 1992; 70: 705–14.

49. Yip R, Sharp TW. Acute malnutrition and high childhood mortality related to diarrhea: lessons from the 1991 Kurdish refugee crisis. JAMA 1993; 270: 587–90.

50. Cohen ML. The epidemiology of diarrheal disease in the United States. Infect Dis Clin North Am 1988; 2: 557–70.

51. Torrens PR. Historical evolution and overview of health services in the United States. In: Williams SJ, ed. Introduction to Health Science, 6th edn. Albany, NY: Delmar, 2002.

52. Carter AO, Borczyk AA, Carlson JA et al. A severe outbreak of Escherichia coli O157:H7-associated hemorrhagic colitis in a nursing home. N Engl J Med 1987; 317(24): 1496–500.

53. Guerrant RL, Van Gilder T, Steiner T et al. Practice guidelines for the management of infectious diarrhea. Clin Infect Dis 2001; 32: 331.

54. Musher DM et al. Contagious acute gastrointestinal infections. N Engl J Med 2004; 350: 2417.

55. Camilleri M. Chronic diarrhea: a review on pathophysiology and management for the clinical gastroenterologist. Clin Gastroenterol Hepatol 2004; 2: 198.

56. Schiller L. Chronic diarrhea. Gastroenterology 2004; 127: 287.

57. Thomas PD, Forbes A, Green J et al. Guidelines for the investigation of chronic diarrhea, 2nd edn. Gut 2003; 52(Suppl 5): v1.

58. Ueno R, Joswicks TR, Wahle A et al. Efficacy and safety of Rubiprostone for the treatment of chronic constipation in elderly patients. Am J Gastroenterol 2005; 100: S324, S328, S329.

59. Ueno R, Panas R, Wahle A et al. The long-term safety and efficacy of lubiprostone for the treatment of chronic idiopathic constipation in elderly and non-elderly patients. Gastroenterology 2006; 130 (A-189): S1262.

CHAPTER 33

Macrovascular complications in the elderly diabetic

Nikiforos Ballian, Mahmoud Malas and Dariush Elahi

Introduction

In the past two decades, diabetes mellitus has earned its place amongst the most significant public health threats worldwide. Obesity and increased life expectancy have been blamed for the growing prevalence of this disease, which is expected to further increase by 23% between 2000 and 2010 in North America.[1] The prevalence of diabetes mellitus is age-dependent, with more than 20% of Americans aged 60–74 years suffering from this disease and another 20% having impaired glucose tolerance, defined by blood glucose levels between 140 and 200 mg/dl 2 hours after an oral glucose load.[2] Diabetes is not only exceedingly common in the elderly, it is also poorly controlled and undertreated. This could be responsible for the increased complication rate in this group.[3]

Whether directly related to aging itself or not, glucose intolerance and diabetes significantly contribute to morbidity and mortality in the elderly male population. Diabetes has a number of effects on the macrovasculature, the most significant being its atherogenic potential. Mortality and morbidity caused by coronary artery disease (CAD) and cerebrovascular disease are the most frequent clinical manifestations of atherosclerotic disease in diabetics and patients with impaired glucose tolerance; nonetheless, lower-extremity peripheral arterial disease (PAD) also leads to substantial morbidity and disability, particularly among the elderly.[4,5] Despite these facts, and significant evidence that elderly diabetics benefit from aggressive atherosclerosis risk factor modification more than non-diabetic patients, it is ironic that this cohort of patients receives suboptimal treatment.[6–8]

Pathophysiology

The role of diabetes mellitus in atherogenesis is still not well understood.[9] Evidence for a causal relationship between diabetes and atherosclerosis has come mostly from epidemiologic studies. A direct pathophysiologic link between chronic hyperglycemia, the major metabolic disturbance in diabetes, and atherosclerosis has been more difficult to establish. This is partly because diabetes results in or co-exists with multiple metabolic abnormalities, including dyslipidemia, insulin deficiency, insulin resistance, altered leptin levels, and obesity, each with their own possible atherogenic effects.[10] A number of animal models of type 1 and type 2 diabetes mellitus have improved our understanding of diabetic atherogenesis, although no animal model perfectly mimics human disease.[9]

The American Heart Association has defined five mechanisms whereby diabetes mellitus contributes to the pathogenesis of atherosclerosis: metabolic factors, increased oxidation/glucoxidation, endothelial dysfunction, vascular inflammation, and induction of a procoagulant state.

Atherogenic metabolic alterations in diabetes mellitus include hyperglycemia, dyslipidemia, insulin resistance, and hyperinsulinemia. Second, increased oxidation/glucoxidation results in the formation of advanced glycation end-products (AGEs) and oxidation of lipids and lipoproteins that lead to foam cell accumulation in the vascular wall. Third, endothelial dysfunction, a result of hyperglycemia, dyslipidemia, hyperinsulinemia, and pre-existing atherosclerosis, contributes to the initiation of atherogenesis. Fourth, vascular inflammation as a result of obesity leads to cytokine release, smooth muscle cell proliferation and migration, and platelet activation. Finally, diabetes induces a prothrombotic state as a result of imbalance between procoagulant and anticoagulant factors.[11] The most important pathophysiologic changes leading to diabetic atherosclerosis are outlined below.

Hyperglycemia

Hyperglycemia is a significant cause of endothelial dysfunction, one of the first steps in the pathogenesis of atherosclerosis. There is evidence that hyperglycemia is directly toxic to the endothelium by reducing the lifespan and increasing the apoptotic rate of endothelial cells.[12] It also has indirect endothelial toxicity through increased intracellular polyol generation, formation of AGEs, protein kinase C (PKC) activation, and generation of reactive oxygen species.[13] Most research on the effects of hyperglycemia on cardiovascular risk has focused on the role of hyperglycemia in initiating and promoting atherosclerosis. Interestingly, some investigators found a significant increase in cardiovascular events in newly diagnosed diabetics, in whom diabetes-induced atherosclerosis has not progressed significantly, leading to the recent hypothesis that hyperglycemia might increase cardiovascular risk via atherosclerosis-independent pathways.[14]

Central to the pathogenesis of atherosclerosis in diabetes mellitus is the formation of AGEs. These are intracellular and extracellular protein or lipid molecules that become non-enzymatically glycated as a result of chronic hyperglycemia and cause atherosclerosis by a combination of numerous extracellular and intracellular effects.[15,16] Their rate of formation depends on the severity and duration of hyperglycemia, making their role more significant in patients with longstanding diabetes, such as the elderly.[15]

Multiple vascular effects of AGEs have been described. AGE formation in the vascular extracellular matrix (ECM) results in vascular stiffness by cross-linking of ECM proteins such as collagen, elastin, vitronectin, and laminin.[17,18] AGEs inhibit the generation and efficacy of nitric oxide (NO), resulting in decreased vasodilation in response to NO, increased endothelial cell proliferation, and formation of reactive oxygen intermediates.[19–23] Intracellular AGEs increase macrophage expression of the scavenger LDL receptor, responsible for accumulation of cholesterol in macrophages, i.e., foam cell formation.[24] Subendothelial AGEs have been shown to stimulate migration of blood monocytes through the endothelium, an important step in atherosclerotic plaque formation.[25] Finally, AGEs have procoagulant properties as a result of altered thrombomodulin activity and tissue factor levels.[17,26]

Epidemiologic studies have not defined the relationship between hyperglycemia and risk of cardiovascular events and mortality.[8] In people without diabetes or impaired glucose tolerance (IGT) there is some evidence that blood glucose levels are associated with macrovascular risk and abnormal glucose metabolism has been shown to correlate with severity of coronary atherosclerosis.[27–29] Although improved glycemic control has shown a trend towards reducing macrovascular disease, studies do not consistently support a link between serum glucose levels and risk of macrovascular disease in type 2 diabetes.[30] In one study, AGEs, high-density lipoprotein (HDL) levels, blood pressure, and other risk factors correlated with CAD risk, which, however, did not vary with progressively worsening glycemia in subjects with normal glucose tolerance, impaired fasting glucose, and diabetes mellitus.[31] Other investigators showed that prevalence of CAD did not differ in diabetic and non-diabetic subjects over 50 years old and that improved glycemic control did not reduce the macrovascular complications of diabetes.[32,33] Hence, it seems that in patients with impaired glucose tolerance and diabetes mellitus, risk factors such as dyslipidemia and hypertension have a greater impact on the incidence of macrovascular complications than glucose levels.

Dyslipidemia

Of all metabolic abnormalities in diabetes mellitus, dyslipidemia is considered the most significant promoter of atherosclerosis.[34] The dyslipidemic profile of diabetes includes elevated serum triglyceride, very low-density lipoprotein (VLDL), and LDL concentrations and reduced levels of HDL.[34] Increased hepatic lipase levels and relative insulin deficiency are thought to be responsible for elevated small dense LDL particles, that are particularly atherogenic.[35,36] On the other hand, other investigators have shown *reduced* levels of hepatic lipase in diabetes, and have shown that these may be responsible for prolonged postprandial lipemia, which has been named 'lipid intolerance' and is also atherogenic.[36,37] Finally, low HDL levels have been attributed to hypertriglyceridemia and poor glycemic control.[34,38]

Evidence from animal models for an underlying pathogenetic link between diabetic dyslipidemia and atherosclerosis is more difficult to obtain. A lack of animal models that closely resemble human disease has probably contributed to this problem.[36] Recently, a new animal model of diabetes has improved understanding of the relative contributions of hyperglycemia and dyslipidemia in diabetic atherosclerosis, suggesting that hyperglycemia initiates atherogenesis, while diabetic dyslipidemia is responsible for lesion progression.[39]

In addition to biochemical evidence, epidemiologic studies have provided further support for a link between diabetic dyslipidemia and atherosclerosis. Risk of fatal and non-fatal CAD is directly proportional to serum LDL concentration and inversely proportional to HDL concentration, even in the 'normal' range.[40] Elevated total cholesterol, hypertriglyceridemia, and low HDL cholesterol are associated with increased stroke risk in diabetic patients.[41] In contrast to improved glycemic control, therapy directed against dyslipidemia has been conclusively shown to decrease CAD events in diabetic patients with and without established CAD and to cause regression of established atherosclerosis.[42–45] Of note, dyslipidemia shows a weaker association with cerebrovascular events than with CAD events. In the United Kingdom Prospective Diabetes Study (UKPDS), dyslipidemia was not a significant predictor of diabetic stroke.[46,47] A recent study showed that elderly diabetics had the highest prevalence of dyslipidemia and were less likely to receive treatment compared to an age-matched population with normal glucose tolerance and impaired fasting glucose. In addition, treatment of dyslipidemia in diabetics was less likely to achieve target LDL levels than in subjects without diabetes mellitus.[8]

Thrombophilia

Diabetes has been recognized as a prothrombotic state, resulting from a combination of abnormal endothelial and platelet function and deregulation of the coagulation and fibrinolytic cascades. Hypercoagulability is an independent risk factor for macrovascular events in diabetics and is also likely to contribute to the pathogenesis of atherosclerosis.[48]

Numerous platelet abnormalities in patients with insulin resistance and diabetes have been described, including decreased anti-aggregating response to insulin and prostacyclin, resistance to the effects of nitrates, reduced nitric oxide synthase activity, and increased thromboxane synthesis and thromboxane receptor activity.[49–54] The net effect of these abnormalities is increased platelet activity that is likely to accelerate progression of existing atheromatous lesions.[55] Importantly, there is evidence that platelet abnormalities precede the development of vascular disease and, therefore, are unlikely to be caused by it.[55]

Alterations in coagulation factor levels also contribute to a thrombotic tendency in patients with diabetes. Fibrinogen is consistently elevated in diabetes and promotes atherogenesis.[48,56,57] Levels of clotting factors VII, VIII, XI, and XII are also elevated, while protein C, an endogenous anticoagulant, is decreased in diabetic patients.[48] Finally, changes in components of the fibrinolytic pathway have been observed in diabetes, such as increased plasminogen activator inhibitor type 1 levels, although the magnitude of this increase was less significant in diabetics with acute stroke.[48,58]

Endothelial dysfunction

A constellation of metabolic abnormalities in diabetes mellitus result in endothelial dysfunction, the first step of atherogenesis.[59] Hyperglycemia and insulin resistance result in multiple abnormalities of NO generation, degradation, and action.[59] Decreased endothelial NO levels result in release of mediators that attract leukocytes and promote subintimal migration of monocytes and smooth muscle cells, which internalize cholesterol, becoming foam cells.[60,61] Lack of NO is also responsible for decreased endothelium-derived vasodilation.[62]

Increased free fatty acid levels in diabetes also cause endothelial dysfunction, directly through reducing endothelial-mediated vasodilation, and indirectly, by increasing serum levels of atherogenic lipoproteins.[59] In addition to endothelial dysfunction resulting from abnormalities in production of and response to NO, diabetes increases levels of endothelium-derived vasoconstrictors including endothelin-1, vasoconstrictor prostanoids, and angiotensin II.[63–65]

Diabetic macrovascular disease

Coronary artery disease

In elderly men, diabetes mellitus significantly increases risk of death from CAD and reduces the chances of survival after myocardial infarction (MI).[66,67] One recent study in subjects over the age of 65 included non-diabetics and two cohorts of diabetics treated with oral hypoglycemic agents or insulin.[66] It showed that CAD mortality in diabetics treated with oral agents and insulin was 2 and 2.5 times higher than in non-diabetics, respectively.[66]

In the US, the prevalence of CAD in diabetic patients over the age of 50 years is 7.5% and increases to 19.2% in the presence of the metabolic syndrome, defined as the simultaneous presence of obesity, hyperlipidemia, diabetes, and hypertension.[32] This is clearly a key factor in the etiology of CAD in the diabetic population as only 13% of diabetics in this age group do not suffer from it.[32] The risk of MI, the most common cause of death in diabetic patients, is equivalent to that of non-diabetic subjects with a previous MI.[9,68] The combination of diabetes and previous MI

would double the risk of major cardiovascular disease, estimated at twice the risk of diabetics without a history of MI.[69]

Importantly, diabetics have a worse prognosis after unstable angina pectoris or non-Q-wave MI, while diabetes increases the risk of in-hospital MI, complications of MI, and mortality.[70] Long-term mortality after coronary events is also worse in patients with diabetes, most likely due to increased rates of heart failure and subsequent MI.[71] Thrombogenic abnormalities in diabetic patients, such as impaired fibrinolysis and increased platelet aggregation, have been blamed for worse outcomes.[68]

However, major epidemiologic studies of patients with diabetes have failed to document decreased mortality from CAD with improved glycemic control.[33,72] A possible interpretation would be that other metabolic disturbances in diabetes, and not hyperglycemia per se, are responsible for coronary atherogenesis and increased cardiovascular mortality. Although there is evidence that diabetes is a stronger risk factor for CAD in women than in men, some authors have shown that any difference is lost when other CAD risk factors are adjusted for.[73–75]

Stroke

Diabetes mellitus is estimated to cause a significant proportion of strokes, estimated at 21% by the Atherosclerosis Risk in Communities Study (ARIS). Diabetes increases stroke risk 2- to 5-fold and contributes to 16% of stroke mortality in men.[76,77] Stroke significantly contributes to the morbidity and mortality in the elderly diabetic male population. Age was an independent risk factor of diabetic stroke in the UKPDS study.[78] Stroke in people aged over 65 is second in incidence among all complications of diabetes after CAD.[79] It is uncertain whether diabetic stroke mortality is greater in men or in women.[58,80]

However, in a recent study of over 23 000 insulin-treated diabetics in the UK, males between the ages of 60 and 84 years were the only cohort in which cerebrovascular mortality rates showed no significant difference to those of the general population.[81] Another study in subjects over the age of 65 years also showed that stroke mortality was not significantly increased in diabetics and found a lower stroke incidence rate in this cohort than that reported in prior decades.[81]

Certain types of stroke seem to be more prevalent in the diabetic population. Specifically, diabetes increases the risk for ischemic but not hemorrhagic stroke.[58] Lacunar infarcts and small vessel atherosclerosis are characteristic in diabetic patients. The risk of transient ischemic attacks (TIAs) is also increased in some but not all studies.[82–85] In addition, infratentorial infarcts are more prevalent in the diabetic population, indicating more frequent atherosclerotic involvement of the vertebrobasilar circulation than in non-diabetics.[86] As with CAD, diabetes is associated with worse outcome after stroke, including disability, prolonged hospital stay, recurrence, dementia, and mortality.[58,76,87,88]

The etiology behind these observations is multifactorial. Risk factors for atherosclerosis such as hypertension and dyslipidemia are more common in diabetics than in the general population.[89] Hypertriglyceridemia and low HDL levels are common in the diabetic population and increase the risk of stroke.[90] Importantly, diabetic stroke incidence remains elevated even after correcting for these factors, indicating that diabetes is an independent risk factor for stroke.[58,91] In the UKPDS, risk factors for diabetic stroke included duration of diabetes, age, sex, smoking, systolic blood pressure, total cholesterol to HDL cholesterol ratio, and atrial fibrillation.[92] Hence, Mankovsky and Ziegler divided the risk factors for diabetic stroke into nonspecific risk factors, such as hypertension and dyslipidemia, and specific, such as hyperglycemia and insulin resistance, that could act independently or by multiplying the effects of non-specific factors.[58] Among patients with established diabetes, complications such as retinopathy, macroalbuminuria, and autonomic neuropathy are also independent risk factors for stroke.[58,93,94]

The role of hyperglycemia in stroke risk remains unclear. Impaired glucose tolerance has been shown to be a risk factor for stroke in men and in patients with subclinical cardiovascular disease, while other investigators did not find such an association.[95–97] Poor glycemic control assessed by elevated HbA1c

levels directly affects risk of stroke and stroke mortality, especially in older diabetics.[80,98,99]

Peripheral arterial disease

Diabetes mellitus causes the same 2- to 4-fold increased risk for PAD as for CAD, and accounts for significant morbidity in the elderly diabetic male population.[68] PAD results in significant disability and functional impairment in the diabetic population and is a marker for CAD and cerebrovascular disease.[100] Peripheral neuropathy caused by diabetes results in a significant increase in the risk of trauma to the feet in the diabetic population. This is simply the result of not being able to feel the object causing the trauma to the foot. Because of the poor blood supply and the anatomic changes to the diabetic foot, heeling of the ulcers caused by trauma is markedly reduced. Infection plays a significant role in these cases. The diabetic traumatized foot has a very high incidence of infection. Because of the absence of feeling, patients present late with fulminate infection that is more likely to result in massive debridement and/or amputation (Figure 33.1).

The prevalence of diabetic PAD increases with age and there is evidence that, amongst diabetics, the cohort on whom PAD has the highest impact is that of elderly males.[100] According to a recent study, diabetic men have higher rates of peripheral revascularization surgery compared to diabetic women and non-diabetic men, that also tends to occur at an older age than in the latter two patient groups.[101] In addition, there is evidence that use of health resources as a result of diabetic PAD in males is increasing.[102] US veterans with diabetes, although comprising only 16% of the veteran service population, undergo one-third of peripheral revascularization procedures and two-thirds of amputations.[102] This patient population, comprised almost exclusively of men, had rates of limb ulceration, peripheral revascularization, and amputation that increased with age.[102]

There are important differences in the epidemiology and pathophysiology of PAD in diabetic patients compared to non-diabetic subjects. PAD incidence and severity correlate with the duration of diabetes. Diabetic patients are more likely to have absent pedal pulses and symptomatic PAD

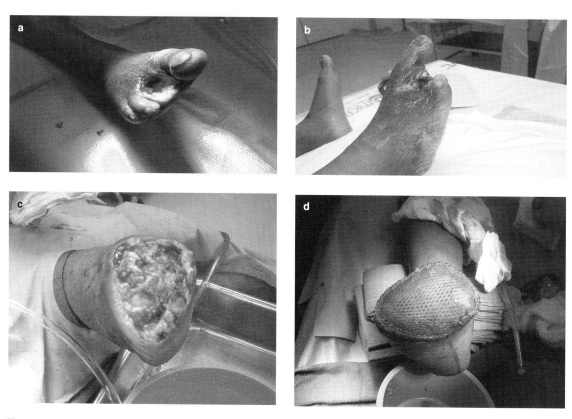

Figure 33.1 *(a) A 63-year-old diabetic patient with prior second toe amputation returned with infected third toe that requires amputation. (b) Patient returns with further infection in the amputated site. (c) Transmetatarsal amputation with revascularization. (d) Split thickness skin grafting was successful in covering the wound.*

than non-diabetic subjects.[68,103] On the other hand, some authors have suggested that reduced pain perception due to peripheral neuropathy could lead to higher rates of asymptomatic PAD and delayed patient presentation compared to non-diabetics.[101,102] This results in peripheral revascularization surgery at an older age with much more extensive disease than in non-diabetics, possibly contributing to lower limb salvage rates in this population.[101] Diabetes also changes the distribution and morphology of atherosclerotic lesions. Diabetics have increased rates of more distal tibial vessel involvement and more plaque calcification compared to non-diabetics. This leads to more complicated distal revascularization procedures. Distal bypasses historically have a much lower patency rate and significant reduction in limb salvage rates.[101–103] The

primary patency rate of above-knee bypass with a vein ranges from 60 to 70% at 5 years with a limb salvage rate of 80–90%. Distal bypass to tibial vessels with a vein has a primary patency of 40–50% at 5 years, with a limb salvage rate of 50–60%. Variables associated with higher limb loss rates include severity of neuropathy, foot ulceration, age, and HbA$_{1c}$. Postoperative complications, including infection and amputation, are also higher in the diabetic population.[101]

Perhaps as a result of these factors, diabetes significantly increases the risk of lower extremity amputation, especially in elderly patients.[104] In a recent study from Taiwan that included over 500 000 diabetics, approximately 40% of them being older than 64 years, men had a higher incidence of lower extremity amputations and peripheral revascularization procedures in all age groups.[101] In addition, the incidence of these end-points in men increased with age up to the 75–84-year-old subgroup. In men, peripheral revascularization incidence peaked in the 65–74-year-old cohort and was higher in elderly males than females, except in the > 84-year-old subjects.

Screening and prevention

The aim of screening for diabetes is to identify asymptomatic individuals who are at high risk of the disease and should receive diagnostic testing. Ideally, this would lead to early diagnosis, treatment, and prevention of diabetic complications. The American Diabetes Association recommends 3-yearly measurement of fasting plasma glucose for diabetes screening in persons over the age of 45 years, reflecting the higher prevalence of this disease with increasing age.[105] Since there is no proven benefit of improved glycemic control in reducing the macrovascular complications of diabetes, the goal of early diagnosis is aggressive treatment of other risk factors for atherosclerosis such as hypercholesterolemia and hypertension.

The American Heart Association (AHA) considers diabetics to be at the same level of risk for CAD as people with established CAD, with obvious implications for risk factor modification.[5] In 2004, the AHA reviewed recommendations for screening asymptomatic diabetic patients for CAD and concluded that, in the absence of relevant clinical trial data, no indication for stress testing or measurement of biochemical markers of CAD can be made.[5] Lack of data in diabetic patients seems to plague other modalities suggested for use in screening for CAD such as ankle-brachial pressure index (ABI) measurements and B-mode ultrasound measurement of carotid intima-media thickness (IMT).

Despite lacking an established role in the estimation of CAD mortality, ABI measurements may aid in detection of subclinical PAD in high-risk populations such as the elderly and patients with diabetes.[106] In its consensus statement on diabetic PAD, the American Diabetes Association recommended the use of ABI as a screening test for PAD

in all diabetic patients over the age of 50 years.[107] The ABI is simple and easy to perform, but can be falsely elevated in patients with calcified vessels, such as elderly diabetics.[107] Toe pressure should be measured during ABI because it would give a more accurate idea of the severity of PAD in diabetic patients. A normal toe-brachial index (TBI) is 0.75.

There is evidence that implementing amputation prevention programs in diabetic patients, including screening for PAD, is both cost-effective and can decrease amputation rates.[108,109]

Patient education is crucial. The physician should alert his diabetic patients with absent pedal pulses or abnormal TBI to the higher incidence of ulceration and tissue loss. Careful podiatry care is highly recommended. Specially fitted diabetic shoes are always a simple but great tool to reduce the incidence of complications. A diabetic patient should never walk bare footed. Since many of these patients are not aware of having an ulcer on the sole of their foot, wearing white socks would alert the patient if any drainage is present. Patients should be educated to promptly see their physician if a new ulcer or drainage is present. Poor glucose control in a patient who had prior good control should alert the patient and physician to possible foot infection in the presence of an ulcer. Early vascular consultation in symptomatic patients with claudication, rest pain, and/or tissue loss is very helpful. The extent of foot infection is always underestimated in diabetic patients (Figure 33.2). An opinion from a vascular surgeon about their care would be valuable in this patient population.

Conclusions

The macrovascular complications of diabetes are a major source of morbidity and mortality in elderly patients. Despite the absence of an established benefit of improved hyperglycemia on macrovascular risk reduction, there is strong evidence for a role of hyperglycemia in the pathogenesis of diabetic atherosclerosis. On the other hand, modification of other risk factors associated with hyperglycemia, such as hypertension and hyperlipidemia, has been shown to significantly reduce the incidence of MI, stroke, and

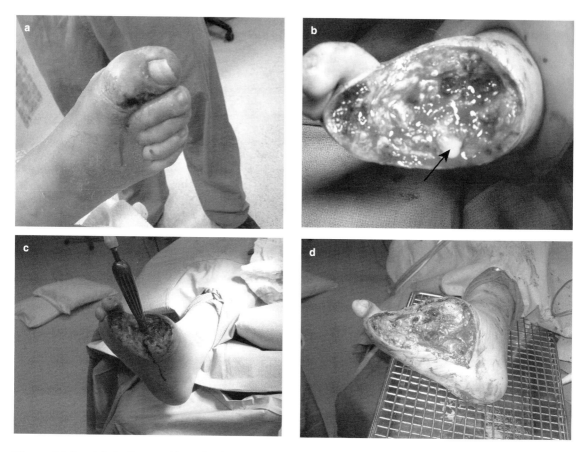

Figure 33.2 *(a) A 48-year-old insulin-dependent diabetic presented with infected foot, sepsis, hypotension, and glucose of 460 mg/dl. (b) Purulent discharge at the planter fascia (arrow). (c) Suction tip inserted in the abscess cavity, demonstrating the extension of the infection (this was underestimated pre-operatively). (d) This patient's foot required four additional debridements and finally a Chopart's amputation, preserving his heel.*

PAD in diabetic patients, especially including the elderly. Importantly, only a small minority of elderly diabetics are receiving adequate treatment and prevention. Physicians have a significant role in improving the macrovascular outcome and reducing the complications in this patient population.[8]

References

1. Zimmet P, Alberti KG, Shaw J. Global and societal implications of the diabetes epidemic. Nature 2001; 414(6865): 782–7.
2. Harris MI, Flegal KM, Cowie CC et al. Prevalence of diabetes, impaired fasting glucose, and impaired glucose tolerance in U.S. adults. The Third National Health and Nutrition Examination Survey, 1988–1994. Diabetes Care 1998; 21(4): 518–24.
3. Smith NL, Heckbert SR, Bittner VA et al. Antidiabetic treatment trends in a cohort of elderly people with diabetes. The Cardiovascular Health Study, 1989–1997. Diabetes Care 1999; 22(5): 736–42.
4. DECODE Study Group, the European Diabetes Epidemiology Group. Glucose tolerance and cardiovascular mortality: comparison of fasting and 2-hour diagnostic criteria. Arch Intern Med 2001; 161(3): 397–405.
5. Redberg RF, Greenland P, Fuster V et al. Prevention Conference VI: Diabetes and Cardiovascular Disease: Writing Group III: risk assessment in persons with diabetes. Circulation 2002; 105(18): e144–52.

6. Jorgensen H, Nakayama H, Raaschou HO, Olsen TS. Stroke in patients with diabetes. The Copenhagen Stroke Study. Stroke 1994; 25(10): 1977–84.

7. Adler AI, Stratton IM, Neil HA et al. Association of systolic blood pressure with macrovascular and microvascular complications of type 2 diabetes (UKPDS 36): prospective observational study. BMJ 2000; 321(7258): 412–19.

8. Smith NL, Savage PJ, Heckbert SR et al. Glucose, blood pressure, and lipid control in older people with and without diabetes mellitus: the Cardiovascular Health Study. J Am Geriatr Soc 2002; 50(3): 416–23.

9. Wu KK, Huan Y. Diabetic atherosclerosis mouse models. Atherosclerosis 2007; 191(2): 241–9.

10. Goldberg IJ. Why does diabetes increase atherosclerosis? I don't know! J Clin Invest 2004; 114(5): 613–15.

11. Grundy SM, Howard B, Smith S et al. Prevention Conference VI: Diabetes and Cardiovascular Disease: executive summary: conference proceeding for healthcare professionals from a special writing group of the American Heart Association. Circulation 2002; 105(18): 2231–9.

12. Duffy A, Liew A, O'Sullivan J et al. Distinct effects of high-glucose conditions on endothelial cells of macrovascular and microvascular origins. Endothelium 2006; 13(1): 9–16.

13. Hammes HP. Pathophysiological mechanisms of diabetic angiopathy. J Diabetes Complic 2003; 17(2 Suppl): 16–19.

14. Smith NL, Barzilay JI, Kronmal R et al. New-onset diabetes and risk of all-cause and cardiovascular mortality: the Cardiovascular Health Study. Diabetes Care 2006; 29(9): 2012–17.

15. Schmidt AM, Hori O, Brett J et al. Cellular receptors for advanced glycation end products. Implications for induction of oxidant stress and cellular dysfunction in the pathogenesis of vascular lesions. Arterioscler Thromb 1994; 14(10): 1521–8.

16. Singh R, Barden A, Mori T, Beilin L. Advanced glycation end-products: a review. Diabetologia 2001; 44(2): 129–46.

17. Goldin A, Beckman JA, Schmidt AM, Creager MA. Advanced glycation end products: sparking the development of diabetic vascular injury. Circulation 2006; 114(6): 597–605.

18. Brownlee M. Advanced protein glycosylation in diabetes and aging. Annu Rev Med 1995; 46: 223–34.

19. Wautier MP, Chappey O, Corda S et al. Activation of NADPH oxidase by AGE links oxidant stress to altered gene expression via RAGE. Am J Physiol Endocrinol Metab 2001; 280(5): E685–94.

20. Bucala R, Makita Z, Vega G et al. Modification of low density lipoprotein by advanced glycation end products contributes to the dyslipidemia of diabetes and renal insufficiency. Proc Natl Acad Sci USA 1994; 91(20): 9441–5.

21. Posch K, Simecek S, Wascher TC et al. Glycated low-density lipoprotein attenuates shear stress-induced nitric oxide synthesis by inhibition of shear stress-activated l-arginine uptake in endothelial cells. Diabetes 1999; 48(6): 1331–7.

22. Bucala R, Tracey KJ, Cerami A. Advanced glycosylation products quench nitric oxide and mediate defective endothelium-dependent vasodilatation in experimental diabetes. J Clin Invest 1991; 87(2): 432–8.

23. Hogan M, Cerami A, Bucala R. Advanced glycosylation endproducts block the antiproliferative effect of nitric oxide. Role in the vascular and renal complications of diabetes mellitus. J Clin Invest 1992; 90(3): 1110–15.

24. Iwashima Y, Eto M, Hata A et al. Advanced glycation end products-induced gene expression of scavenger receptors in cultured human monocyte-derived macrophages. Biochem Biophys Res Commun 2000; 277(2): 368–80.

25. Edelstein D, Brownlee M. Mechanistic studies of advanced glycosylation end product inhibition by aminoguanidine. Diabetes 1992; 41(1): 26–9.

26. Bierhaus A, Illmer T, Kasper M et al. Advanced glycation end product (AGE)-mediated induction of tissue factor in cultured endothelial cells is dependent on RAGE. Circulation 1997; 96(7): 2262–71.

27. Smith NL, Barzilay JI, Shaffer D et al. Fasting and 2-hour postchallenge serum glucose measures and risk of incident cardiovascular events in the elderly: the Cardiovascular Health Study. Arch Intern Med 2002; 162(2): 209–16.

28. Levitan EB, Song Y, Ford ES, Liu S. Is nondiabetic hyperglycemia a risk factor for cardiovascular disease? A meta-analysis of prospective studies. Arch Intern Med 2004; 164(19): 2147–55.

29. Sasso FC, Carbonara O, Nasti R et al. Glucose metabolism and coronary heart disease in patients with normal glucose tolerance. JAMA 2004; 291(15): 1857–63.

30. Schneider CA. Improving macrovascular outcomes in type 2 diabetes: outcome studies in cardiovascular risk and metabolic control. Curr Med Res Opin 2006; 22(Suppl 2): S15–26.

31. Alexander CM, Landsman PB, Teutsch SM. Diabetes mellitus, impaired fasting glucose, atherosclerotic risk factors, and prevalence of coronary heart disease. Am J Cardiol 2000; 86(9): 897–902.

32. Alexander CM, Landsman PB, Teutsch SM, Haffner SM. NCEP-defined metabolic syndrome, diabetes, and prevalence of coronary heart disease among NHANES III participants age 50 years and older. Diabetes 2003; 52(5): 1210–14.

33. UK Prospective Diabetes Study (UKPDS) Group. Intensive blood-glucose control with sulphonylureas or insulin compared with conventional treatment and risk of complications in patients with type 2 diabetes (UKPDS 33). Lancet 1998; 352(9131): 837–53.

34. Taskinen MR. Diabetic dyslipidemia. Atheroscler Suppl 2002; 3(1): 47–51.

35. Syvänne M, Taskinen M-R. Lipids and lipoproteins as coronary risk factors in non-insulin-dependent diabetes mellitus. Lancet 1997; 350(Suppl 1): S20–3.

36. Goldberg IJ. Clinical review 124: Diabetic dyslipidemia: causes and consequences. J Clin Endocrinol Metab 2001; 86(3): 965–71.

37. Taskinen MR. Pathogenesis of dyslipidemia in type 2 diabetes. Exp Clin Endocrinol Diabetes 2001; 109(Suppl 2): S180–8.

38. Drexel H, Aczel S, Marte T et al. Is atherosclerosis in diabetes and impaired fasting glucose driven by elevated LDL cholesterol or by decreased HDL cholesterol? Diabetes Care 2005; 28(1): 101–7.

39. Renard CB, Kramer F, Johansson F et al. Diabetes and diabetes-associated lipid abnormalities have distinct effects on initiation and progression of atherosclerotic lesions. J Clin Invest 2004; 114(5): 659–68.

40. Howard BV, Cowan LD, Go O et al. Adverse effects of diabetes on multiple cardiovascular disease risk factors in women. The Strong Heart Study. Diabetes Care 1998; 21(8): 1258–65.

41. Lehto S, Ronnemaa T, Pyorala K, Laakso M. Predictors of stroke in middle-aged patients with non-insulin-dependent diabetes. Stroke 1996; 27(1): 63–8.

42. Colhoun HM, Betteridge DJ, Durrington PN et al. Primary prevention of cardiovascular disease with atorvastatin in type 2 diabetes in the Collaborative Atorvastatin Diabetes Study (CARDS): multicentre randomised placebo-controlled trial. Lancet 2004; 364(9435): 685–96.

43. Shepherd J, Barter P, Carmena R et al. Effect of lowering LDL cholesterol substantially below currently recommended levels in patients with coronary heart disease and diabetes: the Treating to New Targets (TNT) study. Diabetes Care 2006; 29(6): 1220–6.

44. Haffner SM, Alexander CM, Cook TJ et al. Reduced coronary events in simvastatin-treated patients with coronary heart disease and diabetes or impaired fasting glucose levels: subgroup analyses in the Scandinavian Simvastatin Survival Study. Arch Intern Med 1999; 159(22): 2661–7.

45. Nissen SE, Nicholls SJ, Sipahi I et al. Effect of very high-intensity statin therapy on regression of coronary atherosclerosis: the ASTEROID trial. JAMA 2006; 295(13): 1556–65.

46. Niskanen L, Turpeinen A, Penttila I, Uusitupa MI. Hyperglycemia and compositional lipoprotein abnormalities as predictors of cardiovascular mortality in type 2 diabetes: a 15-year follow-up from the time of diagnosis. Diabetes Care 1998; 21(11): 1861–9.

47. Davis TM, Millns H, Stratton IM, Holman RR, Turner RC. Risk factors for stroke in type 2 diabetes mellitus: United Kingdom Prospective Diabetes Study (UKPDS) 29. Arch Intern Med 1999; 159(10): 1097–103.

48. Carr ME. Diabetes mellitus: a hypercoagulable state. J Diabetes Complic 2001; 15(1): 44–54.

49. Trovati M, Mularoni EM, Burzacca S et al. Impaired insulin-induced platelet antiaggregating effect in obesity and in obese NIDDM patients. Diabetes 1995; 44(11): 1318–22.

50. Kahn NN, Bauman WA, Hatcher VB, Sinha AK. Inhibition of platelet aggregation and the stimulation of prostacyclin synthesis by insulin in humans. Am J Physiol 1993; 265(6 Pt 2): H2160–7.

51. Collier A, Tymkewycz P, Armstrong R et al. Increased platelet thromboxane receptor sensitivity in diabetic patients with proliferative retinopathy. Diabetologia 1986; 29(8): 471–4.

52. Martina V, Bruno GA, Trucco F et al. Platelet cNOS activity is reduced in patients with IDDM and NIDDM. Thromb Haemost 1998; 79(3): 520–2.

53. Anfossi G, Mularoni EM, Burzacca S et al. Platelet resistance to nitrates in obesity and obese NIDDM, and normal platelet sensitivity to both insulin and nitrates in lean NIDDM. Diabetes Care 1998; 21(1): 121–6.

54. Davi G, Catalano I, Averna M et al. Thromboxane biosynthesis and platelet function in type II diabetes mellitus. N Engl J Med 1990; 322(25): 1769–74.

55. Vinik AI, Erbas T, Park TS, Nolan R, Pittenger GL. Platelet dysfunction in type 2 diabetes. Diabetes Care 2001; 24(8): 1476–85.

56. Corrado E, Rizzo M, Muratori I, Coppola G, Novo S. Association of elevated fibrinogen and C-reactive protein levels with carotid lesions in patients with newly diagnosed hypertension or type II diabetes. Arch Med Res 2006; 37(8): 1004–9.

57. Coppola G, Corrado E, Muratori I et al. Increased levels of C-reactive protein and fibrinogen influence the risk of vascular events in patients with NIDDM. Int J Cardiol 2006; 106(1): 16–20.

58. Mankovsky BN, Ziegler D. Stroke in patients with diabetes mellitus. Diabetes Metab Res Rev 2004; 20(4): 268–87.

59. Luscher TF, Creager MA, Beckman JA, Cosentino F. Diabetes and vascular disease: pathophysiology, clinical consequences, and medical therapy: Part II. Circulation 2003; 108(13): 1655–61.

60. Zeiher AM, Fisslthaler B, Schray-Utz B, Busse R. Nitric oxide modulates the expression of monocyte

chemoattractant protein 1 in cultured human endothelial cells. Circ Res 1995; 76(6): 980–6.

61. Nomura S, Shouzu A, Omoto S, Nishikawa M, Fukuhara S. Significance of chemokines and activated platelets in patients with diabetes. Clin Exp Immunol 2000; 121(3): 437–43.

62. Williams SB, Cusco JA, Roddy MA, Johnstone MT, Creager MA. Impaired nitric oxide-mediated vasodilation in patients with non-insulin-dependent diabetes mellitus. J Am Coll Cardiol 1996; 27(3): 567–74.

63. Quehenberger P, Bierhaus A, Fasching P et al. Endothelin 1 transcription is controlled by nuclear factor-kappa in AGE-stimulated cultured endothelial cells. Diabetes 2000; 49(9): 1561–70.

64. Christlieb AR, Janka HU, Kraus B et al. Vascular reactivity to angiotensin II and to norepinephrine in diabetic subjects. Diabetes 1976; 25(4): 268–74.

65. Tesfamariam B, Brown ML, Deykin D, Cohen RA. Elevated glucose promotes generation of endothelium-derived vasoconstrictor prostanoids in rabbit aorta. J Clin Invest 1990; 85(3): 929–32.

66. Kronmal RA, Barzilay JI, Smith NL et al. Mortality in pharmacologically treated older adults with diabetes: the Cardiovascular Health Study, 1989–2001. Public Library of Science Med 2006; 3(10): e400.

67. Wannamethee SG, Shaper AG, Lennon L. Cardiovascular disease incidence and mortality in older men with diabetes and in men with coronary heart disease. Heart 2004; 90(12): 1398–403.

68. Beckman JA, Creager MA, Libby P. Diabetes and atherosclerosis: epidemiology, pathophysiology, and management. JAMA 2002; 287(19): 2570–81.

69. Haffner SM, Lehto S, Ronnemaa T, Pyorala K, Laakso M. Mortality from coronary heart disease in subjects with type 2 diabetes and in nondiabetic subjects with and without prior myocardial infarction. N Engl J Med 1998; 339(4): 229–34.

70. Kjaergaard SC, Hansen HH, Fog L, Bulow I, Christensen PD. In-hospital outcome for diabetic patients with acute myocardial infarction in the thrombolytic era. Scand Cardiovasc J 1999; 33(3): 166–70.

71. Malmberg K, Yusuf S, Gerstein HC et al. Impact of diabetes on long-term prognosis in patients with unstable angina and non-Q-wave myocardial infarction: results of the OASIS (Organization to Assess Strategies for Ischemic Syndromes) Registry. Circulation 2000; 102(9): 1014–19.

72. Effect of intensive diabetes management on macrovascular events and risk factors in the Diabetes Control and Complications Trial (DCCT) Research Group. Am J Cardiol 1995; 75(14): 894–903.

73. Lee WL, Cheung AM, Cape DC, Zinman B. Impact of diabetes on coronary artery disease in women and men. A meta-analysis of prospective studies. Diabetes Care 2000; 23: 962–8.

74. Kanaya AM, Grady D, Barrett-Connor E. Explaining the sex difference in coronary heart disease mortality among patients with type 2 diabetes mellitus: a meta-analysis. Arch Intern Med 2002; 162(15): 1737–45.

75. Huxley R, Barzi F, Woodward M. Excess risk of fatal coronary heart disease associated with diabetes in men and women: meta-analysis of 37 prospective cohort studies. BMJ 2006; 332(7533): 73–8.

76. Tuomilehto J, Rastenyte D, Jousilahti P, Sarti C, Vartiainen E. Diabetes mellitus as a risk factor for death from stroke. Prospective study of the middle-aged Finnish population. Stroke 1996; 27(2): 210–15.

77. Stamler J, Vaccaro O, Neaton J, Wentworth D. Diabetes, other risk factors, and 12-yr cardiovascular mortality for men screened in the Multiple Risk Factor Intervention Trial. Diabetes Care 1993; 16: 434–44.

78. Kothari V, Stevens RJ, Adler AI et al. UKPDS 60: risk of stroke in type 2 diabetes estimated by the UK Prospective Diabetes Study risk engine. Stroke 2002; 33(7): 1776–81.

79. Bertoni AG, Krop JS, Anderson GF, Brancati FL. Diabetes-related morbidity and mortality in a national sample of U.S. elders. Diabetes Care 2002; 25(3): 471–5.

80. Sasaki A, Horiuchi N, Hasegawa K, Uehara M. Mortality from coronary heart disease and cerebrovascular disease and associated risk factors in diabetic patients in Osaka District, Japan. Diabetes Res Clin Pract 1995; 27(1): 77–83.

81. Laing SP, Swerdlow AJ, Carpenter LM et al. Mortality from cerebrovascular disease in a cohort of 23 000 patients with insulin-treated diabetes. Stroke 2003; 34(2): 418–21.

82. Grau AJ, Weimar C, Buggle F et al. Risk factors, outcome, and treatment in subtypes of ischemic stroke: the German stroke data bank. Stroke 2001; 32(11): 2559–66.

83. Gandolfo C, Caponnetto C, Del Sette M, Santoloci D, Loeb C. Risk factors in lacunar syndromes: a case-control study. Acta Neurol Scand 1988; 77(1): 22–6.

84. Fritz VU, Bilchik T, Levien LJ. Diabetes as risk factor for transient ischaemic attacks as opposed to strokes. Eur J Vasc Surg 1987; 1(4): 259–62.

85. Palumbo PJ, Elveback LR, Whisnant JP. Neurologic American Diabetes Association complications of diabetes mellitus: transient ischemic attack, stroke, and peripheral neuropathy. Adv Neurol 1978; 19: 593–601.

86. Iwase M, Yamamoto M, Yoshinari M, Ibayashi S, Fujishima M. Stroke topography in diabetic and nondiabetic patients by magnetic resonance imaging. Diabetes Res Clin Pract 1998; 42(2): 109–16.

87. Luchsinger JA, Tang MX, Stern Y, Shea S, Mayeux R. Diabetes mellitus and risk of Alzheimer's disease

and dementia with stroke in a multiethnic cohort. Am J Epidemiol 2001; 154(7): 635–41.

88. Hankey GJ, Jamrozik K, Broadhurst RJ et al. Long-term risk of first recurrent stroke in the Perth Community Stroke Study. Stroke 1998; 29(12): 2491–500.

89. Stegmayr B, Asplund K. Diabetes as a risk factor for stroke. A population perspective. Diabetologia 1995; 38(9): 1061–8.

90. Pujia A, Gnasso A, Irace C, Colonna A, Mattioli PL. Common carotid arterial wall thickness in NIDDM subjects. Diabetes Care 1994; 17(11): 1330–6.

91. Folsom AR, Rasmussen ML, Chambless LE et al. Prospective associations of fasting insulin, body fat distribution, and diabetes with risk of ischemic stroke. The Atherosclerosis Risk in Communities (ARIC) Study Investigators. Diabetes Care 1999; 22(7): 1077–83.

92. Colagiuri S, Cull CA, Holman RR. Are lower fasting plasma glucose levels at diagnosis of type 2 diabetes associated with improved outcomes?: U.K. prospective diabetes study 61. Diabetes Care 2002; 25(8): 1410–17.

93. Petitti DB, Bhatt H. Retinopathy as a risk factor for nonembolic stroke in diabetic subjects. Stroke 1995; 26(4): 593–6.

94. Fushimi H, Kubo M, Inoue T et al. Peripheral vascular reactions to smoking – profound vasoconstriction by atherosclerosis. Diabetes Res Clin Pract 1998; 42(1): 29–34.

95. Fuller J, Shipley M, Rose G, Jarrett R, Keen H. Mortality from coronary heart disease and stroke in relation to degree of glycaemia: the Whitehall study. BMJ 1983; 287: 867–70.

96. Qureshi AI, Giles WH, Croft JB. Impaired glucose tolerance and the likelihood of nonfatal stroke and myocardial infarction: the Third National Health and Nutrition Examination Survey. Stroke 1998; 29(7): 1329–32.

97. Kuller LH, Velentgas P, Barzilay J et al. Diabetes mellitus: subclinical cardiovascular disease and risk of incident cardiovascular disease and all-cause mortality. Arterioscler Thromb Vasc Biol 2000; 20(3): 823–9.

98. Miettinen H, Haffner SM, Lehto S, Ronnemaa T, Pyorala K, Laakso M. Proteinuria predicts stroke and other atherosclerotic vascular disease events in nondiabetic and non-insulin-dependent diabetic subjects. Stroke 1996; 27(11): 2033–9.

99. Moss SE, Klein R, Klein BE, Meuer SM. The association of glycemia and cause-specific mortality in a diabetic population. Arch Intern Med 1994; 154(21): 2473–9.

100. Marso SP, Hiatt WR. Peripheral arterial disease in patients with diabetes. J Am Coll Cardiol 2006; 47(5): 921–9.

101. Chen HF, Ho CA, Li CY. Age and sex may significantly interact with diabetes on the risks of lower-extremity amputation and peripheral revascularization procedures: evidence from a cohort of a half-million diabetic patients. Diabetes Care 2006; 29(11): 2409–14.

102. Mayfield JA, Reiber GE, Maynard C, Czerniecki J, Sangeorzan B. The epidemiology of lower-extremity disease in veterans with diabetes. Diabetes Care 2004; 27(Suppl 2): B39–44.

103. Jude EB, Oyibo SO, Chalmers N, Boulton AJ. Peripheral arterial disease in diabetic and nondiabetic patients: a comparison of severity and outcome. Diabetes Care 2001; 24(8): 1433–7.

104. Centers for Disease Control and Prevention (CDC) Diabetes-related amputations of lower extremities in the Medicare population – Minnesota, Centers for Disease Control and Prevention (CDC), and 1993–1995. Morb Mortal Wkly Rep 1998; 47(31): 649–52.

105. American Diabetes Association. Standards of medical care in diabetes – 2006. American Diabetes Association Diabetes Care 2006; 29(Suppl 1): S4–42.

106. Smith SC Jr, Greenland P, Grundy SM. AHA Conference Proceedings. Prevention conference V: Beyond secondary prevention: Identifying the high-risk patient for primary prevention: executive summary. American Heart Association. Circulation 2000; 101(1): 111–16.

107. American Diabetes Association. Peripheral arterial disease in people with diabetes. Diabetes Care 2003; 26(12): 3333–41.

108. Lavery LA, Wunderlich RP, Tredwell JL. Disease management for the diabetic foot: effectiveness of a diabetic foot prevention program to reduce amputations and hospitalizations. Diabetes Res Clin Pract 2005; 70(1): 31–7.

109. Ragnarson Tennvall G, Apelqvist J. Prevention of diabetes-related foot ulcers and amputations: a cost-utility analysis based on Markov model simulations. Diabetologia 2001; 44(11): 2077–87.

CHAPTER 34

Upper gastrointestinal complaints

Christopher K Rayner and Michael Horowitz

Introduction

The motor, secretory, and absorptive functions of the upper gastrointestinal tract remain remarkably intact with healthy aging, although aging is associated with an increase in comorbidities that affect the gut, including the use of medications with adverse gastrointestinal effects, and neoplastic disorders. In contrast to the relative preservation of motor and secretory function, visceral perception diminishes even with healthy aging, possibly as a result of neuronal loss in the myenteric plexus.

This chapter summarizes the changes in upper gastrointestinal physiology that occur with healthy aging, followed by discussion of specific upper gut disorders that are of relevance to the aging male. The focus is on the esophagus, stomach, and small intestine, since the oropharynx, hepatobiliary system, pancreas, and large bowel are discussed elsewhere. Most studies of gut function in the healthy elderly have included both males and females, and do not differentiate between the genders. Most of the upper gastrointestinal disorders discussed affect both men and women, although men are disproportionately prone to the complications of gastroesophageal reflux disease (GERD), including Barrett's esophagus and esophageal adenocarcinoma.

Physiologic changes in the aging upper gastrointestinal tract (Table 34.1)

Control of upper gut function

Patterns of contractions involving the circular and longitudinal layers of smooth muscle that extend throughout the gut are coordinated by plexuses of nerves within the gut wall known as the enteric nervous system, which contains an equivalent number of neurons (about 100 million) to the spinal cord.[1] Basic reflex contractile activity, such as that induced by distension, is controlled by the enteric nervous system, but these intrinsic patterns of motility can be modulated by extrinsic neural and humoral signals, including central input conveyed by sympathetic and parasympathetic nerves. Gut sensation is also conveyed to higher centers by both the vagus and spinal afferent nerves, while descending pathways to the spinal cord have the capacity to modulate the transmission of these signals.

Rodent models of aging have demonstrated a substantial reduction in the number of neurons in the enteric nervous system, with about 40% loss in the small intestine and 60% in the colon;[2] comparable neuronal loss is evident in both the esophagus and colon of aging humans. There is comparatively little information as to which neurons are most susceptible, but if the central nervous system is any

Table 34.1 *Changes in upper gastrointestinal physiology with healthy aging*

	Motor function	Sensory function	Secretory function
Esophagus	• More simultaneous contractions • Increased distal but decreased proximal amplitude • Decreased compliance • Secondary peristalsis more difficult to elicit • Impaired acid clearance	• Increased threshold for perception of distension	• Reduced flow of saliva, contributing to impaired acid clearance
Stomach	• Modest delay in emptying • Delayed proximal gastric meal accommodation • Postprandial antral distension	• Reduced perception of proximal gastric distension	• Intact acid secretion • Reduced pepsin and bicarbonate secretion
Small intestine	• Slower propagation of phase III of the MMC • Increase in propagated, clustered contractions • Rate of transit unchanged	• Increased satiation in response to glucose	• Increased CCK release in response to nutrients

guide, it may be anticipated that the loss is selective, rather than global. Indeed, rodents demonstrate preferential loss of sensory neurons, which could result in impairment of stimulus-evoked motor responses. Cholinergic neurons, which serve a range of functions, appear most vulnerable, whereas nitrergic neurons, which mediate inhibitory motor responses, seem to be relatively preserved.[3] Furthermore, the number of vagal fibers innervating the upper gastrointestinal tract does not appear to decline in aging rats. Understanding of the changes in neural control of gut function with age is limited by the relative lack of studies relating to the upper gut, and the paucity of human data.

The fact that gastrointestinal motility is relatively well preserved in the healthy elderly despite apparent substantial neuronal loss suggests that the large number of neurons in the enteric nervous system provides a considerable functional reserve.

Nevertheless, while the rate of upper gut transit appears similar in the healthy elderly and the young, colonic transit is slower in the elderly, where the loss of enteric neurons is greatest.[4] Furthermore, selective loss of intrinsic sensory neurons in the esophagus could explain why the contractile response to distension (so-called 'secondary peristalsis') is elicited less readily in the healthy elderly than the young.[5]

In contrast to the relative preservation of gut motility with aging, gastrointestinal sensation appears to be significantly impaired. In the healthy elderly, the perception of balloon distension in the esophagus,[6] stomach,[7] and rectum[8] is diminished when compared to young adults. Perception of chemical stimuli applied to the esophageal mucosa, such as acid, also decreases with age,[9] suggesting a generalized impairment of gut sensation. As indicated, selective loss of sensory neurons from the enteric nervous system could be responsible, but altered central processing may also contribute, given that the amplitude of brain evoked potentials recorded from scalp electrodes during repeated esophageal distension in older subjects is lower than in the young.[10]

Esophageal function

There are several patterns of esophageal motor activity. 'Primary peristalsis' refers to the coordinated sequence of contraction associated with swallowing, which is propagated aborally, and associated with lower esophageal sphincter (LES) relaxation to allow the swallowed bolus to pass through to the stomach. 'Secondary peristalsis', triggered by distension or reflux of gastric contents, serves to clear the esophagus of acid and bile. 'Tertiary contractions' comprise spontaneous, uncoordinated esophageal motor activity. Both tonic contraction of the LES and its position within the diaphragmatic hiatus provide a barrier to the reflux of gastric contents, although gastric distension, particularly after a meal, triggers transient sphincter relaxations that allow reflux to occur, and these relaxations, rather than low basal LES pressure, represent the most prevalent mechanism of acid reflux in most patients with GERD. Neutralization of acid by saliva, and clearance of refluxate by primary and secondary peristalsis, are important defense mechanisms against gastroesophageal reflux.

The effects of aging have been studied more extensively in the esophagus than any other gastrointestinal region, because it is easily accessible for in vivo studies, and swallowing disorders are relatively prevalent in the elderly. The term 'presbyesophagus' was derived from an early report of radiologic and manometric observations in a group of nonagenarians.[11] Only 2 of 15 subjects had 'normal' esophageal motility, and the barium swallow was characterized by a high prevalence of tertiary contractions, delayed clearance, and esophageal dilatation. Manometric findings included multi-peaked, non-peristaltic pressure waves. However, the subjects in this study had a high prevalence of dementia and other chronic illnesses, and were, accordingly, not representative of the healthy elderly. However, other reports have documented

that esophageal motility is frequently disordered in the very old,[12] whereas subjects less than 80 years of age exhibit little difference in primary peristalsis when compared to the young, albeit with a greater prevalence of simultaneous contractions. The effect of aging on the amplitude of esophageal pressure waves appears to vary by site, with an increase in distal esophageal amplitudes, but decreased amplitude in the proximal esophagus, although the magnitude of these changes is modest.[13] Secondary peristalsis is elicited less consistently by esophageal distension in the healthy elderly compared to the young,[5] both altered biomechanics (increased esophageal stiffness) and impaired sensation (increased threshold for perception of distension) could contribute to this phenomenon.[14]

In the healthy elderly, both the length of the high-pressure zone that constitutes the upper esophageal sphincter (UES) and its resting pressure are less than in the young, but relaxation of this sphincter is delayed,[15] resulting in a prolonged oropharyngeal phase of swallowing, and higher intrabolus pressures in the hypopharynx. In healthy aging, these changes are unlikely to be clinically significant, but should be taken into account when determining an appropriate 'normal range' for swallowing studies in older patients. Reflex UES responses to esophageal stimuli (increased pressure with esophageal balloon distension, and decreased pressure with air distension) remain intact with healthy aging, but reflex UES contraction in response to laryngeal stimulation is impaired,[16] and may predispose to aspiration.

Both the length of the LES and its resting pressure remain intact in the healthy elderly, although the prevalence of hiatus hernia increases with age (around 60% in those over 60 years),[17] and could contribute to GERD. Other predisposing factors include reduced flow of saliva and impaired clearance of acid, which are likely to be important, as the duration of reflux episodes appears to be more prolonged in the elderly than the young, even though their frequency is similar.[18] The frequency of transient LES relaxations has not been specifically studied in the elderly, nor have differences in mucosal repair mechanisms. Despite the impairment of acid clearance, reports relating to total acid exposure are inconsistent, possibly because of variations in the proportion of elderly with atropic gastritis and acid hyposecretion between studies. Even weakly acidic reflux may be important in mucosal injury (e.g. Barrett's mucosa) due to the presence of bile, but this has not been studied specifically in relation to age.[19]

Gastric function

While gastric emptying is only modestly delayed with healthy aging, the perception of gastric distension and the release of gut peptides in response to small intestinal nutrient exposure differ markedly from the young; both could contribute to the 'anorexia of aging', which entails a reduction in nutrient intake out of proportion to declining needs, and represents a major cause of morbidity in the elderly.[20] Furthermore, both the rate of gastric emptying and the small intestinal response to ingested nutrient affect the postprandial fall in blood pressure; therefore postprandial hypotension, which is an important cause of syncope and falls in the elderly,[21] can be regarded in the broadest sense as a gastrointestinal disorder.

The rate of gastric emptying is determined by the coordinated motor activity of proximal and distal gastric regions, under feedback control from neural and humoral signals generated by the interaction of nutrients with the small intestine, which results in the delivery of nutrients from the stomach at a relatively constant rate.[22] The proximal stomach relaxes to accommodate ingested food and fluids, and generates tonic pressure to assist the emptying of liquids, while the distal stomach grinds and mixes ingesta, and pumps chyme across the pylorus in a pulsatile manner; both phasic and tonic pyloric contractions can act as a brake to gastric outflow. The degree of small intestinal feedback can be modulated by previous patterns of nutrient intake, so that gastric emptying is retarded in starvation, and accelerated after dietary glucose supplementation.

Gastric emptying can be measured by scintigraphy, which remains the 'gold standard', and the use of two isotopes allows the behavior of both solids and liquids to be studied concurrently. Furthermore, by defining 'regions of interest' within the stomach, retention in the proximal and distal stomach can also be evaluated. Ultrasound and stable isotope

breath tests are alternative methods of measuring gastric emptying, while manometry allows the frequency, amplitude, and organization of pressures in the antrum, pylorus, and duodenum to be recorded, predominantly in the research setting. The tonic response of the proximal stomach to a meal can be evaluated for research purposes by means of the electronic barostat, which measures the volume of air required to maintain a fixed pressure in an intragastric bag as an index of proximal gastric tone.

In healthy aging, there is a modest slowing of gastric emptying of both solids and nutrient liquids, but in most cases the rate of emptying remains within the normal range for young adults[23–25] (Figure 34.1). This relative slowing of gastric emptying may have implications for appetite regulation, potentially contributing to the 'anorexia of aging' by prolonging both gastric distension and the exposure of the small intestine to the satiating effects of nutrients. Furthermore, slower gastric emptying could delay the absorption of orally administered medications, as has been reported for paracetamol, although absorption of benzodiazepines, tetracycline, or L-dopa does not appear to be significantly affected with healthy aging. Several systemic disorders associated with aging, such as diabetes, are frequently complicated by delayed gastric emptying, while a number of drugs also have potential to slow gastric emptying acutely (Table 34.2).

There are few data regarding altered gastric mechanics associated with aging. Neither fasting nor postprandial antral motor function appeared to be affected by age in patients who were being investigated for unexplained gastrointestinal symptoms.[26] Compliance of the proximal stomach appears similar in healthy elderly and young men in the fasting state, but elderly men demonstrate a marked reduction in the perception of gastric distension,[7] in line with observations in the esophagus and stomach. Furthermore, the relaxation of the proximal stomach in response to a meal is delayed in healthy older men when compared to the young; failure to accommodate ingested food in the proximal stomach might contribute to early satiation. Conversely, the healthy elderly have greater antral distension after a nutrient drink than the young, which is likely to result in increased satiation.[27]

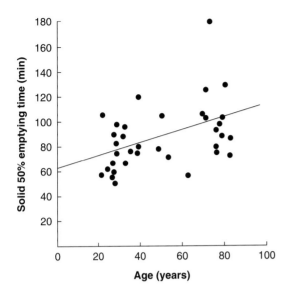

Figure 34.1 Relationship between gastric emptying of a solid meal (50% emptying time) and age in 35 healthy subjects; r = 0.42, P < 0.01. Gastric emptying becomes slower with increasing age, albeit with considerable overlap between older and younger subjects. Adapted from Horowitz et al 1984.[24]

The elderly also potentially differ from the young in their responses to the presence of nutrients in the small intestine. Infusion of identical nutrient loads in each group results in greater cholecystokinin (CCK) release in the healthy elderly, even allowing for the relative elevation of fasting CCK concentrations seen in this group,[20] while intraduodenal glucose is more satiating in the elderly than the young. Such enhancement of small intestinal feedback could contribute to diminution of both the rate of gastric emptying and appetite.

Early reports suggested that acid secretion declines with age, but this is probably confined largely to those with *Helicobacter pylori* infection, which results in gastric atrophy.[28] Most healthy elderly maintain both basal[29] and stimulated[30] acid secretion, although output of pepsin,[30] bicarbonate, and non-parietal fluid secretion[31] may decline. It follows that the elderly remain at risk for GERD and peptic ulcer disease on the basis of their secretory status.

H. pylori infection represents a major risk factor for peptic ulcer, and the prevalence of infection increases with age in developed societies, affecting about 50% of 60-year-olds compared to 10% of young adults in the US.[32] This gradient reflects a decline in transmission of the organism in childhood due to improvements in sanitation, and is not seen in developing nations, where the prevalence is higher in both groups. *H. pylori* infection is characterized by an initial antral gastritis, with subsequent spread to the gastric body, followed ultimately by atropy of the body and intestinal metaplasia of the antrum, which are associated with an increased risk of gastric cancer. Certain strains of *Helicobacter* (CagA positive) appear to be more potent at inducing atropic change.[33] *Helicobacter* eradication therapy appears to be at least as effective in the elderly as in younger adults.[33]

While factors potentially aggressive to the gastroduodenal mucosa persist in older individuals, there is some evidence for a decline in protective factors. In particular, gastroduodenal prostaglandin concentrations decrease with healthy aging,[34] along with a decline in mucus cells and in mucosal glutathione, all of which are elements of gastric mucosal defense. Furthermore, there is limited evidence for a decline in mucosal blood flow with age.[33]

Postprandial hypotension

Older individuals, particularly those with type 2 diabetes, are prone to a marked decrease in blood pressure after meals, which contributes to syncope and falls, and is, therefore, of major clinical concern.[21] Carbohydrate may be the most potent macronutrient for inducing hypotension, though fat is also implicated,[35] and recent studies indicate that the fall in blood pressure is related to the rate at which glucose enters the small intestine.[36] Regulation of splanchnic blood flow and the release of gastrointestinal peptide hormones are likely to be important determinants of the hypotensive response, since it can be attenuated by administration of the somatostatin analog octreotide.[37] Slowing gastric emptying or small intestinal carbohydrate absorption by dietary and pharmacologic approaches, such as with the α-glucosidase inhibitor, acarbose,[38] appears to be a promising strategy to treat this disorder.

Table 34.2 *Medications with potential to affect gastrointestinal motor function*

Decreased motility or decreased rate of gut transit
- Anticholinergics
- Calcium channel antagonists
- Clonidine (an α_2-agonist)
- L-Dopa
- Nitrates
- Opiates
- Phosphodiesterase type 5 inhibitors (e.g. sildenafil)
- Sumatriptan (a 5HT-1P agonist)[*]
- Tricyclic antidepressants

Increased motility or increased rate of gut transit
- Beta-blockers
- Cisapride, tegaserod, and other $5HT_4$ agonists
- Domperidone
- Erythromycin (a motilin analog)[†]
- Metoclopramide
- Selective serotonin reuptake inhibitors

[*]Relaxes the gastric fundus and delays gastric emptying, but increases esophageal motility.
[†]Stimulates gastric emptying but slows small intestinal transit.

Small intestinal function

The motor function of the small intestine does not appear to be altered substantially with healthy aging. During fasting, the small bowel undergoes distinctive periods of activity in cycles lasting about 90 minutes, known as the migrating motor complex (MMC). Each cycle consists of phase I (motor quiescence), phase II (irregular contractions of increasing frequency), and phase III (5–10 minutes of regular contractions that propagate distally and 'sweep' the lumen of debris). Following a meal, this cyclic activity is interrupted by irregular contractions that facilitate digestion and absorption of luminal contents. The cycle length of the MMC is not altered in the healthy elderly when compared with the young, although the velocity of propagation of phase III is slightly slower. The main difference in the elderly is an increase in propagated, clustered contractions during both the fasting and postprandial states;[39] similar patterns are seen in the irritable bowel syndrome, but their functional significance is unclear, since small intestinal transit in the healthy elderly seems to be comparable to the young.[4]

Small intestinal absorptive function also generally remains intact with healthy aging, with the exception of calcium absorption, which may decline due to impaired production of, and intestinal response to, 1,25 hydroxycholecalciferol. Atropic gastritis and the resultant achlorhydria, which are features of longstanding *Helicobacter* infection rather than healthy aging per se, can impair absorption of folate and vitamin B_{12}.[40] Small bowel bacterial overgrowth is uncommon in healthy older individuals,[41] but may be associated with a number of comorbid conditions that affect small intestinal motility (such as diabetes) or acid secretion (atropic gastritis), or with local factors, such as jejunal diverticula, that allow stasis of luminal contents. Bacterial overgrowth represents a potential cause of malnutrition, including B12 deficiency, and diarrhea,[17] and is diagnosed by quantitative culture of duodenal aspirates, or by measurement of breath hydrogen after oral glucose or xylose. Breath tests are, however, reported to have low specificity in the elderly. Treatment consists of a 1–4-week course of an antibiotic such as metronidazole, tetracycline, or a quinolone, and may need to be repeated on a cyclic basis if symptoms are recurrent.

Esophageal disorders in the aging male

Esophageal motor disorders

Disordered esophageal motor function typically presents with dysphagia or chest pain. There is a high prevalence of dysphagia amongst elderly residents of nursing homes (50–60%), and those on general medical wards (10–30%), when patients are questioned specifically.[42] Consequences include aspiration, inadequate nutrient intake, and the potential for impaction of capsules or tablets in the esophagus.

Dysphagia can be classified as 'oropharyngeal' or 'esophageal', depending on whether there is difficulty initiating a swallow or impaired transport of swallowed material, and these can usually be distinguished on history and examination. Potential causes of esophageal dysphagia are listed in Table 34.3. Increasing difficulty in swallowing solids suggests a structural lesion, while difficulty with both liquids and solids is more characteristic of a motility disorder.[43] A prior history of reflux symptoms suggests peptic stricture. Endoscopy is usually indicated, and allows visualization and biopsy of structural lesions, together with the ability to dilate strictures if indicated. Endoscopy can be performed

safely in elderly patients.[44] Contrast videofluoroscopy provides complementary information about structural lesions, and allows some assessment of function. Manometry is of greatest use when a diagnosis of achalasia is being considered.

Disorders of esophageal motility, such as achalasia, diffuse spasm, and nutcracker esophagus, occur over a wide age range. In the case of achalasia, there is a second, smaller peak in incidence in the elderly, following the main peak in early- to mid-adulthood,[13] while many patients with esophageal spasm and with non-specific motility disorders are in the older age group.

Achalasia

Achalasia is characterized by incomplete or absent relaxation of the LES with swallowing, usually combined with an absence of peristalsis in the esophageal body, though in some patients there are high amplitude esophageal pressure waves (so-called 'vigorous' achalasia). The etiology is unknown, but the myenteric plexus shows initial inflammation, followed by ganglion loss and neural fibrosis.[45] Presenting symptoms include dysphagia for both liquids and solids, weight loss, regurgitation, and aspiration;[46] chest pain is reported less often in older patients than in the young.[47]

The barium swallow classically shows a dilated esophageal body, especially in the elderly, with 'bird's beak' or 'rat's tail' tapering at the LES, and delayed emptying of the column of barium. In addition to

---

Table 34.3 *Esophageal causes of dysphagia*

Structural lesions
- Malignancy
- Peptic stricture
- Schatzki ring
- Vascular compression (aortic arch)
- Reflux esophagitis
- 'Pill' esophagitis

Motor disorders
- Achalasia
- Diffuse spasm or 'nutcracker' esophagus
- Non-specific motility disorders
- Systemic disease (e.g. Parkinson's disease, diabetes mellitus)

impaired LES relaxation on swallowing, manometry typically demonstrates simultaneous, low-amplitude pressure waves in the esophageal body, or a total absence of pressure waves. Endoscopy, and sometimes computed tomography (CT) or endoluminal ultrasound, should be performed to exclude 'pseudo-achalasia', which presents with similar features, but is caused by carcinoma of the distal esophagus or cardia, and is suggested by a short history with prominent weight loss.

Achalasia is treated by disrupting the muscle of the LES, either by pneumatic dilatation at endoscopy or by surgical myotomy, which is often performed laparoscopically. A symptomatic response of over 80% is reported for each approach,[48] although the only randomized trial to date favors surgery (95% versus 51% reporting nearly complete symptom relief[49]). Risks include esophageal perforation in about 3% undergoing pneumatic dilatation, and reflux symptoms in about 10%, while repeat dilatations are often required. An antireflux procedure can be performed with surgical myotomy to ameliorate the risk of GERD.

The frail elderly, who are unsuitable for surgery and are less likely to tolerate the potential complications of pneumatic dilatation, can be treated by endoscopic injection of botulinum toxin into the LES. This is reported to achieve adequate symptom relief in only 60%,[48] and has a limited duration of benefit (about 6 months), so that repeat injections are often required. The cost is slightly greater than for pneumatic dilatation, but less than that of surgery.

Diffuse esophageal spasm and 'nutcracker esophagus'

Diffuse esophageal spasm is characterized by simultaneous esophageal pressure waves associated with some but not all swallows,[50] and the barium swallow may have a 'corkscrew' appearance. 'Nutcracker esophagus' describes a pattern of high-amplitude esophageal pressure waves, where peristalsis is maintained. Both disorders may be diagnosed in the setting of chest pain or dysphagia; however, these motor patterns may not be causal, and the outcome of treatment with drugs that relax smooth muscle is frequently disappointing. Drugs that modulate visceral

sensation, such as tricyclic antidepressants, may be more efficacious, though the elderly are prone to adverse effects, including postural hypotension.

Non-specific esophageal motility disorders

In many elderly patients referred for investigation of 'esophageal' symptoms, there are manometric features which are outside the normal range, but do not meet the criteria for the diagnosis of a specific motor disorder, such as achalasia or diffuse spasm. These non-specific abnormalities are evident in more than a third of presentations with dysphagia in patients over 65 years of age, but their relationship to symptoms is uncertain, and there is no specific therapy.

'Pill esophagitis'

Impaction of medications in the esophagus, with resultant mucosal injury and ulceration, represents an important cause of dysphagia and odynophagia in older individuals. Risk factors include polypharmacy, less saliva, delayed esophageal transit, and immobility. Capsules, which have a slower esophageal transit than tablets, present the greater risk, and the most frequently implicated medications include potassium chloride, tetracyclines, aspirin, and non-steroidal drugs, quinidine, theophylline, ferrous sulfate, and alendronate.[51] Typically, small superficial ulcers are seen at endoscopy, while complications include stricture, perforation, and bleeding. Withdrawal of the responsible drug is often sufficient therapy, but sucralfate has been used for severe or persistent disease. Older patients should be advised to drink a full glass of water after taking oral medications.

Gastro-esophageal reflux disease

The prevalence of GERD in older individuals is similar (about 20%) to younger adults, but complications, including erosive esophagitis, are more common,[52] while males are more likely to have erosive disease than females.[53] Delayed acid clearance, or a longer duration of disease, might contribute to complications in older patients.[17] Conversely, the elderly tend to report milder symptoms, and are more likely to present with 'atypical' features including dysphagia, vomiting, respiratory difficulty, weight loss, or anemia, rather than 'typical' symptoms like heartburn. The clinician should be alert to 'alarm symptoms', such as dysphagia, weight loss, or bleeding, which mandate prompt endoscopic investigation to exclude malignancy. 'Extra-esophageal' manifestations of GERD, including chronic cough and asthma, may be difficult to relate to acid reflux with certainty, and a useful diagnostic test is a therapeutic trial of intense acid suppression with a double dose of a proton pump inhibitor (PPI), for up to 8 weeks, depending on symptom frequency.[54]

Healing of esophagitis appears similar in older patients compared to the young, and PPIs appear to maintain their efficacy in this age group, with no need for dosage adjustment to compensate for age-related changes in renal or hepatic function. Given the tendency for elderly GERD patients to have mucosal damage out of proportion to symptoms, the 'step down' approach to PPI dosing, which is guided by symptoms, may be less appropriate than in the young, particularly in the setting of complicated GERD. Long-term acid suppression raises the prevalence of atropic gastritis in individuals infected with *Helicobacter*, theoretically increasing the risk of gastric cancer; therefore, testing for *H. pylori* and eradicating it if present is generally recommended, but this is unlikely to be of significance in the very old. Although maintenance therapy for GERD with long-term PPI administration is likely to be more cost-effective than antireflux surgery in elderly patients, on the basis of the number of years of medical therapy likely to be needed, it should be noted that healthy older individuals have comparable outcomes to the young following laparoscopic fundoplication.[17]

Barrett's mucosa and adenocarcinoma of the esophagus

The incidence of adenocarcinoma of the esophagus is increasing, from less than 5% of esophageal cancers in the 1970s to 50% or more in many developed countries. The increase has been greatest amongst white males, in whom the incidence has been rising by up to 10% annually; moreover, the prevalence increases above 65 years of age.[55,56] Other risk factors include GERD and obesity.

Nevertheless, the absolute incidence of esophageal adenocarcinoma remains relatively low (between 1 and 5 per 100 000 in white males).[57]

The majority of esophageal adenocarcinoma arises from Barrett's mucosa, a condition involving replacement of the normal squamous lining of the distal esophagus by intestinal type columnar mucosa, in association with longstanding reflux disease (Figure 34.2). Barrett's mucosa is found in 10–15% of patients undergoing endoscopy for GERD, but also in 5–10% having endoscopy for other reasons, and autopsy series indicate that the majority of cases are undiagnosed.[58] Males have about a 2-fold increased risk of Barrett's mucosa when compared to females, but their proportional risk of developing adenocarcinoma is 5 times that of women.[53] People reporting reflux symptoms at least once per week have an 8-fold risk of Barrett's esophagus, and the risk appears to increase with the severity and duration of symptoms,[57] although it is not uncommon for Barrett's mucosa to be diagnosed with minimal reflux symptoms, particularly in the elderly.

Barrett's esophagus can be considered a premalignant condition, progressing through low- and high-grade dysplasia to adenocarcinoma. The risk of transition to carcinoma is approximately 0.5% per year, which is about 30–60 times the risk in the general population.[57] Regular endoscopic surveillance with biopsies, typically every 2 years, is widely advocated to detect dysplasia or early carcinoma, but remains controversial.[59] Although surveillance is supported by indirect evidence showing that esophageal adenocarcinoma is diagnosed at an earlier stage in surveyed patients, there are no prospective controlled trials, and cost–benefit data are limited.[58] Surveillance of patients with Barrett's mucosa suffers from sampling error and variations in histologic grading, which limit its sensitivity. New developments offering promise include improvements in endoscopic detection (high-resolution endoscopy, dye staining, and narrow band imaging), alternative sampling techniques (including brushing rather than biopsy), and the use of molecular markers for dysplasia.[60] Screening of all GERD patients for Barrett's mucosa cannot currently be supported on cost–benefit grounds,[58] since the risk

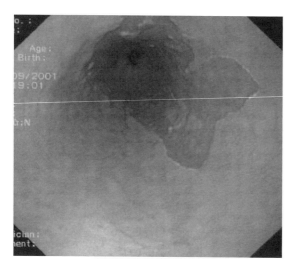

Figure 34.2 *Endoscopic view of Barrett's esophagus, showing the irregular junction between the normal squamous mucosa (pale) and the columnar lined esophagus (darker).*

of adenocarcinoma is relatively low even in those with GERD, and the costs of screening would be high. For example, calculations from Swedish data indicate that 60 obese men aged 50–79 years would need to be followed for 10 years to detect one adenocarcinoma, although the figure may be less in the US, where the incidence of adenocarcinoma is greater.[57] More information is therefore required to select those at high risk. Furthermore, it is unclear to what degree either PPI therapy or antireflux surgery impacts on the development and progression of Barrett's mucosa in patients with GERD.

A further dilemma is the management of patients found to have high-grade dysplasia. Perhaps a quarter will progress to adenocarcinoma over 2 years,[58] but treatment with esophagectomy may have a mortality rate of 5% even in established centers. A number of approaches have been developed to resect or ablate the dysplastic mucosa endoscopically, rather than proceed to surgery, but concerns have been raised regarding remnant foci of columnar cells buried in the mucosa, and such therapies require further evaluation in formal clinical trials.

Squamous cell carcinoma of the esophagus

In contrast to esophageal adenocarcinoma, the incidence of this tumor in aging men is relatively stable in the US, though slightly greater than for women, and the peak incidence occurs in the sixth and seventh decades.[61] Dysphagia is the most common presenting symptom, and endoscopy is the most appropriate investigation, although barium swallow is also recommended if a tracheo-esophageal fistula is suspected on the basis of history (e.g. coughing soon after swallowing fluids).

The disease is staged by CT, with an additional role for endoscopic ultrasound. Surgical resection can be considered for early-stage lesions without nodal metastases, while endoscopic mucosal resection may be an option in patients with early lesions who are poor surgical candidates, including the elderly with comorbidities. Chemoradiotherapy is used for locally invasive disease, while endoscopically placed expanding metal stents have a role in the palliation of dysphagia.[63]

Stomach and duodenal disorders

Peptic ulcer disease

As discussed above, aggressive factors promoting peptic ulceration persist in the elderly, while mucosal defense is diminished. In addition, up to 40% of those over 65 are prescribed non-steroidal anti-inflammatory drugs (NSAIDs),[62] and age has been shown to be an independent risk factor for peptic ulceration in those taking NSAIDs.[63] Regular, long-term use of NSAIDs is not necessarily required to induce peptic ulceration, which can occur after even a relatively brief course of therapy.[33] Selective COX-2 inhibitors are associated with a lower risk of peptic ulceration than the non-selective NSAIDs, but this advantage has not been demonstrated specifically in the elderly, and any selective advantage is lost when these drugs are used in conjunction with aspirin. The interaction of NSAIDs and *Helicobacter* in peptic ulcer disease, and bleeding peptic ulcers in particular, has been a controversial issue in recent years. Aspirin is often implicated in peptic ulceration, and

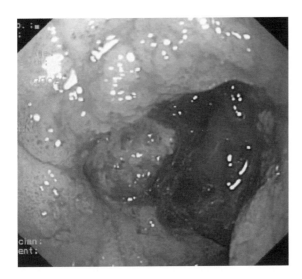

Figure 34.3 *Endoscopic image of a peptic ulcer following a recent bleed. Fresh clot is present in the base of this deep ulcer.*

there is a dose-dependent increase in risk from 300 mg to 1200 mg daily, but even low-dose or enteric-coated preparations entail a 3-fold risk of a bleeding peptic ulcer.[33] Anticoagulants are also a risk factor for upper gastrointestinal bleeding, and this risk appears higher in the elderly than in younger adults.[33]

Peptic ulcer disease in older individuals often presents atypically – abdominal pain is absent in half of those over 60 years,[64] while two-thirds of those over 80 years present with ulcer bleeding in the absence of any abdominal discomfort.[65] Ulcer complications, specifically bleeding and perforation, are also more common in the elderly than the young,[66] and mortality from bleeding is between 4- and 10-fold higher.[67] Endoscopy is the investigation of choice for suspected ulcer disease (Figure 34.3); barium meal has a false negative rate of almost 10%,[68] and does not allow for biopsy or therapeutic procedures.

Upper gastrointestinal bleeding

Patients aged over 60 years make up a disproportionate number of those presenting with hematemesis and/or melena.[69] About 50% of such presentations are due to peptic ulcer disease, with other frequent diagnoses being esophagitis and gastritis (Table 34.4). By contrast, Mallory-Weiss tears and variceal bleeding are more prevalent in the young, and tend to be associated with alcohol abuse.[70] Other causes of upper gastrointestinal bleeding in the elderly include vascular lesions (angiodysplasia, Dieulafoy lesions, and gastric antral vascular ectasia),[70] while aorto-enteric fistula should be suspected in elderly men with a previous aortic graft; a 'herald bleed' often precedes massive bleeding, and the diagnosis is made by endoscopy and CT imaging.[71]

Mortality from upper gastrointestinal bleeding has remained stable at about 10% despite advances in therapy,[72] reflecting an aging population with increasing comorbidities. Eighty-five percent of deaths occur in patients aged over 65 years,[73] while mortality is only about 1% in those under 60 years of age.[74] Indeed, age (but not gender) is one component of a widely used scoring system for evaluating risk in upper gastrointestinal bleeding.[75] Such scores are effective in expediting discharge from hospital in patients at low risk of complications or rebleeding,[76] but not surprisingly, patients receiving a favorable score tend to be younger.[77] In the medical therapy of upper gastrointestinal hemorrhage, caution is needed to avoid fluid overload and overtransfusion, especially in variceal bleeding, where fluid loading is prone to increase portal pressure. Conversely, however, hypovolemia puts elderly patients at risk of myocardial ischemia or infarction. Endoscopic therapy for bleeding upper gastrointestinal lesions is just as efficacious in the elderly as in the young,[78] while the elderly are reported to have higher mortality following both emergency (25% vs 7.5%) and elective (13.6% vs 2%) surgery for gastrointestinal bleeding,[79] although recent data for surgical mortality are not available.

Gastric cancer

Gastric adenocarcinoma is the second most common cancer worldwide, and the incidence increases with age; in men, the incidence peaks at just over 60 years of age.[61] Despite a declining incidence in the developed world over the last 50 years, there has been minimal improvement in survival. Risk factors for gastric cancer include *Helicobacter* infection,

Table 34.4 *Causes of upper gastrointestinal bleeding in the elderly*

Non-variceal bleeding
- Gastric or duodenal ulcer*
- Reflux esophagitis
- Gastritis
- Neoplasia (esophagus, stomach)
- Vascular lesions
    - angiodysplasia
    - Dieulafoy lesions
    - gastric antral vascular ectasia ('watermelon stomach')
- Mallory–Weiss tears
- Aorto-enteric fistula

Variceal bleeding†
- Esophageal varices
- Gastric varices

*Peptic ulcer disease accounts for about 50% of upper gastrointestinal bleeding in the elderly.
†Variceal bleeding is less common in the elderly than in the young to middle-aged group.

with attendant gastric atrophy and intestinal meta-plasia,[80,81] diets high in smoked or salted foods, low fruit and vegetable intake, aflatoxin-contaminated food, and low socio-economic status.[82,83] Other risk factors include familial adenomatous polyposis, pernicious anemia, and a history of gastrectomy.[82,83] For example, there is a 2-fold risk of gastric cancer, as well as a 3-fold risk of esophageal squamous cell carcinoma, in those with pernicious anemia,[84] although the absolute risk would not appear to justify surveillance programs in this population.

Gastric cancer usually presents with weight loss and epigastric pain; anorexia, early satiety, nausea, and vomiting are other common symptoms. 'Alarm features' of weight loss, early satiety, and bleeding or iron deficiency anemia mandate endoscopic examination; barium meal is a less sensitive investigation. Physical signs, such as a mass or succussion splash, are usually indicative of advanced disease.[61] Staging involves abdominal CT imaging, and endoscopic ultrasound can be useful if local staging is required. Survival after gastrectomy actually improves with increasing age, since older patients tend to have less aggressive disease than the young, up to the point where medical comorbidities contribute to higher operative mortality. Amongst those undergoing resection with curative intent, tumor recurrence affects 80% within 5 years. Palliative resection is often beneficial in the setting of gastric outlet obstruction, but expandable metal stents provide an alternative in this setting. Some tumors respond to chemo- or radiotherapy, but without an established survival benefit.

Small intestinal disorders

Celiac disease

Although traditionally thought of as a disease presenting in childhood, celiac disease is increasingly being diagnosed throughout life; undetected celiac disease was found in about 1% of a UK population aged 45–76 years, on the basis of endomyseal antibody testing.[85] Adults present with fewer gastrointestinal symptoms than in the classical descriptions, but complications seem to occur more frequently in the elderly, including T-cell lymphoma and adenocarcinoma of the small intestine, and esophageal carcinoma.[86] However, the risk of malignancy is ameliorated with strict adherence to a gluten-free diet. Osteoporosis and iron deficiency anemia are clues to the diagnosis (60% of elderly celiac patients are anemic).[87] Men may be more severely affected by osteoporosis than women.[88]

Biochemical abnormalities include hypo-albuminemia, -calcemia, and -magnesemia, while abnormal liver function tests are observed in 20% and resolve on a gluten-free diet, but may require investigation to exclude other causes.[87] It is appropriate to screen thyroid function, since there is a strong association with autoimmune thyroid disease. Pancreatic calcification and exocrine pancreatic insufficiency are not uncommon features, and there is also an association with lymphocytic and collagenous colitis; these entities sometimes account for diarrhea that is 'refractory' to a gluten-free diet. Serologic screening of first-degree relatives for endomyseal or transglutaminase antibodies is recommended, since 10% will be affected.

Small intestinal ischemia

While less common than colonic ischemia, which is not discussed here, acute small intestinal ischemia has a high mortality (~60–90%) and affects the elderly predominantly. The causes of acute ischemia include embolus (~50%), thrombosis, or non-occlusive 'low-flow' states affecting the superior mesenteric artery; thrombosis of the superior mesenteric vein; or focal segmental ischaemia.[89] The diagnosis is suggested by abdominal pain that is out of proportion to the abdominal signs; indeed, the presence of definite abdominal tenderness, rebound, or guarding, or radiologic signs of ileus, 'thumb-printing', or intramural air, imply irretrievable intestinal infarction. Leukocytosis and metabolic acidosis are common features, and CT imaging with intravenous contrast is helpful, particularly for demonstrating superior mesenteric vein thrombosis. Immediate management should focus on correction of identifiable causes of low perfusion, such as hypovolemia, hypotension, and arrhythmia, but vasopressors and digoxin are associated with splanchnic vasoconstriction, and are therefore best avoided. Angiography detects emboli and arterial thrombosis, and provides a route for administration of the vasodilator, papaverine, or for thrombolysis in the setting of partial occlusion or emboli distal to

ileocolonic artery origin. Surgical embolectomy is sometimes indicated.[90]

Superior mesenteric vein thrombosis occurs in the setting of hypercoagulable states, local stasis (e.g. cirrhosis or tumor), intra-abdominal inflammation and sepsis, trauma or abdominal surgery, or low-flow states; however, one-third are 'idiopathic'. Anticoagulation is indicated in the absence of any signs of peritonitis.[90]

Chronic mesenteric ischemia is an uncommon condition, characterized by abdominal pain within 10 or 15 minutes of eating ('intestinal angina'). The pain is typically colicky, experienced in the upper abdomen and sometimes in the back, and may persist for an hour or two. Weight loss is often a prominent feature, sometimes with steatorrhea. Angiography demonstrates occlusion or stenosis of at least two major vessels, and therapeutic options include surgical revascularization, or angioplasty with or without stent insertion.

Systemic disorders associated with disturbance of upper gastrointestinal function

While healthy aging is associated with minimal impairment of upper gastrointestinal function, comorbidities with the potential to affect gut function tend to increase with advancing age, and examples of these include Parkinson's disease and diabetes mellitus. Furthermore, numerous medications can affect gastrointestinal motility; some of these are listed in Table 34.2.

Parkinson's disease

Parkinson's disease, which has a slight male preponderance in several US and European studies, is often complicated by gastrointestinal dysfunction.[91] Involvement of the dorsal motor nucleus of the vagus (affecting parasympathetic innervation), and the enteric nervous system (Lewy bodies and loss of dopaminergic neurons), has been documented.

Dysphagia is common, particularly involving the oropharyngeal phase of swallowing, and esophageal transit may also be impaired. Variable effects of L-dopa or anticholinergic therapy have been noted, and swallowing disorders may either improve or deteriorate with these treatments. Gastric emptying may be delayed, either due to Parkinsonism itself, or as a result of L-dopa administration, resulting in a high prevalence of nausea and bloating, together with impaired nutrition and absorption of oral medications. Gastric retention of L-dopa may result in metabolism of the drug to an inactive form, while the rate of gastric emptying may vary with fluctuations in neurologic function, and in this way further contribute to the 'on-off' motor phenomenon that affects a proportion of patients. Metoclopramide is contraindicated in Parkinsonism, but other prokinetic agents such as domperidone (a dopamine antagonist which does not cross the blood–brain barrier to any significant degree) can be used. Patients may have more widespread impairment of gut motility, involving the small intestine, colon, and anorectum, and, in particular, oro-cecal transit time is prolonged compared with age-matched controls.

Diabetes mellitus

The prevalence of type 2 diabetes is increasing dramatically worldwide, and this disorder occurs frequently in older people. Diabetes is associated with disordered motor function involving all segments of the gastrointestinal tract, and gastrointestinal symptoms are common,[92] although there is no information specific to the elderly. Disordered gut function in diabetes has traditionally been attributed to irreversible autonomic neuropathy, but it is now clear that acute changes in the blood glucose concentration have a major, reversible impact on gut motility and sensation.[93]

Abnormalities of esophageal function in diabetes include a reduction in the amplitude of pressure waves, abnormal wave forms, and failure of peristalsis, with delayed esophageal transit.[94] LES pressure may be reduced, and the prevalence of GERD appears to be increased.[95]

Up to 50% of outpatients with longstanding type 1 or type 2 diabetes have delayed gastric emptying for solids or nutrient liquids,[94,96,97] associated with diminished antral motility and impaired propagation of pressure waves from antrum to duodenum, as well as diminished fundic tone. These abnormalities

are more marked during acute hyperglycemia, when compared to euglycemia, and potentially contribute to upper abdominal symptoms, impaired nutrition and absorption of oral medications, and disordered glycemic control. Although a delay in gastric emptying may slow the entry of carbohydrates to the small intestine and actually improve the postprandial blood glucose profile, it is likely to result in a mismatch between glucose absorption and the onset of insulin action in the high, and increasing, proportion of patients requiring exogenous insulin. When associated with symptoms, diabetic gastroparesis is usually treated with a prokinetic drug, such as metoclopramide, domperidone, or erythromycin. Cisapride has been withdrawn in most markets following a number of deaths attributed to cardiac arrhythmias. It is appropriate to screen patients with 'brittle' diabetes for abnormalities of gastric emptying.

Small intestinal motility is often disordered in diabetes mellitus, with a reduction in the MMC cycle length during fasting, and bursts of non-propagated pressure waves after a meal. Transit through the small intestine varies widely, and both diarrhea and constipation appear more common than in healthy individuals. Small bowel bacterial overgrowth, celiac disease, and pancreatic exocrine insufficiency should be excluded in the setting of diarrhea, but if no specific cause is identified, loperamide may be of benefit, as may the α-adrenergic agonist, clonidine.

Functional upper gastrointestinal disorders

Functional gastrointestinal disorders are characterized by recurrent or persistent symptoms referable to the gut, in the absence of organic pathology. This group of disorders includes functional dyspepsia (upper abdominal pain, bloating, or nausea) and non-cardiac chest pain. Irritable bowel syndrome, which involves predominantly lower abdominal discomfort and disturbance of bowel habit, will not be discussed here. Many patients with predominant symptoms of one category of functional disorder have additional symptoms that overlap with other categories.

Functional dyspepsia

In contrast to the irritable bowel syndrome, which appears to remain almost as prevalent in the elderly as it is in the general population, there is little information regarding the prevalence of functional dyspepsia in older individuals; about 15% of adults in Western societies report chronic or recurrent upper abdominal symptoms. Unlike the irritable bowel syndrome, where there is an established bias in favor of women of about 2:1, limited data indicate that there may be a slight male predominance for functional dyspepsia in the community. Nevertheless, amongst those referred for specialist investigation of upper abdominal symptoms, males are more likely than females to have an organic cause identified. Furthermore, both healthy men and those with functional dyspepsia tolerate a greater volume of ingested fluid (the 'water drink' test) than women in each of these categories. Men with functional dyspepsia are also less likely than women to have delayed gastric emptying, suggesting that, in general, men are less prone to derangements of upper gastrointestinal motor and sensory function.[98]

Community-based surveys have found a decrease in dyspeptic symptoms with age, but an increased tendency to consult medical practitioners.[99] It is important to exclude organic diseases such as cancer when gut symptoms arise in older patients, particularly as the prevalence of organic disease is greater than in the young,[100] and the threshold for endoscopic examination should be low. Comorbidities such as Parkinson's disease, medications, thyroid disease, diabetes, depression, and small bowel bacterial overgrowth must also be considered. NSAIDs should be stopped.

Chronic gastrointestinal symptoms impair quality of life, but since many older individuals do not consult their doctors, the impact of these symptoms may go unrecognized. While the elderly appear to be no more prone than the young to depression associated with chronic pain disorders, practitioners should be alert to the possibility that 'gastrointestinal' symptoms, such as anorexia, can be a feature of depression.[100]

Therapies for functional gut disorders must be evaluated in the setting of controlled trials, since there is a very high placebo response rate (between 20 and 70%). However, no clinical trials in patients with functional disorders have focused specifically on the elderly.[101] Current therapies aim to address various possible mechanisms that have been proposed to account for symptoms, including acid sensitivity, delayed gastric emptying, and *Helicobacter* infection.[102] Acid suppression is more likely to be helpful when there is a component of reflux symptoms,[103] while *Helicobacter* eradication is not conclusively effective in the absence of peptic ulcer disease.[104] Antidepressants may be useful when the predominant symptom is pain, and the dose in functional gut disorders is typically lower than standard doses used to treat depression. While selective serotonin re-uptake inhibitors may be better tolerated in the elderly than tricyclics, there are few specific data regarding their efficacy in dyspepsia.

Non-cardiac chest pain

Chest pain is a common symptom, and often presents a diagnostic difficulty, especially in older patients who are at higher risk of ischemic heart disease than the young. Chest pain is often attributed to the esophagus once cardiac causes have been excluded, but musculoskeletal, pulmonary, pericardial, gastric, and biliary disorders should also be considered, and panic disorder is another potential cause.[105]

A narrow majority (50–60%) of patients with non-cardiac chest pain (NCCP) have excessive esophageal acid exposure on pH studies; only a proportion of these will have esophagitis, which limits the diagnostic value of endoscopy. Rather, a trial of double-dose proton pump inhibitor (PPI) for 2 to 8 weeks, with the duration dependent on symptom frequency, is a useful and cost-effective test to determine whether GERD is a likely diagnosis.[106] In patients who respond to the PPI, the dose can be titrated subsequently to the minimum effective dose, while non-responders may be investigated with esophageal manometry and ambulatory pH measurements.

Manometry studies in NCCP patients sometimes reveal diffuse esophageal spasm, 'nutcracker esophagus', or other motility disorders, but a causal relationship between symptoms and abnormal motility is often difficult to establish. Furthermore, medical therapy designed to relax esophageal smooth muscle, such as nitrates, calcium channel antagonists, or sildenafil, has limited efficacy,[107] and is based on the assumption that excessive esophageal contraction is the cause of the pain. As with functional dyspepsia, antidepressants may be useful as pain-modifying agents, and are superior to placebo in non-GERD-related NCCP,[54] although caution should be exercised in the elderly regarding side-effects.

Acknowledgment

The authors wish to thank Associate Professor Peter Devitt, Department of Surgery, University of Adelaide, for providing the images for Figures 34.2 and 34.3.

References

1. Goyal RK, Hirano I. Mechanisms of disease: the enteric nervous system. N Engl J Med 1996; 334: 1106–15.
2. Wade PR. Aging and neural control of the GI tract. I. Age-related changes in the enteric nervous system. Am J Physiol 2002; 283: G489–95.
3. Wade PR, Cowen T. Neurodegeneration: a key factor in the ageing gut. Neurogastroenterol Motil 2004; 16(Suppl 1): 19–23.
4. Madsen JL, Graff J. Effects of ageing on gastrointestinal motor function. Age Ageing 2004; 33: 154–9.
5. Ren J, Shaker R, Kusano M et al. Effect of aging on the secondary esophageal peristalsis: presbyesophagus revisited. Am J Physiol 1995; 268: G772–9.
6. Lasch H, Castell DO, Castell JA. Evidence for diminished visceral pain with aging: studies using graded intraesophageal balloon distension. Am J Physiol 1997; 272: G1–3.
7. Rayner CK, MacIntosh CG, Chapman IM et al. Effects of age on proximal gastric motor and sensory function. Scand J Gastroenterol 2000; 35: 1041–7.
8. Lagier E, Delvaux M, Vellas B et al. Influence of age on rectal tone and sensitivity to distension in healthy subjects. Neurogastroenterol Motil 1999; 11: 101–7.
9. Fass R, Pulliam G, Johnson C et al. Symptom severity and oesophageal chemosensitivity to acid in older and young patients with gastro-oesophageal reflux. Age Ageing 2000; 29: 125–30.
10. Weusten BL, Lam HG, Akkermans LM et al. Influence of age on cerebral potentials evoked by oesophageal balloon distension in humans. Eur J Clin Invest 1994; 24: 627–31.
11. Soergel KH, Zboralske FF, Amberg JR. Presbyesophagus: esophageal motility in nonagenarians. J Clin Invest 1964; 43: 1472–9.
12. Hollis JB, Castell DO. Esophageal function in elderly man. A new look at 'presbyesophagus'. Ann Intern Med 1974; 80: 371–4.
13. Orr WC, Chen CL. Aging and neural control of the GI tract: IV. Clinical and physiological aspects of gastrointestinal motility and aging. Am J Physiol 2002; 283: G1226–31.
14. Rao SS, Mudipalli RS, Mujica VR et al. Effects of gender and age on esophageal biomechanical properties and sensation. Am J Gastroenterol 2003; 98: 1688–95.
15. Shaw DW, Cook IJ, Gabb M et al. Influence of normal aging on oral-pharyngeal and upper esophageal sphincter function during swallowing. Am J Physiol 1995; 268: G389–96.
16. Kawamura O, Easterling C, Aslam M et al. Laryngo-upper esophageal sphincter contractile reflex in humans deteriorates with age. Gastroenterology 2004; 127: 57–64.
17. Firth M, Prather CM. Gastrointestinal motility problems in the elderly patient. Gastroenterology 2002; 122: 1688–700.
18. Smout AJ, Breedijk M, van der Zouw C et al. Physiological gastroesophageal reflux and esophageal motor activity studied with a new system for 24-hour recording and automated analysis. Dig Dis Sci 1989; 34: 372–8.
19. Tack J, Vantrappen G. The aging oesophagus. Gut 1997; 41: 422–4.
20. Chapman IM, MacIntosh CG, Morley JE et al. The anorexia of ageing. Biogerontology 2002; 3: 67–71.
21. Jansen RW, Connelly CM, Kelley-Gagnon MM et al. Postprandial hypotension in elderly patients with unexplained syncope. Arch Intern Med 1995; 155: 945–52.
22. Horowitz M, Dent J. Disordered gastric emptying: mechanical basis, assessment and treatment. Baillieres Clin Gastroenterol 1991; 5: 371–407.
23. Moore JG, Tweedy C, Christian PE et al. Effect of age on gastric emptying of liquid–solid meals in man. Dig Dis Sci 1983; 28: 340–4.
24. Horowitz M, Maddern GJ, Chatterton BE et al. Changes in gastric emptying rates with age. Clin Sci 1984; 67: 213–18.
25. Clarkston WK, Pantano MM, Morley JE et al. Evidence for the anorexia of aging: gastrointestinal transit and hunger in healthy elderly vs. young adults. Am J Physiol 1997; 272: R243–8.
26. Fich A, Camilleri M, Phillips SF. Effect of age on human gastric and small bowel motility. J Clin Gastroenterol 1989; 11: 416–20.
27. Sturm K, Parker B, Wishart J et al. Energy intake and appetite are related to antral area in healthy

young and older subjects. Am J Clin Nutr 2004; 80: 656–67.

28. Katelaris PH, Seow F, Lin BP et al. Effect of age, *Helicobacter pylori* infection, and gastritis with atrophy on serum gastrin and gastric acid secretion in healthy men. Gut 1993; 34: 1032–7.

29. Hurwitz A, Brady DA, Schaal SE et al. Gastric acidity in older adults. JAMA 1997; 278: 659–62.

30. Feldman M, Cryer B, McArthur KE et al. Effects of aging and gastritis on gastric acid and pepsin secretion in humans: a prospective study. Gastroenterology 1996; 110: 1043–52.

31. Feldman M, Cryer B. Effects of age on gastric alkaline and nonparietal fluid secretion in humans. Gerontology 1998; 44: 222–7.

32. Graham DY, Malaty HM, Evans DG et al. Epidemiology of *Helicobacter pylori* in an asymptomatic population in the United States. Effect of age, race, and socioeconomic status. Gastroenterology 1991; 100: 1495–501.

33. Pilotto A. Aging and the gastrointestinal tract. Ital J Gastroenterol Hepatol 1999; 31: 137–53.

34. Cryer B, Lee E, Feldman M. Factors influencing gastroduodenal mucosal prostaglandin concentrations: roles of smoking and aging. Ann Intern Med 1992; 116: 636–40.

35. Visvanathan R, Horowitz M, Chapman I. The hypotensive response to oral fat is comparable but slower compared with carbohydrate in healthy elderly subjects. Br J Nutr 2006; 95: 340–5.

36. O'Donovan D, Feinle C, Tonkin A et al. Postprandial hypotension in response to duodenal glucose delivery in healthy older subjects. J Physiol 2002; 540: 673–9.

37. Jansen RW, Peeters TL, Lenders JW et al. Somatostatin analog octreotide (SMS 201-995) prevents the decrease in blood pressure after oral glucose loading in the elderly. J Clin Endocrinol Metab 1989; 68: 752–6.

38. Gentilcore D, Bryant B, Wishart JM et al. Acarbose attenuates the hypotensive response to sucrose and slows gastric emptying in the elderly. Am J Med 2005; 118: 1289.

39. Husebye E, Engedal K. The patterns of motility are maintained in the human small intestine throughout the process of aging. Scand J Gastroenterol 1992; 27: 397–404.

40. Holt PR. Diarrhea and malabsorption in the elderly. Gastroenterol Clin North Am 2001; 30: 427–44.

41. Mitsui T, Kagami H, Kinomoto H et al. Small bowel bacterial overgrowth and rice malabsorption in healthy and physically disabled older adults. J Hum Nutr Diet 2003; 16: 119–22.

42. Shaker R, Staff D. Esophageal disorders in the elderly. Gastroenterol Clin North Am 2001; 30: 335–61.

43. Lock G. Physiology and pathology of the oesophagus in the elderly patient. Best Pract Res Clin Gastroenterol 2001; 15: 919–41.

44. Cooper BT, Neumann CS. Upper gastrointestinal endoscopy in patients aged 80 years or more. Age Ageing 1986; 15: 343–9.

45. Goldblum JR, Rice TW, Richter JE. Histopathologic features in esophagomyotomy specimens from patients with achalasia. Gastroenterology 1996; 111: 648–54.

46. Ghosh S, Heading RC, Palmer KR. Achalasia of the oesophagus in elderly patients responds poorly to conservative therapy. Age Ageing 1994; 23: 280–2.

47. Eckardt VF, Stauf B, Bernhard G. Chest pain in achalasia: patient characteristics and clinical course. Gastroenterology 1999; 116: 1300–4.

48. Vela MF, Richter JE, Wachsberger D et al. Complexities of managing achalasia at a tertiary referral center: use of pneumatic dilatation, Heller myotomy, and botulinum toxin injection. Am J Gastroenterol 2004; 99: 1029–36.

49. Spiess AE, Kahrilas PJ. Treating achalasia: from whalebone to laparoscope. JAMA 1998; 280: 638–42.

50. Dalton CB, Castell DO, Hewson EG et al. Diffuse esophageal spasm. A rare motility disorder not characterized by high-amplitude contractions. Dig Dis Sci 1991; 36: 1025–8.

51. Levine MS. Drug-induced disorders of the esophagus. Abdom Imaging 1999; 24: 3–8.

52. Mold JW, Reed LE, Davis AB et al. Prevalence of gastroesophageal reflux in elderly patients in a primary care setting. Am J Gastroenterol 1991; 86: 965–70.

53. Cook MB, Wild CP, Forman D. A systematic review and meta-analysis of the sex ratio for Barrett's esophagus, erosive reflux disease, and nonerosive reflux disease. Am J Epidemiol 2005; 162: 1050–61.

54. Wong WM, Fass R. Extraesophageal and atypical manifestations of GERD. J Gastroenterol Hepatol 2004; 19(Suppl 3): S33–43.

55. Cameron AJ, Lomboy CT. Barrett's esophagus: age, prevalence, and extent of columnar epithelium. Gastroenterology 1992; 103: 1241–5.

56. Collen MJ, Abdulian JD, Chen YK. Gastroesophageal reflux disease in the elderly: more severe disease that requires aggressive therapy. Am J Gastroenterol 1995; 90: 1053–7.

57. Lagergren J. Adenocarcinoma of oesophagus: what exactly is the size of the problem and who is at risk? Gut 2005; 54(Suppl 1): i1–5.

58. Sharma P, Sidorenko EI. Are screening and surveillance for Barrett's oesophagus really worthwhile? Gut 2005; 54 (Suppl 1): i27–32.

59. Mashimo H, Wagh MS, Goyal RK. Surveillance and screening for Barrett esophagus and adenocarcinoma. J Clin Gastroenterol 2005; 39: S33–41.

60. Bergman JJ, Tytgat GN. New developments in the endoscopic surveillance of Barrett's oesophagus. Gut 2005; 54(Suppl 1): i38–42.

61. Sial SH, Catalano MF. Gastrointestinal tract cancer in the elderly. Gastroenterol Clin North Am 2001; 30: 565–90.

62. Griffin MR. Epidemiology of nonsteroidal anti-inflammatory drug-associated gastrointestinal injury. Am J Med 1998; 104: 23–9S; discussion 41–2S.

63. Silverstein FE, Graham DY, Senior JR et al. Misoprostol reduces serious gastrointestinal complications in patients with rheumatoid arthritis receiving nonsteroidal anti-inflammatory drugs. A randomized, double-blind, placebo-controlled trial. Ann Intern Med 1995; 123: 241–9.

64. Permutt RP, Cello JP. Duodenal ulcer disease in the hospitalized elderly patient. Dig Dis Sci 1982; 27: 1–6.

65. Wilcox CM, Clark WS. Features associated with painless peptic ulcer bleeding. Am J Gastroenterol 1997; 92: 1289–92.

66. Linder JD, Wilcox CM. Acid peptic disease in the elderly. Gastroenterol Clin North Am 2001; 30: 363–76.

67. Gilinsky NH. Peptic ulcer disease in the elderly. Scand J Gastroenterol Suppl 1988; 146: 191–200.

68. Cotton PB, Shorvon PJ. Analysis of endoscopy and radiography in the diagnosis, follow-up and treatment of peptic ulcer disease. Clin Gastroenterol 1984; 13: 383–403.

69. Cooper BT, Weston CF, Neumann CS. Acute upper gastrointestinal haemorrhage in patients aged 80 years or more. Q J Med 1988; 68: 765–74.

70. Farrell JJ, Friedman LS. Gastrointestinal bleeding in the elderly. Gastroenterol Clin North Am 2001; 30: 377–407, viii.

71. Low RN, Wall SD, Jeffrey RB Jr et al. Aortoenteric fistula and perigraft infection: evaluation with CT. Radiology 1990; 175: 157–62.

72. Friedman LS, Martin P. The problem of gastrointestinal bleeding. Gastroenterol Clin North Am 1993; 22: 717–21.

73. Vellacott KD, Dronfield MW, Atkinson M et al. Comparison of surgical and medical management of bleeding peptic ulcers. BMJ (Clin Res Ed) 1982; 284: 548–50.

74. Rockall TA, Logan RF, Devlin HB et al. Incidence of and mortality from acute upper gastrointestinal haemorrhage in the United Kingdom. Steering Committee and members of the National Audit of Acute Upper Gastrointestinal Haemorrhage. BMJ 1995; 311: 222–6.

75. Rockall TA, Logan RF, Devlin HB et al. Risk assessment after acute upper gastrointestinal haemorrhage. Gut 1996; 38: 316–21.

76. Rockall TA, Logan RF, Devlin HB et al. Selection of patients for early discharge or outpatient care after acute upper gastrointestinal haemorrhage. National Audit of Acute Upper Gastrointestinal Haemorrhage. Lancet 1996; 347: 1138–40.

77. Longstreth GF, Feitelberg SP. Outpatient care of selected patients with acute non-variceal upper gastrointestinal haemorrhage. Lancet 1995; 345: 108–11.

78. Choudari CP, Elton RA, Palmer KR. Age-related mortality in patients treated endoscopically for bleeding peptic ulcer. Gastrointest Endosc 1995; 41: 557–60.

79. Schiller KF, Truelove SC, Williams DG. Haematemesis and melaena, with special reference to factors influencing the outcome. BMJ 1970; 2: 7–14.

80. Parsonnet J, Friedman GD, Vandersteen DP et al. Helicobacter pylori infection and the risk of gastric carcinoma. N Engl J Med 1991; 325: 1127–31.

81. An international association between Helicobacter pylori infection and gastric cancer. The EUROGAST Study Group. Lancet 1993; 341: 1359–62.

82. Fuchs CS, Mayer RJ. Gastric carcinoma. N Engl J Med 1995; 333: 32–41.

83. Neugut AI, Hayek M, Howe G. Epidemiology of gastric cancer. Semin Oncol 1996; 23: 281–91.

84. Ye W, Nyren O. Risk of cancers of the oesophagus and stomach by histology or subsite in patients hospitalised for pernicious anaemia. Gut 2003; 52: 938–41.

85. West J, Logan RF, Hill PG et al. Seroprevalence, correlates, and characteristics of undetected coeliac disease in England. Gut 2003; 52: 960–5.

86. Holmes GK, Stokes PL, Sorahan TM et al. Coeliac disease, gluten-free diet, and malignancy. Gut 1976; 17: 612–19.

87. Freeman H, Lemoyne M, Pare P. Coeliac disease. Best Pract Res Clin Gastroenterol 2002; 16: 37–49.

88. Meyer D, Stavropolous S, Diamond B et al. Osteoporosis in a North American adult population with celiac disease. Am J Gastroenterol 2001; 96: 112–19.

89. Brandt LJ, Boley SJ. AGA technical review on intestinal ischemia. American Gastrointestinal Association. Gastroenterology 2000; 118: 954–68.

90. Greenwald DA, Brandt LJ, Reinus JF. Ischemic bowel disease in the elderly. Gastroenterol Clin North Am 2001; 30: 445–73.

91. Pfeiffer RF. Gastrointestinal dysfunction in Parkinson's disease. Lancet Neurol 2003; 2: 107–16.

92. Horowitz M, O'Donovan D, Jones KL et al. Gastric emptying in diabetes: clinical significance and treatment. Diabet Med 2002; 19: 177–94.

93. Rayner CK, Samsom M, Jones KL et al. Relationships of upper gastrointestinal motor and

sensory function with glycemic control. Diabetes Care 2001; 24: 371–81.

94. Horowitz M, Harding PE, Maddox AF et al. Gastric and oesophageal emptying in patients with type 2 (non-insulin-dependent) diabetes mellitus. Diabetologia 1989; 32: 151–9.

95. Lluch I, Ascaso JF, Mora F et al. Gastroesophageal reflux in diabetes mellitus. Am J Gastroenterol 1999; 94: 919–24.

96. Horowitz M, Maddox AF, Wishart JM et al. Relationships between oesophageal transit and solid and liquid gastric emptying in diabetes mellitus. Eur J Nucl Med 1991; 18: 229–34.

97. Jones KL, Horowitz M, Wishart JM et al. Relationships between gastric emptying, intragastric meal distribution and blood glucose concentrations in diabetes mellitus. J Nucl Med 1995; 36: 2220–8.

98. Chang L. Review article: epidemiology and quality of life in functional gastrointestinal disorders. Aliment Pharmacol Ther 2004; 20(Suppl 7): 31–9.

99. Jones R, Lydeard S. Prevalence of symptoms of dyspepsia in the community. BMJ 1989; 298: 30–2.

100. Bharucha AE, Camilleri M. Functional abdominal pain in the elderly. Gastroenterol Clin North Am 2001; 30: 517–29.

101. Bennett G, Talley NJ. Irritable bowel syndrome in the elderly. Best Pract Res Clin Gastroenterol 2002; 16: 63–76.

102. Cremonini F, Delgado-Aros S, Talley NJ. Functional dyspepsia: drugs for new (and old) therapeutic targets. Best Pract Res Clin Gastroenterol 2004; 18: 717–33.

103. Talley NJ. What the physician needs to know for correct management of gastro-oesophageal reflux disease and dyspepsia. Aliment Pharmacol Ther 2004; 20(Suppl 2): 23–30.

104. Talley NJ. Review article: dyspepsia: how to manage and how to treat? Aliment Pharmacol Ther 2002; 16(Suppl 4): 95–104.

105. Eslick GD, Fass R. Noncardiac chest pain: evaluation and treatment. Gastroenterol Clin North Am 2003; 32: 531–52.

106. Fass R, Fennerty MB, Ofman JJ et al. The clinical and economic value of a short course of omeprazole in patients with noncardiac chest pain. Gastroenterology 1998; 115: 42–9.

107. Richter JE. Oesophageal motility disorders. Lancet 2001; 358: 823–8.

Cardiovascular and Respiratory System

CHAPTER 35

Atherosclerotic risk assessment of androgen therapy in aging men

David Crook

Introduction

Testosterone has traditionally been regarded as a hormone that is harmful to the heart, in the same way that estrogen is perceived as a hormone that is good for the heart.[1] The development of androgen therapies for men has often struggled against the perception that any benefit in terms of improved sexual function or protection from osteoporosis, for example, will be at a cost of myocardial infarction and strokes, in addition to concern over prostatic disease. In fact this has never been a unanimous concern: a vocal minority, increasingly evident on the internet,[2] extols the virtue of androgens as *treatments* for these very same diseases.

Risk–benefit analysis of androgen supplementation in the aging male is essential but cannot proceed until this fundamental uncertainty is resolved. Even minor effects of androgens on coronary heart disease (CHD) risk may have major implications when expressed in large populations of aging men. In the context of clinically hypogonadal men an increased risk of CHD might well be considered acceptable, but if androgens are to be used as a more general supplementation therapy in aging men then such an increased risk may prove to be a major obstacle. Conversely, if the claims that androgen therapies can protect some men from CHD are true, then this benefit could be used to 'fast-track' the wider acceptance of androgen therapies in aging men.

Atherosclerosis: a critical issue in world health

Arterial diseases have come to be regarded as an inevitable consequence of a 'Western' lifestyle – addiction to tobacco, abhorrence of physical activity, and possession of a hunger that can only be sated by processed foods rich in salt and animal fats. Arterial diseases are now the major cause of morbidity and mortality in the USA and much of Europe, with 'hot spots' being seen in Scotland, Northern Ireland, and parts of Scandinavia.

There is an old adage that arterial disease is the leading cause of death in all countries who have achieved such a level of economic progress that they can afford to perform epidemiologic studies. In an unwanted deviation to this pattern, the fallout from the dismantling of the former Soviet Union in the 1980s saw the beginning of an epidemic of arterial disease in Eastern bloc countries. On a more global scale, arterial diseases are likely to become major causes of morbidity and mortality[3] (Figure 35.1). As life expectancy in underdeveloped countries is extended by public health policies, their people survive long enough to enter the age groups in which arterial disease will be prevalent, a trend now exacerbated by the drive to promote tobacco products to these countries.

The underlying pathology of atherosclerosis is believed to represent a preventable process.

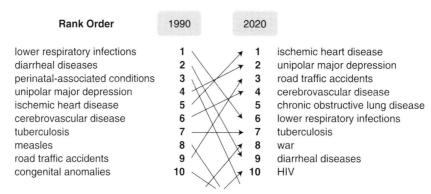

THE GLOBAL BURDEN OF DISEASE PROJECTIONS FOR THE YEAR 2020

'Disability-Adjusted Life Years'

Rank Order	1990		2020	
lower respiratory infections	1		1	ischemic heart disease
diarrheal diseases	2		2	unipolar major depression
perinatal-associated conditions	3		3	road traffic accidents
unipolar major depression	4		4	cerebrovascular disease
ischemic heart disease	5		5	chronic obstructive lung disease
cerebrovascular disease	6		6	lower respiratory infections
tuberculosis	7		7	tuberculosis
measles	8		8	war
road traffic accidents	9		9	diarrheal diseases
congenital anomalies	10		10	HIV

Figure 35.1 *Arterial diseases are predicted to become the major global cause of mortality and morbidity by 2020. Data from reference 3.*

Understanding of the pathogenesis of arterial disease is a surprisingly recent development, originating with the post-World War II investment in medical research in the USA.[4] The discovery of risk factors such as hypertension, cigarette smoking, and dyslipidemia held out the dual possibility of prevention and treatment. More recently, molecular biology has led to major advances in our understanding of that most complex organ, the vascular endothelium. This research supports the proposal by the late Russell Ross[5] that atherosclerosis involves an inappropriate and overenthusiastic inflammatory response by the body to endothelial damage caused by free radicals or other noxious agents. These interlaced phenomena are slowly being unravelled and the list of factors thought to be involved (positively or negatively) in the arterial disease now runs to many hundreds. Steroid hormones are very much a part of this complex scheme.

Steroid hormones and arterial disease

Both estrogens and androgens have been linked to the pathogenesis of arterial disease, originating with the observation that clinically evident CHD is rare in young women compared to young men.[1] The evidence that this gender difference is due to a protective action of estrogen is strong, although final proof – protection of postmenopausal women from CHD in placebo-controlled trials of hormone replacement therapy (HRT) – is still lacking.

The widespread use of estrogens in oral contraception and HRT has meant that the anti-atherogenic potential of estrogen has been studied in depth, while interest in the cardiovascular effects of androgens remains something of a niche area of research. Review articles on androgens and CHD were hard to find until the last decade, but when they did appear they were unusually consistent in their conclusion that treatment of relatively healthy men with modest doses of 'natural' androgens is as likely to reduce CHD risk as it is to increase it.[6–9]

Androgens and arterial disease

The current predictions of the effects of androgen therapies on CHD in men are based on measurement of 'surrogates' such as blood chemistries, animal models of atherosclerosis, and non-invasive evaluations of vascular function. There are no formal randomized controlled trials in which the incidence of myocardial infarction or stroke in men treated with androgens has been compared to that in men given placebo. Such studies are planned but it is unlikely that their results will be available within this current decade.

The prevalence of androgen supplementation in the male population, though increasing in many countries, is unlikely to reach the levels whereby observational epidemiology can be used. This contrasts with the situation in women, in which epidemiologists were able to track the occurrence of diseases such as CHD in large communities of aging women, many of whom were HRT users. It is possible to envisage a time in which androgen replacement therapy in men has become so commonplace in certain countries that such groups of users are easily identifiable, but then a new problem is likely to emerge: the use of different therapies and routes of administration. An interim approach is to break the current published literature into a set of themes relating to androgens and CHD in men.

'Maleness' as a risk factor for CHD

Attempts to discuss androgen therapy in men often flounder at an early stage due to the ingrained popular belief that 'maleness' causes CHD. This is partly due to the heavy promotion of cardiovascular risk assessment strategies that score 'maleness' as a risk factor of similar weight to diabetes or hypertension. What is rarely acknowledged is that the scoring of male gender as a positive factor is essentially an administrative convenience. The term 'femaleness' could just as well be used but there is a convention that such protective factors should be kept out of the equation. Overall it has proved simpler to score male gender as a positive risk factor than to introduce the negative risk factor of female gender.

If the plasma androgen levels associated with being male are responsible for the gender difference in CHD, then castration in men should reduce their CHD risk. The evidence for this is inconclusive.[9]

Arterial disease in men abusing androgenic anabolic steroids

Another widely held view is that androgen therapies in aging men will increase CHD risk because androgenic anabolic steroids (AASs) induce the disease. The evidence for this involves a dozen or so case-reports that describe premature CHD, often of atypical pathology, in young male athletes abusing AASs.[10] However, the toxicity problem highlighted in these case-reports has yet to be validated in formal epidemiologic studies, leading Rockhold[11] to contend that the frequency of such reports is actually lower than would be expected, given the widespread abuse of AASs and the awareness within the medical community of a potential problem.

Parsinnen and colleagues[12] investigated the health of 62 male elite powerlifters who had competed in the Finnish championships in 1977–1982. AAS abuse was commonplace at that time because doping controls had yet to be introduced in Finland. By 1993 eight of these men had died, giving a relative risk of death of 4.6 compared to 1094 population controls (95% confidence interval (CI) 2.0–10.5). Three of these eight deaths were suicides. The authors consider the prevalence of cardiovascular deaths in the two groups to be similar. Even if it is shown that CHD risk is increased in AAS users, could such findings be extrapolated to healthy men taking low doses of androgens under medical supervision? In most studies the AAS abusers were using combinations of oral and injectable steroids, often involving multiple drugs and supplemented with many other agents of unknown arterial safety, such as amfetamines and cocaine. A further complication is the role of strenuous physical exercise in 'triggering' plaque rupture in individuals who may otherwise have peacefully co-existed with their atherosclerotic plaques. Strenuous exertion, as distinct from regular moderate exercise, is strongly linked to acute myocardial infarction events.[13]

The validity of the control subjects used in these studies is also under question. In one study, researchers at the University of Sydney performed a panel of cardiovascular tests in 20 elite body-builders whose self-reporting of AAS abuse was confirmed by urine screening.[14] These men had impaired vascular reactivity and increased carotid intima-media thickness (CIMT) compared with non-bodybuilding sedentary controls, but, critically, such differences were lost when body-builders who denied AAS abuse were used as controls (Figure 35.2). The claim that this latter group was 'clean' must be taken seriously as they belonged to an athletic society in

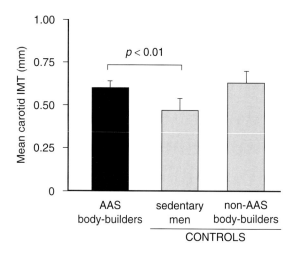

Figure 35.2 *Carotid intima-media thickness (IMT), a surrogate for atherosclerosis, in body-builders who used androgenic anabolic steroids (AAS) Note that these men showed evidence of increased atherosclerosis, but not when compared to body-builders who did not use AAS. Data from reference 14.*

which continued membership relied on repeated negative urine drug screens. However this does not exclude the possibility that these men were previously exposed to AAS and so had some residual arterial damage.

Thus, studies of CHD in AAS abusers pivot on the choice of control group. This uncertainty could be resolved in the setting of a randomized controlled trial, but such a study is unlikely to be commissioned. These studies should alert us to the possibility of an adverse effect of androgen therapy in aging men, but do not in themselves prove that such intervention would be dangerous. Their strength may lie in identifying potential atherogenic mechanisms, such as hypertension, plasma lipoprotein levels, platelet aggregation, myocyte toxicity, or coronary spasm, that can then be investigated in a more clinically relevant population.

Arterial disease in experimental animals treated with androgens

Laboratory animals such as mice, rats, rabbits, and monkeys have been used as a shortcut to understanding drug effects on atherosclerosis. With few exceptions these species do not develop atherosclerosis and

must be fed highly artificial diets rich in saturated fats and crystalline cholesterol in order to induce a gross and atherogenic dyslipidemia. These models are gradually being replaced by genetically engineered animals such as the apoE knockout mouse.

Many such studies find that androgens protect rabbits from diet-induced atherosclerosis (see Chapter 36), with a possible link to induction of androgen receptors in arterial tissue.[15] In contrast, two reports in the cynomolgus monkey have contributed to the fears that androgen administration will induce atherosclerosis.[16,17] Both studies should be regarded with caution as the adverse effects were seen in female animals. There is increasing evidence that androgens may not have the same cardiovascular effects in women as in men. Cynomolgus monkeys have been extensively used for the safety evaluation of HRT and oral contraceptive steroids, but their relevance to human vascular disease is increasingly under question.

Androgens and cardiovascular risk factors

Androgens, like estrogens, affect many aspects of cardiovascular risk (see review by von Eckardstein[18]). The interpretation of these changes is becoming increasingly difficult. Androgens often reduce plasma levels of high density lipoproteins (HDLs) and this change has historically been used to categorize such steroids as 'harmful' to vascular health. But these changes are often seen in parallel with reductions in plasma levels of triglycerides and lipoprotein (a), a pattern that would be considered to reduce CHD risk.[18,19] The effects of androgens on plasma levels of low density lipoproteins (LDLs), the classic metabolic risk factor in men, are difficult to interpret. Some AAS regimens grossly elevate plasma LDL levels, suggestive of an increase in CHD risk,[18] but these levels are often unchanged when considering the doses of androgens being considered for male contraception or androgen replacement[18] and in one study in AAS users LDL levels were reduced.[19]

The increased hemoglobin levels seen with some androgens could be considered to increase CHD risk but in the context of older men may be beneficial.

Studies in AAS abusers suggest an increase in platelet aggregation,[20] especially in older men, and activation of hemostasis as monitored by plasma levels of F1+2 and D-dimer.[21]

There is still no agreement as to which risk factor is the most important in terms of cardiovascular disease and thus there is no way that the complex metabolic data now being generated can be synthesized to produce an estimate of the net effect of a specific androgen therapy on CHD risk. The position is further complicated by emerging evidence from studies in women that steroid-induced changes in plasma levels of CHD risk factors may not reflect changes in underlying pathologic processes.[22,23]

A striking finding from many clinical studies of androgens is the change in body mass, in particular the reduction in fat mass. The status of obesity itself as a CHD risk factor is still controversial: in many studies the relationship disappears once corrections are made for lack of exercise, diet, and diabetes. Obesity, in particular central or 'android' obesity, is linked to insulin resistance and many other CHD risk factors. Without doubt (1) plasma testosterone levels correlate negatively with abdominal fat content, and (2) aging in men is associated with a shift towards central adiposity, but this is likely to reflect a complex interplay between sex hormones, insulin, leptin, growth hormone, changes in physical activity, and so on. Where hypogonadal men have been studied an androgen-induced reduction in android fat mass is quite convincing but the evidence that moderate doses of androgens will have this effect in healthier men is dubious.[24] This issue needs resolution in placebo-controlled clinical trials. In the USA and many Western countries the existence of a 'six-pack' culture makes it likely that any claims that androgens will reduce abdominal fat (and perhaps increase muscle mass) will attract considerable popular interest.

Cardiologic studies of arterial health in androgen users

If androgens are indeed atherogenic (due to changes in plasma lipoproteins or other factors) then men with coronary artery disease would be expected to have higher plasma androgen levels compared to those free of the disease. The epidemiologic evidence fails to support such a contention,[7] but it is the unexpected inverse relationship with angiographically assessed coronary artery disease that has intrigued many cardiologists. The association of low plasma testosterone levels with coronary atherosclerosis first described by Phillips et al[25] has been confirmed by other researchers[26] and has also been shown to exist with plasma DHEA levels.[27] Of particular interest is the subsequent observation by Phillips of a positive relationship between plasma testosterone and angiographically assessed coronary disease in women,[28] reinforcing the theme of a gender difference in the way androgens influence arterial disease.

Testosterone appears to be a vasorelaxant, though one that operates through different and more complex mechanisms than are seen with estradiol.[29] This is an attractive attribute of the steroid, but other aspects of the vascular influence of androgens remain a concern, such as the demonstration of increased monocyte adherence to endothelial cells in culture, at least in part due to overexpression of vascular adhesion molecules.[30]

The true test of the hypothesis that androgens reduce the severity or incidence of arterial diseases will come from placebo-controlled studies using clinical endpoints. The evidence so far – reviewed in Chapter 33 – is encouraging, although it is largely based on the study of men with pre-existing arterial disease.

One issue yet to be addressed is that of androgen resistance in aging men: when testosterone was used to vasodilate rat coronary arteries, it appeared that vessels from older rats were less sensitive to testosterone than were those from young animals.[31]

Conclusions

Over recent years the exciting evidence that androgens might reduce CHD risk has been balanced by some concerns: we simply do not know what any specific androgen supplementation therapy will do in a specific population of men. The experience so far should lead to a wider acknowledgment of the potential of androgens to protect at least some men from arterial disease. The animal data are confusing: androgens appear to be beneficial in some species but harmful in others. The risk factor data are especially difficult to interpret and are overshadowed by the possibility that steroid-induced changes in blood chemistries do not reflect underlying changes in pathologic processes. The present enthusiasm on the part of cardiologists for the beneficial effects of androgen therapy relates to men with established CHD; information on clinical endpoints in men without symptomatic arterial disease is still lacking.

References

1. Godsland IF, Wynn V, Crook D, Miller NE. Sex, plasma lipoproteins and atherosclerosis: prevailing assumptions and outstanding questions. Am Heart J 1987; 114: 1467–503.
2. Kennedy R. http://www.medical-library.net/sites/framer.html?/sites/testerone therapy.html.
3. Lopez AD, Murray CCJL. The global burden of disease: 1990–2020. Nature Med 1998; 4: 1241–3.
4. Braunwald E. Shattuck Lecture – cardiovascular medicine at the turn of the millennium: triumphs, concerns and opportunities. N Engl J Med 1997; 337: 1360–9.
5. Ross R. Atherosclerosis – an inflammatory disease. N Engl J Med 1999; 340: 115–25.
6. Barrett Connor EL. Testosterone and risk factors for cardiovascular disease in men. Diabetes Metabol (Paris) 1995; 21: 156–61.
7. Alexandersen P, Haarbo J, Christiansen C. The relationship of natural androgens to coronary heart disease in males: a review. Atherosclerosis 1996; 125: 1–13.
8. English KM, Steeds R, Jones TH, Channer KS. Testosterone and coronary heart disease: is there a link? Q J Med 1997; 90: 787–91.
9. Crook D. Androgen therapy in the aging male: assessing the effect on heart disease. Aging Male 1999; 2: 1–6.
10. Sullivan ML, Martinez CM, Gennis P, Gallagher EJ. The cardiac toxicity of anabolic steroids. Prog Cardiovasc Dis 1998; 41: 1–15.
11. Rockhold RW. Cardiovascular toxicity of anabolic steroids. Ann Rev Pharmacol Toxicol 1993; 33: 497–520.
12. Parssinen M, Kujala U, Vartiainen E et al. Increased premature mortality of competitive powerlifters suspected to have used anabolic agents. Int J Sports Med 2000; 21: 225–7.
13. Mittleman MA, Maclure M, Tofler GH et al. Triggering of acute myocardial infarction by heavy physical exertion. Protection against triggering by regular exertion. Determinants of Myocardial

14. Infarction Onset Study Investigators. N Engl J Med 1993; 329: 1677–83.
14. Sader MA, Griffiths KA, McCredie RJ et al. Androgenic anabolic steroids and arterial structure and function in male bodybuilders. JACC 2001; 37: 224–30.
15. Hanke H, Lenz C, Hess B et al. Effect of testosterone on plaque development and androgen receptor expression in the arterial vessel wall. Circulation 2001; 103: 1382–5.
16. Adams MR, Williams JK, Kaplan JR. Effects of androgens on coronary artery atherosclerosis and atherosclerosis-related impairment of vascular responsiveness. Arterioscler Thromb Vasc Biol 1995; 15: 562–70.
17. Obasanjo IO, Clarkson TB, Weaver DS. Effects of the anabolic steroid nandrolone decanoate on plasma lipids and coronary arteries of female cynomolgus macaques. Metabolism 1996; 45: 463–8.
18. Von Eckardstein A. Androgens, cardiovascular risk factors and atherosclerosis. In: Nieschlag E, Behre HM, eds. Testosterone. Berlin: Springer, 1998: 229–58.
19. Dickerman RD, McConathy WJ, Zachariah NY. Testosterone, sex hormone binding globulin, lipoproteins and vascular disease risk. J Cardiovasc Risk 1997; 4: 363–6.
20. Ferenchick G, Schwartz D, Ball M, Schwartz K. Androgenic-anabolic steroid abuse and platelet aggregation: a pilot study in weight lifters. Am J Med Sci 1992; 303: 78–82.
21. Ferenchick GS, Hirowaka S, Mammen EF, Schwartz KA. Anabolic-androgenic steroid abuse in weight lifters: evidence for activation of the hemostatic system. Am J Hematol 1995; 49: 282–8.
22. Crook D, Von Eckardstein A, Dieplinger H et al. Tibolone lowers HDL concentrations but does not impair cholesterol efflux from cells. Maturitas 2000; 35: 7–8.
23. Van Kesteren PJ, Kooistra T, Lansink M et al. The effects of sex steroids on plasma levels of marker proteins of endothelial cell functioning. Thromb Haemostasis 1998; 79: 1029–33.
24. Vermeulen A, Goemaere S, Kaufman JM. Testosterone, body composition and aging. J Endocrinol Invest 1999; 22(5 Suppl): 110–16.
25. Phillips GB, Pinkernell BH, Jing T-Y. The association of hypotestosteronemia with coronary artery disease in men. Arterioscler Thromb 1994; 14: 701–6.
26. English KM, Mandour O, Steeds RP et al. Men with coronary heart disease have lower levels of androgens than men with normal coronary androgens. Eur Heart J 2000; 21: 890–4.
27. Adamkiewicz M, Zgliczynski S, Slowinska-Srzednicka J et al. Androgens (testosterone and dehydroepiandrosterone-sulfate) and coronary arteriosclerosis in men.

Presented at III Internationales Grazer Andrologie-Symposion. Graz 2000; 2: 31.

28. Phillips GB, Pinkernell BH, Jing T-Y. Relationship between serum sex hormones and coronary artery disease in postmenopausal women. Arterioscler Thromb Vasc Biol 1997; 17: 695–701.

29. Crews JK, Kahil RA. Antagonistic effects of 17 β-estradiol, progesterone and testosterone on calcium entry mechanisms of coronary vasoconstriction. Atheroscler Thromb Vasc Biol 1999; 19: 1034–40.

30. McCrohon JA, Jessup W, Handelsman DJ, Celermajer DS. Androgen exposure increases human monocyte adhesion to vascular endothelium and endothelial cell expression of vascular cell adhesion molecule-1. Circulation 1999; 99: 2317–22.

31. English KM, Jones RD, Jones TH et al. Aging reduces the responsiveness of coronary arteries from male Wister rats to the vasodilatory action of testosterone. Clin Sci 2000; 99: 77–82.

CHAPTER 36

Male aging: changes in metabolic, inflammatory, and endothelial indices of cardiovascular risk

Ian F Godsland

The development of cardiovascular disease can be understood in terms of exposure to risk factors. These damage the vasculature and, if exposure is chronic, may overwhelm natural repair mechanisms and set in motion processes that ultimately lead to the catastrophic consequences of arterial occlusion, including stroke and heart attack. Risk factor exposure may be external, as with cultural, lifestyle, and environmental influences, or internal, according to the body's physiologic or biochemical characteristics. Sex hormone levels can profoundly influence the latter. External and internal risk factor relationships can interact and, in men, these interactions and interrelationships are exemplified by the changes in risk factor status that accompany aging.

Cardiovascular risk factors

Cigarette smoking, hypertension, and hypercholesterolemia are the classic risk factors for cardiovascular disease. Exposure to tobacco imposes the greatest coronary heart disease burden worldwide,[1] whereas elevated blood pressure is an especially strong indicator of risk of cerebrovascular disease. Each of these risk factors damages the arterial endothelium, but how this damage progresses depends on local conditions and intensity of exposure. For example, cholesterol can be deposited in the subendothelial

space to form atherosclerotic plaque, which can ultimately rupture to expose thrombotic tissue surfaces and oxidized lipid. When this occurs in the coronary arteries, the consequence is angina or myocardial infarction. When the blood supply to the brain is affected, transient ischemic attack or ischemic stroke results. A considerable range of variables may be involved, each of which is in some way linked with the development of the disease, either as a possible cause or as a marker of progressing damage (Figure 36.1). Many of these variables may be measured in serum, in contrast to variables that relate directly to endothelial or arterial structure or function. This chapter will primarily concern such serum-based measures, and how they change as men age.

Measures of cardiovascular risk

Cholesterol metabolism

The role of cholesterol in the development of coronary heart disease (CHD) exemplifies the involvement of metabolic disturbance in atherogenesis. Atherosclerotic plaques contain cholesterol, serum cholesterol concentrations are high in those with CHD, and high serum cholesterol concentrations predict the development of clinical CHD. There are specific inherited defects in cholesterol metabolism

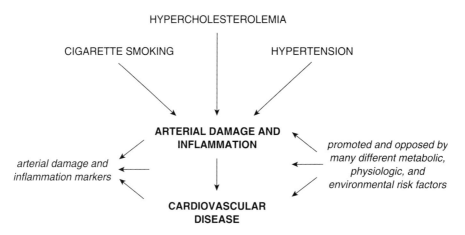

Figure 36.1 *Risk factors and cardiovascular disease.*

associated with a predisposition to CHD and mechanisms have been elucidated whereby cholesterol can enter and be deposited in the subendothelial space. Conclusively, specific pharmacologic interventions have been found which substantially lower both cholesterol concentrations and risk of CHD.

Variation in serum cholesterol concentrations is the net expression of a complex underlying metabolic system, different elements of which can independently affect the development of atherosclerosis. Being insoluble in water, cholesterol must be carried within lipoprotein particles made water soluble by a hydrophilic coating of phospholipid and protein. Three systems of lipoprotein metabolism may be distinguished (Figure 36.2). The endogenous pathway involves the assembly in the liver of triglyceride-rich very-low-density lipoprotein (VLDL) particles. Once released into the circulation, VLDL particles become a substrate for endothelial lipoprotein lipase, which hydrolyzes the core triglycerides and releases non-esterified fatty acids (NEFAs) for oxidation, incorporation into adipose tissue fat depots, or re-incorporation into VLDL triglyceride in the liver. Progressive delipidation of VLDL particles leads to their increasing cholesterol enrichment and the generation of low-density lipoprotein (LDL). LDL is the principal medium through which cholesterol is made available throughout the body, entering tissues via the LDL receptor. Via cholesterol ester transfer

protein (CETP), triglyceride from intermediates in the delipidation of VLDL may be exchanged for cholesterol esters in cholesterol-rich HDL or LDL particles. Triglyceride enrichment of LDL makes it a preferred substrate for lipolysis, resulting in production of a smaller, denser, cholesterol-rich LDL particle. Cholesterol enrichment of intermediates in the delipidation pathway leads to production of cholesterol-rich VLDL remnants.

The exogenous pathway of lipoprotein metabolism performs a similar function, but with freshly absorbed triglycerides and fatty acids from the intestine. Instead of VLDL, the particles produced are the larger triglyceride-rich chylomicrons. Like VLDL, the chylomicrons are acted on by lipoprotein lipase. Intermediates in the delipidation of chylomicrons can provide triglyceride for exchange with cholesterol esters from other lipoprotein particles. The cholesterol-rich chylomicron remnants that are the end product of the exogenous pathway of lipoprotein metabolism are finally removed from the circulation via the hepatic chylomicron remnant receptor.

The third lipoprotein system is reverse cholesterol transport that mediates removal of excess cholesterol from the body via high-density lipoprotein (HDL). Nascent HDL particles are secreted by the liver and intestine and progressively mature with the acquisition of intracellular free cholesterol via

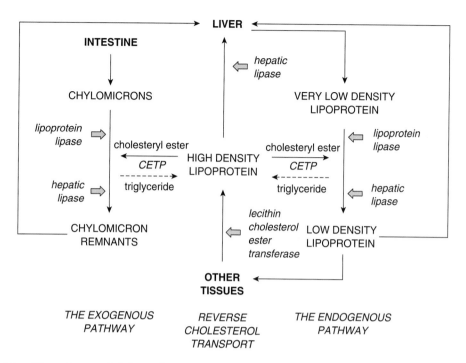

Figure 36.2 *The pathways of cholesterol transport between tissues and lipoproteins, showing the influences of the principal enzymes of lipoprotein metabolism and of cholesterol ester transfer protein (CETP).*

the ATP-binding cassette transporter A1 protein. Free cholesterol in HDL becomes esterified and HDL particles undergo further maturation with the acquisition of apolipoproteins and phospholipid made available during delipidation of VLDL and chylomicrons. HDL thus becomes progressively larger and cholesterol ester enriched and cholesterol esters may be exchanged via CETP for triglycerides from intermediates in VLDL delipidation, ultimately to be removed in LDL by the liver. Triglyceride in the large, cholesterol-rich HDL may be hydrolyzed by hepatic lipase and a smaller, denser HDL particle emerges ready to receive further loads of cholesterol ester.

Disturbances in any one of the elements in the cholesterol transport system may result in elevated cholesterol concentrations and accumulation of cholesterol in the artery wall. A key factor in this appears to be oxidation of LDL that has passed through the endothelium. Oxidized lipid in the subendothelium acts as an endothelial toxin and initiates recruitment of monocytes into the subendothelium, as well as their differentiation into macrophages. Moreover, oxidative modification of the principal apolipoprotein of LDL, apoB, renders the LDL particle less likely to be taken up by the LDL receptor and more likely to be taken up by macrophages. Given sufficient internalization of oxidized lipoprotein, macrophages develop into lipid-laden foam cells which undergo necrosis and release their lipid into the subendothelial space to form the lipid core of the developing atherosclerotic plaque.

The LDL particle, in excess and, possibly, in the absence of sufficient antioxidant activity, therefore provides the vehicle for cholesterol accumulation in the atherosclerotic plaque. VLDL and chylomicron remnants may also provide a similar vehicle. Since the greatest proportion of cholesterol in the circulation is carried on LDL, measurement of total serum cholesterol provides an index of potentially atherogenic LDL levels, with some contribution from cholesterol carried in VLDL and chylomicron remnants. However, a proportion of total cholesterol represents cholesterol in the HDL fraction and, as might be expected from the role of HDL in reverse cholesterol transport, high levels of HDL cholesterol are associated with decreased risk of CHD. In other words, HDL is a negative predictor. The various proteins of HDL also confer other anti-atherogenic effects. ApoAI, the principal apolipoprotein of HDL, can act as a prostacyclin stabilizer, prostacylin having antithrombotic, anti-inflammatory, and vasodilatory actions. HDL also carries antioxidant enzymes, such as paraoxonase. Ideally, therefore, cardiovascular risk assessment as it relates to cholesterol metabolism should include measurement of total and HDL cholesterol.

Insulin resistance and diabetes

Several key control points in lipoprotein metabolism are powerfully affected by insulin. The most sensitive of these is lipolysis of fat stores in adipose tissue, which is acutely suppressed by insulin. Adipose tissue lipolysis provides NEFAs for synthesis of triglycerides by the liver, and NEFA supply to the liver largely determines the rate of synthesis of VLDL. Suppression of lipolysis therefore suppresses VLDL synthesis. Insulin can also suppress VLDL release from the liver and stimulates lipoprotein lipase activity. Insulin, therefore, blocks VLDL secretion and promotes its elimination.

Insulin action is deficient in states of insulin resistance, in which there is a subnormal tissue response to insulin, and in impaired glucose tolerance and diabetes, in which there is impaired insulin secretion. Insulin resistance, impaired glucose tolerance, and diabetes are each associated with increased NEFA supply to the liver, increased output of VLDL, and decreased elimination of VLDL and chylomicrons. An important consequence of the resulting increase in triglyceride-enriched lipoproteins is increased exchange of triglycerides and cholesterol esters via CETP. This results in increased proportions of small dense LDL particles, which are less readily taken up by the LDL receptor, penetrate the subendothelium more readily, and are more susceptible to oxidation. Further consequences include fewer HDL particles available

for reverse cholesterol transport and greater cholesterol enrichment and atherogenicity of VLDL and chylomicron remnant particles.

Beyond these changes in lipid metabolism, deficient insulin action results in further disturbances. These depend on whether insulin deficiency or insulin resistance is primary, the former being characterized by hyperglycemia and the latter by hyperinsulinemia. Fasting hyperglycemia, impaired glucose tolerance, and diabetes have each been linked with the development of cardiovascular disease, possibly through increased release of oxidative free radicals, mitochondrial DNA damage, or protein glycation. The formation of advanced glycation end products is now a well-characterized feature of diabetes and glycation can extend to LDL. Glycation of LDL renders it less able to be taken up by the LDL receptor and more likely to be accumulated in oxidized form in the subendothelium.

Insulin resistance and its accompanying hyperinsulinemia have been linked with increased blood pressure, increased catecholamine levels, increased concentrations of the antifibrinolytic factor plasminogen activator inhibitor-1 (PAI-1), increased fibrinogen, increased uric acid concentrations, impaired endothelial function, and increased markers of subclinical inflammation, each of which may independently promote the atherosclerotic process. It has been suggested that there is an 'insulin resistance syndrome' that encompasses these manifold changes and which may be as critical a factor in cardiovascular risk as hypercholesterolemia.

One uncertainty regarding the syndrome of disturbances centered on insulin resistance is whether it can exist independently of increased body fat accumulation, particularly in the visceral or central region of the body. Central body fat is highly lipolytic and is consequently a particularly rich source of NEFAs. It is also a source of inflammatory cytokines, one of which, tumor necrosis factor alpha, can induce insulin resistance and promote triglyceride release. It is also a negative regulator of the adipose tissue-derived cytokine adiponectin, which acts to reduce insulin resistance. The possibility that visceral fat deposition rather than insulin resistance is the primary disturbance has led to the 'metabolic syndrome' concept, which – in contrast to the

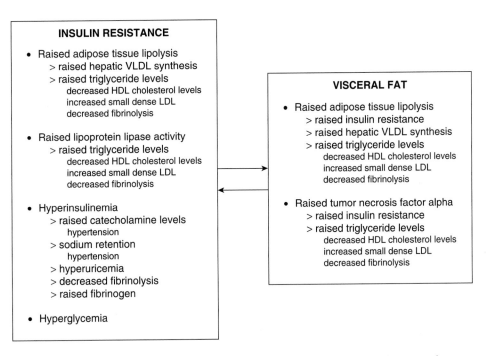

INSULIN RESISTANCE

- Raised adipose tissue lipolysis
  > raised hepatic VLDL synthesis
  > raised triglyceride levels
    decreased HDL cholesterol levels
    increased small dense LDL
    decreased fibrinolysis

- Raised lipoprotein lipase activity
  > raised triglyceride levels
    decreased HDL cholesterol levels
    increased small dense LDL
    decreased fibrinolysis

- Hyperinsulinemia
  > raised catecholamine levels
    hypertension
  > sodium retention
    hypertension
  > hyperuricemia
  > decreased fibrinolysis
  > raised fibrinogen

- Hyperglycemia

VISCERAL FAT

- Raised adipose tissue lipolysis
  > raised insulin resistance
  > raised hepatic VLDL synthesis
  > raised triglyceride levels
    decreased HDL cholesterol levels
    increased small dense LDL
    decreased fibrinolysis

- Raised tumor necrosis factor alpha
  > raised insulin resistance
  > raised triglyceride levels
    decreased HDL cholesterol levels
    increased small dense LDL
    decreased fibrinolysis

Figure 36.3 *Interrelated disturbances of the metabolic syndrome. First-level effects that are a direct consequence of insulin resistance or visceral fat are bulleted. Second-level effects resulting from these first-level effects are arrowed. Third-level effects resulting from the second-level effects are shown in smaller type.*

insulin resistance syndrome – includes among its features disturbances which may cause, as well as be caused by, insulin resistance. This concept provides a convenient way of referring to co-associated risk factor disturbances and several international health organizations have proposed working definitions. Whether use of such definitions improves existing algorithms for cardiovascular risk assessment remains controversial, however. The contributions of insulin resistance and visceral fat to a range of intercorrelated metabolic disturbances linked with cardiovascular disease are illustrated in Figure 36.3.

Markers of inflammation and vascular damage

An important feature of atherosclerosis is inflammation, which is one aspect of the normal healing response to injury, but may become chronic, causing further damage beyond the original lesion that initiated the inflammatory process. Leukocyte count,

globulin concentrations, and erythrocyte sedimentation rate are among the traditional indices of inflammation that have been joined more recently by the so-called 'acute phase markers' such as C-reactive protein (CRP), fibrinogen, serum amyloid A, and lipoprotein-associated phospholipase A2. These measures are markedly elevated in clinical conditions associated with inflammation. However, relatively minor, subclinical elevations may be present in the early stages of atherosclerosis and there is now substantial evidence from prospective studies confirming that elevations in these measures can indeed predict subsequent cardiovascular disease.

Inflammatory cytokines can influence the synthesis of lipoprotein (a) which is present in high concentrations at sites of vascular inflammation. The role of lipoprotein (a) in this respect is uncertain, although one possibility is that it is providing cholesterol for membrane synthesis at sites of vascular damage. Lipoprotein (a) bears a structural resemblance to LDL, but also resembles tissue plasminogen activator (tPA) and may act as a competitive inhibitor of tPA action, thus inhibiting fibrinolysis. This could be the principal influence underlying the association between high lipoprotein (a) levels and CHD, seen both in prospective studies in humans and in transgenic animals in which the apolipoprotein (a) gene has been inserted.

As described above, insulin resistance and obesity are accompanied by subclinical inflammation, which may relate to early atherosclerosis. A surrogate index of more advanced stages of endothelial damage is provided by microalbuminuria, measured as the albumin/creatinine ratio (upper limit in men 2.5 mmol/mg) in an early morning urine sample. Hypertension and diabetes are its most common clinical correlates although, interestingly, there is an association between microalbuminuria, insulin resistance, and cardiovascular disease in non-diabetic individuals. Also associated with microalbuminuria in diabetes are elevated homocysteine levels. Homocysteine predicts cardiovascular disease in patients with diabetes, although in normoglycemic individuals, homocysteine may be raised in cardiovascular disease but is not a predictor, which suggests that it may be a marker of existing vascular disease rather than an active agent.

Changes in risk factor status with age in men

Puberty and adolescence

Puberty in boys is accompanied by a rise in testosterone levels and a fall in HDL cholesterol concentrations, possibly as a result of induction of the sex-hormone-sensitive enzyme of lipoprotein metabolism, hepatic lipase.[2] It is at puberty that HDL levels fall in males, thus establishing one of the principal risk factor differences that may underlie the higher age-standardized CHD rates in men compared with women. Puberty is also accompanied by a transient increase in insulin resistance on account of the increase in growth hormone levels taking place at the time.[3] However, the increase in both androgen and growth hormone levels combines to induce a substantial increase in lean body mass. Since muscle is one of the principal sites of

action of insulin, this net increase in insulin-sensitive metabolic tissue as boys pass from puberty to adulthood restores whole-body insulin sensitivity to levels which are probably somewhat higher than those seen in women.

Adulthood

Although the rise in testosterone in boys at puberty is associated with a decrease in HDL levels, in men there is a positive correlation between testosterone and HDL. This may reflect the predominance of a further effect of testosterone on HDL metabolism, beyond induction of hepatic lipase, namely stimulation of hepatic synthesis of apoAI.[4]

HDL does not appear to change appreciably in adult males in passing from youth to middle age, but most other risk indices deteriorate. To what extent this is due to lifestyle and environmental influences or to factors intrinsic to the aging process is unclear, but both are likely to be operating. Excessive calorie intake and an increasingly sedentary lifestyle in men can combine to promote the deposition of visceral fat, a process which becomes increasingly noticeable as middle age approaches. As described above, visceral fat has manifold adverse metabolic effects which could contribute to the tendency for cardiovascular disease to manifest in mid life in men. The chronic insulin resistance associated with central fat deposition may be a precursor of maturity onset, or type 2 diabetes, thus further compounding the impairment of insulin action associated with insulin resistance.

Diet in men may be suboptimal, not only in relation to total caloric intake but to the quality of food as well. Prospective epidemiologic studies of cardiovascular disease have included increasingly accurate evaluation of dietary composition, particularly in terms of vitamin and fruit and vegetable intake, and there is increasing evidence that these can reduce cardiovascular risk.[5-7] Total cholesterol levels, too, increase steadily with age. Again lifestyle influences may contribute, but there is also progressive impairment of cholesterol elimination.[8] Protein turnover decreases with increasing age, and proteins involved in lipoprotein metabolism, such as apoB and the LDL receptor, are therefore more likely to undergo glycation or oxidative modification.

Late life

Risk factor status worsens with increasing age, although different rates of change may be detected for some factors in men and women. For example, the age-related increase in procoagulatory factor VII may be significantly less in men.[9] Beyond maturity, the rate of adverse change in risk factor profiles appears to diminish. Much of the information relating to risk factor changes later in life comes from cross-sectional studies. It could, therefore, be argued that those susceptible to adverse risk factor changes have already died, leaving a population with somewhat healthier intrinsic risk factor characteristics. Nevertheless, although risk factor changes may diminish, the clinical consequences of earlier disturbances do not. By this time, irrevocable damage may already have been done in terms of the onset of diabetes and vascular disease and there may be additional factors, in particular declining testosterone concentrations, which exacerbate the effects of such damage.

Age and declining testosterone concentrations in men

In men, testosterone levels start to decline after 20 years of age,[10] and this leads to an appreciable deficit in testosterone beyond about 50 years.[10-13] This could be part of an intrinsic physiologic process,[14-16] but there may be some communities in which these changes are not apparent,[17] which suggests an important contribution from psychosocial and lifestyle factors.[18]

Causes of the age-related decline in testosterone levels

Associations between low testosterone levels and cigarette smoking, alcohol intake, and obesity indicate the potential importance of lifestyle factors. Both longitudinal[19] and cross sectional studies[20-22] have found evidence for lower testosterone levels, or a more rapid decline in testosterone levels with age in cigarette smokers, although not all cross-sectional studies support these findings.[10,23-27] Nevertheless, reductions in testosterone levels would be expected on the basis of animal experimental data showing a dose-dependent reduction in testosterone levels

in response to cigarette smoking[28,29] or to the components of cigarette smoke.[30]

Evidence regarding the effects of alcohol intake on testosterone levels is also inconsistent. Chronic alcoholism[31] and acute intake[32] have been linked with reduced gonadal function. However, with regard to moderate alcohol intake, no association has been observed with testosterone levels.[19,26,33,34]

There is consistent evidence relating obesity to low total testosterone levels. This association is apparent over a broad range of degrees of over-weight,[35,36] and a causative association is suggested by the decreases in testosterone levels that accompany weight loss.[24] Moreover, there is evidence from both cross-sectional and prospective studies that the association may be particularly strong with abdominal obesity.[37-40] When free testosterone levels are considered, however, the evidence is less strong since an obesity-related increase in sex hormone-binding globulin (SHBG) may confound the relationship and be responsible for the associations seen with total testosterone.[41]

Type A personality classification could also contribute to the age-related decline in testosterone levels,[42,43] as might be expected since the increased cortisol levels in type A individuals could suppress testosterone levels in men.[19]

Risk factor changes associated with low testosterone levels

In adult men, low testosterone levels have been linked with low HDL cholesterol, both cross-sectionally[44] and longitudinally.[19] An association between low testosterone and high blood pressure has also been reported,[40,45,46] although not consistently.[19,47,48] Other associations with a low testosterone level have included elevated plasma insulin concentrations,[49,50] suggesting an association between low testosterone concentrations and insulin resistance, and this is supported by the observation that low testosterone levels can predict the development of type 2 diabetes.[51] Studies in which insulin sensitivity has been measured show either a strong positive relationship between insulin sensitivity and testosterone levels,[52,53] or no relationship.[54] One recent positive study found that the relationship between low insulin sensitivity and low testosterone levels could be explained statistically by the degree of adiposity.[53] Potentially adverse changes in factors of the hemostatic system have also been linked with low testosterone levels. These include elevated fibrinogen and factor VII antigen[47,55] and PAI-1.[56] One exception, however, may be adiponectin. Low rather than high levels of this negative risk factor for diabetes and cardiovascular disease are seen in association with high free testosterone.[57] Testosterone and adiponectin appear to have mechanistic interactions independent of their associations with insulin sensitivity, as suggested by the in vitro observation that testosterone can specifically inhibit adiponectin secretion from isolated adipocytes.[58]

The strongest risk factor correlates of a low testosterone level therefore appear to be central obesity, low HDL cholesterol, and increased insulin concentrations. The resemblance of these changes to the classic metabolic syndrome is striking, and it is noteworthy that low testosterone concentrations are linked with elevated leptin levels,[59-61] another potential feature of the metabolic syndrome.[62] These associations could be augmented by the decreasing muscle mass associated with increasing age and decreasing testosterone levels, which diminishes available metabolizing tissue.

Associations between hypogonadism and features of the metabolic syndrome are being increasingly reported,[63,64] and appear to be independent of body composition and SHBG. Moreover, there is evidence that low testosterone levels precede the development of features of the metabolic syndrome and can independently predict their emergence.[65] Risk factor correlates of a low testosterone level are listed in Table 36.1.

Not all studies of risk factor associations with testosterone included measurement of free, bioavailable testosterone. As with associations between obesity and testosterone, SHBG could confound these relationships. Insulin resistance is associated with low SHBG concentrations in humans,[66] and in experimental studies SHBG secretion is reduced by insulin and increased by testosterone.[67] Although not entirely consistent, associations with free testosterone or associations independent of SHBG have been reported for HDL cholesterol,[44] blood

Table 36.1 *Risk factor correlates of a low testosterone level in adult men*

- Central obesity
- Low HDL cholesterol concentrations
- Increased insulin concentrations
- Decreased insulin sensitivity
- Type 2 diabetes
- Increased leptin concentrations
- Increased fibrinogen and factor VII concentrations

pressure,[46] and insulin.[49] Moreover, low free testosterone levels are an independent predictor of the development of type 2 diabetes.[51]

Statistical analysis designed to identify independent associations between risk factors is problematic when applied to the co-associations of the metabolic syndrome. For example, it has recently been observed that the inverse association between testosterone and insulin resistance is independent of SHBG and can be explained statistically by variation in body fat.[68] The mechanistic interrelationships between the various features of the metabolic syndrome and its correlates are such that no definite conclusions can be drawn regarding causation. The interdependencies of risk factor variation could account for the observation that, although testosterone levels correlate negatively with severity of coronary disease measured angiographically,[69-71] low testosterone levels do not independently predict CHD.[45,72-74] This would be expected if low testosterone was either an initiating or exacerbating factor in interrelated changes, each of which independently promoted the development of CHD; statistically it will be these changes that emerge as significant in multivariate analysis rather than testosterone itself.

Effects of reversing the age-related decline in testosterone concentrations

In the continuum of risk factor disturbances, prescribed interventions only exist for the most extreme manifestations: hypertension, hyperlipidemia, and diabetes. A range of pharmacologic strategies, which generally act by inhibiting a key step in the processes involved, are available for dealing with these, e.g. the angiotensin converting enzyme inhibitors in the case of hypertension or the HMG CoA reductase inhibitors in the case of hypercholesterolemia. Treatment strategies for diabetes generally involve stimulation either of insulin sensitivity or of insulin secretion, but this may be combined with therapies for any accompanying hypertension or dyslipidemia.

Although, in deteriorating beyond diagnostic limits, risk factor disturbances become disease entities around which systems of clinical practice develop, the relationship between risk factor disturbances and the development of cardiovascular disease is, if not always linear, then at least continuous. In other words, there is no such thing as a completely safe risk factor level. Many of the consequences of subclinical disturbances in risk factor levels in men have hitherto been regarded simply as the inevitable accompaniments of aging, as has the progressive rise in rates of cardiovascular disease and diabetes with age. But if risk factor impact could be minimized throughout the male lifespan, such apparent inevitabilities might be effectively prevented.

For men, there are several specific areas in which risk factor modification may be expected to have particular benefits. In addition to the independent effects of cigarette smoking, the complex of smoking, poor living conditions, and respiratory infection has the potential for increasing cardiovascular risk.[75] A further complex may be found in decreasing physical activity, increased central body fat, and the decreasing testosterone levels seen in the aging male. In contrast to the analogous changes in estrogens in postmenopausal women, endogenous testosterone levels are highly variable and there is considerable overlap in the range between older and younger men.[11] Therefore, it remains to be established whether, in aging men, the combination of low testosterone level and central obesity, or even low testosterone in itself, could constitute a distinct clinical entity.

However, the complexes of changes that could particularly affect the aging male do offer points of intervention at all levels. Decreased cigarette smoking and increased physical activity are clearly the most straightforward of these, and the latter could, in itself, diminish fat deposition and increase testosterone levels. Physical activity can also increase growth hormone levels. Given the strong association observed between increased adiposity and reduced testosterone levels, reducing fat stores might be expected to increase testosterone levels. Given that the age-related fall in testosterone levels may be an intrinsic physiologic change, analogous to the menopause in women, replacement administration of testosterone might be of value.

Effects of testosterone replacement on body composition

Testosterone replacement in healthy, middle-aged men would be expected to increase muscle mass and reduce central fat. In a recent meta-analysis of randomized, controlled trials of the effects of testosterone in such men, Isidori and colleagues identified 14 studies in which effects on total fat mass had been measured.[76] A significant reduction was apparent overall, with an equivalent effect in study groups with an average plasma testosterone concentration within and below the reference range. Fifteen studies evaluated effects on fat-free mass and a significant increase was apparent overall in response to testosterone. This meta-analysis did not evaluate effects on central body fat, but the weight of evidence from individual studies suggests that the reduction in total fat mass seen with testosterone or androgen administration is concentrated in central fat.[77,78] Testosterone administration has also been shown to be effective in reducing central body fat in middle-aged men with type 2 diabetes.[79]

Effects of testosterone replacement on lipid metabolism

The classic effects of androgens on lipid and lipoprotein levels include a reduction in HDL cholesterol concentrations and no change or an increase in LDL cholesterol.[80] In their meta-analysis of randomized clinical trials of testosterone in apparently healthy middle-aged men, Isidori and colleagues identified 16, 11, and 13 studies in which total cholesterol, LDL cholesterol, and HDL cholesterol, respectively, had been measured. Testosterone significantly reduced total cholesterol concentrations, particularly in men with low initial testosterone levels. No change in LDL cholesterol was detectable and there was a reduction in HDL cholesterol, specifically in those with high initial testosterone concentrations. There is some evidence that the reduction in HDL cholesterol relates more to the cholesterol-poor, HDL_3 subfraction rather than the cholesterol-rich, HDL_2 subfraction.[81] The latter has been linked more strongly with CHD, but the clinical consequences of testosterone-induced changes in HDL cholesterol levels and its subfraction distribution will need to be studied in depth before any conclusions can be drawn regarding the importance of these changes.

Effects of testosterone replacement on insulin resistance and the metabolic syndrome

If testosterone replacement reduces central body fat, an accompanying improvement in insulin sensitivity would be expected and this is apparent in the few studies in which insulin sensitivity has been measured.[77,78,82] An improvement in insulin sensitivity in response to testosterone has also been reported in hypogonadal men with type 2 diabetes.[79] It should be noted, however, that improvements in insulin sensitivity could be a direct consequence of testosterone administration rather than a secondary effect of loss of central fat, since strong relationships have been identified between short-term changes in testosterone levels and insulin sensitivity.[83] Beneficial effects of testosterone administration in healthy men have also been demonstrated with regard to variables that are adversely affected by insulin resistance, including fibrinogen and PAI-1.[84] Moreover, raised leptin levels in hypogonadal men have been shown to fall in response to testosterone.[85]

Potentially beneficial effects of testosterone replacement in healthy, older men, therefore, include reductions in central adiposity, increased fat-free mass, and increased insulin sensitivity, with associated improvements in a range of correlates of

Table 36.2 *Risk factor changes that accompany testosterone administration in healthy, older men*

- Decreased central obesity
- Increased fat-free mass
- Decreased total cholesterol concentrations
- Decreased HDL cholesterol concentrations
- Increased insulin sensitivity
- Decreased leptin concentrations
- Increased fibrinogen and factor VII concentrations
- Decreased adiponectin concentrations

insulin sensitivity. Potentially adverse effects include decreased HDL cholesterol concentrations and, very likely, a reduction in adiponectin concentrations. These effects are summarized in Table 36.2. The improvements in central body fat, insulin sensitivity, and some correlates of insulin sensitivity, have led some to promote the possibility that testosterone therapy might be effective in alleviating the metabolic syndrome and preventing its consequences.[86] However, in a review, Alexandersen and Christiansen concluded that there was still insufficient trial evidence for there to be any degree of certainty regarding the effects of testosterone replacement on risk factors related to lipid and carbohydrate metabolism, inflammation, and coagulation and fibrinolysis.[87]

Not all the risk factor changes induced by testosterone administration to older men are potentially beneficial and this is an area where considerable research will be needed to establish when, or even if, such intervention is appropriate. Studies evaluating the relative merits of interventions at the lifestyle or hormonal level will be needed to establish the most effective approach to diminishing the impact of the age-related metabolic syndrome of low testosterone and increased visceral fat in men and will need a sufficient duration of follow-up to establish whether there is, ultimately, any reduction in the emergence of clinical cardiovascular disease.

Conclusions

There are several key areas in which our knowledge is now sufficiently advanced to justify and provide effective interventions in the aging male. Use of pharmacologic agents, in addition to diet, to alleviate the risk factor disturbances in hypercholesterolemia and diabetes is now well established. Dietary strategies long believed to be of benefit, particularly increased fruit and vegetable consumption, are receiving increasing support from epidemiologic studies. The causes and consequences of obesity are increasingly well understood and emphasize the adverse cardiovascular consequences of excessive calorie intake. Further areas in which intervention may be of value are being identified, particularly insulin resistance and the various manifestations of the metabolic syndrome, chronic low-grade inflammation, and the correlated changes that accompany aging and declining testicular function. Testosterone administration to older men carries the potential for achieving a broad range of risk factor improvements, but considerable work will be needed to establish the context in which such an intervention is optimally effective; the age of the individual, their general health, their prevailing testosterone level, and the mode of testosterone administration could all be important in decision-making. Further characterization of the risk factor changes induced by testosterone will be needed, particularly with regard to areas in which changes appear to conflict, for example, reductions in both total and HDL cholesterol and in insulin resistance and adiponectin. Ultimately, any recommendations will need to be based on long-term clinical outcomes.

References

1. Teo KK, Ounpuu S, Hawken S et al. Tobacco use and risk of myocardial infarction in 52 countries in the INTERHEART study: a case-control study. Lancet 2006; 368: 647–58.
2. Tan KCB, Shiu SWM, Kung AWC. Alterations in hepatic lipase and lipoprotein subfractions with transdermal testosterone replacement therapy. Clin Endocrinol 1999; 51: 765–9.
3. Amiel SA, Sherwin RS, Simonson DC, Lauritano AA, Tamborlane WV. Impaired insulin action in puberty. N Engl J Med 1986; 315: 215–19.
4. Tang J, Srivastava RAK, Krul ES et al. In vivo regulation of apolipoprotein A-I gene expression by estradiol and testosterone occurs by different mechanisms in inbred strains of mice. J Lipid Res 1991; 32: 1571–85.
5. Steffen LM, Jacobs DRJ, Stevens J et al. Associations of whole-grain, refined-grain, and fruit and vegetable consumption with risks of all-cause mortality and incident coronary artery disease and ischemic stroke: the Atherosclerosis Risk in Communities (ARIC) Study. Am J Clin Nutr 2003; 78: 383–90.
6. Tucker KL, Hallfrisch J, Qiao N et al. The combination of high fruit and vegetable and low saturated fat intakes is more protective against mortality in aging men than is either alone: the Baltimore Longitudinal Study of Aging. J Nutr 2005; 135: 556–61.
7. Dauchet L, Amouyel P, Dallongeville J. Fruit and vegetable consumption and risk of stroke: a meta-analysis of cohort studies. Neurology 2005; 65: 1193–7.
8. Ericsson S, Eriksson M, Vitols S et al. Influence of age on the metabolism of plasma low density lipoproteins in healthy males. J Clin Invest 1991; 87: 591–6.
9. Ariens RA, Coppola R, Potenza I, Mannucci PM. The increase with age of the components of the tissue factor coagulation pathway is gender-dependent. Blood Coagul Fibrinolysis 1995; 6: 433–7.
10. Simon D, Preziosi P, Barrett-Connor E et al. The influence of aging on plasma sex hormones in men: the Telecom Study. Am J Epidemiol 1992; 135: 783–91.
11. Vermeulen A, Rubens R, Verdonck L. Testosterone secretion and metabolism in male senescence. J Clin Endocrinol Metab 1972; 34: 730–5.
12. Gray A, Feldman HA, McKinlay JB, Longcope C. Age, disease, and changing sex hormone levels in middle-aged men: results of the Massachusetts Male Aging Study. J Clin Endocrinol Metab 1991; 73: 1016–25.
13. Harman SM, Metter EJ, Tobin JD, Pearson J, Blackman MR. Longitudinal effects of aging on serum total and free testosterone levels in healthy men. J Clin Endocrinol Metab 2001; 86: 724–31.
14. Rubens R, Dhont M, Vermeulen A. Further studies on Leydig call function in old age. J Clin Endocrinol Metab 1974; 39: 40–5.
15. Takahashi J, Higashi Y, LaNasa JA et al. Studies of the human testis XVIII. Simultaneous measurement of nine intratesticular steroids: evidence for reduced mitochondrial function in testis of elderly men. J Clin Endocrinol Metab 1983; 56: 1178–87.
16. Harman SM, Tsitouras PD, Costa PT, Blackman MR. Reproductive hormones in aging men. II Basal

pituitary gonadotropins and gonadotropin responses to luteinizing hormone-releasing hormone. J Clin Endocrinol Metab 1982; 54: 547–51.

17. Ellison PT, Bribiescas RG, Bentley GR et al. Population variation in age-related decline in male salivary testosterone. Hum Reprod 2002; 17: 3251–3.

18. Valenti G. The pathway of partial androgen deficiency of aging male. J Endocrinol Invest 2005; 28(11 Suppl Proc): 28–33.

19. Zmuda JM, Cauley JA, Kriska A et al. Longitudinal relation between endogenous testosterone and cardiovascular disease risk factors in middle-aged men: a 13-year follow-up of former multiple risk factor intervention trial participants. Am J Epidemiol 1997; 147: 609–27.

20. Briggs MH. Cigarette smoking and infertility in men. Med J Aust 1973; 1: 616–7.

21. Shaarawy M, Mahmoud KZ. Endocrine profile and semen characteristics in male smokers. Fertil Steril 1982; 38: 255–7.

22. Sofikitis N, Miyagawa I, Dimitriadis D et al. Effects of smoking on testicular function, semen quality, and sperm fertilising capacity. J Urol 1995; 154: 1030–4.

23. Barrett-Connor E, Khaw K-T. Cigarette smoking and increased endogenous estrogen levels in men. Am J Epidemiol 1987; 126: 187–92.

24. Dai WS, Gutai JP, Kuller LH, Cauley JA. Cigarette smoking and serum sex hormones in men. Am J Epidemiol 1988; 128: 796–805.

25. Deslypere JP, Vermeulen A. Leydig cell function in normal men: effect of age, life-style, residence, diet and activity. J Clin Endocrinol Metab 1984; 59: 955–62.

26. Field AE, Colditz GA, Willett WC, Longcope C, McKinlay JB. The relation of smoking, age, relative weight, and dietary intake to serum adrenal steroids, sex hormones, and sex-hormone-binding globulin in middle-aged men. J Clin Endocrinol Metab 1994; 79: 1310–16.

27. Vogt HJ, Heller WD, Borelli S. Sperm quality of healthy smokers, ex-smokers, and never-smokers. Fertil Steril 1986; 45: 106–10.

28. Mittler JC, Pogach L, Ertel NH. Effects of chronic smoking on testosterone metabolism in dogs. J Steroid Biochem 1983; 18: 759–63.

29. Yardimci S, Atan A, Delibasi T, Sunguroglus K, Guven MC. Long-term effects of cigarette smoke exposure on plasma testosterone, luteinizing hormone and follicle stimulating hormone levels in male rats. Br J Urol 1997; 79: 66–9.

30. Yeh J, Barbieri RL, Friedman AJ. Nicotine and cotinine inhibit rat testis androgen biosynthesis in vitro. J Steroid Biochem 1989; 33: 627–30.

31. Irwin M, Dreyfus E, Baird S, Smith TL, Schuckit M. Testosterone in chronic alcoholic men. Br J Addict 1988; 83: 949–53.

32. Gordon CG, Altman K, Southren AL, Rubin E, Lieber CS. Effect of alcohol (ethanol) administration on sex-hormone metabolism in normal men. N Engl J Med 1976; 295: 793–7.

33. Sparrow D, Bosse R, Rowe JW. The influence of age, alcohol consumption, and body build on gonadal function in men. J Clin Endocrinol Metab 1980; 51: 508–12.

34. Dai WS, Kuller LH, LaPorte RE et al. The epidemiology of plasma testosterone levels in middle aged men. Am J Epidemiol 1981; 114: 804–16.

35. Glass AR, Swerdloff RS, Bray GA, Dahms WT, Atkinson RL. Low serum testosterone and sex-hormone-binding-globulin in massively obese men. J Clin Endocrinol Metab 1977; 45: 1211–19.

36. Zumoff B, Strain GW, Miller LK et al. Plasma free and non-sex-hormone-binding-globulin-bound testosterone are decreased in obese men in proportion to their degree of obesity. J Clin Endocrinol Metab 1990; 71: 929–31.

37. Haffner SM, Karhapaa P, Mykkanen L, Laakso M. Insulin resistance, body fat distribution and sex hormones in men. Diabetes 1994; 43: 212–19.

38. Khaw K-T, Barrett-Connor E. Lower endogenous androgens predict central adiposity in men. Ann Epidemiol 1992; 2: 675–82.

39. Seidell JC, Bjorntorp P, Sjostrom L, Kvist H, Sannerstedt R. Visceral fat accumulation in men is positively associated with insulin, glucose, and C-peptide levels, but negatively with testosterone levels. Metabolism 1990; 39: 897–901.

40. Simon D, Charles MA, Nahoul K et al. Association between plasma total testosterone and cardiovascular risk factors in healthy adult men: the Telecom Study. J Clin Endocrinol Metab 1997; 82: 682–5.

41. Mohr BA, Bhasin S, Link CL, O'Donnell AB, McKinlay JB. The effect of changes in adiposity on testosterone levels in older men: longitudinal results from the Massachusetts Male Aging Study. Eur J Endocrinol 2006; 155: 443–52.

42. Zumoff B, Rosenfeld RS, Friedman M et al. Elevated daytime urinary excretion of testosterone glucuronide in men with the type A behavior pattern. Psychosom Med 1984; 46: 223–5.

43. Nilsson PM, Moller L, Solstad KA. Adverse effects of psychosocial stress on gonadal function and insulin levels in middle-aged males. J Intern Med 1995; 237: 479–86.

44. Barrett-Connor EL. Testosterone and risk factors for cardiovascular disease in men. Diabetes Metab 1995; 21: 156–61.

45. Barrett-Connor E, Khaw KT. Endogenous sex hormones and cardiovascular disease in men. A prospective population-based study. Circulation 1988; 78: 539–45.

46. Khaw KT, Barrett-Connor E. Blood pressure and endogenous testosterone in men: an inverse relationship. J Hypertens 1988; 6: 329–32.

47. Bonithon-Kopp C, Scarabin PY, Bara L et al. Relationship between sex hormones and haemostatic

factors in healthy middle-aged men. Atherosclerosis 1988; 71: 71–6.

48. Dai WS, Gutai JP, Kuller LH et al. Relation between plasma high-density lipoprotein cholesterol and sex hormone concentrations in men. Am J Cardiol 1984; 53: 1259–63.

49. Haffner SM, Valdez RA, Mykkanen L, Stern MP, Katz MS. Decreased testosterone and dehydroepiandrosterone sulfate concentrations are associated with increased insulin and glucose concentrations in nondiabetic men. Metabolism 1994; 43: 599–603.

50. Simon D, Preziosi P, Barrett-Connor E et al. Interrelation between plasma testosterone and plasma insulin in healthy adult men: the Telecom Study. Diabetologia 1992; 35: 173–7.

51. Stellato RK, Feldman HA, Hamdy O, Horton S, McKinlay JB. Testosterone, sex hormone binding globulin, and the development of type 2 diabetes in middle-aged men: prospective results from the Massachusetts male ageing study. Diabetes Care 2000; 23: 490–4.

52. Pasquali R, Macor C, Vicennati V et al. Effects of acute hyperinsulinaemia on testosterone concentrations in adult obese and normal-weight men. Metabolism 1997; 46: 526–9.

53. Pitteloud N, Mootha VK, Dwyer AA et al. Relationship between testosterone levels, insulin sensitivity, and mitochondrial function in men. Diabetes Care 2005; 28: 1636–42.

54. Ebeling P, Stenman UH, Seppala M, Koivisto VA. Acute hyperinsulinaemia, androgen homeostasis and insulin sensitivity in healthy man. J Endocrinol 1995; 146: 63–9.

55. Glueck CJ, Glueck HI, Stroop D et al. Endogenous testosterone, fibrinolysis, and coronary heart disease risk in hyperlipidaemic men. J Lab Clin Med 1993; 122: 412–20.

56. Caron P, Benet A, Camare R, Louvet JP. Plasminogen activator inhibitor in plasma is related to testosterone in men. Metabolism 1988; 38: 1010–15.

57. Gannage-Yared MH, Khalife S, Semaan M et al. Serum adiponectin and leptin levels in relation to the metabolic syndrome, androgenic profile and somatotropic axis in healthy non-diabetic elderly men. Eur J Endocrinol 2006; 155: 167–76.

58. Xu A, Chan KW, Hoo RL et al. Testosterone selectively reduces the high molecular weight form of adiponectin by inhibiting its secretion from adipocytes. J Biol Chem 2005; 280: 18073–80.

59. Vettor R, DePergola G, Pagano C et al. Gender differences in serum leptin in obese people: relationships with testosterone, body fat distribution and insulin sensitivity. Eur J Clin Invest 1997; 27: 1016–24.

60. Baumgartner RN, Waters DL, Morley JE et al. Age-related changes in sex hormones affect the sex difference in serum leptin independently of changes in body fat. Metabolism 1999; 48: 378–84.

61. Soderberg S, Olsson T, Eliasson M et al. A strong association between biologically active testosterone and leptin in non-obese men and women is lost with increasing (central) adiposity. Int J Obes Relat Metab Disord 2001; 25: 98–105.

62. Leyva F, Godsland IF, Ghatei M et al. Hyperleptinaemia as a component of a metabolic syndrome of cardiovascular risk. Arterioscler Thromb Vasc Biol 1998; 18: 928–33.

63. Laaksonen DE, Niskanen L, Punnonen K et al. Sex hormones, inflammation and the metabolic syndrome: a population-based study. Eur J Endocrinol 2003; 149: 601–8.

64. Muller M, Grobbee DE, den Tonkelaar I, Lamberts SW, van der Schouw YT. Endogenous sex hormones and metabolic syndrome in aging men. J Clin Endocrinol Metab 2005; 90: 2618–23.

65. Laaksonen DE, Niskanen L, Punnonen K et al. Testosterone and sex hormone-binding globulin predict the metabolic syndrome and diabetes in middle-aged men. Diabetes Care 2004; 27: 1036–41.

66. Haffner SM. Sex hormone-binding protein, hyperinsulinemia, insulin resistance and noninsulin-dependent diabetes. Horm Res 1996; 45: 233–7.

67. Plymate SR, Matej LA, Jones RE, Friedl KE. Inhibition of sex hormone-binding globulin production in the human hepatoma (Hep G2) cell line by insulin and prolactin. J Clin Endocrinol Metab 1988; 67: 460–4.

68. Tsai EC, Matsumoto AM, Fujimoto WY, Boyko EJ. Association of bioavailable, free, and total testosterone with insulin resistance: influence of sex hormone-binding globulin and body fat. Diabetes Care 2004; 27: 861–8.

69. Barth JD, Jansen H, Hugenholtz PG, Birkenhager JC. Postheparin lipases, lipids and related hormones in men undergoing arteriography to assess atherosclerosis. Atherosclerosis 1983; 48: 235–41.

70. Chute CG, Baron JA, Plymate SR et al. Sex hormones and coronary artery disease. Am J Med 1987; 83: 853–9.

71. Phillips GB, Pinkernell BH, Jing TY. The association of hypotestosteronaemia with coronary artery disease in men. Arterioscler Thromb 1994; 14: 701–6.

72. Cauley JA, Gutai JP, Kuller LH, Dai WS. Usefulness of sex steroid hormone levels in predicting coronary artery disease in men. Am J Cardiol 1987; 60: 771–7.

73. Phillips GB, Yano K, Stemmermann GN. Serum sex hormone levels and myocardial infarction in the Honolulu Heart Program. Pitfalls in prospective studies on sex hormones. J Clin Epidemiol 1988; 41: 1151–6.

74. Yarnell JW, Beswick AD, Sweetnam PM, Riad-Fahmy D. Endogenous sex hormones and ischaemic heart disease in men. The Caerphilly prospective study. Arterioscler Thromb 1993; 13: 517–20.

75. Grimes DS, Hindle E, Dyer T. Respiratory infection and coronary heart disease: progression of a paradigm. QJM 2000; 93: 375–83.

76. Isidori AM, Giannetta E, Greco EA et al. Effects of testosterone on body composition, bone metabolism and serum lipid profile in middle-aged men: a meta-analysis. Clin Endocrinol (Oxf) 2005; 63: 280–93.

77. Marin P, Holmang S, Jonsson L et al. The effects of testosterone on body composition and metabolism in middle aged men. Int J Obes Relat Metab Disord 1992; 16: 991–7.

78. Schroeder ET, Zheng L, Ong MD et al. Effects of androgen therapy on adipose tissue and metabolism in older men. J Clin Endocrinol Metab 2004; 89: 4863–72.

79. Kapoor D, Goodwin E, Channer KS, Jones TH. Testosterone replacement therapy improves insulin resistance, glycaemic control, visceral adiposity and hypercholesterolaemia in hypogonadal men with type 2 diabetes. Eur J Endocrinol 2006: 899–906.

80. Godsland I, Wynn V, Crook D, Miller N. Sex, plasma lipoproteins, and atherosclerosis: prevailing assumptions and outstanding questions. Am Heart J 1987; 114: 1467–503.

81. Tan KCB, Shiu SWM, Pang RWC, Kung AWC. Effects of testosterone replacement on HDL subfractions and apolipoprotein A-1 containing lipoproteins. Clin Endocrinol 1998; 48: 187–94.

82. Simon D, Charles MA, Lahlou N et al. Androgen therapy improves insulin sensitivity and decreases leptin level in healthy adult men with low plasma total testosterone: a 3-month randomized placebo-controlled trial. Diabetes Care 2001; 24: 2149–51.

83. Pitteloud N, Hardin M, Dwyer AA et al. Inhibition of sex hormone-binding globulin production in the human hepatoma (Hep G2) cell line by insulin and prolactin. J Clin Endocrinol Metab 2005; 90: 2636–41.

84. Anderson RA, Ludlam CA, Wu FC. Haemostatic effects of supraphysiological levels of testosterone in normal men. Thromb Haemostas 1995; 74: 693–7.

85. Jockenhovel F, Blum WF, Vogel E et al. Testosterone substitution normalizes elevated serum leptin levels in hypogonadal men. J Clin Endocrinol Metab 1997; 82: 2510–13.

86. Makhsida N, Shah J, Yan G, Fisch H, Shabsigh R. Hypogonadism and metabolic syndrome: implications for testosterone therapy. J Urol 2005; 174: 827–34.

87. Alexandersen P, Christiansen C. The aging male: testosterone deficiency and testosterone replacement. An up-date. Atherosclerosis 2004; 173: 157–69.

CHAPTER 37

Androgens: studies in animal models of atherosclerosis

Peter Alexandersen

Introduction

Animals are extensively used as in vivo models of human atherosclerosis since it was first demonstrated by Anitschkow more than eight decades ago that atheroma lesions can be induced in rabbits by a cholesterol-rich diet.[1] At present, many species besides rabbits are used in atherosclerosis research, such as rodents, dogs, and monkeys. Data from the non-primate cynomolgus monkey model are sometimes extrapolated to the human situation (because the monkey has a 28-day menstrual cycle, undergoes menopause, has changes in plasma lipoprotein concentrations at menopause, and has responses to estrogen/progestogen replacement therapy (HRT) similar to those observed in postmenopausal women, etc.) but in fact in terms of hard endpoints there are no data to indicate that these changes reflect what takes place in humans. Accumulating evidence suggests, however, that the monkey and the rabbit produce very similar and consistent results, at least regarding the effect of HRT on atherosclerosis. The rabbit model, however, has certain drawbacks, particularly with respect to the lipid and lipoprotein profile during cholesterol feeding and HRT, which differ from the human situation. Another drawback is the degree of heterogeneity in plaque size (or accumulation of cholesterol) among rabbits as a result of a fat-rich diet, increasing the number of animals needed in a study to obtain statistical differences between treatment groups.

Nevertheless, this relatively inexpensive rabbit model (compared to the monkey model) is frequently used as atherogenesis can reliably be induced dietarily within weeks (which in the monkey typically requires several months), and because the rabbit is easy to handle and house.

The influence of androgen replacement therapy on cardiovascular risk factors and atherogenesis in an animal model was not studied until the late 1960s. However, despite considerable evidence from human and animal studies, the effect – beneficial or detrimental – of androgen replacement on cardiovascular risk and development of atherosclerosis (particularly coronary heart disease and stroke) in men currently remains a subject of intense debate. In view of the high morbidity and mortality due to cardiovascular disease in both genders in industrialized countries, the androgen issue seems more important than ever. Published human data are not ubiquitous, but experimental animal studies have several advantages. First, the effect on a specific end point (i.e., atherosclerosis) can be evaluated which is otherwise difficult to study. Second, it is possible to eliminate (or at least significantly reduce) bias from differences in food intake, hormone doses, and external confounding factors. Third, direct mechanisms of hormone action in terms of cardiovascular risk factors or atherogenesis may be investigated, for instance by vascular rings or by cell/tissue cultures. Animal studies may thus provide some indications to the effect(s) of androgens that might be anticipated in humans, and ultimately as to whether androgens are beneficial or detrimental in men at risk of cardiovascular disease.

Experimental studies of exogenous androgens in fat-fed animals

Table 37.1 summarizes the 16 experimental studies of cholesterol-fed (or fat-fed) male (and/or female) animals treated with exogenous androgens in order to study their effect on atherogenesis. Most studies have focused on natural androgens, such as testosterone (T) from the testis or the weaker dehydroepiandrosterone (DHEA) from the adrenal gland. Other studies have investigated the effect of synthetic androgens (stanozolol and nandrolone). The effects of exogenous androgens on the vascular system have been determined in a number of ways:

- by direct determination of the accumulation of cholesterol/cholesteryl esters
- determination of intimal plaque size or thickening (atheroma) developed in the vascular wall
- indirect measurement of the amount of certain compounds generated (e.g. collagen) believed to be related to the atherogenic process.

In a well-conducted study, Gordon and colleagues studied the effect of oral DHEA treatment on atherogenesis in 34 cholesterol-fed male rabbits.[6] In order to enhance aortic atherogenesis, endothelial balloon injury was performed in two of the groups. After 12 weeks of therapy resulting in supraphysiologic plasma DHEA concentrations, aortic plaque size was found to be inhibited by approximately 50% compared with cholesterol-fed control animals ($P = 0.006$), which was consistent with what was observed in other regions. The reduction in plaque size was furthermore found to correlate inversely with the plasma DHEA concentrations.[6] However, the inhibitory DHEA effect on atherogenesis appeared to be lipid and lipoprotein independent.

DHEA was also used as oral androgen treatment in another study of cardiac transplantation,[10] which also used cholesterol-fed male rabbits. However, the

rabbits received donor-heart implants which had been anastomosed to the abdominal aorta. In this way, an animal model of accelerated atherosclerosis was obtained. Trans-sectional cuts of coronary arteries from native and transplanted animals showed a marked and significant reduction in atherogenic plaque formation compared with control animals (62 and 45%, respectively; $P < 0.05$), and overall (transplanted and non-transplanted) the number of stenosed vessels was reduced by 50% compared with controls ($P < 0.05$). No significant changes in the lipid profile occurred, suggesting that a non-lipid mechanism was involved. However, there were no mechanistic data reported to account for the effect of DHEA observed, and a substantial number of animals died during surgery.[10]

In another study, testosterone enanthate (TE) was given twice weekly for 17 weeks to castrated cholesterol-clamped male rabbits in an experimental placebo-controlled study.[11] The authors did not report any statistically significant difference in aortic accumulation of cholesterol between the TE-treated and the placebo-treated animals at necropsy. Therefore, they concluded that T does not promote atherogenesis in castrated, cholesterol-fed male rabbits. However, methodologic problems in terms of absorption and/or metabolism of T may have influenced the results of that study, since half of the animals showed only modest increases in serum total cholesterol concentrations compared with the remaining half, despite individual feeding.[11]

In a later, very interesting study,[14] castrated cholesterol-fed male and female rabbits were treated with either T (given intramuscularly as enanthate), estradiol, or a combination of both for 12 weeks. An untreated group served as controls. Morphometric analysis of the intimal thickening of the proximal aorta showed a significant ($P < 0.05$) reduction in plaque size in male rabbits treated with T (and in female rabbits treated with estrogen (E)). In groups treated with a combination of the two sex hormones, plaque size was significantly smaller than in control animals ($P < 0.05$), and the effects were independent of plasma lipids and lipoproteins.[14] Interestingly however, plaque size was significantly increased in female animals treated with T compared with males ($P < 0.05$) (Figure 37.1), which is

Table 37.1 *Published studies on cholesterol-fed animals to investigate the effect of exogenous androgens on atherogenesis*

Species	Authors	Year	No of animals	Duration of study	Androgen(s)	Influence of androgen(s)
Female dogs	Sirek et al[2]	1977	22	11 weeks	T	↔
Cockerels	Copeman et al[3]	1984	36	87 days	T	→
Male chicks	Toda et al[4]	1984	24	7 weeks	T	←
Female rabbits	Fischer et al[5]	1985	54*	10 weeks	T	←
Male rabbits	Gordon et al[6]	1988	34	12 weeks	DHEA	→
Male rabbits	Wojcicki et al[7]	1989	20	12 weeks	T	→
Male and female rabbits	Arad et al[8]	1989	15 (2 m + 13 f)	8 weeks	DHEA	↕
Male rabbits	Fogelberg et al[9]	1990	17	12 weeks	STAN	↔/↓
Male rabbits	Eich et al[10]	1993	48	5 weeks	DHEA	←
Male rabbits	Larsen et al[11]	1993	36	17 weeks	TE	←
Female cynomolgus monkeys	Adams et al[12]	1995	64	32 months	T	→
Female cynomolgus monkeys	Obasanjo et al[13]	1996	59	2 years	NAN	→
Male and female rabbits	Bruck et al[14]	1997	64 (32 m + 32 f)	12 weeks	T	→
Male rabbits	Alexandersen et al[15]	1998	100	30 weeks	TE, TU, DHEA	→
Female rabbits	Hayashi et al[16]	1999	48	10 weeks	DHEA	→
Male mice	Nathan et al[17]	2001	57	8 weeks	T, E, AN	→

AN, anastrozole; DHEA, dehydroepiandrosterone; NAN, nandrolone decanoate; STAN, stanozolol; T, testosterone; TE, testosterone enanthate; TU, testosterone undecanoate.
m denotes males, f denotes females, ↑, ↓, and ↔ indicate an increase, decrease, or no change, respectively, in atherogenesis vs control animals.
*The number is estimated as the exact number is not given by the authors (52 ≤ n ≤56).

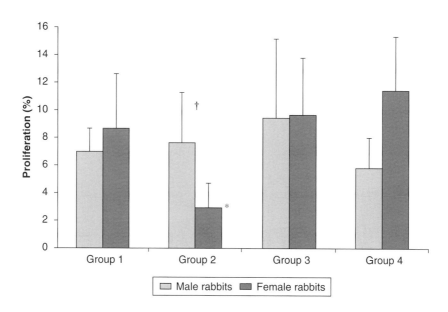

Figure 37.1   *Mean extent of neointimal thickening from three serial cross-sections of the aortic arch in male and female cholesterol-fed rabbits (0.5%). Group 1: control group, no hormone treatment; group 2: estradiol valerate (1 mg); group 3: testosterone enanthate (25 mg); group 4: estradiol valerate (1 mg) and testosterone enanthate (25 mg), each per kg body weight/week during the 12-week study period. In females, plaque development was inhibited by estrogen or estrogen + testosterone compared with controls (P<0.05). In males, plaque development was inhibited by testosterone or estrogen + testosterone compared with controls (P<0.05). *Between hormone-treated groups and control group for each gender. † Between corresponding male and female rabbits with regard to their respective control groups. Adapted from reference 14.*

in line with two studies of female cynomolgus monkeys treated with T.[12,13] Similarly, plaque size was increased 2-fold in male animals treated with E compared with females (although this was not statistically significant). These data suggest that some sex hormones (i.e., T and E) may possess gender-specific effects in terms of atherogenesis.

An atheroprotective effect of both DHEA and T (both oral and parenteral) was found in a larger study of castrated, cholesterol-fed male rabbits.[15] However, in that study the effect of androgens could for a large part be contributed to modifications in lipoprotein concentrations, except for treatment with intramuscular T (that resulted in supraphysiologic T concentrations), thus indicating a non-lipid-mediated anti-atherogenic effect for this treatment. Castration per se also resulted in a significant (P<0.01) reduction in the aortic accumulation of cholesterol.[15]

New studies using transgenic animals have helped to further investigate the impact of exogenous androgens on atherogenesis. Particularly interesting in this context has been the study by Nathan et al,[17] who took it a step further as they investigated the role of aromatization of T to E to account for the observed protective effects of T replacement. Using an LDL-receptor knockout (LDLR$^{-/-}$) mouse model, 57 male animals were stratified into two groups, castration or sham operation. Castrated mice were treated with either T, T + anastrozole (AN) (a potent and selective aromatase inhibitor), E, or placebo, whereas sham animals were treated with AN or placebo. During the 8 weeks of treatment all animals were fed a fat-rich 'Western' diet to induce atherosclerosis. The authors reported that sham animals had similar aortic atherosclerotic lesions compared to castrated and T-treated animals and to castrated E-treated animals, indicating a significant T-induced reduction in atherogenesis in these animals. Furthermore, sham AN-treated animals were found to have twice the amount of atherosclerosis compared to the sham mice (testicular intact) ($P < 0.05$), but not statistically significantly different from either castrated placebo-treated mice or from castrated T + AN-treated animals. Because administration of E to castrated fat-fed mice thus also attenuated atherosclerosis to the same extent as T, and because AN when given together with T completely inhibited the anti-atherogenic effect of T alone, the results collectively pointed towards an anti-atherogenic effect of T due to its conversion to E.[17]

Androgenic mechanism of action

Evidence of a protective effect of exogenous androgens on early atherogenesis in male animals is rapidly accumulating (Table 37.1), suggesting that both DHEA and T may inhibit the deposition of cholesterol in the arterial wall in males of most species. In females, in contrast, T, but not DHEA, seems to favor atherogenesis rather than delaying it. Table 37.2 lists experimental studies using male and/or female animals to investigate mechanisms responsible for the androgenic effects observed on atherogenesis. Taken together, a little more than half of these studies (23 of 43 studies published) dealing with more mechanistic aspects of androgenic effects on the vasculature suggest that natural androgens in general (and T and DHEA in particular) have a favorable influence on the vasculature leading to a decreased risk of coronary heart disease. This thus supports the in vivo studies of fat-fed animals (Table 37.1), of which some have investigated mechanisms themselves.[17]

However, in many of the 'mechanistic' studies no discrimination was made as to the sex of cells used in the cell/tissue cultures or of the vascular rings studied. Often a mixture of males and females was used (Table 37.2), which may be crucial in terms of the genomic effects of androgens. For DHEA, the mechanistic studies consistently indicate a favorable effect of this androgen on cardiovascular risk factors (Table 37.2). Another important issue relates to the androgen exposure of the tissue(s) studied. Acute effects may be mediated via non-genomic effects (e.g. calcium channels[33]) and thus do not reflect effects caused by long-term (or chronic) androgen

therapy. Thus, as acute androgen treatment/exposure is often used in cell/tissue cultures, the mechanism(s) involved may not reflect the clinical outcome in male patients receiving long-term androgen replacement.

An important study by Hayashi and colleagues[16] tested the hypothesis that the beneficial effect of DHEA on atherogenesis is mediated through the conversion to estradiol via aromatase (Figure 37.2). Despite the fact that the study used female animals, they reported evidence that some of the anti-atherogenic effect of DHEA was mediated via its conversion to estradiol, and that in part an endothelium-dependent increase in the synthesis of nitric oxide (NO) occurred.[16] If these results are confirmed by others, it is tempting to speculate that indeed all aromatizable androgens may use this pathway and that local estrogen synthesis at the vascular level may in part be responsible for an atheroprotective effect of androgens. This mechanism of action, if also of biologic importance for T in men, may counteract the seemingly deleterious effects of T (Table 37.2), but this still remains to be investigated. Non-aromatizable androgens (e.g., dihydrotestosterone and synthetic compounds) may therefore work through alternative mechanisms of action. The lack of intact sympathetic and parasympathetic nerve fibers to the vascular smooth muscle cells in ring preparations should also be kept in mind when evaluating these data. For instance, it has been shown for estradiol that it affects the muscarinic receptors of vascular smooth muscle cells, and androgens themselves or by conversion into E may have similar influences.

The route of androgen administration in terms of vascular effects is also an issue that needs much more study. Only one study has looked into this.[15] In that study of fat-fed male rabbits, T was given either orally or intramuscularly, and despite the fact that an anti-atherogenic effect was observed for both modalities, the serum concentrations obtained and thus the exposure of vascular tissue to T differed between groups, which may be important regarding the accumulation of cholesterol.[15] Although transdermal T patches are becoming available in still more countries, to date no studies comparing the various routes of administration

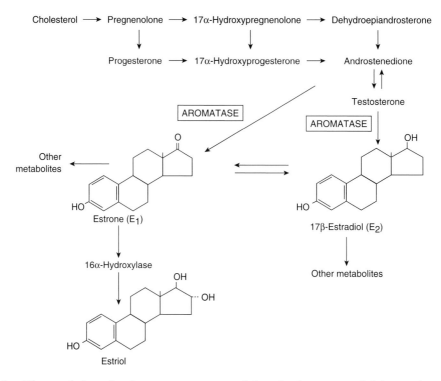

Figure 37.2 *The metabolism of androgens to estrogens and the role of aromatase. Inhibitors of aromatase block this enzyme, thus inhibiting the conversion of androgens to estrogens, termed aromatization. The molecular structure is also shown for dehydroepiandrosterone and testosterone. Adapted from reference 16.*

have been performed to assess cardiovascular risk factors or atherogenesis.

Finally, the influence of androgens on the hemostatic system has only been investigated by a few groups in an animal model or in animal cell/tissue culture (Table 37.2). With human cell/tissue cultures easily available, most data on this subject come from these and clinical studies.

Summary and conclusions

Experimental animal studies have been and still are used to investigate the effect of androgen exposure on atherogenesis and suggest which effect could be expected in men treated with androgens. Moreover, they are useful to investigate the mechanism(s) involved in the androgenic effects observed (mechanistic studies using various cell cultures, vascular

rings, or studying in vivo vascular reactivity or other measurable variable in the animal). Unfortunately, despite the fact that several in vivo studies have been performed to date, these animal studies vary considerably in experimental design and differ with respect to species, which may account for the inconsistency of the data available (Table 37.1). It seems that T replacement therapy is associated with an increase in plaque formation in *female* macaques,[12,13] which is in accordance with studies of T in *female* rabbits.[5,14] Most early studies of T were done in *female* animals (Table 37.1). The lack of studies of androgen replacement in *male* cynomolgus monkeys is striking!

In general, caution should be made when it comes to extrapolating the results from animals studies to the human situation. Enzymatic processes may show subtle differences across species and this contributes to differences in terms of clinical

Table 37.2 In vitro studies of androgen effects on isolated cell cultures or vascular rings and experimental in vivo studies on vascular resistance, inflammatory markers, or serum lipoproteins

Species	Authors	Year	Type of study or cell culture used	Androgen(s)	Influence of androgen(s)	Comment
Male and female cats	Bhargava et al[18]	1967	In vivo	T	Blood pressure ↑	Effect considered unfavorable
Male rats	Fisher and Swain[19]	1972	In vivo	T	Vascular connective tissue ↑	Effect considered unfavorable
Male rats	Wolinsky[20]	1972	In vivo	T	Vascular connective tissue ↑	Effect considered unfavorable
Male and female dogs	Greensberg et al[21]	1974	In vivo	T	Vasoconstriction	Effect considered unfavorable
Male and female rats	Baker et al[22]	1978	In vivo	T	Blood pressure ↑	Effect considered unfavorable
Male rats	Nakao et al[23]	1981	Aortic VSMCs	T	Prostacyclin synthesis ↓	Effect considered unfavorable
Male and female rats and rabbits	Karanian et al[24]	1982	Aortic rings	T	Vasoconstriction	Effect considered unfavorable
Male (?) calves	Bronson et al[25]	1987	Aorta VSMCs	T	Lysyl oxidase activity ↑	Effect considered unfavorable
Male and female rats and rabbits	Wakasugi et al[26]	1989	Rat aortic rings, rabbit aortic VSMCs	T	Prostacyclin synthesis ↔ in males but ↓ in females	Effect considered unfavorable
Male rats	Masuda et al[27]	1991	Aortic VSMCs	T	TxA$_2$ receptors ↑	Effect considered unfavorable
Male rats	Hölmang and Björntorp[28]	1992	In vivo	T	Insulin resistance ↑	Effect considered favorable
Male cynomolgus monkeys	Weyrich et al[29]	1992	In vivo	T	TxB$_2$ ↑, HDL-C ↓	Effect considered unfavorable

(Continued)

Table 37.2 (Continued)

Species	Authors	Year	Type of study or cell culture used	Androgen(s)	Influence of androgen(s)	Comment
Female rats	Mohan and Jacobsen[30]	1993	Peritoneal Mφ	DHEA, T	Superoxide generation ↓*	Effect considered favorable
Male rats	Fujimoto et al[31]	1994	Aortic VSMCs	T, DHT	Androgen receptor expression ↑, proliferation of VSMCs ↑	Effect considered unfavorable
Male guinea pigs	Schror et al[32]	1994	Coronary artery VSMCs	T	Vasoconstriction	Effect considered unfavorable
Male and female rabbits	Yue et al[33]	1995	Vascular rings	T	Vasorelaxation	Effect considered favorable
Male and female pigs	Farhat et al[34]	1995	Coronary artery rings	T	Vasoconstriction	Effect considered unfavorable
Male dogs	Chou et al[35]	1996	In vivo	T	Vasodilatation	Effect considered favorable
Male (?) mice†	Taniguchi et al[36]	1996	Mφ	DHEA	Cholesteryl ester accumulation ↓	Effect considered favorable
?	Mohan and Benghuzzi[37]	1997	Endothelial cells	DHEA	Proliferation ↑	Effect considered favorable
Male rabbits	Hutchison et al[38]	1997	Aortic rings	T	Endothelium-dependent relaxation ↓	Effect considered unfavorable
Male (?) rabbits†	Furutama et al[39]	1998	VSMCs	DHEA	Proliferation ↑ and migration ↓	Effect considered favorable
Male and female pigs	Quan et al[40]	1999	Coronary artery rings	T	Vasorelaxation ↓	Effect considered unfavorable
Male (?) rats (normotensive + spontaneously hypertensive)	Honda et al[41]	1999	Aortic rings	T	Vasorelaxation	Effect considered favorable

(Continued)

Table 37.2 *(Continued)*

Species	Authors	Year	Type of study or cell culture used	Androgen(s)	Influence of androgen(s)	Comment
Male rats	Stokes et al[42]	2000	Plasma TC	T, DHT, AED	Plasma TC $\downarrow$	Effect considered favorable
Male and female pigs	Teoh et al[43]	2000	Coronary artery rings	T, E	Vasoconstriction by T (vasodilatation by E)	Effect considered unfavorable
Male (?) mice	Friedl et al[44]	2000	Mϕ	T	iNOS $\downarrow$	Effect considered favorable
Male (?) pigs	Deenadayalu et al[45]	2001	Coronary artery SMC	T, DHT	Vasorelaxation	Effect considered favorable
Male rats	Ding and Stallone[46]	2001	Vascular rings	T	Vasorelaxation	Effect considered favorable
Male rats	English et al[47]	2002	Vascular rings	T	Vasorelaxation	Effect considered favorable
Male rats	Pugh et al[48]	2002	Vascular rings	T	Vasorelaxation	Effect considered favorable
Male rats	Ter-areenan et al[49]	2003	Aortic rings	T	Vasorelaxation	Effect considered favorable
Male and female mice	Nishizawa et al[50]	2002	Adipocytes	T	Adiponectin synthesis and secretion $\downarrow$	Effect considered unfavorable
Female rats	Simoncini et al[51]	2003	Aortic endothelial cells	DHEA	eNOS synthesis and expression restored	Effect considered favorable
Male rats and male mice	Xu et al[52]	2005	Adipocytes in vivo and in vitro	T	Adiponectin synthesis and secretion $\downarrow$ from adipocytes	Effect considered unfavorable
Male rats	Karbowska and Kochan[53]	2005	In vivo and in vitro	DHEA	PPARγ mRNA expression $\uparrow$; adiponectin gene expression $\uparrow$	Effect considered favorable

(Continued)

Table 37.2 (Continued)

Species	Authors	Year	Type of study or cell culture used	Androgen(s)	Influence of androgen(s)	Comment
Male rabbits	Aydilek and Aksakal[54]	2005	In vivo	T	TC ↓, HDL-C ↓, LDL-C ↔, TG ↔, fibrinogen ↔	Effect considered unfavorable
Male rats	Iwasaki et al[55]	2005	In vitro	DHEA	Type I collagen from cardiac fibroblasts ↓	Effect considered favorable
Male rhesus monkeys	Mishra et al[56]	2005	Intracoronary infusion in vivo; vascular rings	DHT	Vasoconstriction in vivo; thromboxane prostanoid receptor expression ↑ in vivo and in vitro	Effect considered unfavorable
Male rats	Razmara et al[57]	2005	In vivo and in vitro	T, E	Inflammatory markers (COX2 and iNOS) ↑ by T	Effect considered unfavorable
Male and female pigs	Hutchison et al[58]	2005	In vivo and in vitro	T, DHEAS	Coronary blood flow ↑; vasorelaxation of vascular rings	Effect considered favorable
Male rats	Vasudevan et al[59]	2006	In vivo (blood pressure) and in vitro (artery rings)	T	Endothelial dysfunction ↑	Effect considered unfavorable
Male rats	Liu et al[60]	2006	In vitro	T	Heat shock protein 70 showed viability ↑ and expression ↑	Effect considered favorable

AED, androstenedione; COX2, cyclooxygenase-2; DHEA(S), dehydroepiandrosterone (sulfate); DHT, dihydrotestosterone; E, estradiol; eNOS, endothelial nitric oxide synthase; HDL-C, high-density lipoprotein cholesterol; HUVEC, human umbilical endothelial cells; iNOS, inducible nitric oxide synthase; LDL-C, low-density lipoprotein cholesterol; Mφ, macrophages; PPARγ, peroxisome proliferator-activated receptor gamma; SMC, smooth muscle cells; T, testosterone; TC, total cholesterol; TG, triglycerides; Tx, thromboxane; VSMCs, vascular smooth muscle cells.

*The inhibition of superoxide generation was found to be minimal for T.

↑, ↓, and ↔ indicate an increase, decrease, or no change, respectively in atherogenesis vs control animals.

[†] The gender of the animals used is not reported.

response to treatment. Also, some species (e.g. the rabbit) seem to be particularly sensitive to sex hormone replacement therapy resulting in an outcome which may not reflect the clinical situation. Nevertheless, despite these limitations, animal models may be useful in screening drugs for potential beneficial effects in humans, and may also be of value in elucidating mechanisms of action of sex hormones on the vasculature.

To assess the efficacy and safety of long-term treatment with exogenous androgens in men at risk of coronary heart disease, prospective, randomized, placebo-controlled and double-blind studies are needed. Because such data will probably not be available for some time yet, further animal research (particularly secondary prevention studies and more mechanistic studies) is clearly of the utmost relevance, regarding both 'old', well-known androgens and also new 'designer' androgens, which perhaps some day may be of benefit to the health of men at risk of coronary heart disease.

References

1. Anitschkow N. Über die Atherosklerose der Aorta beim Kaninchen und über deren Entstehungsbedingungen. Beitr path Anatomie allgem Pathologie 1914; 59: 306–48.
2. Sirek OV, Sirek A, Fikar K. The effect of sex hormones on glycosaminoglycan content of canine aorta and coronary arteries. Atherosclerosis 1977; 27: 227–33.
3. Copeman HA, Papadimitriou JM, Watson IG. Hormonal effects on prevention or regression of atheroma. Adv Exp Med Biol 1984; 168: 51–84.
4. Toda T, Toda Y, Cho BH, Kummerow FA. Ultrastructural changes in the comb and aorta of chicks fed excess testosterone. Atherosclerosis 1984; 51: 47–57.
5. Fischer GM, Bashey RI, Rosenbaum H, Lyttle CR. A possible mechanism in arterial wall for mediation of sex difference in atherosclerosis. Exp Mol Pathol 1985; 43: 288–96.
6. Gordon GB, Bush DE, Weisman HF. Reduction of atherosclerosis by administration of dehydroepiandrosterone. A study in the hypercholesterolemic New Zealand White rabbit with aortic intimal injury. J Clin Invest 1988; 82: 712–20.
7. Wojcicki J, Tustanowski S, Samochowiec L. Endocrine function in atherosclerotic rabbits. Pol J Pharmacol Pharm 1989; 41: 109–13.
8. Arad Y, Badimon JJ, Badimon L, Hembree WC, Ginsberg HN. Dehydroepiandrosterone feeding prevents aortic fatty streak formation and cholesterol accumulation in cholesterol-fed rabbit. Arteriosclerosis 1989; 9: 159–66.
9. Fogelberg M, Björkhem I, Diczfalusy U, Henriksson P. Stanozolol and experimental atherosclerosis: atherosclerotic development and blood lipids during anabolic steroid therapy of New Zealand White rabbits. Scand J Clin Lab Invest 1990; 50: 693–6.
10. Eich DM, Nestler JE, Johnson DE et al. Inhibition of accelerated coronary atherosclerosis with dehydroepiandrosterone in the heterotopic rabbit model of cardiac transplantation. Circulation 1993; 87: 261–9.
11. Larsen BA, Nordestgaard BG, Stender S, Kjeldsen K. Effect of testosterone in atherogenesis in cholesterol-fed rabbits with similar plasma cholesterol levels. Atherosclerosis 1993; 99: 79–86.
12. Adams MR, Williams JK, Kaplan JR. Effects of androgens on coronary artery atherosclerosis and atherosclerosis-related impairment of vascular responsiveness. Arterioscler Thromb Vasc Biol 1995; 15: 562–70.
13. Obasanjo IO, Clarkson TB, Weaver DS. Effects of the anabolic steroid nandrolone decanoate on plasma lipid and coronary arteries of female cynomolgus macaques. Metabolism 1996; 45: 463–8.
14. Bruck B, Brehme U, Guel N et al. Gender-specific differences in the effects of testosterone and estrogen on the development of atherosclerosis in rabbits. Arterioscler Thromb Vasc Biol 1997; 17: 2192–9.
15. Alexandersen P, Haarbo J, Byrjalsen I, Lawaetz H, Christiansen C. Natural androgens inhibit male atherosclerosis: a study in castrated, cholesterol-fed rabbits. Circ Res 1999; 84: 813–19.
16. Hayashi T, Esaki T, Muto E et al. Dehydroepiandrosterone retards atherosclerosis formation through its conversion to estrogen: the possible role of nitric oxide. Arterioscler Thromb Vasc Biol 2000; 20: 782–92.
17. Nathan L, Shi W, Dinh H et al. Testosterone inhibits early atherogenesis by conversion to estradiol: critical role of aromatase. Proc Natl Acad Sci USA 2001; 98: 3589–93.
18. Bhargava KP, Dhavan KN, Saxena RC. Enhancement of noradrenaline pressor responses in testosterone-treated cats. Br J Pharmacol 1967; 31: 26–31.
19. Fisher GM, Swain ML. Effect of sex hormones on blood pressure and vascular connective tissue in castrated and noncastrated male rats. Am J Physiol 1977; 232: H617–21.
20. Wolinsky H. Effects of androgen treatment on the male rat aorta. J Clin Invest 1972; 51: 2552–5.
21. Greensberg S, George WR, Kadowitz PJ, Wilson WR. Androgen-induced enhancement of vascular reactivity. Can J Physiol Pharmacol 1974; 52: 14–22.

22. Baker PJ, Ramey E, Ramwell PW. Androgen-mediated sex differences of cardiovascular responses in rats. Am J Physiol 1978; 235: H242–6.

23. Nakao J, Change WC, Murota SI, Orimo H. Testosterone inhibits prostacyclin production by rat aortic smooth muscle cells in culture. Atherosclerosis 1981; 39: 203–9.

24. Karanian JW, Sintetos AL, Moran FM, Ramey ER, Ramwell PW. Androgenic regulation of vascular responses to prostaglandins. In: Herman AG, Vanhoutte PM, Denolin H, Goossens A, eds. Cardiovascular Pharmacology of the Prostaglandins. New York: Raven Press, 1982: 245–58.

25. Bronson RE, Claaman SD, Traish AM, Kagan HM. Stimulation of lysyl oxidase (EC 1.4.3.13) activity by testosterone and characterization of androgen receptors in cultured calf aorta smooth muscle cells. Biochem J 1987; 244: 317–23.

26. Wakasugi M, Noguchi T, Kazama YI, Kanemaru Y, Onaya T. The effects of sex hormones on the synthesis of prostacyclin (PGI2) by vascular tissues. Prostaglandins 1989; 37: 401–10.

27. Masuda A, Mathur R, Halushka PV. Testosterone increases thromboxane A_2 receptors in cultured rat aortic smooth muscle cells. Circ Res 1991; 69: 638–43.

28. Hölmang A, Björntorp P. The effects of testosterone on insulin sensitivity in male rats. Acta Physiol Scand 1992; 146: 505–10.

29. Weyrich AS, Rejeski WJ, Brubaker PH, Parks JS. The effects of testosterone on lipids and eicosanoids in cynomolgus monkeys. Med Sci Sports Exerc 1992; 24(3): 333–8.

30. Mohan PF, Jacobson MS. Inhibition of macrophage superoxide generation by dehydroepiandrosterone. Am J Med Sci 1993; 306: 10–15.

31. Fujimoto R, Morimoto I, Morita E et al. Androgen receptors, 5 alpha-reductase activity and androgen-dependent proliferation of vascular smooth muscle cells. J Steroid Biochem Mol Biol 1994; 50: 169–74.

32. Schror K, Morinelli TA, Masuda A et al. Testosterone treatment enhances thromboxane A2 mimetic induced coronary artery vasoconstriction in guinea pigs. Eur J Clin Invest 1994; 24(Suppl 1): 50–2.

33. Yue P, Chatterjee K, Beale C, Poole-Wilson PA, Collins P. Testosterone relaxes rabbit coronary arteries and aorta. Circulation 1995; 91: 1154–60.

34. Farhat MY, Wolfe R, Vargas R, Foegh ML, Ramwell PW. Effect of testosterone treatment on vasoconstrictor response of left anterior descending artery in male and female pigs. J Cardiovasc Pharmacol 1995; 25: 495–500.

35. Chou TM, Sudir K, Hutchison SJ et al. Testosterone induces dilation of canine coronary conductance and resistance arteries in vivo. Circulation 1996; 94: 2614–19.

36. Taniguchi S, Yanase T, Kobayashi K, Takayanagi R, Nawata H. Dehydroepiandrosterone markedly inhibits the accumulation of cholesteryl ester in mouse macrophage J774–1 cells. Atherosclerosis 1996; 126: 143–54.

37. Mohan PF, Benghuzzi H. Effect of dehydroepiandrosterone on endothelial cell proliferation. Biomed Sci Instrum 1997; 33: 550–5.

38. Hutchison SJ, Sudhir K, Chou TM et al. Testosterone worsens endothelial dysfunction associated with hypercholesterolemia and environmental tobacco smoke exposure in male rabbit aorta. J Am Coll Cardiol 1997; 29: 800–7.

39. Furutama D, Fukui R, Amakawa M, Ohsawa N. Inhibition of migration and proliferation of vascular smooth muscle cells by dehydroepiandrosterone sulfate. Biochim Biophys Acta 1998; 1406: 107–14.

40. Quan A, Teoh H, Man RY. Acute exposure to a low level of testosterone impairs relaxation in porcine coronary arteries. Clin Exp Pharmacol Physiol 1999; 26: 830–2.

41. Honda H, Unemoto T, Kogo H. Different mechanisms for testosterone-induced relaxation of aorta between normotensive and spontaneously hypertensive rats. Hypertension 1999; 34: 1232–6.

42. Stokes KI, Benguzzi HA, Cameron JA. Physiological responses associated with sustained delivery of T, DHT, and AED in male rats. Biomed Sci Instrum 2000; 36: 209–14.

43. Teoh H, Quan A, Man RY. Acute impairment of relaxation by low levels of testosterone in porcine coronary arteries. Cardiovasc Res 2000; 45: 1010–18.

44. Friedl R, Brunner M, Moeslinger T, Spieckermann PG. Testosterone inhibits expression of inducible nitric oxide synthase in murine macrophages. Life Sci 2000; 68: 417–29.

45. Deenadayalu VP, White RE, Stallone JN, Gao X, Garcia AJ. Testosterone relaxes coronary arteries by opening the large-conductance, calcium-activated potassium channel. Am J Physiol Heart Circ Physiol 2001; 281: H1720–7.

46. Ding AQ, Stallone JN. Testosterone-induced relaxation of rat aorta is androgen structure specific and involves K+ channel activation. J Appl Physiol 2001; 91: 2742–50.

47. English KM, Jones RD, Jones TH, Morice AH, Channer KS. Testosterone acts as a coronary vasodilator by a calcium antagonistic action. J Endocrinol Invest 2002; 25: 455–8.

48. Pugh PJ, Jones RD, Jones TH, Channer KS. Intrinsic responses of rat coronary arteries in vitro: influence of testosterone, calcium, and effective transmural pressure. Endocrine 2002; 19: 155–61.

49. Ter-areenan P, Kendall DA, Randall MD. Testosterone-induced vasorelaxation in the rat mesenteric arterial bed is mediated predominantly

via potassium channels. Br J Pharmacol 2002; 135: 735–40.

50. Nishizawa H, Shimomura I, Kishida K et al. Androgens decrease plasma adiponectin, an insulin-sensitizing adipocyte-derived protein. Diabetes 2002; 51: 2734–41.

51. Simoncini T, Mannella P, Fornari L et al. Dehydroepiandrosterone modulates endothelial nitric oxide synthesis via direct genomic and non-genomic mechanisms. Endocrinology 2003; 144: 3449–55.

52. Xu A, Chan KW, Hoo RL et al. Testosterone selectively reduces the high molecular weight form of adiponectin by inhibiting its secretion from adipocytes. J Biol Chem 2005; 280: 18073–80.

53. Karbowska J, Kochan Z. Effect of DHEA on endocrine functions of adipose tissue, the involvement of PPAR gamma. Biochem Pharmacol 2005; 70: 249–57.

54. Aydilek N, Aksakal M. Effects of testosterone on lipid peroxidation, lipid profiles and some coagulation parameters in rabbits. J Vet Med A Physiol Pathol Clin Med 2005; 52: 436–9.

55. Iwasaki T, Mukasa K, Yoneda M et al. Marked attenuation of production of collagen type I from cardiac fibroblasts by dehydroepiandrosterone. Am J Physiol Endocrinol Metab 2005; 288: E1222–8.

56. Mishra RG, Hermsmeyer RK, Miyagawa K et al. Medroxyprogesterone acetate and dihydrotestosterone induce coronary hyperreactivity in intact male rhesus monkeys. J Clin Endocrinol Metab 2005; 90: 3706–14.

57. Razmara A, Krause DN, Duckles SP. Testosterone augments endotoxin-mediated cerebrovascular inflammation in male rats. Am J Physiol Heart Circ Physiol 2005; 289: H1843–50.

58. Hutchison SJ, Browne AE, Ko E et al. Dehydroepiandrosterone sulfate induces acute vasodilation of porcine coronary arteries in vitro and in vivo. J Cardiovasc Pharmacol 2005; 46: 325–32.

59. Vasudevan H, Nagareddy PR, McNeill JH. Gonadectomy prevents endothelial dysfunction in fructose-fed male rats, a factor contributing to the development of hypertension. Am J Physiol Heart Circ Physiol 2006; 291: H3058–64.

60. Liu J, Tsang S, Wong TM. Testosterone is required for delayed cardioprotection and enhanced heat shock protein 70 expression induced by preconditioning. Endocrinology 2006; 147: 4569–77.

CHAPTER 38

Androgens and blood pressure in men

Guy Lloyd

Introduction

Hypertension amongst men is a major public health issue, with a rate nearly double that of pre-menopausal women (Figure 38.1). Hypertension confers a significantly higher chance of cardiovascular disease, with the risk of myocardial infarction being doubled and that of stroke increased 4-fold. Modern treatment strategies have led to a decline in hypertensive mortality over the last 20 years, but despite this hypertension was responsible for over 17 000 deaths in the USA for the year 1997 alone. Different ethnic groups, in particular those of Afro-Caribbean origin, are particularly at risk and in some populations 30% of hypertensive males die as a result of their blood pressure.[1]

Traditional therapy for hypertension controlled the risk of stroke but was less successfull at reducing coronary disease. This was particularly evident in the early randomized controlled trials. In the Medical Research Council trial men and women with systolic blood pressure up to 209 mmHg were randomized to either diuretics or β-blockade, or placebo. Stroke was reduced by 25% but coronary events by only 19%, confined to the patients treated with diuretics.[2] Subsequent studies using newer drugs such as calcium channel antagonists in high-risk populations have confirmed a cardiac benefit.[3,4] More recently, large scale randomized trials have confirmed the usefulness of thiazide diuretics[5] and angiotensin receptor antagonists[6] in reducing both heart disease and stroke, and when combination treatment is required a non-atenolol-based regimen is preferred.[7]

Other than the first-line use of β-blockers (which for hypertensives without other β-blocker indications can no longer be recommended) the choice of antihypertensive agent may be less important than the absolute risk of disease at baseline and the efficacy of the intervention (in terms of blood pressure reduction). Guidelines now focus on achieving an optimal blood pressure of below 140/85 with more aggressive targeting of diabetic subjects who are at special risk.[8]

Whilst much research energy has been directed at assessing the impact of estrogen and other female sex hormones on cardiovascular disease, adrenal and testicular androgens continue to have an enigmatic relationship with cardiovascular diseases. The attraction of female sex hormones as cardioprotective agents is intuitive, based on the low incidence of disease in premenopausal women compared to age-matched males, together with a (less convincing) increase in disease following the menopause. The corollary of this relationship – that androgens are harmful, perhaps due to adverse effects on plasma lipids – has also achieved widespread acceptance. However, in men plasma androgen levels do not show a rapid and steep decline as seen in women at menopause. There is no analogous acute 'deficiency syndrome' although some time-trends are now acknowledged. Men show an age-dependent decrease

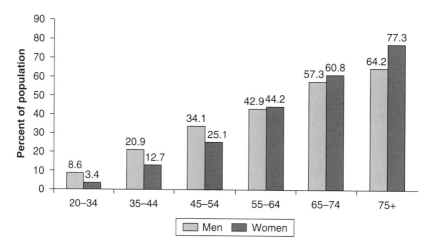

Figure 38.1 *The percentage of the American population with hypertension according to age and gender. Note the lower incidence of hypertension among premenopausal women. (Reproduced with permission from reference 1.)*

in sex hormones, particularly testosterone. This decline predates the decline in women, starting as early as 21 years, and continues in a near linear manner into old age (Figure 38.2).[9] The rate of fall of free testosterone concentrations is around 1.2% per year and is heavily influenced by other factors, most particularly body weight.[10]

Cross-sectional studies show lower (not higher) plasma androgen levels in patients with coronary artery disease,[11] indicating that androgens, far from being deleterious, may share a role similar to that hypothesized for estrogen, in maintaining vascular integrity in men. Thus, the age-dependent decline in plasma testosterone levels may be an important cofactor in the development of cardiovascular diseases such as hypertension and atherosclerosis. This chapter covers the relationship between androgens and blood pressure in both experimental and in vivo settings, and discusses whether androgens may modulate cardiovascular risk in hypertensive men.

Relationship between androgens and hypertension

Animal models
Much of our understanding of the influence of androgens on blood pressure is derived from the salt-sensitive, spontaneous hypertensive (Sprague-Dawley) rat model of hypertension. In this model testosterone clearly has a pivotal role in mediating blood pressure. Males develop significantly higher arterial blood pressure than females, but when castrated this difference is lost in both sexes (Figure 38.3). Furthermore, subcutaneous testosterone implants resulting in physiologic male plasma concentrations in females raise their blood pressure to that of non-castrated males. Adding back testosterone to castrated animals results in blood pressure equivalent to that of intact animals, while treatment of non-castrated animals with estrogen results in lower pressures.[12] The renin/angiotensin system appears to be a major determinant of this hormone-dependent gender dimorphism: enalapril treatment equally reduces blood pressure across male, female, castrated, and testosterone-replaced animals.[13] In the same model intact males and ovariectomized females treated with testosterone have a significantly lower incremental renal sodium excretion in response to increases in blood pressure compared to castrated males or intact females.[14] This androgenic influence on blood pressure is receptor-mediated, as it can be inhibited by the androgen receptor antagonist flutamide.[15] However, finasteride, an inhibitor of 5α-reductase, does not antagonize this hypertensive response. This suggests that a direct testosterone/

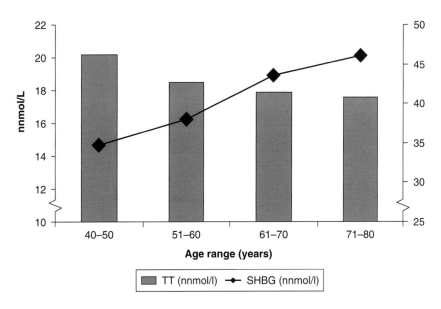

Figure 38.2 *Changes in total testosterone (TT) and SHBG (sex hormone-binding globulin) with increasing age. (adapted from reference 10).*

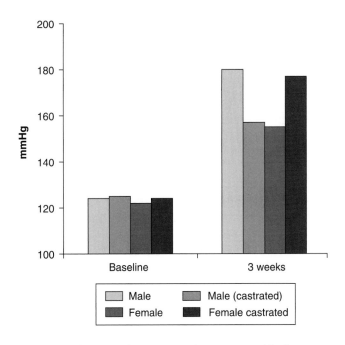

Figure 38.3 *The influence of modifying endogenous sex hormones on blood pressure in the Sprague-Dawley salt-sensitive rat model (adapted from reference 12).*

receptor effect is responsible, rather than a conversion to the active metabolite dihydrotestosterone as with many 'testosterone effects' such as benign prostatic hypertrophy and male pattern baldness.

Animal models have also helped explain how testosterone might regulate cardiac hypertrophy in response to hypertension. Morano and colleagues[16] report that in spontaneously hypertensive rats the reduction in blood pressure seen in response to castration was linked to an increased expression of the β-myosin heavy chain gene, while testosterone replacement (3 mg/day of dihydrotestosterone) favors the expression of α-heavy chain gene. This switch in gene regulation would be expected to lead to cardiac hypertrophy. This phenomenon has been observed in an alternative model based on the denervated rat model (Wistar strain). Subcutaneous testosterone propinate treatment (0.5 pg/kg) after castration resulted in increased blood pressure in the rats and a significantly increased left ventricular weight at necropsy, when compared to intact animals.[17]

Available evidence from limited animal models therefore suggests that testosterone should have a negative influence on blood pressure and the left ventricular reaction to hypertension. Epidemiologic evidence from male populations and studies in human subjects suggest an alternative hypothesis.

Blood vessel behavior

Endothelial dysfunction is seen in most hypertensives and may represent an early stage in the pathophysiology of their condition. Estrogen administration improves the function of the endothelium in both women[18] and men,[19] but the effect of androgens is unclear. When testosterone at doses ranging from sub- to grossly supraphysiologic is introduced into the coronary arteries of men during angiography, it causes a dose-dependent increase in vessel diameter and coronary blood flow, similar to that seen with estradiol administration.[20] This suggests that testosterone improves endothelial function. Conversely, in female-to-male transsexuals, testosterone treatment reduced flow-mediated forearm blood flow, an endothelium-dependent process.[21] Surgically or chemically castrated prostate cancer patients have an enhanced brachial artery reactivity, suggesting enhanced nitric oxide release.[22]

In the classic aortic ring system testosterone relaxes preconstricted rabbit arterial rings.[23] In a landmark study the relaxation was significantly greater in the coronary artery rings than in the aortic rings, perhaps explaining the negative findings in the forearm investigations outlined above. What is fascinating about these experiments is that the testosterone-dependent vasodilatation did not seem to be acting through any of the well-recognized pathways for sex steroid action. The dilatation was not dependent on an intact endothelium nor was it influenced by nitric oxide synthase inhibitors; the dose-dependent contraction in response to calcium was unchanged, suggesting that calcium antagonism was not responsible; and testosterone receptor blockade did not affect the response, suggesting a direct effect on the arterial wall.

Effects of DHEAS and adrenal androgens on blood pressure

The effect of the endogenous adrenal androgens androstenedione and dihydroepiandrostenedione sulfate (DHEAS) on blood pressure is unclear and the literature is divided. Schunkert and colleagues[24] examined a group of 646 men and in this population DHEAS concentrations in middle-aged men were significantly higher in the hypertensive individuals. This was also associated with, but independent of, higher levels of aldosterone. A recent large American cohort, however, demonstrated an opposite finding with a clear association between DHEAS and increasing arterial stiffness and its various surrogate parameters, although this was not an independent association and was at least in part co-correlated with age.[25] Furthermore, in patients with established hypertension, low levels of DHEAS are associated with a reduction in diurnal blood pressure variation, generally considered to be an indication of adverse outcome.[26]

Testosterone

In the Rancho–Bernardo study with 1132 men a negative association was seen between plasma testosterone levels and blood pressure[27] (Figure 38.4). The relationship with lower plasma testosterone was true across all the quintiles of blood pressure and was independent of other factors

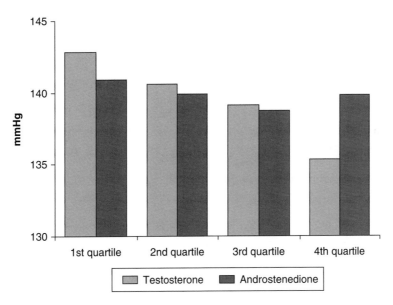

Figure 38.4 *The relationship between increasing quartiles of testosterone and androstenedione and systolic blood pressure in the Ranch–Bernardo study (from reference 27).*

including obesity. No relationship was seen with estrogens or adrenal androgens. In a small study of hypertensive men, hypertension was associated with reduced levels of both total and free testosterone.[28] In contrast, the women in this study showed a positive correlation with testosterone, suggesting that the effects of testosterone on blood pressure may be gender-dependent. In a small group of men evaluated for the association between blood pressure and erectile dysfunction, testosterone levels were lower in the hypertensive men, although conventional measures of erectile dysfunction were similar in both groups.[29] Further studies of varying designs have also supported the association, such as the Telecom Study, where blood pressure was significantly higher in the low testosterone group as were other markers of insulin sensitivity.[30] In the Tromso Study there was a weak association between total testerone and both systolic and diastolic blood pressure, but this relationship was significantly weakened after allowing for BMI and alchol drinking habits.[31] In this study the development of left ventricular hypertrophy was also associated with low testosterone levels, a finding which runs contrary to some of the data presented below.

There is, however, little agreement in the literature. Data from the Multiple Risk Factor Intervention Trial substudy[32] suggest that the reduction in testosterone levels with time may not be directly related to the development of hypertension. In 66 participants in the study mean total testosterone declined by a mean 41 ng/dl. When analyzed using multivariate analysis the change in testosterone levels was associated with a rise in triglyceride and a fall in high-density lipoprotein (HDL) cholesterol, but not with changes in either systolic or diastolic blood pressure.[28] In a large Danish study testosterone and sex hormone-binding globulin concentrations were strongly associated with a range of metabolic parameters, but not blood pressure.[33] In a further small study of 30 men and 30 women, plasma testosterone did not correlate with blood pressure in men although, once more, a positive relationship was seen in women.[34] Amongst black subjects in South Africa, testosterone concentrations were higher in the hypertensives than in the normotensives.[35] Testosterone may also have important effects in women; in a cross-sectional study of women attending an endocrine clinic for menstrual irregularity, an elevated testosterone level (>30 ng/dl) predicted central obesity and to some extent hypertension. The odds ratios for systolic and diastolic blood pressure were 2.4 (1.0–6.2) and 2.7 (0.8–8.8), respectively. The combination of hyperandrogenemia and obesity was a powerful predictor of the presence of hypertension.[36]

It is difficult to explain the variety of findings from the observational literature. The relationship between testosterone and obesity, which in itself is strongly related to blood pressure, may be a confounding variable and may also explain why different populations behave differently. The androgen association may, in these circumstances, have a causal association or simply be an innocent bystander. It is well recognized that hypertension represents the final common pathway of a number of mechanisms and therefore subjects in whom blood pressure is closely related to fluctuations in the renin/angiotensin system may be more sensitive to androgens, and thus may respond differently to populations where the renin/angiotensin system is relatively less important.

Exogenous androgens and blood pressure

Testosterone and derivatives
Studies designed to investigate the influence of androgen administration on blood pressure in healthy men are rare. Whitworth and coworkers[37] carried out a small trial in which a synthetic androgen (testosterone undecanoate, 120 mg/day) was administered to 14 normotensive males. No increase in blood pressure or plasma volume was noted with this large dose over 5 days. However, the study was small and might not have had the statistical power to detect any changes. Similarly, a randomized crossover study of 20 men treated with intravenous testosterone in either physiologic (twice normal) or supraphysiologic doses (six times normal) found no obvious effects on blood pressure.[38] Administration of 'physiologic' doses of testosterone by various regimens including depot and transdermal to obese men has resulted in no change in blood pressure but improved insulin sensitivity.[39]

Many small studies have evaluated the use of various androgen replacement regimens in partial androgen deficiency; none of the studies is adequately powered to give a full answer, but although most have reported no change some have reported a reduction in blood pressure.[40]

Anabolic androgenic steroids
In contrast to the findings with testosterone, the high doses of anabolic androgenic steroids used in sport do seem to increase blood pressure. In an early randomized control trial of 13 athletes given methandrostenolone, a small but significant increase in blood pressure was observed, although clinical hypertension developed in only one individual.[41] In an observational Dutch study, self-administration of anabolic steroids was associated with elevated blood pressure, an effect sustained at an average of 5 months of follow-up.[42] In a randomized trial of 21 weight-lifters, testosterone enanthate resulted in a reversible 10 mmHg increase in systolic blood pressure.[43] Conversely, Palatini and colleagues[44] demonstrated no overall effect of steroid abuse on blood pressures measured in the clinic setting. However, a reduction in nocturnal dipping was observed, and this loss of day/night variability on 24-hour blood pressure monitoring is an early hypertensive change. Nandrolone also appears to induce a rise in diastolic blood pressure that reverts to normal within 6 weeks,[45] and the effects of other steroids appear to be relatively short-lived after stopping therapy.[46]

Biologically effective doses of anabolic steroids appear to have an opposite and reversible effect on vascular function, when compared to physiologic androgens. Endothelial-independent (response to glycerol trinitrate) dysfunction is observed in users whereas endothelial function remains intact.[47]

One important covariate that must be considered is changes in body habitus associated with anabolic steroid use, particularly an increase in the circumference of the arm, which may influence blood pressure measurement. Riebe and colleagues[48] found that systolic and diastolic pressures both at rest and after various forms of exercise were raised compared with non-users and sedentary controls (Figure 38.5). However, after the inclusion of biceps

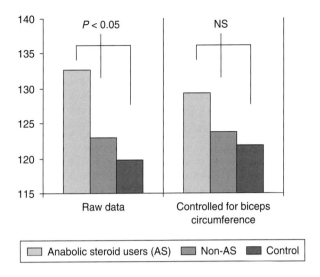

Figure 38.5 *The effect of anabolic steroid use and exercise training on systolic blood pressure before and after controlling for biceps circumference (adapted from reference 48).*

size in the statistical model, these differences were no longer significant.

Left ventricular hypertrophy (LVH) is a common finding in patients with hypertension and predicts an adverse prognosis. Among athletes in training, left ventricular hypertrophy is also a common finding and relates to increased myocardial work. In vitro work in hypertensive rats has demonstrated that treatment with anabolic steroids results in a decrease in myocardial compliance.[49] This absence of an influence on experimental LVH has, however, been observed with other steroids such as nandrolone.[50] Indirect evidence for an additive effect of steroids on LVH comes from the retrospective arm of a study by Dickerman and colleagues,[51] where LVH on echocardiography was found in 43% of body-builders compared with 100% of those who used anabolic steroids in addition to exercise. In a further study by di Bello and coworkers,[52] there was a trend towards highest left ventricular mass among steroid users, although that was not statistically significant. However, other observational studies have failed to replicate these findings.[53–55] Most studies appear to agree that diastolic relaxation of the left ventricle is not affected by the presence of LVH,

whether or not steroids are used. Recently, the use of more sensitive tissue Doppler echocardiographic techniques has revealed possible early evidence of stiffening of the left ventricle with a reduction in the velocity of early diastolic relaxation.[56]

Anabolic steroids seem to induce hypertension and may increase LVH; their use should therefore be discouraged. Users should be monitored closely for the development of hypertension, and if it develops all steroid use should cease. Clearly anabolic derivatives of testosterone should never be used for the purposes of physiologic replacement.

Conclusions

Lessons learnt from the study of the relationship between female sex hormones and cardiac pathology should warn against the overinterpretation of hypotheses and the relationship between androgens and hypertension remains far from clear. Evidence from existing animal models suggests that testosterone administration has the potential to induce hypertension and increase the hypertrophic response of the left ventricle to hypertension. Conversely, in

507

vivo testosterone appears to act as a coronary and possibly peripheral vasodilator, acting through endothelium-dependent and -independent mechanisms. Certainly testosterone levels appear to be lower in patients with both hypertension and coronary artery disease and it remains an attractive hypothesis that sex steroids in both sexes are important in maintaining vascular integrity. However, the large number of covariates, including smoking, lipid changes, and weight in particular, makes the epidemiologic evidence difficult to evaluate. Administration of physiologic dose testosterone to hypogonadal men or those more loosely classified as being andropausal does not seem to be associated with any hypertensive effect and can be considered 'safe', although in hypertensive subjects suitable monitoring should continue. The abuse of anabolic steroids in sport may induce small, reversible rises in blood pressure and close observation of these individuals is prudent. If hypertension develops, then subjects should be strongly advised to stop using these drugs, especially because of the potential role of these steroids in mediating the development of LVH. For men with hypertension the cornerstone of therapy remains the evidence-based strategies of aggressive blood pressure reduction and risk-factor modulation.

References

1. American Heart Association. 2001 Heart and Stroke Statistical Update. Dallas, TX: AHA, 2000.
2. The MRC Working Party. Medical research council trial of treatment of hypertension in older adults: principal results. BMJ 1992; 304: 405–12.
3. Staessen J, Fagard R, Thijs L et al. Randomised double-blind comparison of placebo and active treatment for older patients with isolated systolic hypertension. The Systolic Hypertension in Europe (Syst-Eur) Trial Investigators. Lancet 1997; 350: 757–64.
4. Wang J, Staessen J, Gong L, Liu L. Chinese trial on isolated systolic hypertension in the elderly. Systolic Hypertension in China (Syst-China) Collaborative Group. Arch Intern Med 2000; 160: 211–20.
5. ALLHAT Officers and Coordinators for the ALLHAT Collaborative Research Group. The Antihypertensive and Lipid-Lowering Treatment to Prevent Heart Attack Trial. Major outcomes in high-risk hypertensive patients randomized to angiotensin-converting enzyme inhibitor or calcium channel blocker vs diuretic: The Antihypertensive and Lipid-Lowering Treatment to Prevent Heart Attack Trial (ALLHAT). JAMA 2002; 288(23): 2981–97.
6. Dahlof B, Devereux RB, Kjeldsen SE et al. LIFE Study Group. Cardiovascular morbidity and mortality in the Losartan Intervention For Endpoint reduction in hypertension study (LIFE): a randomised trial against atenolol. Lancet 2002; 359(9311): 995–1003.
7. Dahlof B, Sever PS, Poulter NR et al. ASCOT Investigators. Prevention of cardiovascular events with an antihypertensive regimen of amlodipine adding perindopril as required versus atenolol adding bendroflumethiazide as required, in the Anglo–Scandinavian Cardiac Outcomes Trial–Blood Pressure Lowering Arm (ASCOT-BPLA): a multicentre randomised controlled trial. Lancet 2005; 366(9489): 895–906.
8. Ramsay L, Williams B, Johnston G et al. Guidelines for management of hypertension: report of the third working party of the British Hypertension Society. J Hum Hypertens 1998; 13: 569–92.
9. Zumoff B, Strain G, Kream J et al. Age variation of the 24-hour mean plasma concentrations of androgens, estrogens and gonadotrophins in normal adult men. J Clin Endocrinol Metab 1982; 54: 534–8.
10. Muller M, den Tonkelaar I, Thijssen JH, Grobbee DE, van der Schouw YT. Endogenous sex hormone levels in men aged 40–80 years. Eur J Endocrinol 2000; 149: 583–9.
11. English K, Mandour O, Steeds R et al. Men with coronary artery disease have lower levels of androgens than men with normal coronary angiograms. Eur Heart J 2000; 21: 890–4.
12. Crofton J, Share L. Gonadal hormones modulate deoxycorticosterone–salt hypertension in male and female rats. Hypertension 1997; 29: 494–9.
13. Reckelhoff J, Zhang H, Srivastava K. Gender differences in development of hypertension in spontaneously hypertensive rats. Role of the renin–angiotensin system. Hypertension 2000; 35: 480–3.
14. Reckelhoff J, Zhang H, Granger J. Testosterone exacerbates hypertension and reduces pressure-natiuresis in male spontaneously hypertensive rats. Hypertension 1998; 31: 435–9.
15. Reckelhoff J, Zhang H, Srivastava K, Granger J. Gender differences in hypertension in spontaneously hypertensive rats, role of androgens and androgen receptor. Hypertension 2000; 34: 920–3.
16. Morano I, Gerstner J, Ruegg J et al. Regulation of myosin heavy chain expression in the hearts of hypertensive rats by testosterone. Circ Res 1990; 66: 1585–90.
17. Cabral A, Vasquez E, Moyses MR, Antonio A. Sex hormone modulation of ventricular hypertrophy in sinoaortic denervated rats. Hypertension 1988; 11: I-93–I-97.

18. Collins P, Rosano G, Sarrel P et al. 17 beta-Estradiol attenuates acetylcholine-induced coronary arterial constriction in women but not men with coronary artery disease. Circulation 1995; 92: 24–30.

19. New G, Timmins K, Duffy S et al. Long-term estrogen therapy improves vascular function in male to female transsexuals. J Am Coll Cardiol 1997; 29: 1437–44.

20. Webb C, McNeill J, Hayward C et al. Effects of testosterone on coronary vasomotor regulation in men with coronary heart disease. Circulation 1998; 100: 1960–6.

21. McCredie R, McCrohon J, Turner L et al. Vascular reactivity is impaired in genetic females taking high-dose androgens. J Am Coll Cardiol 1998; 32: 1331–5.

22. Herman S, Robinson J, McCredie R et al. Androgen deprivation is associated with enhanced endothelium-dependent dilatation in adult men. Arterioscler Thromb Vasc Biol 1997; 17: 2004–9.

23. Yue P, Chatterjee K, Beale C et al. Testosterone relaxes rabbit coronary arteries and aorta. Circulation 1998; 91: 1154–60.

24. Schunkert H, Hense H, Andus T et al. Relation between dehydroepiandrosterone sulphate and blood pressure levels in a population-based sample. Am J Hypertens 1999; 12: 1140–3.

25. Hougaku H, Fleg JL, Najjar SS et al. Relationship between androgenic hormones and arterial stiffness, based on longitudinal hormone measurements. Am J Physiol Endocrinol Metab 2006; 290(2): E234–42.

26. Barna I, Feher T, de Chatel R. Relationship between blood pressure variability and serum dehydroepiandrosterone sulphate levels. Am J Hypertens 1998; 11: 532–8.

27. Khaw K, Barrett-Connor E. Blood pressure and endogenous testosterone in men: an inverse relationship. J Hypertens 1988; 6: 329–32.

28. Hughes G, Mathur R, Margolius H. Sex steroid hormones are altered in essential hypertension. J Hypertens 1989; 7: 181–7.

29. Jaffe A, Chen Y, Kisch E et al. Erectile dysfunction in hypertensive subjects. Assessment of potential determinants. Hypertension 1996; 28: 859–62.

30. Simon D, Charles M, Nahoul K et al. Association between plasma total testosterone and cardiovascular risk factors in healthy adult men: the Telecom Study. J Clin Endocrinol Metab 1997; 82: 682–5.

31. Svartberg J, von Muhlen D, Schirmer H et al. Association of endogenous testosterone with blood pressure and left ventricular mass in men. The Tromso Study. Eur J Endocrinol 2004; 150(1): 65–71.

32. Zmuda J, Cauley J, Glynn N et al. Longitudinal relation between endogenous testosterone and cardiovascular risk factors in middle-aged men. A 13-year follow-up of former Multiple Risk Factor Intervention Trial participants. Am J Epidemiol 1997; 146: 609–17.

33. Gyllenborg J, Rasmussen SL, Borch-Johnsen K et al. Cardiovascular risk factors in men: the role of gonadal steroids and sex hormone-binding globulin. Metabolism 2001; 50(8): 882–8.

34. Lundberg U, Wallin L, Lindstedt G, Frankenhaeuser M. Steroid sex hormones and cardiovascular function in healthy males and females: a correlation study. Pharmacol Biochem Behav 1990; 37: 325–7.

35. Huisman HW, Schutte AE, Van Rooyen JM et al. The influence of testosterone on blood pressure and risk factors for cardiovascular disease in a black South African population. Ethn Dis 2006; 16(3): 693–8.

36. Ayala C, Steinberger E, Sweeney A et al. The relationship of serum androgens and ovulatory status to blood pressure in reproductive-age women. Am J Hypertens 1999; 12: 772–7.

37. Whitworth J, Scoggins B, Andrews J et al. Haemodynamic and metabolic effects of short term administration of synthetic sex steroids in humans. Clin Exp Hypertens A 1992; 14: 905–22.

38. White C, Ferraro-Borgida M, Moyna N et al. The effects of pharmacokinetically guided intravenous testosterone administration on electrocardiographic and blood pressure variables. J Clin Pharmacol 1999; 39: 1038–43.

39. Marin P, Krothiewski M, Bjorntorp P. Androgen treatment of middle-aged, obese men: effects on metabolism, muscle and adipose tissues. Eur J Med 1992; 1: 329–36.

40. Li JY, Zhu JC, Dou JT et al. Effects of androgen supplementation therapy on partial androgen deficiency in the aging male: a preliminary study. Aging Male 2002; 5(1): 47–51.

41. Freed D, Banks A, Longson D, Burley D. Anabolic steroids in athletics: crossover double-blind trial on weightlifters. BMJ 1975; 31: 471–3.

42. Lenders J, Demacker P, Vos J et al. Deleterious effects of anabolic steroids on serum lipoproteins, blood pressure and liver function in amateur body builders. Int J Sports Med 1988; 9: 19–23.

43. Giorgi A, Weatherby R, Murphy P. Muscular strength, body composition and health responses to the use of testosterone enanthate: a double blind study. J Sci Med Sport 1999; 2: 341–55.

44. Palatini P, Giada F, Garavelli G et al. Cardiovascular effects of anabolic steroids in weight-training subjects. J Clin Pharmacol 1996; 12: 1132–40.

45. Kuipers H, Wijnen J, Hartgens F, Willems S. Influence of anabolic steroids on body composition, blood pressure, lipid profile and liver function in body builders. Int J Sports Med 1991; 12: 413–18.

46. Hartgens F, Kuipers H, Wijnen J, Keizer H. Body composition, cardiovascular risk factors and liver function in long-term androgenic-anabolic steroids using bodybuilders three months after drug withdrawal. Int J Sports Med 1996; 6: 429–33.

47. Lane HA, Grace F, Smith JC et al. Impaired vasore-activity in bodybuilders using androgenic anabolic steroids. Eur J Clin Invest. 2006; 36(7): 483–8.

48. Riebe D, Fernhall B, Thompson P. The blood pressure response to exercise in anabolic steroid users. Med Sci Sports Exerc 1992; 24: 633–7.

49. LeGros T, McConnell D, Murray T et al. The effects of 17 alpha-methyltestosterone on myocardial function in-vitro. Med Sci Sports Exerc 2000; 32: 897–903.

50. Phillis B, Irvine R, Kennedy J. Combined cardiac effects of cocaine and the anabolic steroid, nandrolone, in the rat. Eur J Pharmacol 2000; 398: 263–72.

51. Dickerman R, Schaller F, McConathey W. Left ventricular wall thickening does occur in elite power athletes with or without anabolic steroid use. Cardiology 1998; 90: 145–8.

52. di Bello V, Giorgi D, Bianchi M et al. Effects of anabolic-steroids on weight-lifters' myocardium: an ultrasonic videodensitometric study. Med Sci Sports Exerc 1999; 31: 514–21.

53. Salke R, Rowland T, Burke E. Left ventricular size and function in body builders using anabolic steroids. Med Sci Sports Exerc 1985; 17: 701–4.

54. Thompson P, Sadaniantz A, Cullinane E et al. Left ventricular function is not impaired in weight-lifters who use anabolic steroids. J Am Coll Cardiol 1992; 19: 278–82.

55. Yeater R, Reed C, Ullrich I et al. Resistance trained athletes using or not using anabolic steroids compared to runners: effects on cardiorespiratory variables, body composition and plasma lipids. Br J Sports Med 1996; 30: 11–14.

56. Nottin S, Nguyen LD, Terbah M, Obert P. Cardiovascular effects of androgenic anabolic steroids in male bodybuilders determined by tissue Doppler imaging. Am J Cardiol 2006; 97(6): 912–15.

CHAPTER 39

Androgens and arterial disease

Carolyn M Webb and Peter Collins

Introduction

Historically androgens have been considered a risk factor for coronary artery disease in men, since postmenopausal women have a lower incidence of coronary heart disease and myocardial infarction than men of a similar age. However, there has been no direct evidence linking physiologic concentrations of androgens to an increased incidence of coronary heart disease and myocardial infarction, and recent evidence suggests that the reverse may be true. In a study examining the effect of risk factors (including estradiol and testosterone) on predicting myocardial infarction in males who had not had a previous myocardial infarction, Phillips and coworkers[1] raised the possibility that hypotestosteronemia in men may be a risk factor for coronary atherosclerosis. Serum total and free testosterone levels were negatively correlated with degree of risk of coronary artery disease and with risk factors for myocardial infarction. These findings have been confirmed by other studies.[2,3] Decreased total and free testosterone levels have been shown to be associated with ischemic stroke in men,[4] further implicating testosterone in the pathophysiology of vascular diseases. Declining levels of the androgen dehydroepiandrosterone sulfate (DHEAS) have been associated with an increased risk of vascular disease.[5] Confusion arises from data concerning the use of high doses of androgens (anabolic steroids) to increase muscle mass and athletic performance, where there is a well-documented increase in incidence of cardiovascular events.[6]

Androgens and the coronary and peripheral circulations

Testosterone is known to affect the coronary circulation in animals[7,8] and humans.[9] In men with coronary artery disease, physiologic concentrations of testosterone infused directly into the coronary arteries induced coronary dilatation and enhancement of coronary blood flow (Figure 39.1).[9] There was no effect on vasomotor or flow responses to acetylcholine before versus after testosterone administration, indicating a possible endothelium-independent mechanism.

The direct effects of testosterone on coronary arteries, increasing blood flow, may explain the observed effects of testosterone administration on signs of exercise-induced myocardial ischemia. Reports from the 1940s suggested that testosterone therapy in men has a beneficial effect on angina pectoris.[10–13] This was confirmed and extended in the 1970s in a double-blind study carried out in 50 men who had ST segment depression after exercise.[14] It was shown that, after 4–8 weeks' treatment with testosterone or placebo, there was a significant decrease in the exercise-induced extent of ST segment depression by testosterone when compared to placebo. The mechanism by which testosterone decreased postexercise ST segment depression was not established. This study may have been confounded by the fact that the presence of significant coronary artery disease was not confirmed. Recent studies have demonstrated an acute and longer-term beneficial effect of testosterone on myocardial

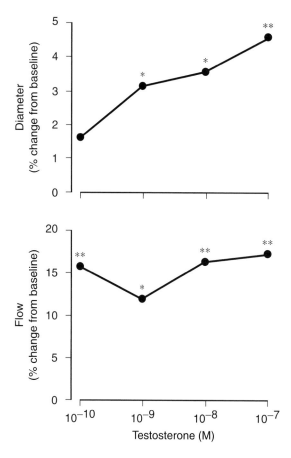

Figure 39.1 *Testosterone-induced increases in coronary artery diameter (a) and blood flow (b).*P < 0.05 and **P < 0.01 compared with baseline. Reproduced with permission from Lippincott, Williams & Wilkins. Webb CM, McNeill JG, Hayward CS et al. Effects of testosterone on coronary vasomotor regulation in men with coronary heart disease. Circulation 1999; 100(16): 1690–6.[9]*

infusion; however, the study of Rosano and co-workers[15] also showed a benefit on total exercise time and rate–pressure product (an indicator of myocardial work). Transdermal testosterone patches, given for 12 weeks in addition to current anti-anginal medication, has been shown to significantly increase time to 1 mm ST segment depression on the electrocardiogram in men with coronary artery disease.[17] Interestingly, the magnitude of the response was greater in men with lower baseline testosterone levels.

Acute testosterone-induced increases in flow-mediated brachial artery diameter changes have been demonstrated in men with coronary artery disease, suggesting that in this vascular bed testosterone may have a beneficial effect on endothelium-dependent responses (Figure 39.2).[18] This differs from a study which suggested an improvement in vasoreactivity in men undergoing treatment for prostatic cancer, who were orchidectomized or given anti-androgen therapy, compared to controls.[19] In this publication the endothelium-dependent dilatation response of the control group was only 2–3%, an unusually low value, and interestingly this response was not significantly associated with cholesterol levels. This is different from similar reports by these investigators.[20,21] Also, hormone withdrawal may not necessarily be expected to have inverse effects to hormone supplementation, especially in a different population of men such as those with coronary heart disease. As is shown with the varying effects of steroid hormones on lipid levels, extrapolation of hormonal effects outside study parameters cannot be assumed.[22]

ischemia in men with established coronary artery disease.[15–17] In the studies performed by both Rosano and Webb and their colleagues, acute intravenous testosterone or placebo was given in a crossover design to men withdrawn from cardioactive medication, and the study of Webb and colleagues[16] included men with baseline testosterone levels below or at the lower end of the normal range. Both studies showed an enhancement in exercise time to myocardial ischemia 30 minutes after testosterone

Androgens and atherosclerosis

Large doses of testosterone can increase coronary artery atheroma progression in female animals but preserve endothelial function in coronary arteries in these animals.[23] A study in rabbits demonstrated a sex-specific atheroprotective effect of testosterone in male animals, independent of changes in lipid profile.[24] Intimal thickening in the proximal aortic arch was significantly inhibited by testosterone in these male animals.

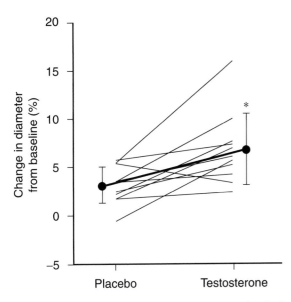

Figure 39.2 *Flow-mediated reactivity in individual patients 60 minutes after an intravenous infusion of 2.3 mg of testosterone. Bold line indicates mean change from baseline, *P = 0.005. Reproduced with permission from Excerptor Medica Inc. Testosterone enhances flow-mediated brachial artery reactivity in men with coronary artery disease. Am J Cardiol 2000; 85: 269–72.*

There is no evidence that physiologic levels of testosterone increase the risk of myocardial infarction, in contrast to data from men taking high doses of anabolic steroids who are known to be at increased risk for myocardial infarction and stroke.[6] High doses of androgens have been associated with advanced atheroma progression,[23] and detrimental effects on plasma lipid profile[25] and hemostatic factors.[26,27]

Androgens and vasoreactivity: lessons from studies in women

There is evidence from studies in women that testosterone may have favorable effects on arterial endothelial function. Preliminary evidence indicates an increase in flow-mediated dilatation of the brachial artery induced by testosterone implants in postmenopausal women already receiving hormone replacement therapy (12 women were taking a cyclical progestin in addition to a non-standardized estrogen).[28] In female-to-male transsexuals, high-dose androgen treatment is associated with impaired vascular reactivity in the brachial artery.[29] Compared to untreated age- and cigarette smoking-matched controls (9 of 12 subjects in each group were smokers), transsexuals had the same endothelium-dependent responses, but significantly impaired response to the endothelium-independent vasodilator glyceryl trinitrate. These studies highlight the importance of dose of androgen treatments in determining a beneficial or detrimental vasomotor effect.

Androgens and atherosclerosis

The influence of androgens on atherogenesis in women is unclear and relatively unexplored. Endogenous androgens, DHEAS in particular, have been shown to correlate with a lower risk of carotid artery atherosclerosis in women,[30,31] but not coronary atherosclerosis.[32] There is evidence to suggest that premenopausal women with coronary artery disease, a relatively rare disease in women before the menopause, may have decreased DHEAS levels,[33] indicating that DHEAS may in some way be atheroprotective.

Sex differences in foam cell formation, known to play a key role in atherogenesis, have recently been identified. Lipid loading of macrophages isolated from women was not affected by the androgen dihydrotestosterone, whereas macrophages from men showed a dose-dependent and androgen receptor-mediated increase in macrophage cholesteryl ester content.[34]

Conclusions

Contrary to previous assumptions, physiologic levels of androgens appear to be associated with arterial health in men. Findings of recent studies indicate the need for further investigation of the cardiovascular effects of androgens in men.

513

References

1. Phillips GB, Pinkernell BH, Jing TY. The association of hypotestosteronemia with coronary artery disease in men. Arterioscler Thromb 1994; 14: 701–6.

2. Chute CG, Baron JA, Plymate SR et al. Sex hormones and coronary artery disease. Am J Med 1987; 83: 853–9.

3. English KM, Mandour O, Steeds RP et al. Men with coronary artery disease have lower levels of androgens than men with normal coronary angiograms. Eur Heart J 2000; 21: 890–4.

4. Jeppesen LL, Jorgensen HS, Nakayama H et al. Decreased serum testosterone in men with acute ischemic stroke. Arterioscler Thromb Vasc Biol 1996; 16: 749–54.

5. Barrett-Connor E. Sex differences in coronary artery disease. Why are women so superior? The 1995 Ancel Keys Lecture. Circulation 1997; 95: 252–64.

6. Bagatell CJ, Bremner WJ. Androgens in men – uses and abuses. N Engl J Med 1996; 334: 707–14.

7. Yue P, Chatterjee K, Beale C et al. Testosterone relaxes rabbit coronary arteries and aorta. Circulation 1995; 91: 1154–60.

8. Chou TM, Sudhir K, Amidon TM et al. Testosterone-induced coronary conductance and resistance vessel relaxation in vivo: potential mechanisms of action. J Am Coll Cardiol 1995; 14A (abstr).

9. Webb CM, McNeill JG, Hayward CS et al. Effects of testosterone on coronary vasomotor regulation in men with coronary artery disease. Circulation 1999; 100: 1690–6.

10. Hamm L. Testosterone propionate in the treatment of angina pectoris. J Clin Endocrinol 1942; 2: 325–8.

11. Sigler LH, Tulgan J. Treatment of angina pectoris by testosterone propionate. NY State J Med 1943; 43: 1424–8.

12. Walker TC. The use of testosterone propionate and estrogenic substance in the treatment of essential hypertension, angina pectoris and peripheral vascular disease. J Clin Endocrinol 1942; 2: 560–8.

13. Lesser MA. Testosterone propionate therapy in one hundred cases of angina pectoris. J Clin Endocrinol 1946; 6: 549–57.

14. Jaffe MD. Effect of testosterone cypionate on postexercise ST segment depression. Br Heart J 1977; 39: 1217–22.

15. Rosano GMC, Leonardo F, Pagnotta P et al. Acute anti-ischemic effect of testosterone in men with coronary artery disease. Circulation 1999; 99: 1666–70.

16. Webb CM, Adamson DL, de Ziegler D, Collins P. Effect of acute testosterone on myocardial ischemia in men with coronary artery disease. Am J Cardiol 1999; 83: 437–9.

17. English KM, Steeds RP, Jones TH et al. Low-dose transdermal testosterone therapy improves angina threshold in men with chronic stable angina: a randomized, double-blind, placebo-controlled study. Circulation 2000; 102: 1906–11.

18. Ong PJL, Patrizi G, Chong WCF et al. Testosterone enhances flow-mediated brachial artery reactivity in men with coronary artery disease. Am J Cardiol 2000; 85: 14–17.

19. Herman SM, Robinson JT, McCredie RJ et al. Androgen deprivation is associated with enhanced endothelium-dependent dilatation in adult men. Arterioscler Thromb Vasc Biol 1997; 17: 2004–9.

20. Celermajer DS, Sorensen KE, Gooch VM et al. Noninvasive detection of endothelial dysfunction in children and adults at risk of atherosclerosis. Lancet 1992; 340: 1111–16.

21. Celermajer DS, Cullen S, Deanfield JE. Impairment of endothelium-dependent pulmonary artery relaxation in children with congenital heart disease and abnormal pulmonary hemodynamics. Circulation 1993; 87: 440–6.

22. Hulley S, Grady D, Bush T et al. Randomized trial of estrogen plus progestin for secondary prevention of coronary heart disease in postmenopausal women. JAMA 1998; 280: 605–12.

23. Adams MR, Williams JK, Kaplan JR. Effects of androgens on coronary artery atherosclerosis and atherosclerosis-related impairment of vascular responsiveness. Arterioscler Thromb Vasc Biol 1995; 15: 562–70.

24. Bruck B, Brehme U, Gugel N et al. Gender-specific differences in the effects of testosterone and estrogen on the development of atherosclerosis in rabbits. Arterioscler Thromb Vasc Biol 1997; 17: 2192–9.

25. Thompson PD, Cullinane EM, Sady SP et al. Contrasting effects of testosterone and stanozolol on serum lipoprotein levels. JAMA 1989; 261: 1165–8.

26. Ajayi AA, Mathur R, Halushka PV. Testosterone increases human platelet thromboxane A2 receptor density and aggregation responses. Circulation 1995; 91: 2742–7.

27. Heller RF, Meade TW, Haines AP et al. Interrelationships between factor VII, serum testosterone and plasma lipoproteins. Thromb Res 1982; 28: 423–5.

28. Worboys S, Kotsopoulos D, Teede H et al. Evidence that parenteral testosterone therapy may improve endothelium-dependent and independent vasodilation in postmenopausal women already receiving estrogen. J Clin Endocrinol Metab 2001; 86: 158–61.

29. McCredie RJ, McCrohon JA, Turner L et al. Vascular reactivity is impaired in genetic females taking high-dose androgens. J Am Coll Cardiol 1998; 32: 1331–5.

30. Bernini GP, Sgro M, Moretti A et al. Endogenous androgens and carotid intimal–medial thickness in women. J Clin Endocrinol Metab 1999; 84: 2008–12.

31. Bernini GP, Moretti A, Sgro M et al. Influence of endogenous androgens on carotid wall in postmenopausal women. Menopause 2001; 8: 43–50.

32. Herrington DM, Gordon GB, Achuff SC et al. Plasma dehydroepiandrosterone and dehydroepiandrosterone sulfate in patients undergoing diagnostic coronary angiography. J Am Coll Cardiol 1990; 16: 862–70.

33. Slowinska-Srzednicka J, Malczewska B, Srzednicki M et al. Hyperinsulinaemia and decreased plasma levels of dehydroepiandrosterone sulfate in premenopausal women with coronary heart disease. J Intern Med 1995; 237: 465–72.

34. McCrohon JA, Death AK, Nakhla S et al. Androgen receptor expression is greater in macrophages from male than from female donors. A sex difference with implications for atherogenesis. Circulation 2000; 101: 224–6.

CHAPTER 40

Androgenic influences on ventilation and ventilatory responses to oxygen and carbon dioxide during wakefulness and sleep

Christopher P Cardozo

Effects of androgens on ventilatory control

Gender-dependent differences in ventilation and ventilatory control have been observed in several reports.[1-3] As compared to women, men at rest were found to have greater ventilation, lower ventilation per milliliter of CO_2 produced, higher tidal volumes, and lower respiratory rates. Respiratory responses of men had greater sensitivity to both hypoxia and hypercapnea.[1] The greater ventilation in men was associated with a higher metabolic rate.[3]

There is evidence that the sex steroids testosterone, estrogen, and progesterone contribute to these differences. Administration of testosterone to hypogonadal men raised both resting ventilation and metabolic rate in hypogonadal men. Because end-tidal partial pressure of carbon dioxide (pCO_2) did not change with testosterone treatment, these investigators proposed that the increased metabolic rate stimulated the increase in ventilation. An increase in metabolic rate has been observed in one other study in which testosterone was administered to hypogonadal men,[4] and ventilation correlates well with metabolic rate. In contrast, Matsumoto and coworkers found no change in metabolic rate

after administration of testosterone to hypogonadal men for 6 weeks.[5] Studies in cats have demonstrated that when neutered male cats were treated with testosterone, resting ventilation and CO_2 production increased whereas end-tidal pCO_2 was unchanged,[5] in agreement with the results of White and colleagues.[1] The reason for these conflicting results is unclear.

The reported effects of testosterone on hypoxic (HVR) and hypercapnic ventilatory responses (HCVR) are conflicting. White and colleagues reported an augmented HVR and HCVR after testosterone replacement in hypogonadal men.[6] Similarly, testosterone treatment of neutered male cats raised HVR.[7] By contrast, testosterone did not alter HCVR in animals, and Matsumoto and co-workers found in humans that HVR was decreased by testosterone whereas HCVR was unchanged.[5] On balance therefore, the literature suggests that testosterone increases sensitivity to hypoxic respiratory stimuli with unclear effects on hypercapneic stimuli.

An interesting aspect of the studies of the effects of testosterone replacement in cats[6] and humans[6] was that there was a poor correlation between testosterone levels, which varied widely, and changes in respiratory control. On the one hand, one might have expected greater effects with higher concentrations. Support for the major alternative, that there is a plateau for respiratory effects of testosterone, comes from the observation that administration of testosterone to a subject later found to be eugonadal had no appreciable change in respiratory control.[6]

While not specifically tested, one likely explanation for the effect of testosterone on resting metabolic rate is the increase in skeletal muscle mass that is stimulated by this hormone.[8-11] Mechanisms whereby testosterone might alter chemoreceptor sensitivity or processing of chemoreceptor signals by the central nervous system are less clear. It remains possible that testosterone affects either or both of these components of respiratory control. Testosterone is well recognized for its role in stimulating gender-specific changes of the central nervous system, such as influencing the death of certain neurons or promoting or inhibiting the formation of synapses.[12,13]

The physiological receptor for testosterone is the androgen receptor (AR) a member of the steroid hormone receptor family of nuclear receptors. The classical view is that AR resides in the cytoplasm bound to a complex formed around heat shock protein 90, and is liberated once bound by testosterone. Free AR–testosterone complexes migrate to the nucleus where they bind specific DNA sequences and alter gene expression.[14] While variations on this theme exist, the end result is testosterone-induced alterations in gene expression mediated by interactions of the AR with chromatin.

Influence of testosterone on breathing during sleep

A strong link exists between male gender and sleep hypopneas, apneas, and desaturations.[15,16] Evidence of a link between testosterone levels and sleep-disordered breathing came initially from case-reports. In a study of obese males, all but one (who was hypogonadal) had sleep apnea.[17] Others observed the development of sleep apnea in one man and one woman who were administered testosterone; sleep apnea resolved upon discontinuation of this hormone.[18,19]

Several small prospective studies also support a link between sleep apnea and testosterone. Administration of testosterone to 11 hypogonadal males significantly increased the numbers of apneas and hypopneas, resulting in a more than 2-fold increase in disordered breathing events.[20] Testosterone did not alter respiratory rhythm, sleep distribution, or airflow. A more recent prospective, randomized, placebo-controlled crossover study found that for one night of sleep, testosterone reduced total time asleep by 1 hour, increased disruptions to sleep by 7 events an hour, and increased the duration of hypoxemia by 5 minutes.[21] These changes in sleep quality did not correlate with upper airway dimensions, driving ability, or scores on Epworth or Stanford sleepiness scales.

Although these findings link testosterone levels to alterations in breathing during sleep, they are not sufficient to determine whether testosterone, or more importantly, testosterone replacement in hypogonadal men, increases the risk of developing sleep apnea. Some insight into this question comes from a meta-analysis of 19 studies in which testosterone was administered to men with low testosterone levels in randomized trials. The analysis examined data from 651 testosterone-treated and 433 placebo-treated men.[22] Testosterone replacement did not significantly alter the risk of sleep apnea. Nevertheless, the Endocrine Society clinical guide to practice advises against beginning testosterone in patients with untreated obstructive sleep apnea,[23] and prudence suggests that patients should be asked about symptoms of sleep-disordered breathing prior to and after starting testosterone.

Insights into possible mechanisms underlying these effects of testosterone come from studies that administration of testosterone to premenopausal women raised their hypocapnic apnea threshold,[24] suggesting effects on chemoreceptors, central processing of chemoreceptor signals, or both. Studies of the effects of increased respiratory loading concluded that differences in predisposition to sleep apnea between men and women related to greater collapsability of airways in men, and that central control of breathing in response to increased respiratory loads was unaffected by gender.[25] In this study, the two subjects with greater numbers of dysrhythmic episodes while administered testosterone tended to have a higher supraglottic resistance and lower mean pharyngeal airway size. Consistent with this speculation, in a case-report, administration of testosterone to a woman known to snore resulted in the development of sleep apnea associated with the development of elevated supraglottic resistance, all of which normalized with withdrawal of testosterone.[19]

Neither the site nor mechanisms by which testosterone promotes sleep apnea are known. As noted above, testosterone has multiple effects on the central nervous system. It remains possible that this hormone could alter central control of respiration or upper airway caliber or collapsibility. Testosterone has direct effects on muscle, resulting in increased muscle size and strength, and increased expression of insulin-like growth factor-1, a potent stimulus for muscle hypertrophy. Whether testosterone changes muscle mechanical properties to facilitate collapse of the upper airway remains unknown.

Conclusions

Androgen administration increases resting ventilation, metabolic rate, and hypoxic and chemoreceptor responsiveness in the awake state. In contrast, androgens may cause or act to accentuate apnea and hypopnea during sleep. Neither the site of action nor the mechanism by which these effects are mediated is understood.

Acknowledgment

This work was supported by the Department of Veterans Affairs Rehabilitation Research and Development Service (B4162C, B3347K).

References

1. White DP et al. Sexual influence on the control of breathing. J Appl Physiol 1983; 54: 874–9.
2. Regensteiner JG et al. Possible gender differences in the effect of exercise on hypoxic ventilatory response. Respiration 1988; 53: 158–65.
3. Aitken ML et al. Influence of body size and gender on control of ventilation. J Appl Physiol 1986; 60: 1894–9.
4. Gibney J et al. Growth hormone and testosterone interact positively to enhance protein and energy metabolism in hypopituitary men. Am J Physiol Endocrinol Metab 2005; 289: E266–71.
5. Matsumoto AM et al. Testosterone replacement in hypogonadal men: effects on obstructive sleep apnoea, respiratory drives, and sleep. Clin Endocrinol (Oxf) 1985; 22: 713–21.
6. White DP et al. Influence of testosterone on ventilation and chemosensitivity in male subjects. J Appl Physiol 1985; 59: 1452–7.
7. Tatsumi K et al. Influences of gender and sex hormones on hypoxic ventilatory response in cats. J Appl Physiol 1991; 71: 1746–51.
8. Urban RJ et al. Testosterone administration to elderly men increases skeletal muscle strength and protein synthesis. Am J Physiol 1995; 269: E820–6.
9. Mauras N et al. Testosterone deficiency in young men: marked alterations in whole body protein kinetics, strength, and adiposity. J Clin Endocrinol Metab 1998; 83: 1886–92.
10. Ferrando AA et al. Testosterone administration to older men improves muscle function: molecular and physiological mechanisms. Am J Physiol Endocrinol Metab 2002; 282: E601–7.
11. Bhasin S et al. Older men are as responsive as young men to the anabolic effects of graded doses of testosterone on the skeletal muscle. J Clin Endocrinol Metab 2005; 90: 678–88.
12. Morris JA, Jordan CL, Breedlove SM. Sexual differentiation of the vertebrate nervous system. Nat Neurosci 2004; 7: 1034–9.
13. DonCarlos LL et al. Novel cellular phenotypes and subcellular sites for androgen action in the forebrain. Neuroscience 2006; 138: 801–7.
14. Gelmann EP. Molecular biology of the androgen receptor. J Clin Oncol 2002; 20: 3001–15.
15. Block AJ et al. Sleep apnea, hypopnea and oxygen desaturation in normal subjects. A strong male predominance. N Engl J Med 1979; 300: 513–17.
16. Bresnitz EA, Goldberg R, Kosinski RM. Epidemiology of obstructive sleep apnea. Epidemiol Rev 1994; 16: 210–27.
17. Harman E et al. Sleep-disordered breathing and oxygen desaturation in obese patients. Chest 1981; 79: 256–60.
18. Sandblom RE et al. Obstructive sleep apnea syndrome induced by testosterone administration. N Engl J Med 1983; 308: 508–10.
19. Johnson MW, Anch AM, Remmers JE. Induction of the obstructive sleep apnea syndrome in a woman by exogenous androgen administration. Am Rev Respir Dis 1984; 129: 1023–5.
20. Schneider BK et al. Influence of testosterone on breathing during sleep. J Appl Physiol 1986; 61: 618–23.

21. Liu PY et al. The short-term effects of high-dose testosterone on sleep, breathing, and function in older men. J Clin Endocrinol Metab 2003; 88: 3605–13.
22. Calof OM et al. Adverse events associated with testosterone replacement in middle-aged and older men: a meta-analysis of randomized, placebo-controlled trials. J Gerontol A Biol Sci Med Sci 2005; 60: 1451–7.
23. Bhasin S et al. Testosterone therapy in adult men with androgen deficiency syndromes: an Endocrine Society clinical practice guideline. J Clin Endocrinol Metab 2006; 91: 1995–2010.
24. Zhou XS et al. Effect of testosterone on the apneic threshold in women during NREM sleep. J Appl Physiol 2003; 94: 101–7.
25. Pillar G et al. Airway mechanics and ventilation in response to resistive loading during sleep: influence of gender. Am J Respir Crit Care Med 2000; 162: 1627–32.

CHAPTER 41

The role of androgens in respiratory function

Ann M Spungen

Introduction

This chapter will review the muscles of breathing, the effect of endogenous and exogenous testosterone or anabolic steroid agents on peripheral skeletal muscle, and the animal and limited human literature on the effect of anabolic steroid administration on respiratory function. Only 'androgens', such as testosterone or any of its synthetic anabolic steroid derivatives, will be discussed in this section. Other anabolic agents, such as ß2-agonists or growth hormone, which also promote anabolism but are not androgens, will be excluded from discussion.

Muscles of breathing

The muscles of breathing comprise three main groups: the diaphragm, intercostal/accessory muscles, and the abdominal wall group. These muscles are unique from the other skeletal muscles in three aspects: (1) they are both involuntary and voluntary; (2) they overcome resistive and elastic loads rather than inertial loads; and (3) they must contract regularly without prolonged rest throughout life.[1] The respiratory muscles work as either prime movers or stabilizers of the chest wall to promote inspiration and exhalation. The inspiratory muscles of breathing function in a coordinated effort to enlarge the thoracic cavity, creating a negative intrapleural pressure and inflating the lung. The diaphragm is the primary muscle responsible for inspiration during quiet breathing (tidal breathing). Exhalation during quiet breathing is largely passive. The inspiratory action of the diaphragm is dependent on its configuration and the presence of abdominal resistance. In patients with pulmonary compromise, the diaphragm may flatten, weakening its ability to inspire. The diaphragm is innervated at cervical level 3, 4, and 5 (Figure 41.1). The accessory muscles include the scalenes, sternocleidomastoids, and trapezius; these muscles contribute minimally to inhalation during tidal breathing. DeTroyer et al.[2] speculated that the scalenes may play an active role by stabilizing the rib cage during quiet breathing. In cases of cervical paralysis, such as that seen in those with tetraplegia, the pectoralis major has been shown to participate in expiration.[3] The intercostal muscles are primarily responsible for forced efforts of inhalation (external intercostals) and exhalation (internal intercostals); these muscles are innervated at thoracic level 1 to 12 (Figure 41.1) and are recruited to assist with deep inspirations and forceful exhalations. The abdominal wall group consists of the recti, external and internal obliques, and the transverse abdominis. These muscles are innervated at thoracic level 1 to lumbar level 2 and they primarily contract to participate in exhalation at higher levels of ventilation, such as during exercise or stress and during explosive exhalation (cough). The abdominal wall group is relatively inactive during quiet breathing.

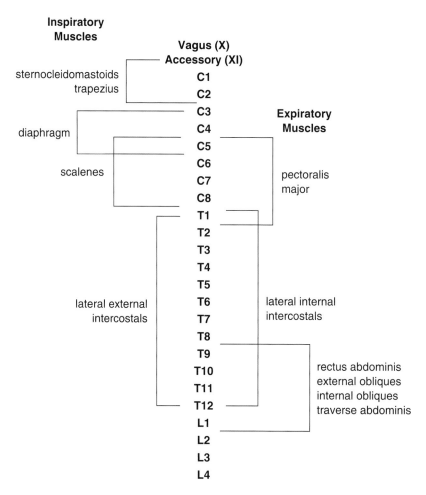

Figure 41.1 *The innervation of the muscles of breathing.*

Morgan and colleagues[1] describe three major etiologies responsible for respiratory failure and muscle fatigue manifesting themselves in three ways: (1) lack of central neurologic drive; (2) mechanical disorders of the chest wall; and (3) failure of the muscles to generate the required force, that is fatigue. Anabolic therapies are postulated to have the most significant impact on the third mechanism, muscle fatigue, by their effect to strengthen respiratory muscles. Following is a discussion of the mechanisms of anabolic therapies and their effect on respiratory muscles.

Effects of testosterone on skeletal muscle

Testosterone administration increases muscle protein synthesis in normal men.[4] Hypogonadism in non-elderly men is associated with reductions in lean body muscle mass, with testosterone replacement therapy increasing lean body tissue and muscle strength.[5–9] Mauras and colleagues[8] addressed the specific effects of androgens on body composition and protein metabolism in six healthy men (23.2 ± 0.5 (SE) years of age). Gonadal suppression was achieved with a long-acting gonadotropin releasing factor analog (Lupron, TAP Pharmaceuticals, IL, USA) to produce prepubertal levels of serum testosterone. After 10 weeks of suppressive therapy, all subjects demonstrated a decrease in fat-free mass and an increase in fat mass; muscle strength of the legs was decreased.[8] Thus, in men with hypogonadism or in young men who were chemically ablated for endogenous androgens, muscle mass and strength were clearly deficient.

Normal aging is associated with a decline in serum testosterone levels.[10,11] It has been controversial as to whether the fall in serum testosterone levels with advancing age is due to aging, chronic illness, or medication use. Gray and colleagues[10] conducted a cross-sectional survey of a population of men aged 39 to 70 years who were either completely healthy ($n = 415$) or who had a medical condition or were on prescription medications ($n = 1294$). The less healthy men had 10 to 15% lower levels of androgens than those who were healthy. However, regardless of health status, the rates of decline of total testosterone, free testosterone, or major androgens and metabolites were similar.[10] As part of the Baltimore Longitudinal Study, Harman and coworkers[11] performed serum testosterone measurements in a population of men ($n = 890$) over 20 years. The incidence of hypogonadism, based upon total testosterone concentration, increased from 20% of men over the age of 60 to 30% over 70 and 50% over 80. Because of the potential of testosterone replacement to prevent or partially reduce the age-related changes in body composition, muscle strength, functional impairment, and quality of life, such hormonal therapy may be indicated in those men with the lowest serum testosterone concentrations.

Several reports have studied testosterone replacement in elderly men.[12–15] Urban and colleagues[12] investigated the effects of physiologic testosterone administration for 4 weeks in six healthy older men (67 ± 2 (SE) years of age). Leg muscle strength increased, as did fractional synthetic rate of muscle protein by a stable-isotope infusion technique. Other reports have generally noted an increase in lean body tissue and muscle strength, and decreased fat mass in response to testosterone replacement therapy.[13–15] Muscle loss

attributed to secondary causes of androgen deficiency, such as that occurring in hypogonadal men with acquired immunodeficiency syndrome (AIDS) and a wasting myopathy, have been shown to correlate with testosterone levels and respond to androgen therapy.[9,16,17]

Individuals with spinal cord injury occupy the lowest end of the activity spectrum and have been considered to be a model of immobilization and premature aging.[18,19] The level of pulmonary impairment is closely related to the level of spinal cord lesion. Chronic spinal cord injury is associated with a continuous loss in lean body tissue mass.[19] Tsitouras and colleagues[20] noted that persons with spinal cord injury had significantly lower levels of serum total and free testosterone compared with able-bodied subjects. In larger groups of subjects, Bauman and coworkers[21] found that those with spinal cord injury also had lower serum total testosterone levels, which declined at 9% per decade compared with 5% per decade in the able-bodied controls.

Supraphysiologic administration of testosterone has been demonstrated to have a pronounced effect on muscle mass. Bhasin and colleagues[22] administered 600 mg of testosterone enanthate or placebo weekly for 10 weeks. Even in the absence of strength training, supraphysiologic testosterone doses produced increased muscle mass of the arms and legs, associated with increased strength; this effect was further augmented with strength training.[22] Anabolic steroid therapy in the higher dose ranges would be expected to have a similar effect on muscle mass to that seen with supraphysiologic testosterone administration.

Effects of anabolic steroids on the diaphragm

Several animal studies have been performed to investigate the effect of synthetic anabolic steroid and/or testosterone administration on respiratory muscles. In a study of healthy postpubescent female and male rats, Bisschop and co-workers[23] investigated the effect of 5 weeks of low-dose (1.5 mg/kg) and high-dose (7.5 mg/kg) nandrolone decanoate (a testosterone derivative administered im with a moderately high anabolic-to-androgenic ratio) on histochemical, contractile, and fatigue properties of the diaphragm. In the nandrolone decanoate-treated groups compared with the control group, the cross-sectional area of type IIx/b fibers was increased ($P < 0.05$), whereas those of type I and type IIa fibers were not significantly altered. Time-to-peak tension and half-relaxation time decreased in the two treatment groups ($P < 0.05$ and $P < 0.01$, respectively), whereas maximal twitch tension, maximal tetonic tension, and the ratio did not change significantly with treatment. Force-frequency curves and fatigue properties were not affected by nandrolone decanoate treatment. No gender bias was found for any of the diaphragm properties measured. The significant changes in muscle function found in this study were consistent with diaphragm muscle hypertrophy. Prezant and colleagues[24] investigated the use of testosterone propionate (2.5 mg/day; 5 days/week) in healthy male and female rats during short-term (2.5 weeks) and long-term (10 weeks) administration. In females, but not males, testosterone treatment produced significant increases in body weight, costal diaphragm weight, and contractility and significant decreases in fatigue resistance indexes. One explanation for the lack of a significant finding in male rats was that the dose of testosterone administered was too low to elicit an effect. In both sexes, no significant difference in fiber type proportions or areas was observed, regardless of treatment duration or the baseline circulating androgen level. When all rats were analyzed together, significant improvements were found for diaphragm contractility and fatigue resistance. The authors noted that these were healthy, normally breathing animals and that in a more compromised breathing model, greater testosterone-related changes may occur.

Van Balkom and colleagues[25] studied the effect of anabolic steroid administration on respiratory muscle function in pulmonary compromised animal models. One study was designed to investigate whether anabolic steroid administration could block the loss of diaphragm force caused by long-term use of methylprednisolone. Adult male rats were administered low-dose methylprednisolone

(0.2 mg/kg/day for 9 months) with saline or with saline and nandrolone decanoate (1 mg/kg/week im during the final 3 months). The methylprednisolone-only group experienced a reduction in diaphragm force of 10%. This effect was completely antagonized in the group that received nandrolone decanoate. In a similar study by these same investigators, using an emphysematous hamster model, the addition of nandrolone decanoate in a clinically relevant dose completely reversed myosin heavy chain type IIa and IIx diaphragm muscle atrophy caused by the glucocorticoid agent. In both in vitro and in vivo rat studies, anabolic steroid agents have been demonstrated to competitively displace corticosteroids from their cytoplasmic receptors in muscle.[26] At low stimulation frequencies in the emphysematous hamsters, the improvement in force generation in the diaphragm from the anabolic steroid addition was to the level of the control animals.[27]

Compared with other skeletal muscles, the diaphragm has a higher cytosol androgen receptor density[28] and participates in continuous cyclic contraction, theoretically increasing its potential to benefit from anabolic steroid administration. These animal studies lend support to the concept that anabolic steroid administration may significantly impact respiratory skeletal muscle fatigue. Patients with pulmonary compromise, such as emphysema, chronic obstructive pulmonary disease (COPD), tetraplegia, and other neuromuscular disorders, may benefit from anabolic steroid administration. To date, there is a scarcity of investigation performed in this area. However, it may be speculated that anabolic steroid therapy has the potential to improve diaphragmatic strength and endurance in patients with respiratory failure.

Effects of anabolic steroids on pulmonary function

Only a few studies exist in humans that have investigated the role of anabolic steroids to improve respiratory muscle function and/or general pulmonary function. However, patients with chronic obstructive pulmonary disease (COPD) often experience moderate to severe weight loss in association with decreases in pulmonary function and their general ability to breathe. Ferreira and coworkers[29] investigated the effect of oral anabolic steroids on body mass index (BMI), lean body mass, anthropometric measures, respiratory muscle strength, and functional exercise capacity in subjects with COPD in a prospective, randomized, double-blind, placebo-controlled study. The study group received testosterone (250 mg im) and oral stanozolol (12 mg/day) for 27 weeks. The control group received placebo injection and an oral placebo tablet. Seventeen of 23 subjects completed the study (10 in the treatment group and 7 controls). Anabolic treatment was associated with increases in BMI, lean body mass, and anthropometric measures of arm and thigh circumference, with no significant changes in endurance exercise capacity. A trend was evident in the treatment group for maximal inspiratory mouth pressure (PI_{max}) to increase by an average of 41%, but this was not statistically different from the control group (who demonstrated a 20% increase in PI_{max}). The authors reported that administration of an oral anabolic steroid for 27 weeks to malnourished male subjects with COPD was free of clinical or biochemical side-effects.

In another study, by Schols and colleagues,[30] 217 patients with COPD participated in a placebo-controlled, randomized trial investigating the physiologic effects of nutritional intervention alone for 8 weeks or combined with an anabolic steroid, nandrolone decanoate, injected im over 8 weeks (on days 1, 15, 29, and 43 at doses of 25 mg in women or 50 mg in men). Maximal inspiratory mouth pressure improved for the nutrition-only and the anabolic steroid plus nutrition groups in the first 4 weeks of treatment. After week 8 of treatment, only those in the nandrolone decanoate plus nutrition group were significantly greater than the placebo group for maximal inspiratory pressure ($P < 0.03$). The nutrition group had a significant weight gain that was predominantly due to an expansion of fat mass ($P < 0.03$). In contrast, the weight gain in the nandrolone decanoate plus nutrition group resulted from more favorable relative changes in fat-free mass, as well as other measures of muscle mass ($P < 0.03$).

Pulmonary complications are a major cause of morbidity and mortality among individuals with cervical spinal cord lesions, primarily due to paralysis of the muscles of respiration. Strengthening of the remaining intact respiratory musculature may reduce these complications and improve pulmonary function. An open-label pilot study was performed to investigate the effect of 1 month of treatment with oxandrolone (an anabolic steroid with the highest anabolic-to-androgenic ratio) on weight gain and pulmonary function. Ten healthy adult male subjects with complete motor tetraplegia of greater than 1-year's duration participated in this study. Spirometry, maximal inspiratory and expiratory pressures, and resting self-rating of dyspnea (Borg scale) were measured at baseline and repeated again at the end of 1 month of oxandrolone therapy (20 mg/day). On average, the subjects gained 1.4 ± 1.5 kg, a $2 \pm 2\%$ increase in weight ($P = 0.01$). A significant $9 \pm 2\%$ improvement was found in the combined measures of spirometry ($P < 0.005$). Maximal inspiratory pressure improved by an average of $10 \pm 7\%$ ($P < 0.001$). Maximal expiratory pressure improved by $9 \pm 13\%$ (non-significant). Subjective self-rating of dyspnea decreased by an average of $37 \pm 28\%$ ($P < 0.01$). In healthy subjects with tetraplegia, the use of oxandrolone was associated with significant improvements in weight and pulmonary function, and a subjective reduction in breathlessness.[31] In the absence of any clinical studies, it may be speculated that anabolic steroid administration be considered in the therapy of individuals with tetraplegia in an effort to strengthen respiratory musculature during respiratory insufficiency precipitated by intercurrent infectious pulmonary illness.

Association of male gender with greater airway inflammation and airway responsiveness

In a study designed to investigate the influence of gender on lung function, airway inflammation, and airway responsiveness to provocative challenge in naïve laboratory mice, Card et al reported significant gender differences.[32] Several experiments were performed. In the first, no gender differences were found for baseline conditions of breathing frequency and tidal volume. Following administration of aerosolized methacholine (cholinergic stimulation), peak values for resistance and elastance were significantly greater in males compared with females. Overall, the airways of male mice were more hyperresponsive than female mice after challenge. In mice treated with lipopolysaccharide (LPS), a known airway inflammatory agent, male mice had significantly increased bronchoalveolar lavage (BAL) fluid cells compared with saline-treated and female LPS-treated mice. LPS-treated female mice were not different from saline-treated mice. LPS-treated male mice were also found to have higher BAL fluid indices of inflammation and histopathologic scores for inflammation than saline- and LPS-treated female mice. The experiment was repeated in gonadectomized male and ovariectomized female mice. In the castrated male mice treated with LPS, there was an attenuation of airway inflammation, while the ovariectomy had no effect. Testosterone administration to female mice increased their responsiveness to LPS and methacholine challenge. It was concluded that male sex hormones appear to play a role in promoting airway hyperresponsiveness to cholinergic challenge and to the inflammatory response to LPS challenge.[32] In a second publication by this same group, the authors provide further evidence that male sex hormones are associated with vagally mediated airway responsiveness.[33] As yet, no such findings of an association of testosterone or other male hormones with airway hyperresponsiveness have been demonstrated in humans. However, because of the potential use of testosterone replacement therapy for hypogonadism the effects on airway reactivity should be investigated.

Summary

The respiratory musculature may have an augmented potential to respond to anabolic steroid therapy compared with other skeletal muscles to improve in size, strength, and contractility and delay the onset of fatigue. For the pulmonary compromised patient, there is an obvious need for further investigation in this area. Studies to determine the optimal dosing regimens of anabolic steroids combined with nutrition and/or exercise training are needed. Potential applications to accelerate ventilator weaning are also of considerable importance.

Acknowledgments

This work was supported by the Department of Veterans Affairs Rehabilitation Research and Development Service.

References

1. Morgan MDL, Silver JR, William SJ. The respiratory system of the spinal cord patient. In: Bloch RF, Basbaum M, eds. Management of Spinal Cord Injury. Baltimore, MD: Williams & Wilkins, 1986: 78–116.
2. DeTroyer A, Kelly S, Zin WA. Mechanical action of the intercostal muscles on the ribs. Science 1983; 220: 87–8.
3. DeTroyer AD, Estenne M. The expiratory muscles in tetraplegia. Paraplegia 1991; 29: 359–63.
4. Griggs RC, Kingston W, Jozefowicz RF et al. Effect of testosterone on muscle mass and muscle protein synthesis. J Appl Physiol 1989; 66: 498–503.
5. Forbes GB, Reina JC. Adult lean mass declines with age: some longitudinal observations. Metabolism 1970; 19: 653–63.
6. Brodsky IG, Balagopal P, Nair KS. Effects of testosterone replacement on muscle mass and muscle protein synthesis in hypogonadal men. J Clin Endocrinol Metab 1996; 81: 3469–75.
7. Bhasin S, Storer TW, Berman N et al. Testosterone replacement increases fat-free mass and muscle size in hypogonadal men. J Clin Endocrinol Metab 1997; 82: 407–13.
8. Mauras N, Hayes V, Welch S et al. Testosterone deficiency in young men: marked alterations in whole body protein kinetics, strength, and adiposity. J Clin Endocrinol Metab 1998; 83: 1886–92.
9. Grinspoon S, Cororan C, Lee K et al. Loss of lean body mass and muscle mass correlates with androgen levels in hypogonadal men with acquired immunodeficiency syndrome wasting. J Clin Endocrinol Metab 1996; 81: 4051–58.
10. Gray A, Feldman HA, McKinlay JB et al. Age, disease, and changing sex hormone levels in middle-aged men: results of the Massachusetts Male Aging Study. J Clin Endocrinol Metab 1991; 73: 1016–25.
11. Harman SM, Metter EJ, Tobin JD et al. Longitudinal effects of aging on serum total and free testosterone levels in healthy men. J Clin Endocrinol Metab 2001; 86: 724–31.

12. Urban RJ, Bodenburg YH, Gilkison C et al. Testosterone administration to elderly men increases skeletal muscle strength and protein synthesis. Am J Physiol 1995; 269: E820–6.

13. Tenover JS. Effects of testosterone supplementation in the aging male. J Clin Endocrinol Metab 1992; 75: 1092–8.

14. Snyder PJ, Peachey H, Hannoush P et al. Effect of testosterone treatment on body composition and muscle strength in men over 65 years of age. J Clin Endocrinol Metab 1999; 84: 2647–53.

15. Wang C, Swerdlof RS, Iranmanesh A et al. Transdermal testosterone gel improves sexual function, mood, muscle strength, and body composition parameters in hypogonadal men. J Clin Endocrinol Metab 2000; 85: 2839–53.

16. Berger JR, Pall L, Hall CD et al. Oxandrolone in AIDS-wasting myopathy. AIDS 1996; 10: 1657–62.

17. Bhasin S, Storer TW, Asbel-Sethi N et al. Effects of testosterone replacement with a nongenital, transdermal system, Androderm, in human immunodeficiency virus-infected men with low testosterone levels. J Clin Endocrinol Metab 1998; 83: 3155–62.

18. Bauman WA, Spungen AM. Disorders of carbohydrate and lipid metabolism in veterans with paraplegia or quadriplegia: a model of premature aging. Metabolism 1994; 43: 749–56.

19. Spungen AM, Wang J, Pierson RN Jr et al. Soft tissue body composition changes from immobilization determined from a monozygotic twin model: one with spinal cord injury. J Applied Physiol 2000; 88: 1310–15.

20. Tsitouras PD, Zhong YG, Spungen AM et al. Serum testosterone and insulin-like growth factor-I/growth hormone in adults with spinal cord injury. Horm Met Res 1995; 27: 287–92.

21. Bauman WA, Zhong YG, Spungen AM. Depressed serum testosterone levels in subjects with SCI. J Spinal Cord Med 2001; 24: S20.

22. Bhasin S, Storer TW, Berman N et al. The effects of supraphysiological doses of testosterone on muscle size and strength in normal men. N Engl J Med 1996; 335: 1–7.

23. Bisschop A, Gayan-Ramirez G, Rollier H et al. Effects of nandrolone decanoate on respiratory and peripheral muscles in male and female rats. J Appl Physiol 1997; 82: 1112–18.

24. Prezant DJ, Valentine DE, Gentry EI et al. Effects of short-term and long-term androgen treatment on the diaphragm in male and female rats. J Appl Physiol 1993; 75: 1140–9.

25. Van Balkom RH, Dekhuijzen PN, Folgering HT et al. Anabolic steroids in part reverse glucocorticoid-induced alterations in rat diaphragm. Appl Physiol 1998; 84: 1492–9.

26. Mayer M, Rosen F. Interaction of anabolic steroids with glucocorticoid receptor sites in rat muscle cytosol. Am J Physiol 1975; 229: 1381–6.

27. Van Balkom RH, Dekhuijzen PN, van der Heijden HF et al. Effects of anabolic steroids on diphragm impairment induced by methylprednisolone in emphysematous hamsters. Eur Respir J 1999; 13: 1062–9.

28. Eggington S. Effects of an anabolic hormone on aerobic capacity of rat striated muscle. Pflugers Arch 1987; 410: 356–62.

29. Ferreira IM, Verreschi IT, Nery LE et al. The influence of 6 months of oral anabolic steroids on body mass and respiratory muscles in undernourished COPD patients. Chest 1998; 114: 19–28.

30. Schols AM, Soeters PB, Mostert R et al. Physiologic effects of nutritional support and anabolic steroids in patients with chronic obstructive pulmonary disease. A placebo-controlled randomized trial. Am J Respir Crit Care Med 1995; 152: 1268–74.

31. Spungen AM, Grimm DR, Strakhan M et al. Treatment with an anabolic agent is associated with improvement in respiratory function in persons with tetraplegia: a pilot study. Mt Sinai J Med 1999; 66: 201–5.

32. Card JW, Carey MA, Bradbury JA et al. Gender differences in murine airway responsiveness and lipopolysaccharide-induced inflammation. J Immunol 2006: 177: 621–30.

33. Card JW, Voltz JW, Ferguson CD et al. Male sex hormones promote vagally-mediated reflex airway responsiveness to cholinergic stimulation. Am J Physiol Lung Cell Mol Physiol 2007; 292(4): L908–14.

Central Nervous System and Psyche

CHAPTER 42

Changes in libido/sex life

Syed H Tariq

Introduction

Decline in sexual activity, interest, and desire has been reported by a number of investigators.[1–5] Advanced age has a significant negative effect on sexual desire, but there is no difference in sexual enjoyment and satisfaction between young and older persons.[6] About 50% of older adults express sexual desire in the ninth decade and about 15% are sexually active.[7] Pfeiffer et al[8] reported that in their study 95% of the men aged 46 to 50 years had weekly intercourse, which decreased to 28% at the age of 66 to 71. Kinsey et al[9] reported reduced frequency of intercourse to once every 10 weeks by age 80. Sexual activity is reported to decrease in older married couples from 53% at the age of 60 to 24% over the age of 76.[10] In one study of older adults between the ages of 80 and 102 years who were sexually active, 83% of men were reported touching and caressing without intercourse, and 72% of men engaged in masturbation.[11] Janus and Janus[12] reported a decrease in frequency of masturbation after the age of 65 years.

Erectile dysfunction affects about 10 to 20 million men in the United States.[13] Kinsey et al[14] reported an increase in erectile dysfunction with age, 27% at the age of 70 years, 55% at the age of 75 years, and about 75% at the age of 80 years.

In the USA there are about 3.5 million gay people over the age of 60.[15,16] Older gay men are a diverse population, with many aging successfully, living a healthy and satisfying lifestyle.[17] All older gay persons have in common, at least in the USA, an experience of living in a society where the gay lifestyle is oppressed, and there is a general failure to recognize and affirm loving relationships among the same gender. Most of the older homosexual men will not reveal their sexual feelings in public. They face the same sort of problems with relationships that older heterosexual men experience. Older homosexual men suffer additional problems of stress when they hide their sexual preferences or attempt to find a partner, especially in the nursing homes. Gay-oriented long-term care facilities are currently not available.

A support group called 'Gay and Lesbians Older and Wiser' (GLOW) has been established in Ann Arbor, Michigan.[18] The GLOW service is provided by a university-based geriatric clinic, staffed by professional social workers who provide social support. The GLOW initiative and others have shown that older gay men who are integrated into the gay community develop extended relationships, which serve as a surrogate family.[19,20]

Recent advances in the physiology of aging have made it possible to understand the effects of aging on sexuality, and the effects of disease and drugs on sexual/erectile dysfunction. Today there are more treatment options available that are non-invasive and are efficacious. The media play a major role in advertising the newly available commercial products that place the burden on the primary care physician to identify and treat sexual problems. Patients expect physicians to help maintain quality of life in the seventh decade and beyond. Men with erectile dysfunction have an impaired quality of life compared with healthy individuals as sexual activity contributes to the quality of life of couples or individuals.[21]

Physiology of penile erection

Sexual activity consists of libido and potency. Libido comprises sexual desire/drive, thoughts and fantasies, satisfaction and pleasure. Potency is the ability to attain and maintain erection and to ejaculate. Penile erection is obtained in three different ways. The first pathway is through local genital stimulation, causing afferent sensations in the sensory receptors of the penile shaft and glans penis that are carried to the spinal cord by the somatic pudendal nerve. The sensory perception is then carried to the higher centers, and efferent impulses leave the spinal cord via the sacral parasympathetic center to the pelvic plexus and the cavernous nerves into the corpus cavernosum. The second pathway is psychogenic stimulation that occurs through visual or auditory stimuli; this is more complex and less well understood. The third type of penile erection is seen during rapid eye movement (REM) sleep, the physiology of which is not known.

In the flaccid state, sympathetic activity causes vasoconstriction of the arteries, arterioles, and sinusoidal spaces within the corpora cavernosa. During erection the adrenergic-induced vasoconstriction of the sinusoidal spaces is overcome by the vasodilatation of the parasympathetic nervous system. The vasodilatation leads to an increase in arterial blood flow causing an increased pressure in the cavernosal spaces, which occludes the venous system and leads to penile erection. After ejaculation or termination of the erotic stimuli, the sympathetic nerve terminals release catecholamines. The catecholamines cause contraction of the smooth muscles around the sinusoids and arterioles, resulting in a decrease in blood inflow and expulsion of blood out of the sinusoidal spaces, resulting in a flaccid state.

A number of neurotransmitters play an important role in penile erection. Nitric oxide is released during sexual stimulation by endothelial cells and cavernous nerves. Nitric oxide, along with other agents such as prostaglandins E_2 and E_1, vasoactive intestinal peptide, neuropeptide Y, and acetylcholine, causes smooth muscle relaxation and penile erection. Smooth muscle contraction is caused by prostaglandin $F_{2\alpha}$, substance P, histamine, and norepinephrine.

Physiologic changes with age in the male

There are four stages of the sexual response cycle: excitement, plateau, orgasm, and resolution. Masters and Johnson described changes in these cycles with aging.[22] During the excitement phase there is delay in erection, decrease in the erectile strength, and decrease in scrotal congestion and testicular elevation with advanced age. There is a prolongation of the plateau phase along with a decrease in preejaculatory secretion. The orgasmic phase is shorter with diminished prostatic and urethral contractions and a decrease in ejaculatory force. The ejaculation time is longer compared to young adults with longer periods of coitus. In the resolution phase there is rapid detumescence and rapid testicular descent. The refractory period is also prolonged with age.

The sensitivity of the penis to stimulation decreases with age and it takes longer to achieve erection.[23] Erection becomes more dependent on physical stimulation of the penis and less responsive to visual, non-genital, and psychologic stimulation. Although penile rigidity decreases with age it generally remains adequate for vaginal penetration, although in some men the capability for penetration is lost.[14]

Nocturnal penile tumescence is impaired and is considered an indicator of erectile dysfunction. Schiavi et al reported that, in married couples or those in stable relationships between the ages of 45 and 75, sexual desire, arousal, coital frequency, and prevalence of erectile problems correlated with nocturnal penile tumescence measures.[6] Furthermore in healthy older men there is a decrease in frequency and degree of erection obtained during sleep.[24–26]

In normal older adults there are individual variations in circulating testosterone levels, which are not associated with individual variations in sexual drive or behavior.[27] With the onset of middle age there is a gradual decrease in sexual desire or libido.[28,29] Libido in men is linked to testosterone[30] and when testosterone is replaced in hypogonadal men there is an increase in sexual thoughts and sexual desire.[31–33] In men a male 'menopause', 'viropause', or 'andropause' occurs, similar to the menopause in women. It is characterized by a decrease in total as well as bioavailable testosterone, but without a concomitant increase in luteinizing hormone levels.[34–37] Schiavi et al[6] reported that bioavailable testosterone is related to sexual desire but not to coital frequency. The mechanism of action of androgens on sexual drive is yet to be determined in humans, but there are data from animal studies that indicate that the median preoptic hypothalamus area and associated limbic structures are involved in sexual behavior.[38]

Other agents that have been suggested by others to be involved in sexual desire and arousal in men are estrogen, prolactin, and endogenous opiate peptides.[39,40] Elevated prolactin levels can be associated with low sexual desire independently from androgen levels and probably act directly or via reduced central dopaminergic activity.

Psychologic problems can be attributed to sexual problems in both young and older adults. Psychologic conditions such as depression and psychosocial stresses (divorce, death of spouse, loss of social status, loss of job, health-related family problems) are prevalent in older adults and contribute to sexual problems.[40] Sexual dissatisfaction is also related with marital relationship problems, which vary from interpersonal problems and inadequate communication of sexual needs to poor sexual techniques. Other issues such as problems of commitment, power struggle, and lack of trust may all reflect dissatisfaction on the partner's behalf and may relate to sexual problems.[40–42] Older men may develop 'widower's syndrome', which is characterized by failure of erection after the death of a spouse.[43,44]

Evaluation of the decrease in sexual drive/libido

A thorough and careful history will help differentiate difficulty in erection from a decreased desire in sex or libido; early-morning erection can be seen in persons with both organic and psychogenic problems. A detailed history with the partner will help uncover some of the problems within a relationship. Risk factors for erectile dysfunction can also be assessed in the history, such as vascular disease, hormonal problems (thyroid, diabetes) neurologic dysfunction, medication, past surgery, or trauma; and psychologic and social factors, including evaluation for depression. A detailed examination of medication is important, since a number of medications are associated with decreased libido, as shown in Table 42.1. The standard depression assessment tools such as the Beck Depression Inventory or Yesavage Geriatric Scale can be used. Tools are also available to screen patients for androgen deficiency such as that developed by Saint Louis University, the Androgen Deficiency in Aging Males (ADAM) questionnaire (Table 42.2) A positive answer to question 1 or 7 or any other three questions is considered to have a high likelihood of having low testosterone. The ADAM questionnaire has a sensitivity of 88% and a specificity of 60%, validated in 310 Canadian physicians. There is clear improvement in the ADAM questionnaire results after treatment with testosterone.[45] The ADAM questionnaire also helps to identify patients with symptoms of depression and hypothyroidism. It is advisable to exclude both depression and hypothyroidism prior to initiating work-up for hypogonadism and erectile dysfunction.

Physical examination should include an assessment of secondary sexual characteristics along with a detailed examination for vascular and neurologic problems. Local penile shaft examination is also important to rule out Peyronie's disease.

The laboratory evaluation will help to look for the etiology of erectile dysfunction, such as tests for diabetes, renal function, lipid profile, thyroid function, prolactin levels, and penile brachial pressure index. The single most important test for a decrease in sexual drive or libido is to check bioavailable testosterone (non-sex-hormone-bound testosterone) if the calculated total testosterone level is between 300 and 500 ng/dl. The bioavailable testosterone level measured in the saliva of patients has recently been shown to correlate well with the bioavailable testosterone measured in plasma.

Most cross-sectional studies[35,46–49] have demonstrated that testosterone levels decease with age, although the Baltimore Longitudinal Aging Study

Table 42.1 *Drugs that may affect sexual desire in men*

Drugs that may increase sexual desire
Androgens (in androgen deficit states)
Baclofen (possible anti-anxiety effect)
Benzodiazepines (anti-anxiety effect)
Haloperidol (indirect effect due to improved sense of well-being)

Drugs that may decrease sexual desire
Antihistamines/barbiturates/benzodiazepines
Tricyclic antidepressants
Diuretics
   spironolactone
   hydrochlorothiazide
   acetazolamide
   methazolamide
Antihypertensives
   reserpine
   propranolol
   clonidine
   alpha-methyldopa
   prazosin
Cimetidine
Hormones
   estrogen
   medroxyprogesterone
Clofibrate
Digoxin
Lithium

Table 42.2 *Saint Louis University ADAMS questionnaire*

1. Do you have a decrease in libido (sex drive)?
2. Do you have a lack of energy?
3. Do you have a decrease in strength and/or endurance?
4. Have you lost height?
5. Have you noticed a decreased 'enjoyment of life'?
6. Are you sad and/or grumpy?
7. Are your erections less strong?
8. Have you noted a recent deterioration in your ability to play sports?
9. Are you falling asleep after dinner?
10. Has there been a recent deterioration in your work performance?

Adapted from Morley et al. Validation of a screening questionnaire for androgen deficiency of aging males. Metabolism 2000; 49: 1239–42.[45]

failed to find a decrease in testosterone in cross-sectional data.[50] Morley et al[51] demonstrated a fall in testosterone levels of 100 ng/dl per decade in a longitudinal study of older males in the New Mexico Aging Process Study. Just as free testosterone level declines with aging, a number of studies have reported a decline in bioavailable testosterone with aging.[35–37,52,53] Bioavailable and free testosterone decline earlier than the total testosterone with aging.[54] A decline in bioavailable testosterone is seen in 50% of men by 50 years of age.[36] Luteinizing hormone levels fail to increase appropriately in response to the decreasing testosterone levels with age, suggesting failure of hypothalamic–pituitary axis and hence secondary hypogonadism.[35,36,55,56]

Treatment of decreased sexual drive

The choice of treatment in men with a decrease in sexual drive or libido is guided by the possible cause and the treatment options available. If the history suggests any marital discord or psychiatric problems such as depression or anxiety, appropriate counseling should be provided or medical treatment should be offered for depression. This is discussed elsewhere in this section. If the decrease in sexual desire is related to medication use it should be stopped. If the problem is secondary to testosterone deficiency, then testosterone replacement therapy is indicated. A number of options are available for administration of testosterone.

Intramuscular injections
Intramuscular injections of testosterone enanthate or cypionate are the two available forms. Injection of either 100 mg or 200 mg can be given every 7 to 21 days, but in clinical practice it is usually given every 14 days. It is cheap compared to other preparations but is contraindicated in patients who are on warfarin therapy.

Transdermal preparations

Three transdermal preparations are available. Testoderm (Alza Pharmaceuticals, Palo Alto, CA) is a patch that is applied to the scrotum (with a prerequisite of shaving). The absorption is good, a normal physiologic level of circulating testosterone is achieved, and it is successfully used in older persons.[58,59] The initial dose of Testoderm is 6 mg/day, applied to the scrotal skin for 22 to 24 hours. Serum levels are determined after 3–4 weeks of daily application. If the desired levels are not achieved in 6–8 weeks of therapy another form of testosterone should be considered.

The second preparation is Androderm (SmithKline Beecham, Pittsburgh, PA), which is placed on any area of the skin except the scrotum and is associated with higher levels of allergic reactions.[60,61] It is applied for 24 hours. Clinical studies of transdermal systems demonstrate their efficacy in providing adequate testosterone replacement therapy.[62–64] Skin irritation may be associated with the use of transdermal systems; however, Testoderm and Testoderm TTS caused significantly less topical skin irritation than Androderm in two separate clinical studies.[65,66]

Testosterone is also available in a form of a gel called Androgel and Testim. It has the advantage of not being visible and maintains patient privacy.

Testosterone pellets

Testosterone pellets are a slow-release preparation, lasting for 3 months, implanted under the skin. The major disadvantage is difficulty in removing the pellets.

Oral preparations

Oral preparations are potentially toxic to the liver with the exception of testosterone undecanoate (Ondrol®), which is absorbed through the lymphatics. It can be used as an alternative to intramuscular injections for testosterone replacement therapy. Both modified and unmodified oral testosterone preparations are available. Unmodified testosterone is rapidly absorbed by the liver, making satisfactory serum concentrations difficult to achieve. Modified 17α-alkyltestosterones, such as methyltestosterone or fluoxymesterone, also require relatively large doses that must be taken several times a day. An intranasal spray of testosterone is in the process of development.

Monitoring patients on testosterone replacement

Patients on testosterone replacement therapy should be monitored to ensure that testosterone levels are within normal levels. Serum testosterone levels should be checked 3 to 12 hours after application of a transdermal delivery system. For patients on injectable testosterone, nadir testosterone levels should normally be obtained at three to four months prior to the next injection. Levels that exceed 500 ng/dL or are less than 200 ng/dL require adjustment of the dose or frequency. A digital rectal examination (DRE) and prostate specific antigen (PSA) test should be repeated at approximately 3 to 6 months, and then annually in men >40 years of age. An abnormal DRE, a confirmed increase in PSA >2 ng/ml, or a total PSA >4.0 ng/ml requires urologic evaluation that usually consists of transrectal ultrasonography and prostate biopsy. The hematocrit level should also be checked at 3 to 6 months, and then annually. A hematocrit >55% warrants evaluation for hypoxia and sleep apnea and/or a reduction in the dose of testosterone therapy.[67–69]

Polycythemia and testosterone replacement

Replacement of testosterone appears to stimulate erythropoiesis. A rise in hematocrit is generally beneficial in anemia; elevation above the normal range may have grave consequences, resulting in coronary or cerebrovascular accidents.[69–72] An increase in hemoglobin is associated with the route of testosterone replacement. Injections have been reported to increase the hematocrit by 44%, the transdermal non-scrotal patch to increase it by 15%,[73] and the scrotal patch to increase it by 5%.[74] Wang et al[75] reported a direct relationship between testosterone dosage and the incidence of erythrocytosis. Erythrocytosis was reported in 2.8% of men on 5 mg of non-scrotal patches, and in 11% using 50 mg/day and 18% using 100 mg/day gel, respectively.

Table 42.3 *Effects of testosterone replacement in older hypogonadal men*

- Increase in libido
- Increase in visual-spatial cognition
- Increased facial recognition
- Increased beard growth
- Gynecomastia
- Increased hematocrit
- Increase in muscle mass
- Increase in muscle strength
- Increase in protein synthesis
- Increase in bone mineral density
- Decrease in hip fracture
- Decrease in leptin (decrease in visceral fat)
- ? Decrease in atherosclerosis (minimal effects on lipids)
- ? Enhanced potency
- Worsening of metastatic prostate cancer

Benign prostatic hypertrophy

It is a well-established fact that androgens induce benign prostatic hypertrophy (BPH), and that it decreases with a decrease in serum testosterone. However, a number of studies have failed to show that testosterone replacement exacerbated urinary retention or the voiding symptoms of BPH compared to placebo.[73,76–81]

Prostate cancer and testosterone replacement

Case reports have suggested that testosterone replacement therapy may convert occult cancer into a clinically apparent lesion.[82,83] To date, prospective studies have demonstrated a low frequency of prostate cancer in association with testosterone replacement therapy. A compilation of published prospective trials of testosterone replacement therapy showed prostate cancer in 5 of 461 men (1.1%) followed for 6 to 36 months,[73,75,81] a prevalence rate very similar to that of the general population. There is some concern that the underlying prevalence of occult prostate cancer in men with low testosterone levels appears to be substantial.[84] Despite decades of research there is no compelling evidence that testosterone has a causative role in prostate cancer.[79,80,85–88] Other side-effects are outlined in Table 42.3.

References

1. Bachman GA. Sexual issues at menopause. Ann NY Acad Sci 1988; 87: 87–94, 123–33.
2. Kaiser FE. Sexuality and impotence in aging men. Clin Geriatr Med 1991; 7: 63–72.
3. Kellet JM. Sexuality in later life. Rev Clin Gerontol 1993; 3: 309–14.
4. Ludeman K. The sexuality of older persons: Review of the literature. Gerontology 1981; 21: 203–8.
5. Morley JE, Kaiser FE. Sexual function with advancing age. Med Clin North Am 1989; 73: 1483–5.
6. Schiavi RC, Schreiner-Engel P, Mandeli J. Healthy aging and male sexual function. Am J Psychiatry 1990; 147: 766–71.
7. Mulligan T, Katz G. Erectile failure in the aged: evaluation and treatment. J Am Geriatr Soc 1988; 36: 54–62.
8. Pfeifer E, Verwoerdt A, Wang HS. Sexual behavior in aged men and women. Arch Gen Psychiatry 1968; 19: 735–58.
9. Kinsey AC, Pomeroy WB, Martin CE. Sexual behavior in the human male. Philadelphia, PA: WB Saunders, 1953.
10. Marsiglio W, Donnelly D. Sexual relations in later life: a national study of married persons. J Gerontol 1991; 46: S338–44.
11. Catalan J, Hawton K, Day A. Couples referred to a sexual dysfunction clinic. Psychological and physical morbidity. Br J Psychiatry 1990; 156: 61–7.
12. Janus SS, Janus CL. The Janus report on Sexual Behavior. New York, John Wiley & Sons, 1993.
13. NIH consensus development panel on impotence. JAMA 1993; 270: 83–90.
14. Kinsey AC, Pomeroy WB, Martin CE. Sexual behavior in the human male. Philadelphia, PA: WB Saunders Co, 1948.
15. Dawson K. Serving the older gay community. SIECUS, Report, 5–6, November 1982.
16. Gwenwald M. The sage model for serving older lesbians and gay men. J Social WorkHum Sexuality 1984; 2(2/3): 53–61.
17. Quam JK, Whiteford GS. Adaptation and age-related expectations of older gay and lesbian adults. Gerontol 1992; 32: 367–74.
18. Slusher MP, Mayer CJ, Dunkle RE. Practice concepts: gay and lesbians older and wiser (GLOW): a support group for older gay people. Gerontology 1996; 36:1; 118–23.
19. Bell AP, Weinberg MA. Homosexuality: a study of diversity among men and women. New York: Simon and Schuster 1978.
20. Francher JS, Henkin J. The menopausal queen: adjustment to aging and the male homosexual. Am J Orthopsychiatry 1973; 43: 670–4.
21. John M, Moon T, Brannan W. The effect of age, ethnicity and geographic location on impotence and quality of life. Br J Urol 1995; 75: 651–5.

22. Masters WH, Johnson VE. Human sexual response. Boston, MA: Little, Brown, 1970.

23. Edward AE, Husted J. Penile sensitivity, age, and sexual behavior. J Clin Psychol 1976; 32: 697–700.

24. Kahn E, Fisher C. REM sleep and sexuality in the aged. J Geriatr Psychiatry 1969; 2: 181–99.

25. Karacan I, William RL, Thornby JI. Sleep related penile tumescence as a function of age. Am J Psychiatry 1975; 132: 932–7.

26. Schiavi RC, Schreiner-Engel P. Nocturnal penile tumescence in healthy aging men 1988; 43: M146–50.

27. Schiavi RC, White D. Androgen and male sexual function. A review of human studies. J Sex Marital Ther 1976; 3: 214.

28. Pardridge WM, Gorski RA, Lippe BM. Androgen and sexual behavior. Ann Intern Med 1982; 96: 488–501.

29. Verwoerdt A, Pfeiffer E, Wang HS. Sexual behavior in senescence. Patterns of sexual activity and interest. Geriatrics 1969; 24: 137–54.

30. Segraves RT. Hormone and libido. In: Leiblum SR, Rosen RC, eds. Sexual Desire Disorders. New York: Guildford Press, 1988: 271.

31. Davidson JM, Kwan M, Greenleaf WJ. Hormonal replacement and sexuality. Clin Endocrinol Metab 1982; 11: 599.

32. Kwan M, Greenleaf WJ, Mann J. The nature of androgen on men's sexuality: a combined laboratory/ self reported study on hypogonadal men. J Clin Endocrinol Metab 1983; 57: 557.

33. Skakkeoaek NE, Bancroft J, Davidson DW. Androgen replacement with oral testosterone undecanoate in hypogonadal men. A double blinded control study. Clin Endocrinol 1981; 14: 49.

34. Kaiser FE, Morley JE. Gonadotropin, testosterone, and the aging male. Neurobiol Aging 1994; 15: 559–63.

35. Kaiser FE, Viosca SP, Morley JE. Impotence and aging: clinical and hormonal factors. J Am Geriatr Soc 1988; 36: 511–19.

36. Korenman SG, Morley JE, Mooridian AD. Secondary hypogonadism in older men: its relationship to impotence. J Clin Endocrinol Metab 1990; 71: 963–9.

37. Tenover JS, Matsumoto AM, Plymate SR. The effect of aging in normal men on bioavailable testosterone and luteinizing hormone secretion: response to clomiphene citrate. J Clin Endocrinol Metab 1987; 65: 1118–26.

38. Everitt BJ, Bancroft J. Of rats and men: the comparative approach to male sexuality. Ann Rev Sex Res 1991; 2: 77.

39. Bancroft J. Endocrinology of sexual function. Clin Obstet Gynecol 1980; 7: 253.

40. Cole MJ. Psychological approach to treatment. Edinburgh, Churchill Livingstone, 1993.

41. Kaplan HS. The New Sexual Therapy. New York, Brunner/Mazel, 1974.

42. LoPiccolo J, Stock W. Treatment of sexual dysfunctions. J Consult Clin Psychol 1986; 54:158–67.

43. Dunn ME. Psychological perspectives of sex and aging. Am J Cardiol 1988; 61: 24–6H.

44. Morley JE, Korenman SG, Mooradian AD. UCLA geriatric rounds: sexual dysfunction in the elderly male. J Am Geriatr Soc 1987; 35: 1014–22.

45. Morley JE, Charlton E, Patrick P, Kaiser FE, Perry HM. Validation of a screening questionnaire for androgen deficiency in aging males. Metabolism 2000; 49: 1239–42.

46. Gray A, Feldman HA, McKinlay JB. Age, disease, and changing sex hormone levels in middle-aged men: results of Massachusetts Male Aging Study. J Clin Endocrinol Metab 1991; 73: 1066–1025.

47. Gray A, Berlin JA, McKinlay JB. An examination of research design effects on association of testosterone and male aging: results of meta-analysis. J Clin Epidemiol 1991; 44: 671–84.

48. Deslypere JP, Vermeulen A. Leydig cell function in normal men: effect of age, life style, residence, diet, and activity. J Clin Endocrinol Metab 1984; 59: 955–62.

49. Baker HW, Burger HG, De Kretser DM. Changes in the pituitary–testicular system with age. Clin Endocrinol (Oxf) 1976; 5: 349–72.

50. Harman SM, Tsitouras PD. Reproductive hormones in aging men. Measurement of sex steroids, basal luteinizing hormone and Leydig cell response to human chorionic gonadotropin. J Clin Endocrinol Metab 1980; 51: 35–40.

51. Morley JE, Kaiser FE. Longitudinal changes in testosterone luteinizing hormone and follicular stimulating hormone in healthy older males. Metabolism 1997; 46: 410–14.

52. Baker HW, Hudson B. Changes in the pituitary–testicular axis with age. Clin Endocrinol 1983; 25: 71–83.

53. Nakin HR, Calkins JH. Decreased bioavailable testosterone in aging normal and impotent men. J Clin Endocrinol Metab 1986; 63: 1418–20.

54. Nahoul K, Roger M. Age-related decline of plasma bioavailable testosterone in adult men. J Steroid Biochem 1990; 35: 293–9.

55. Vermeulen A, Deslypere JP, DeMeirleir K. A new look to the andropause: altered function of the gonadotrophs. J Steroid Biochem 1989; 32: 163–5.

56. Tennekoon KH, Karunanayake EH. Serum FSH, LH, and testosterone concentrations in presumably fertile men: effect of age. Int J Fertil 1993; 38: 108–12.

57. Kaufman JM, Deslypere JP, Giri M. Neuroendocrine regulation of pulsatile luteinizing hormone secretion in elderly men. J Steroid Biochem Mol Biol 1990; 37: 421–30.

58. Jankowsky JS, Oviatt SK, Orwoll ES. Testosterone influences spatial cognition in older men. Behav Neurosci 1994; 108: 325–32.

59. Orwall ES. Osteoporosis in men. Endocr Rev 1995; 16: 87–116.

60. Arver S, Dobs AS, Meikle AW. Improvement of sexual function in testosterone deficient men treated for 1 year with a permeation enhanced testosterone transdermal patch. J Urol 1996; 155: 1604–8.

61. Meikle SW, Arver S, Dobs AS. Pharmacokinetics and metabolism of a permeation enhanced testosterone transdermal system in hypogonadal men: influence of application site – a clinical research center study. J Clin Endocrinol Metabol 1996; 81: 1832–40.

62. Cofrancesco J, Dobs AS. Transdermal testosterone delivery systems. Endocrinol 1996; 6: 207.

63. Yu Z, Gupta SK, Hwang SS et al. Testosterone pharmacokinetics after application of an investigational transdermal system in hypogonadal men. J Clin Pharmacol 1997; 37: 1139.

64. Yu Z, Gupta SK, Hwang SS et al. Transdermal testosterone administration in hypogonadal men: comparison of pharmacokinetics at different sites of application and at the first and fifth days of application. J Clin Pharmacol 1997; 37: 1129.

65. Jordan W. Allergy and topical irritation associated with transdermal testosterone administration: a comparison of scrotal and nonscrotal transdermal systems. Am J Contact Derm 1997; 8(2): 103.

66. Jordan WP, Atkinson LE. Comparison of the skin irritation potential of two testosterone transdermal systems: an investigational system and a marketed product. Clin Ther 1998; 20(1): 80.

67. Tariq SH, Haren MT, Kim MJ, Morley JE. Andropause: Does the emperor have no clothes. Rev Endocr Metab Disord 2005; 6 (2): 77–84.

68. Morley JE, Tariq SH. Sexuality and disease. Clin Geriatr Med 2003; 19: 563–73.

69. Tariq SH, Haleem U, Omran ML et al. Erectile dysfunction: etiology and treatment in young and older patients. Clin Geriatr Med 2003; 19: 539–51.

70. Sih R, Morley JE. Testosterone replacement in older hypogonadal men: a 12 month randomized controlled trial. J Clin Endocrinol Metab 1997; 82: 1661–7.

71. Basaria S, Dobs AS. Risks versus benefits of testosterone therapy in elderly men. Drugs Aging 1999; 15: 131–42.

72. The Endocrine Society. Clinical bulletins in andropause: benefits and risks of treating hypogonadism in the aging male. Endocr Rep 2002; 2: 1–6.

73. Dobs AS, Meikle AW, Arver S et al. Pharmacokinetics, efficacy, and safety of a permeation-enhanced testosterone transdermal system in comparison with bi-weekly injections of testosterone enanthate for the treatment of hypogonadal men. J Clin Endocrinol Metab 1999; 84: 3469–78.

74. Leifke E, Gorenoi V, Wichers C. Age related changes in serum sex hormones, insulin-like growth factor and sex-hormone binding globulin levels in men; cross sectional data from a healthy male cohort. Clin Endocrinol 2000; 53: 689–95.

75. Wang C, Swerdloff RS, Iranmanesh A et al. Transdermal testosterone gel improves sexual function, mood, muscle strength, and body composition parameters in hypogonadal men. J Clin Endocrinol Metab 2000; 85: 2839–53.

76. Comhaire FH. Andropause: hormone replacement therapy in the aging male. Eur Urol 2000; 38: 655–62.

77. Krieg M, Nass R, Tunn S. Effect of aging on endogenous level of 5(alpha)-dihydrotestosterone, testosterone, estradiol, and estrone in epithelium and stroma of normal and hyperplastic human prostate. J Clin Endocrinol Metab 1993; 77: 375–81.

78. Pechersky AV, Mazurov VI, Semiglazov VF et al. Androgen administration in middle-aged and ageing men: effects of oral testosterone undecanoate on dihydrotestosterone, oestradiol and prostate volume. Int J Androl 2002; 25: 119–25.

79. Marcelli M, Cunningham GR. Hormonal signaling in prostatic hyperplasia and neoplasia. J Clin Endocrinol Metab 1999; 84: 3463–8.

80. Slater S, Oliver RTD. Testosterone: its role in development of prostate cancer and potential risk from use as hormone replacement therapy. Drugs Aging 2000; 17: 431–9.

81. Snyder PJ, Peachey H, Hannoush P et al. Effect of testosterone treatment on bone mineral density in men over 65 years of age. J Clin Endocrinol Metab 1999; 84: 1966–72.

82. Curran MJ, Bihrle W III. Dramatic rise in prostate-specific antigen after androgen replacement in a hypogonadal man with occult adenocarcinoma of the prostate. Urol 1999; 53: 423–4.

83. Loughlin KR, Richie JP. Prostate cancer after exogenous testosterone treatment for impotence. J Urol 1997; 157: 1845.

84. Morgentaler A, Bruning CO III, DeWolf WC. Occult prostate cancer in men with low serum testosterone levels. JAMA 1996; 276: 1904–6.

85. Carter HB, Pearson JD, Metter EJ et al. Longitudinal evaluation of serum androgen levels in men with and without prostate cancer. Prostate 1995; 27: 25–31.

86. Heikkila R, Aho K, Heliovaara M et al. Serum testosterone and sex hormone-binding globulin concentrations and the risk of prostate carcinoma: a longitudinal study. Cancer 1999; 86: 312–15.

87. Hsing AW. Hormones and prostate cancer: what's next? Epidemiol Rev 2001; 23: 42–58.

88. Kamel NS, Caracci JM, Tariq SH. Emerging treatment modalities for erectile dysfunction. In: Kohli K, Gupta M, Tejwani S, eds. Contemporary Perspectives on Clinical Pharmacotherpeutics, 1st edn. Elsevier. 2006; 38: 431–42.

CHAPTER 43

Depression

Margaret-Mary G Wilson

The agony they do not show,
the suffocating sense of woe …

Lord Byron (1788–1824)
Prometheus, Works: 1832

Introduction

The pervading trend of global consumerism threatens the positive concept of durability by emphasizing the hazards of antiquity. The perception of aging by modern society is affected by this trend. Western cultures propagate the impression that the aging process is merely the descent along a gradual slope that inevitably leads to death. Viewed in this manner, it is not surprising that depression is erroneously considered a natural reaction to the aging process. Available evidence indicates that this bias exists even among health-care professionals.[1] Such attitudes pose obstacles to the provision of adequate, well-coordinated care to a segment of the population at risk from a life-threatening disease.

In the USA one million people over the age of 65 years are diagnosed with major depression and 5 million others experience depressive symptoms. Annual health-care costs related to depression are estimated at 43 billion dollars. Within the next two decades these figures are expected to increase by more than 50%.[2–4] The prevalence of depression among community-dwelling older adults ranges from 1 to 3%, with depressive symptoms occuring in 8–16% of this population.[5,6] Although similar figures are reported for the younger segment of the community-dwelling population, older adults are more likely to commit suicide as a result of depression than younger adults.[7] Across the life cycle depression occurs in men at half the frequency with which it occurs in women. Similarly, older men are less likely than older women to be diagnosed with depression. However, following diagnosis the incidence of recurrent episodes is similar between the genders.[8] Gender differences have also been observed in the frequency of suicide, which is higher in men. This gender difference increases with age and peaks among the oldest old.[9] However, suicide attempts, the majority of which are unsuccessful, occur with greater frequency among women.[10] Older, white men commit suicide at a higher rate than any other cohort in society. However, the rate of suicide among African-American men is rising at a faster rate. Between 1980 and 1986, suicide rates among white men increased by 23% compared with an increase of 42% among African-American men.[9] Several explanations have been proffered for the gender and age-related variations in the frequency of suicide. Older men are more likely to use more violent methods of suicide, such as hanging and gunshots. The higher rates of substance abuse and the relatively lean social support systems of older men constitute additional risk factors for suicide in the depressed older man.[10,11]

The relatively high prevalence of depression in the institutionalized setting may be a reflection of the significant medical comorbidity associated with depression in the older adult.[12,13] Major depression

539

is diagnosed in approximately 30% of long-term care residents, with a similar frequency between the genders.[4,14] The older man is less likely than the older woman to report depressive symptoms or seek psychiatric help. However, available data indicate that depression is a marker for increased use of hospital services among older men. A similar relationship does not occur in older women.[9,15] These characteristics may jeopardize prompt clinical detection and treatment of depression in the older man, thereby increasing the risk of morbidity and mortality associated with this disease.

Pathophysiology

The pathophysiology of depression has not been fully elucidated. Even less well understood are the observed age and gender differences in the manifestations of depression. The role of neurotransmitters has been extensively explored. Current theories implicate a reduction in central nervous system serotoninergic activity. Decreased levels of 5-hydroxyindoleacetic acid (5-HIAA) have been identified in the cerebrospinal fluid (CSF) of depressed persons. Bryer and colleagues[16] measured the concentrations of CSF monoamine metabolites in patients with a recent cerebrovascular infarct. They found significantly lower concentrations of 5-HIAA in the subgroup of patients with depression compared with non-depressed patients. They also demonstrated a significant correlation between 5-HIAA levels and the distance of the infarct from the frontal lobe. Additional studies of post-stroke patients identified a correlation between depression and the anatomic location of the infarct. Review of these studies supports a lateralized effect, but restricts this correlation to the left hemisphere only.[17–19] More recent studies in support of these findings show that left anterior hemisphere lesions are significantly associated with a higher incidence of depression. However, this association was restricted to one month following the stroke, after which anatomic correlation to depressive symptoms can no longer be demonstrated.[20] Neurochemical imaging studies showed that among patients with left hemisphere strokes, 5-hydroxytryptamine receptor binding was significantly lower

in the left temporal cortex of depressed patients.[21] These studies lend credence to the occurrence of depression as a biochemical response to structural brain injury. The location of the injury and its consequent impact on the neuronal circuits may determine the extent of the mood disorder. Among older adults, 85% of persons with ischemic white matter changes on magnetic resonance imaging (MRI) suffered from depression. Depressed persons with leuko-encephalopathic changes identified on MRI also demonstrated greater apathy and manifested with fewer cognitive symptoms of depression. The increased frequency of these lesions in older men may be relevant to the age and gender differences observed in the clinical manifestations of depression.[22]

Functional imaging studies may ultimately provide a more unified theory regarding the pathogenesis of depression. Positron emission tomography (PET) studies have identified hypometabolic areas in caudate and frontal cortical regions in depressed persons.[23,24] These findings have proved consistent using both glucose metabolism and cerebral blood flow as physiologic variables. More recent studies using this modality have been able to correlate PET findings with disease activity, familial traits, and therapeutic response. Prefrontal and subgenual hypometabolism have been identified in groups of non-depressed persons with a history of familial depression.[25] Additionally, depressed persons with areas of caudate hypometabolism manifest with increased caudate metabolism following initiation of antidepressant therapy. The presence of anterior cingulate hypometabolism has been found by some workers to be a marker for a poor response to therapy.[24,26]

Earlier theories implicated dysregulation of the hypothalamic – pituitary – adrenal (HPA) axis as a central theory in the pathogenesis of depression. This was based on the observation that persons with hypercortisolism were found, in some studies, to have an increased incidence of depression.[27] Consequently, age-related dysregulation of the HPA axis was proffered as a possible explanation for depression in the elderly.[28] Definitive evidence in support of this theory is lacking. Furthermore it fails to provide an explanation for age- and gender-related differences in the manifestations of depression.

Neuroendocrine theories are favored as most logical in terms of defining gender differences in the manifestations of depression. Such theories appear to be validated by the occurrence of mood disturbances in association with the menopause and menstruation. However, the validity of biologic theories as the sole explanation for depression in the older adult is challenged by the persistence of gender differences despite the physiologic blunting of gonadal function that occurs with aging.[12] Based on current research, depression is most probably a syndrome that stems from a complex interplay of biologic and psychosocial factors.

Cognitive and behavioral theories remain attractive and offer a psychosocial basis for gender differences in the manifestations of late-life depression. With aging, deteriorating functional status and changing social roles may have a negative impact on the older man's self-image, self-esteem, and self-worth. As his adult offspring start their own families and spousal illness or bereavement occurs, the older man may place unrealistic expectations on himself if he fails to recognize that his role as primary provider is no longer critical to family cohesion. The inevitable redistribution of leadership roles within the family may be misconstrued by the aging man as a reflection of his inadequacy or failure, rather than the natural progression of social events. Consequently, the older man may develop a dislocation in his 'sense of belonging'. The latter is a recognized psychologic concept which has been shown to correlate with depression. A robust sense of belonging is nurtured by energy, motivation, and the perceived possession of shared group characteristics. Retirement, age-related reduction in physical activity, and consequent trimming of the older adult's social support mechanisms may have a negative impact on these vital 'sense of belonging' antecedents. A low 'sense of belonging' is significantly associated with an increased frequency of depression, and current data indicate that this may be a better predictor of depression than social isolation or lack of social support.[29,30] Behavioral and cognitive theorists also emphasize the role of age-related distorted thinking in the genesis of depression. Isolated events in which the individual's performance falls short of personal expectations are often regarded as measures of overall ability and a reflection of the person's social standing and value. The dynamic interplay of these psychosocial cognitive processes may transform into a permanent formalized thought scheme which forms the substrate for the interpretation of life events. Insignificant life events, when viewed within this substrate, may assume greater significance and precipitate or perpetuate depression.[12,31,32]

There is currently no convincing evidence to indicate that these theories are gender-specific. It is likely that the difference in social roles and thus perceived expectations may affect the magnitude of these changes. As social equality between genders becomes increasingly widespread, it is likely that gender differences may yield to individual variation and idiosyncratic differences. In support of this hypothesis is the lack of a demonstrable gender difference in the prevalence of depression among older African-Americans. Sociologists attribute this observation to the relatively even distribution of social roles relating to employment and child care among this generation of African-Americans.

Risk factors

Recognized risk factors for depression in the older adult include female sex, poverty, inadequate social support and divorce, separation, and single marital status. Adverse life events are also effective stressors and may precipitate or perpetuate depression in the older adult.[33] The association of significant comorbidity, cognitive dysfunction, and functional impairment with late-onset depression has been confirmed in several studies which show that depressed older adults are more likely to have a higher burden of physical illness than non-depressed persons.[34,35] Additionally, severity of medical illness has been shown to correlate with an increased risk of depression.[36,37] A wide variety of medical illnesses are associated with depression (Table 43.1).[33] The adverse effects of chronic disease on functional status provide a plausible explanation for depressive symptoms in such cases. Conversely, alternative theories suggest that depression may have an immunosuppressive effect, thereby increasing vulnerability to certain illnesses.

Table 43.1 *Some medical illnesses associated with depression*

Endocrine/metabolic
Thyroid disease
Cushing's disease
Hypoadrenalism
Diabetes mellitus
Porphyria
Hyperparathyroidism

Central nervous system
Dementia
Parkinson's disease
Cerebrovascular disease
Intracranial neoplasms
Multiple sclerosis
Complex partial seizures

Cardiopulmonary disease
Congestive cardiac failure
Chronic obstructive pulmonary disease
Pulmonary fibrosis
Coronary artery disease
Fibromgalgia

Connective tissue disease
Systemic lupus erythematosus
Rheumatoid arthritis
Temporal arteritis

Miscellaneous
Chronic pain syndromes
Chronic hepatitis
AIDS
Cancer

In older adults a positive association has been identified between the extent of cortical and subcortical atropy, number of cortical infarcts, pituitary volume, and the risk of depression. Older adults with an increased ventricular–brain ratio are also more likely to be depressed.[38] Similar neuroanatomic correlates have not been identified in younger adults. Additional risk factors for depression include advancing age, low educational achievement, co-existing psychiatric illness, and alcohol abuse.[37] The actual mechanism whereby comorbidity increases the risk of depression is unclear. However, favored theories include the possible adverse effects of such illnesses on psychosocial

well-being and self-esteem. The structure of available social support systems may be altered by the perception of a real or imagined increase in the burden of illness.[39–41] It is conceivable that the older adult's perception of self within a redefined social network may be adversely affected by such changes.

Available evidence indicates that genetics may be a less significant factor in the pathogenesis of depression in the older adult. Relatives of patients who develop late-life major depression have a lower risk of developing depression compared with relatives of depressed middle-aged adults. Additionally, current data do not support genetic theories as a plausible explanation for gender differences in the incidence of late-life depression.[42,43] Previous hypotheses suggested that depression may be transmitted in an X-linked dominant fashion, thus accounting for the higher incidence of depression in women. Related theories suggested that depression and alcoholism may be clinical expressions of the same gene with manifestations determined by gender. This would account for the increased incidence of alcoholism in the male offspring of depressed persons, while the female offspring demonstrated an increased incidence of depression.[44] To date, objective substantiation of these genetic theories is lacking.

Clinical features

The diagnostic criteria for depression are well defined (Table 43.2). However, self-reporting of depressive symptoms occurs infrequently among older adults. This may be attributed to the perceived stigma of the disease by the elderly. The intrinsic negativism peculiar to the disease is an additional obstacle to self-reported symptomatology. Consequently, depressive illness in the older adult may be shrouded in a mesh of somatic complaints which often defy physical diagnosis despite elaborate investigations. The attribution of such symptoms to a psychologic cause is often fiercely resisted by the patient. Data exist to show that patients who manifest with somatic symptoms are often much less likely to admit to a depressed mood.[45,46] Clinical suspicion of depression should be heightened when dealing with the older adult who expresses inappropriate pessimism with regard to

Table 43.2 *Summary of DSM IV criteria for the diagnosis of major depression*

A. At least five of the following symptoms over a 2-week period; at least one of the symptoms is either depressed mood or anhedonia:

- Depressed mood
- Anhedonia
- Unexplained weight loss or weight gain
- Insomnia or hypersomnia
- Psychomotor agitation or retardation
- Fatigue
- Persistent feelings of guilt or worthlessness
- Poor concentration
- Recurrent thoughts of death or suicidal ideation

B. Symptoms result in significant distress or impairment in social functioning

C. Symptoms are not due to the direct physiologic effect of any substance or underlying general medical condition

D. Symptoms can not be accounted for by bereavement

their physical illness or functional status. Older adults who experience apparent satisfaction with remaining in the sick role and display helplessness inconsistent with their physical status should be screened carefully for depression. Such persons usually display behavior counterproductive to the defined therapeutic management plan.[47,48] Noncompliance and poor personal hygiene and self-care should also prompt evaluation for depressive symptoms. Generalized anxiety, irritability, and preoccupation with memory and cognitive function may also serve as diagnostic clues to late-life depression. Anxiety, apprehension, or panic attacks may be accompanied by physical correlates of inappropriate tachycardia, tremors, lightheadedness, or dizziness. These result from inappropriate activation of the autonomic nervous system.[49]

Evidence indicates that late-life depression associated with cerebrovascular disease is more likely to present with cognitive impairment, an association that does not occur in younger adults. Proponents of the 'vascular depression' hypothesis postulate that cerebral ischemic disease may cause late-onset depression. Cerebral atherosclerosis, which is a recognized cause of progressive cognitive decline with aging, may provide a common pathophysiologic pathway for these two syndromes.[33,38] However, a clear distinction needs to be made between cognitive dysfunction associated with 'vascular depression' and 'pseudodementia'. The latter syndrome refers to the cognitive impairment which is a direct outcome of the patient's depressed mood. Pseudodementia frequently resolves with effective antidepressant therapy. Additionally, patients with pseudodementia often display a characteristic reluctance to undergo any form of cognitive evaluation, despite the fact that they retain good insight into their illness. Poverty of facial expression and bradykinesia, hallmarks of Parkinson's disease, are recognized features of depression and may confound the early diagnosis of depression in older adults. The recognition of depression may be further thwarted by the co-existence of depression in 30% of persons with dementia and Parkinson's disease.[50]

Weight loss in the older adult is a prime index of underlying depression. Available data indicate that depression may be the underlying cause of weight loss and low body weight in one third of older adults with weight problems.[51] Sleep disturbances are another common manifestation of depression in the elderly. The depressed older adult often complains of difficulty in falling asleep at night or frequent awakenings.[49] The peculiarities inherent in the presentation of late-life depression justify the use of the term 'masked depression' in describing this syndrome.[52] Evidence indicates that older adults who present with masked depression exhibit a greater degree of functional impairment and significantly increasing morbidity.[53] Health professionals must be cognizant of the myriad symptoms which may indicate depression, as early detection, particularly in the older man, is crucial (Table 43.3). Older depressed men have fewer severe melancholic symptoms. Nevertheless, approximately half of these patients will admit to some form of suicidal ideation. Five percent of older men with depression have active suicidal ideation with a definite plan or a history of attempted suicide.[37] Older men who may be depressed must be directly questioned regarding active and passive suicidal ideation.

Table 43.3 *Atypical features of depression in the older adult*

Anorexia
Weight loss
Bradykinesia
Memory dysfunction
Irritability
Dizzyness
Anxiety
Paranoid delusions
Multiple unexplained somatic complaints
Increased physical and social dependence
Non-compliance with therapeutic regimens
Poor personal hygiene

The presentation of depression varies with the clinical setting. Hospitalized medically ill patients are less likely to present with delusions and suicidal ideation. However, anhedonia, anxiety, helplessness, and pessimism may predominate in this patient population.[37] The intuitive expectation of differences in the prevalence of depression between cultures and ethnic groups cannot be supported by objective data. Several studies failed to find any significant difference in the prevalence of depression between Caucasian and African-American older adults. However, presenting symptoms may differ between ethnic groups. Older African-Americans are more likely to present with paranoid features, psychomotor disturbance, and appetite dysregulation. Older Caucasian Americans report an increased frequency of sleep disturbance, feelings of guilt, and suicidal ideation.[54]

The diverse manifestations of depression place the diagnostic burden almost exclusively on the discerning health professional. The physician should be sensitive to counter-transference of feelings of helplessness. These may invoke an unjustifiable empathic response thereby resulting in acceptance of the patient's despair as an appropriate response to the perceived physical or psychosocial burden. Depression in the older adult is a persistent and chronic disorder even when it occurs in the setting of an obviously stressful life event. Thus, substituting protracted clinical observation for aggressive intervention merely constitutes harmful paternalistic inactivity in the management of a potentially deadly disease.

Diagnosis

Studies indicate that depression frequently remains undetected in the older adult. In one study non-psychiatric house staff recognized clinical depression in less than 10% of depressed hospitalized older adults.[55] Recognition rates within the community-dwelling population range from 19 to 94%, emphasizing the wide variability in the ability of physicians to recognize depression.[56] Evidence indicates that most older adults opt to receive antidepressant therapy from their primary care physician, rather than to undergo formal evaluation and management by a psychiatrist. Thus, 75% of older depressed adults present initially to their primary care physician.[3] However, 75% of depressed older persons who commit suicide have visited a primary care physician in the preceding month, yet eluded diagnosis and treatment.[13,57] Older men are less likely than women to report a depressed mood and more reluctant to attribute dysphoric symptoms to stressful life events.[12] These attributes increase the risk of undertreatment in this cohort of patients.

Clinical diagnosis of depression based on judgement and subjective interpretation of the patient's medical history is unreliable and ineffective in prompting intervention. Studies indicate that health professionals are more likely to intervene if a positive score is identified on a screening instrument.[58] Routine screening is therefore recommended and highly desirable in the development of an effective therapeutic approach toward combating depression. Several self-rating and examiner-rating scales are available (Table 43.4).[59–64] Self-rating scales should not be used in persons with impaired cognitive function. The Cornell scale, which utilizes care-givers as surrogate reporters of depressive symptoms, has been well validated as an effective screening tool for depression in persons with dementia.[63] The Geriatric Depression Scale (GDS) is frequently used in clinical geriatric evaluation. This tool should be reserved for persons with minimal impairment of cognitive function. In persons with a Folstein's

Table 43.4 *Depression scales*

Self-rating scales

- Geriatric Depression Scale[59]
- Zung Scale[60]
- Center for Epidemiological Studies Depression Scale[61]

Examiner-rating scales

- Hamilton Depression Rating Scale[62]
- Cornell Scale for Depression in Dementia[63]
- Comprehensive Psychopathological Rating Scale[64]

Mini-mental score above 15, the GDS has a sensitivity of 84% and a specificity of 91%. Evidence indicates that despite the relative paucity of somatic items on the GDS questionnaire, co-existent medical illness may confound accurate interpretation of the results.[36] Few rating scales have been standardized for use in the acutely ill older adult. However, the GDS is less affected by acute hospitalization and the clinical course of disease compared with other rating scales, such as the Hamilton Depression Rating Scale (HDRS).

Increasing age, psychomotor retardation, somatization, and severity of illness compromise the predictive value of rating scales.[65,66] The effects of these multiple confounding factors on the diagnosis of depression are minimized if rating scales are used solely for screening and initial evaluation. Rating scales should not be utilized as a substitute for formal psychiatric evaluation. Health professionals should also be wary of using the rating score to refute the diagnosis of depression in cases where clinical suspicion of depression is substantial.

Management

Antidepressant therapeutic options include psychosocial and biologic modalities. The latter comprise pharmacologic and biologic treatments. Therapeutic outcome measures, as these relate to remission and relapses, should be defined for each patient, prior to initiating therapy.

Pharmacotherapy

Treatment with antidepressant therapy should be initiated in the older man with severe depression. Selective serotonin reuptake inhibitors (SSRIs) have emerged as the drugs of first choice in the management of depression. These agents are comparable in efficacy to tricyclic antidepressants (TCAs), but have a more favorable side-effect profile. Several classes of antidepressants are available which may be suitable for use in the older man (Table 43.5). However, the choice of antidepressant should be individualized with due consideration given to the side-effect profile. Monotherapy is preferred and treatment should be initiated using the lowest beneficial dose. Physicians should be aware that older adults may not exhibit significant improvement for 6–12 weeks after initiation of therapy. Thus, objective evaluation of clinical response should be deferred for a corresponding period.[67] Drug compliance must be closely monitored, as 70% of patients take less than 50% of their medication.[41] Patients who fail to respond to initial therapy with adequate doses of one antidepressant should be switched to another antidepressant of a different class. Referral to a psychiatrist should be considered if the patient fails to respond to or tolerate two different antidepressants, or if suicidal ideation is suspected.

The risk of recurrence of depression increases from 50% after the first episode of major depression to 90% after the third recurrent episode. Thus, older men who exhibit a satisfactory response to pharmacotherapy should be continued on full-dose maintenance therapy for 6–9 months after remission from a first episode. Following recurrent episodes maintenance therapy should be continued for at least one year. This strategy has been shown to reduce the risk of a relapse by 80%.[2] When the decision is made to discontinue an antidepressant, gradual tapering of the dose is recommended to reduce the risk of withdrawal symptoms. These often include anxiety, headache, myalgia, and flu-like symptoms.[68] However, older men with an initial onset of depression very late in life have a risk of relapse which equals that of men with recurrent episodes of depression. In these groups of patients it may be prudent to continue life-long full-dose maintenance therapy.[69]

Table 43.5 *Pharmacotherapy in older men: comparison of selected medications*

Drug	Advantages	Disadvantages
Tricyclic antidepressants Desipramine Nortriptyline Protriptyline Amoxapine	Inexpensive Once-daily dosing	Anticholinergic side-effects Multiple drug interactions Delirium Cardiotoxic
Selective serotonin reuptake inhibitors Sertraline Paroxetine Fluoxetine Citalopram	Safer in overdosage Once daily dosing	Sexual dysfunction Nausea Seizures Headache Cytochrome P450 interactions
Serotonin antagonist reuptake inhibitors Trazodone Nefazodone	Few drug interactions Once daily dosing	Sexual dysfunction Priapism Possible cardiotoxicity
Serotonin–norepinephrine reuptake inhibitors Venlafaxine	Favorable side-effect profile	Hypertension Sexual dysfunction Hyperlipidemia Multiple daily dosing
Mirtazapine	Appetite stimulant	Sexual dysfunction Blood dyscrasias Dependence potential
Dopamine reuptake inhibitors Bupropion	Safer in overdose Minimal cardiotoxicity	Seizures

Electroconvulsive therapy

Evidence indicates that electroconvulsive therapy (ECT) is underused in the management of depression.[33] However, this therapeutic modality is utilized more often in the treatment of older men than in their younger counterparts. This is attributed to the reluctance of older men to undergo pharmacotherapy for depression.[12] ECT is a safe and effective form of antidepressant therapy; studies show a 75–80% efficacy rate in the treatment of medically ill, depressed older adults. Specific indications for the use of ECT include refractory, psychotic, or life-threatening depression.[70–72] Cardiovascular and neuropsychiatric complications occur most often, although serious complications are infrequent (Table 43.6). ECT causes death in 2–4 persons/100 000 treatments.[73] As ECT may be lifesaving in certain situations, there are no absolute contraindications to this procedure. However, the American Psychiatry Association (APA) task force considers certain conditions to be indicators of increased risk (Table 43.7).[74]

Table 43.6 *Complications of ECT therapy in older men*

Cardiovascular
Cardiac arrhythmias
Hypertension
Cardiac ischemia
Hypoxia

Neurologic

Amnesia–retrograde and antegrade
Headache
Delirium
Gait instability

Table 43.7 *Conditions associated with an increase in the morbidity of ECT*

Elevated intracranial pressure
Severe cardiovascular disease
Severe pulmonary disease
Recent cerebral hemorrhage/infarction
Unstable cerebral vascular malformation
Anesthetic risk (ASA class IV)

ASA, American Society of Anesthesiologists.

With the rising cost of medication ECT is becoming increasingly cost-effective. Older adults frequently undergo ECT as an outpatient procedure, eliminating the cost of acute hospitalization which was associated with its utilization in the past. Maintenance ECT is recommended for patients who respond satisfactorily to the index treatment. Available studies indicate a significant reduction in rehospitalization and relapse rates in patients receiving maintenance ECT compared with patients on maintenance pharmacotherapy.[75]

Psychotherapy

Therapeutic intervention with a combination of pharmacotherapy and psychotherapy is the most effective strategy for the treatment of moderate to severe depression in older men. Interpersonal therapy facilitates effective role transition and allows for the definition of realistic expectations. Exploration of the quality of interpersonal relationships and social interaction is also enhanced by this form of therapy. Cognitive therapy is an alternative psychotherapeutic model. Theoretically, this model allows for conceptualization of the psychologic reasoning of the depressed adult. Areas of conflict are identified and resolution strategies are developed that may facilitate effective treatment.[32,76,77]

Conclusions

Depression is the commonest psychiatric disorder in the older adult. Effective intervention is frequently compromised by delayed diagnosis and inadequate treatment. These factors constitute major obstacles to positive outcomes in the management of depression. Health professionals must develop comprehensive treatment strategies to combat depression in older adults. Ideally, these should include efficient screening methods, appropriate psychologic intervention, and prompt pharmacotherapy where indicated. The aggressive institution of such strategies tailored to the individual patient is a pivotal weapon in battling this deadly disease.

References

1. Callahan CM, Dittus RS, Tierney WM. Primary care physicians' medical decision making for late-life depression. J Gen Intern Med 1996; 11: 218–25.
2. Hirschfield RM, Keller MB, Panico S et al. The National Depressive and Manic-Depressive Association consensus statement on the undertreatment of depression. JAMA 1997; 277: 333–40.
3. Boswell EB, Stoudemire A. Major depression in the primary care setting. Am J Med 1996;101(6A):3–9S.
4. Reynolds CF. Depression: making the diagnosis and using SSRIs in the older patient. Geriatrics 1996; 51(10): 28–34.
5. Blazer D, Hughes DC, George LK. The epidemiology of depression in an elderly community population. Gerontologist 1987; 27: 281–7.
6. Weissman MM, Leaf PJ, Tischler GL et al. Affective disorders in five United States communities. Psychol Med 1988; 18: 141–53.
7. Dorpet T, Ripley H. A study of suicide in the Seattle area. Compr Psychiatry 1960; 1: 349–59.
8. Kessler RC, McGonagle KA, Swartz M et al. Sex and depression in the national co-morbidity survey: 1.

Lifetime prevalence, chronicity and recurrence. J Affect Disord 1993; 29: 85–96.

9. Meechan P, Salsman L, Satin R. Suicide among older United States residents: epidemiological characteristics and trends. Am J Public Health 1991; 81: 1198–200.

10. Blazer DG, Bachar JR, Manton KG. Suicide in later life. J Am Geriatr Soc 1986; 34: 519–25.

11. Adamek M, Kaplan M. Firearm suicide among older men. Psychiatr Serv 1996; 47: 304–6.

12. Blazer D. Depression and the older man. Med Clin North Am 1999; 83(5): 1305–16.

13. Ganzini L, Smith DM, Fenn DS et al. Depression and mortality in medically ill older adults. J Am Geriatr Soc 1997; 45(3): 307–12.

14. Parmelee PA, Katz IR, Lawton MP. Depression among institutionalized aged: assessment and prevalence estimation. J Gerontol 1989; 44: M22–9.

15. Huang B. Depression and Use of Health Services in the Elderly. Master of Public Health thesis, University of North Carolina, Chapel Hill, 1998.

16. Bryer JB, Starkstein SE, Votypka V et al. Reduction of CSF monoamine metabolites in post-stroke depression. J Neuropsychiatry Clin Neurosci 1992; 55: 377–82.

17. Morris PLP, Robinson RG, Carvalho ML et al. Lesion characteristics and depressed mood in the stroke data bank study. J Neuropsychiatry Clin Neurosci 1996; 8: 153–9.

18. Herrmann M, Bartles C, Wallesch C-W. Depression in acute and chronic aphasia: symptoms, pathoanatomical–clinical correlations and functional implications. J Neurol Neurosurg Psychiatry 1993; 56: 672–8.

19. Astrom M, Adolfsson R, Asplund K. Major depression in stroke patients: a 3-year longitudinal study. Stroke 1993; 24: 976–82.

20. Shimoda K, Robinson RG. The relationship between post-stroke depression and lesion location in long-term follow-up. Biol Psychiatry 1999; 45: 187–92.

21. Mayberg HS, Robinson RG, Wong DF et al. PET imaging of cortical S_2-serotonin receptors after stroke: lateralized changes and relationship to depression. Am J Psychiatry 1988; 145: 937–43.

22. Krishnan KR, Hays JC, Blazer DG. MRI-defined vascular depression. Am J Psychiatry 1997; 154: 519–22.

23. Drevets WC, Videen TO, Price JL et al. A functional anatomic study of unipolar depression. J Neurosci 1992; 12: 3628–41.

24. Martinot JL, Hardy P, Feline A et al. Left prefrontal glucose hypometabolism in the depressed state: a confirmation. Am J Psychiatry 1990; 147: 1313–17.

25. Drevets WC, Price JL, Simpson JR et al. Subgenual prefrontal cortex abnormalities in mood disorders. Nature 1997; 386: 824–7.

26. Mayberg HS, Brannan SK, Mahurin RK et al. Cingulate function in depression. Neuroreport 1997; 8: 1056–61.

27. McEwen BS. Protective and damaging effects of stress mediators. N Engl J Med 1998; 338: 171–9.

28. Veith R, Raskin M. The neurobiology of aging: does it predispose to depression? Neurobiol Aging 1988; 9: 101–17.

29. Hagerty BMK, Williams RA, Coyne JC, Early MR. Sense of belonging and indicators of social and psychological functioning. Arch Psychiatr Nursing 1996; 10(4): 235–44.

30. Hagerty BM, Williams RA. The effects of sense of belonging, conflict, and loneliness on depression. Nurs Res 1999; 48(4): 215–19.

31. Vezina J, Bourque P. The relationship between cognitive structure and symptoms of depression in the elderly. Cogn Ther Res 1984; 8: 29–36.

32. Blazer D. Depression in Late Life, 2nd edn. St Louis, MO: Mosby, 1993.

33. National Institutes of Health Consensus Development Panel on Depression in Late-life. Diagnosis and treatment of depression in late life. JAMA 1992; 268: 1018–24.

34. Jones BN, Reifler BV. Depression co-existing with dementia: evaluation and treatment. Med Clin North Am 1994; 78(4): 823–40.

35. Koenig HG, Meador KG, Cohen HJ et al. Depression in hospitalized patients with medical illness. Arch Intern Med 1988; 148: 1929–36.

36. Koenig HG, Meador KG, Cohen HJ et al. Screening for depression in hospitalized elderly medical patients: taking a closer look. J Am Geriatr Soc 1992; 40: 1013–17.

37. Koenig HG, Meador KG, Shelp F et al. Major depressive disorder in hospitalized medically ill patients: an examination of young and elderly male veterans. J Am Geriatr Soc 1991; 39: 881–90.

38. Leuchter AF. Brain structural and functional correlates of late life depression. Presented at the National Consensus Conference on the diagnosis and treatment of depression in late life, National Institutes of Health, Bethesda, MD: 1991.

39. Murphy E. Social origins of depression in old age. Br J Psychiatry 1982; 141: 135–42.

40. Rodin G. Depression in the medically ill: an overview. Am J Psychiatry 1986; 143: 696–705.

41. Beck DA, Koenig HG, Beck JS. Depression. Clin Geriatr Med 1998; 14(4): 765–83.

42. Rice J, McGuffin P. Genetic etiology of schizophrenia and affective disorders. In: Michels R, ed. Psychiatry. Philadelphia, PA: JB Lippincott, 1990.

43. Slater EVC. The Genetics of Mental Disorders. London: Oxford University Press, 1971.

44. Winokur G, Clayton P. Family history studies: II. Sex differences and alcoholism in primary affective illness. Br J Psychiatry 1967; 113: 973–9.

45. Bridges K, Goldberg D, Evans B, Sharpe T. Determinants of somatization in primary care. Psychol Med 1991; 21: 473–83.

46. Ban T. Chronic disease and depression in the geriatric population. J Clin Psychiatry 1984; 45: 18–23.

47. Fava GA, Zielezny M, Pilowsky I et al. Patterns of depression and illness behavior in general hospital patients. Psychopathology 1984; 17: 105–9.

48. Simon RI. Silent suicide in the elderly. Bull Am Acad Psychiatry Law 1989; 17: 83–95.

49. Gareri P, Falconi U, De Fazio P, De Sarro G. Conventional and new anti-depressants in the elderly. Prog Neurobiol 2000; 61: 353–96.

50. Starkstein SE, Petracca G, Chemerinski E et al. Depression in classic versus akinetic-rigid Parkinson's disease. Movement Dis 1998; 13(1): 29–33.

51. Wilson MMG, Vaswani S, Liu D et al. Prevalence and causes of undernutrition in medical outpatients. Am J Med 1998; 104: 56–63.

52. Reugg RG, Zissok S, Swerdlow NR. Depression in the aged: an overview. Psychiatr Clin North Am 1988; 11: 83–99.

53. Broadhead WE, Blazer DG, George LK et al. Depression, disability days, and days lost from work in a prospective epidemiologic survey. JAMA 1990; 264: 2524–8.

54. Blazer DG, Landerman LR, Hays JC et al. Symptoms of depression among community-dwelling elderly African-Americans and White older adults. Psychol Med 1998; 28: 1311–20.

55. Rapp SR, Walsh DA, Parisi SA et al. Detecting depression in elderly medical inpatients. J Consult Clin Psychol 1988; 56: 509–13.

56. Callahan CM, Dittus RS, Tierney WM. Primary care physicians' decision making for late life depression. J Gen Intern Med 1996; 11(4): 218–25.

57. Centers for Disease Control and Prevention. Suicide among older persons: United States, 1980–1992. Morbidity and Mortality Weekly Review 1996; 45(1): 3–6.

58. German PS, Shapiro S, Skinner EA et al. Detection and management of mental health problems of elderly patients by primary care providers. JAMA 1987; 257: 489–93.

59. Yesavage JA, Brink TL, Rose TL et al. Development and validation of a geriatric depression screening scale: a preliminary report. J Psychiatr Res 1983; 17: 37–49.

60. Zung WWK. A self-rating depression scale. Arch Gen Psychiatry 1965; 12: 63–70.

61. Radloff LS. The CES-D scale: a self-report depression scale for research in the general population. J Appl Psychol Measures 1977; 1: 385–401.

62. Hamilton M. A self-rating scale for depression. J Neurol Neurosurg Psychiatry 1960; 23: 56–62.

63. Alexopolous GS, Abrams RC, Young RC, Shamoian CA. Cornell scale for depression in dementia. Biol Psychiatr 1988; 23: 271–84.

64. Asberg M, Montgomery SA, Perris C et al. A comprehensive psychopathological rating scale. Acta Psychiatr Scand (Suppl) 1978; 271: 5–27.

65. Kurlowicz LH. Depression in hospitalized medically ill elders: evolution of the concept. Arch Psychiatr Nurs 1994; 8: 124–36.

66. Kitchell MA, Barnes RF, Veith RC et al. Screening for depression in hospitalized geriatric medical patients. J Am Geriatr Soc 1982; 30: 174–7.

67. Georgotas A, McCue R. The additional benefit of extending an antidepressant trial past seven weeks in the depressed elderly. Int J Geriatr Psychiatry 1989; 4: 191–5.

68. Sussman N, Stahl S. Update in the pharmacotherapy of depression. Am J Med 1996; 101(6A): 26–36S.

69. Alexopoulos GS. Affective disorders. In Sadavoy J, Lazarus LW, Jarvik LF et al, eds. Comprehensive Review of Geriatric Psychiatry – II. Washington, DC: American Psychiatric Association Press, 1996.

70. Rifkin A. ECT versus tricyclic antidepressants in depression: a review of the evidence. J Clin Psychiatry 1988; 49: 3–7.

71. Burke WJ, Rubin EH, Zorumski CF et al. The safety of ECT in geriatric practice. J Am Geriatr Soc 1987; 35: 516–21.

72. Williams JH, O'Brien JT, Cullum S. Time course of response to electroconvulsive therapy in elderly depressed subjects. Int J Geriatr Psychiatry 1997; 12: 563–66.

73. Abrams R. The mortality rate with ECT. Convuls Ther 1997; 13: 125–7.

74. American Psychiatric Association. The Practice of Electroconvulsive Therapy: Recommendations for Treatment, Training and Privileging. Washington DC: APA Press, 1990.

75. McDonald WM, Phillips VL, Figiel GS et al. Cost effective maintenance treatment of resistant geriatric depression. Psychiatr Ann 1998; 28: 47–52.

76. Reynolds CF III, Frank E, Perel JM et al. High relapse rate after discontinuation of adjunctive medication for elderly patients with recurrent major depression. Am J Psychiatry 1996; 153: 1418–22.

77. Sholomskas A, Chevron E, Prusoff B et al. Short-term interpersonal therapy with the depressed elderly: case reports and discussions. Am J Psychother 1983; 37: 552–65.

CHAPTER 44

Testosterone, depression, and cognitive function

John E Morley

For it is the semen, when possessed of vitality which makes us to be men, hot, well-braced in limbs, well voiced, spirited, strong to think and act

Aretaeus, *The Cappadocian*, AD 150

What is, therefore, the cause that castrates slow down in their whole vitality?

Galen, *Peri Spermatas*

Introduction

The above citations from ancient times suggest that testosterone plays a role in behavior. Despite these early anecdotes, with the exception of studies on libido, there are few well-controlled studies examining the effect of testosterone on behavior. This is in contrast to the relatively large literature on estrogen in women, linking it to cognitive behaviors and perhaps to playing a role in Alzheimer's disease.[1,2] While testosterone has been strongly associated with the mythologic concept of the aggressive male, studies examining the effects of testosterone on behavior have yielded mixed results. Schaal et al[3] found that high testosterone levels were more likely to be a marker of social success than to be associated with physical aggression. On the other hand, in free-ranging adolescent male non-human primates, cerebrospinal fluid levels of testosterone were associated with overall aggressiveness but not impulsivity.[4] Administration of moderately high doses of testosterone for contraception has failed to reveal adverse effects on male sexual and aggressive behavior.[5] In a controlled trial supraphysiologic doses of testosterone failed to increase angry behavior in healthy eugonadal males.[6] In males rendered hypogonadal with a GNRH antagonist there was not only a decrease in sexual desire and fantasies, but also a trend to increased aggression.[7] In contrast, using a similar approach, Loosen et al[8] found a reduction in outward-directed anger and no change in inward-directed behavior in hypogonadal males. Burris et al[9] found that hypogonadal men were more angry than eugonadal men and that this anger decreased with testosterone therapy. A 48XXYY hypogonadal male had a reduction in long-standing aggressive fantasies and behaviors towards women.[10]

The reason for the inability to find convincing effects of testosterone on aggressive behavior in males is multifactorial. Most studies have utilized total testosterone rather than free or bioavailable testosterone. The effect of testosterone is small, perhaps in the neighborhood of 1%, which would require sample sizes of around 1000 males to demonstrate a clearly significant effect. The reported studies have been much smaller than this. Aggressive behaviors tend to cause a decrease in testosterone either directly within the central nervous system or secondary to increases in cortisol. For example, salivary testosterone levels decreased 15 minutes after watching a stressful movie on dental surgery;[11] high psychologically stressed males had lower testosterone levels than their low-stress counterparts;[12] and male internal medicine residents have markedly decreased testosterone levels.[13] It is possible that there is an optimal level of testosterone related to appropriate aggressive behaviors and higher or lower levels may create a U-shaped dose–response curve. Finally, in measuring aggression, the environment and the lifetime learning experience will result in greatly modified responses to any given hormone level.

The rest of this chapter will summarize the meager data available on the effects of testosterone on general behavior, depression, and memory in the middle-aged and older male.

Testosterone and behavior in the older male: an overview

A syndrome of male 'menopause' was first reported in the 1940s (Table 44.1).[14] In 1979, Greenblatt et al,[15] based on a large clinical experience, suggested that testosterone replacement in the male 'climacteric' improved fatigue, depression, headaches, and libido. More recently we reported a screening questionnaire for androgen deficiency in aging males that included a number of psychologic symptoms (Table 44.2).[18] We used low bioavailable testosterone as our 'gold standard'. The questionnaire was developed in 316 Canadian physicians aged 40 to 82 years of age. The questionnaire had acceptable reproducibility. The Androgen Deficiency in Aging Males (ADAM) questionnaire had an 88% sensitivity and a 60% specificity. Persons with dysphoria were the most likely to produce false positives on the questionnaire. When males with a positive ADAM were treated improvement was seen in 18/21 patients.

Wu et al[17] analyzed the male andropause in males over 50 years of age (Table 44.1). They found that a number of psychologic symptoms similar to those in the ADAM questionnaire were related to the andropause. These included decreased libido (91%), lack of energy (89%), erection problems (79%), falling asleep after dinner (77%), memory impairment (77%), sad or grumpy mood changes (68%), decreased endurance (66%), and deterioration in work performance (51%).

The Massachusetts Male Aging Study examined psychologic factors associated with androgen levels in 1709 males aged 39 to 70 years.[20] They found that males with a high 'availability of androgens' were more likely to display a dominant profile with some associated aggressive behavior. They went on to characterize a testosterone deficiency pattern that included 'low dominance'[19] (Table 44.1).

Overall these studies suggest that the fall in testosterone that occurs in older men is associated with a syndrome of behavioral changes in addition to the physical effects of decreased strength, decreased bone mineral density, increased adiposity, and decreased hematocrit. The characteristics of the behavioral syndrome of the andropause are decreased enthusiasm for sex, lack of energy, dysphoria, decreased cognition, fatigue, decreased work and sports performance, falling asleep after dinner and low dominance. Besides the ability of testosterone to reverse the effects on libido, its effects on the rest of this complex of symptoms remain to be proven.

Dysphoria and depression

Approximately 70% of men receiving testosterone have an enhanced sense of well-being. Women are more than twice as likely to have major depression compared to men. Based on these two factors, it seems likely that testosterone may play a role in mood disorders.

Epidemiologic studies have reported varying relationships between testosterone and dysphoria. Barrett-Connor et al,[21] in a study of 856 men aged 50 to 89 years, found a significant inverse relationship between the Beck Depression Inventory and bioavailable testosterone as well as dihydrotestosterone. Seidman et al[22] reported that depression as measured by the Center for Epidemiologic Studies Depression Scale was more common in men with shorter androgen receptor cytosine, adenine, guanine (CAG) repeat length and low testosterone, but this relationship was not seen in men with moderate or shorter CAG repeat length. T'Sjoen et al[23] could not find a relationship between CAG repeat length or free testosterone and depression in a group of men aged 70 years and older. Delhez et al,[24] in a group of

Table 44.1 Attempts to characterize an andropause syndrome which includes behavioral factors

Author:	Werner[14]	Greenblatt et al[15]	Heinemann et al[16]	Wu et al[17]	Morley et al[18]	Smith et al[19]
Source:	JAMA	JAGS	Aging Male	Chang-Keng	Metabolism	Clin Endocrinol
Year:	1946	1979	1999	2000	2000	2000
Behavioral factors:	Nervousness	Decreased libido	Decreased general well-being	Decreased libido	Decreased libido	Low dominance
	Decreased libido	Fatigue	Joint pain	Lack of energy	Lack of energy	Headaches
	Decreased potency	Depression	Muscular aches	Erection problems	Decreased strength/endurance	Sleeplessness
	Irritability	Headaches	Fatigue	Falling asleep after dinner	Loss of height	Excessive sweating
	Depression		Sleep problems	Memory impairment	Decreased enjoyment of life	
	Memory problems		Tiredness	Sad or grumpy	Sad or grumpy	
	Sleep disturbances		Irritability	Decreased work performance	Decreased work performance	
	Numbness and tingling		Nervousness	Decreased endurance		
	Hot flashes		Anxiety	Loss of pubic hair		
			Physical exhaustion	Loss of axillary hair		
			Decreased muscular strength	Decreased ability to play sports		
			Depressive mood	Decreased strength of erections		
			Feeling past your peak	Falling asleep after dinner		
			Feeling burnt out			
			Decrease in beard growth			
			Decreased ability to perform sexually			
			Decreased libido			
			Decrease morning erections			

Table 44.2 *The Androgen Deficiency in Aging Male (ADAM) questionnaire: a positive answer represents 'yes' to 1 or 7 or any three other questions*

(Circle one)

Yes	No	1.	Do you have a decrease in libido (sex drive)?
Yes	No	2.	Do you have a lack of energy?
Yes	No	3.	Do you have a decrease in strength and/or endurance?
Yes	No	4.	Have you lost height?
Yes	No	5.	Have you noticed a decreased enjoyment of life?
Yes	No	6.	Are you sad and/or grumpy?
Yes	No	7.	Are your erections less strong?
Yes	No	8.	Have you noticed a recent deterioration in your ability to play sports?
Yes	No	9.	Are you falling asleep after dinner?
Yes	No	10.	Has there been a recent deterioration in your work performance?

men aged 50 to 70 years, found a negative correlation between severity of depression as assessed by the Carroll Rating Scale and free testosterone levels. Morley et al[25] could not show a relationship between dysphoria and bioavailable testosterone.

Schweiger et al,[26] utilizing frequent sampling over a 24-hour period in 15 male depressed patients and 24 control subjects, found the depressed subjects to have lower daytime, night-time, and 24-hour mean testosterone secretion. Luteinizing hormone (LH) pulse frequency tended to be decreased in the depressed males.

Booth et al[27] examined the interaction of social behavior and dysphoria in 4393 men. In males with a below average testosterone level there was an inverse relationship between testosterone and dysphoria, whereas, in those with above average testosterone levels, testosterone was directly related to dysphoria. This supports a parabolic model for the relationship of testosterone to dysphoria. In men with higher testosterone levels, the relationship is no longer maintained when antisocial and risk-taking behavior as well as protective factors such as marriage and steady employment are taken into account.

Kaneda and Fujii[28] could find no association between total testosterone and depression. Given the complexities of the factors involved in the pathogenesis of depression, it is perhaps not surprising that a clear relationship between androgens and depression has not emerged in epidemiologic studies.

In a small study of 11 men, Kenny et al[29] found no effect of intramuscular testosterone (200 mg every 3 weeks) on the Geriatric Depression Scale. This is similar to the failure of Sih et al,[30] who used 200 mg of testosterone every 2 weeks to find an effect on dysphoria. Cavallini et al[31] studied 120 patients, of whom one-third were randomized to receive oral testosterone undecanoate 160 mg daily. The mean age of the men was 66 years with a range of 60 to 74 years. Testosterone improved the scores on both the Depression Melancholia Scale Score and Fatigue Scale Score. Haren et al,[32] using low doses of oral testosterone, also found similar positive effects.

Grinspoon et al,[33] in a large study of HIV-infected males, found a higher Beck Depression Inventory score in the hypogonadal compared to eugonadal males. Testosterone therapy resulted in a significant decrease in the Beck Depression Score. There was a strong relationship between decreased dysphoria and weight gain. Seidman and Rabkin[34] added testosterone to the treatment regimen of five men who had failed SSRI treatment for depression. Testosterone augmentation produced a rapid improvement in depressive symptoms.

Overall, the available data support the concept that depression is a stress state that results in a decline in testosterone levels. Whether or not testosterone replacement improves depressive symptoms will require large controlled trials. Preliminary and anecdotal data suggest that testosterone may be a useful adjuvant therapy for depression.[35]

Cognition

In rodents androgens have major effect on brain structure and function. The effects of testosterone in enhancing memory retention in mice appear to involve both its aromatization to estrogen and an effect of dehydrotestosterone. The SAMP8 mouse is a spontaneous animal model of Alzheimer disease.[36] These mice develop early acquisition and retention deficits that are related to overproduction of β-amyloid.[37] SAMP8 mice also develop low testosterone; replacement results in a reversal of the acquisition and memory deficits.[38] This reversal is associated with a rapid reduction in amyloid precursor protein levels in the limbic system.

While it is recognized that human males and females display different learning abilities for different tasks, a clear relationship between testosterone and memory has been elusive to demonstrate. This is most probably because the relationship between cognitive performance and testosterone is nonlinear. In general, testosterone in younger men has been related to spatial but not verbal cognitive tasks.[39,40]

Carlson and Sherwin[41] suggested that higher estradiol levels in older males may protect against the declines in explicit memory associated with normal aging. Morley et al[42] reported that across the lifespan bioavailable testosterone was the steroid hormone that best predicted a variety of cognitive performance tests.

Aleman et al[43] found that testosterone was associated with a composite measure of fluid intelligence performance, but not with crystallized intelligence, nor verbal long-term memory in 25 elderly men with a mean age of 69 years. In another study of 79 men (aged 61 to 72 years) higher total testosterone levels were associated with speed of information processing and high estradiol levels with spatial span performance.[44] In the Massachusetts Male Aging Study log free testosterone was associated with better functioning, but this was not found in their adjusted model.[45] Muller et al[46] assessed

cognitive function in 400 independently living men aged 40 to 80 years. They found that lower bioavailable testosterone was related to lower scores on processing capacity/speed and executive function. The relationship tended to be curvilinear. Moffat et al[47] examined the correlations between free testosterone index and a variety of memory tests in participants in the Baltimore Longitudinal Study of Aging aged 59 to 91 years of age. Men who were hypogonadal had lower scores on memory and visuospatial performance and a greater rate of decline in visual memory over 10 years.

A decline in serum testosterone in men (mean age 65 years) receiving androgen deprivation therapy was reported to lead to visuomotor slowing, slowed reaction times, and impaired delayed recall and recognition speed of letters.[48] Some of these findings appear to be more associated with estradiol than testosterone decline.[49] Beer et al[50] found that immediate and delayed verbal memory were significantly worse in patients with prostate cancer on androgen deprivation therapy than in age-matched healthy controls. Estradiol replacement improved verbal memory performance. Almeida et al[51] followed 40 men with prostate cancer who received androgen blockade therapy for 36 weeks, followed by discontinuation for 18 weeks. The Cambridge Cognitive Assessment – Revised (CAMCOG) and word list scores improved significantly after withdrawal of androgen blockade. Visuospatial scores were not affected. The changes in word list scores were associated with a decrease in serum amyloid-beta levels.

Janowsky et al[52] studied a relatively large group of healthy elderly men who received testosterone in a double-blind trial for 3 months. They found an improvement in spatial cognition, but no effect on verbal and visual memory, motor speed, cognitive flexibility, or mood. Sih et al,[30] using a battery of cognitive tests which did not include a spatial task, found no effect of testosterone replacement on memory in older men who were treated for a year. In another study, Janowsky et al[53] found that testosterone enhanced working memory as measured by the Subject Ordered Pointing Test in older men. Wolf et al[54] found that a single injection of testosterone blocked the practice effect in verbal fluency, but had no effect on spatial or verbal memory.

Cherrier et al[55] treated 25 healthy men aged 50 to 80 years with 100 mg testosterone weekly for 6 weeks in a randomized, double-blind, placebo-controlled trial. Testosterone improved spatial memory (recall of a walking pathway), spatial ability (block construction), and verbal memory (recall of short story). Others have failed to show improved block construction.[56] In another study, Cherrier et al found improvement of spatial memory in hypogonadal men receiving either testosterone or dehydrotestosterone.[57] They then examined the effect of blocking the conversion of testosterone to estradiol using an aromatase inhibitor, viz anastrozole.[58] Spatial memory was improved significantly with both testosterone treatment and in the persons where aromatization to estrogen was blocked. Verbal memory, however, was only improved in the group in which the aromatase inhibitor was not given. Azad et al[59] showed that testosterone enhanced cerebral perfusion in hypogonodal men in the midbrain and superior frontal gyrus (Brodman area 8).

A number of studies have examined the association between testosterone and dementia. Gillett et al[60] found that lower calculated free testosterone levels were associated with increasing levels of amyloid beta peptide 40. Hogervorst et al[61] compared 83 persons with dementia of the Alzheimer's type (DAT) with 103 cognitively normal older persons. Men with DAT had lower levels of serum testosterone compared to controls. In another study they found the effect of testosterone was more pronounced in persons with the APOE epsilon 4 genome.[62] In mice there is evidence that APOE4 is associated with lower cytosolic androgen receptors in the neocortex and that androgen treatment improves memory in these mice.[63] Persons with younger onset DAT appear to have predominantly secondary hypogonadism,[64] while LH levels are elevated in older DAT patients.[65] Paoletti et al[66] found a lower free androgen index in lean subjects with DAT compared to lean controls without DAT. Low free testosterone levels have been demonstrated to be an independent risk factor for DAT.[65,67] One small study failed to show the correlation of low testosterone with DAT.[68]

Testosterone increases the non-amyloidogenic amyloid precursor protein fragment derived from alpha secretase activity while reducing the secretion of amyloidogenic beta-amyloid peptides from neuronal cultures.[69] This effect is mediated by aromatization of testosterone to estrogen and activation of the mitogen-activated protein kinase signaling pathway.[70] Non-aromatizable testosterone protects neurons against apoptosis.[71,72] Testosterone increases heat shock protein 70 to inhibit Abeta 1–42 induced cell death.[73] Testosterone also prevents the hyperphosphorylation of tau by inhibiting the heat shock-induced overactivation of the glycogen kinase-3 beta pathway.[74]

Three studies have shown that testosterone can improve cognition in older patients with Alzheimer's disease. Tan and Pu[75] found improvement in Alzheimer's Disease Assessment Scale – Cognition (ADASCog), Mini-Mental status examination, and clock drawing in DAT patients treated for one year with intramuscular testosterone (200 mg every 2 weeks). Cherrier et al[76] reported improvements in spatial and verbal memory as well as constructional abilities in men with DAT and/or mild cognitive impairment receiving 100 mg of testosterone every week intramuscularly. Lu et al[77] reported improvements in the scores for the caregiver version of the quality of life scale in patients with DAT receiving testosterone. It is important to recognize that all three studies were very small and these results, while exciting, must be viewed as preliminary. A single study showed that aggressive behavior in a 78-year-old male with DAT was successfully treated by lowering testosterone activity with a synthetic gonadotropin-releasing hormone analog.[78]

While cross-sectional data in older men suggest an effect of testosterone on cognition, the results of testosterone replacement tests have not been conclusive. In many cases it would appear that there is an optimal level of testosterone for enhancing cognition and that higher and lower levels are less effective. Testosterone may improve spatial and working memory in older persons. There are interesting data emerging on the effects of testosterone on cognition in persons with Alzheimer's disease.

Conclusions

Overall, the effects of testosterone on behavior, while significant, are relatively small. Testosterone appears to have effects on mood, dominance, sleep, and cognition. Further studies are necessary to determine whether there exists an optimal range of testosterone to produce behavioral effects or whether supraphysiologic and physiologic levels of testosterone are equally effective.

References

1. Almeida OP. Sex playing with the mind. Effects of oestrogen and testosterone on mood and cognition. Arquivos de Neuro-Psiquiatria 1999; 57: 701–6.
2. LeBlanc ES, Janowsky J, Chan BKS, Nelson HD. Hormone replacement therapy and cognition – systematic review and meta-analysis. JAMA 2001; 285: 1489–99.
3. Schaal B, Tremblay RE, Soussignan R, Susman EJ. Male testosterone linked to high social dominance but low physical aggression in early adolescence. J Am Acad Child Adolesc Psychiatr 1996; 35: 1322–30.
4. Higley JD, Mehlman PT, Poland RE et al. CSF testosterone and 5-HIAA correlate with different types of aggressive behaviors. Biol Psychiatr 1996; 40: 1067–82.
5. Bahrke MS, Yesalis CE IV, Wright JE. Psychological and behavioural effects of endogenous testosterone and anabolic-androgenic steroids. An update. Sports Med 1996; 22: 367–90.
6. Tricker R, Casaburi R, Storer TW et al. The effects of supraphysiological doses of testosterone on angry behavior in healthy eugonadal men – a clinical research center study. J Clin Endocrinol Metab 1996; 81: 3754–8.
7. Bagatell CJ, Heiman JR, Rivier JE, Bremner WJ. Effects of endogenous testosterone and estradiol on sexual behavior in normal young men. J Clin Endocrinol Metab 1994; 78: 711–16.
8. Loosen PT, Purdon Se, Pavlou SN. Effects on behavior of modulation of gonadal function in men with gonadotropin-releasing hormone antagonists. Am J Psychiatr 1994; 151: 271–3.
9. Burris AS, Banks SM, Carter CS, Davidson JM, Sherins RJ. A long-term, prospective study of the physiologic and behavioral effects of hormone replacement in untreated hypogonadal men. J Andrology 1992; 13: 297–304.
10. Sourial N, Fenton F. Testosterone treatment of an XXYY male presenting with aggression: a case report. Can J Psychiatry 1988; 33: 846–50.
11. Hellhammer DH, Hubert W, Schurmeyer T. Changes in saliva testosterone after psychological stimulation in men. Psychoneuroendocrinology 1985; 10: 77–81.
12. Francis KT. The relationship between high and low trait psychological stress, serum testosterone, and serum cortisol. Experientia 1981; 37: 1296–7.
13. Singer F, Zumoff B. Subnormal serum testosterone levels in male internal medicine residents. Steroids 1992; 57: 86–9.
14. Werner AA. Male climacteric: report of 273 cases. JAMA 1946; 132: 188–94.
15. Greenblatt RB, Nexhat C, Roesel RA, Natrajan PK. Update on the male and female climateric. J Am Geriatr Soc 1979; 27: 481–90.
16. Heineman AJ, Zimmermann T, Vermeulen A, Thiel C. A new aging male's symptoms (AMS) rating scale. Aging Male 1999; 2: 105–14.
17. Wu Cy, Yu TJ, Chen MJ. Age related testosterone level changes and male andropause syndrome. Chang-Ken I Hsueh Tsa Chih 2000; 23: 348–53.
18. Morley JE, Charlton E, Patrick P et al. Validation of a screening questionnaire for androgen deficiency in aging males. Metabolism Clin Exp 2000; 49: 1239–42.
19. Smith KW, Feldman HA, McKinlay JB. Construction and field validation of a self-administered screener for testosterone deficiency (hypogonadism) in ageing men. Clin Endocrinol 2000; 53: 703–11.
20. Gray A, Jackson DN, McKinlay JB. The relation between dominance, anger, and hormones in normally aging men: results from the Massachusetts Male Aging Study. Psychosom Med 1991; 53: 375–85.
21. Barrett-Connor E, Von Muhlen DG, Kritz-Silverstein D. Bioavailable testosterone and depressed mood in older men: the Rancho Bernardo Study. J Clin Endocrinol Metab 1999; 84: 573–7.
22. Seidman SN, Araujo AB, Roose SP, McKinlay JB. Testosterone level, androgen receptor polymorphism, and depressive symptoms in middle-aged men. Biol Psychiatr 2001; 50: 371–6.
23. T'Sjoen GG, De Vos S, Goemaere S et al. Sex steroid level, androgen receptor polymorphism and depressive symptoms in healthy elderly men. J Am Geriatr Soc 2005; 53: 636–42.
24. Delhez M, Hansenne M, Legros JJ. Andropause and psychopathology: minor symptoms rather than pathological ones. Psychoneuroendocrinology 2003; 28: 863–74.
25. Morley
26. Schweiger U, Deuschle M, Weber B et al. Testosterone, gonadotropin, and cortisol secretion in male patients with major depression. Psychosom Med 1999; 61: 292–6.
27. Booth A, Johnson DR, Granger DA. Testosterone and men's depression: The role of social behavior. J Health Soc Behav 1999; 40: 130–40.

28. Kaneda Y, Fujii A. No relationship between testosterone and depressive symptoms in aging men. Eur Psychiatr 2002; 17: 411–13.

29. Kenny Am, Fabregas G, Song C, Biskup B, Bellantonio S. Effects of testosterone on behavior, depression, and cognitive function in older men with mild cognitive loss. J Gerontol Med Sci 2004; 59A: 75–8.

30. Sih R, Morley JE, Kaiser FE et al. Testosterone replacement in older hypogonadal men: a 12-month randomized controlled trial. J Clin Endocrinol Metab 1997; 82: 1661–7.

31. Cavallini G, Caracciolo S, Vitali G, Biagiotti G. Carnitine versus androgen administration in the treatment of sexual dysfunction, depressed mood, and fatigue associated with male aging. Urology 2004; 63: 641–6.

32. Haren MT, Wittert GA, Chapman IM, Coates P, Morley JE. Effect of oral testosterone undecanoate on visuospatial cognition, mood and quality of life in elderly men with low-normal gonadal status. Maturitas 2005; 50: 124–33.

33. Grinspoon S, Corcoran C, Stanley T et al. Effects of hypogonadism and testosterone administration on depression indices in HIV-infected men. J Clin Endocrinol Metab 2000; 85: 60–5.

34. Seidman SN, Rabkin JG. Testosterone replacement therapy for hypogonadal men with SSRI-refractory depression. J Affect Disord 1998; 49: 157–61.

35. Seidman SN, Walsh BT. Testosterone and depression in aging men. Am J Geriatr Psychiatr 1999; 7: 18–33.

36. Flood JF, Morley JE. Learning and memory in the SAMP8 mouse. Neurosci Biobehav Rev 1998; 22: 1–20.

37. Morley JE, Kumar VB, Bernardo AE et al. Beta-amyloid precursor polypeptide in SAMP8 mice affects learning and memory. Peptides 2000; 21: 1761–7.

38. Flood JF, Farr SA, Kaiser FE, Laregina M, Morley JE. Age-related decrease of plasma testosterone in SAMP8 mice – replacement improves age-related impairment of learning and memory. Physiol Behav 1995; 57: 669–73.

39. Neave N, Menaged M, Weightman DR. Sex differences in cognition: the role of testosterone and sexual orientation. Brain Cogn 1999; 41: 245–62.

40. Moffat SD, Hampson E. A curvilinear relationship between testosterone and spatial cognition in humans: possible influence of hand preference. Psychoneuroendocrinology 1996; 21: 323–37.

41. Carlson LE, Sherwin BB. Higher levels of plasma estradiol and testosterone in healthy elderly men compared with age-matched women may protect aspects of explicit memory. Menopause 2000; 7: 168–77.

42. Morley JE, Kaiser F, Raum WJ et al. Potentially predictive and manipulable blood serum correlates of aging in the healthy human male – progressive decreases in bioavailable testosterone, dehydroepiandrosterone sulfate, and the ratio of insulin-like growth factor 1 to growth hormone. Proc Natl Acad Sci USA 1997; 94: 7537–42.

43. Aleman A, de Vries WR, Koppeschaar HP et al. Relationship between circulating levels of sex hormones and insulin-like growth factor-1 and fluid intelligence in older men. Exp Aging Res 2001; 27: 283–91.

44. Hogervorst E, De Jager C, Budge M, Smith AD. Serum levels of estradiol and testosterone and performance in different cognitive domains in healthy elderly men and women. Psychoneuroendocrinology 2004; 29: 405–21.

45. Fonda SJ, Bertrand R, O'Donnell A, Longcope C, McKinlay JB. Age, hormones, and cognitive functioning among middle-aged and elderly men: cross-sectional evidence from the Massachusetts Male Aging Study. J Gerontol Med Sci 2005; 60: 385–90.

46. Muller M, Aleman A, Grobbee DE, De Haan EH, Van der Schouw YT. Endogenous sex hormone levels and cognitive function in aging men: is there an optimal level? Neurology 2005; 64: 866–71.

47. Moffat SD, Zonderman AB, Metter EJ, Blackman MR, Harman SM, Resnick SM. Longitudinal assessment of serum free testosterone concentration predicts memory performance and cognitive status in elderly men. J Clin Endocrinol Metab 2002; 87: 5001–7.

48. Salminen EK, Portin RI, Koskinen A, Helenius H, Nurmi M. Associations between serum testosterone fall and cognitive function in prostate cancer patients. Clin Cancer Res 2004; 10: 7575–82.

49. Salminen EK, Portin RI, Koskinen AI, Helenius HY, Nurmi MJ. Estradiol and cognition during androgen deprivation in men with prostate carcinoma. Cancer 2005; 103: 1381–7.

50. Beer TM, Bland LB, Bussiere JR et al. Testosterone loss and estradiol administration modify memory in men. J Urology 2006; 175: 130–5.

51. Almeida OP, Waterreus A, Spry N, Flicker L, Martins RN. One year follow-up study of the association between chemical castration, sex hormones, beta-amyloid, memory and depression in men. Psychoneuroendocrinology 2004; 29: 1071–81.

52. Janowsky JS, Oviatt SK, Orwoll ES. Testosterone influences spatial cognition in older men. Behav Neurosci 1994; 108: 325–32.

53. Janowsky JS, Chavez B, Orwoll E. Sex steroids modify working memory. J Cogn Neurosci 2000; 12: 407–14.

54. Wolf OT, Preut R, Hellhammer DH et al. Testosterone and cognition in elderly men: a single testosterone injection blocks the practice effect in verbal fluency, but has no effect on spatial or verbal memory. Biol Psychiatr 2000; 47: 650–4.

55. Cherrier MM, Asthana S, Plymate S et al. Testosterone supplementation improves spatial and verbal memory in healthy older men. Neurology 2001; 57: 80–8.

56.

57. Cherrier MM, Craft S, Matsumoto AH. Cognitive changes associated with supplementation of testosterone

or dihydrotestosterone in mildly hypogonadal men: a preliminary report. J Andrology 2003; 24: 568–76.

58. Cherrier MM, Matsumoto Am, Amory JK et al. The role of aromatization in testosterone supplementation: effects on cognition in older men. Neurology 2005; 64: 290–6.

59. Azad N. Pitale S, Barnes WE, Freidman H. Testosterone treatment enhances regional brain perfusion in hypogonadal men. J Clin Endocrinol Metab 2003; 88: 3064–8.

60. Gillett MJ, Martins RN, Clarnette RM et al. Relationship between testosterone, sex hormone binding globulin and plasma amyloid beta peptide 40 in older men with subjective memory loss or dementia. J Alzheimer's Dis 2003; 5: 267–9.

61. Hogervorst E, Williams J, Budge M et al. Serum total testosterone is lower in men with Alzheimer's disease. Neuroendocrinol Lett 2001; 22: 163–8.

62. Hogervorst E, Lehmann DJ, Warden DR, McBroom J, Smith AD. Apolipoprotein E epsilon4 and testosterone interact in the risk of Alzheimer's disease in men. Int J Geriatr Psychiatr 2002; 17: 938–40.

63. Raber J, Bongers G, LeFevour A, Buttini M, Mucke L. Androgens protect against apolipoprotein E4-induced cognitive deficits. J Neurosci 2002; 22: 5204–9.

64. Hogervorst E, Combrinck M, Smith AD. Testosterone and gonadotropin levels in men with dementia. Neuroendocrinol Lett 2003; 24: 203–8.

65. Hogervorst E, Bandelow S, Combrinck M, Smith AD. Low free testosterone is an independent risk factor for Alzheimer's disease. Exp Gerontol 2004; 39: 1633–9.

66. Paoletti AM, Congia S, Lello S et al. Low androgenization index in elderly women and elderly men with Alzheimer's disease. Neurology 2004; 62: 301–3.

67. Okun MS, DeLong MR, Hanfelt J, Gearing M, Levy A. Plasma testosterone levels in Alzheimer and Parkinson diseases. Neurology 2004; 62: 411–13.

68. Pennanen C, Laakso MP, Kivipelto M, Ramberg J, Soininen H. Serum testosterone levels in males with Alzheimer's disease. J Neuroendocrinology 2004; 16: 95–8.

69. Gouras GK, Xu H, Gross RS et al. Testosterone reduces neuronal secretion of Alzheimer's beta-amyloid peptides. Proc Natl Acad Sci USA 2000; 97: 1202–5.

70. Goodenough S, Engert S, Behl C. Testosterone stimulates rapid secretory amyloid precursor protein release from rat hypothalamic cells via the activation of the mitogen-activated protein kinase pathway. Neurosci Lett 2000; 296: 49–52.

71. Hammond J, Le Q, Goodyer C et al. Testosterone-mediated neuroprotection through the androgen receptor in human primary neurons. J Neurochem 2001; 77: 1319–26.

72. Pike CJ. Testosterone attenuates beta-amyloid toxicity in cultured hippocampal neurons. Brain Res 2001; 919: 160–5.

73. Zhang Y, Chapagne N, Beitel LK et al. Estrogen and androgen protection of human neurons against intracellular amyloid beta 1–42 toxicity through heat shock protein. J Neurosci 2004; 24: 5315–21.

74. Papasozomenos SC, Shanavas A. Testosterone prevents the heat shock-induced overactivation of glycogen synthase kinase-3 beta but not of cyclin-dependent kinase 5 and c-Jun NH2-terminal kinase and concomitantly abolishes hyperphosphorylation of tau: implications for Alzheimer's disease. Proc Natl Acad Sci USA 2002; 99: 1140–5.

75. Tan RS, Pu SJ. A pilot study on the effects of testosterone in hypogonadal aging male patients with Alzheimer's disease. Aging Male 2003; 6: 13–17.

76. Cherrier MM, Matsumoto AM, Amory JK et al. Testosterone improves spatial memory in men with Alzheimer disease and mild cognitive impairment. Neurology 2005; 64: 2063–8.

77. Lu PH, Masterman DA, Mulnard R et al. Effects of testosterone on cognition and mood in male patients with mild Alzheimer disease and healthy elderly men. Arch Neurol 2006; 63: 177–85.

78. Rosin RA, Raskind MA. Gonadotrophin-releasing hormone agonist treatment of aggression in Alzheimer's disease: a case report. Int Psychogeriatr 2005; 17: 313–18.

CHAPTER 45

Modern antidepressants

Margaret-Mary G Wilson

He who is of calm and happy nature will hardly feel the pressure of age . . .

Plato, (428BC–348BC)
The Republic

Introduction

Late-life depression is a major contender in the battle to achieve successful aging. Epidemiologic studies estimate the prevalence of major depression at 2–7% in community-dwelling older adults.[1,2] Additionally, 15–30% of community-dwelling older adults report depressive symptoms or a notably depressed mood. Among older adults in the acute care setting, the prevalence of major depression ranges from 30 to 45%. Within the nursing home setting, major depression occurs in 15–25% of residents.[3] Available data indicate a significant increase in morbidity, functional disability, and mortality associated with depression, especially in the frail older adult.[4–6] Efficient screening and early clinical recognition are critical to improving the prognosis of adults with late-life depression. However, the prompt initiation of the correct therapeutic strategy maximizes the potential for complete recovery. Current evidence indicates that depression is often undertreated in the older adult.[7–9] The incidence of initiation of pharmacotherapy is less than 1.5% each year, with older depressed men being half as likely to be treated with antidepressants as women.[10]

A working knowledge of the mechanism of action of available antidepressants is crucial to the definition of an objective treatment strategy. A favored unitary hypothesis links depression with a central and perhaps cytokine-mediated disturbance in the metabolism of the monoamines, noradrenaline (NA), 5-hydroxytryptamine (5-HT), and dopamine. In support of this pathogenetic theory, most effective antidepressant agents tend to result in an increase in either 5-HT or NA neurotransmission. Tricyclic antidepressants affect either NA and 5-HT, or NA alone. Similarly, selective serotonin re-uptake inhibitors (SSRIs) act primarily to inhibit 5-HT uptake and also exert some inhibitory effect on NA uptake.[11,12]

A wide variety of effective antidepressants are available (Table 45.1). However, age-related changes in pharmacodynamics and pharmacokinetics are major determining factors in the use of these medications in the older adult. Furthermore, the limited data specifically relating to the safety and efficacy of newer agents in the treatment of depression in the older adult mandates caution. Optimal characteristics of an antidepressant for the older adult include not only a rapid onset of action and optimal efficacy, but limited potential for side-effects and drug interactions (Table 45.2). Once daily administration and the availability of the pharmaceutic agent in tablet, liquid, and parenteral forms enhance patient compliance. Drugs proven to be non-fatal in toxic doses possess the advantage of a reduced risk of death from attempted suicide.

Table 45.1 *Classification and mode of action of selected newer antidepressants*

Class	Mode of action	Drug
Selective serotonin reuptake inhibitors	Inhibits presynaptic neuronal reuptake of 5-HT	Fluoxetine Paroxetine Sertraline Fluvoxamine Citalopram
Serotonin antagonists reuptake inhibitors	Antagonize 5-HT receptors and block 5-HT reuptake	Trazodone Nefazodone
Serotonin-norepinephrine reuptake inhibitors	Inhibit 5-HT and norepinephrine uptake. Weak inhibition of dopamine reuptake	Venlafaxine Mirtazapine
Selective norepinephrine reuptake inhibitors	Inhibits reuptake of norepinephrine	Reboxetine
Dopamine reuptake inhibitors	Inhibits reuptake of norepinephrine and dopamine. Negligible effect on serotonin reuptake	Bupropion
Monoamine oxidase inhibitors	Selective and reversible inhibition of monoamine oxidase	Transdermal selegiline Moclobemide
Alternative herbal therapy	Undefined	*Hypericum perforatum* (St. John's wort) S-adenosyl-l-methionine

Thus, despite the advent of numerous effective newer antidepressants, health professionals must remain cognizant of the fact that basic principles of geriatric prescribing must still be applied.

Selective serotonin re-uptake inhibitors

SSRIs have emerged as first-choice antidepressants in the older adult. In depressed patients, there is an upregulation of postsynaptic receptors due to a deficiency in 5-HT availability. Postsynaptic upregulation affects both the terminal and the somatodendritic autoreceptors. Animal studies indicate that the administration of SSRIs causes an increase in 5-HT levels due to blockade of the 5-HT transport pump. This occurs initially in the midbrain raphe, which harbors predominantly neuronal soma. The increase in 5-HT levels leads to downregulation of the somatodendritic receptors, thereby disrupting 5-HT autoregulation. Consequently, the magnitude of neuronal impulse transmission and terminal axonal 5-HT release increases. This sequence of events suggests that SSRIs exert their effect via a cascading mechanism that induces an exponential response, when triggered. Intact dopaminergic limbic and cortical systems are critical to the maintenance of hedonia. SSRIs may also exert an effect by modulating serotoninergic receptor-mediated dopamine release in the limbic areas of the brain.[13,14]

Compared to tricyclic antidepressants (TCAs), SSRIs are equally effective in the short-term treatment of depression. Evidence-based studies comparing efficacy of two agents in the long-term treatment of depression have yielded conflicting results.[15,16]

Table 45.2 *Characteristics of the ideal antidepressant for the older adult*

- Effective
- Minimal side-effects
- Low potential for drug interactions
- Safe in over-dosage
- Once daily administration
- Rapid onset
- Tablet and liquid formulations
- Enteral and parenteral formulations

Prior to the advent of SSRIs, the TCAs and traditional monoamine oxidase inhibitors (MAOIs) were the mainstays of antidepressant drug therapy.

However, despite the efficacy of these agents patient compliance was adversely affected by the myriad of adverse effects associated with their use. The subsequent development of antidepressants of comparable efficacy, but with better safety profiles, has relegated these older medications to second-choice agents in the management of depression (Table 45.3). SSRIs possess the advantage of exerting a notably reduced effect on histamine, cholinergic, and alpha-adrenergic receptors, thereby minimizing the side-effects that result from blockade of these receptors (Table 45.4). Available data also indicate that patients receiving SSRIs have lower withdrawal rates than those receiving TCAs.[17,18]

Table 45.3 *Comparative side-effect profile of selected newer antidepressants*

Drug	Sedation	Orthostatic hypotension	Anticholinergic
• Citalopram	+	−	−
• Fluoxetine	−	+	−
• Fluvoxamine	−	−	−
• Mirtazapine	+	−	−
• Nefazodone	+	+	+
• Paroxetine	−	+	−
• Sertraline	+	+	−
• Trazodone	++	++	++
• Venlafaxine	++	−	−
• Reboxetine	−	+	−

Table 45.4 *Antidepressant adverse effects related to receptor blockade*

Receptor blockade	Adverse effects
• Muscarinic	Urinary retention
	Overflow incontinence
	Constipation
	Delirium
	Blurred vision
	Xerostomia
	Anorexia
• Histamine	Sedation
	Delirium
	Weight gain
• Alpha-adrenergic	Orthostatic hypotension
	Inappropriate tachycardia
	Priapism (penile and clitoral)

Fluoxetine

Fluoxetine is the prototypical agent of the SSRI antidepressant group and is still very widely prescribed in the United States.[18] Following oral administration, fluoxetine is almost completely absorbed. However, bioavailability is reduced by first-pass hepatic metabolism. Fluoxetine is highly protein bound, has a large volume of distribution, and is renally excreted. Oxidative metabolism and conjugation result in the production of several metabolites. More than 90% of the parent compound is inactivated. However, active metabolites are also produced. Norfluoxetine is the primary desmethylated active metabolite produced by action of the cytochrome P2D6 (CYP2D6) in the liver and has a half-life of 3–20 days. This exceeds the half-life of fluoxetine which ranges from 1 to 3 days.

Thus, steady-state plasma concentrations may not be achieved for 12–42 days.[19] Due to the nonlinear pharmacokinetic profile of fluoxetine, cautious use is advised in patients with hepatic impairment.

Although the usual starting dose of fluoxetine is 20 mg daily, in the older adult the recommended starting dose is 5–10 mg daily.[20] Due to age-related changes in the cytochrome P450 enzyme system, fluoxetine and the active metabolite norfluoxetine have even longer half-lives and steady-state therapeutic levels are achieved much more slowly in older adults. Thus dosage increases should not be made during the first 4 to 6 weeks of therapy.[21] Consequently, the dose should be cautiously increased, in small increments, to a maximum dose of 40 mg. Preliminary studies examining the feasibility of therapeutic drug monitoring (TDM) of fluoxetine may alter the safety profile of this drug.[22]

Initial concerns that initiation of SSRI therapy may enhance motivation and increase the risk of impulsive acts, including suicide, have not been borne out by evidence-based data. Various groups, including the Food and Drug Administration's Psychopharmacological Drugs Advisory Committee, have failed to demonstrate any scientifically objective causal association between the use of fluoxetine and suicidal ideation. On the contrary, data have identified a reduced risk of attempted suicide in older depressed patients treated with SSRIs.[23]

Recognized adverse effects of fluoxetine include activating symptoms such as anxiety, insomnia, agitation, and tremors. Gastrointestinal adverse events such as nausea, vomiting, diarrhea, weight loss, and anorexia may occur.[24] Reduced libido and anorgasmia may occur and compromise patient compliance with therapy. Anorgasmia has been linked to fluoxetine-mediated reduction in tactile sensitivity.[25] Headaches and lethargy may also complicate fluoxetine use.[26] As with other SSRIs, the occurrence of these symptoms, especially in older adults, mandates exclusion of hyponatremia due to the SSRI-induced syndrome of inappropriate antidiuretic hormone secretion (SIADH).[27]

Drug interactions must be given careful consideration when fluoxetine is prescribed.[28] Serotoninergic syndrome is a potentially fatal condition resulting from the use of fluoxetine in conjunction with other serotoninergic agents, notably MAOI, lithium, chlorimipramine, and tryptophan. This syndrome, attributed to elevated central nervous system levels of serotonin, presents with hyperthermia, neuromuscular irritability, delirium, and psychomotor agitation. The long half-life of fluoxetine mandates a long wash-out period of about 5 weeks between cessation of fluoxetine and institution of an MAOI.[29,30]

Paroxetine

Paroxetine hydrochloride is a highly selective serotonin reuptake inhibitor. Therapeutic efficacy comparable to tricyclic antidepressants (TCAs) has been demonstrated in several studies. Paroxetine has a predictable half-life of 24 hours and is highly protein bound. Following absorption, paroxetine undergoes partial first-pass hepatic metabolism. Renal excretion of inactive metabolites follows subsequent hepatic transformation. Effective clearance of paroxetine is markedly impaired by renal insufficiency. Dosage reduction is therefore recommended in patients with a creatinine clearance < 60 ml/minute.

Compared with other SSRIs, paroxetine is a highly potent inhibitor of cytochrome P450 2D6, which is involved in the metabolism of a wide range of drugs. Paroxetine also possesses the added disadvantage of high affinity for muscarinic receptor blockade, resulting in a corresponding increase in the incidence of anticholinergic side-effects. Additional side-effects of paroxetine include nausea, insomnia, diaphoresis, tremors, and ejaculatory dysfunction. Recent data indicate that, unlike fluoxetine, paroxetine may cause a notable decrease in anxiety and is less likely to cause psychomotor agitation. Paroxetine is therefore an appropriate choice in the treatment of depressed persons with prominent features of anxiety or agitation. Therapeutic efficacy has been demonstrated in older depressed adults in doses ranging from 10 to 30 mg daily.[31–33] As with fluoxetine, controlled-release formulations of paroxetine are just as effective in the treatment of depression and well tolerated. Indeed, available data indicate that recipients of paroxetine CR may experience significantly less nausea.[34]

Sertraline

Sertraline hydrochloride is comparable in efficacy to tricyclic agents and has been shown to have a much safer side-effect profile in older adults. Sertraline has a half-life of approximately 24 hours. Hepatic methylation produces a weakly active metabolite, N-demethyl-sertraline, which has a half-life of 66 hours. Regardless, a steady state is produced after about 7 days. Sertraline is non-sedating with minimal cardiotoxicity and anticholinergic potential. Clinically apparent side-effects usually involve the gastrointestinal tract, causing nausea, vomiting, or diarrhea. However, the occurrence of these adverse events may be reduced by administration with food. A notable advantage to the use of sertraline is the reduced potential for drug interactions, as sertraline displays the least P450 2D6 inhibition compared with other commonly used SSRIs. A starting dose of 12.5 mg/day is recommended for older adults. If tolerated, the dose may subsequently be increased in increments of 12.5 to 25 mg to a maximum of 150 mg/day. An added advantage of sertraline therapy in older adults is that cessation of therapy is associated with a lower burden of moderate to severe discontinuation symptoms.[35]

Fluvoxamine

Fluvoxamine maleate is a selective inhibitor of presynaptic serotonin neuronal re-uptake. Initially approved for the treatment of obsessive-compulsive disorders, fluvoxamine possesses antidepressant efficacy comparable to SSRIs, such as sertraline and fluoxetine, and older antidepressants including imipramine, desimipramine, amitriptyline, and dothiepin.[36,37] Fluvoxamine is well absorbed following oral administration and has a half-life of 19–22 hours. Following hepatic metabolism, 90% of the dose is converted to inactive metabolites. Steady-state levels are usually achieved within 10–14 days. Fluvoxamine is relatively well tolerated, although administration of large doses has been associated with an increased incidence of nausea.[38,39]

Fluvoxamine is especially beneficial in severely depressed adults with suicidal ideation. Although the effective dose of fluvoxamine may range from 50 to 200 mg daily, the recommended initial daily dose is 100 or 150 mg. Available data indicate that patients on the latter dose are more likely to respond to treatment. Factors predictive of a positive response to fluvoxamine include age younger than 50 years and no prior history of depression.[40] As the cumulative percentage of positive responders exceeds 80% at 6 weeks, failure to improve after 6 weeks of fluvoxamine should warrant consideration of alternative therapeutic options.[41]

Citalopram

Citalopram is an SSRI used in the treatment of depression. Animal studies show a reduction in the release of excitatory amino acid neurotransmitters, glutamate and aspartate, by the involvement of the inhibitory neuromodulator adenosine.[42] This agent is well tolerated by older patients and is of comparable efficacy to older antidepressants.[43–46] Citalopram is well absorbed orally, 80% protein bound, and has a half-life of 35 hours. Hepatic demethylation results in the production of less active metabolites that undergo both renal and fecal excretion. Available data support minimal inhibition of cytochrome P450 2DS and consequently limited potential for drug interactions. Citalopram has minimal effects on the cardiovascular system and has a much better safety profile than TCAs. This agent may be a suitable choice in the older depressed adult with cardiovascular disease or comorbid conditions that predispose to autonomic instability.[47,48]

Escitalopram

Escitalopram oxalate (S-citalopram), the S-enantiomer of citalopram, is also an SSRI and an effective antidepressant. Escitalopram binds with high affinity to the human serotonin transporter and is approximately 30-fold more potent than citalopram at this transporter. Pharmacokinetic studies show that escitalopram has a very predictable dose–response ratio and negligible effects on cytochrome P450 enzyme systems, thereby minimizing the potential for adverse drug interactions. Escitalopram has been shown to be equally as effective as earlier SSRIs and may be especially effective in patients with major depressive disorder associated with pronounced symptoms of anxiety. Escitalopram is dosed once daily and patients may experience a clinically relevant response much earlier compared to their peers on citalopram. Side-effects of escitalopram include nausea, insomnia, ejaculation disorder, diarrhea, dry mouth, and somnolence.[49,50] Drug-induced delirium is a frequent concern when antidepressant therapy is started in patients with Alzheimer's disease. Escitalopram has been shown to be a safe and effective antidepressant in patients with dementia.[51,52]

Serotonin antagonist re-uptake inhibitors

Serotonin antagonist re-uptake inhibitors (SARIs) mediate their antidepressant action through a combination of 5-HT2 receptor blockade and 5-HT re-uptake inhibition. The additional mechanism of 5-HT2 receptor blockade prevents non-specific activation of receptors by the increase in 5-HT produced by serotonin re-uptake inhibition. Indeed, data indicate that the SARIs may have a lower incidence of agitation, anxiety, and sexual dysfunction compared with SSRIs.[53,54]

Trazodone

Trazodone is a phenylpiperazine derivative with weak antidepressant activity. It is frequently, although inappropriately, used as an anxiolytic or sedative in older adults. Trazodone inhibits 5-HT reuptake and antagonizes histamine and α_1-adrenoreceptors, resulting in an increased incidence of adverse effects, such as drowsiness, dizziness, and orthostatic hypotension.[55] Additionally, priapism is an infrequent, but particularly troublesome, side-effect of trazodone which may discourage the use of this agent in older men. Trazodone-induced priapism is attributed to pronounced alpha-1 adrenergic blockade.[56] Current evidence indicates that trazodone may be a useful agent in patients with major depressive disease and disturbing insomnia. Administration at night in such patients improves sleep and eliminates the need for adjunctive hypnotic therapy.[57]

Nefazodone

Nefazodone is also a phenylpiperazine derivative that inhibits serotonin re-uptake and blocks 5-HT receptors. In contrast to trazodone, nefazodone has less α_1-adrenergic receptor blockade with minimal effect on muscarinic and histamine receptors.[43] This may account for the improved side-effect profile associated with the use of nefazodone compared

with trazodone. Orthostatic hypotension and sedation occur with much less frequency in persons who use nefazodone. As with trazodone, priapism has been described as a rare side-effect of nefazodone is moderate. Additionally, several reports have emerged of drug-induced clitoral priapism in association with both drugs.[58,59]

Nefazodone is rapidly absorbed after oral administration, reaching a peak plasma concentration 2 hours after administration. However, first-pass metabolism reduces bioavailability to approximately 20%. Subsequent hepatic metabolism results in the production of active metabolites. Altered pharmacokinetics in older adults result in plasma concentrations that may be twice as high as levels in younger adults. Older men tend to have lower levels than older women. Regardless, available data do not indicate an increased likelihood of adverse effects in older subjects. The recommended starting dose in older adults is 50 mg twice a day, with slow incremental titration of 100 mg/day every 2 weeks. The recommended maximum total daily dose is 600 mg. Nefazodone inhibits the metabolism of drugs metabolized by the CYP 3A3-4 isoenzyme, thereby increasing the potential for drug interactions. Increased levels of benzodiazepines and carbamazepine may result when these drugs are given in combination with nefazodone. Of particular concern is the potentially fatal interaction that may result from cardiac arrhythmias, characteristically torsades de pointes, when nefazodone is taken with terfenadine, astemizole, or cisapride. Less serious side-effects of nefazodone include nausea, sedation, constipation, and dizziness.

The inhibiting effect of nefazodone on postsynaptic serotonin receptors makes it a useful choice in the depressed anxious patient. Additionally, the preservation of normal sleep architecture is often useful in the management of depressed persons with insomnia.[60–62]

Serotonin–norepinephrine re-uptake inhibitors

Venlafaxine

Venlafaxine, the prototypical agent of this group, exerts a greater effect on 5-HT re-uptake than norepinephrine re-uptake. Studies have shown that venlafaxine does not demonstrate significant binding to 5HT, norepinephrine, dopamine, muscarinic, cholinergic, α_1-adrenergic, or histamine receptors. This accounts for the rarity of side-effects related to blockade of these receptors. Hepatic metabolism results in the production of active metabolites with a half-life of 9–12 hours compared to 3–5 hours for the parent drug. Venlafaxine is excreted through the kidneys. Clinically significant age-related changes in pharmacokinetics have not been documented. Thus, dose adjustment for age is not necessary, unless there is evidence of renal or hepatic impairment. The recommended starting dose is 75 mg/day in two or three daily divided doses to a maximum of 375 mg/day. Venlafaxine is comparable in therapeutic efficacy to TCAs and SSRIs.[63–65]

Adverse effects of venlafaxine are more likely to occur at the onset of treatment and tend to subside with continued use. These include anorexia, dry mouth, sleep disturbance, headaches, and sweating. At high doses, sexual dysfunction has been reported in 9% of patients. Dose-related diastolic hypertension complicating therapy has been reported in 3–13% of patients, mandating routine blood pressure monitoring in persons on this drug.[66–68] Additionally, venlafaxine, though effective, may be poorly tolerated in frail elders.[69–71]

Mirtazapine

Mirtazapine blocks presynaptic α_2-adrenergic receptors and postsynaptic 5-HT2 and 5-HT3 receptors. Mirtazapine has a half-life of 20–40 hours, permitting once daily administration. This drug is extensively metabolized by the CYP 450 system and clearance may be reduced in persons with hepatic disease. The administration of mirtazapine with drugs that are co-metabolized by CYP 1A2, CYP 2D6, and CYP 3A4 should be avoided to reduce the risk of competitive inhibition and unwanted side-effects. Comparative studies show that mirtazapine is equally as effective as fluoxetine, amitriptyline, trazodone, and chlorimipramine. Studies also show that mirtazapine has fewer anticholinergic side-effects compared with TCAs. Commonly reported unwanted adverse effects associated with the use of mirtazapine include somnolence, dizziness, and sexual dysfunction. Paradoxically, other common side-effects, namely increased appetite and weight gain, may serve as a clinical advantage in the older depressed person with anorexia and weight loss. Similarly, the relatively high affinity of mirtazapine for histamine receptors has proven useful in the management of patients with anxiety, agitation, and insomnia.[72,73] Pharmacokinetic studies support dosage adjustments in renal failure. Older adults have also been shown to have relatively higher serum levels. Regardless, available evidence does not support dosage adjustment in older adults with normal renal and hepatic function. The recommended starting dose is 15 mg at bedtime with slow titration upwards every 2 weeks to a maximum of 45 mg/day. Although dose adjustments have not been recommended for the older adult, it is reasonable to start at a lower dose of 7.5 mg at bedtime and titrate upwards after observing for tolerance.[72]

Selective noradrenaline re-uptake inhibitors

Reboxetine

Reboxetine is a selective norepinephrine inhibitor that has been shown to be just as effective as SSRIs in the treatment of depression. Reboxetine is highly protein bound and less than 10% of the dose is cleared renally. The primary route of reboxetine elimination appears to be through hepatic metabolism. Reboxetine is metabolized by cytochrome P450 (CYP) 3A4. CYP 2D6 is not involved, thereby limiting the risk of drug interactions with agents such as ketoconazole that share this cytochrome metabolic pathway.[74] Reboxetine plasma concentrations are increased in elderly individuals and in those with hepatic or renal dysfunction. A specific advantage of reboxetine is the minimal effect on sexual function and libido, rendering it a reasonable choice for patients at risk for sexual dysfunction with SSRIs.[75,76] Higher rates of remission may be achieved with reboxetine compared to traditional SSRIs. This has been attributed to more effective noradrenergic suppression resulting in better control of associated anxiety symptoms.[77]

Dopamine re-uptake inhibitors

Bupropion

Bupropion is an aminoketone that exerts its effect by selective inhibition of the re-uptake of dopamine and norepinephrine. Bupropion has a therapeutic half-life of 18 hours and undergoes hepatic metabolism and renal excretion. Studies indicate that bupropion is an effective activating antidepressant and is well tolerated in older adults. The absence of significant anticholinergic, cardiovascular, or sedating side-effects renders this agent a favorable choice for the older patient. There are no reports of sexual dysfunction complicating the use of this agent. This is attributed to the minimal serotoninergic effect associated with the use of this agent.[78–80]

Bupropion reduces the seizure threshold and is associated with an increased frequency of grand mal seizures. Additionally, bupropion has a low therapeutic index and requires multiple dosing, thereby increasing the risk of overdosage, which frequently presents with tremors and seizures.

The recommended starting dose of bupropion is 50 mg orally twice daily for both the immediate-release and sustained-release preparations. The sustained-release preparation may be associated with lower peak plasma levels and a reduction in the frequency of side-effects. The maximum daily dose should not exceed 400 mg daily. Nocturnal dosing should be avoided as this may result in insomnia.[81,82] There may be an increased risk for accumulation of bupropion and its metabolites in the elderly, mandating close monitoring for toxicity in older patients.[83]

Monoamine oxidase inhibitors

Although MAOIs possess antidepressant activity, the marked potential for food and drug interactions discouraged use of these agents. Recently more selective MAOIs with reversible inhibition have been identified.

Selegiline

Selegiline, a selective monoamine oxidase B inhibitor, originally approved for the treatment of Parkinson's disease, is also an effective antidepressant at higher doses. By inhibiting MAO-B, selegiline increases dopamine levels in the substantia nigra. Selegiline also blocks dopamine re-uptake from the synaptic cleft, thereby increasing dopamine concentrations in the brain. However, at high doses oral selegiline is less selective, thereby increasing the potential for tyramine interactions.

Recently, transdermal selegiline was approved for the treatment of depression. Transdermal administration of selegiline avoids the first-pass effect, resulting in increased drug delivery to the brain and reduced production of peripherally acting metabolites such as desmethylselegiline, which also possess some MAO-B inhibitory property. Transdermal selegiline thus inhibits central nervous system monoamine oxidase isoenzymes with minimal effects on hepatic and gastrointestinal MAOI systems, thereby reducing the risk of interactions with tyramine-rich foods.[84–86]

Moclobemide is another reversible inhibitor of monoamine oxidase A that has been shown to be as effective in the treatment of depression as tricyclic antidepressants and SSRIs. Moclobemide has also been shown to be effective in the treatment of subtypes of depression that tend to occur more often in older adults, such as atypical, agitated, and retarded depression.[87,88]

Newer agents

Notable advances in the neurobiology of depression have prompted exploration of several therapeutic alternatives in the management of depression. CRF antagonists, glucocorticoid receptor antagonists, substance P receptor antagonists, and NMDA glutamate receptor antagonists are being explored. 'Triple' re-uptake inhibitors that inhibit the re-uptake of norepinephrine, serotonin, and dopamine look promising.[89,90]

Unopposed clearance of serotonin by dopaminergic neurons may reduce the efficacy of SSRIs in the treatment of depression. Theoretically, triple re-uptake inhibitors, by providing additional pharmacologic inhibition of the dopamine receptors, should induce a synergistic increase in serotonin levels.[91,92] Studies exploring these novel antidepressant therapies are ongoing.

Complementary and alternative therapy

With the growing use of alternative and complementary medicine, several therapeutic options are being touted for the treatment of depression. Depressed persons may attach negative connotations to conventional antidepressants. Such patients may opt for 'natural remedies', which often do not labor under the traditional stigma of psychiatric medication. According to the 1994 Dietary Supplement Health Education Act, herbal products are classified as foods and are not subject to the stringent quality-control regulations as are standard pharmaceuticals. However, patients have unrestricted and unregulated access to these products. The lack of standardization, regulation, and sufficient evidence-based information regarding the safety of these products precludes formal prescription of these agents by orthodox health practitioners. Nevertheless, patients may choose to use these preparations of their own volition. Consequently, the onus is on all health-care providers to become familiar with marketed integrative therapies in order to function effectively as patient advocates and counselors.

St John's wort (*Hypericum perforatum*)

Hypericum perforatum is a flowering plant which was traditionally used in medieval England during the feast of John the Baptist. The term 'wort' is the old English word for plant. *Hypericum* extracts have been used for medicinal purposes for several centuries, mainly as a treatment for vaguely characterized 'nervous conditions' and insomnia.[62] *Hypericum* extract contains several biologically active substances, several of which have been shown to inhibit 5-HT and monoamine oxidase re-uptake. Over the past two decades, St John's wort has become an increasingly popular alternative treatment for depression, with annual sales increasing from $20 million to $200 million between 1995 and 1997 (Table 45.5).[63] Review of available data from randomized controlled trials

Table 45.5 *St. John's wort* (Hypericum perforatum extract): *Biologically active ingredients.*

Hypericin
Pseudohypericin
Monoterpenes
Xanthones
β-sitosterol
Quercetin
Catechin

examining the efficacy of St John's wort reveals conflicting results, which vary significantly with the *Hypericum* extract used.[93,94]

Available data indicate that St John's wort is well tolerated in the majority of patients, with side-effects occurring in 2–8% of adults. Nausea, lethargy, and skin rash are the most common side-effects reported. Rarely, photosensitivity complicates the use of St John's wort.[95] Additionally, St John's wort is an inducer of cytochrome P450 (CYP) 3A enzymes and is therefore associated with an increased risk of drug interactions with agents that share this same pathway. Inconsistent efficacy data, lack of regulatory oversight, and absence of stringent standardization criteria constitute major drawbacks to the use of this preparation.[96]

S-Adenosylmethionine

S-Adenosyl-l-methionine (SAMe) is a naturally occurring transmethylating compound that occurs within the brain. Studies examining the short-term effect of SAMe indicate a possible role in the treatment of major depression in adults. Although the pharmacokinetics and pharmacodynamics of SAMe are unclear, available evidence suggest that at oral dosages of less than 1600 mg/day, SAMe is significantly bioavailable and lacks notable toxic effects. Nevertheless, further studies are needed to confirm efficacy and define the precise role of this supplement in the treatment of depression.[97]

Conclusions

Depression is a common problem in older adults. Inadequate treatment has grave consequences. The choice of antidepressant, as with all medications prescribed for the older adult, is often based on several factors. These include age-related changes in pharmacodynamics and pharmacokinetics and the kinetic profile of the prescribed agent. Other considerations include cost, dosing intervals, patient compliance, associated medical conditions, and drug interactions. Specifically, with regard to antidepressants, the patient's response to previous antidepressant therapy should be considered.

Available evidence indicates that most antidepressants are of comparable efficacy. However, they differ significantly with regard to their side-effect profile. Geriatric health professionals often display justifiable caution in prescribing new drugs as these agents have frequently not been well evaluated in the older population. Antidepressants are one of the few exceptions to this rule. The emergence of newer drugs has not only expanded the armamentarium of pharmacologic therapeutic options, but also reduced the risk of adverse effects traditionally associated with the treatment of late-life depression.

References

1. Mojtabai R, Olfson M. Major depression in community-dwelling middle-aged and older adults: prevalence and 2- and 4-year follow-up symptoms. Psychol Med 2004; 34: 623–34.
2. Blazer DG. Depression in late life: review and commentary. J Gerontol A Biol Sci Med Sci 2003; 58: 249–65.
3. Jongenelis K et al. Prevalence and risk indicators of depression in elderly nursing home patients: the AGED study. J Affect Disord 2004; 83: 135–42.
4. Jongenelis K et al. Prevalence and risk indicators of depression in elderly nursing home patients: the AGED study. J Affect Disord 2004; 83: 135–42.
5. Yaffe K, Edwards ER, Covinsky KE, Lui LY, Eng C. Depressive symptoms and risk of mortality in frail, community-living elderly persons. Am J Geriatr Psychiatry 2003; 11: 561–7.
6. Katz IR. Depression and frailty: the need for multidisciplinary research. Am J Geriatr Psychiatry 2004; 12: 1–6.
7. Undertreatment of depression and comorbid anxiety translates into costly mismanagement of resources and poor patient outcomes. Manag Care 2005; 14: 1–12.
8. Collins KA, Westra HA, Dozois DJ, Burns DD. Gaps in accessing treatment for anxiety and depression: challenges for the delivery of care. Clin Psychol Rev 2004; 24: 583–616.
9. Charlson M, Peterson JC. Medical comorbidity and late life depression: what is known and what are the unmet needs? Biol Psychiatry 2002; 52: 226–35.
10. Blazer D. Depression and the older man. Med Clin North Am 1999; 83: 1305–16, vii.
11. Hayley S, Poulter MO, Merali Z, Anisman H. The pathogenesis of clinical depression: stressor- and cytokine-induced alterations of neuroplasticity. Neuroscience 2005; 135: 659–78.
12. Blier P. Crosstalk between the norepinephrine and serotonin systems and its role in the antidepressant response. J Psychiatry Neurosci 2001; 26(Suppl): S3–10.
13. Dremencov E, Weizmann Y, Kinor N, Gispan-Herman I, Yadid G. Modulation of dopamine transmission by 5HT2C and 5HT3 receptors: a role in the antidepressant response. Curr Drug Targets 2006; 7: 165–75.
14. Millan MJ. Serotonin 5-HT2C receptors as a target for the treatment of depressive and anxious states: focus on novel therapeutic strategies. Therapie 2005; 60: 441–60.
15. Cipriani A et al. Fluoxetine versus other types of pharmacotherapy for depression. Cochrane Database Syst Rev 2005; CD004185.
16. Geddes JR, Freemantle N, Mason J, Eccles MP, Boynton J. SSRIs versus other antidepressants for depressive disorder. Cochrane Database Syst Rev 2000; CD001851.
17. Mottram P, Wilson K, Strobl J. Antidepressants for depressed elderly. Cochrane Database Syst Rev 2006; CD003491.
18. Wilson K, Mottram P. A comparison of side effects of selective serotonin reuptake inhibitors and tricyclic antidepressants in older depressed patients: a meta-analysis. Int J Geriatr Psychiatry 2004; 19: 754–62.
19. Mandrioli R, Forti GC, Raggi MA. Fluoxetine metabolism and pharmacological interactions: the role of cytochrome P450. Curr Drug Metab 2006; 7: 127–33.
20. Tierney J. Practical issues in geriatric psychopharmacology. J Ind Med Assoc 1999; 97: 145–7.
21. Harvey AT, Preskorn SH. Fluoxetine pharmacokinetics and effect on CYP2C19 in young and elderly volunteers. J Clin Psychopharmacol 2001; 21: 161–6.
22. Mandrioli R, Forti GC, Raggi MA. Fluoxetine metabolism and pharmacological interactions: the role of cytochrome p450. Curr Drug Metab 2006; 7: 127–33.
23. Cipriani A et al. Fluoxetine versus other types of pharmacotherapy for depression. Cochrane Database Syst Rev 2005; CD004185.
24. Brambilla P, Cipriani A, Hotopf M, Barbui C. Side-effect profile of fluoxetine in comparison with other SSRIs, tricyclic and newer antidepressants: a meta-analysis of clinical trial data. Pharmacopsychiatry 2005; 38: 69–77.

25. Frohlich P, Meston CM. Fluoxetine-induced changes in tactile sensation and sexual functioning among clinically depressed women. J Sex Marital Ther 2005; 31: 113–28.

26. Brambilla P, Cipriani A, Hotopf M, Barbui C. Side-effect profile of fluoxetine in comparison with other SSRIs, tricyclic and newer antidepressants: a meta-analysis of clinical trial data. Pharmacopsychiatry 2005; 38: 69–77.

27. Romerio SC, Radanowicz V, Schlienger RG. [SIADH with epileptic seizures and coma in fluoxetine therapy.] Schweiz Rundsch Med Prax 2000; 89: 404–10.

28. Gourion D, Perrin E, Quintin P. [Fluoxetine: an update of its use in major depressive disorder in adults.] Encephale 2004; 30: 392–9.

29. Gury C, Cousin F. [Pharmacokinetics of SSRI antidepressants: half-life and clinical applicability.] Encephale 1999; 25: 470–6.

30. Morales-Molina JA, Mateu-de AJ, Grau CS, Marin CM. [Likely serotoninergic syndrome from an interaction between amitryptiline, paroxetine, and linezolid.] Farm Hosp 2005; 29: 292–3.

31. Ackermann RT, Williams JW Jr. Rational treatment choices for non-major depressions in primary care: an evidence-based review. J Gen Intern Med 2002; 17: 293–301.

32. Loosbrock DL, Tomlin ME, Robinson RL, Obenchain RL, Croghan TW. Appropriateness of prescribing practices for serotonergic antidepressants. Psychiatr Serv 2002; 53: 179–84.

33. Crown WH, Treglia M, Meneades L, White A. Long-term costs of treatment for depression: impact of drug selection and guideline adherence. Value Health 2001; 4: 295–307.

34. Bang LM, Keating GM. Paroxetine controlled release. CNS. Drugs 2004; 18: 355–64.

35. Sir A et al. Randomized trial of sertraline versus venlafaxine XR in major depression: efficacy and discontinuation symptoms. J Clin Psychiatry 2005; 66: 1312–20.

36. Rossini D et al. Sertraline versus fluvoxamine in the treatment of elderly patients with major depression: a double-blind, randomized trial. J Clin Psychopharmacol 2005; 25: 471–5.

37. Dalery J, Honig A. Fluvoxamine versus fluoxetine in major depressive episode: a double-blind randomised comparison. Hum Psychopharmacol 2003; 18: 379–84.

38. Gerstenberg G et al. Relationship between clinical effects of fluvoxamine and the steady-state plasma concentrations of fluvoxamine and its major metabolite fluvoxamino acid in Japanese depressed patients. Psychopharmacology (Berl) 2003; 167: 443–8.

39. Schwarzenbach F et al. Antidepressant response and fluvoxamine plasma concentrations: a pilot study. Pharm World Sci 2003; 25: 27–9.

40. Morishita S, Arita S. Possible predictors of response to fluvoxamine for depression. Hum Psychopharmacol 2003; 18: 197–200.

41. Morishita S, Arita S. Suitable dose and duration of fluvoxamine administration to treat depression. Psychiatry Clin Neurosci 2003; 57: 177–81.

42. Blardi P et al. Activity of citalopram on adenosine and serotonin circulating levels in depressed patients. J Clin Psychopharmacol 2005; 25: 262–6.

43. de Mendonca Lima CA et al. Effect of age and gender on citalopram and desmethylcitalopram steady-state plasma concentrations in adults and elderly depressed patients. Progr Neuropsychopharmacol Biol Psychiatry 2005; 29: 952–6.

44. Blardi P et al. Activity of citalopram on adenosine and serotonin circulating levels in depressed patients. J Clin Psychopharmacol 2005; 25: 262–6.

45. Galecki P et al. [Efficiency and safety of citalopram and venlafaxine in treatment of depressive disorders in elderly patients.] Pol Merkuriusz Lek 2004; 17: 621–4.

46. Rocca P et al. Citalopram versus sertraline in late-life nonmajor clinically significant depression: a 1-year follow-up clinical trial. J Clin Psychiatry 2005; 66: 360–9.

47. Rush AJ, Bose A, Heydorn WE. Naturalistic study of the early psychiatric use of citalopram in the United States. Depress Anxiety 2002; 16: 121–7.

48. Sidhu J et al. Steady-state pharmacokinetics of the enantiomers of citalopram and its metabolites in humans. Chirality 1997; 9: 686–92.

49. Burke WJ. Escitalopram. Expert Opin Invest Drugs 2002; 11: 1477–86.

50. Murdoch D, Keam SJ. Spotlight on escitalopram in the management of major depressive disorder. CNS Drugs 2006; 20: 167–70.

51. Rao V et al. An open-label study of escitalopram (Lexapro) for the treatment of 'Depression of Alzheimer's disease' (dAD). Int J Geriatr Psychiatry 2006; 21: 273–4.

52. Rausch JL, Corley KM, Hobby HM. Improved potency of escitalopram on the human serotonin transporter: demonstration of an ex vivo assay technique. J Clin Psychopharmacol 2004; 24: 209–13.

53. Almasi J, Rihmer Z. [Review of antidepressants from the TCAs to the third generation drugs.] Neuropsychopharmacol Hung 2004; 6: 185–94.

54. Feighner JP. Mechanism of action of antidepressant medications. J Clin Psychiatry 1999; 60(Suppl 4): 4–11.

55. Mendelson WB. A review of the evidence for the efficacy and safety of trazodone in insomnia. J Clin Psychiatry 2005; 66: 469–76.

56. Correas Gomez MA et al. [Trazodone-induced priapism.] Actas Urol Esp 2000; 24: 840–2.

57. Mashiko H et al. Effect of trazodone in a single dose before bedtime for sleep disorders accompanied by a

depressive state: dose-finding study with no concomitant use of hypnotic agent. Psychiatry Clin Neurosci 1999; 53: 193–4.

58. Brodie-Meijer CC, Diemont WL, Buijs PJ. Nefazodone-induced clitoral priapism. Int Clin Psychopharmacol 1999; 14: 257–8.

59. Pecknold JC, Langer SF. Priapism: trazodone versus nefazodone. J Clin Psychiatry 1996; 57: 547–8.

60. Dunner DL et al. Six-year perspectives on the safety and tolerability of nefazodone. J Clin Psychiatry 2002; 63(Suppl 1): 32–41.

61. Schatzberg AF et al. Clinical use of nefazodone in major depression: a 6-year perspective. J Clin Psychiatry 2002; 63(Suppl 1): 18–31.

62. DeVane CL, Grothe DR, Smith SL. Pharmacology of antidepressants: focus on nefazodone. J Clin Psychiatry 2002; 63 (Suppl 1): 10–17.

63. Olver JS, Burrows GD, Norman TR. The treatment of depression with different formulations of venlafaxine: a comparative analysis. Hum Psychopharmacol 2004; 19: 9–16.

64. Masand PS, Gupta S. Long-term side effects of newer-generation antidepressants: SSRIs, venlafaxine, nefazodone, bupropion, and mirtazapine. Ann Clin Psychiatry 2002; 14: 175–82.

65. Dewan MJ, Anand VS. Evaluating the tolerability of the newer antidepressants. J Nerv Ment Dis 1999; 187: 96–101.

66. Masand PS, Gupta S. Long-term side effects of newer-generation antidepressants: SSRIs, venlafaxine, nefazodone, bupropion, and mirtazapine. Ann Clin Psychiatry 2002; 14: 175–82.

67. Dewan MJ, Anand VS. Evaluating the tolerability of the newer antidepressants. J Nerv Ment Dis 1999; 187: 96–101.

68. Ansseau M. [Pharma-Clinics. The drug of the month. Venlafaxine (Efexor).] Rev Med Liege 1998; 53: 106–8.

69. Shelton C, Entsuah R, Padmanabhan SK, Vinall PE. Venlafaxine XR demonstrates higher rates of sustained remission compared to fluoxetine, paroxetine or placebo. Int Clin Psychopharmacol 2005; 20: 233–8.

70. Oslin DW et al. Probing the safety of medications in the frail elderly: evidence from a randomized clinical trial of sertraline and venlafaxine in depressed nursing home residents. J Clin Psychiatry 2003; 64: 875–82.

71. Staab JP, Evans DL. Efficacy of venlafaxine in geriatric depression. Depress Anxiety 2000; 12(Suppl 1): 63–8.

72. Anttila SA, Leinonen EV. A review of the pharmacological and clinical profile of mirtazapine. CNS Drug Rev 2001; 7: 249–64.

73. Stimmel GL, Dopheide JA, Stahl SM. Mirtazapine: an antidepressant with noradrenergic and specific serotonergic effects. Pharmacotherapy 1997; 17: 10–21.

74. Fleishaker JC. Clinical pharmacokinetics of reboxetine, a selective norepinephrine reuptake inhibitor for the treatment of patients with depression. Clin Pharmacokinet 2000; 39: 413–27.

75. Brambilla P, Cipriani A, Hotopf M, Barbui C. Side-effect profile of fluoxetine in comparison with other SSRIs, tricyclic and newer antidepressants: a meta-analysis of clinical trial data. Pharmacopsychiatry 2005; 38: 69–77.

76. Clayton AH et al. Lack of sexual dysfunction with the selective noradrenaline reuptake inhibitor reboxetine during treatment for major depressive disorder. Int Clin Psychopharmacol 2003; 18: 151–6.

77. Eker SS, Akkaya C, Akgoz S, Sarandol A, Kirli S. [Comparison of reboxetine and sertraline in terms of efficacy and safety in major depressive disorder.] Turk Psikiyatri Derg 2005; 16: 153–63.

78. Ross S, Williams D. Bupropion: risks and benefits. Expert Opin Drug Safety 2005; 4: 995–1003.

79. Tomarken AJ, Dichter GS, Freid C, Addington S, Shelton RC. Assessing the effects of bupropion SR on mood dimensions of depression. J Affect Disord 2004; 78: 235–41.

80. Haustein KO. Bupropion: pharmacological and clinical profile in smoking cessation. Int J Clin Pharmacol Ther 2003; 41: 56–66.

81. Jefferson JW, Pradko JF, Muir KT. Bupropion for major depressive disorder: pharmacokinetic and formulation considerations. Clin Ther 2005; 27: 1685–95.

82. Zwar N, Richmond R. Bupropion sustained release. A therapeutic review of Zyban. Aust Fam Physician 2002; 31: 443–7.

83. Sweet RA et al. Pharmacokinetics of single- and multiple-dose bupropion in elderly patients with depression. J Clin Pharmacol 1995; 35: 876–84.

84. Patkar AA, Pae CU, Masand PS. Transdermal selegiline: the new generation of monoamine oxidase inhibitors. CNS Spectr 2006; 11: 363–75.

85. Mahmood I. Clinical pharmacokinetics and pharmacodynamics of selegiline. An update. Clin Pharmacokinet 1997; 33: 91–102.

86. Gordon MN et al. Oral versus transdermal selegiline: antidepressant-like activity in rats. Pharmacol Biochem Behav 1999; 63: 501–6.

87. Bonnet U. Moclobemide: therapeutic use and clinical studies. CNS Drug Rev 2003; 9: 97–140.

88. Sogaard J et al. A 12-week study comparing moclobemide and sertraline in the treatment of outpatients with atypical depression. J Psychopharmacol 1999; 13: 406–14.

89. Beer B et al. DOV 216,303, a 'triple' reuptake inhibitor: safety, tolerability, and pharmacokinetic profile. J Clin Pharmacol 2004; 44: 1360–7.

90. Holtzheimer PE III, Nemeroff CB. Advances in the treatment of depression. NeuroRx 2006; 3: 42–56.
91. Mossner R, Simantov R, Marx A, Lesch KP, Seif I. Aberrant accumulation of serotonin in dopaminergic neurons. Neurosci Lett 2006.
92. Holtzheimer PE III, Nemeroff CB. Advances in the treatment of depression. NeuroRx 2006; 3: 42–56.
93. Linde K, Mulrow CD, Berner M, Egger M. St John's wort for depression. Cochrane Database Syst Rev 2005; CD000448.
94. Linde K, Berner M, Egger M, Mulrow C. St John's wort for depression: meta-analysis of randomised controlled trials. Br J Psychiatry 2005; 186: 99–107.
95. Linde K, Mulrow CD, Berner M, Egger M. St John's wort for depression. Cochrane Database Syst Rev 2005; CD000448.
96. Hall SD et al. The interaction between St John's wort and an oral contraceptive. Clin Pharmacol Ther 2003; 74: 525–35.
97. Williams AL, Girard C, Jui D, Sabina A, Katz DL. S-Adenosylmethionine (SAMe) as treatment for depression: a systematic review. Clin Invest Med 2005; 28: 132–9.

CHAPTER 46

Sleep disorders

Hosam K Kamel

Introduction

Sleep disorders are estimated to affect more than 50% of community-dwelling elderly and more than 65% of institutionalized elderly.[1] Older individuals with sleep disorders may complain of waking tired, difficulty falling asleep, difficulty maintaining wakefulness during the day, or abnormal behavior associated with sleep. Although sleep requirements do not decrease with advancing age, older adults are less able to sleep.[2] Individuals with sleep disorders may complain of difficulty sustaining attention, slowed response time, difficulty with memory, and decreased performance. Many sleep disturbances in the elderly remain undiagnosed and untreated as they are mistakenly attributed to aging.[1] Epidemiologic studies of older adults found an association between sleep complaint and the presence of chronic illness, mood disturbances, decreased physical activity, and physical disability.[3-5] Older women are more likely than older men to report sleep complaints.[6]

Age-related changes in sleep patterns

Aging is associated with multiple changes in sleep patterns (Table 46.1). While stages 1 and 2 (the lighter stages of sleep) increase or remain the same, stages 3 and 4 (the deeper stages of sleep) decrease with advancing age. Rapid eye movement (REM) sleep occurs earlier during the sleep cycle, with the percentage of REM sleep remaining the same.[7] Older adults have decreased sleep efficiency (time asleep over time in bed), decreased sleep time, and an increased sleep latency (time to fall asleep). Additional findings include earlier bedtime and earlier morning awakening, more arousal during sleep, and more daytime napping compared to younger adults. After a period of sleep deprivation, older adults show less daytime sleepiness, less evidence of decline in performance measure, and recover their normal sleep structure more rapidly than younger adults. Older persons, however, have more sleep disturbances with jet lag and shift work than younger persons.[8]

Evaluation of sleep in older persons

The National Institutes of Health Consensus Statement on the Treatment of Sleep Disorders in Older People suggested three simple questions for clinicians to screen for sleep disorders in the elderly.[9] First, is the person satisfied with his/her sleep? Second, does sleep or fatigue intrude into daytime activities? And third, does the bed partner or others complain of unusual behavior during sleep, such as snoring, interrupted breathing, or leg movement?

In general, transient sleep disturbances (less than 4 weeks) are usually situational; persistent sleep problems, on the other hand, often require detailed evaluation. To aid the assessment of sleep complaints, it is helpful to ask patients to keep a 'sleep

Table 46.1 *Age-related changes in sleep*

- Decrease in stages 3 and 4 sleep
- Increased night-time awakenings
- Increased sleep latency (time to fall asleep)
- Decreased sleep efficiency (time asleep over time in bed)
- Increased daytime napping
- Earlier morning awakening
- Earlier onset of REM sleep in night
- Decreased total REM sleep

REM: rapid eye movement.

log' in which, each morning, they record their time in bed, their estimated amount of sleep, number of awakenings, time of morning awakenings, and any symptoms that occur during the night (Table 46.2).[10] This should be supplemented by information from the bed partner when possible. Patients should have a general physical examination that includes mental status assessment and depression screening.

In addition to sleep logs, there are several tools available that can help assess for possible sleep disorders. Polysomnography is indicated when a primary sleep disorder, such as sleep apnea or periodic limb movement in sleep, is suspected. A wrist actigraph is another tool that utilizes a monitor to estimate sleep versus wakefulness time based on wrist activity. Its utility may be limited in individuals with tremor, dyskinesia, or myoclonus. Overnight use of pulse oximetry allows direct monitoring of oxygen saturation for evidence of hypoxemia that might indicate the presence of sleep apnea. Another measure of sleep that has been developed for home sleep monitoring is a pressure-sensitive pad that reports signals from respiration and movement.

Insomnia

Insomnia is defined as difficulty in initiating or maintaining sleep. Insomnia can be primary when it does not occur exclusively during the course of another sleep or mental disorder, nor is it due to a direct physiologic effect of substance or alcohol abuse or a general medical condition.[11] Primary insomnia is uncommon in the elderly. Insomnia in

this patient population is usually secondary to a psychiatric or medical illness.[12]

Causes

Psychiatric disorders have been reported to be responsible for more than 50% of cases of insomnia in this patient population. Depression is the most common condition involved and is characterized by early awakening, increased sleep latency, and more night-time wakefulness. In depressed elderly with sleep disturbances, treatment of depression has been reported to improve sleep abnormality, with changes in sleep electroencephalography towards a more normal sleep structure. Anxiety and stress may be associated with difficulty in initiating sleep. Older caregivers report more sleep complaints than do similarly aged healthy adults. In one study about 40% of older women who were family caregivers of older adults with dementia reported using a sleeping medication in the previous months.[13]

Drug and alcohol use account for another 10 to 15% of cases of insomnia. Chronic use of sedatives may cause light and fragmented sleep. Alcohol abuse is often associated with lighter and shorter duration of sleep. The use of alcohol to treat insomnia should be discouraged. Although alcohol may cause an initial drowsiness, it can impair sleep later in the night as blood alcohol levels decrease.

Pain from arthritis and other medical conditions, cough, dyspnea from cardiac or pulmonary illness, gastroesophageal reflux, and night-time urination can impair sleep. In addition, sleep can be impaired by certain medications/substances taken near bedtime such as diuretics and stimulating agents (for example caffeine, sympathomimetics, and bronchodilators). Certain medications, such as some antidepressants, antiparkinsonian agents, and antihypertensives (such as propranolol), may cause nightmares and impair sleep.

Management

A trial of improved sleep hygiene is usually the recommended initial approach to the management of insomnia. Short-term hypnotic therapy may be appropriate in conjunction with improved sleep hygiene in some cases of transient, situational insomnia such as periods of temporary acute stress.

Table 46.2 *Suggested items of a sleep log*[10]

- Date and day of the week
- Activities during the day
- Timing of meals and quantity of food eaten
- Timing and medications taken (prescription and non-prescription)
- Alcohol and caffeine consumption (including caffeinated beverages)
- Activities before bedtime (e.g. taking a bath, watching TV, or reading)
- Time of going to bed
- Time needed to fall asleep
- Quality of sleep (including awakening periods and nightmares)
- Dreams, snoring, or unusual movement during sleep
- Time of wakening in the morning
- Feelings on waking in the morning (well rested or tired)
- Daytime naps

In chronic insomnia (insomnia lasting 30 days or more), the clinician should rule out primary sleep disorders (e.g. sleep apnea, restless leg syndrome) and review medications and other medical conditions that may be contributory. Non-pharmacologic interventions are the recommended choice of treatment for chronic insomnia.[14]

Several non-pharmacologic interventions can be quite effective in improving sleep in older persons. Behavioral interventions have been shown to produce multiple therapeutic benefits including improved sleep efficiency, sleep continuity and satisfaction with sleep, and decreased hypnotic use.[15,16] Stimulus control[17] and sleep restriction therapy[18] have been shown to be helpful for older persons with insomnia. Cognitive and educational interventions have been shown to be superior to pharmacologic therapy in producing sleep improvements that are better sustained over time.[19]

The effects of exposure to bright light (either natural sunlight or commercially available boxes) on sleep in older persons with insomnia have been tested in multiple studies.[20,21] Positive effects on sleep have been demonstrated with light exposure of various intensities for various durations and at various times during the day. Evening light exposure was particularly useful in older persons with an advanced sleep phase. Even short durations of bright light exposure in the morning have been shown to improve sleep complaints in healthy older

adults. Taking a warm bath before sleep has been demonstrated to enhance the quality of sleep in older people. Moderate intensity exercise has also been shown to improve sleep in healthy sedentary people aged 50 years and older who reported moderate sleep complaints at baseline.[22]

Pharmacologic therapy of insomnia usually consists of a benzodiazepine with a short half-life or a short-acting non-benzodiazepine. Table 46.3 lists pharmacologic agents commonly used to treat insomnia. Benzodiazepines should only be used for short periods, and if used for longer than a week they should be used for more than three nights a week. Short-acting agents are recommended for problems with sleep maintenance. Short-acting agents are less likely to be associated with falls and hip fractures. Rebound insomnia after cessation of a short-acting agent is frequent and can be reduced by tapering the dosage prior to discontinuing the drug. Temazepam has an intermediate half-life and no known active metabolites, and its metabolism is not affected by aging. However, daytime sedation may occur with this agent. Estazolam is a benzodiazepine with rapid onset and intermediate duration of action, so it may be effective in both initiating and maintaining sleep. This agent has a weak active metabolite. The most common adverse effects reported with this agent are somnolence and hypokinesia. Estazolam is thought to have little effect on daytime psychomotor performance. Long-acting

Table 46.3 *Pharmacologic agents commonly used to treat insomnia*

Drug	Suggested dose (mg/day)	Time to onset of action (min)	Half-life (hours)
Non-benzodiazepines			
Eszopiclone	1–2	45–60	6
Ramelteon	8	<30	1–2
Zaleplon	5–10	<30	1
Zolpidem	5–10	30	1.5–4.5
Benzodiazepines			
Estazolam	1–2	15–30	8–24
Flurazepam	15–30	30–60	10–15
Lorazepam	1–4	30–60	8–24
Temazepam	15–30	45–60	3–25
Triazolam	0.125–0.25	15–30	1.5–5
Others			
Trazodone	25–50	30–60	5–9
Mirtazapine	15–30	60–120	20–40
Melatonin	3	60–120	0.5–0.75

benzodiazepines should not be used in older people because of associated daytime sedation, lethargy, ataxia, and cognitive and psychomotor impairment.[23]

Short-acting non-benzodiazepine hypnotics that are currently approved by the US Food and Drug Administration (FDA) for the treatment of insomnia include zolpidem, zaleplon, eszopiclone, and ramelteon. Although zolpidem, zaleplon, and eszopiclone are structurally unrelated to benzodiazepines, they share some of the pharmacologic properties such as interacting with the central nervous system γ-amino butyric acid (GABA) receptor complex at benzodiazepine (GABA-BZ) receptors. Ramelteon, on the other hand, belongs to a new class of drugs, selective ML-1 receptor agonists that mimic the action of the naturally occurring hormone melatonin. All four drugs have a rapid onset of action and should be taken within 30 minutes of bedtime or after the individual has gone to bed and has been unable to fall asleep. These agents have been shown to have little effect on daytime performance of cognitive and psychomotor tests. Eszopiclone was the first sleeping agent approved by

the FDA (in December 2004) for long-term use. Nightly treatment with eszopiclone 2 mg for 2 weeks was shown in a randomized controlled trial to effectively induce and maintain sleep in 231 older subjects with primary insomnia. Overall, the drug was well tolerated. Dosage adjustment is necessary for individuals with severe liver disease, but not for those with renal impairment.[24,25]

Ramelteon (approved in July 2005) is the first sleep medication not to be designated a controlled substance by the US Drug Enforcement Administration. Like eszopiclone, ramelteon is approved by the FDA for long-term use. Results from a randomized placebo-controlled study involving 829 older adults with chronic insomnia were reported at the American Geriatric Society's annual scientific meeting in May 2005 and showed patients who received ramelteon 4 mg or 8 mg at bedtime for 5 weeks had decreased sleep latency (time needed to fall asleep) compared to the placebo group.[26] The drug was well tolerated. Ramelteon is contraindicated in patients with severe liver disease. Low doses of sedating antidepressants such as trazodone or mirtazapine may also be used as a sleeping aid.

Melatonin is a hormone that is secreted by the pineal gland and appears to have a role in regulating the circadian and seasonal biorhythms in humans and other mammals. Its synthesis and release are stimulated by darkness and inhibited by light. Thus, the diurnal rhythm of melatonin secretion closely follows the day–night cycle. This circadian rhythm, however, may be affected by changes in environmental lighting. Although plasma melatonin levels undergo a continuous decline after peaking at the age of 2 to 5 years, night-time plasma levels of the hormone remain greater than those during the day throughout the life-span.[27]

There is evidence that links the age-related decline in melatonin plasma levels to the development of insomnia in later years of life. The administration of melatonin to older adults with insomnia at doses sufficient to raise night-time plasma levels to those of younger adults restored normal sleep patterns in these individuals.[28] In another study the administration of melatonin to older persons with insomnia decreased sleep latency and wake time after the onset of sleep, and increased sleep efficiency (time asleep over time in bed).[29] On the other hand, melatonin supplementation had no effect on sleep patterns in older adults who did not have insomnia in spite of the presence of low melatonin plasma levels.

Sleep apnea

Sleep apnea refers to a periodic reduction in ventilation during sleep. Patients with sleep apnea often complain of excessive daytime sleepiness. Sleep apnea may be central (simultaneous cessation of breathing efforts and nasal and oral airflow), obstructive (impaired airflow), or mixed. Most older patients with sleep apnea have obstructive sleep apnea. In this condition, patients usually present with hypersomnolence and are typically unaware of the frequent arousals associated with reduction in ventilation. Patients are often obese and may have morning headaches and personality changes. They may also complain of poor memory, confusion, and irritability. Other symptoms include loud snoring, cessation of breathing, and choking sounds during sleep.

The prevalence of sleep apnea increases with age. The reported prevalence of sleep apnea among older adults varies from 20 to 70% depending on the population studied. The most important predictor of sleep apnea is large body mass.[30] Other predictors identified include falling asleep at inappropriate times, male gender, and frequent daytime napping. Alcoholism is an important risk factor for sleep apnea, and sleep-disordered breathing is a significant contributor to sleep disturbances in men with alcohol abuse who are over the age of 40 years. Sleep apnea has been linked to dementia. In one study among institutionalized elderly, the presence of sleep apnea was linked to dementia and there was a positive correlation between the severity of sleep disturbances and the severity of dementia.[31] Individuals suspected of having sleep apnea should be referred to a sleep laboratory for evaluation. Patients with sleep apnea should be encouraged to lose weight, avoid alcohol and sedative use, and avoid the supine sleeping position. Continuous positive airway pressure (CPAP) is the treatment of choice for patients with sleep apnea. Older patients generally tolerate CPAP well. For those who fail or are unable to tolerate CPAP treatment, surgery may be considered. Surgical procedures vary from laser-assisted uvuloplasty (effective in 30% of patients) to mandibular-maxillary advancement (effective in 90% of patients).

Periodic limb movements in sleep and 'restless legs syndrome'

Periodic limb movements in sleep (PLMS, or nocturnal myoclonus) are a condition of repetitive, stereotypical leg movements occurring in non-REM sleep. The leg movements occur every 20 to 40 seconds and can last much of the night, which may interfere with sleep. The prevalence of PLMS increases with age and it is estimated to affect about 20–60% of older adults.[32] PLMS may present as difficulty maintaining sleep or excessive daytime sleepiness. A bed partner may be aware of the leg movements, or these movements may remain occult until identified in a sleep laboratory.

'Restless leg syndrome' (RLS) is a condition of uncontrollable urges to move one's legs at night. The diagnosis is made based on the patient's description of symptoms, and the sleep complaint is usually difficulty in initiating sleep. There may be a family history of the condition and, in some cases, an underlying medical disorder (such as renal, neurologic, or cardiovascular disease). The prevalence of RLS increases with age. A large community-based study estimated the prevalence of RLS at 10.6%. In this study female sex was an independent predictor of RLS diagnosis.[33] Many patients with RLS also have PLMS. In older patients with PLMS or RLS, dopaminergic agents are the initial treatment of choice for both conditions (for example, an evening dose of carbidopa/levodopa, pergolide, or ropinirole). Benzodiazepines or opiates have also been used for these conditions.

REM sleep behavior disorder

REM sleep behavior disorder is characterized by excessive motor activity during sleep, with the pathologic absence of the normal muscle atonia during REM sleep. The presenting symptoms are usually vigorous sleep behaviors associated with vivid dreams. These behaviors may even result in injury to the patient or the bed partner. This condition is more common in older men than women and may be acute or chronic. Acute transient REM sleep behavior disorders have been associated with toxic-metabolic abnormalities, primarily drug or alcohol withdrawal or intoxication. The chronic form of REM sleep behavior disorder is usually idiopathic or associated with a neurologic abnormality (for example, drug intoxication, vascular disease, tumor, infection, degenerative disorder, or trauma). Polysomnography is recommended to establish the diagnosis. Clonazepam is the treatment of choice for REM sleep behavior disorder. Pharmacologic therapy should be accompanied by environmental safety interventions, such as removing dangerous objects from the bedroom, and putting cushions on the floor around the bed.

Disturbances in the sleep–wake cycle

Disturbances in the sleep–wake cycle may be transient, as in jet lag, or associated with an obvious cause (for example shift work). Some patients have persistent disturbances with either a delayed sleep phase (in which they fall asleep late and wake up late) or an advanced sleep phase (in which they fall asleep early and wake up early). The advanced sleep phase is particularly common in older individuals. Problems related to an advanced sleep phase may respond to timed exposure to bright light. Patients with a significant sleep-phase cycle disturbance should be referred to a sleep laboratory for evaluation.

References

1. Mazza M, Della Merca G, De Risio S et al. Sleep disorders in the elderly. La Clinica terapeutica 2004; 155(9): 391–4.
2. Ancoli-Israel S. Sleep and aging: prevalence of disturbed sleep and treatment consideration in older adults. J Clin Psychiatry 2005; 66(Suppl 9): 24–30.
3. Roberts RE, Shema SJ, Kaplan GA, Strawbridge WJ. Sleep complaints and depression in an aging cohort: a prospective perspective. Am J Psychiatry 2000; 157(1): 81–8.
4. McCrae CS, Rowe MA, Tierney CG et al. Sleep complaints, subjective and objective sleep patterns, health, psychological adjustment, and daytime functioning in community-dwelling older adults. J Gerontol B Psychol Sci Soc Sci 2005; 60(4): P182–9.
5. Foley DJ, Monjan AA, Masaki KH et al. Associations of symptoms of sleep apnea with cardiovascular disease, cognitive impairments, and mortality among older Japanese American men. J Am Geriatr Soc 1999; 47(5): 524–8.
6. Fukuda N, Honma H, Kohsaka M et al. Gender differences of slow wave sleep in middle aged and elderly subjects. Psychiatry Clin Neurosci 1999; 53(2): 151–3.
7. Avidan AY. Sleep disorders in the older patient. Primacy Care 2005; 32(2): 563–86.
8. Moline ML, Pollak CP, Monk TH et al. Age-related differences in recovery from simulated jet lag. Sleep 1992; 15(1): 28–40.
9. National Institutes of Health Consensus Development Conference Statement: the treatment of sleep disorders of older people. Sleep 2001; 14: 169–77.

10. Susman JL. Sleep. In: Ham RJ, Sloan PD, Warshaw GA, eds. Primary Care Geriatrics: A Case-Based Approach. St. Louis, MO: Mosby Inc, 2002: 437–44.

11. American Psychiatric Association. Diagnostic and Statistical Manual of Mental Disorders, 4th edn. Washington, DC: American Psychiatric Publishing Inc, 1994: 551–607.

12. Ancoli-Israel S, Cooke JR. Prevalence and comorbidity of insomnia and effect on functioning in elderly population. J Am Geriatric Society 2005; 53(7 Suppl): S264–71.

13. Roberts RE, Shema SJ, Kaplan GA, Strawbridge WJ. Sleep complaints and depression in an aging cohort: a prospective perspective. Am J Psychiatry 2000; 157(1): 81–8.

14. Morin CM, Colecchi C, Stone J et al. Behavioral and pharmacological therapies for late-life insomnia: a randomized controlled trial. JAMA 1999; 47: 430–8.

15. Morin CM, Mimeault V, Gagne A. Non-pharmacological treatment of late-life insomnia. J Psychosom Res 1999; 46(2): 103–16.

16. Ancoli-Israel S. Sleep and aging: prevalence of disturbed sleep and treatment consideration in older adults. J Clin Psychiatry 2005; 66(Suppl 9): 24–30.

17. Schnelle JF, Alessi CA, Al-Samarrai NR et al. The nursing home at night: effects of an intervention on noise, light and sleep. J Am Geriatric Soc 1999; 47: 430–8.

18. Hoch CC, Reynolds CF III, Bysse DJ et al. Protecting sleep quality in later life: a pilot study of sleep restriction and sleep hygiene. J Gerontol B Psychol Sci Soc Sci 2001; 56(1): P52–9.

19. Alessi CA, Martin JL, Webber AP et al. Randomized controlled trial of a nonpharmacological intervention to improve abnormal sleep/wake patterns in nursing home residents. J Am Geriatr Soc 2005; 53(5): 803–10.

20. Dowling GA, Hubbard EM, Mastick J et al. Effect of morning bright light treatment for rest-activity disruption in institutionalized patients with severe Alzheimer's disease. Int Psychogeriatr 2005; 17(2): 221–36.

21. Lack L, Wright H, Kemp K, Gibbon S. The treatment of early-morning awakening insomnia with 2 evenings of bright light. Sleep 2005; 28(5): 616–23.

22. Alessi CA, Yoon E, Schnle JR et al. A combined physical activity and environmental intervention in nursing home residents: do sleep and agitation improve? J Am Geriatr Soc 1999; 47: 784–0/ 789–91.

23. McCall WV. Diagnosis and management of insomnia in older people. J Am Geriatr Soc 2005; 53(7 Suppl): S272–7.

24. Scharf M, Erman M, Rosenberg R et al. A 2-week efficacy and safety study of eszopiclone in elderly patients with primary insomnia. Sleep 2005; 28(6): 720–27.

25. Melton ST, Wood JM, Kirkwood CK. Eszopiclone for insomnia. Ann Pharmacother 2005; 39(10): 1659–66.

26. Roth T, Seiden D, Zee P et al. Phase III outpatient trial of ramelteon for the treatment of chronic insomnia in elderly patients. Abstract A21. Presented at the American Geriatric Society annual scientific meeting, Orlando, FL, 13 May 2005.

27. Brown GH, Young SN, Gruthler S et al. Melatonin in human cerebrospinal fluid in daytime: its origin and variation with age. Life Sci 1979; 25: 929–36.

28. Wurtman RJ, Zhdanova I. Improvement of sleep quality by melatonin (letter). Lancet 1995; 346: 1491.

29. Van Reeth O, Weibel L, Olivares E et al. Melatonin or a melatonin agonist corrects age-related changes in circadian response to environmental stimuli. Am J Physiol Regul Integr Comp Physiol 2001; 280(5): R1582–92.

30. Resta O, Bonfitto P, Sabato R et al. Prevalence of obstructive sleep apnea in a sample of obese women: effect of menopause. Diabetes Nutr Metab 2004; 17(5): 296–303.

31. Ancoli-Israel S, Klanber MR, Butters N et al. Dementia in institutionalized elderly: relation to sleep apnea. J Am Geriatr Soc 1991; 39: 258–63.

32. Lesage S, Hening WA. The restless legs syndrome and periodic limb movement disorder: a review of management. Semin Neurol 2004; 24(3): 249–59.

33. Hogl B, Kiechl S, Willeit J et al. Restless legs syndrome: a community-based study of prevalence, severity, and risk factors. Neurology 2006; 64(11): 1920–4.

CHAPTER 47

Cognitive changes in aging

Syed H Tariq and John E Morley

Introduction

Cognition is defined as the various thinking processes through which knowledge is gained, stored, manipulated, and expressed. Although many cognitive skills decline with age, the extent and pattern of decline vary both at individual level and with the type of function. Some individuals age successfully and maintain a similar cognitive function to that of the young, and some functions may even improve with aging. Other individuals may have some intact cognition functions (e.g. long-term memory, complex motor skills) while there is a decline in other areas of cognition (e.g. learning new information).

Cognitive function is affected by a number of variables such as demographic factors (age, education), work and leisure activities, and individual differences.[1,2] Psychiatric problems such as depression and substance abuse also affect cognition.

In this chapter we will discuss the epidemiology of cognitive impairment, different methods involved in studying cognition, normal age-associated cognitive decline, and the disease process involved in causing changes in cognition (dementia), diagnostic strategies, and available treatments.

Epidemiology of cognitive impairment in old age

The prevalence of dementia is 5% in persons of 65 years of age[3] and increases to 22% between the ages of 85 and 89 years. When persons with mild cognitive impairment are included the prevalence is almost doubled.[4] Alzheimer's disease (AD) is the most common type of dementia and affects 4 million people in the USA. Epidemiologists project the number of patients with AD to be 14 million by 2040.[5,6] Males less commonly develop AD than do females. Minor cognitive decline is seen in the normal elderly; two out of three of the intact elderly have some sort of impairment on psychologic testing, which increases with aging.[7]

Conceptual issues in the study of cognitive function

Studying cognitive impairment is a difficult task. When studying cognition one should have in mind that cognitive tests are affected by educational level, culture, language usage, prior experience, emotional and physical status, and measurement error. This makes it difficult to differentiate differences in cognitive score as a result of these factors from those due to disease processes. In contrast to clinical studies, in epidemiologic studies it is very important to consider a wide range of cognition, from the upper end of normal to the lower end of the disease process. Similarly there is a need for uniform measurement of cognition in all subjects along with restrictions on time and subject burden.

Published epidemiologic data have relied upon cognitive testing at one point in time, which is a direct approach but influenced by a number of factors other than disease process, such as education, which is easily measured, and others which are difficult to define or measure. The easy way to find cognitive decline is by analyzing change over a period of time. The timing between tests should be long enough to provide time for change.

There are a number of challenges that limit a change in cognitive function as an outcome in epidemiologic studies. First the test should examine the entire range of cognitive function in the population to be studied, since it is difficult to develop brief tests for cognitive function measurement, which usually has some degree of floor and ceiling effect. Second, the observed difference in cognitive function is usually very small compared to the entire range of function, which requires the development of tests that are of sufficient sensitivity to measure small changes and which are more reliable. Unfortunately reliability data on most of the tests are not available. Third, to measure cognitive change it is important to use the same test at multiple end-points. Some people do well over time because of the learning effect and the size of the effect may vary among the risk group, thereby changing the estimates.[8]

In modeling the association between risk factors and change in cognitive function, the analytic issues are complicated by the need for time to be considered in the analysis. The methods that are most effective include advanced longitudinal analysis.

Multiple outcome models, such as multivariate regression methods, including random effect models and generalized estimating questions (GEEs), can be used with three or more risk factors over time. These methods can use all the observations and estimate the association of risk factor with level of cognitive function and with rates of change. A mixed model of fixed and random effect is the model of choice, when the cognitive scores are approximately within normal limits.[9] It also allows for individual variation, i.e., the random effect. The main limitations of this method are that it requires continuous data and multiple assumptions need to be made. The GEEs are used when the cognitive scores are not randomly distributed.[10,11] GEEs have the same benefits as the random effects models except that they do not allow for differences in individual rates of decline. Another

approach is to use a linear regression model and compute the change in cognitive score over time. These linear slopes are then used to determine the outcome variables in another linear regression model. The main limitation is that the individual slopes are treated as true slopes rather than estimates. There is a chance of finding an association where there is none, because some of the risk factors are underestimated.

It is important to include age and education in these models. When building models for change in cognitive function, both age and education need careful consideration. They are both associated with many other potential risk factors, so these effects should be carefully modeled when investigating other risk factors.[12] When assessing score over time one should take into account the differential effects of learning on age and education.[8]

When cognitive decline is used as a categoric variable, i.e. decline in cognition or no decline, this approach limits the statistical power and introduces the potential of deriving wrong associations by providing cut-off values. Similarly when individuals are combined into groups (persons showing improvement and those showing no improvement), it is possible for an exposure group with more variation to appear to have more decline even though in fact it experienced more improvement. When a certain score defines dementia, rather than a change in score, many other variables are ignored. For example, a person with a low educational level may score close to the cut-off point of dementia as compared to one of high educational status, but a small change in the latter's score may be required to fall into the group of patients with dementia on follow-up. This approach becomes limited by the way in which the ability to distinguish between the initial level and change is lost.

Sometimes tests are combined to reduce the skewed distribution between the floor and ceiling effects. When selecting a method for combining tests, the investigator should give careful consideration to how different tests are weighted and to what assumption this implies about the relationships among the tests.[13] In conclusion, advanced statistical and longitudinal designs should be used in any studies aimed at age-associated changes.[12]

Decline in cognitive functions with aging, or primary cognitive decline

The cognitive domains are intelligence, attention, language, memory, learning, visuospatial ability, psychomotor ability and speed, and executive functions.

Intelligence

Intelligence is a multifactorial construct; intellectual performance peaks at the age of 30 years, plateaus through the fifties and sixties and then declines after that, but there is a sharper decline in the late seventies.[14] Changes in intelligence as a function of age may be confounded by cohort effects as shown in many cross-sectional studies,[15] while longitudinal studies may either overestimate or underestimate changes in intelligence.[16] Four decades ago Horn and Cattell[17] introduced the concept of crystallized and fluid intelligence. 'Crystallized intelligence' presents an individual's accumulated knowledge base, which is obtained and can be expanded throughout the lifespan. 'Fluid intelligence' is the ability to solve new problems in everyday life and requires new knowledge and skills. With this concept in mind studies have shown that fluid intelligence deteriorates more with aging as compared to crystallized intelligence.[18,19] Czaja and Sharit[20] compared the abilities of 65 subjects to learn new computer tasks in the age range of 25–70 years; the older age subjects had more errors and longer response times. Similarly, in another study elderly skilled typists did not show any slowing in their motor abilities, but the elderly unskilled typists were slower than young unskilled typists, demonstrating the effects of fluid intelligence. Some slowing in the central processing may be responsible for the decline in fluid intelligence in old age.[21–23]

The Wechsler Adult Intelligence Scale (WAIS) is the standard test used for testing intelligence.[24] There is an earlier and age-related decline observed on the verbal subsets of this scale. Hultsch et al[25] examined a non-institutional sample of the population and reported that the age-related decline occurred in the working memory, verbal fluency, and world knowledge, when the sample was controlled for differences in individual effects of aging. In a meta-analysis of 65 studies, there was no clear relationship between age and work performance; but these studies did not show the nature of the jobs and the experience of the individuals performing them.[26] It is also reported that experience at a job leads to an increase in crystallized intelligence, which in fact does not decline with age but can increase.

Performance speed

Speed of performance is usually not regarded as a cognitive function on its own, but it operates in many aspects of cognition. Performance speed decline is evident in a decrease in the speed of walking[27] and in the finger-tapping test.[28] Slowing of cognition or reaction time is also recognized by psychologic testing with advancing age.[21,22,29] The WAIS has shown that there is more age-related decline in the performance subsets scores as compared to the verbal subsets scores.[24,30] The decline in the performance subset is not because of motor slowing but it involves perceptual and integrative processes. The latter is evident by the relationship of P300 event-related latencies and age. The P300 and other evoked potentials directly measure the central processing time.[31]

Memory and learning

Memory and learning are the general set of functions associated with the acquisition, storage, and retrieval of new information. Thirty-one percent of elderly living in the community without cognitive impairment and 47% of those with cognitive impairment complain of memory problems.[32] This self-reported memory loss is valid for current memory function as well as a predictor of impending cognitive decline.[32–35]

There are three types of memory that are affected by age in different ways. Primary memory or working memory is a temporary storage capacity, which is time limited and is maintained only through practice. One example of primary memory is to hold a telephone number in mind while one uses it to dial a number, or to hold a number while one scans for the address. Craik[36] reported that older people might be slower in accessing information from primary stores, though tasks on digit span are performed equally well in the young and old age groups.[37]

Secondary memory is the ability to acquire new information and seems to be susceptible to aging. Age-dependent impairment in secondary memory is somewhat more apparent during tasks such as free recall rather than crude recall or recognition.[38,39] Furthermore, episodic memory (e.g. recall of specific words on a list displayed 5 minutes earlier) declines substantially with age, whereas semantic memory (e.g. retrieval from one's vocabulary or general knowledge base) declines modestly.[40,41] If one takes into account educational attainment, decrement in semantic memory almost does not exist.[42] Some investigators reported that explicit memory (conscious attempts to recall specific information) declines more than implicit memory (skills acquired through previous experience).[43,44] It is hypothesized that the decreased ability to learn new information might be related to degeneration of the hippocampus and a decrease in efficacy or abundance of acetylcholine.[45] Numerous age-related differences are found with both the encoding and the retrieval of new information in long-term memory. Older adults are more sensitive to distraction on attention tasks,[36] quick pacing of materials,[46] and the amount of material presented at one time.[47] When older people are provided with memory-encoding strategies, they do well on memory performance, provided they continue using these techniques.[48] Perhaps reinforcement paradigms that emphasize rehearsal and use of these new learned skills would prove beneficial. It has been shown that learning in older adults might be less effective because they are more likely to learn peripheral information, while the younger are more task oriented.[49] In addition to encoding, retrieval is also more difficult for older people. It is very difficult to understand whether older adults apply less effort to retrieve information or whether weakly encoded material by definition is difficult to retrieve.

Tertiary or remote memory is a type of memory that is stored and consolidated over time (examples are one's wedding anniversary or birthday or a historic event). Clinicians have long been aware that remote memories are clearer and more readily accessible to older adults than more recent memories.

Older adults do better on remembering things over a 50-year period as compared to their younger counterparts. Elderly people do as well as young on skills learned long ago, e.g. reading and spelling. In fact the performance of the elderly on these tests generally is consistent with or higher than their previous academic achievement.

Language

Difficulty with spoken language (speech) is a common complaint in older individuals.[50] Disability in communication is reported by older adults to affect the quality of life.[51] Most of the studies in older adults have reported that peripheral auditory impairment accounts for most of the variance in speech perception scores. This is considered as the primary contributor to age-related decline in understanding speech.[52,53] Humes and Watson[52] reported that hearing loss accounted for 75% of the variance in identification of scores among older subjects listening in a quiet environment; when background noise was added only 50% of the variance could be explained by the person's absolute sensitivity. The input side of language involves perception of the letters and speech sounds that make up words, and comprehension of meaning of the words and sentences. These input-side processes remain remarkably stable in old age, independent of sensory deficits and decline in the ability to encode new information.[54] The technique used to measure the processing of word meanings and their organization in semantic memory is the semantic priming paradigm (e.g. the reduction in the time required to identify a target word). The semantic priming effect is similar in both young and older adults as evidence for the integrity of this important comprehension process in old age.[55] The semantic selection process during sentence comprehension remains constant across the age groups.[54] Off-line task measures comprehension processes by examining what people remember about the meaning of a paragraph presented earlier. Age differences invariably appear in such tasks,[56] but may have less to do with initial comprehension than with the process of encoding and recall of comprehended information.[57] Wingfield et al[58] asked younger and older adults to repeat sentences that were produced at different speaking rates in two levels of semantic context. The first sentences were semantically and syntactically meaningful (e.g. he walked along the path), while the second sentences were syntactically correct but semantically meaningless (e.g. fruitless brown dreams sleep curiously). Performance was significantly poorer for both age groups when sentences did not include semantic information. However, when the semantic context was added to the syntax context, older adults performed better than the younger adults.[59,60] Studies indicate that at least two cognitive abilities are essential for processing spoken language, which become impaired as function of old age. First is the ability to maintain perceptual constancy with speech signals that vary because of vocal-tract differences among talkers. Second is the ability to distinguish phonetically similar words. These are referred as talker normalization and lexical discrimination, respectively. They are part of the earliest stages of speech perception and have been shown to be important for recognizing spoken words.[61,62]

Words produced by a man, a women, and a child will have different acoustic properties because of differences in physical characteristics of the speaker.[63] Sommers[61] has shown that there is a significant age-related reduction in the ability to carry out perceptual normalization of talker differences. In this study both young and older adults were asked to identify words against a background noise. In the first part, all the words were produced by a single speaker, and in the second 10 different speakers produced the words. There was no difference in the speech recognition performance with a single speaker, but in the second part of the test both groups performed worse. However, the decline from single to multiple speakers was significantly greater for older adults. The multiple speakers had greater effect on the perception of speech in the older adults. This finding suggests that one of the factors that may contribute to age-related impairment in speech understanding is a reduced ability to maintain perceptual constancy by compensating for acoustic-phonetic changes that result from differences in speaker (vocal-tract) characteristics.

Lexical, as in 'lexicon', refers to the structure of meaning and its representation in words. Intact lexical functions include the ability to access and recognize words on demand. Sommers[61] measured the speech identification score for two types of words as a function of age. The first type was lexically 'easy' words. The second type of stimulus, lexically 'hard' words, was, in contrast, phonetically similar to other common English words. There was no difference in the identification of easy words between the two groups (70%), but the performance on hard words in both groups was poor. The older group exhibited significantly lower scores in identification of lexically hard words compared to young adults. A multiple regression model indicated that the performance on lexically difficult words was not correlated with a measure of absolute sensitivity. Thus, independently of hearing status, older subjects had greater difficulty in identifying words that were phonetically similar to others stored in their long-term memory.

Visuospatial functioning

Visuospatial function is the ability to perceive objects and subsequently manipulate visual, rather than non-verbal, information. The magnification hypothesis model predicts that individual differences (between young and older adults) will increase systematically with task difficulty. When both young and older adults performed visuospatial information tasks, the response times yielded a single principal component with a similar composition in both age samples. For both samples, response time for fast and slow subgroups for the seven tasks (18 conditions) on the corresponding mean of response time for their age group accounted for 99% of the variance. These findings suggest that individual differences in processing time were largely task independent. The response times of slower individuals are more affected by aging than those of faster individuals.

It is also hypothesized that aging and hemispheric laterality interact to produce relatively greater decrements in older individuals in right hemispheric-dominant (visuospatial) than left hemispheric-dominant (verbal) tasks. Twenty-four early middle-aged males (mean age 37.6 years) and 24 older males (mean age 71.2 years) – of equal educational status – were given a task. The Shark test is a verbal and visuospatial paired-associated learning task and is sensitive to left and right hemispheric dysfunction, respectively. The subjects were also given the Shipley Institute for Living Scale and the Memory-for-Designs Test. No group differences were present on the Shipley verbal age scale, but the older group had significantly lower Shipley abstraction ages and memory-for-designs scores. They made more errors than the middle-aged group on both the verbal and visuospatial learning tasks. These data do not support the notion of a laterality effect associated with aging.

A cross-sectional analysis of community residents aged 65 and older found a decrease in visuospatial ability and speed of execution as age increased. There was also poor performance among female subjects and those with lower levels of education. A convenience sample of 59 people (35 women and 24 men) with mild dementia of the Alzheimer type, 66 (39 women and 27 men) with mild dementia of the Alzheimer type, and 146 healthy non-demented individuals (90 women and 56 men) was studied. The participants' ages ranged from 51 to 96 years. Dementia severity was staged by means of the Clinical Dementia Rating. In this sample, visuospatial deficit was more apparent in very mild dementia of the Alzheimer type. Individuals with both very mild and mild dementia of the Alzheimer type made more errors involving peripheral figures and rotation of a major figure than did healthy, non-demented individuals.

Executive function

Executive functions are cognitive processes that orchestrate complex, goal-directed activities.[64] The American Psychiatric Association added executive function to its list of the cognitive domains that can be used to establish the diagnosis of dementia.[65] Executive function has been associated with the frontal cortex, but is thought to be more of a product of the frontal cortico-subcortical system.[66] Impairment in executive function is linked to age-related frontal cortical atrophy and decline in frontal perfusion among healthy people.[67,68] Executive impairment undermines a patient's independence by interfering with the direction, planning, execution, and supervision of behavior.[69] The

prevalence of executive function impairment is unknown in older adults in the community. It is reported that decline in executive function can be detected in healthy adults as young as 45–65 years of age compared to educationally and sex-matched adults aged 20–35 years.[67] Executive function can be measured by the Wisconsin Card Sorting Test (WCST), Executive Interview (EXIT-25), Mini-Mental State Examination (MMSE), and Clock Drawing Task (CLOX). The EXIT-25 correlated with other measures of executive control including the WCST ($r=0.54$), Trail Marking Part B ($r=0.64$), the test of sustain attention (time, $r=0.82$; errors, $r=0.83$), and Lezak's Tinker Toy Test ($r=0.57$). The EXIT-25 is more sensitive than the MMSE to early cognitive impairment and non-cortical dementia in elderly subjects.[70,71] The MMSE is a very familiar instrument,[72] but insensitive in early dementia and poorly educated subjects.[73] CLOX, when administered to healthy and demented elderly as an executive function, was closely correlated with EXIT-25 and MMSE.[74] This association persists after adjusting for age and education.[75]

Neuropsychologic data show that age-related frontal lobe changes are most significant compared to other cortical structures.[76] These changes vary across individuals and are evident after 65 years of age. One theory of aging links impairment in executive function to cognitive decline in memory and attention, which in turn is associated with frontal lobes.[77] Executive memory supervises the content of working memory, where information from long-term memory is integrated with information in the immediate present to plan, initiate, and carry out a course of action.[78] Cognitive impairment recognized by the MMSE or by the Dementia Rating Scale is associated with impairment on complex, instrumental activities of daily living.[79] In the early stages of dementia patients under-report difficulties in daily activities; this inaccuracy is correlated with cognitive impairment.[80] Executive function plays an important role in daily motor functions of the elderly, and many of them report difficulty in one or more activities of daily living (ADLs). Executive abilities are necessary to recognize, initiate, and carry out consequences of actions, and may well be the critical skills that regulate performance of many ADLs, particularly high-order ADLs (the operation of tools or instruments requires more steps for successful completion than do the basic ADLs). One study examined the association of cognition and physical function with the least disabilities, in community dwellers in East Baltimore with a mean age of 74 years. In this sample it was found that old age, lower education, and African-American race were all associated with poor physical performance. Impairments in executive function – flexibly planning and initiating a course of action – were selectively associated with slower performance of high-order tasks such as the instrumental activities of daily living tests, relative to other domains of cognition, in high-functioning community elders.[81]

Executive dysfunction also helps to determine the care received by older retirees in a retirement community. In one study in such a community, residents were provided with services at three levels of care: independent living apartments (level 1), residential care where laundry, house cleaning, meals, and supervision of medication were provided (level 2), and skilled nursing units (level 3) in which residents were provided with assistance in ADLs, nursing care, and medication. Several tests (EXIT-25, [the executive interview], MMSE [general cognition], Geriatric Depression Scale short form [mood], the Nursing Home Behavior Problem Scale [problem behavior], and the Cumulative Illness Rating Scale [physical disability]) as well as age, educational level, and number of medications prescribed were used to examine the effect on the need for the perceived level of care given. In this small sample it was found that impaired executive function contributed the most to the variance of care in this retirement community. The other markers of general cognition, depression, and physical illness contributed relatively little additional variance. The strongest contribution to the level of care was from EXIT-25, which accounted for 70% of the observed variance in care. In this sample it was also found that 55% of the residents who scored greater than or equal to 24 on the MMSE failed the EXIT-25 at 15/50, suggesting that the MMSE is not as sensitive as the EXIT-25.[82]

Attention

Attention is the ability to concentrate on tasks. Attention can be divided into two: divided attention and sustained attention. Divided attention is the ability to differentiate between two different stimuli, such as different auditory stimuli presented to each ear; this begins to decline in the fourth decade. Sustained attention is the ability to focus on single tasks; examples are series of numbers differing by 7 (e.g., 100, 93, 86, 79, 72 . . .) or spelling 'world' backwards. Sustained attention is maintained and does not decline before the age of 80 years.

Primary dementing illness

Dementia is a general term used to describe a significant decline in two or more areas of cognitive functioning, usually associated with cognitive decline. Dementia is not synonymous with aging because the cognitive changes are progressive and disabling and not an inherent part of aging. Table 47.1 provides a list of the possible etiologies of dementia.

Alzheimer's disease

Alzheimer's disease (AD) usually affects people after the age of 60 years. It rarely affects people before this age. The disease process is gradual and progressive; the average life expectancy after the first symptom is 8–10 years. AD is seen in 6–8% of all persons after the age of 65 years and the prevalence doubles every 5 years after the age of 60 years, so that at the age of 85 years this increases to 30%.[83–85] Alzheimer's is a disease characterized by amyloid plaques and neurofibrillary tangles. It has been genetically associated with chromosome 21 (Down's syndrome and beta amyloid gene), chromosomes 14 and 1, and chromosome 19 (apolipoprotein E_4).

The risk factors for Alzheimer's disease are outlined in Table 47.2. AD is a major burden on society and in the USA costs about $100 billion each year, which accounts for medical, long-term care, home care, and loss of productivity for caregivers.[86,87] AD also causes emotional toll on the caregivers and 50% of the families develop some form of psychological distress.[88]

Table 47.1 *Disorders that may cause dementia*

Primary dementing illness	Secondary dementing illness

Primary dementing illness
- Alzheimer's disease
- Pick's disease
- Frontotemporal dementia
- Huntington's disease
- Parkinson's disease
- Progressive supranuclear palsy
- Cortical Lewy-body disease

Drugs and toxins
- Alcohol-induced dementia
- Drug-induced dementia

Intracranial conditions
- Brain tumors
- Brain abscesses
- Hydrocephalus
- Subdural hematoma

Trauma to the head

Infections
- Creutzfeldt–Jakob disease
- AIDS
- Neurosyphilis
- Chronic meningitis

Secondary dementing illness
- Vascular dementias
- Thrombotic disorders
- Embolic disease
- Inflammatory vascular conditions
- Systemic lupus erythematosus
- Temporal arthritis

Metabolic and endocrine disturbances
- Hypothyroidism/hyperthyroidism
- Hypoadrenalism/hyperadrenalism
- Hypoparathyroidism and hyperparathyroidism
- Hypoglycemia/hyperglycemia
- Vitamin B_{12} deficiency
- Pellagra
- Uremic/dialysis encephalopathy
- Aluminum

Psychiatric disorders
- Depression
- Mania
- Schizophrenia

Table 47.2 *Risk factors and protective factors for Alzheimer's disease*

Risk factors
Age
Family history
Early age (genetic mutation on chromosomes 1, 14, 21)
Late onset (apolipoprotein E*$_4$ allele on chromosome 19)
Down's syndrome
Head trauma
Female gender
Lower educational achievement

Protective factors
Estrogen use
Higher educational level
Anti-inflammatory drug use
Apolipoprotein E*$_2$ allele
Antioxidant use

The Diagnostic and Statistic Manual of Mental Disorders (DSM) IV has developed criteria for the level of dementia in AD. The cognitive deficit manifested by both memory impairment and at least one of the following cognitive disturbances – aphasia, apraxia, agnosia, and disturbance in executive functions – causes impairment in social and occupational function. These symptoms should arise because of other conditions or drugs that cause impairment in cognition. The onset is gradual and there is a progressive decline in cognition, with sparing of motor and sensory functions, until late in the disease. The average course of AD ranges from 3 to 20 years from the onset of the first symptom to death. Memory impairment is present in the early stages of the disease and the person has difficulty learning new information and even retaining it for a shorter period.

Cognitive impairment may also affect activities of day-to-day living: problems with meal planning,

Table 47.3 *Differences between delirium and dementia*

Characteristics	Delirium	Dementia
Onset	Sudden	Gradual over months to years
Reversibility	Usually reversible	Irreversible and progressive
Disorientation	Early and profound	Later during the disease
Consciousness	Clouded, fluctuating	Not usually affected
Language	Uses wrong words, vocabulary intact	Worsens with advanced disease
Attention span	Strikingly short	Not affected
Speech	Incoherent	Coherent
Sleep–wake cycle	Hour to hour variability	Day–night reversal
Psychomotor changes	Marked*	None until late

*Hyperactive or hypoactive.

Table 47.4 *Differences between depression and Alzheimer's disease (AD)*

Characteristic	Depression	AD
Onset	Rapid, relatively short duration	Gradual, long duration
Mood	Flat or depressed (anxiety, suicidal)	Apathetic to irritable (memory loss occurs first)
Intellectual function	Doesn't know answers	Confident but inaccurate answers
Memory	Loss of short- and long-term memory	Recent memory most impaired
Other symptoms	Impaired concentration	Impaired orientation
Self-image	Poor	Normal
Personal/family history	Depression more common	Depression less common

managing medication and finances, telephone use, and driving problems. In mild to moderate AD many of the activities of daily living as well as social skills are intact until late in the disease. Changes occur in mood and behavior, such as personality changes, irritability, anxiety or depression, delusions, and hallucinations,[89] which is very troubling for the family and frequently leads to nursing home placement.[90] It is very hard to identify dementia in the setting of either delirium or depression and sometimes they coexist in hospital settings.[91] It is very important to differentiate delirium and depression from dementia; Tables 47.3 and 46.4 outline the important differences, respectively. Dementia is a risk factor for delirium and contributes to the higher prevalence of delirium in the elderly.[91] Fifty percent of reversible causes of dementia and depression can lead to irreversible dementia in 5 years.[92]

Pick's disease

Pick's disease is characterized by a preponderance of atropy in the frontotemporal region in contrast to AD, where the distribution is parietal-temporal distribution. Pick's disease constitutes 5% of all irreversible dementias. In Pick's disease the earliest changes are related to personality such as socially inappropriate behavior and frontal lobe disinhibition. Patients with Pick's disease have early onset of language disturbances and Klüver–Bucy syndrome (hyperphagia, emotional blunting, hypersexuality,

Table 47.5 *Differences between cortical and subcortical dementias*

Characteristics	Cortical dementia	Subcortical dementia
Language	Early aphasia	No aphasia
Memory	Both recall and recognition impaired	Recall more impaired than recognition
Abstraction	Impaired	Impaired on difficult tasks
Mood	Normal	Depressed
Personality	Normal	Apathetic
Speech	Affected late	Dysarthric
Posture	Upright	Extended
Coordination	Normal but affected late	Impaired
Motor function	Normal	Slow
Site of disease	Hippocampus and associated cortex	Basal ganglion, thalamus, brain stem
Disease	AD and FTD	Parkinson's disease, Huntington's disease, progressive supranuclear palsy

AD, Alzheimer's disease; FTD, frontotemporal dementia.

and visual and auditory agnosia), but there is sparing of memory, visuospatial abilities, and the ability to calculate.[93] The CT scan shows frontotemporal atropy, and histology shows Pick bodies, inflated cells, white matter gliosis, and loss of dendritic spines. There is no known etiology and therefore no specific treatment.

Other frontal lobe degeneration dementias are: frontal lobe degeneration without Pick's pathology, amyotropic lateral sclerosis, progressive subcortical gliosis, stroke involving the anterior cerebral artery, multiple sclerosis, hydrocephalus, and syphilis.

Mendaz et al[94] investigated the cognitive estimations test (CET) in subjects with frontotemporal dementia (FTD) and AD. The CET was administered to 31 FTD subjects, 31 AD subjects, and 31 normal elderly controls. Both dementia groups gave significantly more extreme estimates on the CET than did the controls. AD patients gave more extreme estimates than did FTD patients. It was concluded that the CET may be particularly impaired in AD because it reflects impaired memory and numeric ability, and impaired judgment and reasoning.

On tasks of construction and calculation FTD patients performed significantly better than the AD patients. In addition to personality and neuroimaging features, relatively preserved performance of elementary drawings and calculations in FTD suggests additional features for distinguishing FTD patients from comparably demented AD patients.[95]

Dementia with extrapyramidal disorders

Dementia with extrapyramidal disorders is different from AD or frontal lobe disease. The descriptive terms 'cortical' and 'subcortical' dementia are used to differentiate between the two dementias, and are outlined in Table 47.5.

Huntington's disease

Huntington's disease is idiopathic degenerative disease characterized by dementia and chorea. It is an autosomal dominant trait with 50% penetration and the gene is located on chromosome 4. The age at onset is usually 35 to 40 years, but it can occur after the age of 50 years. It is characterized by dementia and affective disorders, and a considerable number of patients develop a schizophrenic-like disorder.[96] There is atropy of the caudate nucleus on both CT scan and PET scans; there is also a decrease in gamma amino butyric acid.[97] No specific treatment is available; however, the associated psychiatric disorders respond to treatment.

Parkinson's disease

Parkinson's disease is a disease of middle-aged and older adults; 80% of the people affected are between the ages of 60 and 79 years.[98] The prevalence of dementia in Parkinson's disease is 8–80%.[99] Parkinson's disease is manifested by resting tremor, rigidity, bradykinesia, and loss of righting reflexes. Intellectual impairment is more common in older patients with akinesa and a prolonged disease course. There is a deficiency of dopamine, with variable loss of epinephrine, serotonin, acetylcholine, and selected neuromodulators. Pathologically, there is cell loss and gliosis in the substantia nigra, and some portion of Lewy bodies in the remaining neurons. It is reported that some patients with Parkinson's disease have classical Alzheimer's lesions.[98,99] Fetal tissue implants are being investigated as a treatment for the motor symptoms.[100]

Cortical Lewy-body disease

A subgroup of patients with dementia has Lewy bodies (hyaline inclusion bodies) associated with neuronal loss in certain nuclei, e.g. the nucleus basalis and brain stem nuclei.[101] It is been suggested that in Lewy-body disease there is dopamine deficiency and cholinergic deficiency.[99] The older neuroleptic medications are likely to worsen the motor symptoms of Parkinson's disease and cause psychotic symptoms, but the newer neuroleptic drugs such as clozapine or risperidone may be useful. Persons with Lewy-body dementia tend to present with behavioral symptoms before they develop cognitive symptoms.

In a community-based study of 135 subjects with dementia, from whom autopsy and brain tissue was available, there were 48 patients with AD, 65 with LB and AD, and 22 with LBD. There were no significant differences between groups demographically or on performance in the MMSE or Dementia Rating Scale. AD patients performed worse than the LBD patients on memory measures and a naming test. LBD patients were more impaired than AD patients on executive function and attention tasks. Decline in MMSE and Dementia Rating Scale scores over time were greatest in the patients with AD/LBD.[102]

Progressive supranuclear palsy

This illness is more common in men than in women, affects people in the sixth or seventh decade, and

the average length of time until death is 5–10 years. Progressive supranuclear palsy is characterized by an extrapyramidal syndrome and dementia. Clinically there is more rigidity in midline structures and erect posture with extension of the neck. It is most often associated with sleep disturbances and depression.[103] Progressive supranuclear palsy involves the subthalamic nucleus, red nucleus, globus pallidus, substantia nigra, and dentate nucleus. Pathologically, there is granulovacuolar degeneration, neurofibrillary tangles, and cell loss. A variety of drugs have been used to treat these patients, such as L-dopa, amantadine, benztropine, and amitriptyline.[104–106]

Secondary dementing illness

Vascular dementia

Vascular dementia is the second most common cause of dementia and occurs more in people aged 55 or older. The criteria for the diagnosis of vascular dementia are multiple cognitive deficit manifested by both memory impairment and one of the following: aphasia, apraxia, agnosia, or disturbances in executive functioning along with focal neurologic signs that are judged to be etiologically related to the disturbances (DSM-IV). The risk factors for vascular dementia are hypertension and other cardiovascular risk factors.[107] The differences between vascular dementia and Alzheimer's disease are outlined in Table 47.6.

A neuropathologic classification of vascular dementia has been provided, determined by the cause of vascular disease, size of the vessel affected, and region of the brain affected.[108] Small vessel disease may cause subcortical damage resulting in subcortical dementia, or may affect the white matter of the frontal lobes, producing a frontal lobe syndrome.

Binswanger's disease is also known as subcortical atherosclerotic encephalopathy. It is characterized by multiple small infarcts of the white matter; lacunar infarcts are also seen in Binswanger's disease.[108] In the past it was considered less common but with the availability of sophisticated techniques such as magnetic resonance imaging it is diagnosed more commonly these days.

Table 47.6 *Differences between vascular dementia (VaD) and Alzheimer's disease (AD)*

Characteristic	VaD	AD
Onset	Sudden; may be stroke related	Gradual
Progression	Stepwise; sudden cognitive declines, fluctuates	Gradual decline in cognition and function
Neurologic findings	Focal deficit	No focal deficit
Neuroimaging	One or more infarcts in the area affecting cognition	May appear normal
Gait	Disturbed early in dementia	Usually normal
Cerebrovascular history	History of TIA, remote stroke, or vascular risk factors	Less common

The elderly represent 12% of the population and consume about 30% of all the prescribed medications, and 70% of them use over-the-counter medications.[108] Any drug can potentially cause cognitive or behavioral changes; some drugs are ore common as causative agents than others and can be easily remembered by the mnemonic: 'ACUTE CHANGE IN MS' outlined in Table 47.7.[109–111]

Table 47.7 *Drugs associated with dementia*

A: Antiparkinsonian drugs
C: Corticosteroids
U: Urinary incontinence drugs
T: Theophylline
E: Emptying drugs (e.g. metoclopramide)

C: Cardiovascular drugs (digoxin, clonidine, methyldopa, procainamide)
H: H$_2$ blockers
A: Antimicrobials (rare but case-reports exist)
N: Narcotics
G: Geropsychiatric drugs
E: ENT drugs

I: Insomnia drugs
N: NSAIDs

M: Muscle relaxants
S: Seizure drugs

ENT, ear nose throat drugs; NSAIDs, non-steroidal anti-inflammatory drugs.

Dementia associated with toxic substances

Alcoholism is one of the most important health problems in the USA.[112] It has a bimodal distribution, with the second peak occurring between the seventh and eighth decades of life.[113] Long-term alcohol consumption produces dementia syndrome with frontal lobe dysfunction, and apathy independent of head injury, malnutrition, and hepatic failure.[114,115] Alcoholic dementia is usually mild and slowly progressive and may partially remit if abstinence can be maintained for several months.[115] There is evidence that alcohol primarily causes white matter atropy because of its toxic effect on myelin. New-onset alcoholism may occur in older persons.

Exposures to some metals, e.g. lead, arsenic, mercury, manganese, nickel, bismuth, and tin, can cause dementia. Aluminum has been associated with dialysis-induced dementia in patients with long-term dialysis.[116] Patients with dialysis-induced dementia present with personality changes, myoclonus, and seizures. Treatment includes reducing the exposure and treating with the chelating agent deferoxamine.

Neoplasms causing dementia

Neoplasms are common in the elderly and must be considered in the differential diagnosis of dementia. Brain tumors may cause different symptoms depending on the location. They can cause mental status changes, increase intacranial pressure, focal weakness, personality changes, intellectual changes, and sensory and visual defects. Dementia occurs in 70% of patients with frontal lobe tumors, e.g. meningiomas, gliomas, or metastatic tumors.[117,118]

Dementia caused by infectious diseases
HIV encephalopathy
Acquired immunodeficiency syndrome is caused by the human immunodeficiency virus that attacks the immune system and impairs patient response to infections. HIV encephalopathy is the leading infectious cause of dementia.[118] The HIV invades the brain, shortly afterwards causing systemic infection, and remains latent for long periods.[119] HIV encephalopathy has subcortical features, such as apathy, impaired concentration and memory, indifference, and poor motivation.[120] The Center for Disease Control (CDC), in a longitudinal study, reported no decline in neuropsychologic profile among patients with stage 2 or 3 disease for one year, but in another study 25% of the patients developed clinically significant dementia at 9 months and an additional 25% at 1 year.[121,122] Azidothymidine (AZT) may improve cognitive functions in patients with encephalopathy, and methylphenidate or dextroamfetamine may improve apathy, poor motivation, and attention deficit.[123,124]

Creutzfeldt–Jakob disease
This condition was first described by Creutzfeldt in 1920 and by Jakob in 1921. The incidence is one in one million. This disorder is sporadic in 85% of cases and is caused by a virus or 'prion' (a proteinaceous infectious agent). About 5 to 10% of cases are familial in nature.[125] An autosomal dominant form is described in families with abnormalities in chromosome 20 in about 10% of cases. Creutzfeldt–Jakob disease (CJD) typically starts in the sixth or seventh decade of life and is rapidly progressive, with 50% of the patients dying in 6–9 months. The disease is particularly common in persons who received growth hormone extracted from the pituitary when they were children. Clinically, CJD manifests in three stages. In stage 1 there is fatigue, insomnia, depression, anxiety, and unpredictable behavior. In the next stage dementia, myoclonic jerks, cerebellar ataxia, aphasia, blindness, and brain stem involvement are evident, and in

the final stage the patient enters into a vegetative state, coma, and finally death. The CT may show cortical atropy or no significant change, while EEG shows a characteristic pattern, with periodic bursts of polyspike and wave activity, enabling the clinician to make a correct diagnosis.[126] Pathologic findings include prominent astrocytes and spongiform changes involving the cerebral cortex. CJD has been shown to be infectious, and can be transmitted by corneal grafts.[127]

Meningitis
Chronic meningitis – bacterial, parasitic, or fungal – may present with a dementia syndrome, cranial nerve palsies, and raised intacranial pressure.[128] Diagnosis is made by cerebrospinal fluid examination and treatment is according to the specific agent identified.

Normal pressure hydrocephalus
The etiology of the disease is not known, but there is a history of subarachnoid bleeding (ruptured aneurysm) in one-third of patients. The classic presentation is a triad of dementia, gait abnormality, and urinary incontinence. Normal pressure hydrocephalus is associated with depressive symptoms and apathy, and rarely with psychosis.[129,130]

On CT scan there is ventricular enlargement with disproportionate enlargement of frontal and temporal horns compared to the posterior and lateral horns. There are no randomized control trials for shunt placement but there are some case-reports. Thomas and Borgeson[131] reported a better outcome if the cause of normal pressure hydrocephalus is known, and there is a short history and an absence of gyral atropy. Persons whose gait improves after removal of 120 ml of cerebrospinal fluid also do better after shunting.

Dementia caused by head injury
Traumatic brain injury causes dementia in both young and older adults. About 500 000 individuals are hospitalized in the USA for head injuries. About 70 000 to 90 000 of these will develop long-term disabilities.[132] Dementia after head injury results from diffuse axonal injury from shearing

forces, focal contusion, hemorrhage, laceration, and hypoxic insults. Even patients without loss of consciousness after head injury develop cognitive impairment.[133] Traumatic contusion affects the anterior temporal and inferior frontal lobes, while diffuse axonal injury affects the subcortical white matter, the mesencephalon, and the diencepahalon.

In boxers dementia occurs because of repeated head blows. This dementia is associated with ataxia and is termed dementia pugilistica.[134] Pathologic findings include diffuse brain atrophy, ventricular dilatation, and deep pigmentation of the substantia nigra. Neuroimaging is important to identify the pathologic condition of most dementia secondary to trauma.

Evaluation

The components of evaluation include history and physical examination and laboratory tests. If these are inconclusive specialized testing is indicated.

History and physical examination are important parts of the diagnostic assessment.[135,136] Historical information should be obtained from the patient, family members, nurses in case of nursing homes, and social workers. The history should document the onset of the dementing illness and a detailed past medical history, including specific diseases, injuries, operations, hospitalizations, psychiatric disorders, alcohol and substance abuse, nutrition, and exposure to environmental toxins. It is important to obtain a family history in patients who have symptoms of dementia or depression or any other psychiatric problems. Social history should be obtained, with regard to specific events that may affect the emotional state of the patient. It is very important to obtain a detailed history of medications, both prescription and over-the-counter medications. It is good practice to ask a patient to bring all their medications for each clinic visit. It is important to recognize and treat reversible causes of dementia by adding a complete blood count, battery of chemical tests, and thyroid function test to the history and physical examination.[135] In approximately 90% of cases the diagnosis of AD is made on general medical and psychiatric evaluation.[137] Tools such as the Functional Activity Questionnaire[138] and Revised

Memory and Behavior Problem Checklist[139] are two important instruments that help determine lapses in memory and language use, and the ability to read and retain new information, handle complex information, and demonstrate sound judgment.

The physician should also perform a comprehensive physical examination including a neurologic and mental status examination. A brief screening of cognitive function can be performed, using for example the Saint Louis University Mental Status Examination (SLUMS),[140] the MMSE,[72] or the Informant Questionnaire on Cognition.[141] Patients with a lower educational level will score low on the MMSE and a higher educational level may give normal scores even if the patient is impaired. It is well known that the MMSE is not very sensitive in detecting mild neurocognitive disorder. The SLUMS has been validated and it is a more effective screening tool in detecting mild neurocognitive disorder and dementia. It is probably important to consider neuropsychologic testing in patients with a higher educational level and minimum cognitive impairment. It is also important to look for depression in the elderly population using a geriatric depression scale, as depression can mimic dementia; use of the Cornell Scale of Depression is recommended for the demented patient.[142] Delirium is also common in elderly hospitalized patients with dementia, thus an episode of delirium should prompt an evaluation for dementia.[91,143] Causes of delirium can be remembered using the mnemonic: D-E-L-I-R-I-U-M-S:

Drugs
Emotions (depression)
Low O_2 states (myocardial infarction, pulmonary embolism, CVA)
Infection
Retention of urine or feces
Ictal (seizure)
Undernutrition, dehydration, electrolyte disorders
Metabolic disorders (thyroid, vitamin B_{12}, massive organ failure)
Subdural hematoma

Laboratory evaluation generally includes a complete blood count, blood chemistry, liver function tests, serological test for syphilis, and determination of thyroid function testing and B$_{12}$ levels.[144] Other laboratory tests should be ordered as indicated by history and physical examination. Elevated serum homocysteine levels are considered by some to be a sensitive indicator for cognitive impairment[145,146] but in a cross-sectional study increased homocysteine levels were found to be very common in centenarians, probably because of vitamin deficiencies and decreased renal clearance, but they were not associated with cognitive impairment.[147] Apolipoprotein E genotyping does not provide sufficient sensitivity or specificity to be used alone as a diagnostic test for Alzheimer's disease.[148] Other laboratory tests should be ordered when directed by history and physical examination, e.g. HIV testing would be appropriate if the patient has risk factors for HIV infection.

Imaging studies are optional but recommended by most experts. A non-contrast CT scan of the head is adequate in most instances, especially if no reversible causes of dementia can be identified and there are focal neurologic signs of short duration. Magnetic resonance imaging is better for vascular dementia but white matter changes revealed by T$_2$-weighted images are not generally related to dementia and should not be overinterpreted.[135,136,149] Vascular dementia is probably overdiagnosed.[150] If the initial work-up is negative and there is progressive cognitive decline a repeat assessment is recommended in 6 months. Functional imaging studies, such as positron emission tomography and single-photon emission CT (SPECT), may show the characteristic parietal and temporal deficits in AD or widespread irregular deficits in vascular dementia,[151,152] and are usually recommended when CT/MRI is/are negative and the diagnosis of AD is still suspected.[153] Some patients diagnosed with vascular dementia are found on autopsy to have AD. However, cerebrovascular disease may contribute to the severity of the cognitive symptoms of AD.[154] Potentially reversible dementias are uncommon.[155]

Pharmacologic treatment

Cholinesterase inhibitors

Tacrine is a centrally acting aminoacridine with reversible non-specific cholinesterase inhibitor activity. In approximately 2000 patients with mild to moderate AD, between 20 and 30% showed an observable improvement compared with placebo, representing on average 6 months of deterioration.[156] The side-effects were frequent gastrointestinal distress and cholinergic effects, and 30% had elevation of serum transaminase.[157] The starting dose is 10 mg four times a day to a maximum of 40 mg four times a day. This drug is no longer recommended for use.

Donepezil, a second-generation cholinesterase inhibitor, has a longer duration of inhibitory activity and greater specificity for brain tissue. There have been eight randomized control trials involving 2664 participants. In selected patients with mild to moderate AD treated for a period of 12, 24, or 54 weeks, donepezil produced modest improvement in cognitive function. No improvement was present in patients' self-assessed quality of life. A 5 mg dose of donepezil was better tolerated than 10 mg in these trials.[158] One study addressed the cost-effectiveness of donepezil and showed it to be cost neutral over a 6-month period.[142]

Rivastigmine is a cholinesterase inhibitor and is used in 60 countries. There have been seven randomized control trials involving 3370 participants. Rivastigmine is associated with mild to moderate improvement in AD. Improvement is seen in cognitive functions, activities of daily living, and severity of dementia with daily dose of 6 to 12 mg. Adverse effects are mostly cholinergic in nature.[159] Studies have shown rivastigmine to be cost saving with regard to the direct cost of caring for patients with AD after 2 years of treatment.[160,161]

Galantamine is a specific, competitive, and reversible aceylcholinesterase inhibitor, and is currently available in Sweden and Austria. Seven randomized control trials have been carried out, with six being phase II or III industry-sponsored multicenter studies. In all these trials 8 mg of galantamine was consistently associated with significant benefits. Galantamine has shown positive effects in trials of 3 months, 5 months, and 6 months. There is evidence demonstrating the efficacy of galantamine on global rating, cognitive function, activities of daily living, and behavior. The cognitive effects of donepezil, rivastigmine, and tacrine are comparable.

The main side-effects are cholinergically mediated gastrointestinal side-effects, but the whole side-effect profile is not available.[162]

N-Methyl-D-aspartase receptor antagonist

Memantine is an antagonist to glutamate N-methyl-D-aspartase (NMDA) receptors, and may prevent excitatory neurotoxicity in dementia. A meta-analysis by the Cochrane Database suggested a small beneficial effect of memantine at 6 months in moderate to severe AD. This effect was seen in the areas of cognition, activities of daily living, and behavior, supported by a clinical impression of change. The beneficial effect on cognition in patients with mild to moderate vascular dementia was not detectable on global assessment at 6 months. The effect of memantine on mild to moderate AD is unknown.[163]

Antioxidants

There has been one randomized control trial of vitamin E.[164] The primary outcome used in this study of 341 participants was survival time to the first of four end-points: death, institutionalization, loss of two out of three basic activities of daily living, or severe dementia, defined as a global Clinical Dementia Rating of 3. There appeared to be some benefit from vitamin E with fewer participants reaching end-point – 58% (45/77) of completers compared with 74% on placebo. However, more participants taking vitamin E suffered a fall (15.6% compared with 5%). It was not possible to interpret the reported results for specific end-points or for secondary outcomes of cognition, dependence, behavioral disturbance, and activities of daily living. There is insufficient evidence of efficacy of vitamin E in the treatment of people with AD. The one published trial[164] was restricted to patients with moderate disease, and the published results are difficult to interpret, although there is sufficient evidence of possible benefit to justify further studies. There was an excess of falls in the vitamin E group compared with placebo that requires further evaluation. Animal studies suggest that alpha-lipoic acid may be more effective antioxidant than vitamin E for treating persons with dementia. A recent review

by the Cochrane Database has suggested that there is insufficient evidence of the efficacy of vitamin E in the treatment of people with AD.[165]

Alpha lipoic acid

Alpha lipoic acid (ALA) is an endogenous antioxidant that interrupts cellular oxidative processes in both its oxidized and reduced forms. These properties might qualify ALA for a modulator role in the treatment of people with dementia. A systematic search by the Cochrane Group concluded that there are no randomized double-blind placebo-controlled trials investigating ALA for dementia. Currently no evidence exists of the exploration of any potential effects, thus at this time ALA cannot be recommended for people with dementia.[166]

Selective monoamine oxidase-B inhibitors

In a meta-analysis of 15 trials, most of them examined the effect of selegiline on cognition and 12 of them also explored mood and behavioral aspects. The data showed improvement in cognitive function, mood, and behavior, although the global rating scale showed no effects of selegiline. The conclusion from the analysis was that selegiline has beneficial effects on patients with AD but there is still not enough evidence to recommend its use in routine clinical practice.[167]

Other agents
Hydergine for dementia

Currently hydergine is used almost exclusively for treating patients with either dementia or age-related cognitive decline. In a meta-analysis of 19 trials, hydergine was well tolerated by 78% of the randomized subjects who were available for analysis. In this review it was concluded that hydergine showed significant treatment effects when assessed by global rating or comprehensive rating scales. There is a limited number of trials available for subgroup analysis to identify significant moderating effects. The main limitation with the randomized control trials was that most of the data were published before 1984 when there were no standardized diagnostic criteria. As a result uncertainty remains regarding the use of hydergine.[168,169]

Gingko biloba *extract*

In a 52-week, randomized, double-blind, placebo-controlled, parallel-group, multicenter study, mild to severely demented outpatients with AD or multi-infarct dementia, without other significant medical conditions, received either treatment with *Gingko biloba* extract (120 mg/day) or placebo. *Gingko biloba* extract was safe and appears capable of stabilizing and, in a number of cases, improving the cognitive performance and the social functioning of demented patients for 6 months to 1 year.[170]

In a 26-week trial for the treatment of AD and multi-infarct dementia a dose of 120 mg of *Gingko biloba* extract (EGb) was used. Intent to treat analysis was performed. The primary outcome measures included the Alzheimer's Disease Assessment Scale-Cognitive Subscale (ADAS-Cog), Geriatric Evaluation by Relative's Rating Instrument (GERRI), and Clinical Global Impression of Change. Of 309 patients, 244 (76% for placebo and 73% for EGb) actually reached the 26th week visit for intent to treat analysis. Mean treatment differences favored EGb with 1.3 and 0.12 points, respectively, on the ADAS-Cog ($P=0.04$) and the GERRI ($P=0.007$). In the group receiving EGb, 26% of the patients achieved at least a 4-point improvement on the ADAS-Cog, compared to 17% with placebo ($P=0.04$). On the GERRI, 30% of the EGb group improved and 17% worsened, while the placebo group showed an opposite trend, with 37% of patients worsening and 25% improving ($P=0.006$). Regarding safety, no differences between EGb and placebo were observed.[171]

Overall there is promising evidence of improvement in cognition and function associated with *Ginkgo*. However, the three later trials show inconsistent results. There is a need for a large trial using modern methodology and permitting an intent to treat analysis to provide robust estimates of the size and mechanism of any treatment effects.[172]

Nimodipine

The usefulness of nimodipine in patients with AD, vascular dementia, or unspecified dementia is still controversial. Two trials have included patients with AD, nine trials included patients with CVD (cerebrovascular disease), and three trials included patients with AD, CVD, and mixed disease. Nine trials (2492 patients) covered the domains of cognitive function, activities of daily living, global clinical state, safety, and tolerability. By pooling available data from all trials, a benefit was found to be associated with nimodipine (90 mg/day at 12 weeks) compared with placebo on clinical global impression and cognitive function scales, but not on scales assessing activities of daily living. This effect was seen with both AD an vascular dementia trials. The short-term benefits of nimodipine do not qualify this drug for long-term use in dementia. New research must focus on longer-term outcomes.[173]

Melatonin

It has been suggested that there is a relationship between decline of melatonin function and the symptoms of dementia. The Cochrane Database reviewed three studies which met the inclusion criteria and showed non-significant effects from the pooled estimates of changes in MMSE and ADAS-Cog scores. Individual study estimates for treatment effect demonstrated a significant improvement for melatonin compared with placebo in behavioral and affective symptoms with 2.5 mg/day (SR) melatonin, but not with 10 mg/day. The remainder of the treatment affects behavior, and activities of daily living were non-significant. Currently there is insufficient evidence to support the effectiveness of melatonin in managing the cognitive and non-cognitive sequelae of dementia.[174]

Estrogen

There is little evidence regarding the effect of HRT (hormonal replacement therapy) or ERT (estrogen replacement therapy) on overall cognitive function in healthy postmenopausal women. There is an effect in young women and surgically menopausal women on some verbal memory functions (immediate recall), on a test of abstract reasoning, and on a test of speed and accuracy. It is not known at this time whether factors such as older age, type of menopause (surgical or natural) and type of treatment (E_2 with or without a progestagen), mode of delivery (transdermal, oral, or intramuscular), dosage, and duration (>3 months) can alter the effect on memory functions to a clinically relevant level.[175]

Propentofylline

Propentofylline is a novel therapeutic agent for dementia that readily crosses the blood–brain barrier and acts by blocking the uptake of adenosine and inhibiting the enzyme phosphodiesterase. Currently there is limited evidence that propentofylline might benefit cognition, global function, and activities of daily living of people with AD and/or vascular dementia.[176]

Lecithin

Patients with AD have been found to lack the enzyme responsible for converting choline into acetylcholine within the brain. Lecithin is a major dietary source of choline, so extra consumption may reduce the progression of dementia. A meta-analysis by the Cochrane group suggested that the evidence from randomized trials does not support the use of lecithin in the treatment of patients with dementia at this time.[177]

Acetyl-l-carnitine

Acetyl-l-carnitine (ALC) is derived from carnitine and is described as having several properties which may be beneficial in dementia, such as activity at cholinergic neurons, membrane stabilization, and enhancing mitochondrial function. ALC has a beneficial effect on the clinical global impression scale as a categoric measure and on the MMSE at 24 weeks, but there is no evidence from objective assessments in any other area of outcome. At present there is no evidence to recommend its routine use in clinical practice.[178]

Other drugs

The use of non-steroidal anti-inflammatory drugs (NSAIDs) and estrogen for the treatment of AD is supported by epidemiologic studies but not confirmed by prospective trials. There are no generally accepted benefits for lecithin, chelation therapy, or choline.

Currently most clinicians use aspirin for cognitive impairment in vascular dementia, though the literature lacks any evidence to support the effectiveness of aspirin in the treatment of vascular dementia. Further research is required to assess the effectiveness of aspirin on cognition, behavior, and quality of life.[179]

Antidepressants are recommended when depressive symptoms are present. Treatment of depression includes non-pharmacologic and pharmacologic approaches. The choice of antidepressant should be used based on the side-effect profile and the patient's general and medical condition. Selective serotonin re-uptake inhibitors, tricyclic antidepressants, and monoamine oxidase A inhibitors can be used. All have different side-effect profiles.

In the middle or later stages of dementia about 50% of patients exhibit agitation,[180] while psychosis is less common. A meta-analysis has shown that antipsychotic drugs can produce modest improvement in some behavioral symptoms in dementia[181] and may be most effective in psychotic symptoms.[182] Evidence suggests that risperidone and clozapine are effective at very low doses in the treatment of agitation and psychosis in elderly patients.[183,184] Some of the newer atypical antipsychotics are sertindole, quetiapine, and ziprazadone. Clinical trials show comparable efficacies among the antipsychotic drugs, therefore clinicians should base the use of such drugs on their side-effect profile. The high-potency antipsychotic drugs should be used with caution because they can cause parkinsonian symptoms, sedation, postural hypotension, and anticholinergic effects. Tardive dyskinesia and neuroleptic malignant syndrome are reported with typical antipsychotics and risperidone, but not with clozapine.[185] However, clozapine can cause anticholinergic effects and requires blood monitoring for agranulocytosis.

Benzodiazepines are also used for the treatment of behavioral symptoms, particularly anxiety, associated with dementia. The short-acting benzodiazepines such as oxazepam and lorazepam are preferred over the long-acting benzodiazepines, but the latter are associated with adverse affects.[186] Other drugs used include the anticonvulsants carbamazepine[187] and valproate;[188] the hydroxytryptophan modulator trazodone;[189] buspirone;[190] and SSRIs.[191]

Role of testosterone replacement and cognition

In a randomized, double-blind, placebo-controlled study, Cherrier et al studied the efficacy of testosterone supplementation on cognition in men with

AD or mild cognitive impairment (MCI).[192] The age range was from 63 to 85 years; 15 subjects had AD and 17 had MCI. The duration of the study was 6 weeks, with weekly intramuscular injections of 100 mg testosterone enanthate ($n=19$) or placebo ($n=13$). A battery of neuropsychologic tests was conducted at baseline, week 3, and week 6 of treatment, and again after 6 weeks. The testosterone replacement group showed improvements in spatial memory, constructional abilities, and verbal memory. No changes were noted for selective and divided attention or language.

Cherrier et al also studied the effect of the conversion of testosterone to estradiol on cognitive processing in healthy older men who received testosterone supplementation.[193] The study comprised sixty community-dwelling volunteers aged 50 to 90 years. Participants were randomized to receive weekly intramuscular injections of 100 mg testosterone enanthate plus a daily oral placebo pill ($n=20$), 100 mg testosterone enanthate plus 1 mg daily of anastrozole, an aromatase inhibitor that blocks the conversion of testosterone to estradiol ($n=19$), or saline injection and a placebo pill ($n=21$) for 6 weeks. Batteries of neuropsychologic tests were conducted at baseline, week 3, and week 6 of treatment, and after 6 weeks of wash-out. It was concluded from this study that, in healthy older men, improvement in verbal memory induced by testosterone administration depends on the aromatization of testosterone to estradiol, whereas improvement in spatial memory occurs in the absence of increases in estradiol.

Transcutaneous electrical nerve stimulation

Transcutaneous electrical nerve stimulation (TENS) is the application of an electrical current through electrodes attached to the skin. The commonest clinical application of TENS is in pain control, but it is also used occasionally for the treatment of a range of neurologic and psychiatric conditions including drug and alcohol dependence, headaches, and depression. TENS is rarely used for the treatment of dementia. However, a number of studies carried out in the Netherlands and in Japan suggest that TENS applied to the back or head may improve cognition and behavior in patients with AD or multi-infarct dementia. The Cochrane Group Database review suggests that TENS may produce short-lived improvements in some neuropsychologic or behavioral aspects of dementia.[194] The currently available data from these studies do not allow definite conclusions to be made on the possible benefits of this intervention – larger studies are needed.

Non-pharmacologic treatment

It is important that dementia patients take regular exercise and maintain adequate caloric intake.[195,196] Techniques proposed to restore cognitive dysfunction include reality orientation and memory retraining.[197] Individual and group therapies focused on emotional aspects such as pleasant events and stimulation-oriented treatment are examples of psychosocial treatments that may influence depressive symptoms.

Managing patients with Alzheimer's disease is a great challenge and importance should be given to a safe environment and functional independence. The most important principles are to keep regular follow-up appointments, review medication, screen for sleep problems, identify early behavioral and medical problems, and work closely with the family or caregivers. It is very important to discuss with the family and patient early in the disease the treatment options, including the need for a 'living will' and advance directives as well as long-term care placement. It is helpful for the family to be aware of the progression of the disease, including memory problems, and emotional and behavioral symptoms. Studies have shown that information and emotional support enhance the quality of life for the patient and caregivers, and delays placement in long-term care facilities.[198] Programs should be established to improve patient behavior and mood and they should be encouraged to attend family events on a regular basis. Environmental modulation is important and moderate stimulation is the best. It is necessary to explain to the family that overstimulation can cause agitation and understimulation can cause withdrawal. For the mildly demented individual it is important to be in contact with the world by electronic media and reminders of time can be achieved by displaying the time and calendars and list of daily tasks. Close attention should be paid to safety to prevent injury by the use of electronic alarm guards and door locks to prevent wandering. It is also important to have a discussion with the family regarding driving skills; if the patient is getting lost in familiar surroundings this may signal that driving is unsafe. Incontinence is also a great burden and frequent toileting and prevention of bedsores need to be addressed. Most family members are unaware of the concept of hospice, which needs to be addressed early in the course of the disease. Finally, the family should be made aware of the available resources, including specialist careworkers such as gerontologists, neurologists, geriatric psychiatrists, psychologists, and social workers.

References

1. Mejia S, Pineda D, Alvarez LM. Individual differences in memory and executive function abilities during normal aging. Int J Neurosci 1999; 95: 271–84.
2. Butler SM, Ashford JW, Snowdon DA. Age, education, and changes in the Mini-Mental State Exam score of older women: findings from the Nun Study. Am J Geriatr Soc 1996; 44: 675–81.
3. Jorm AF, Korten AE, Henderson AS. The prevalence of dementia: a quantitative integration of the literature. Acta Psychiatr Scand 1987; 76: 465.
4. Ganguli M, Seaberg E, Belle S. Cognitive impairment and the use of health services in an elderly rural population: the MoVIES project. J Am Geriatr Soc 1993; 41: 1065.
5. Advisory Panel on Alzheimer's disease. Alzheimer's disease related dementias: acute and long-term care services. NIH Publication 96-4136. Washington, DC: US Dept of Health and Human Services, 1996.
6. Evans DA. Estimated prevalence of Alzheimer's disease in the US. Milbank Q 1990; 68: 267–89.
7. Benton AL, Eslinger PJ, Damasio R. Normative observation on neuropsychological tests performance in old age. J Clin Neuropsychol 1981; 3: 33.
8. Jacqmin-Gadda H, Fabrigoule C, Commenges D. A 5 year longitudinal study of Mini-Mental State Examination in normal aging. Am J Epidemiol 1997; 145: 498–506.
9. Laird NM, Ware JH. Random-effects models for longitudinal data. Biometrics 1982; 38: 963–74.
10. Liang KY, Zeger SL. Longitudinal data analysis using generalized. Biometrika 1986; 73: 13–22.
11. Zeger SL, Liang KY. Longitudinal data analysis for discrete and continuous outcomes. Biometrics 1986; 42: 121–30.
12. Morris MC, Evans DA, Hebert LE. Methodological issues in the study of cognitive decline. 1999; 149: 9: 789–93.
13. Guildford JP, Fruchter B. Fundamental Statistics in Psychology and Education, 6th edn. New York: McGraw-Hill Book Company, 1978.
14. Cunningham WR. Intellectual abilities and age. In: Schaie KW, ed. Annual Review of Gerontology and Geriatrics. New York: Springer, 1987: 117–134.
15. Eisdorfer C, Wilke F. Intellectual changes with advancing age. In: Jarvik LF, Eisdorfer C, eds. Intellectual Functioning in Adults. New York: Springer, 1973: 21–9.
16. Schaie KW. Internal validity threats in studies of adult cognitive development. In: Howe ML, ed. Cognitive Development in Adulthood: Progress in Cognitive Development Research. New York: Springer-Verlag, 1988: 241–72.
17. Horn JL, Cattell RB. Age differences in fluid and crystallized intelligence. Acta Psycho Biol 1967; 26: 107.
18. Christensen H, Mackinnon A, Jorm AF. Age differences and interindividual variation in cognition in community-dwelling elderly. Psychol Aging 1994; 9: 381.
19. Kaufman AS, Horn JL. Age changes on test of fluid and crystallized ability for women and men on the Kaufman Adolescent and Adult Intelligence Test (KAIT) at age 17–94 years. Arch Clin Neuropsychol 1996; 11: 97.
20. Czaja SJ, Sharit J. Age differences in the performance of computer-based work. Psychol Aging 1993; 8: 59–67.
21. Birren JE, Fisher LM. Aging and slowing of behavior: consequences for cognition and survival. Nebr Symp Motiv 1991; 38: 1.
22. Fleishmann UM. Cognition in humans and the borderline to dementia. Life Sci 1994; 55: 2051.
23. Salthouse TA. The processing-speed theory of adult age differences in cognition. Psychol Rev 103: 104, 1996
24. Wechsler B. Manual for the Wechsler Adult intelligence Scale – Revised. New York: The Psychological Corp, 1981.
25. Hultsch DF, Hertzog C, Small BJ. Short-term longitudinal changes in cognitive performance in later life. Psychol Aging 1992; 7: 571–84.
26. McEvoy GM, Casico WF. Cumulative evidence of the relationship between employee age and job performance. J App Psychol 1989; 74: 11–17.
27. Bohannon RW. Comfortable and maximum walking of adults aged 20–79 years. Reference values and determinants. Age Ageing 1997; 26: 15.

28. Ruff RM, Parker SB. Gender- and age-specific changes in motor speed and eye–hand coordination in adults: normative values for finger tapping and grooved Pegboard test. Percept Mot Skills 1993; 76: 1219.

29. Lorge I. The influence of the test upon the nature of mental decline as a function of age. J Educ Psychol 1936; 27: 100.

30. Anderer P, Semlitsch HV, Saletu B. Multichannel auditory event-related brain potentials: Effects of normal age on the scalp distribution of N1, P2, N2 and P300 latencies and amplitudes. Electroencephalogr Clin Neurophysiol 1996; 99: 458.

31. Gilmore R. Evoked potentials in the elderly. J Clin Neurophysiol 1993; 12: 132.

32. Schofield PW, Marder K, Dooneief G. Association of subjective memory complaints with subsequent cognitive decline in community-dwelling elderly individuals with baseline cognitive impairment. Am J Psychiatry 1997; 154: 609.

33. Small GW, La Rue A, Komo S. Mnemonics usage and cognitive decline in age-associated memory impairment. Int Psychogeriatr 1997; 9: 47.

34. Jonker C, Launer LJ, Hooijer C. Memory complaints and memory impairment in older individuals. J Am Geriatr Soc 1996; 44: 44.

35. Barker A, Prior J, Roy J. Memory complaints in attenders at a self-referral memory clinic: the role of cognitive factors, affective symptoms and personality. Int J Geriatr Psychiatry 1995; 10: 777.

36. Craik FIM. Age differences in human memory. In Handbook of the Psychology of Aging. Birren JE, Schaie KW, eds. New York, Van Nostrand Reinhold, 1997; 384–20.

37. Botwinick J. Intellectual abilities. In Handbook of the Psychology of Aging. Birren JE, Schaie KW, eds. New York, Van Nostrand Reinhold, 1997; 580–05.

38. Craik FIM, Byrd M. Patterns of memory loss in three elderly samples. Psychol Aging 1987; 2: 79.

39. Wahlin A, Beckman L. Free recall and recognition of slowly and rapidly presented words in very old age: a community-based study. Exp Aging Res 1995; 21: 251.

40. Nilsson L-G, Backman L. The Betula prospective cohort study: memory, health, and aging. Aging Neuropsychol Cogn 1997; 4: 1.

41. Perlmutter M. What is memory aging the aging of ? Dev Psychol 1978; 14: 330.

42. Backman L, Nilsson L-G. Semantic memory functioning across the adult life span. Eur Psychol 1996; 1: 27.

43. Jelicic M, Craik FIM, Moscovitch M. Effects of aging on different explicit and implicit memory tasks. Eur J Cogn Psychol 1996; 8: 225.

44. Schugens MM, Daum I, Spinder M. Differential effects of aging on explicit and implicit memory. Aging Neuropsychol Cogn 1997; 4: 33.

45. La Rue A, Bank L. Health in old age: how do physicians rating and self-rating compare? J Gerontol 1979; 8: 108.

46. Monge R, Hultsch D. Paired associate learning as a function of age and length of anticipation and inspection intervals. J Gerontol 1971; 26: 157–62.

47. Light LL, Zelinski EM, Moore M. Adult age difference in reasoning from new information. J Exp Psychol Learn Cognition 1982; 8: 435–47.

48. Scogin F, Bienas JL. A three year follow up of older adults participating in a memory skills training program. Psychol Aging 1988; 3: 334–37.

49. Boyarsky RE, Eisdorfer C. Forgetting in older persons. J Gerontol 1988; 27: 254–58.

50. CHABA. Speech understanding and aging. J Acoust Soc Am 1988; 83: 859–895.

51. Jacobs-Condit L, ed. Gerontology and Communication Disorders. Rockville MD: American Speech-Language-Hearing Association, 1984.

52. Humes LE, Watson BU. Factors associated with individual differences in clinical measures of speech recognition among the elderly. J Speech Hear Res 1994; 37: 464–74.

53. Humus LE. Speech understanding in the elderly. J Am Acad Audiol 1996; 7: 161–7.

54. Madden DJ. Adult age differences in the effects of sentence context and stimulus degradation during visual word recognition. Psychol Aging 1988; 3: 167–72.

55. Laver GD, Burke DM. Why do semantic priming effects increase in old age? A meta-analysis. Psychol Aging 1993; 8: 34–43.

56. Hartley J. Aging and individual differences in memory for written disclosure. In: Language, Memory and Aging. New York: Cambridge University Press, 1988: 36–57.

57. Burke DM, Harrold RM. Automatic and effortful semantic process in old age. Experimental and naturalistic approaches. In: Language, Memory and Age. New York: Cambridge University Press, 1988: 100–16.

58. Wingfield A, Alexander AH, Cavigelli S. Does memory constrain utilization of top-down information in spoken word recognition? Evidence from normal aging. Lang Speech 1994; 37: 221–35.

59. Pichora-Fuller MK, Scheider BA. How young and old adults listen to noise. J Acoust Soc Am 1995; 97: 593–608.

60. Hutchinson KM. Influence of sentence context on speech perception in young and older adults. J Gerontol 1989; 44: 36–44.

61. Sommers MS. The structural organization of the mental lexicon and its contribution to age-related

changes in spoken word recognition. Psychol Aging 1996; 11: 333–41.

62. Mullennix JW, Pisoni DB, Martin CS. Some effects of talker variability on spoken word recognition. J Acoust Soc Am 1989; 85: 365–78.

63. Peterson GE, Barney HL. Control methods used in a study of the vowels. J Acoust Soc Am 1952; 24: 175–84.

64. Lezak MD. The problem of accessing executive functions. Int J Psychol 1981; 17: 281–97.

65. American Psychiatric Association. Diagnostic and Statistics Manual of Mental Disorders, 4th edn. Washington, DC: American Psychiatric Association, 1994.

66. Mega MS, Cummings JL. Frontal-subcortical circuits and neuropsychiatric disorders. J Neuropsychiatry 1994; 6: 358–70.

67. Daigneault S, Brian CMG. Early effects of normal aging on preservatives and non-preservatives pre-frontal measures. Dev Neuropsychol 1992; 8: 99–114.

68. Kuhl DE. The effects of normal aging patterns of local cerebral glucose utilization. Ann Neurol 1984; 15: 133–7.

69. Fogel BS, Brock D, Goldscheider F. Cognitive dys-function and the need for long term care: implica-tion for public policy. Washington, DC: American Association of Retired Persons, 1994.

70. Royall DR, Mahurin RK. Bedside assessment of dementia type using qualitative evaluation of dementia (QED). Neuropsychiatry Neuropsychol Behav Neurol 1993; 6: 235–44.

71. Royall DR, Mahurin RK, Gray K. Bedside assess-ment of executive cognitive impairment. The exec-utive interview (EXIT). J Am Geriatr Soc 1992; 40: 1221–6.

72. Folstein M, Folstein S, McHugh PR. Mini-mental state: a practical method for grading the cognitive state of patients for the clinicians. Psychiatry Res 1975; 12: 89–98.

73. Nelson A, Fogel BS, Faust D. Bedside cognitive screening instruments: a critical assessment. J Nerv Ment Dis 1986; 174: 73–84.

74. Royall DR, Cordes JA, Polk M. CLOX: an execu-tive clock drawing test. J Neurol Neurosurg Psychiatry 1998; 64: 588–94.

75. Ainslie NK, Murden RA. Effect of education on the clock drawing dementia screen in non-demented elderly persons. J Am Geriatr Soc 1993; 41: 249–52.

76. Shaw TG, Mortel KF, Meyer JS. Cerebral blood flow changes in benign aging and cerebrovascular dis-ease. Neurology 1995; 34: 855–62.

77. Dempster FN. The rise and fall of inhibitory mech-anism: towards a unified theory of cognitive devel-opment and aging. Develop Rev 1992; 12: 45–75.

78. Cummings JL. Subcortical Dementia. New York: Oxford University Press, 1990.

79. Lemsky CM, Smith G, Malec JF. Identifying risk for functional impairment using cognitive measures: an application of CART modeling. Neuropsychology 1996; 10: 368–75.

80. DeBettignies FN, Mahurin RK. Insight for impair-ment in independent living skill in Alzheimer's dis-ease and multi-infarct dementia. J Clin Exp Neuropsychol 1990; 12: 355–63.

81. Carlson MC, Linda FP. Association between executive attention and physical performance in community-dwelling old women. J Gerontol 1999; 54; 5: S262–70.

82. Royall DR, Cabello M. Executive dyscontrol: an important factor affecting the level of care received by older retirees. J Am Geriatr Soc 1998; 46: 1519–24.

83. Ritchie K, Kildea D. Is senile dementia age related or aging related? Evidence from meta-analysis of dementia prevalence in the oldest old. Lancet 1995; 346: 931–34.

84. Bachman DL, Wolf PA, Linn RT. Incidence of dementia and probable Alzheimer's disease in a gen-eral population: the Framingham study. Neurology 1993; 43: 515–19.

85. Jorm AF. The epidemiology of Alzheimer's disease and related disorders. London: Chapman & Hall: 1990.

86. National Institute of Aging. Progress Report on Alzheimer's Disease 1996. Bethesda, MD: NIH Publication 1996; 96-4137.

87. Ernst RL, Hay JW. The US economic and social cost of Alzheimer's disease revisited. Am J Pub Health 1994; 84: 1261–64.

88. Schulz R, O'Brien AT. Psychiatric and physical morbidity effects of dementia caregiving: preva-lence, correlates, and causes. Gerontologist 1995; 35: 771–91.

89. Mega MS, Cummings JL. The spectrum of behav-ioral changes in Alzheimer's disease. Neurology 1996; 46: 130–35.

90. Stern Y, Alpert M. Utility of extrapyramidal signs and psychosis as a predictor of cognitive and func-tional decline, nursing home admission and death in Alzheimer's disease: prospective analysis from the Predictors Study. Neurology 1994; 44: 2300–7.

91. Lerner AJ, Hedera P, Koss E. Delirium in Alzheimer's disease. Alzheimer's Dis Assoc Disord 1997; 11: 16–20.

92. Alexopoulos GS, Meyers BS. The course of geriatric depression with reversible dementia: a controlled study. Am J Psychiatry 1993; 150: 1693–99.

93. Jung R, Solomon K. Psychiatric manifestation of Pick's disease. Int Psychogeriat 1993; 5: 187–202.

94. Mendez MF, Doss RC, Cherrier MM. Use of the cognitive estimations test to discriminate fronto-temporal dementia from Alzheimer's disease. Geriatr Psychiatry Neurol 1998; 11(1): 2–6.

95. Mendez MF, Cherrier M, Perryman KM et al. Frontotemporal dementia versus Alzheimer's disease: differential cognitive features. Neurology 1996; 47(5): 1189–94.

96. Caine ED, Shoulson I. Psychiatric syndromes in Huntington's disease. Am J Psychiatry 1983; 140: 727–33.

97. Hayden MR, Martin AJ. Positron emission tomography in the earlier diagnosis of Huntington's disease. Neurology 1986; 36: 888–94.

98. Martilla RJ. Epidemiology. In: Koller WC, ed. Handbook of Parkinson's Disease. New York: Marcel Dekker, 1976.

99. Cummings JL. Intellectual impairment in Parkinson's disease: clinical, biochemical and pathologic correlates. J Geriatr Psychiatr Neurol 1988; 1: 24–36.

100. Lewin R. Dramatic results with brain graft. Science 1987; 237: 245–7.

101. Forstl H, Burns A, Luthert P. The Lewy-body variant of Alzheimer's disease. Clinical and pathological findings. Br J Psychiatry 1993; 162: 385–92.

102. Kraybill ML, Larson EB, Tsuang DW et al. Cognitive differences in dementia patients with autopsy-verified AD, Lewy body pathology, or both. Neurology 2005; 64(12): 2069–73.

103. Aldrich MS, Foster NL, White RF. Sleep abnormalities in progressive supranuclear palsy. Ann Neurol 1989; 25: 477–581.

104. Mendell JR, Chase TN, Engel WK. Modification by L-dopa of case progressive supranuclear palsy. Lancet 1970; 1: 593–94.

105. Haldman S, Goldman JW, Hyde J. Progressive supranuclear palsy computed tomography, and response to antiParkinson's drugs. Neurology 1982; 31: 442–59.

106. Newman GC. Treatment of progressive supranuclear palsy with tricyclic antidepressants. Neurology 1985; 35: 1189–93.

107. Ermini-Funfschilling D, Stahelin HB. Is prevention of dementia possible? Z Gerontol 1993; 26: 446.

108. Roman GC, Tatemichi TK, Erkinjuntti T. Vascular dementia. diagnostic criteria for research studies. Neurology 1993; 43: 259–60.

109. Thompson TL, Moran MG. Psychotropic drug use in elderly. N Engl Med 1993; 308: 134–8.

110. Flaherty JH. Commonly prescribed and over the counter medication: causes of confusion. Clin Geriatr Med 14(1): 101–27.

111. Cummings JL. Dementia: A Clinical Approach, 2nd edn. Stoneham, MA: Weinemann-Butterworths, 1992.

112. West LJ. Alcoholism. Ann Int Med 1984; 100: 405.

113. Zimberg S. Alcohol abuse among the elderly. In: Carstenson B, Edelstein B, eds. Handbook of Clinical Gerontology. New York: Pergamon, 1987: 57.

114. Cutting J. The relationship between Korsakov's syndrome and alcohol dementia. Br J Psychiatry 1978; 132: 240–51.

115. Ron MA. Brain damage in chronic alcoholism: a neuropathological, neuroradiological, and psychological review. Psychol Med 1977; 7: 103–12.

116. Mach J, Korchik W, Mahowald M. Dialysis dementia, in treatment consideration of Alzheimer's disease and related dementing illness. In: Clinical Geriatric Medicine. Philadelphia, PA: WB Saunders, 1988: 853–68.

117. Avery TL. Seven cases of frontal tumor with psychiatric presentation. Br J Psychiatry 1971; 119: 19–23.

118. Price RW, Brew B, Sidtis J. The brain in AIDS: central nervous system HIV-1 infection and AIDS dementia complex. Science 1987; 239: 586–92.

119. Resnick L, Berger JR. Early blood brain barrier penetration by HIV. Neurology 1988; 38: 9–14.

120. Navia BA, Jordan BD. The AIDS dementia complex, I: clinical features. Ann Neurol 1986; 19: 517–24.

121. Selnes OA, Miller E, McArther J. HIV infection: no evidence of cognitive decline during the asymptomatic stages. Neurology 1990; 40: 204–8.

122. Sidtis JJ, Thaller H, Brew BJ. The interval between equivocal and definite neurological signs and symptoms in the AIDS dementia complex. In abstract of the Fifth International Conference on AIDS. International Development Research Center, Montreal, 1989.

123. Yarchoan R, Berg G, Brouwer P. Responses of human immunodeficiency virus-associated neurological disease to 3-azido-3-deoxythymidine. Lancet 1987; 1: 132–35.

124. Fernandez F, Adams F. Cognitive impairment due to AIDS, related complex, and its response to psychostimulants. Psychosomatics 1988; 29: 38–46.

125. Collings J, Palmer MS. Prion diseases in humans and their relevance to other neurodegenerative diseases. Dementia 1993; 4: 178–85.

126. Brown P, Cathala F, Castaigne P. Creutzfeldt–Jakob disease: clinical analysis of a consecutive series of 230 neuropathologically verified cases. Ann Neurol 1986; 20: 597–602.

127. Gajdusek DC. Unconventional viruses and the origin and the disappearance of kuru. Science 197: 943–60.

128. Mahler ME, Cummings JL. Treatable dementias. West J Med 1987; 146: 705–12.

129. Price TRP, Tucker GJ. Psychiatric and behavioral manifestation of normal pressure hydrocephalus. J Nerv Ment Dis 1977; 164: 51–5.

130. Dewan MJ, Blick A. Normal pressure hydrocephalus and psychiatric patients. Biol Psychiatry 1985; 20: 1127–31.

131. Thomsen AM, Borgeson SE. Prognosis of dementia in normal pressure hydrocephalus after shunt operation. Ann Neurol 1986; 20: 304–10.

132. Goldstein M. Traumatic brain injury, a silent epidemic. Ann Neurol 1990; 27: 327.

133. Cummings JL, Benson DF. A Clinical Approach. Boston, MA: Butterworth-Heinemann, 1992.

134. Corsellis JAN. Post-traumatic dementia. In: Katzman R, Terry RD, eds. Aging: Alzheimer's Disease: Senile Dementia and Related Disorders. New York: Raven Press, 1973: 1.

135. Larson EB. Diagnostic tests in the evaluation of dementia. A prospective study of 200 elderly outpatients. Arch Intern Med 1986; 146: 1917–22.

136. Van Creval H. Early diagnosis of dementia: which tests are indicated? What are their costs? J Neurol 1999; 246: 73–8.

137. Rasmusson DX, Brandt J, Steele C. Accuracy of clinical diagnosis of Alzheimer's disease and clinical features of non-Alzheimer's neuropathology. Alzheimer's Dis Assoc Discord 1996; 10: 180–8.

138. Pfeffer RI, Kurosaki TT. Measurement of functional activities in older adults in the community. J Gerontol 1982; 37: 323–9.

139. Teri L, Truax P, Logsdon R. Assessment of behavior problems in dementia: the revised memory and behavior problems checklist. Psychol Aging 1992; 7: 622–31.

140. Tariq SH, Tumosa N, Chibnall JT, Perry III MH, Morley JE. The Saint Louis University Mental Status (SLUMS) Examination for Detecting Mild Cognitive Impairment and Dementia is more sensitive than Mini Mental Status Examination (MMSE) – a pilot study. J Am Geriatr Psych (in press).

141. ACP Journal Club. Mini-Mental State Examination and the Informant Questionnaire on cognitive decline were efficient screening tests for dementia. Jan-Feb 1997; 2: 25.

142. Alexopoulos GS. Cornell scale for depression in dementia. Biol Psych 1988; 23(3): 271–184.

143. Francis J, Kapoor WN. Prognosis after hospital discharge of older medical outpatients with delirium. J Am Geriatr Soc 1992; 40: 601–6.

144. American Academy of Neurology. Practice parameter for diagnosis and evaluation of dementia: report of the Quality Standards Subcommittee of the American Academy of Neurology. Neurology 1994; 44: 2203–6.

145. Clarke R. Folate, vitamin B-12, and serum total homocysteine levels confirmed Alzheimer's disease. Arch Neurol 1998; 55(1): 1449–55.

146. McCaddon A. Total serum homocysteine in senile dementia of Alzheimer's type. Int Geriatr Psychiatry 1998; 13(4): 235–39.

147. Ravaglia G, Forti P, Maioli F. Elevated plasma homocysteine levels in centenarians are not associated with cognitive impairment. Mech Ageing Dev 2001; 20: 121(1–3): 251.

148. Gertrude H. Utility of the apolipoprotein E genotype in the diagnosis of Alzheimer's disease. Alzheimer's Disease Centers Consortium on Apolipoprotein E and Alzheimer's Disease. N Engl J Med 1998; 338(8): 506–11.

149. Scheltens P. Early diagnosis of dementia: neuroimaging. J Neurol 1990; 246(1): 16–20.

150. Brust JC. Vascular dementia: still over diagnosed. Stroke 1983; 14: 298–300.

151. Herholz K, Adams R, Kesseler J. Criteria for the diagnosis of Alzheimer's disease with positron emission tomography. Dementia 1990; 1: 156–64.

152. Kippenhan JS, Barker WW, Pascal S. Evaluation of neural-network classifier for PET scans of normal and Alzheimer's disease subjects. J Nucl Med 1992; 33: 1459–69.

153. Tamaki N. Image analysis in patients with dementia. Hokkaido Igaku Zasshi 1996; 71(3): 303–7.

154. Snowdon DA, Greiner LH. Brain infarction and the clinical expression of Alzheimer's disease. The Nun Study. JAMA 1997; 277: 813–17.

155. Arnold SE, Kumar A. Reversible dementias. Med Clin North Am 1993; 77: 215–30.

156. Schneider LS. Clinical pharmacology of aminoacridines in Alzheimer's disease. Neurology 1993; 43: S64–S79.

157. Watkins PB, Zimmerman HJ, Knapp MJ. Hepatotoxic effects of tacrine administration in patient with Alzheimer's disease. JAMA 1994; 271: 992–8.

158. Birk JS, Melzer D, Beppu H. Donepezil for mild and moderate Alzheimer's disease. Cochrane Database System Rev, Issue 1, 2006.

159. Birk JS, Grimley Evans J, Iakovidou. Rivastigmine for Alzheimer's disease. Cochrane Database System Rev, Issue 1, 2006.

160. Hauber AB. Saving in the cost of caring for patients with Alzheimer's disease in Canada: an analysis of treatment with rivastigmine. Clin Therapeutic 2000; 22: 439–51.

161. Hauber AB. Potential saving in the cost of caring for Alzheimer's disease: treatment with rivastigmine. Pharmacoeconomics 2000; 17: 351–60.

162. Olin J, Schneider L. Galantamine for Alzheimer's disease. Cochrane Database System Rev, Issue 1, 2001.

163. Areosa Sastre A, Sherriff F, McShane R. Memantine for dementia. Cochrane Database System Rev, Issue 1, 2006.

164. Sano M. A Controlled trial of selegiline, alpha-tocopherol, or both as treatment of Alzheimer's disease. N Engl J Med 1997; 336: 17: 1216–22.

165. Tabet N, Birks J, Grimley Evans J et al. Vitamin E for Alzheimer's disease. Cochrane Database System Rev, Issue 1, 2006.

166. Sauer J, Tabet N, Howard R. Alpha lipoic acid for dementia. Cochrane Database System Rev, Issue 1, 2006.

167. Brick J, Flicker L. Selegiline for Alzheimer's disease. Cochrane Database System Rev, Issue 1, 2001.

168. Olin J, Schneider L. Hydergine for dementia. Cochrane Database System Rev, Issue 1, 2001.

169. Olin J, Schneider L, Novit A, Luczak S. Hydergine for dementia. Cochrane Database System Rev, Issue 1, 2006.

170. Le Bars PL. A. placebo-controlled, double blinded, randomized trial of an extract of *Ginkgo biloba* for dementia. JAMA 1997; 278(16): 1327–32.

171. Le Bars PL, Kieser M, Itil KZ. A 26-week analysis of a double-blind, placebo-controlled trial of *Ginkgo biloba* extract Egb 761 in dementia. Dement Geriatr Cogn Disord 2000; 11: 4: 230–7.

172. Birks J, Grimley Evans J. *Ginkgo biloba* for cognitive impairment and dementia. Cochrane Database System Rev, Issue 1, 2006.

173. Lopez-Arrieta, Birks J. Nimodipine for primary degenerative, mixed and vascular dementia. Cochrane Database System Rev, Issue 1, 2006.

174. Jansen SL, Forbes DA, Duncan V, Morgan DG. Melatonin for cognitive impairment. Cochrane Database System Rev, Issue 1, 2006.

175. Hogervorst E, Yaffe K, Richards M, Huppert F. Hormone replacement therapy for cognitive function in postmenopausal women. Cochrane Database System Rev, Issue 1, 2006.

176. Frampton M, Harvey RJ, Kirchner V. Propentofylline for dementia. Cochrane Database of System Rev, Issue 1, 2006.

177. Higgins JPT, Flicker L. Lecithin for dementia and cognitive impairment. Cochrane Database System Rev, Issue 1, 2006.

178. Hudson S, Tabet N. Acetyl-l-carnitine for dementia. Cochrane Database System Rev, Issue 1, 2006.

179. Williams PS, Rands G, Orell M, Spector A. Aspirin for vascular dementia. Cochrane Database System Rev, Issue 1, 2001.

180. Patterson MB, Bolger JP. Assessment of behavioral symptoms in Alzheimer's disease. Alzheimer's Dis Assoc Disord 1994; 8: S3: 4–20.

181. Schneider LS, Pollock VE. A meta-analysis of controlled trials of neuroleptic treatment in dementia. J Am Geriatr Soc 1990; 28: 553–63.

182. Rada RT, Kellner R. Thiothixene in the treatment of geriatric patients with chronic organic brain syndrome. J Am Geriatr Soc 1976; 24: 105–7.

183. Madhusoodanan S, Brenner R, Aruja L. Efficacy of risperidone treatment for psychosis associated with schizophrenia, bipolar disorder or senile dementia in geriatric patients: a case series. J Clin Psychiatry 1995; 56: 514–18.

184. Salzman C. Clozapine in older patients with psychosis and behavioral disturbance. Am J Geriatr Psychiatry 2006; 14: 11: 900–10.

185. Jesto DV, Eastham JH. Management of late life psychosis. J Clin Psychiatry 1996; 57: S3: 39–45.

186. Grad R. Benzodiazepines for insomnia in community dwelling elderly: a review of benefits and risks. J Fam Pract 1995; 41: 473–81.

187. Tariot PN, Erb R, Leibovici A et al. Carbamazepine treatment for agitation in nursing home patients with dementia. J Am Geriatr Soc 1994; 42: 1160–6.

188. Mellow AM, Solano-Lopez C, Davis S. Sodium valproate in the treatment of behavioral disturbance in dementia. J Geriatr Psychiatry Neurol 1993; 6: 205–9.

189. Sultzer DL, Gray KF. A double-blinded comparison of trazodone and haloperidol for treatment of agitation in patients with dementia. Am J Geriatr Psychiatry 1997; 5: 60–9.

190. Sakauye KM, Camp CJ. Effects of buspirone on agitation associated with dementia. Am J Geriatr Psychiatry 1993; 1: 894–901.

191. Nyth AL, Gottfries CG. A controlled multicenter clinical study of citalopram and placebo in elderly depressed patients with and without concomitant dementia. Acta Psychiatr Scand 1992; 86: 138–45.

192. Cherrier MM, Matsumoto AM, Amory JK et al. Testosterone improves spatial memory in men with Alzheimer disease and mild cognitive impairment. Neurology 2005; 64(12): 2063–8.

193. Cherrier MM, Matsumoto AM, Amory JK et al. The role of aromatization in testosterone supplementation: effects on cognition in older men. Neurology 2005; 64(2): 290–6.

194. Cameron M, Lonergan E, Lee H. Transcutaneous electrical nerve stimulation (TENS) for dementia. Cochrane Database System Rev, Issue 1, 2006.

195. Broe GA. Health habits and risk of cognitive impairment and dementia in old age. A prospective study on the effect of exercise, smoking and alcohol consumption. Aust N Z J Pub Health 1998; 22(5): 621–3.

196. Spinder AA. Nutritional status of patients with Alzheimer's disease: a 1 year study. J Am Diet Assoc 1996; 96: 10: 1013–18.

197. Baines S, Saxby P. Reality oriented and reminiscence therapy: a controlled cross over study of elderly confused people. Br J Psychiatry 1987; 151: 222–31.

198. Mittelman MS, Ferris SH, Shulman E. A family intervention to delay nursing home placement of patients with Alzheimer's disease: a randomized, control trial. JAMA 1996; 276: 1725–31.

Skeletal System

CHAPTER 48

Bone loss and osteoporotic fracture occurrence in aging men

Steven Boonen and Dirk Vanderschueren

Osteoporosis in men: the size of the problem

Incidence of osteoporotic fractures in men

In men over the age of 65, the annual hip fracture incidence is 4–5/1000 compared to 8–10/1000 in women.[1,2] Although age-specific incidence rates in men are about half those in women, only about 25–30% of all hip fractures occur in men because of differences in life expectancy.[3–5] In both sexes, the incidence of these fractures rises exponentially with aging, the majority of fractures occurring in men over the age of 80 years. With continued aging of the population, the annual number of fractures in men is expected to rise dramatically in coming decades. Mortality after sustaining a hip fracture is twice as high in men as in women.[6] This difference is only partially explained by differences in comorbidity, suggesting that male gender is a major risk factor for hip fracture-associated mortality. Additionally, almost 50% of men with hip fractures will have to be institutionalized because of the fracture, and up to 80% of those who survive fail to regain their prefracture level of functional independence.

Overall, symptomatic vertebral fractures have similar incidences to those for hip fractures, but occur more in middle-aged men than in the very old. In men, vertebral fractures often result from severe trauma, whereas moderate trauma is more often reported in women. In addition to clinically symptomatic fractures, aging men may develop silent vertebral deformities as revealed by radiologic screening. The reported prevalences of these vertebral deformities vary considerably.[7] Their health impact is important, especially in men with multiple severe deformities resulting in disabling back pain.

There are age-related increases not only for hip and spine fractures in men but also for fractures of the proximal humerus, pelvis, and ankle. Similarly, the incidence of distal forearm fractures increases with age, although incidence rates remain lower than in women. Importantly, distal forearm fractures in men are also a risk factor for other osteoporotic fractures.

Prevalence of osteoporosis in men

In women, bone densities at either the lumbar spine or the proximal femur of at least 2.5 standard deviations (SD) below the young adult mean are proposed by the World Health Organization (WHO) as thresholds for osteoporosis. These thresholds, however, have hardly been validated as markers for fracture risk in men. It remains unknown, therefore, whether a similar approach can be taken for the diagnosis of osteoporosis in men as in women. A key issue in this regard is whether it would be more appropriate to use gender-specific normative values of bone mass in the evaluation of osteoporosis in men, or whether the same level of absolute bone mass should determine diagnostic categorization in both men and women. This issue is currently quite unclear, and technical, pathophysiologic, and public-health considerations influence the decision. Not surprisingly, the prevalence of osteoporosis is greater using male-specific ranges. According to male cut-off data from the third National Health and Nutrition Examination Survey (NHANES III), the prevalence of osteoporosis in elderly men is 3–6%.[8] For comparison, the prevalence would be only 1–4% when using female standards.

Clinical presentation of osteoporosis in men

Most fractures occur in older age, in men as in women, and result from the (poorly understood) process of age-related bone loss that has inevitably occurred by that stage of life. This relatively common form of osteoporosis is referred to as 'age-associated' osteoporosis. Fractures resulting from age-associated osteoporosis are most frequent among men over the age of 70. This type of osteoporosis is quite distinct from the unexpected appearance of osteoporosis in a younger man, a syndrome referred to as 'idiopathic' osteoporosis. Idiopathic osteoporosis is much less common than age-associated osteoporosis and will mostly be diagnosed in men between the ages of 30 and 60 years. The diagnosis of 'idiopathic' osteoporosis (in men younger than 70 years) or 'age-associated' osteoporosis (in men older than 70 years) should only be applied if careful screening reveals no potential underlying cause of bone fragility (such as alcohol abuse, glucocorticoid excess, or hypogonadism) indicating 'secondary' osteoporosis, a form of osteoporosis seen much more frequently among men than among women.

Age-associated osteoporosis

Aging is the major determinant of fracture incidence, not only in women but also in men. Although men do not experience a well-defined equivalent of the menopause, there is increasing evidence for a relationship between age-related endocrine changes and osteoporosis in men as well.

In particular, changes in sex steroid secretion, in the growth hormone–insulin-like growth factor-I (GH–IGF-I) axis, and in the vitamin D–parathyroid hormone (25(OH)D–PTH) system may be associated with osteoporosis and osteoporotic fracture occurrence in men.[9] Recent evidence suggests that bone loss in aging men may be particularly related to declining levels of (bioavailable) estradiol, rather than to other age-associated hormonal changes (such as the partial androgen deficiency associated with normal aging). Even low concentrations of estradiol may be critically important in determining the rate of bone loss, not only in postmenopausal women but also in men.[10,11] However, it remains to be clarified whether and to what extent these hormonal changes act independently of age to increase the risk of skeletal fragility.

Most studies in aging men have addressed the potential impact of hormonal changes on bone density (as a surrogate marker for fracture risk) and have used a cross-sectional design. These studies have reported either the presence or the absence of an association between selected potential endocrine determinants (using different assays) and measurements of bone density (using different methodologies and sites), mostly in a small number of subjects with a wide variation of age ranges. This heterogeneity, in terms of both methodology and study population, and the inconsistent results make it difficult to interpret the findings of these studies. Moreover, some investigations failed to adjust for concomitant changes in body mass index or age, and, thus, do not allow independent associations between hormonal changes and bone loss to be established. Even more important, most studies do not take into account the complex interactions that exist between testosterone, estradiol, IGF-I, sex hormone-binding globulin, and/or PTH, which may significantly confound reported associations.

Secondary osteoporosis

If one surveys a typical population of men with osteoporosis, several etiologies will surface frequently. They are alcohol abuse, glucocorticoid excess (either endogenous – Cushing's syndrome – or, more commonly, chronic glucocorticoid therapy), and hypogonadism. In addition, other etiologies are important to consider, including primary hyperparathyroidism, excessive thyroid hormone exposure (hyperthyroidism or overtreatment with thyroid hormone), multiple myeloma and other malignancies, anticonvulsant use, gastrointestinal disorders, and high-dose chemotherapeutics.

Glucocorticoid excess is probably the major cause of secondary osteoporosis in men, found in about 20%. The main mechanism in this type of osteoporosis is osteoblast insufficiency. Additionally, glucocorticoids may induce muscular atropy and secondary hypogonadism.

Numerous reports have clearly documented that male hypogonadism is associated with reduced bone density, especially when present before puberty. The extreme delay of skeletal maturation in men suffering from estrogen deficiency as the result of a mutation in either the estrogen receptor or the aromatase enzyme suggests that part of the androgen action on the male skeleton is mediated by estrogens. Hypogonadism (either primary or secondary) is reported in 15–20% of cases with spinal osteoporosis. In case–control studies of male fracture patients, varying prevalences of hypogonadism have been reported, but the use of different and insufficiently validated thresholds for both total and free testosterone makes it difficult to compare different studies. These discrepancies emphasize the need to establish cut-offs to define hypogonadism, based on the impact of different degrees of androgen deficiency on the musculoskeletal or other systems.

Alcohol abuse can be revealed in about 15–20% of osteoporotic men, and is probably an underestimated cause of skeletal fragility in men. Bone loss is increased in men with alcohol intake above the median, and recent findings indicate that alcohol abuse may even be associated with an increase in fracture risk.

Finally, a particular secondary cause of osteoporosis in men is idiopathic hypercalciuria. Hypercalciuria (more than 0.1 mmol/kg per day or 4 mg/kg per day), if present, may in part be due to increased intestinal absorption of calcium resulting from alterations in vitamin D metabolism, but the exact underlying mechanism remains to be established. In our experience, the prevalence of hypercalciuria in osteoporotic men may amount to up to 15%.

Idiopathic osteoporosis

Idiopathic osteoporosis is an uncommon syndrome, the estimated incidence being only four new cases per 100 000 persons per year. Nevertheless, the number of men whose osteoporosis remains unexplained after a routine evaluation is approximately 50% in most series. However, many series come from referral centers that tend to attract more unusual patients, and might therefore overestimate the proportion of men with unexplained disease. The diagnosis of idiopathic osteoporosis should be applied only to men under the age of 70 years. By that stage of life, it is more likely that the disease is at least the result of the cumulative effects of the process of age-related bone loss and of factors that affected skeletal health earlier in life (for example, failure to achieve adequate peak bone mass and calcium undernutrition) but which are no longer identifiable.

The overwhelming majority of patients with idiopathic osteoporosis is symptomatic and presents with fractures. Fractures are most often at the vertebrae, although cortical fractures may occur as well, including stress fractures of the lower extremities or hip fractures. The predominant presenting symptom is back pain. Bone mass measurements in these men reveal markedly reduced bone mineral density. Typically, lumbar spine density T-scores in these men are below −2.5 SD. In our experience, the mean T-score is even less than −3.0. By definition, biochemical screening shows no abnormalities. The natural course of idiopathic osteoporosis is not well documented, but available data seem to indicate that – even with conservative measures – bone loss is not accelerated, suggesting that most of these men failed to reach normal peak bone density.

The pathogenesis of idiopathic osteoporosis is unknown. Both abnormalities in the GH–IGF-I system and alterations in the metabolism or activity of androgens have been suggested as potential etiologies. By no means, however, have they been established as causes.

Diagnosis of osteoporosis in men

The diagnosis of osteoporosis requires assessment of bone mineral density (BMD). In men as in women, diagnostic thresholds have been best validated with dual-energy X-ray absorptiometry (DXA).

There is overall agreement that bone density measurement using DXA should be performed in all men who present with findings that suggest the presence of osteoporosis (such as low trauma fractures or radiographic criteria indicating bone loss), and who are considered to be at increased risk for an atraumatic fracture because of specific medical conditions (hypogonadism, hyperthyroidism, excessive alcohol intake).

The use of T-scores requires a comparison with measurements in a young reference population. Although fracture risk varies between populations, there is insufficient knowledge at present to recommend that local reference ranges be used. It is recommended, therefore, that the NHANES III database be used as an international reference until further research changes this view. There is some ongoing controversy as to whether gender-specific T-scores should be used or not. Most, but not all, cross-sectional data support the use of female reference values, but some authors propose using young normal mean levels derived from a male reference population. However, in men, the risk of fracture is substantially lower for a bone mineral measurement within their own reference range, so a more stringent criterion seems to be needed to yield the same risk as in women. The most effective approach to the resolution of this problem would be prospective observation in men of the relationship between measures of bone density and future fracture risk. Those data becoming available suggest that absolute BMD rather than gender-specific diagnostic criteria may be more appropriate. For the time being, it might therefore be most appropriate to define osteoporosis in men as a BMD of 2.5 SD or more below the reference range for young women.

In men as in women, spine measurements in older individuals may be confounded by osteoarthritis, whereas the hip is very much less affected. In men over the age of 65–70 years, BMD assessment should therefore include a measurement taken from the hip region.

Clinical evaluation of men with osteoporosis

Clinical assessment

The medical history should include a family and a fracture history and should address calcium intake, medications, alcohol intake, and tobacco use. The clinical examination should particularly focus on signs of hypogonadism (especially testicular atropy and span length for early hypogonadism), alcohol abuse, and glucocorticoid excess. Body length should be monitored as a marker of osteoporosis. Dorsal kyphosis may indicate severe vertebral deformities. Low body mass index should be considered a risk factor.

Biochemical measures

The biochemical evaluation should include a complete blood count, serum levels of calcium, phosphate, alkaline phosphatase, albumin, creatinine, 25(OH)D, and ferritin (to detect hemochromatosis and alcoholic liver disease), liver function tests, and serum protein electrophoresis (to exclude multiple myeloma, in particular in older individuals). A 24-hour urine calcium and creatinine excretion level is needed to exclude hypercalciuria (>300 mg/day). Hypocalciuria (<100 mg/day) should raise suspicion of markedly reduced dietary calcium absorption (due to vitamin D deficiency, bowel disease, or malnutrition).

Measurement of serum intact PTH is indicated whenever serum calcium, phosphate or, 25(OH)D levels are abnormal (to detect primary or secondary hyperparathyroidism). In all patients, we would recommend measurement of serum testosterone and thyroid-stimulating hormone (TSH) to exclude hypogonadism and hyperthyroidism, especially in older individuals. Total testosterone should be measured in a morning sample, because testosterone concentrations fluctuate according to a circadian pattern. Some controversy remains as to whether free testosterone, bioavailable testosterone, or sex hormone-binding globulin should be assessed in all patients. Some authors even advocate the routine measurement of estradiol. In men with androgen deficiency, serum levels of luteinizing hormone (LH) and prolactin should be measured to allow differentiation between primary and secondary hypogonadism and to detect a potential prolactinoma. A 24-hour cortisoluria test is indicated whenever there is clinical suspicion of Cushing's disease.

The added value of biochemical markers of bone turnover, such as serum osteocalcin or urinary collagen cross-links, in the clinical management of osteoporotic men remains to be demonstrated. Therefore, the routine measurement of bone markers in men with osteoporosis cannot be recommended.

Therapeutic options for men with osteoporosis

Life-style measures and dietary recommendations

Whether and to what extent risk-factor modification will reduce fracture rates remains unknown, in men as well as in women. Nevertheless, adequate exercise should be recommended and excessive alcohol intake or smoking discouraged. Medications that potentially increase the risk of falling, such as psychotropic drugs, should be reconsidered, particularly in frail elderly men.

Dietary supplementation of calcium and vitamin D also reduces the rate of bone loss in elderly men with low calcium intake, and may even have an effect on fracture incidence. In line with the recommendations of the National Institutes of Health, dietary calcium intake should be at least 1200 mg/day. In men older than 65 years, a calcium intake of 1500 mg and a vitamin D intake of 800 IU daily are required.

Current pharmacologic options

None of the currently available therapeutic options has proven antifracture efficacy as documented in properly designed, randomized, placebo-controlled fracture-endpoint trials. Such studies are difficult to perform because of the low fracture incidence in men. They would require a large study group and long-term follow-up. Therefore, the question arises to what extent data available in women may be extrapolated to men. One possibility is to use bone density as a surrogate marker for fracture risk as primary end-point, rather than fracture end-points. Agents with proven antifracture efficacy in postmenopausal women particularly should be considered for use in male osteoporosis, if clinical trials in men document favorable effects on bone mass of similar magnitude to those shown to result in reduced fracture rates in women.

Androgen replacement has been documented to prevent bone loss in hypogonadal men, but the extent to which this type of replacement would be beneficial in normal elderly men with partial androgen deficiency and low bone density remains to be clarified. According to a recent randomized trial, no significant gain in lumbar BMD is observed in older men with borderline low serum testosterone concentrations and low bone density, when compared with calcium supplementation alone.[12] Only in those with low pretreatment testosterone levels will testosterone replacement be associated with a moderate gain in bone density. In addition to information on the potential benefit of androgen replacement in normal elderly men, there is an urgent need for data regarding the long-term safety of this type of therapy.

In postmenopausal osteoporosis, bisphosphonates have become one of the treatments of choice. Recent evidence suggests that they may be equally useful in male patients. In men suffering from glucocorticoid osteoporosis, bisphosphonate therapy is associated with similar increases in bone density to those in women. In a randomized placebo-controlled trial with alendronate, significant improvements of both lumbar and femoral bone density were observed in osteoporotic men with or without hypogonadism.[13] The chief entry criteria were a BMD at the femoral neck of at least 2 SD below the mean value in normal young men or a BMD at the femoral neck of at least 1 SD below the mean value in normal young men, and at least one vertebral deformity or a history of an osteoporotic fracture. Over a period of 2 years, the use of alendronate was associated with an increase in lumbar spine BMD of approximately 7% and a gain in total hip BMD of 2.5%. The incidence of vertebral fractures was lower in the alendronate group than in the placebo group (0.8% vs 7.1%). In line with these radiographic findings, alendronate-treated men showed no decrease in height, whereas men taking placebo lost height significantly. The effects of alendronate were independent of baseline serum free testosterone, suggesting that bisphosphonate therapy may be useful in both androgen-replete and androgen-deficient men. More importantly, the benefits of alendronate therapy in men with osteoporosis were similar to those in postmenopausal women, suggesting that bisphosphonate therapy might be equally effective in men and women with osteoporosis. Further evidence for this concept comes from studies with risedronate. In male patients on corticosteroid therapy, risedronate increased lumbar spine and hip BMD, along with a (statistically significant) reduction in the incidence of vertebral fractures.[14] Positive results from a similarly designed study with risedronate in men with idiopathic osteoporosis are about to be reported (S Boonen, personal communication).

Antiresorptives act primarily by inhibiting osteoclast-mediated bone loss and may be associated with an increase in bone density by filling in of resorption cavities and increased deposition of mineral into existing bone matrix. The concept of a bone anabolic agent is based upon stimulation of bone formation, a physiologic process opposite to that of inhibiting bone resorption. Inherent to this concept is the ability for an anabolic agent, such as teriparatide, to restore bone microarchitecture. In a recent study in men with low BMD, teriparatide was found to significantly increase BMD and to reduce the risk of fracture,[15] supporting the notion that teriparatide is effective in treating osteoporosis and reducing the risk of fracture regardless of gender.

Male osteoporosis: a practical approach

There is increasing evidence that the approaches developed to diagnose and treat the disorder in women may be equally useful for similar problems in men. Nevertheless, the evaluation and treatment of men suffering from osteoporosis remains a clinical challenge, despite recent advances in the understanding of the male osteoporotic syndrome. In most countries (including the USA) there are currently no approved therapies for male osteoporosis. Moreover, there is some ongoing controversy about the reference values that should be used to derive T-scores, as indicated above.

All men with low bone density should be investigated (both clinically and biochemically) for secondary causes of bone loss, and should be informed regarding life-style measures and dietary calcium intake. In line with recent recommendations from the International Osteoporosis Foundation, we would recommend that the same diagnostic thresholds be used in men – namely a BMD at the hip that lies 2.5 SD below the reference range for young women – until further research changes this view. Because the relationship between BMD and fracture risk seems to be similar in men and women (although the data are scanty), we would recommend treating all men with osteoporosis as defined by female reference values with calcium, vitamin D (when appropriate), and an antiresorptive agent. In view of recent evidence, bisphosphonate therapy might be the treatment of choice. A BMD measurement value more than 2.5 SD below the young male reference may not warrant antiresorptive treatment (except if there is history of an osteoporotic fracture), but it warrants further investigation to exclude secondary causes of bone loss as well as general recommendations regarding life-style measures and appropriate dietary intake of calcium.

Key messages

1. There is increasing evidence that the approaches developed to diagnose and treat osteoporosis in women may be equally useful in approaching similar problems in men. In particular, bisphosphonates are likely to become an important strategy to increase bone density and reduce fracture risk in osteoporotic men.
2. In men with osteoporosis, it remains critical to exclude underlying pathologic causes as these are much more likely to occur than in women.
3. The extent to which age-associated endocrine deficiencies contribute to bone loss and fracture

predisposition in men remains to be established. In particular, it is not yet clear whether the partial androgen deficiency associated with normal aging has implications for skeletal maintenance.

Acknowledgments

Dr S Boonen and Dr D Vanderschueren are both Senior Clinical Investigators of the Fund for Scientific Research, Flanders, Belgium (FWO-Vlaanderen). Dr S Boonen is holder of the Leuven University Chair in Metabolic Bone Diseases, supported by Roche & GSK.

References

1. Bilezikian JP. Osteoporosis in men. J Clin Endocrinol Metab 1999; 84: 3431–4.
2. Orwoll ES, Klein RF. Osteoporosis in men. Endocr Rev 1995; 16: 87–116.
3. Cooper C, Campion G, Melton LJ III. Hip fractures in the elderly: a world-wide projection. Osteoporosis Int 1992; 2: 285–9.
4. de Laet CE, van Hout BA, Burger H et al. Bone density and risk of hip fracture in men and women: cross sectional analysis [Published erratum appears in BMJ 1997; 315: 916]. BMJ 1997; 315: 221–5.
5. Jones G, Nguyen T, Sambrook PN et al. Symptomatic fracture incidence in elderly men and women: the Dubbo Os Epidemiology Study (DOES). Osteoporosis Int 1994; 4: 277–82.
6. Poor G, Atkinson EJ, Lewallen DG et al. Age-related hip fractures in men: clinical spectrum and short-term outcomes. Osteoporosis Int 1995; 5: 419–26.
7. O'Neill TW, Felsenberg D, Varlow J et al. The prevalence of vertebral deformity in European men and women: the European Vertebral Osteoporosis Study. J Bone Min Res 1996; 11: 1010–18.
8. Looker AC, Orwoll ES, Johnston CC Jr et al. Prevalence of low femoral bone density in older US adults from NHANES III. J Bone Min Res 1997; 12: 1761–8.
9. Boonen S, Vanderschueren D, Geusens P, Bouillon R. Age-associated endocrine deficiencies as potential determinants of femoral neck (type II) osteoporotic fracture occurrence in elderly men. Int J Androl 1997; 20: 134–43.
10. Khosla S, Melton LJ III, Atkinson EJ et al. Relationship of serum sex steroid levels and bone turnover markers with bone mineral density in men and women: a key role for bioavailable estrogen. J Clin Endocrinol Metab 1998; 83: 2266–74.
11. Vanderschueren D, Boonen S, Bouillon R. Action of androgens versus oestrogens in male skeletal homeostasis. Bone 1998; 23: 391–4.
12. Amory JK, Watts NB, Easley KA et al. Exogenous testosterone or testosterone with finasteride increases bone mineral density in older men with low serum testosterone. J Clin Endocrinol Metab 2004; 89(2): 503–10.
13. Orwoll ES, Ettinger M, Weiss S et al. Alendronate for the treatment of osteoporosis in men. N Engl J Med 2000; 343: 604–10.
14. Reid DM, Adami S, Devogelaer J-P, Chiness AA. Risedronate increases bone density and reduces vertebral fracture risk within one year in men on corticosteroid therapy. Calcif Tissue Int 2001; 69: 242–7.
15. Kaufman JM, Orwoll E, Goemaere S et al. Teriparatide effects on vertebral fractures and bone mineral density in men with osteoporosis: treatment and discontinuation of therapy. Osteoporos Int 2005; 16: 510–16.

Sensory Organs

CHAPTER 49

Aging and the eye

Ali R Djalilian and Hamid R Djalilian

Introduction

Visual function is an important determinant of the quality of life in older individuals. An older patient with visual impairment is at significantly greater risk for injuries and accidents.[1] Furthermore, loss of vision can lead to the loss of independence by losing the ability to drive and perform activities of daily living. Visually impaired patients may subsequently become depressed and socially isolated.

The incidence of visually significant eye diseases rises dramatically with increasing age. In the USA, the most common age-related conditions responsible for visual loss in the elderly are macular degeneration, glaucoma, and cataract. This chapter deals primarily with these three visually significant disorders, although less threatening age-related conditions such as presbyopia, dry eyes and vitreous degeneration are also briefly discussed (Table 49.1).[2] Diabetic retinopathy, which is another important cause of blindness in both older and younger patients, will not be discussed and the reader is referred to other excellent reviews.[3]

Presbyopia

One of the earliest signs of aging in the eye is loss of accommodation. This occurs universally and is manifested by the inability to focus at near distance. The person will initially try to compensate by holding reading material further from the eye, but eventually is no longer able to read fine print.

The typical age of onset is 40–45 years, with progressive loss of accommodation continuing until the age of 60–65 years, when essentially all accommodation is lost. Physiologically, presbyopia is thought to be due to the gradual hardening of the lens, which limits its flexibility. Specifically, the lens can no longer change its shape to increase its power, which is necessary for focusing on near objects. Although frustrating for the patient, presbyopia is benign, and readily treatable with the use of reading glasses or bifocals.

Dry eyes

Advancing age is associated with a physiologic decrease in tear production. Dry eye symptoms are one of the most common ocular complaints in older patients. At least 10% of patients over the age of 65 develop some degree of symptoms related to dry eyes.[4] The most commonly reported symptoms are grittiness and foreign body sensation (like feeling sand in the eye). Other complaints may include burning, photophobia, and intermittent blurry vision. Women are affected more often than men partly due to declining levels of sex hormones, which appear to be important for tear production.[4,5] Besides inadequate production, dry eye symptoms may also be due to increased evaporation of tears. Increased evaporation occurs typically when there is increased exposure (inadequate blink, or lid retraction) or insufficient oil film resulting from plugging of the meibomian glands (as in patients with blepharitis).

Table 49.1 *Typical age-related changes in the eye[2]*

Structure	Age-related change
Eyelids	Increased laxity, atrophy of orbit fat leading to enophthalmus, prolapse of orbital fat leading to dermatochalasis, levator dehiscence causing ptosis
Lacrimal gland	Decreased tear production in part due to declining sex hormones
Cornea	Arcus senilis (lipid deposit in peripheral cornea), gradual decrease in endothelial cells
Lens	Gradual hardening leading to loss of accommodation, loss of clarity and increased yellowish color, increase in size (anterior–posterior diameter)
Vitreous gel	Gradual condensation and collapse leading to posterior vitreous detachment, floaters
Retina	Gradual decrease in number of photoreceptors and ganglion cells, accumulation of unmetabolized debris (drusen)

Moderate to severe dry eyes can be vision threatening. Autoimmune diseases such as Sjögren's syndrome can lead to immunologic destruction of the lacrimal gland, as well as the salivary glands. Sjögren's syndrome can occur primarily, or secondary to collagen vascular diseases such as rheumatoid arthritis or lupus. Patients with severe tear deficiency are at risk for developing corneal ulcers, infections, and perforations with ultimate loss of the eye.

Dry eyes are treated symptomatically with ocular lubricants. A number of preparations are available over the counter. Patients who require the use of artificial tears more than four times a day are best served by using preservative-free drops, which limits the toxicity due to the preservative. These patients may also benefit from occlusion of the punta, using plugs or cauterization. Immunomodulatory therapy appears to be important for patients with inflammation associated with dry eyes. The role of hormonal therapy in dry eyes is currently under investigation.[5,6]

Vitreous degeneration

The vitreous gel that normally fills the posterior cavity (Figure 49.1) gradually begins to liquefy in late middle age. Functionally, degeneration of the vitreous has no effect on the eye, since the vitreous is primarily important during the development of the eye. In most people the vitreous continues to

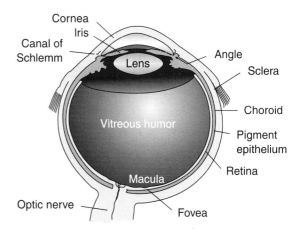

Figure 49.1 *Schematic diagram of the human eye.*

condense, and eventually separates posteriorly from the retina. This is known as a posterior vitreous detachment. Patients with vitreous condensation or detachment will frequently notice a few floaters, which represent opacities in the vitreous. While irritating to the patient, if stable and only a few in number, these vitreous floaters do not require any specific treatment beyond regular examination of the retina.

Occasionally, as the vitreous detaches from the retina it may cause a tear in the retina. Patients may experience a sudden increase in the number of floaters owing to hemorrhage from the tear. Traction on the retina by the vitreous can also cause the patient to experience light flashes. Any patient who experiences an increase in floaters or recurrent light flashes requires an urgent dilated examination of the retina, since untreated retinal tears can lead to the development of a retinal detachment. Most retinal tears can be treated readily with laser. Patients with high degrees of nearsightedness, a family history of retinal detachment, or a history of eye surgery or trauma are at greater risk for developing such tears.

Cataract

A cataract is by definition any opacity of the crystalline lens. It is the third most common cause of visual impairment among the elderly in the USA, and the leading cause of blindness worldwide. The incidence rises significantly with increasing age. The Framingham Study found a 17.6% incidence in people under the age of 65, 47.1% in 65–74-year-olds and 73.3% in those older than 75 years.[7,8] In addition to age, exposure to ultraviolet light, smoking, low intake of antioxidants, medications (e.g. steroids), and systemic diseases (e.g. diabetes) are known risk factors for the development of cataracts. Decreased estrogen levels in females may also contribute to the development of age-related cataracts.

Diagnosis

In the early stages, cataracts do not cause any visual symptoms. However, as the lens opacity increases, there is a gradual decline in the visual acuity. Typically, in age-related cataracts the distance vision is affected more than the near vision. In addition to blurry vision, patients frequently complain of glare, especially in bright lights. Driving at night can become very difficult for some patients owing to scattering of the light from oncoming cars.

Diagnosis can be readily made by examination. Although the slit lamp is the standard tool for examining the lens, in the primary-care setting a direct ophthalmoscope may also be used to detect changes in the lens opacity. Adequate visualization of the lens can be difficult in an undilated pupil. The most common finding is a yellowish discoloration of the lens. The view of the fundus is likewise degraded according to the degree of lens opacification. Patients with diabetes or a history of steroid use are prone to developing a posterior subcapsular cataract. These patients may see better under dim light, which allows the pupil to dilate.

Treatment

The treatment for a visually significant cataract is surgical removal. However, the timing of surgery depends mainly on the patient's life-style and the extent to which their vision prevents them from participating in their usual activities. For many patients, the ability to drive has the most significant impact on their decision. Before surgery, some of these patients may benefit from tinted glasses or an antireflective coating to reduce their glare symptoms from the cataract. Except in unusual situations, delaying cataract extraction generally does not put the eye at any significant risk.

The earlier techniques for cataract extraction involved removing the whole lens in one piece, which required a 10–12-mm incision. The latest techniques employ an incision which is only 3–4 mm in length, and the lens is fragmented into small pieces using ultrasound before it is aspirated from the eye (phacoemulsification). Unlike the earlier techniques, phacoemulsification does not require the cataract to be 'ripe', and surgery can be done any time the patient feels functionally impaired by the cataract. Placement of an intraocular lens is now a standard part of modern cataract surgery. Adequate anesthesia can be achieved in most patients with the use of only topical drops, although some patients or surgeons may prefer to have a retrobulbar or peribulbar injection. Using these latest techniques, cataract surgery has excellent visual results with low complication rates and minimal stress to the patient.

Although the visual impairment due to cataracts is treatable, life-style modifications may play an important role in preventing or delaying the onset of cataracts. These include the use of ultraviolet protection outdoors, adequate dietary intake of fruits and vegetables high in antioxidants, and avoiding smoking. In the USA, cataract is still an

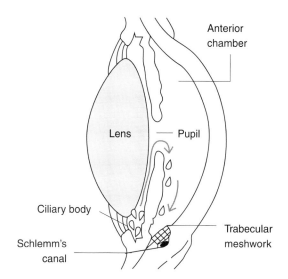

Figure 49.2 *Schematic diagram of the anterior segment, demonstrating the flow of aqueous humor from the ciliary body to the trabecular meshwork.*

important cause of visual impairment either due to lack of access or because patients may consider their visual decline to be a natural part of aging. Primary-care physicians can make a significant difference by educating their patients, and ensuring that all aging patients receive regular eye examinations.

Glaucoma

Glaucoma is the second most common cause of blindness in the USA and the leading cause of blindness among African-Americans. Nearly 10% of African-Americans over age 70 have glaucoma, compared with 2–3% of Caucasians. Fewer than half of all patients with glaucoma in the USA have been diagnosed, and the rest are unaware of their disease.[9] Therefore, the role of primary-care physicians is of the utmost importance in detecting and managing patients with glaucoma.

Normally, aqueous humor is produced by the ciliary body, which passes through the pupil and drains through the trabecular meshwork into Schlemm's canal (Figure 49.2). Any resistance to the outflow of aqueous through the trabecular meshwork can lead to increased intraocular pressure (IOP). This

elevated pressure can be transmitted to the optic nerve, resulting in damage to the nerve fibers. The mechanism of this damage may be mechanical or ischemic, or programmed cell death.

Risk factors

The most important risk factors for the development of glaucoma are increased IOP, age, family history, and race. Previously, an elevated IOP (>22 mmHg) was thought to be a prerequisite for the diagnosis of glaucoma. It is now known that a specific IOP cannot be relied on for the diagnosis of glaucoma. Generally, the range of IOP in 'normal' adult subjects is 10–22 (i.e. 95% of patients without glaucoma fall into this range). However, up to one-fifth of patients with glaucoma will have an IOP of less than 22 ('low tension glaucoma'). Likewise, many patients with an IOP of greater than 22 will never develop glaucoma.[10] Therefore, there is no cut-off pressure, and each patient will vary as to the pressure their eye can withstand. Nonetheless, the higher is the IOP the greater is the likelihood that the patient will have glaucoma. Similar to the case with blood pressure, patients are usually unaware and cannot feel the elevation in their IOP. The exception is when the IOP increases very suddenly (such as acute angle closure).

Age is also a consistent risk factor for development of glaucoma. The prevalence in patients under 40 is about 0.1%, while in those over the age of 70 it may be as high as 2–3%.[11] Racial differences are also striking, with African-Americans having a five times higher chance of developing glaucoma and losing vision, compared with white races. Having a first-degree relative with glaucoma likewise increases the risk significantly. Hypertension, diabetes, and myopia (nearsightedness) have also been identified as associated risk factors for glaucoma.

Diagnosis

Besides intraocular pressure, the diagnosis of glaucoma relies heavily on examination of the optic nerve. One of the characteristic findings is an increase in the central depression (cup) of the optic nerve head (Figure 49.3). Although there is no absolute number, the risk of glaucoma is generally less when the cup-to-disk ratio is below 0.5 (i.e. the

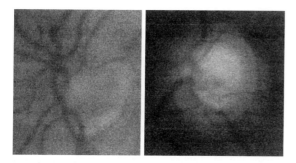

Figure 49.3 *A normal optic nerve (left) from a patient with light pigmentation and a cup-to-disk ratio of 0.3. The optic nerve from an African-American patient with glaucoma and a cup-to-disk ratio of 0.75 (right).*

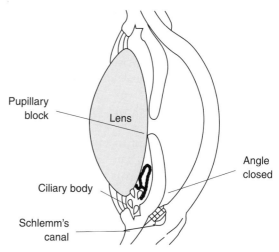

Figure 49.4 *Schematic diagram of the anterior chamber in angle closure due to pupillary block. Aqueous humor is trapped behind the iris and pushes it forward to close the angle.*

diameter of the cup is less than one-half the diameter of the disk). Actual progression in the cup-to-disk ratio over time is definitive evidence for the presence of glaucoma. Other optic nerve findings include vertical elongation or notching of the cup, thinning of the neural rim, or displacement of vessels to the margin.

In addition to the optic nerve, examination of the visual field is an integral part of the diagnosis and the follow-up of glaucoma. The visual loss in glaucoma begins primarily in the periphery and progresses gradually towards the center. Thus, the patient may have significant damage from glaucoma and not realize it, because good central vision can be maintained until the final stages. Patients with severe field loss who have less than 20° remaining in their better eye are legally considered blind. These patients are at significant risk for accidental injuries. If untreated, most of these patients will eventually lose their central vision as well.

Classification

In general, glaucoma is classified into open angle and closed angle. Open angle refers to all cases in which the anterior chamber angle (between the iris and cornea) is open, and aqueous can readily reach the trabecular meshwork. In this case the resistance to outflow is within the structure of the trabecular meshwork. In closed-angle glaucoma, the peripheral iris has come forward to close the angle, and is preventing the flow of aqueous from reaching the trabecular meshwork. In the USA, more than 90% of cases are of the open-angle type. Closed-angle glaucoma can develop gradually (chronic) or acutely. In acute-angle closure, the initial event is usually pupillary block, whereby the aqueous cannot flow into the anterior chamber and is trapped behind the iris. This trapped aqueous then pushes the peripheral iris forward, which subsequently closes the angle (Figure 49.4). Patients will usually present with acute pain, redness, and decreased vision. Since acute elevation of intraocular pressure may also cause nausea and vomiting, patients with angle closure have presented with clinical pictures that were mistakenly diagnosed as myocardial ischemia, or appendicitis. Patients with intermittent acute-angle closure may also complain of intermittent halos and blurriness, owing to edema of the cornea.

In patients with narrow angles, medications with anticholinergic or sympathomimetic effects (for example over-the-counter cold medications) can induce an attack of angle closure by causing the pupil to dilate. The warning label seen on many medications regarding patients with glaucoma refers only to this subset of patients with narrow angles, and otherwise the great majority of patients with open-angle glaucoma should have no problem with such medications. Asian patients and patients with hyperopia are most likely to have narrow angles. The risk of angle closure also increases with age owing to enlargement of the lens in the anterior–posterior direction. In patients with a narrow angle, shining a pen-light parallel to the iris from the lateral side may cast a shadow on the medial iris.

Overall, acute-angle closure occurs very infrequently in Caucasians and African-Americans. When it does occur, the intraocular pressure should be lowered immediately with medications. The definitive treatment for acute-angle closure or markedly narrow angles is to create a bypass for the aqueous to reach the anterior chamber. This is commonly done in the clinic by making a hole in the peripheral iris using a laser (peripheral iridotomy).

Treatment

The medical treatment of glaucoma is currently aimed at lowering the intraocular pressure. Although this does not cure glaucoma, it can significantly slow the progression of the disease. Topical drops are the mainstay of treatment. The most important consideration for the primary-care physician is awareness of the potential systemic side-effects due to these medications. Currently, the most widely used medications are beta-blockers such as timolol or levobunolol, which decrease the production of aqueous. Beta-blockers are actually the most likely drops to have significant systemic side-effects, including bronchospasm, bradycardia, depression, and impotence. The other topical medications including alpha-adrenergic agonists (bromonidine (Alphagan®)), carbonic anhydrase inhibitors (dorzolamide (Trusopt®), brinzolamide (Azopt®)), and prostaglandin analogs (latanoprost (Xalatan®)) are much less likely to cause any significant systemic problems. Cholinergic agonists (pilocarpine), which are used less frequently these days, may cause headaches and other cholinergic side-effects. Oral medications such as carbonic anhydrase inhibitors (acetazolamide (Diamox®)), and methazolamide (Neptazane®) are not tolerated well by most patients and cannot be used for long-term therapy. In addition to malaise, anorexia, and paresthesia, the use of oral carbonic anhydrase inhibitors may occasionally lead to the development of kidney stones.

When medical treatments fail to control the IOP adequately then surgical therapy is considered. Laser trabeculoplasty is an office procedure in which a laser is used to induce structural changes in the trabecular meshwork. In most patients this causes a mild to moderate reduction in the IOP, but the effect usually degrades over the course of several years. The most common surgical technique is a trabeculectomy, whereby a small section of the trabecular meshwork is removed in the operating room. The aqueous then drains through this hole and is collected in a 'bleb' under the conjunctiva, from where it is absorbed into the venous system. In most cases the trabeculectomy is done superiorly; thus, the fluid drains under the superior conjunctiva and is hidden by the upper lid. An important consideration in patients who have undergone a trabeculectomy is that any eye infection such as conjunctivitis should be treated aggressively (with topical antibiotics), given the risk of bacteria entering the eye through this hole and causing an endophthalmitis. An alternative technique to trabeculectomy is using a tube with one end in the anterior chamber and the other end (usually a plate) buried under the conjunctiva.

In patients with established glaucoma, severe loss of vision is rare if the condition is diagnosed early and the patient is compliant with the therapy. The most common reason for loss of vision due to glaucoma is not failure of therapy, but instead delay in the diagnosis. As mentioned earlier, nearly half of all the patients with glaucoma are unaware of their disease. Primary-care physicians play a critical role by referring patients for regular eye examinations, particularly those with risk factors including African-Americans and patients with a family history of glaucoma. In those with established glaucoma, one should remain aware of the side-effects from the medical therapy, while working to control disorders such as diabetes and hypertension that may potentially exacerbate the glaucoma through vascular problems.

Macular degeneration

Age-related macular degeneration (AMD) is the leading cause of visual loss among Americans of age

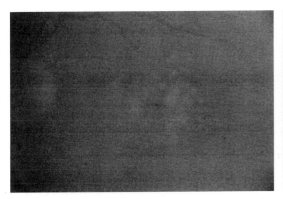 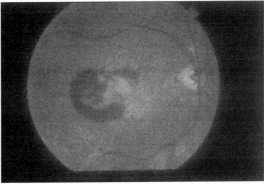

Figure 49.5 *A patient with early macular degeneration demonstrating multiple drusen in the macula (left). A patient with exudative macular degeneration and hemorrhage due to neovascularization (right).*

65 or older. Its prevalence increases significantly with age. In a US population-based study, the incidence of late AMD was 0.1% among people 43–54 years old compared with 7.1% among those aged 75 years or older.[12] The most important risk factors identified besides age include family history, smoking, hypertension, and low dietary intake of antioxidants. It is more common among white races, and probably more common among females. Increased exposure to sunlight, and having light-colored irises may also be potential risk factors.

The pathologic basis of AMD is the gradual loss of function in the center of the retina, namely, the macula. The macular region includes the central foveal area, which provides the sharp visual acuity necessary for tasks such as reading, driving and recognizing faces (Figure 49.1). The primary cells affected by AMD appear to be the retinal pigment epithelial cells, which are in close contact with the photoreceptors and are important for maintaining their health.

Diagnosis

Clinically, AMD can be divided into early and late stages. During the early stage, the visual acuity is relatively well maintained. The initial and most characteristic finding is the presence of drusen in the macula (Figure 49.5). Drusen are small yellow extracellular deposits of unmetabolized debris from retinal pigment epithelial cells. The prevalence of

ophthalmoscopically identifiable drusen increases with age, especially after the sixth decade. Eyes without drusen are generally not considered to have AMD. Typically, drusen do not affect the vision significantly; however, larger and more extensive drusen seem to be associated with an increased risk of central visual acuity loss. In addition to drusen, pigment abnormalities are also a common sign of early AMD.[13]

The late stage of AMD is divided into dry (atropic) and wet (exudative) forms. The dry form, which represents 90% of cases, involves gradual loss and atropy of retinal pigment epithelium and photoreceptors in the macular region. Patients experience a slow decline in their central vision. While in many cases a small area of central acuity may be relatively preserved, patients can still be functionally limited in their ability to read or drive owing to blind spots or distortions. Patients who develop 'geographic atrophy', involving the foveal region, experience more severe loss of vision.

Exudative or wet AMD represents only 10–15% of cases, but it accounts for more than 80% of cases with severe visual loss. The hallmark of the exudative form is the presence of neovascularization. The new blood vessels arise from the choroids and grow under the macula, and can cause leakage, hemorrhage, and ultimately scarring (Figure 49.5). Compared with dry AMD, the visual loss is more acute and devastating. The symptoms noted by the

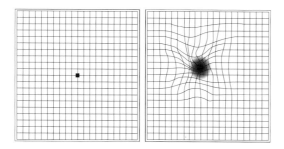

Figure 49.6 *Amsler's grid as seen normally (left) and as seen by a patient with exudative macular degeneration (right).*

patient may be distortions, whereby straight lines appear as curved, or the presence of a new blind spot. The use of a grid pattern (Amsler's grid) may help patients to recognize these changes earlier (Figure 49.6). Patients who develop these changes require urgent evaluation for possible treatment. If left untreated, many of these cases lead eventually to scarring of the macula with irreversible and severe loss of central vision.

Treatment

Unfortunately, at this time there is no effective treatment to prevent the development or the progression of AMD. The only therapies available are for patients with wet AMD. Laser photocoagulation, the gold standard, can be used in 10–15% of cases in which the neovascular lesions are small and well defined. However, recurrences are common after laser treatment. Furthermore, in many cases where the neovascularization involves the fovea, the laser treatment actually destroys most or part of the patient's central vision. Therefore, laser treatment only benefits a small subset of patients with wet AMD. Many new treatments such as photodynamic therapy and transpupillary thermotherapy are under investigation for patients with exudative AMD. Likewise, surgical procedures such as submacular surgery and retinal translocation are also under study. These therapies are likely to provide some benefit to the majority of cases of exudative AMD that are currently untreatable.[13]

At present there is no proven treatment for dry AMD. A number of observational studies have found an association between low dietary intake of foods containing antioxidants and the risk of developing AMD.[14] In other studies, lutein, zeaxanthin, and zinc have been suggested to be protective against visual loss from AMD.[15] Currently, there are no definitive data proving or disproving that dietary supplement of vitamins or minerals can slow the progression of AMD. This subject is under investigation in the Age-Related Eye Disease Study sponsored by the National Eye Institute.[16] This study has enrolled 3640 patients 55–80 years old to study the clinical course of AMD as well as cataracts. It will attempt to identify factors that influence their development and progression, and evaluate the potential efficacy of high-dose vitamins and zinc in arresting or retarding their progression.

The natural history of AMD is not of relentless progression. While usually bilateral, it is frequently asymmetric with variable and unpredictable progression. Many patients experience only mild to moderate changes in their visual function. Patients with severe loss of central vision usually maintain their peripheral vision, which allows them to ambulate. All patients should be encouraged to seek low-vision services that can provide them with various aids and optical devices, along with training for visual rehabilitation.

A very important consideration for all physicians is to be aware of depression in patients with recent loss of vision from AMD. Losing the ability to drive and perform certain activities of daily living has a profound impact on the person's ability to function independently. Many patients will go through a period of grievance that may result in clinical depression. While most patients eventually learn to adjust to their visual impairment, they may require treatment for the depression in the meantime. The social and family support network plays a critical role in this adjustment process.

Currently, AMD remains a significant public-health problem. Controlling risk factors such as smoking and hypertension while encouraging diets high in fruits and vegetables are the primary preventive measures at this time. With advances in genetics and molecular biology, future treatments may provide the ability to institute preventive therapies long before the onset of the disease.

Summary

Visual impairment is a significant problem in the elderly. At least one-third of all patients over the age of 65 have problems with their vision. The leading causes of blindness among older Americans are macular degeneration, glaucoma, cataract, and diabetic retinopathy. More than half of the visual loss in these patients is preventable or treatable. Physicians can maximize their patients' quality of life by enquiring about their visual health, recommending regular eye examinations, and referring those with decreased vision.

References

1. Ivers RG, Cummings RG, Mitchell P, Attebo K. Visual impairment and falls in older adults: the Blue Mountain Eye Study. J Am Geriatr Soc 1998; 46: 58–64.

2. Faye EE, Stuen CS, eds. The Aging Eye and Low Vision: A Study Guide for Physicians, 2nd edn. New York: The Lighthouse Inc, 1995: 7.

3. Flynn HW, Smiddy WE, eds. Diabetes and Ocular Disease. Past, Present, and Future Therapies. Ophthalmology Monographs 14. San Francisco, CA: The Foundation of the American Academy of Ophthalmology, 2000.

4. Schein OD, Munoz B, Tielsch JM et al. Prevalence of dry eye among the elderly. Am J Ophthalmol 1997; 124: 723–8.

5. Mathers WD, Stovall D, Lane JA et al. Menopause and tear function: the influence of prolactin and sex hormones on human tear production. Cornea 1998; 17: 353–8.

6. Nelson JD, Helms H, Fiscella R et al. A new look at dry eye disease and its treatment. Adv Ther 2000; 17: 84–93.

7. Lee DA, Higginbotham EJ, eds. Clinical Guide to Comprehensive Ophthalmology. New York: Thieme, 2000.

8. Liebowitz HM, Kruege DE, Maunder LR, et al. The Framingham Eye Study Monograph: an ophthalmologic and epidemiologic study of cataract, glaucoma, diabetic retinopathy, macular degeneration and visual acuity in a general population of 2631 adults. Surv Ophthalmol Suppl 1980; 24: 335–610.

9. Quigley HA. Open angle glaucoma. N Engl J Med 1993; 328: 1097–106.

10. Leisgang TJ. Glaucoma: changing concepts and future directions. Mayo Clin Proc 1996; 71: 689–94.

11. Chaudhry I, Wong A. Recognizing glaucoma: a guide for the primary care physician. Postgrad Med 1996; 99: 247–64.

12. Klein R, Klein BE, Linton KL. Prevalence of age related maculopathy. The Beaver Dam Eye Study. Ophthalmology 1992; 99: 933–43.

13. Fine SL, Berger JW, Maguire MG, Ho AC. Drug therapy: age-related macular degeneration. N Engl J Med 2000; 342: 483–92.

14. Mares-Perlman JA, Lyle BJ, Klein R et al. Vitamin supplement use and incident cataracts in a population-based study. Arch Ophthalmol 2000; 118: 1556–63.

15. Mares-Perlman JA, Klein R, Klein BE et al. Association of zinc and antioxidant nutrients with age-related maculopathy. Arch Ophthalmol 1996; 114: 991–7.

16. Age-related Eye Disease Study Research Group. The Age-Related Eye Disease Study: a clinical trial of zinc and anti-oxidants – AREDS report No 2. J Nutr 2000; 130: 1516S–19S.

CHAPTER 50

Aging and inner ear dysfunction

Emiro Caicedo, Diego Preciado, George Harris, and Frank Ondrey

Introduction

As humans age, there is a gradual dysfunction of nearly all organ systems. It is said that communication is both what the message is and the manner in which it is interpreted. Hearing is a key part of this communication in man. However, cochlear dysfunction is often an overlooked entity which can seriously affect the quality of life as one ages. It is estimated by the National Institutes of Health (NIH) in the USA that between 40 and 50 million Americans will experience a disorder of communication during their lifetime, the vast majority of which is hearing loss. While not completely debilitating, hearing problems may result in fear and anxiety, and may also bring up feelings of one's own mortality and aging. This chapter is designed to give the physician a point of reference for diagnosis and treatment of hearing and balance disorders that are more common as one ages.

Auditory perception and cochlear anatomy

Hearing relies upon several chief components to maintain quality of life in people of all ages. The ear has three basic parts: the external ear, the middle ear, and the inner ear.

The external ear includes the pinna (or auricle) and the external auditory meatus (the auditory canal). The pinna has a limited function to direct sound into the auditory canal. The auditory canal curves somewhat upward, and is about 25 mm long. Inside the outer portion of the canal are modified sweat glands that secrete cerumen (wax), and small hairs line this portion. The inner portion of the canal is hairless and smooth, and is lined by portions of the temporal bone. The medial border of the auditory canal is the tympanic membrane (TM) at the annulus.

The TM marks the beginning of the middle ear. The middle ear is normally an air-filled space. Within the middle ear lie the ossicles: the malleus, the incus, and the stapes. The last of these, the stapes, contacts the fluid-filled portion of the cochlea, via the oval window. The middle ear contacts the nasopharynx via the eustachian tube.

The inner ear contains the bony and membranous labyrinth, forming the cochlea and vestibule. The bony portion begins where the stapes contacts the vestibule via the oval window. The vestibule leads into the scala vestibuli, which spirals its way through the cochlea for 2¾ turns; it then passes through the helicotrema (where it begins to return back down the cochlea) and continues to spiral as the scala tympani, until it reaches the round window. The membranous portion of the cochlea is the cochlear duct (scala media), which is bordered by three structures: the basilar membrane, Reissner's membrane, and the stria vascularis. All three chambers (the scala vestibuli, scala media, and scala tympani) are filled with fluid. The scala vestibuli and the scala tympani are filled with perilymph. The components of perilymph are quite similar to cerebrospinal fluid. On the other hand, the scala media contains endolymph, which has a high K^+ concentration (145 mM) and a low Na^+ concentration (2 mM, similar to intracellular fluid). The stria vascularis is the blood and oxygen supply to the cochlea.

Hearing mechanics

When the TM is induced to move inward by sound waves reaching it from the surroundings, movement of the ossicles results in transduction of that wave into motion of the stapes footplate at the oval window. The fluid in the vestibule is displaced, resulting in a pressure wave that travels down the scala vestibuli, through the helicotrema, and continues to the scala tympani, where it displaces the round (cochlear) window. The resulting pressure wave is transmitted to the basilar membrane of the cochlea. The basilar membrane contacts both scalae and the organ of Corti. The organ of Corti is the means by which the oscillations of the basilar membrane result in mechanical displacement of the hair cells' stereocilia, which then either depolarizes or hyperpolarizes the hair cell. Depolarization of the hair cell results in firing of specific branches of the cochlear portion of the vestibulocochlear nerve (CN VIII). The displacement of the basilar membrane results in movement of the organ of Corti, and with it movement of the stereocilia of the inner and outer hair cells relative to the tectorial membrane. The stereocilia of the hair cells are not of one set length, but instead progressively lengthen, establishing an axis of polarization (a sense of direction). Simply put, when the stereocilia of the hair cell are deflected toward the taller stereocilia, the cell depolarizes and fires. When deflected away, the cell hyperpolarizes. There are 15 000 outer hair cells and 3500 inner hair cells. Most of the neural supply is to the inner hair cells (there are usually multiple afferents per cell). The place theory of hearing states that the basilar membrane affects the organ of Corti differently at different places along the cochlea. It is possible to map the portion of the cochlea stimulated by different frequencies, from 20 Hz near the apex (wide region) to about 20 000 Hz near the base (narrow region).

The neural pathway for these signals is as follows: the hair cells in the cochlea synapse with cells of the spiral ganglion (located in the wall of the cochlea) and become the cochlear nerve. This portion of CN VIII may enter either the dorsal or ventral cochlear nucleus of the pons. Here the fibers synapse and either head to the contralateral side or ascend directly to the midbrain. In the midbrain, they synapse with the inferior colliculus, where they may cross via the commissural neurons, and head to the medial geniculate body, where they synapse again and follow the auditory radiations to the auditory center in the superior temporal gyrus, under the lateral fissure of the brain.

The vestibular (or balance) system is closely linked with the hearing system. The main organ of balance is the vestibular labyrinth. There are three canals, the superior, the posterior, and the horizontal semicircular canals, and two otolith organs (the utricle and saccule). They are continuous with each other and are filled with endolymph, while they are surrounded by perilymph. The sensory epithelium of the semicircular canals contains a ridge in which hair cells are embedded. The vestibular branch of CN VIII innervates these hair cells. The stereocilia of the hair cells are embedded in a structure called the cupula, which moves when the head is experiencing angular acceleration in some plane, but because the cupula has the same specific gravity as the endolymph, it does not move in response to linear acceleration (like gravity). Instead the sensory epithelium in the otolith organs (the utricle and the saccule), called the macula utriculi and sacculi, have hair cells in a gel mass that contains many small stones of calcium carbonate. These stones increase the specific gravity of the epithelium, known as the otolithic membrane, and are responsive to linear acceleration.

CN VIII is responsible for carrying the information from these hair cells to the brain. The pathway is multileveled. Inputs from the semicircular canals travel in the vestibulocochlear nerve (the cell bodies are in the vestibular ganglion in the mastoid) to the vestibular nuclei in the floor of the fourth ventricle. There are four vestibular nuclei on each side: the superior, the inferior, the lateral, and the medial, where the incoming neurons may synapse; other fibers continue to the cerebellum.

From the above description and redundancy of eighth nerve pathways in the brain, one quickly realizes that peripheral disorders of both the end organs (vestibule and cochlea) should be much more common than central disorders of hearing and balance from cortical or brain stem pathologies. Clearly this is the case. It is rare for central nervous system processes to manifest themselves as a simple hearing or balance problem.[1]

Objective testing of hearing function

Audiometric testing

Formal audiometry in a sound booth is a part of the physical evaluation for any symptom referable to the ear including problems with hearing, tinnitus, and imbalance. A basic understanding of the audiogram is most helpful for any caretakers of patients presenting otologic symptoms. An audiogram can be ordered by any physician and is performed by an audiologist with a masters or PhD degree in a hearing science that allows the individual to become licensed to administer complete audiograms. These facilities may be part of hospitals, clinics, or otolaryngology offices, or free-standing. An overview of the basic portions of the audiogram is provided in this section to assist non-otolaryngologists with the basic interpretation of audiograms.

Components of an audiogram

The audiogram is arranged on a series of horizontal and vertical axes (Figure 50.1). The horizontal axes represent the threshold, in decibels (dB), that a pure tone is recognized by the examinee. The vertical axes represent the frequency, in Hz, that the tones are typically presented, from 125 to 8000 Hz. Tones are typically presented at the frequencies designated along the upper portion of the axes. Frequencies can be tested above 8000 Hz in special situations, but not routinely. Typically tones are presented at a reasonably high level at first, to help the patient recognize the sound of the tone, then they are presented at decreasing levels until the threshold value is reached for that frequency. The presentation level of each tone is varied in 5 dB increments until the patient's threshold is ascertained. The test/retest reliability of this system is typically less than 15 dB variance. The speech frequencies most important for normal conversation are in the 500 to 4000 Hz range, and patients with deficits in this range will have conversational difficulties, particularly in noisy environments like restaurants. Hearing loss is typically rated as mild, moderate, severe, or profound. Mild hearing loss is that which occurs from a 21–40 dB loss from the threshold. Losses greater than 40 dB but less than 60 are rated as moderate, severe in the range 61–80 dB, and profound losses are greater than 80 dB. Presenting tones accurately above 80 dB can be a challenge for some audiometers.

If there are abnormalities in the pure tones tested by air conduction testing, the audiologist will then screen the bone conduction thresholds to test for abnormalities in the conduction system to the cochlea. Air conduction thresholds may be in error for any reason that would affect the sound transmission through the ossicles. At the level of the external ear canal, plugging of the canal with cerumen or a foreign body may affect perception. At the level of the TM, scarring, perforation, or prior surgery are common reasons why air conduction may be affected. At the level of the middle ear, abnormalities of the ossicles including sclerosis, fibrosis, and trauma and disconnection may affect air conduction. In the middle ear, the presence of fluid or negative pressure are common causes of conductive hearing losses. Fixation of the stapes footplate to the oval window membrane, as observed in otosclerosis, will also affect conduction. This type of audiometric testing is performed with a microphone that sits directly over the mastoid air cells and transmits sound by bypassing the middle ear structures. A simpler screen for middle ear disturbances would be testing for sound lateralization with a Weber test with a 512 Hz tuning fork. Lateralization of the perceived sound to one ear when the vibrating tuning fork is placed on the forehead will indicate a conductive loss in the ear to which the sound lateralizes. A Rinne test can then

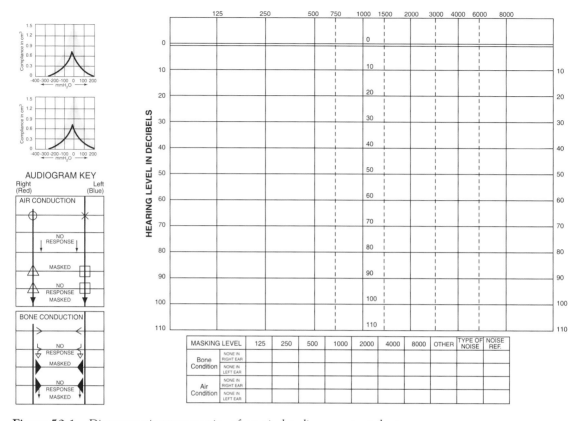

Figure 50.1 *Diagrammatic representation of a typical audiogram report sheet*

be followed up to examine whether bone conduction is greater than air conduction in the affected ear. Testing for conductive losses and severe asymmetric losses can be complicated by hearing the sound in the better functioning ear. The trained audiologist can compensate for these asymmetries by use of the technique of masking the better hearing ear. A discussion of masking is beyond the scope of this text.

Speech audiometry

A second form of testing that comprises a complete audiogram would be the testing of speech and word recognition. In this testing spondaic words are read to a patient at levels 25 dB above the average of 500, 1000, and 2000 Hz. The level of presentation is modulated until a patient scores 50% of the words correctly. This would be the speech reception

threshold. Next a standard word list consisting of 25 or 50 items is read to the patient at a level about 30 dB above the threshold. The items are then scored and the percentage of words repeated correctly is determined. If a significant asymmetry exists between the right and left ears (a 20% point or greater difference) the cause must be established, particularly if pure tone differences are small. Causes for this asymmetry could be retrocochlear lesions including acoustic neuroma.

Immitance audiometry

Tympanometry is the most common immitance measure utilized and is routinely tested. Typically a seal is developed over the ear canal and a pressure gradient from − 400 to + 200 kP of water is delivered during a 220 Hz tone. This test measures the volume of the ear canal and the compliance of the TM, as well as its

Table 50.1 *Causes of hearing loss*

Category	Examples
Developmental/ hereditary	Waardenburg's, Alport's, Usher's syndrome, Mondini deformity
Infectious	bacterial labrynthitis, herpes, cytomegalovirus, syphilis, Lyme disease
Toxicity	aminoglycosides, diuretics, salicylates, platinum
Trauma	head trauma, blast injury, noise, perilymph fistula, radiation
Neurologic	multiple sclerosis, vertebral basilar insufficiency, atherosclerosis
Immune	Cogan's syndrome, Wegener's granulomatosis, autoimmune inner ear disease
Bone disorders	Paget's disease, otosclerosis
Neoplasms	acoustic neuroma, meningioma, metastases, primary malignancy of temporal bone
Presbycusis	
Endolymphatic hydrops	
Sudden SNHL	

integrity. It can therefore indicate negative pressure within the middle ear, scarring or perforations of the TM, or eustachian tube dysfunction. The tympanograms are classified as type A (normal), B (flat), or C (negative pressure).[2]

Other tests

Acoustic reflexes

A test is utilized on occasion to measure the phenomenon of loud sounds causing a reflex contraction of the stapedial muscle. Reflexes should be bilateral when the tone is presented to either ear. If they are absent then one may be experiencing a pathology of the eighth cranial nerve, like acoustic neuroma.

Auditory evoked potentials

This test has several names including acoustic brain stem response (ABR) and brain stem auditory evoked response (BAER). In this test tones are presented to the patient by ear canal microphone and then auditory thresholds are established from scalp electrode recordings similar to those used in electroencephalography (EEG). These tests are helpful when the patient cannot cooperate for standard testing. Additionally, they are highly sensitive measures for screening for acoustic neuromas.

Caveats in testing hearing function in the elderly

Typically hearing function decreases with age, therefore it is important for the audiologist to take the time necessary to establish accurate thresholds in patients who are experiencing decreased hearing as a function of their age. Additionally, the specialized tests, including the ABR, acoustic reflexes, and some of the word discrimination tests, are less accurate when hearing levels and thresholds decline significantly.

Sensorineural hearing loss

In the aging patient, the cause of hearing loss is most frequently due to deterioration of peripheral and/or central auditory pathways. There is a relatively large differential diagnosis associated with sensorineural hearing loss (SNHL). Diseases from several categories can cause hearing loss and must be ruled out for optimal patient care. The most common causes are detailed within this chapter, but for reasons of developing a clear differential refer to Table 50.1.

Establishing causes of hearing loss

One must develop a clear differential diagnosis for hearing loss associated with aging. It is easy to attribute all hearing loss in males over 50 to presbycusis, but other diseases associated with hearing loss must be excluded. Therefore, a thorough history should be established. Important questions about the hearing loss would include the length of symptom onset, presence of tinnitus and its character, and any sudden or fluctuating changes in hearing or balance as well as any precipitating or associated events for the same. A past medical history of any diseases that would be associated with hearing loss, including diabetes, thyroid dysfunction, atherosclerosis, immune diseases, or other metabolic disease (otosclerosis, Paget's disease), should be taken. A family history of hearing loss in parents or older relatives to establish a potential familial pattern of presbycusis onset and progression is often helpful. Further family history of syndromic and congenital diseases associated with loss of hearing should be questioned. Whether or not the patient experienced significant otitis media as a child or young adult and experienced some level of hearing dysfunction secondary to these infections should be established. A history of toxic medicine exposures including aminoglycoside antibiotics, cancer chemotherapy agents, trauma to the temporal bone, or previous otologic surgery as part of the medical history should be established. Clearly, occupational exposures in males over the age of 50 need to be established. Regulations for hearing conservation in the workplace are more recent developments and most workers in factories have experienced levels of industrial noise in excess of current guidelines. The use of power tools, rifle hunting, smoking, and combat noise exposure should be established as part of the social history.

Once these items are clearly addressed, examination of the ear can proceed. Abnormalities of the pinna, ear canal, and TM may guide the physician to a diagnosis associated with any of a number of the conditions aforementioned. Once examination is concluded an audiogram should be performed. If a gradual sloping onset of symmetric hearing loss above 2 kHz is demonstrated with good discrimination scores, the patient likely has presbycusis, provided that the patient has described a gradual onset to his symptoms, and the TM is normal in appearance. Occasionally, a 'notch' is noted in the audiogram at a particular frequency and this may signify a significant noise-induced loss at that frequency. Asymmetries in pure tone hearing, conductive hearing, and speech discrimination will require further work-up to establish an underlying cause. Clearly an entity such as an acoustic tumor should not be missed because an unusual hearing loss was attributed to an entity such as combat noise exposure.

Presbycusis

Decreased hearing normally occurs as a function of aging. After the age of 40, the average threshold of the highest frequency speech sounds (4 kHz) is already beyond the normal range in the male population. At the age of 60, all of the speech frequencies demonstrate at least a mild hearing loss, on average (Table 50.2). Typically, people develop compensation mechanisms so that communication is not affected as aging causes mild losses. The classic hearing complaint of an aging male patient would be that he is experiencing difficulty understanding conversation with females or children when in situations with a significant background noise (e.g. restaurant dining). At this point it would not be unusual for the affected individual to have abnormal auditory thresholds in the moderate to severe range at the frequencies associated with speech (0.5–4 kHz).

Presbycusis is the most common cause of hearing loss in the elderly population. Presbycusis is defined as the hearing loss that is caused by the degenerative changes of aging. These changes can be pathologically demonstrated in several areas of the cochlea and can involve hair cell loss, neuronal loss, and decreased blood supply through cochlear microvasculature. It is defined as SNHL that is usually symmetric and presents in patients over the age of 60. It is characterized by a slowly progressive hearing loss, which is worse at frequencies above 2000 Hz. Although the exact pathophysiology remains ill defined, it appears to be a multifactorial process related to hereditary factors, diet, metabolism, noise exposure, and stress. It may also result from heart disease, high blood pressure, diabetic vascular conditions, or other circulatory problems involving perfusion of the nerve or any of the related structures, including the auditory centers in the brain, i.e.

Table 50.2 *Age adjusted normalized hearing thresholds for men at various frequencies*

Mean age (years)	Hearing thresholds (dB) at the indicated frequency (kHz)			
	0.5	1.0	2.0	4.0
25	10	5	5	10
27.5	10	10	10	15
30	15	10	10	20
32.5	15	10	10	20
35	15	10	15	25
37.5	15	15	15	30
40	15	15	20	30
42.5	20	15	20	35
45	20	20	20	40
47.5	20	20	25	40
50	20	20	25	45
52.5	25	25	30	50
55	25	25	30	50
57.5	25	25	35	55
60	25	30	35	55
62.5	30	30	40	60
65	30	30	40	65
67.5	30	35	45	65
70	30	35	45	70
72.5	35	40	50	70
75	35	40	50	75
77.5	35	40	55	75
80	40	45	55	80
82.5	40	45	60	80
85	40	50	60	80
87.5	45	50	65	85
90	45	50	65	85

stroke.[3,4] Studies have failed to clearly link any of these factors individually to presbycusis. Efforts to prevent presbycusis need to be investigated further.

Aural rehabilitation

Aural rehabilitation in the form of hearing aids helps most elderly people with presbycusis. Currently, there are numerous strategies under development for the further improvement of hearing aid technology. Typically, most hearing losses can now be treated with hearing aids that fit within the ear or ear canal. Many of these hearing aids also come in both digital and programmable variations

that allow the end user to customize their aid for different listening environments. Certain strategies, such as opening the venting of the ear mold, and digitizing the signal, may be useful in selectively amplifying the high frequencies. If the hearing loss is profound enough to not be helped even with the most powerful hearing aid, cochlear implantation remains an option. The passage of the 'Americans with Disabilities Act' has provided for enhanced quality of life for hearing impaired individuals with the addition of FM listening assistance devices for public gatherings at theaters, churches, and public forums.

Tinnitus

Definition

Tinnitus (from the Latin *tinnire*, which means to ring or to tinkle) is the perceived sensation of sound in the absence of acoustic stimuli. Tinnitus is a manifestation of malfunction in the processing of auditory signals involving both perceptual and psychologic components and should be differentiated from auditory hallucinations, which are considered to be a symptom of psychiatric or neurologic disorders.[5] Auditory hallucinations are more complex sounds such as voices or music. An abnormal neural activity of the auditory pathway is erroneously interpreted as true sound by the central auditory system of the patient suffering from tinnitus. A majority of tinnitus cases can be related to cochlear dysfunction, which could involve central modifications.[6]

Tinnitus is not a recent entity; it was reported as early as 2500 BC in Egyptian papyri which refer to 'the treatment of the bewitched ear'.[7] Over 10% of the US population have a complaint of tinnitus. Approximately 20% of these individuals rate their tinnitus as being severe enough to significantly decrease their quality of life. The age range of patients suffering from tinnitus is between 40 and 80 years; however, tinnitus may occur at any age. The prevalence of tinnitus has been shown to increase with age, and males and females are affected equally.[8]

Causes of tinnitus

Various hypotheses have addressed the mechanisms that could underlie tinnitus, but none has yet been determined. Researchers have tracked the origin of tinnitus using positron emission tomography (PET). They found activated sites in the temporal lobe opposite to the affected ear and unexpectedly they found that the hippocampus was activated too. This hippocampal activation could explain the adverse psychologic effects that patients with tinnitus often experience.[9] When talking about tinnitus we must keep in mind that it is a symptom not an illness.

Some causes of tinnitus are:[5]

1. inner ear pathology associated with hearing impairment: noise-induced hearing loss, presbycusis, Meniere's disease, etc.

2. middle ear pathology often associated with hearing impairment: chronic suppurative otitis media, otosclerosis
3. cerumen in the ear canal
4. drug ingestion
5. cardiovascular or neurologic disorders
6. emotional response to stimulus furthered by stress or depression, and
7. neoplasm: acoustic neuroma, temporal lobe tumors.

Classification

There are several ways to classify tinnitus. A common classification is objective versus subjective tinnitus. Objective tinnitus refers to a tinnitus that a physician can hear by placing a stethoscope over the patient's external auditory canal or by placing his ear against the patient's ear. An identifiable cause is usually found when objective tinnitus is present. Consequently, a successful treatment will be implemented. Table 50.3 shows the causes of objective tinnitus. On the other hand, subjective tinnitus cannot be heard by the physician. It is more common and less understood than objective tinnitus. Table 50.3 also lists the causal factors associated with subjective tinnitus.[8] Additionally, tinnitus can be classified in accordance with time of presentation. Chronic tinnitus lasts for more than 3 months without signs of spontaneously resolving. A distinction should be made between chronic tinnitus occurring after acute tinnitis and chronic tinnitus of insidious onset. Tinnitus sounds may be continuous or intermittent, fluctuating or non-fluctuating in loudness.[10]

Patient evaluation

A complete history is necessary in the work-up of a patient with tinnitus. It is crucial to address age of onset and whether the tinnitus began gradually or suddenly. Characteristics of the tinnitus must be obtained. These include pitch (high or low), location of the tinnitus, pattern (continuous, intermittent, or pulsatile), and intensity. Associated symptoms such as hearing loss, vertigo, aural fullness, and otorrhea should be explored. Approximately one-third to one-half of patients seeking help for tinnitus are depressed. Mood disorders, especially major depression, are

Table 50.3 *Causes of tinnitus*[8]

Objective tinnitus
Clonic muscular contractions
   Tensor veli palatini muscle spasm
   Levator veli palatini muscle
   Tensor tympani muscle spasm
Patulous eustachian tube
Vascular disease
   Arterial bruits
      carotid stenosis
      high-riding carotid artery
      persistent stapedial artery
      vascular loop
Arteriovenous aneurysm
Arteriovenous fistula
Arteriovenous shunt
Benign intracranial hypertension
Carotid occlusive disease
Eagle's syndrome
Glomus tumor
Paget's disease
Venous hum
   Dehiscent jugular bulb

Subjective tinnitus
Acoustic neuroma
Anxiety
Autoimmune disease
   Arthritis
   Cervical spondylosis
   Multiple sclerosis
Bell's palsy
Chronic suppurative otitis media
Cranial nerve VII compression
Depression
Ear wax impaction
Foreign body in auditory external canal
Head trauma
Heavy metals
   Arsenic
High-output anemia
Hypertension
Iatrogenic secondary to ear surgery
Lyme disease
Metabolic
   Diabetes mellitus
   Hypothyroidism
   Hyperthyroidism
   Hyperlipidemia

Table 50.3 *(continued)*

   Trace metal deficiency
      copper
      iron
      zinc
   Vitamin deficiency
Middle ear cholesteatoma or inflammation
Noise-induced hearing loss
Otosclerosis
Perilymph fistula
Pharmacologic agents
   Aminoglycoside antibiotics
   Antipsychotic drugs
   Aspirin and aspirin-containing compounds
   Carbamazepine
   Heterocyclic antidepressants
   Lithium
   Loop diuretic
   Non-steroidal anti-inflammatory drugs
   Quinine containing compounds
   Tetracycline antibiotics
Presbycusis
Temporal lobe neoplasms
Temporomandibular joint disorders

related to patients suffering from tinnitus.[8] Consequently, tinnitus patients should be asked about depressive symptoms. Past medical history of cardiovascular, neurologic, and metabolic disorders (i.e. diabetes mellitus, hypothyroidism, hyperthyroidism, and hyperlipidemia) is important in the evaluation. Drug ingestion (acetyl salicylates and quinine) should be ruled out. An essential part of the history is the family history, past head trauma, previous ear surgery, prior ear infections, and an exposure to ototoxic drugs (e.g. aminoglycosides and loop diuretics).

A complete otoneurologic and head and neck examination must be done. Inspection of the auricle, external auditory canal, and TM is important. Pneumatic otoscopy and tuning fork tests should be done. Auscultation of the mastoid tip, neck, ear, and skull needs to be performed. Neurologic examination focusing on cranial nerves V, VII, and VIII is crucial to detect acoustic neuroma in an early stage. All patients should have their blood pressure evaluated in both arms.

Audiometry should be performed on the patient to evaluate air and bone conduction and speech discrimination. If tinnitus is persistent and annoying, the patient should be referred to an ear, nose, and throat clinic, tinnitus clinic, or audiology department for further examination.

The information obtained by history, physical examination, and initial tests will determine the next step in the patient's evaluation. An arteriogram, MR angiogram, or transcranial Doppler should be ordered if a vascular abnormality is suspected. Patients with positive cranial nerve findings in the physical examination and complaints of unilateral constant tinnitus with progression to hearing loss and vertigo should be evaluated for a posterior fossa tumor by MRI. When medical or metabolic problems are suspected a battery of laboratory studies may be required. These studies include hematocrit, complete blood count, fasting blood glucose levels, thyroid function tests, a lipid battery, and a serologic test for syphilis. Tinnitus is a symptom in chronic Lyme disease. Patients with a suspected history of exposure to *Borrelia burgdorferi* should be tested for antibodies again this bacterium.[5]

Management and treatment

The treatment for tinnitus begins in primary practice with a thorough explanation of the basic physiology and psychologic mechanisms involved in the perception of tinnitus. Patients have to be reassured of the benign nature of their problem. Patients who look for medical help are those who cannot habituate to their tinnitus. Relevant examination and reassurance typically helps 80% of the patients referred to otolaryngology clinics. The patient has to be informed that there is no cure for tinnitus. First, any reversible otologic or medical condition causing tinnitus should be treated. Second, an evaluation of medications the patient is taking is crucial, and an attempt should be made to eliminate all agents known to produce tinnitus.

There are two modalities to relieve tinnitus. Masking the tinnitus is one of the measures. Masking of tinnitus means that an external sound is applied to the ear, and the sound completely blocks out the tinnitus. These features are pitch and intensity of the tinnitus, and minimal masking levels.

The masking can be performed by using hearing aids, tinnitus maskers, or simple measures such as increasing background noise in the environment (e.g. radio). The second modality treatment is drug therapy. The pharmacologic treatment of tinnitus has progressed little in the past few decades. Since 1937 the intravenous administration of local anesthetics has been used. Many studies have shown the benefit of using lidocaine, but it is of limited value due to its instability in vivo and the potentially life-threatening cardiac side-effects, as well as nausea, dizziness, and parenthesis. Attempts using oral analogs have been unsuccessful (i.e. tocainide and mexiletene). Some studies have focused on the intratympanic instillation of local anesthetics, but this method of administration has not been shown to increase the number of positive responses and it is accompanied by extreme side-effects that affect the vestibular system. The use of anxiolytics, sedatives, and hypnotics is probably the most successful therapy in tinnitus. Nortriptyline was found to reduce tinnitus loudness, but the effect was more evident in patients who were depressed. Alprazolam, a triazolo-benzodiazepine, was reported to be effective in tinnitus, but the highly addictive features limit its clinical use.[7]

Vasodilators have been used for the treatment of tinnitus with the hypothesis that the increase in blood flow would result in increased oxygenation of peripheral and central auditory structures. Among these drugs are channel antagonists (i.e. nimodipine), B-histine, for which the effectiveness is limited to Meniere's syndrome, and prostaglandin analogs such as misoprostol. *Ginkgo biloba*, an extract from the Chinese Maidenhair tree, has shown vasodilator effects. This extract has been studied in different clinical trials that have failed to show any particular efficacy.[7,11]

Conclusion

Patients presenting with tinnitus need a thorough examination of current health, an otoaudiologic examination, and a psychologic evaluation. It is important to give a clear explanation to the patient about their tinnitus. Patients should not just be told they will have to live with their tinnitus, although this is basically true, and the physician should spend more time reassuring the patient. Patients who are depressed or have psychologic problems should be identified as such and treated. All patients should be encouraged to join the American Tinnitus Association.[8]

Balance disorders

Dizziness, disequilibrium, and vertigo are common complaints in the elderly population. The sense of balance depends on a multitude of physiologic systems that need to function cohesively. Interaction of inputs from the vestibular, visual, and proprioceptive systems is necessary to maintain a sense of orientation in space. Dizziness may result with impairment of any of these three systems. Therefore, thorough evaluations of visual, neurologic, and musculoskeletal status are necessary before diagnosing vestibular pathology as the source of dizziness. Cardiac dysfunction must also be investigated. Pure labyrinthine dysfunction rarely, if ever, causes syncope. Orthostatic side-effects should also be considered. Lightheadedness on standing is not typical of vestibular dysfunction. Despite the multiplicity of disease states that may cause dizziness in the elderly, a specific cause can be found in up to 85% of patients with appropriate evaluation and work-up.[12]

Peripheral vestibular disorders are the most common cause of dizziness in the elderly. Up to 50% of aged patients complaining of disequilibrium have peripheral vestibular pathology. Peripheral vertigo is often distinguishable from central vertigo both on history and/or physical examination. Peripheral vertigo is often positional. It causes rotational nystagmus that has latency, is fatigable, and may be repressed by visual fixation. Central nystagmus more commonly is purely vertical, constant, and not repressed by visual fixation. Furthermore, certain types of peripheral vestibular pathologies may be associated with SNHL. Table 50.4 lists common causes of central and peripheral vertigo in the elderly.

Benign positional paroxysmal vertigo (BPPV) is certainly one of the most common etiologies of peripheral vertigo, even in the elderly. It is characterized by sudden attacks of vertigo precipitated by

Table 50.4 *Common causes of central and peripheral vertigo in the elderly*

Peripheral vertigo disorders	Central vertigo disorders
Meniere's disease	Stroke
Benign paroxysmal positional vertigo (BPPV)	Vertebrobasilar insufficiency
Ototoxicity	Intracranial tumors
Perilymphatic fistula	Multiple sclerosis
Vestibular neuronitis	Migraine
Acoustic neuroma	
Oscillopsia	
Temporal bone fracture/trauma	

certain head positions. The attacks are prompted usually by moving the head to the right or left, or by looking upward. Classically, BPPV has been thought to be secondary to otolith deposits onto the cupula of the posterior semicircular canal. Therapy is aimed at redirecting these otoliths into the utricle via head turning treatments called 'Epley repositioning maneuvers'. Other causes of BPPV include previous head trauma, vascular occlusion, and ear surgery. It may occur spontaneously in patients aged over 40 years. Other than Epley repositioning maneuvers treatment should consist of symptomatic control and reassurance as BPPV remits in the vast majority of cases.

Meniere's disease is another frequent cause of vertigo in the elderly. It is characterized by episodes of severe vertigo lasting hours, accompanied by aural fullness, hearing loss (typically low-frequency SNHL), and low-pitched tinnitus. The symptom complex occurs in concert and is fluctuating. The disorder is thought to occur secondary to increased pressure within the endolymphatic chamber, and is thus also named endolymphatic hydrops. Although the process is usually unilateral, the other side may become involved in about 15% of patients. The natural history of the disease is of complete remission in about 60% of patients.

Other causes of peripheral vertigo include perilymphatic fistula (PLF), vestibular neuronitis, and oscillopsia. Patients with a PLF often have a history of preceding trauma or barotraumas. A sneeze or vigorous nose blowing may be the inciting event. PLFs are not typically age related. Vestibular neuronitis typically begins with a viral illness followed by a period of vertigo lasting up to 6 weeks. Severe attacks may last days to weeks. Again, vestibular neuronitis is not thought to be related specifically to aging. Finally, oscillopsia is also known as vestibular ataxia and is described as inability to maintain the horizon level while walking. It is secondary to severe bilateral vestibular dysfunction. It may also result from degeneration of vestibulo-proprioceptive interconnections.

Vestibular function testing is used to help in distinguishing central from peripheral pathologies and to quantify the degree of unilateral or bilateral vestibular dysfunction. Quantitative testing includes electronystagmograms (ENGs), rotational testing, and posturography. Results of vestibular testing are unfortunately not specific to a particular disorder or condition and are typically normal for patients with central vascular insufficiency or stroke. Also, in the elderly, caloric responses frequently show declines in response, making ENG testing somewhat less sensitive in this population. Often ENG testing is most useful in pinpointing a specific hypofunction in one of the labyrinths, which may guide rehabilitative, medical, or surgical therapy. The specific vestibular disorder is not diagnosed with testing alone, but with a compilation of the findings obtained in the clinical history, physical examination, and ancillary tests.

Treatment of the elderly patient with vertigo consists of medical, surgical, and rehabilitative modalities. The treatment of peripheral vertigo is often the same in the elderly as it is in younger patients. It is important to note, however, that elderly patients have a more difficult time compensating to treatment when compared to younger patients.

Vestibular rehabilitation consists of exercises aimed at developing alternate balance mechanisms to compensate for the vestibular dysfunction. They are most useful in the setting of unilateral vestibular hypofunction. Alternative balance strategies include visual and proprioceptive inputs to stabilize the visual and postural environments. Many of these exercises were introduced by Cawthorne in the

1940s and remain as mainstays of vertigo treatment in the elderly.

Medical therapies mainly consist of vestibular suppressive therapies in the form of antihistamines (such as meclizine) and long-acting benzodiazepenes (such as diazepam). Often medical vestibular ablative therapy is tried when a unilateral vestibular pathology is diagnosed on ENG. Maintenance of balance sensation is easier for patients with unilateral vestibular input compared to disparate bilateral inputs secondary to hypofunction of one of the vestibules. For this reason, therapy can be aimed at ablating the pathologic side. The level of hearing in the pathologic side must be taken into account prior to ablation. Recently, topical gentamicin in the middle ear has been used as a vestibulotoxic agent in order to wipe out pathologic vestibular function. Importantly, gentamicin may cause SNHL in about 10–20% of cases. If this risk of hearing loss is not acceptable to the patient, then alternate treatment therapies must be sought. Obviously, ablative therapy is simpler in cases where the hearing has been affected by the pathologic process.

Surgical management of the patient with vertigo is aimed at removing the vestibular input from the dysfunctional side in cases of unilateral vestibular dysfunction. If the hearing has not been affected by the disease process and is stable, then the procedure of choice is vestibular nerve section. Either a middle cranial fossa or occipital craniotomy approach is taken to identify the 7th and 8th nerve complex as it enters the internal acoustic meatus. The vestibular nerve fibers are identified and cut, leaving the cochlear fibers intact. If the hearing has been affected, then the entire labyrinth may be surgically removed, effectively destroying any residual cochlear or vestibular function.

It is important for elderly patients who have undergone these types of surgical ablative treatments to enroll in intensive rehabilitative programs in order to assist with compensation of vestibular function.

Finally, surgery should not be withheld in elderly patients solely on the basis of age if medical therapies have failed and progressive vestibular dysfunction has been identified. Persistent ataxia after treatment is common. Patients should be counseled to move slowly and deliberately, often with the assistance of canes or other devices. Ultimately, the goal of treatment of vertigo in the elderly should be directed at preventing falls, as these are a significant source of morbidities in the elderly.[13] Hip fractures are potential life-threatening complications of falls. Certainly, control of vestibular symptoms in the elderly should be directed at preventing these complications.

References

1. Cummings CW, Fredrickson JM, Harker LA et al., eds. Ear and cranial base. In Otolaryngology, Head and Neck Surgery, Vol 4. St Louis, MO: Mosby, 1993.
2. Laufer W, Gabbay MS, Gold S, Katz J, eds. Handbook of Clinical Audiology, 4th edn. Philadelphia, PA: Lippincott, Williams and Wilkins, 1994.
3. Shuknecht HF. Pathology of the Ear, 2nd edn. Philadelphia, PA: Lea and Febiger, 1993.
4. Schuknecht HF. Further observations on the pathology of presbycusis. Arch Otolaryngol 1964; 80: 369–75.
5. Vesterager V. Fortnightly review: tinnitus – investigation and management. BMJ 1997; 314: 728.
6. Norena A, Cransac H, Chery-Croze S. Towards an objectification by classification of tinnitus. Clin Neurophysiol 1999; 110: 666–75.
7. Simpson JJ, Davies WE. Recent advances in the pharmacological treatment of tinnitus. Trends Pharmacol Sci 1999; 20: 12–18.
8. Peifer KJ, Rosen GP, Rubin AM. Tinnitus, etiologia and management. Clin Geriatr Med 1999; 15: 193–204.
9. Voelker R. Tracking tinnitus. JAMA 1998; 279: 574.
10. Erlandsson SI, Hallberg LR-M. Prediction of quality of life in patients with tinnitus. Br J Audiol 2000; 34: 11–20.
11. Drew S, Davies E. Effectiveness of Ginkgo biloba in treating tinnitus: double blind, placebo-controlled trial. BMJ 2001; 322: 73–5.
12. Koopmann CF, Goldestein JC. Geriatrics otolaryngology. In Johnson JT, Blitzer A, Ossoff R, Thomas JR, eds. Instructional Courses. American Academy of Otolaryngology – Head and Neck Surgery. St Louis, MO: Mosby, 1988: 21–26.
13. Rubenstein LZ, Robins AS, Schulman BL et al. Falls and instability in the elderly. J Am Geriatr Soc 1988; 36: 266–75.

CHAPTER 51

Smell and taste

Weiru Shao and Frank Ondrey

Introduction

The chemical sensations of food, smoke, and dangerous fumes play an important role in our daily life, nutrition, and survival. Olfactory and gustatory dysfunction is associated with a broad range of common diseases and anomalies, including Alzheimer's and Parkinson's diseases. In addition, taste and smell show physiologic deterioration as part of the natural aging process. Physicians treat thousands of patients every year for taste and smell dysfunction. For patients such as cooks, professional food and wine tasters, firemen, natural gas workers, chemists, and many industrial workers, livelihood or immediate safety is dependent upon a normal gustatory and olfactory function.[1,2] Treating gustatory and olfactory dysfunction should be a priority for these patients. In this chapter, the anatomy, physiology, pathology, evaluation, and treatment of taste and smell complaints common to primary-care offices are presented.

Olfaction

Anatomy and physiology

The olfactory epithelium is located high in the nasal vault with an area of $2-10\,cm^2$. It covers the majority of the cribriform plate and superior septum, and some of the superior turbinates. It is a pseudostratified columnar epithelium and consists of olfactory receptor cells, supporting cells, basal cells, and Bowman's glands (the primary source of olfactory mucus).[3] The basal cells are small stem cells in contact with the underlying basement membrane. They have a unique propensity to regenerate into olfactory receptor cells and supporting cells after their damaged.[4]

Odorants, most of which are hydrophobic, dissolve and bind to odorant binding proteins in the olfactory mucus. The bipolar olfactory receptor cells project cilia to the mucosa, which dramatically increases the surface area of the olfactory epithelium. The odorant–protein complexes then bind to special receptors located primarily on the cilia, leading to action-potential firing of the receptor cells. These receptor cells are first-order neurons that send unmyelinated axons directly into the cranial cavity without synapse. Viruses and toxins may invade the central nervous system directly through these conduits of nerve fibers.[4]

The axons of olfactory receptor cells penetrate through small perforations in the cribriform plate of the ethmoid bone to the olfactory bulb (Figure 51.1), where they synapse with dendrites of second-order neurons such as mitral cells and tufted cells in intricate microscopic structures called 'glomeruli'.[3] About 15 000 olfactory receptor cells converge on one mitral cell or tufted cell in one glomerulus. Numerous periglomerular cells, granular cells, and short axon cells interconnect the glomeruli. Consequently, caudal projection of the olfactory signal becomes divergent. Unlike the visual and somatosensory systems, the olfactory system does not demonstrate point-to-point accuracy.[5]

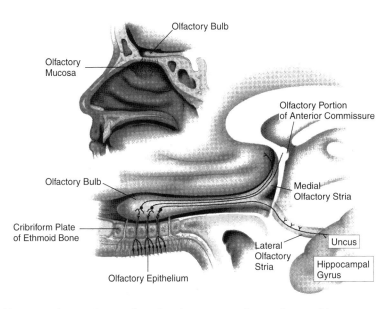

Figure 51.1 *Olfactory pathway. Figure adapted with permission from reference 21.*

The myelinated axons of mitral or tufted cells form the olfactory tract that gives off medial, intermediate, and lateral striae. The medial stria projects to the anterior olfactory nucleus, olfactory tubercle, perpiriform cortex, and amygdala – part of the limbic system which processes emotion and memory. Through the lateral stria, olfactory information reaches the hypothalamus, which controls appetite. The intermediate stria projects to the intermediate olfactory area. Its role in olfactory perception is probably insignificant in the human.[6,7]

Pungency is generally not regarded as a smell, but a different sense related to nociception. It is mediated by the trigeminal nerve, and has a threshold much higher than that of normal smell.[8,9] It has its use in the evaluation of olfaction.

Olfactory disorders

The National Institute on Deafness and Other Communication Disorders estimated that more than 2.7 million adults in the USA (1.4% of the population) have chronic olfactory impairment.[10] The most commonly cited impairments were of the ability to detect spoiled food, gas leaks, or smoke, and in eating and cooking. Major olfactory disorders include the following: anosmia (absence of smell), hyposmia (diminished smell sensitivity), dysosmia (distorted smell perception), hyperosmia (abnormally acute smell function), and phantosmia (olfactory hallucination).

The most frequent complaints seen in a primary-care office are anosmia and hyposmia. The etiologies include a multitude of causes (Table 51.1) or occur as a consequence of normal aging. In diagnosing olfactory disorders, it helps to consider two major categories: conductive vs sensorineural loss.[4] In conductive loss, the access of olfactory stimuli to the olfactory epithelium is obstructed by conditions such as nasal polyps, thickened or excessive mucus overlying the epithelium, edema within the epithelium due to nasal or paranasal sinus disease, severe septal deviation, intranasal tumors, lack of airflow due to laryngectomy, and others. In sensorineural loss, lesions are located proximal to the olfactory receptor cells. They may include loss of receptor cells from viral invasion, shear injury of receptor cell axons as they penetrate the cribriform plate in head trauma, intracranial mass lesions, and effects of environmental and industrial pollutants on the receptor epithelium, radiation injury, and so on. Other causes such as adverse drug

Table 51.1 *Medical conditions that affect smell*

Nervous
Korsakoff's syndrome
Parkinson's disease
Head trauma
Multiple sclerosis
Intranasal tumors

Endocrine
Adrenal cortical insufficiency
Primary amenorrhea
Pseudohypoparathyroidism
Cushing's syndrome
Hypothyroidism
Diabetes mellitus
Gonadal dysgenesis (Turner's syndrome)
Hypogonadotropic hypogonadism
  (Kallman's syndrome)

Nutritional
Vitamin B12 deficiency
Chronic renal failure
Liver disease including cirrhosis

Local
Allergic rhinitis and atopy
Bronchial asthma
Leprosy
Ozena
Sinusitis and polyposis
Sjögren's syndrome

Other
Familial (genetic)
Laryngectomy
Olfactory sarcoidosis

effects, nutritional deficits, and central nervous system (CNS) degenerative and congenital diseases are often overlooked during the diagnostic work-up.[4]

In many cases, there is a combination of conductive and sensorineural losses, as blockage of olfactory stimuli to the receptor cells and damage to the central elements of the olfactory pathway can be presented at the same time. Nevertheless, the utility in the two diagnostic categories is that we are able to treat many conductive losses, yet the majority of sensorineural losses remain at present untreatable.[4] According to a study of 750 consecutive patients at a major smell and taste center, upper respiratory infection, head trauma, and nasal and paranasal sinus disease accounted for 60% of cases.[11]

Upper respiratory infection

Upper respiratory infection (URI) is one of the most common causes of temporary hyposmia and, rarely, anosmia. Inflammation from URI causes edema in and around the olfactory cleft, and blocks olfactory stimuli from binding to the olfactory receptors. Symptoms typically resolve or lessen in 3–5 days.[4] However, a small group of patients, mostly middle-aged and healthy women, have persistent symptoms. Possible culprits have been suggested to include viral invasion and destruction of the olfactory fibers and other central olfactory components.[3] Only one-third of these patients recover after a number of years.[12]

Nasal and paranasal sinus disease

The airstream that carries olfactory stimuli to the olfactory epithelium has been shown to be medial to the anterior portion of the middle turbinate. Because of its close proximity to the anterior ethmoid sinus, the site most prone to sinusitis, anatomic changes in this area such as mucosal swelling and polyposis from chronic infectious or allergic sinusitis can impair olfaction. The progression of symptoms is usually gradual, and prognosis is good if the underlying condition is treated. Relief with a 1–2-week course of oral steroids is diagnostic as well as therapeutic.[3]

Medication

Drugs – oral, intravenous, or topical – have all been reported to cause olfactory dysfunction (Table 51.2).[13] The possible mechanisms are diverse, and may involve altered receptor site binding, diminished cellular renewal at the olfactory epithelium, change of neurotransduction, and general CNS toxicity. Sometimes it is almost impossible to differentiate drug effects from the concomitant medical illness that the medication is taken for. Overall, only a small group of patients complain of these olfactory-drug adverse effects, which can be

Table 51.2 *Examples of medications that affect olfaction*[13]

Local anesthetic	cocaine hydrochloride
Antihypertensives	nifedipine, diltiazem, propranolol
Antimicrobials	clarithromycin, ciprofloxacin, ampicillin
Antithyroids	carbimazole, thiouracil
Opiates	codeine, morphine
Antidepressants	amitriptyline, clozapine
Sympathomimetics	amfetamines
Amebicides and anthelmintics	metronidazole, nizidazole
Immunosuppressants	methotrexate, azathioprine
Antirheumatics	gold, colchicine, allopurinol
Antihistamines	loratadine, pseudoephedrine

temporary or permanent.[3] Discontinuing the offending medication and changing to another kind may be helpful.

Medical disease

Adrenal insufficiency, hypophyseal insufficiency, hypothyroidism, and uremia all affect receptor cell turnover rate, and have all been associated with olfactory dysfunction. Niacin and zinc deficiency can have a similar effect.[3] Intranasal neoplasms, such as inverted papilloma, squamous cell carcinoma, adenocarcinoma and olfactory neuroblastoma, may obstruct the olfactory airflow. Intracranial meningiomas, pituitary adenomas and gliomas may cause local neurodestruction.[4] Approximately 25% of temporal lobe tumors produce an olfactory disturbance.[3]

Laryngectomy and other iatrogenic causes

Total laryngectomy results in breathing through a cervical stoma, bypassing the upper airway. The lack of nasal airflow and, hence, lack of intranasal odorants cause a decrease in olfactory perception.[3] It also diminishes retronasal airflow behind the soft palate,

reducing the many so-called tastes that are actually smelled, such as chocolate, coffee, tea, and meat.[8] Previous nasal and paranasal surgery can affect olfaction by nasal airway obstruction with postoperative adhesions, direct trauma to the olfactory epithelium, and axonal damage by cribriform plate fracture.[3]

Head trauma

The severity of head injury correlates with olfactory loss, although even minor trauma can produce total anosmia. The mechanism involves shearing of the olfactory receptor axons as they penetrate the cribriform plate. As the body heals over time, the perforations in the cribriform plate may be scarred, which prevents regenerating axons from reaching the olfactory bulb to reinnervate.[8,14] Frontal blows frequently result in olfactory loss; however occipital blows, in themselves less common, are five times more likely to result in total anosmia,[12] possibly by a contra-coup mechanism. Olfactory loss is usually immediate, and recovery occurs in less than 10% of patients. Major recovery, if there is any, usually starts within 3 months and occurs within 6 months. Amnesia following head trauma for more than 24 hours indicates a poor prognosis.[15]

Environmental exposure

Both direct and passive smoking are associated with olfactory loss.[16] The unique exposure of olfactory receptors to the external environment renders them vulnerable to inhaled chemicals. Physiologic and anatomic damage, even modification of neurotransmitter levels, can be induced by brief or prolonged exposure to pollutants.[14,16]

Congenital

Children begin to discern odors, tastes, and pungency at around age 8. Congenital anosmia can be partial to a particular chemical or complete as pananosmic. Females are twice as likely as males to be affected. Kallman's syndrome is associated with olfactory bulb ageneis and hypogonadotropic hypogonadism.[17] Congenital anosmia is also associated with Turner's syndrome, premature baldness, and vascular headaches in some patients. These patients have been reported to avoid fragrance for fear of overuse.[18] The diagnosis is by exclusion.[18]

Psychiatric

In the 'olfactory reference syndrome' the patient is so obsessively concerned with minor bodily smell that she/he bathes frequently and overuses perfume. Patients with 'Marcel Proust syndrome' often dramatically conjure up memories of odors which interfere with daily routines.[3] In addition, disturbance of the limbic to hypothalamic pathways in depressive states may also lead to olfactory dysfunction.[19] On the other hand, dysfunction itself may affect patients psychologically, as those with dysosmia and dysgeusia are 1.5 times more prone to depression using the Beck Depression Inventory scoring system.[10,20]

Neurodegeneration and aging

It has been found that more than 75% of people over the age of 80 have major difficulty detecting and identifying odors.[21] Yet patients with Alzheimer's disease score lower on olfactory tests than do age-matched controls, even when mild levels of dementia are taken into account.[22,23] The presence of relatively high levels of neuritic plaques and neurofibrillary tangles has been noted in olfactory pathways, including the anterior olfactory nucleus, olfactory bulb, prepiriform cortex, prefrontal cortex, and the dorsomedial thalamic nucleus. It has been suggested that olfactory dysfunction is among the first signs of Alzheimer's disease.[23]

In Parkinson's disease, olfactory dysfunction is also found early in its development, however the dysfunction is unrelated to neurologic signs, disease stage, or duration.[20] Anosmia is rare in multiple sclerosis.[24]

Gustation

Anatomy and physiology

The sensation of taste begins with the presentation of a taste stimulus to taste buds that are scattered primarily on the dorsal surface of the tongue, lateral tongue margin, and base of the tongue. Taste buds are also found on the soft palate, pharynx, larynx, epiglottis, uvula, and upper third of the esophagus. Food stimulates taste buds during chewing and swallowing, and while being pressed on the palate by the tongue.[21]

Taste buds are ovoid clusters of receptor cells, supporting cells and precursor cells arranged in segments like those of an orange. Taste receptor cells have a limited lifespan of around 10 days.[1] They are susceptible to malnutrition, radiation, and medications that impair cell renewal.[25] Lingual taste buds are found in taste papillae, which give the tongue its bumpy appearance.

There are four kinds of taste papillae: filiform, fungiform, foliate, and circumvallate. The filiform papillae are the most numerous, but they have little role in the human's sense of taste. The fungiform papillae are located mostly on the tip and the edges of the anterior two-thirds of the tongue. The density diminishes towards the center. They are visible as small red dots on the tongue. Each of them contains 1–18 taste buds. The foliate papillae appear deep red from the surrounding mucosa at the posterior lateral sides of the tongue. They are better seen with the mouth wide open and the tongue moved to one side. The circumvallate papillae are slightly elevated and circular. They are located on the rear part of the tongue, with the largest mostly around the midline.[25]

The idea of a tongue map – a picture of taste distribution with sweet at the tip of the tongue, sour along the edges, bitter at the back, while salty at all locations – is misleading yet has been tenacious to correction. In 1901, Hänig measured the thresholds for the four basic tastes on the tongue. He noted lower thresholds, although very small differences, to the four tastes on the four loci and generated the tongue map. The truth is that all four primary tastes are independent of each other, and every taste bud has some degree of sensitivity to all four tastes. They can be perceived anywhere on the tongue as long as taste buds are located there.[25]

In a taste bud the sensory receptor cells, also called type III cells, taper to form apical microvilli projecting into the taste pore. At the base of the receptor cells there are synaptic vesicles with

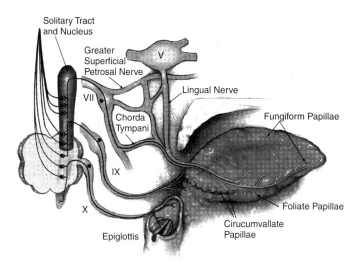

Figure 51.2 *Gustatory pathway. Figure adapted with permission from reference 21.*

associated afferent gustatory nerve endings. A single taste bud is innervated by about 50 nerve fibers. Taste stimuli can reach the receptor cells via two means. First, taste elements released during chewing and swallowing reach the microvilli in the taste pore and interact with ion channels (most often salt and acid stimuli) or membrane receptors (bitter stimuli). The subsequent signals lead to activation of the neural synapses at the base of the receptor cells. The biochemical mechanism for sweetness is still unknown, but has been suggested to involve more than one receptor mechanism. Second, blood-borne substances diffuse through capillary walls and stimulate sensitive sites at the base of receptor cells directly. This phenomenon, called venous taste, may be a source of altered taste associated with certain intravenous medications.[8,25]

Three nerves carry taste information from taste receptor cells to the brain: facial (cranial nerve, CN VII), glossopharyngeal (CN IX) and, less importantly, vagus (CN X) nerves (Figure 51.2). Two branches of the facial nerve are involved. The chorda tympani nerve innervates the taste buds in the fungiform papillae on the anterior two-thirds of the tongue and some in the foliate papillae.[6]

Running along the lingual nerve (CN V_3), which supplies sensation to the same area, the chorda tympani nerve joins the parasympathetic fibers from the submandibular ganglion, which innervates the submandibular and sublingual glands. Coursing cephalad, the nerve reaches the infratemporal fossa between the medial pterygoid muscle and the angle of the mandible, where it leaves the lingual nerve. The chorda tympani penetrates the petrotympanic fissure (Hunguier's canal) of the petrous temporal bone and enters the middle ear at the superior lateral aspect. The nerve is then suspended in the superior quadrants of the middle ear space. The freely suspended section of the chorda tympani nerve is susceptible to damage from middle ear pathology such as ear infection. The nerve exits the middle ear through a bony canaliculus posteriorly, just medial to the fibrous annulus of the tympanic membrane. It then joins the motor portion of the facial nerve in the mastoid. Together they travel towards the internal auditory canal (IAC).[25]

The greater superficial petrosal nerve (GSPN), another branch of the facial nerve, supplies taste to the palate.[6] Nerves that innervate the palatal taste buds travel through the lesser palatine foramina, greater palatine canal, pterygopalatine fossa, and pterygoid canal where they become the GSPN. It crosses the foramen lacerum into the middle cranial fossa before it enters the petrous temporal bone at the facial hiatus. The GSPN finally joins the facial nerve at the geniculate ganglion immediately distal to the IAC.[25]

The glossopharyngeal nerve innervates the foliate and the circumvallate papillae at the posterior tongue.[6] It runs deep in the tonsillar bed, where it may be vulnerable during difficult tonsillectomy. It eventually enters the jugular foramen and reaches the retro-olivary area of the medulla through the cerebellopontine angle.[25]

The superior laryngeal nerve, a branch of the vagus nerve, innervates the taste buds on the laryngeal surface of the epiglottis and possibly the upper third of the esophagus.[6] It also enters the jugular foramen and reaches the medulla. Its role in taste perception is unknown.[25]

The taste fibers of all three cranial nerves project to the rostral portion of the nucleus solitary tract in the medulla. From there it further projects to the thalamus, hypothalamus, amygdala, and stria terminalis. From the thalamus, it also runs separate projections to the primary gustatory cortex and then secondary cortex on the orbitofrontal surface.[6]

Gustatory disorders

Gustatory impairment classification is similar to its olfactory counterpart: ageusia (absence of taste), hypogeusia (diminished taste), dysgeusia (distorted taste), and phantogeusia (more commonly called 'taste phantom').[25]

Gustatory loss (Table 51.3) seems to be a rare complaint overall. One reason is the multiple peripheral innervation to the gustatory system, which provides a safety net against complete ageusia. Another is the intrinsic self-inhibitory mechanism among gustatory nerves. It has been observed clinically that when a chorda tympani nerve is anesthetized unilaterally by transtympanic membrane injection of lidocaine, tastes innervated by the glossopharyngeal nerve are intensified, with the contralateral bitter taste being the greatest. Painting a topical anesthetic on the contralateral tongue can then abolish the intensified bitterness.

Table 51.3 *Medical conditions that affect taste*

Nervous
Bell's palsy
Damage to chorda tympani
Head trauma
Multiple sclerosis

Endocrine
Adrenal cortical insufficiency
Congenital adrenal hyperplasia
Pseudohypoparathyroidism
Panhypopituitarism
Cushing's syndrome
Cretinism
Hypothyroidism
Diabetes mellitus
Gonadal dysgenesis (Turner's syndrome)

Nutritional
Cancer
Chronic renal failure
Liver disease including cirrhosis
Niacin (vitamin B3) deficiency
Zinc deficiency
Thermal burn

Local
Facial hypoplasia
Glossitis and other oral disorders
Leprosy
Oral Crohn's disease
Radiation therapy
Sjögren's syndrome

Other
Hypertension
Influenza-like infection

This suggests that the taste phantom results from abnormal spontaneous excitation because of the release of active inhibition from the disabled side.[25]

'Supertasters' have higher sweet (but not in relation to all artificial sweeteners) and bitter taste sensations for a variety of stimuli than do medium tasters and non-tasters. This is suspected to involve two codominant traits. Supertasters may have more taste buds than medium tasters, and medium tasters more than non-tasters.[25] It is noted that women are more likely than men to be supertasters, and Asians more than Caucasians. Clinically supertasters assign higher bitter intensity scores when given 6-n-propylthiouracil than do non-tasters. It is likely that supertasters complain more than do non-tasters of oral pain, involving taste bud areas, connected with mucositis and aphthous ulcers. Supertasters also perceive fat to be more creamy than do non-tasters (fat has no taste or smell). In a sample of postmenopausal women, supertasters had lower body mass indices (weight/height^2) than non-tasters.[25]

Chorda tympani injury

Acute or chronic otitis media is the most common middle ear pathology, and has been recognized as an important source of damage to the gustatory system. The chorda tympani nerve is susceptible to inflammatory or direct infectious injury, as it is completely exposed traveling through the middle ear cavity.[8] However, chronic otitis media patients actually experience enhanced tastes from some stimuli. This is partly due to increased activity in some nerves as the result of lessened self-inhibition by damaged nerves.[25]

During ear surgeries, such as middle ear exploration, stapedectomy, tympanoplasty, and mastoidectomy, the chorda tympani nerve may be stretched or cut leading to temporary or permanent taste loss. Although it renders the ipsilateral anterior tongue completely devoid of taste, the most common complaint is not loss of taste but rather a metallic phantom.[26,27] Even washing the ear canal has been reported to produce a similar taste phantom.

Glossopharyngeal trauma

The CN IX, including its lingual and pharyngeal branches, is vulnerable during tonsillectomy.[25] Unfortunately, many tonsillectomy patients have a history of recurrent or chronic ear infection, and may have damaged chorda tympani preoperatively. Because of its insidious nature, the taste change due to chorda tympani damage may be barely noticeable subjectively. Nevertheless, the addition of a glossopharyngeal loss leaves no reserve, such that patients complain of complete loss of taste in the affected tongue area.

Viral injury

Bell's palsy (herpes simplex mononeuritis) and Ramsay Hunt syndrome (herpes zoster oticus) are associated with taste dysfunction as well as unilateral facial paralysis.[8] Interestingly, a natural course of Ramsay Hunt syndrome was carefully documented by Carl Pfaffmann, a pioneer chemosensory researcher who contracted the illness himself. Initially, the affected left side was completely devoid of taste, while the right side produced heightened sense of taste. Daily taste experience was not affected. Over the next 3 years of recovery on the left, the right side taste gradually lessened towards normal.[25]

In Lyme disease, about 10% of patients are affected with unilateral or bilateral facial paralysis. Its mechanism is unknown.[8,25]

Mass lesion

Temporal bone tumors such as glomus jugulare, facial nerve neuroma, and squamous cell carcinoma may affect chorda tympani before facial paresis manifests. Cerebellopontine angle tumors such as acoustic neuroma and meningioma can produce isolated taste loss by involving the nervus intermedius.[25]

'Jugular foramen syndrome', also named Vernet syndrome, is the paralysis of all nerves that traverse the jugular foramen (CNs IX, X, and XI) from lesions directly involving the skull base at the jugular foramen (glomus jugulare, schwannoma, squamous cell carcinoma). Symptoms include taste loss from CNs IX and X, ipsilateral vocal cord paralysis, and ipsilateral shoulder drop. When a tumor extends deep into the foramen magnum causing ipsilateral tongue paralysis, it becomes Collet–Sicard syndrome. If the tumor compromises the sympathetic trunk in addition to all of the above, it is termed Villaret syndrome. Patients also exhibit Horner's syndrome.[25]

Oral cavity and oropharyngeal tumors do not present with taste loss alone. Lack of gag reflex would be more noticeable.[25]

Central nervous system

Pontine hemorrhage and damage to the rostral insular cortex may lead to ipsilateral taste loss. Temporal lobe epilepsy occasionally presents a metallic taste prior to a seizure.[25]

In head trauma, the incidence of taste loss is 0.4–0.5% by report.[25]

Medication

Medications passing through the capillary walls can stimulate taste receptors in taste buds directly. This may be the origin of dysgeusia for many chemotherapy agents.[25] Patients receiving levothyroxine complain of taste loss more frequently, but their taste identification test scores are not lower than those of controls.[4]

Some medications have been associated with metallic dysgeusia in some patients. They include tetracycline, lithium, penicilliamine, and captopril. Cisplatin and bleomycin are reported to cause hypogeusia, especially at high doses.[28]

Clinical evaluation of olfactory and gustatory disorders

To taste or to smell – that is the question

The distinction between taste and smell is vague among the general public. Odorants that are sniffed into the nose are identified as smells without confusion. Yet most people wrongly label odorants entering the nose through the nasopharynx during eating as part of taste.[8] One report showed that of 750 patients complaining of taste loss, fewer than 4% had measurable gustatory deficit; in contrast, 71% had absent or diminished olfactory function.[11]

Gustatory loss is much less common than olfactory loss, considering that gustation has multiple innervations over a large area of tongue while olfaction has a single innervation by CN I over a limited area in the olfactory cleft. In addition, olfactory neurons are receptor cells exposed vulnerably to the external environment, while gustatory neurons are buried deep in the taste buds, protected from potential toxins.

True taste loss signifies a loss in the ability to taste saltiness, sweetness, sourness, and bitterness.[8] In a primary-care setting, it is often helpful to ask patients whether they can taste the sweetness of sugar, the sourness of grapefruit juice, the bitterness of strong coffee, and the saltiness of potato chips. Affirmative answers to all of the above usually preclude general gustatory dysfunction.[8] An olfactory loss should be considered, especially if patients report weak tastes to the above items.

In general, a thorough history and physical examination is necessary as an initial evaluation to smell and taste disorders. Much information and clinical clues are generated from the medical and surgical history alone. A careful examination of the posterior tongue and intranasal mucosa requires special instruments, such as reflective mirror, nasal endoscope, and sometimes flexible laryngoscope. Special imaging studies, such as sinus computed tomography, are justified and cost-effective only after physical examination is concluded. They are indispensable in diagnosing sinusitis, examining the integrity of the cribriform plate, or locating a posterior mass. Sinus plain X-ray films lack specificity, and are generally discouraged.[4] Early referral to otolaryngology specialists is preferred when symptoms persist.

Olfactory and gustatory tests

In a primary-care office, a rapid and reliable alcohol sniff test (AST) can be used to screen olfactory dysfunction.[9] Developed at the University of California, San Diego, the test involves a standard 70% isopropyl alcohol preparation pad found in most clinics. The pad is opened such that 0.5 cm of the pad is visible. The alcohol pad is then placed beneath the patient's nostrils while the patient inspires twice to become familiarized with the alcohol odor. The pad is then withdrawn and the threshold test is ready to begin. The patient is asked to close the mouth and eyes, breathe normally and indicate when the odor is detected. Active sniffing and deep inspiration are discouraged. The alcohol pad is placed 30 cm below the nose and, with each expiration, is moved 1 cm closer to the nares until the patient detects the presence of the odor. The distance from the anterior nares to the alcohol pad is measured in centimeters where the odor is first detected. The procedure is repeated four times and the mean distance defines the threshold. A distance of more than 10 cm at mid-chest is found in normosmia, 5–10 cm in hyposmia, and less than 5 cm in anosmia (private communication with the authors).

The mechanism of the AST is that odor thresholds for alcohol are two or more orders of magnitude lower than the trigeminal pungent threshold for the same stimulus. In anosmia, alcohol odor stimulates the trigeminal nerve only when it is very close to the nose. The test is simple and takes only 5 minutes. Note that the AST is not designed to rule out malingering.

For more accurate and objective information, there are seven smell and taste tests used by special chemosensory centers. Owing to the specialized materials required, associated costs and the length of the tests, their usage is limited:[11]

1. University of Pennsylvania smell identification test (UPSIT): a standardized 40-stimulus microencapsulated 'scratch-and-sniff' odor identification test.
2. Phenyl ethyl alcohol (PEA) test: a forced-choice single-staircase rose-like odor detection threshold test that has little or no intranasal trigeminal stimulation properties at any concentration.
3. Suprathreshold taste quality identification of sucrose, citric acid, caffeine, and sodium chloride.
4. Taste intensity rating test: uses different concentrations of the tastants mentioned in 3.
5. Taste threshold test: detects the minimal concentration of detection of the four tastes.
6. Regional taste quality identification test: identifies unilateral, anterior, or posterior tongue deficit that is innervated by different nerves.
7. Electrogustometric threshold test: differentiates the sensitivity of the two sides of the anterior portion of the tongue to minute electric currents.

Treatment

Currently, no effective treatments for smell dysfunction other than those associated with nasal/sinus

disease have been identified. Antibiotics for acute and chronic infection can decrease mucosal inflammation. Nasal decongestants, oral and topical with short-term use, can treat mucosal edema. Topical steroids are frequently used for long-term maintenance of nasal mucosa. Sinonasal surgery may eradicate chronic sinus infection and correct intranasal anatomic anomalies.

For metallic dysgeusia induced by certain medications, most reports indicate quick resolution with termination of the offending agents; but with captopril, it has been reported to persist for months in some patients.[28]

Impact of aging on smell and taste

Age-related decline in both sensory functions demonstrates progressively diminished sensitivity, with that of smell worse than that of taste. These losses begin around age 60 and become more severe at age 70.[6] Such deficits adversely affect nutritional intake, immunologic defense, and a variety of biochemical measures in the elderly, such as insulin and other pancreatic enzyme secretion. There is no proven pharmacologic treatment, and the prognosis for recovery of smell and taste sensation is generally poor.[6] Nevertheless, preventive measures and compensatory methods are available.

Many elderly patients have decreased salivary flow due to dehydration, medication, head and neck irradiation, sialithiasis, or vitamin deficiencies. Treating these conditions and ensuring adequate fluid intake may increase saliva flow and help tastants reach taste buds.[29] Sialogogs can be prescribed to stimulate saliva glands if their function is intact.

Tongue brushing twice a day may increase taste acuity by removing thick white mucoid coats on the dorsal tongue.[29] Smoking not only diminishes the taste of food, but also makes flavorful food taste flat and unappetizing.[6,29] Both direct and passive smoking are associated with olfactory loss.[16]

Sensory interventions to intensify the taste and odor of food can compensate for certain perceptual loss. It has been shown that sour and bitter are less affected by aging than salty and sweet.[6] To enhance food flavor efficiently, excessive sugar and salt intake should be avoided. Instead, flavoring agents to enhance taste acuity in other aspects should be added, such as vanilla, orange, strawberry, caraway, chilli powder, chives, cinnamon, cloves, curry, garlic (not garlic salt), ginger, lemon juice, mint, dry mustard, peppers, sage, tarragon, and vinegar.[29]

For patients who complain that 'food doesn't taste the way it used to', i.e. when they were young, elevating concentrations of flavor may offset their loss in smell and taste. For example, adding chicken flavor while cooking chicken may amplify its aroma. Bacon, cheese flavor, tomato, and pea can also be added to soups and vegetables.[6] In 13 cancer patients, preferences for food increased from 8–31% to 69–92% after flavoring agents were added.[30]

Dietary supplements with zinc, vitamin A, or niacin have been tried in the past, but evidence for their effectiveness is not compelling.[11]

Dietary use of monosodium glutamate

Recent research into monosodium glutamate (MSG) has shown that food intensified with MSG and other flavors increases food acceptance and intake in the elderly, and improves their immune status by enhanced T and B cell levels and immunoglobulin A (IgA) secretion.[30]

Monosodium glutamate is the sodium salt of the amino acid, glutamic acid. Its average daily intake is estimated to be 0.3–1.0 g in industrialized countries.[31] Functioning as a flavoring agent, glutamate is added to food during cooking as MSG. Glutamate also occurs naturally in a variety of foods, such as tomatoes, cheese, meat, and fish, and in soups where glutamate is released by cellular breakdown and protein hydrolysis, and adds much flavor.[32] Although not widely appreciated in Western culture, glutamate has been a key flavoring ingredient in Asian cuisine for ages. The Chinese call MSG WeiJing, the spirit of taste. The Japanese name it Umami, distinct from the basic four tastes.[33] A variety of testing techniques have demonstrated that the taste quality of MSG does not fall within the qualitative taste range defined by the traditional

four tastes of sweet, sour, salt, and bitter.[6] It has been suggested that Umami, since Western culture does not have a name for it, is the fifth essential taste.[30]

Both central and peripheral actions from glutamate sensors have been identified. After applying MSG to the tongue, selective responding neurons in the hypothalamus, important in appetite control, and the orbital prefrontal cortex, important in taste and smell perception, have been demonstrated.[34,35] There are also glutamate receptors in the oral cavity and small intestine that are found to be capable of inducing a reflex activation of efferent fibers from the brain to the pancreas and elsewhere via the vagus nerve. It is conceivable that glutamate ingestion might facilitate food digestion and nutrient absorption and distribution.[36] Commercially available MSG often contains a mixture of 5′-ribonucleotides including inosine-5′-monophosphate (IMP) and guanosine-5′-monophosphate (GMP). These compounds have potent synergistic effects with MSG, which lower the MSG threshold level.[30]

Safety of dietary monosodium glutamate

Once glutamate enters the gut, it is preferentially metabolized by the intestine. Up to half of the energy consumed by the intestine during digestion comes from glutamate.[37] The rest of it participates in a variety of important biochemical pathways in the body, such as gluconeogenesis, transamination and deamination of other amino acids, and hepatic nitrogen elimination via the urea cycle.[32] The fact that a large amount of glutamate is consumed for energy in the gut and as a metabolic substrate in the liver before entering the systemic circulation may help to explain why glutamate concentrations in the blood rise only moderately after large MSG or glutamate doses are ingested by adults, either as MSG added to food or as glutamate contained in food proteins.[38]

In 1988 a joint expert committee from the World Health Organization and the Food and Agriculture Organization of the United Nations published its safety evaluation of MSG. The committee noted that intestinal and hepatic metabolism results in elevated levels of MSG in the systemic circulation only after extremely high doses are given by gavage (> 30 mg/kg body weight). The committee allocated an 'acceptable daily intake not specified' to glutamic acid and its salts. The Scientific Committee for Food of the European Commission reached a similar recommendation in 1991.[39] In 1989 the Food and Drug Administration (FDA) affirmed the safety of MSG at levels normally consumed by the general population. In 1991 it again concluded that there is no evidence linking current MSG food use to any serious, long-term medical problems in the general population.[39]

The FDA did acknowledge the existence of some evidence of dose-dependent, mild reactions to MSG in a small group of the general population. The 'Chinese-restaurant syndrome' is a complex of symptoms following ingestion of a Chinese meal. It consists of numbness at the back of the neck and arms, weakness, flushing, and palpitations.[31] In addition, there have been preliminary reports associating asthma attacks with oral MSG challenge without simultaneous food intake.[40] Nevertheless, double-blind, placebo-controlled human studies have failed to confirm an involvement of MSG in Chinese-restaurant syndrome.[39] The existence of MSG-induced asthma, even in patients with a positive history, has not been replicated in well-designed studies.[40]

In the mammalian CNS and especially in the retina, glutamate is the principal excitatory neurotransmitter whose extracellular level is tightly regulated. Excessive levels lead to neuroexcitotoxicity, which has been implicated in the pathogenesis of many neurologic and ophthalmic diseases, including stroke, trauma, epilepsy, dementia, and glaucoma.[41] Under normal conditions, glutamate is stored in neurons and released at neurosynapses for very brief periods in localized areas. Specialized glutamate receptors found in the CNS rapidly transport glutamate back into the intracellular space and thus maintain physiologic concentrations. Because functional glutamate transporters should timely restore its homeostatic levels, glutamate transporter malfunction has been strongly implicated in glutamate receptor-mediated neuroexcitotoxicity. In fact, transient release of glutamate is found to be not associated with a significant elevation in extracellular glutamate in some neurologic diseases mentioned above, and a decreased level of glutamate transporters is identified in human glaucoma with retinal ganglion cell death.[41]

More evidence will emerge over the next decade about the safety of MSG in humans. At present, moderate use of MSG as a food-flavoring agent should be considered safe. In the neonatal mouse the oral effective dose (ED_{50}) for producing noticeable lesions in the hypothalamus where there is a lack of blood–brain barrier is ~500 mg MSG/kg body weight by gavage, whereas the largest palatable dose for humans is ~ 60 mg/kg body weight. In a 70-kg man this is about 12 teaspoons or four tablespoons of MSG – with higher doses causing nausea. Thus, voluntary ingestion should not exceed this level.[39]

Conclusions

Smell and taste dysfunction can impact substantially on our psychological well-being, impede performance in some occupations, and lead to nutritional deficiency. It may render patients vulnerable to hazardous environments, toxic fumes, and spoiled food. The elderly are at greater risk, as smell and taste acuity declines naturally with age. Although treatment options for olfactory impairment remain limited, especially in sensorineural loss, thorough evaluation is needed, particularly with regard to safety issues and other related conditions such as depression and nutritional deficit. Adding food-flavoring agents and MSG are proven methods to improve oral intake and immune status in the elderly.

References

1. Schiffman SS. Taste and smell in disease. N Engl J Med 1983; 308: 1275–9, 1337–43.
2. Doty RL. A review of olfactory dysfunctions in man. Am J Otolaryngol 1979; 1: 57–79.
3. Jones N, Rog D. Olfaction: a review. J Laryngol Otol 1998; 113: 11–24.
4. Deems DA, Doty RL, Hummel T, Kratskin IL. Olfactory function and disorders. In: Bailey BJ, ed. Head and Neck Surgery – Otolaryngology, 2nd edn. Philadelphia, PA: Lippincott-Raven, 1998: 317–31.

5. Mori K, Yoshihara Y. Molecular recognition and olfactory processing in the mammalian olfactory system. Prog Neurophysiol 1995; 45: 585–619.

6. Schiffman SS. Taste and smell losses in normal aging and disease. JAMA 1997; 278: 1357–62.

7. Wilson-Pauwels L, Akesson EJ, Stewart PA. Olfactory nerve. In: Sandoz, ed. Cranial Nerves – Anatomy and Clinical Comments. New York: BC Decker, Inc, 1988.

8. Weiffenbach JM, Bartoshuk LM. Taste and smell. Clin Geriatr Med 1992; 8: 543–55.

9. Davidson TM, Murphy C. Rapid clinical evaluation of anosmia – the alcohol sniff test. Arch Otolaryngol Head Neck Surg 1997; 123: 591–4.

10. Miwa T, Furukawa M, Tsukatani T et al. Impact of olfactory impairment on quality of life and disability. Arch Otolaryngol Head Neck Surg 2001; 127: 497–503.

11. Deems DA, Doty RL, Settle GS et al. Smell and taste disorders, a study of 750 patients from the University of Pennsylvania Smell and Taste Center. Arch Otolaryngol Head Neck Surg 1991; 117: 519–28.

12. Hendriks APJ. Olfactory dysfunction. Rhinology 1988; 26: 229–51.

13. Schiffman SS. Clinical physiology of taste and smell. Annu Rev Nutr 1993; 13: 405–36.

14. Cowart BJ, Young IM, Feldman RS, Lowry LD. Clinical disorders of smell and taste. Occup Med 1997; 12: 465–83.

15. Mott AE. Disorders of taste and smell. Med Clin North Am 1991; 75: 1321–53.

16. Frye RE. Dose related effects of cigarette smoking on olfactory function. JAMA 1990; 263: 1233–6.

17. Singh N, Grewal MS, Austin JH. Familial anosmia. Arch Neurol 1970; 22: 40–4.

18. Leopold DA, Hornung DE, Schwob JE. Congenital lack of olfactory ability. Ann Otol Rhinol Laryngol 1992; 101: 229–36.

19. Jesberger JA. Brain output dysregulation induced by olfactory bulbectomy: an approximation in the rat of major depressive disorder in human? Int J Neurosci 1988; 38: 241–65.

20. Ward CD, Hess WA, Calne DB. Olfactory impairment in Parkinson's disease. Neurology 1983; 33: 943–6.

21. Schiffman SS. Taste and smell losses in normal aging and disease. JAMA 1997; 278: 1357–62.

22. Nordin S, Murphy C. Odor memory in normal aging and Alzheimer's disease. Ann NY Acad Sci 1998; 855: 686–93.

23. Doty R. Olfactory capacities in aging and Alzheimer's disease. Ann NY Acad Sci 1991; 640: 20–7.

24. Doty RL, Shaman P, Damm M. Development of the University of Pennsylvania smell identification test: a standardized microencapsulated test of olfactory function. Physiol Behav 1984; 32: 489–502.

25. Kveton JF, Bartoshuk LM. Taste. In Bailey BJ, ed. Head and Neck Surgery – Otolaryngology, 2nd edn. Philadelphia, PA: Lippincott-Raven, 1998: 609–26.

26. Bull TR. Taste and the chorda tympani. J Laryngol Otol 1965; 79: 479–93.

27. Moon CN, Pullen EW. Effects of chorda tympani section during middle ear surgery. Laryngoscope 1963; 73: 392–405.

28. Frank ME, Hettinger TP. The sense of taste: neurobiology, aging, and medication effects. Crit Rev Oral Biol Med 1992; 3: 371–93.

29. Winkler S, Garg AK, Trakol M et al. Depressed taste and smell in geriatric patients. JAMA 1999; 130: 1759–65.

30. Schiffman SS. Intensification of sensory properties of foods for the elderly. J Nutr 2000; 130: 927S–30S.

31. Geha RS, Beiser A, Ren C et al. Review of alleged reaction to monosodium glutamate and outcome of a multicenter double-blind placebo-controlled study. J Nutr 2000; 130: 1058–62S.

32. Fernstrom JD. Second international conference on glutamate: conference summary. J Nutr 2000; 130: 1077–9S.

33. Yamaguchi S, Ninomiya K. Umami and food palatability. J Nutr 2000; 130: 921–6S.

34. Nishijo H, Ono T, Uwano T et al. Hypothalamic and amygdalar neuronal responses to various tastant solutions during ingestive behavior in rats. J Nutr 2000; 130: 954–9S.

35. Rolls ET. The representation of umami taste in the taste cortex. J Nutr 2000; 130: 960–5S.

36. Nijima A. Reflex effects of oral, gastrointestinal and hepatoportal glutamate sensors on vagal nerve activity. J Nutr 2000; 130: 971–3S.

37. Reeds PJ, Burrin DG, Stoll B, Jahoor F. Intestinal glutamate metabolism. J Nutr 2000; 130: 978–82S.

38. Tsai PJ, Huang PC. Circadian variation in plasma and erythrocyte glutamate concentrations in adult men consuming a diet with and without added monosodium glutamate. J Nutr 2000; 130: 1002–4S.

39. Walker R, Lupien JR. The safety evaluation of monosodium glutamate. J Nutr 2000; 130: 1049–52S.

40. Stevenson D. Monosodium glutamate and asthma. J Nutr 2000; 130: 1067–73S.

41. Naskar R, Vorwerk CK, Dreyer EB. Concurrent downregulation of a glutamate transporter and receptor in glaucoma. Invest Ophthalmol Vis Sci 2000; 41: 1940–4.

Skin and Hair

CHAPTER 52

Healthy skin aging

Walter Krause

Introduction

The skin is subjected to relevant alterations during aging. 'Intrinsic aging' describes the morphologic and functional alterations due to aging itself. The resulting phenomena are similar to those in other organs, such as a reduction in epidermal growth, synthesis of collagen and elastic fibers, and immune competence. 'Extrinsic aging' means the sum of exogenous influences, since the skin as the body cover is exposed to environmental pollutions and toxins more than any other organ during life. The most important burden is the sunlight, which causes a broad spectrum of visible alterations such as skin folds, atropy, and pigment inconsistencies. The most hazardous consequences are the development of malignancies of epidermal and melanocytic cells. More than 1 000 000 new skin cancers are diagnosed per year in the USA, and nearly 10 000 people will die from the disease. The incidence of melanoma tripled between 1980 and 2000 in spite of intense education on the hazards of skin exposure to UV light. On the other hand, sunlight itself is essential for the production of vitamin D as the main factor for calcium homeostasis and bone density.

The skin is also a target organ of several hormones. Primarily, androgens are essential for skin function, driving the development, maintenance, and regression of masculinity throughout life. The body contour and the terminal hairs are the most remarkable expressions of androgens; they grow with increasing masculinity, and they change with the regression in the aging male. Androgens also induce skin diseases like acne, which do not occur in men lacking androgen production. A number of other hormones also act on the skin, changing the effects of androgens or inducing specific diseases. The most important hormones in this respect are growth hormone, thyroid hormones, corticosteroids, estrogens, and insulin. The balance of all of them contributes to normal appearance and function as well as to aging and malfunction of the skin.

In addition, the skin is a prominent organ within the immune system. Many of the functions of the immune system are restricted to the skin, producing specific pathomechanisms. The changing resistance to infections, the increase in reactions to drugs, and the broad field of autoimmune diseases of the skin are signals of the changes in the immune system throughout life.

Disorders of the peripheral vascular system cause another important group of disease entities. The life-long insufficiency of the veins of the lower extremities leads to chronic diseases, which account for a severe burden in the individual, but also for large economic costs for the general population. Hair diseases, on the other hand, are not life-threatening and do not cause severe changes in the capacity to work. However, they significantly change the esthetic aspect of a man and cause discomfort and decrease self-esteem. They are thus of great relevance for the quality of life.

Altogether, the maintenance of an intact skin and avoidance of skin diseases is an important postulate of healthy aging in men.

Acanthosis nigricans

Acanthosis (acantho meaning thorn) nigricans (black) is a reactive skin pattern seen in association with diabetes mellitus type 2, obesity, cancer, and other systemic disorders. It is a rare disease due to the hyperactivity of different growth factors. It may preceed diabetes mellitus type 2; the prevalence increases with age.[1] The association with obesity is presumably via the insulin resistance and the enhanced production of the insulin-like growth factors (IGFs) IGF-1 and IGF-2. Acanthosis nigricans is often a symptom of a malignant tumor, mainly in the gastrointestinal tract; however it has also been linked with other tumors, e.g. of the endometrium.[2] It may preceed the clinical diagnosis of the tumor, and it regresses after extirpation. It is unknown, however, whether a relapse of acanthosis nigricans also indicates a relapse of the tumor. It has also been observed following bone marrow transplantation in lymphoblastic lymphoma, in which case it is likely that it was a graft-versus-host reaction.

The disease occurs in mutations of the receptors of epidermal growth factors (EGFs) and fibroblast growth factors (FGFs), or by mutations of the ligands themselves. On a molecular basis, the common pathogenic pathway of the diseases is the activation of tyrosine kinases, which exert mitogenic and anti-apoptotic effects on the keratinocytes.[3] The earlier classification of acanthosis nigricans into malignant and benign types is not justified, as the clinical features are common in all causes.

The lesions are gray-brown to black, rough, with thickened plaques and prominent skin lines, and occur most commonly in flexural areas (e.g., axillae, back and sides of neck, inguinal creases, and inframammary folds) (Figure 52.1). Palms and soles may also show amplified relief as 'tripe palms and soles'. Histologically, there is hyperkeratosis, epidermal papillomatosis, and increased numbers of melanocytes. Acanthosis nigricans is frequently asymptomatic, but patients may present with lesions that are painful, disfiguring, malodorous, or macerated.

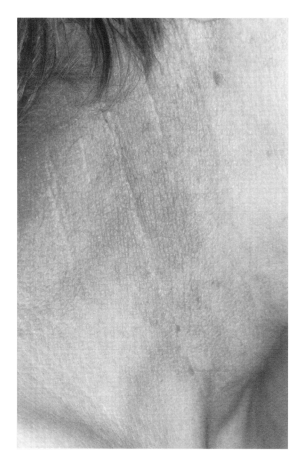

Figure 52.1 *Acanthosis nigricans: gray-brown to black lesions, rough, thickened plaques, and prominent skin lines.*

Treatment is difficult. Skin abradation and topical calcipotriol have been recommended.[4] Treatment of the underlying disease (obesity, diabetes mellitus, instestinal tumor) is essential.

Androgens

Physiology

Testosterone is an important growth factor for the terminal hairs, sebaceous glands, follicle epithelia, fibroblasts, and melanocytes. It is thus the hormone with the most prominent effects on the skin. The biochemical and molcular biological bases of the

Table 52.1 *Effects of testosterone in skin diseases*

Improvement	Impairment
Elasticity, water-binding capacity	Acne, androgenetic alopecia
Venous system	Acne fulminans
Keloids	Course of melanoma
	Systemic sclerosis

clinical effects are well understood. The skin and its appendages are capable of intense androgen metabolism. Nearly all the enzymes necessary for the metabolism of steroids to testosterone and those managing the degradation of testosterone are found in the skin. Of particular importance is 5α-reductase, since the reduced form of testosterone, 5α-dihydrotestosterone, is a closer ligand to the androgen receptor in the skin than testosterone itself.[5]

Testosterone is essential for the development of distinct skin diseases (Table 52.1).

In addition, some clinical parameters indicate a normal androgen supply in the male:

- The thickness of the skin is associated with the bone mineral density (BMD). Thus the determination of skin thickness, which is easily achieved by ultrasound measurement, may serve as a prognostic factor in osteoporosis instead of the direct measurement of BMD, which requires other techniques.[6]
- Measurement of a standardized skin fold allows an estimate of the lean body mass (LBM). LBM is negatively correlated to testosterone levels.[7]

Androgen deficiency (hypogonadism)

If hypogonadism is already present in the prepubertal male, no pubertal signs occur during growth. In these men, the aging skin remains thin and smooth, the pores remain small, which is particularly evident in the face. The periocular wrinkles are notably small and crinkling (Figure 52.2). The beard and other terminal hairs (axillae, pubes) are lacking. The reduction of scalp hairs is delayed. Specific skin diseases do not occur.

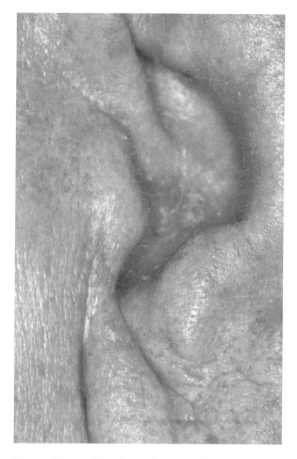

Figure 52.2 *The skin in hypogonadism. The skin is thin and smooth, wrinkles are notably small and crinkling.*

The normal decline of testosterone levels in the aging male is associated with a thinning of the skin. The skin becomes atropic and loses elasticity; the surface becomes dry and produces fewer lipids. Sebum secretion declines; the cells of the sebaceous glands, which are holocrine glands, increase their life cycle. However, hyperplasia of the glands also occurs, as a consequence of the decreasing collagen synthesis. The terminal hairs do not regress, but they turn gray. In men supplemented with testosterone the signs appear to a lesser extent. However, there are no controlled studies demonstrating the effect of testosterone substitution in the aging skin. The reduction of scalp hairs is also triggered by androgens.

Carcinoid syndrome

Carcinoid cells originate from the Kulchitsky cells of Lieberkuehns crypts (Glandulae intestinalis) of the small intestine. Carcinoid tumors can spread to large parts of the intestine, stomach, and bronchus; they may metastasize to lymph nodes and the liver.[8]

The pathophysiologic basis of the syndrome is an excessive secretion of serotonin and a malfunction of tryptophan metabolism. In normal metabolism, 1% of the daily intake of tryptophan is metabolized to serotonin, but in the carcinoid syndrome this amount increases to about 60%. As a consequence, a trypophan deficiency of other organs occurs. In the skin, this results in a pellagra-like appearance. Serotonin induces vasoconstriction and dilation of the arterioles, which appears clinically as the typical flush. In addition, histamine, kallikrein, prostaglandins, and some vasoactive peptides may be produced by the carcinoid tumor, which intensifies the clinical symptoms.

Episodic flushing is the clinical hallmark of the carcinoid syndrome, and occurs in 85% of patients (Figure 52.3). The typical flush begins suddenly and lasts for 20 to 30 seconds. It primarily involves the face, neck, and upper chest. As the disease progresses, the episodes may last longer and the flushing may be more diffuse and cyanotic. Most flushing episodes occur spontaneously, but they can be provoked by eating, drinking alcohol, defecation, emotional events, palpation of the liver, and anesthesia. Due to prolonged and repeated vasodilation, venous telangiectasias may occur. The most debilitating component of the syndrome is the diarrhea. Some patients develop pellagra-like lesions with pigmentation and hyperkeratosis in the legs or the arms. These alterations respond well to the application of niacin.[9]

The diagnosis is made by the demonstration of a significantly increased urinary excretion of 5-hydroxyindol acetic acid (5-HIAA), up to 1000 mg per day.[10] The therapy for the syndrome is extirpation of the tumor. If this is not possible, long-acting somatostatin analogs are the treatment of choice. Corticoids and beta-adrenoreceptor inhibitors are ineffective for symptomatic improvement.

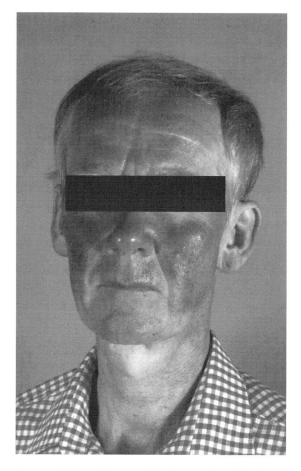

Figure 52.3 *The typical flush, the clinical hallmark of the carcinoid syndrome, begins suddenly and lasts for 20 to 30 seconds. It primarily involves the face, neck, and upper chest. (Courtesy of Prof Dr Arnold, Marburg.)*

Corticosteroids

Physiology

Nearly all cells of the organism need glucocorticoids for the maintenance of normal function.[11] The concentrations of cellular binding proteins (glucocorticoid receptors (GRs)) in the skin show large variations between different sites. This possibly reflects the varying sensitivity of different skin areas to topically applied glucocorticoids (e.g. the foreskin is highly sensitive, while the abdominal skin

Table 52.2 *Clinical signs in Cushing's disease*

Epidermis	Dermis	Blood vessels	Skin appendages	Subcutis
Atropic, smooth, translucent, wound healing defective	Flaccid, anelastic, vulnerable, defective immune reactions, striae distensae	Hematomas, ecchymoses, telangiectasias	Increasing vellus hairs, general hypertrichosis, frontal alopecia, altered pigmentation	Increase of fat in cheeks, neck: 'moon facies', 'buffalo hump'

has low and the face has moderate sensitivity). Cultivated keratinocytes or fibroblasts from different areas also show different receptor densities. Corticosteroid receptors are also present in the endothelial cells of the skin vessels. The blanching effect due to vascular constriction exerted by different glucocorticoids parallels the receptor affinity of the compounds.[12]

After binding of glucocorticoids to the receptors, the complexes bind to distinct DNA sequences and modulate the activity of certain genes.[13] Some studies have suggested a positive association between obesity, hypertension, and insulin resistance and alleles at the GR gene. Also distinct mutations in the GR gene have been postulated as being relevant to progression to type 2 diabetes and cardiovascular diseases, but as yet they have not been fully elucidated.[14]

Addison's disease

The consequence of a hyposecretion of glucocorticoids (adrenal insufficiency) is Addison's disease. Usually, this is due to a primary insufficiency of the adrenal gland following inflammation or autoimmune disease. The typical sign at the skin is hyperpigmentation, due to an increased pituitary secretion of proopiomelanotropincorticotropin (POMC) peptides (see the section on 'Vitiligo and melanocytes', below). The pigmentation is generalized, similar to sunburn, and more pronounced in scars, skinfolds, palmae, nipples, perineum, genitalia, and the linea alba. Sometimes the pigmentation occurs in the form of freckles. The hairs become darker and the nails show dark bands. Existing nevi also become darker. With sufficient treatment the pigmentation resolves. The pigmentation may occur before signs of adrenal insufficiency are visible; 12% of patients show a vitiligo.

Cushing's disease

Cushing's disease is a consequence of hypersecretion of the adrenal gland. The cause of the hypersecretion may be primary (adrenal) or secondary (hypophyseal). The typical signs are listed in Table 52.2. Cushing's disease may also include hepatic steatosis, disease of the gallbladder, pulmonary insufficiency, osteoarthitis, proteinuria, increased hemoglobin concentration, and immune incompetence.

Systemically applied corticosteroids at a dose above the daily production of endogenous cortisol (more than 20 mg) usually lead to a clinical picture identical to endogenous hypersecretion. The clinical appearance is indistinguishable without data on the medical history.

Diseases due to topical corticosteroid overdosage

Following long-term application of topical glucocorticoids striae distensae, thinning of the skin, telangiectasias and – in the face – a rosacea-like dermatitis may occur (Figure 52.4). These unwanted side-effects are inseparably connected to the anti-inflammatory effects of glucocorticoids. They are always more pronounced in the face than in other areas of the body,

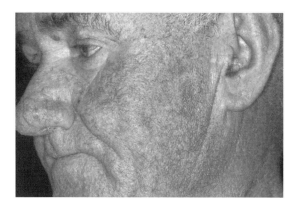

Figure 52.4 *Topical overdosage of corticosteroids. Following long-term application the development of telangiectasias and a rosacea-like dermatitis may occur, in particular on the face.*

since they increase the degradation of collagen and elastic fibers induced by sunlight. Thus aging skin is at higher risk than younger skin.

One of the aims of the continuing development of topical steroids is to improve the anti-inflammatory and immune suppressive effect by avoiding stronger side-effects. However, as yet the ideal steroid has not been found. Such a steroid should permeate well through the stratum corneum and penetrate the skin, but without leading to raised concentrations in the blood serum. In order to reach this goal, the lipid solubility of steroids was increased by esterification, however, other changes in the molecular structure which resulted in an improvement in the efficacy mostly also caused more pronounced side-effects. Examples of typical compounds are betamethasone-dipropionate and clobetasol-propionate. Novel steroids such as budesonide, mometasone-furoate, prednicarbate, 17,21-hydrocortisone-aceponate, hydrocortisone-17-butyrate-21-propionate, methyl-prednisolone-aceponat, alclometason-dipropionate, and fluticasone-propionate have a good anti-inflammatory effect and lower side-effects.[15]

Dehydroepiandrosterone

The quantitatively largest secretory product of the adrenal gland is esterified dehydroepiandrosterone-sulfate (DHEAS). In young men, the serum concentration amounts to 5000 ng/ml or more, but it decreases constantly throughout life. It is one of the few serum parameters which correlate with age. In severe diseases, in particular in diseases of the cardiovascular system, the decline is more pronounced. Smokers, however, have higher mean levels. From these data, a causative role of low DHEAS levels and cardiovascular disease was inferred, and the compound was used as a drug. DHEAS was assumed to be a 'youth hormone', which should also exert improvement on skin function. From controlled studies, however, no such effects could be concluded (Table 52.3).

The effect of DHEAS at the cellular level is unclear. Receptor-like structures were not found in any of the studies. In an experimental study on human fibroblasts, an influence on the extracellular matrix was demonstrated.[18] This may indicate a benefit of DHEAS application to skin aging. After systemic (oral) application of DHEAS its serum levels increase, as do the levels of testosterone and estradiol. As a consequence, virilization may take place in women. An alteration of the serum lipid profile was also observed.[19]

Diabetes mellitus

Diabetic dermopathy

Skin diseases in diabetes mellitus are the consequence of several influences, dependent on the duration of diabetes and the quality of insulin therapy:

1. The skin of the patient with diabetes is characterized by the risk for bacterial and mycotic infections. If such diseases occur frequently in aging men, the exclusion of diabetes mellitus is mandatory. The frequency of skin diseases in diabetic patients is illustrated by the following. By dermatologic investigation of 500 diabetic outpatients, Wozniak and Bar[20] found obesity in 54% (273 persons), and in 83.6% (418 persons) they observed lesions on the skin or mucous membranes. Signs of infection are erythema, warmth, tenderness, swelling, and abscess.[21]

Table 52.3 *Effects of DHEA application for 6 months in controlled studies*

	Morales et al[16]	Baulieu et al[17]
Body weight	No change	No change
Body mass index	No change	
Lean body mass	No change	
Well-being	Improvement	No change
IGF-1 levels	Increase	
Testosterone levels		No change
Bone metabolism		No change
Skin lipids and humidity		No change
Sexual functions		No change

IGF-1, insulin-like growth factor-1.

2. The diabetic microangiopathy originates from the modification of blood flow characteristics. Histologically, capillaries and arterioles show thickening of the intima, focal deposits of PAS-positive material, and extravasation of erythrocytes and leukocytes. The metabolism of the vascular walls is altered due to changes in the collagen types and the decreased water-binding capacity. The permeation of granulocytes through the vascular wall is inhibited, and the phagocytic activity of leukocytes is decreased. Subsequently, wound healing is also impaired. Diabetic dermopathy is often associated with angiopathy of other vascular areas.[22] Screening for vascular disease includes peripheral pulses, skin temperature, skin thickness, and skin color.[21]

3. Neuropathy leads to decreased pain sensations and to changes in pressure and temperature sensation. Screening for diabetic neuropathy includes a detailed history and physical examination (vibration, pressure, pain, and temperature sensation), and may result in a quantitative signs score.[21]

The diabetic foot

The main focus of skin diseases is the feet (Figure 52.5). The diabetic foot occurs in both types of diabetes and involves up to 10% of diabetic patients. Skin defects and subsequent ulcers result from an interaction of a number of causes. The vulnerability

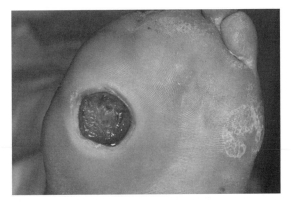

Figure 52.5 *The diabetic foot: chronic inflammation of the skin with defects and subsequent ulcer, showing recurrent infection.*

of the diabetic skin promotes infection. Peripheral vascular disease appears to be more frequent in type 2 diabetes, and the risk increases with the duration of the disease. Neuropathy is present in over 80% of patients with foot ulcers; it promotes ulcer formation by decreasing pain sensation and perception of pressure as well as by causing muscle imbalance.

Bacterial infections are mostly caused by *Staphylococcus aureus*, and also by enterococcae and *E. coli* to a lesser degree. It is not unusual that multiple bacterial species are found; in a number of cases no common antibiotic is available. In up to 80% of severe infections anaerobic bacteria are

Table 52.4 *Diabetic foot care*

Disease	Risks	Treatment	Prevention
Pruritus	Scratching, skin defects	Ointments	Avoiding skin dryness and fissure
Vulnerability	Skin defects, infections	Bandage, warm and comfortable footwear	Accurate cleaning, accurate drying after washing, no barefoot walking
Poor wound healing	Ulcers	Avoid dents	Accurate filing of nails, band aid also in small wounds
Tinea (onychomycosis)	Bacterial infections	Antimycotics	Avoid constricting clothes and shoes, avoid cooling
Bacterial infections	Sepsis, osteomyelitis, amputation, Pay attention for MRSA, anerobics	Due to antibiotic testing, topical treatment only in slight to moderate infection, wound debridement	Avoid dents and clavus, no sharp-edged instruments
Diabetic ulcers	Sepsis, osteomyelitis, amputation	Systemic antibiotics, amputation	Avoid dents, soft sandals, shoe-lifts

found; they may be accompanied by general symptoms ('diabetic foot flu'). Treatment should be related to the bacterial species and sensitivity. Wound debridement is mandatory. Topical treatment is allowed only in slight or moderate infections, in all other cases, which are risks for a possible amputation (cellulitis, lymphangitis, deep ulceration, necrosis, gangrene, osteomyelitis), only systemic antibiotics should be used. Foot infections and ulcers are risk factors for subsequent amputations. Osteomyelitis is frequent in diabetic feet; in particular, those patients in whom bone is visible in the ulcer are jeopardized.

In order to prevent ulcers the rules for foot care in diabetes should be strictly followed (Table 52.4). If foot care education in patients is sufficient and skin changes are intensively treated, patients have a significantly lower incidence of disease. Training of the health personnel also significantly improved skin health in the diabetics under observation.[23,24]

The incidence of tinea and onychomycosis in the diabetic foot is increased. The treatment is oral antimycotics, which are well tolerated and without diabetes-specific side-effects. They are far more effective than topical antimycotics, even if the nail substance is mechanically reduced.[25]

Necrobiosis lipoidica diabeticorum

The pathogenesis of necrobiosis lipoidica diabeticorum (NLD) is not known. Immunohistologic studies suggest the involvement of immunologic mechanisms. The extent of the association of diabetes mellitus and NLD is under debate. In one study,[22] only 10% of 171 patients did not have diabetes when NLD was observed. In rare cases, NLD occurs as part of a syndrome.

The lesion in NLD begins as a dark red, elevated nodule with an irregular border. Later, the skin becomes atropic. The lesion becomes yellowish-brown, only the margin maintains the red color (Figure 52.6). The epidermis is thin and shows *geringe* scaling. Enlarged vessels may be seen through the translucent skin. New lesions of NLD may be observed as a Koebner phenomenon. Subjective sensations are not reported. No sufficient treatment is known; corticosteroids and cryotherapy with liquid nitrogen are applied. Systemic application of small doses of ASS was assumed to be successful.

Adverse skin reactions to insulin
Insulin itself may have side-effects on the skin. Local itching, edema, stinging, pain, or warmth and redness at the injection site may occur, as well as generalized urticaria. Lipatrophy and lipohypertrophy are frequently seen. They may be caused by altered kinetics of the injected insulin. The risk increases if the injection site is not frequently changed. Rapidly resorbed insulins may decrease the risk, but a regular change of injection site is mandatory. Liposuction of the altered fat deposits is not effective. There may also be allergic constituents of insulin medications.[26]

Estrogens

Estrogen deficiency
Estrogens are essential for the structure and function of normal skin. The decrease in circulating estrogens in the female climacteric leads to specific alterations. Estrogen levels also decrease in the aging male, but it is unknown whether similar alterations are also due to a lack of estrogens:[27]

- The lifespan of keratinocytes declines.
- The epidermal water loss increases.
- The activity of sebaceous glands and sweat glands declines.
- The epidermis becomes atropic and wrinkles arise ('aging skin').
- The skin becomes more irritable to temperature, moisture, and mechanical trauma.

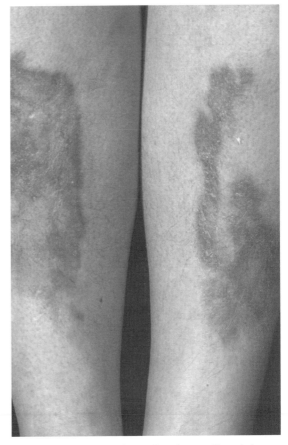

Figure 52.6 *Necrobiosis lipoidica: yellowish-brown lesions with a red margin. The epidermis is thin and shows little scaling; ulceration is common.*

- The water-binding capacity of the cutis declines, the skin loses tone.
- The collagen content of the cutis decreases by 1% per year of age.
- The collagen fibers disentangle; the skin becomes flaccid, thin, and translucent.
- Skin fold thickness declines. This effect is increased when diabetes is present.
- The amount and complexity of elastic fibers decline.

Gynecomastia
Gynecomastia is the consequence of increased estrogen action in the male. The male breast tissue

is estrogen sensitive, as in women. In this respect, not only are enhanced estrogen levels significant, but an altered relationship of testosterone to estrogens is also of relevance.

Gynecomastia appears at different ages with different frequencies. At the age of 14, about 40% of boys have gynecomastia, this figure rises to 60% in aging men.[28] Usually, in both groups gynecomastia is associated with obesity, but a particular cause has not been found. The risk of gynecomastia is enhanced in several groups:

- men using drugs with an estrogen-like action or promoting the aromatization of androgens
- tumors from the testis or from other organs producing human chorionic gonadotropin
- hyperprolactinemia induced by prolactinoma or by dopamine-inhibiting drugs.

The clinical appearance of gynecomastia in the range of a palpable tumor under the areola up to a large pendulous breast with a significant submammary fold is independent of the pathogenesis (Figure 52.7). In the development of gynecomastia often pressure pain is the first symptom. The areola is enlarged to more than 2.5 cm and hyperpigmented. The differential diagnosis from male breast carcinoma is essential, although its incidence is only 1% of the incidence of breast cancer in women. One-sided gynecomastia is suspicious, it should be clarified using mammography and fine-needle puncture.

The therapy of choice in gynecomastia, in particular if no endocrine or pharmacologic causes are found, comprises surgical intervention. Usually, the skin is opened by a circular incision along the margin of the areola and then the gland is removed or extracted by suction. The intervention is simple to perform. A relapse may occur, if the cause of the gynecomastia is still active. In male breast carcinoma, a radical excision including axillary lymph nodes is necessary.

Glucagonoma syndrome

Glucagonoma syndrome is a rare disease resulting from a nearly always malignant pancreatic tumor.

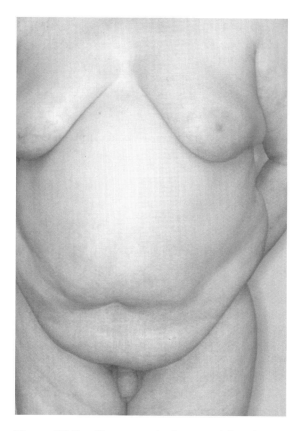

Figure 52.7 *Gynecomastia: large pendulous breasts with significant submammary folds in a patient with Klinefelters' syndrome.*

As a skin disease, the necrolytic migratory erythema is often one of the first presenting symptoms (Figure 52.8). Cutaneous eruptions occur mainly in the groin, extremities, thighs, buttocks, and perineum. They begin as erythematous papules or plaques. Central clearing then occurs, leaving bronze-colored, indurated areas centrally, with blistering, crusting, and scaling at the borders. The affected areas are often pruritic and painful. Skin biopsies obtained from the edges of the lesions reveal superficial necrolysis with separation of the outer layers of the epidermis and perivascular infiltration with lymphocytes and histiocytes. Also the mucous membranes are affected, resulting in glossitis, angular cheilitis, stomatitis, and blepharitis.[29] The patients also suffer from weight loss and diabetes mellitus (75%) and normochromic anemia (90%). Further symptoms are thromboembolism (30%) and neuropsychiatric disorders. Gastrointestinal symptoms include diarrhea or constipation, which may lead to the development of vitamin B deficiencies and aggravation of the dermatosis.[30] Finally, glucagonomas may produce multiple hormones in addition to glucagon, including VIP, gastrin, serotonin, insulin, calcitonin, pancreatic polypeptide, and ACTH.

The diagnosis is established by typical clinical findings in association with hyperglucagonemia.[31] However, a serum glucagon concentration below 500 pg/ml does not exclude a glucagonoma, because pathologic molecular weight forms of glucagon may not be measured by the immunoassays used. On the other hand, concentrations above 1000 pg/ml are virtually diagnostic of glucagonoma. The underlying tumor has to be diagnosed by specific imaging procedures.

The therapy consists of surgical removal of the pancreatic tumor. Near complete resolution of the skin disease is often seen only one week after surgery. However, since the glucagonoma is a malignant tumor, further growth of the tumor and recurrence of the necrolytic migratory erythema is not unlikely.[32]

Growth hormone

Growth hormone (GH)-regulated gene expression contributes to many of the effects of GH on cellular metabolism, growth, and differentiation. Studies of model systems have revealed several mechanisms by which GH regulates gene expression and transcription factors. Several genes are also sexually dimorphically expressed. GH-regulated STAT 5 has also been implicated in the regulation of other physiologically important genes, including those encoding components of the IGF-1 axis and insulin.[33]

The IGFs form a family of ligands with specific binding proteins and receptors. They are important in both the development of the organism and the maintenance of the normal function of many cells. The system also has powerful anti-apoptotic effects. Specific signaling pathways emanating from the

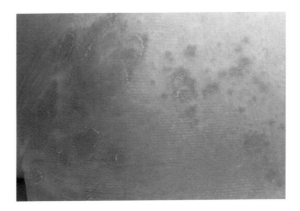

Figure 52.8 *Necrolytic migratory erythema in glucagonoma: bronze-colored, indurated areas with blistering, crusting, and scaling at the borders.*

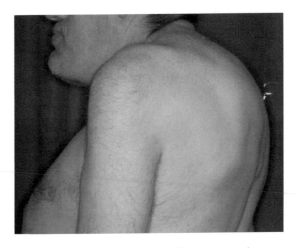

Figure 52.9 *Acromegaly: thickening and pasty consistency of the skin, thickening of skin folds, thickening of lips and eyelids, hypertrichosis, bushy eyebrows, growth of bones, enlargement of the ears, protrusion of zygoma, mandible, and chin.*

IGF-1 receptor affect cancer cell proliferation, adhesion, migration, and cell death.[34]

Hypersecretion of growth hormone induces the disease acromegaly (Table 52.5, Figure 52.9). The pasty edema of the skin is a consequence of increased levels of glycosaminoglycans and collagen in the dermis. The water storage is also increased due to the increase in hydrophilic compounds of the

Table 52.5 *Clinical signs in acromegaly*

Skin	Skin appendages	Pigmentation	Skeleton
Thickening, pasty consistency, thickening of skin folds, thickening of lips and eyelids	Widening of follicle ostia, thickening and hardening of the nails, increased secretion of eccrine and apocrine sweat glands, acne inversa, generalized hypertrichosis, bushy eyebrows	Moderate hyperpigmentation of all skin areas, numerous skin tags	Growth of bones and cartilage, elongation of the nose, enlargement of the ears, protrusion of zygoma, mandible, and chin

dermal matrix. The epidermis and the skin appendages become hyperplastic. As a consequence of the concomitant hypersecretion of melanocyte-stimulating hormone, hyperpigmentation occurs. Sweating in heat and under physical stress is reduced. Patients with acromegaly describe a sense of decreased well-being in controlled studies; the questionnaires indicated a decreased quality of life.

The secretion of growth hormone and IGF-1 decrease with age, as does IGF, which is produced under the influence of growth hormone. An administration of hGH in aging men therefore appears to be plausible. This has already been performed in several studies, and regulation of dysfunction to a certain extent was observed. However, uncontrolled treatment was often started without first proving a lack of growth hormone secretion. In these cases, the physiologic levels were often exceeded, and side-effects were observed. These side-effects were, particularly in elderly and obese patients, hyperinsulinemia, sodium and water retention, weight gain, edema in the lower extremities, carpal tunnel syndrome, increase in intracranial pressure, papillary edema, arthralgies, and myalgies. As the most severe side-effect, a growth enhancement of malignant tumors was observed.[35] All the side-effects were reversible once growth hormone application was stopped.

Due to the side-effects described, uncritical use of growth hormone as a 'youth hormone' should be urgently discouraged.

Thyroid hormones

Hypothyroidism (myxedema)

The thyroid hormones thyroxine (T_4) and tri-iodothyronine (T_3) are important for the growth and function of most tissues. Transport to the hormone target organs requires binding to thyroid-hormone-binding globulin (TBG) in the blood. In the cell there are binding proteins for T_4 and T_3 in the cytosol, which transport the hormones to the DNA-bound thyroid hormone receptor. Receptors of an α- and a β-type were identified in many cells. They express three major functional domains, one binding DNA, one binding ligand, and two major domains regulating RNA transcription.[36]

In the general deficiency of thyroid hormones the skin changes to the characteristic myxedema. The skin is pasty and voluminous and shows a non-impressible edema, which is not position dependent (Figure 52.10). The skin is dry, cool, and pale. This appearance is the consequence of the decreased vascular flow and the decreased reaction to heat. Also the mucous membranes become dry and the tongue becomes fissured. The epidermis is thin, raspy, and hyperkeratotic (shark skin). The texture of the cornea is altered. The hairs are dry, fragile, and raspy. Sometimes localized alopecia or a diffuse effluvium occurs. The nails grow slowly and become brittle. Wound healing slows down.

Myxedema is a consequence of the storage of large amounts of proteoglycans, which are also

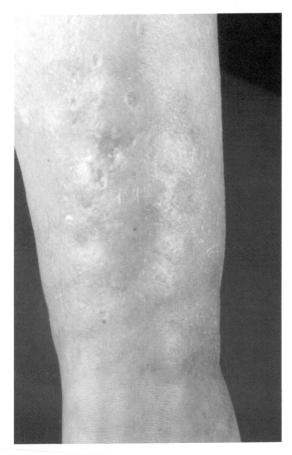

Figure 52.10 *Myxedema: pasty and voluminous skin, non-impressible and position-independent edema.*

responsible for the yellowish color. After substitution of the thyroid hormones the pathologic proteoglycan deposits are quickly mobilized again.[37]

Hyperthyroidism

In hyperthyroidism, which may result from autochthonal hyperfunction of the gland or from increased stimulation by pituitary TSH, the skin is warm, tender, and wet with a soft turgor, resembling infantile skin. This originates from peripheral vasodilation with increased blood flow, particularly in the face. The patients have a tendency to increased sweating, especially in plantae and palmae. The hairs are thin and tender, the nails have a normal appearance. Pigmentation is unaltered.

Hyperthyroidism may also be caused by stimulation of the TSH receptors by antibody-like proteins (Graves' disease, Basedow's disease[38]). Autoimmune thyroid disease may be associated with other diseases of the immune system, e.g. with chronic urticaria. Its prevalence is quoted to be between 12% and 29% of urticaria cases. If thyroid antibodies are demonstrated in chronic urticaria, the functional status of the thyroid gland should be analysed. Most patients are euthyroid. If hypothyroidism is diagnosed, a substitution should be performed. Improvement of chronic urticaria is achieved best with L-thyroxine in euthyroid patients. The blood levels of thyroxin should be monitored in order to avoid hyperthyroidism, in particular in elderly patients.[38]

Vitamin D

Vitamin D ('soltriol') is a phylogenetically ancient steroid hormone with effects on multiple organs and organ systems. The effect on bone metabolism and the maintenance of calcium homeostasis of the body is its most important function, but it is also indispensable in reproduction, in the parathyroid gland, in skin, in the differentiation of muscle cells, and in cancer growth.

Provitamin D is formed from 7-dehydrocholesterol in the skin under the influence of sunlight. Wavelengths of the UV spectrum at about 300 nm are particularly effective.[39] Once formed, vitamin D_3 is metabolized in the liver to 25-hydroxyvitamin D_3 and then in the kidney to its biologically active form, 1,25-dihydroxyvitamin D_3. The melanocytes of the skin play an important role in the synthesis of vitamin D. It is well known that men with dark skin color have a higher BMD than Caucasians, and they have a lower calcium excretion.

1,25-Dihydroxyvitamin D_3 binds, similarly to other steroid hormones, to the so-called vitamin D-responsive elements (VDREs) of the DNA, thus influencing the transcription of certain genes. Among others, the activity of phospholipase D1 is specifically enhanced. This leads to the hydrolysis of phospholipids, whereby lipids as second messengers are formed, e.g. diacylglycerin (DAG). DAG

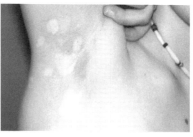
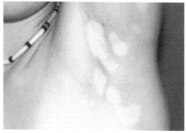

pretreatment

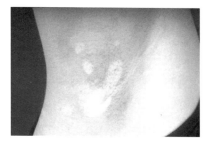
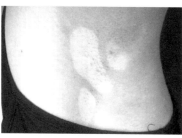

posttreatment

Figure 52.11 *Vitiligo: local loss of skin pigmentation due to the malfunction or loss of melanocytes. After 3 months' treatment with tacrolimus, lesion size has decreased.*

again activates several protein kinases, which are of relevance in the terminal differentiation of the keratinocytes.[40] In this way the effects of vitamin D in psoriasis may be explained.[41] The metabolite calcipotriol is less effective in calcium metabolism than the original vitamin D. Calcipotriol is possibly effective in all skin diseases with abnormalities of keratinocyte differentiation.

Vitamin D deficiency is a consequence of too low uptake and too low sun exposure. Vitamin D deficiency has been associated with increased risks of deadly cancers, cardiovascular disease, multiple sclerosis, rheumatoid arthritis, and type 1 diabetes mellitus. Although chronic excessive exposure to sunlight increases the risk of non-melanoma skin cancer, the avoidance of all direct sun exposure increases the risk of vitamin D deficiency, which can have serious consequences.[42]

Vitiligo and melanocytes

Vitiligo describes a local loss of skin pigmentation due to the malfunction or loss of melanocytes. Vitiligo is a frequent disease, worldwide about 0.5%

of men suffer from it. The causes are unclear – genetic factors, autoimmunity to melanocytes, toxic compounds, nerve disorders, and defective melanocyte growth factors have been considered.[43] Huang et al[44] interpreted vitiligo as a manifestation of apoptosis. This is more likely than necrosis of melanocytes, which is rarely observed. Apoptosis may be induced by UV light, by cytokines from the keratinocytes, or by environmental pollutants, e.g. hydroquinone. Since corticosteroids and other immunosuppressants are able to influence apoptosis, it is plausible that these compounds have a certain effect in vitiligo.

However, there is no specific treatment for vitiligo. In the literature trials have been reported, using UV-B (narrowband 311 nm), UV-A in combination with 5-methoxypsoralen, topical corticoids, and topical calcineurin antagonists (tacrolimus and pimecrolimus). Randomized controlled studies are not available; the application was not controlled and used in only few cases (Figure 52.11). Surgical methods have also been applied, including autotransplantation of blister skin or cultivated melanocytes. In expanded vitiligo decoloration of the pigment residues is advisable. After unsuccessful therapy, camouflage (make-up) should be recommended. In each case reliable sun protection is essential.

A similar mechanism to vitiligo is assumed to be the basis of depigmentation in malignant melanoma, which is suggested to be a good prognostic sign. Insight into humoral and cellular immune reactions affecting normal and malignant melanocytes could lead to strategies for therapeutic modalities in vitiligo as well as in melanoma.[45]

α-melanocyte-stimulating hormone (α-MSH) stimulates the production of melanin, predominantly the eumelanin as well as the dendricity of melanocytes. The hormone is secreted by the intermediate lobe of the pituitary gland. The melanocytes themselves and other epidermal cells of the skin also produce MSH. It is part of the so-called pro-opiomelanotropincorticotropin (POMC) peptide. Melanocytes express the melanocortin 1 receptor (MC1-R). Mutations of MRC-1 are not infrequent; these melanocytes do not respond to α-MSH stimulation, and they are highly sensitive to UV irradiation. The loss-of-function mutations are associated with red hair and an increased risk of skin cancer.[46]

Melanocytes secrete a number of compounds into their cellular environment, such as signaling molecules, cytokines, POMC peptides, catecholamines, and nitric oxide. By these secretions they influence the function of keratinocytes, lymphocytes, fibroblasts, mast cells, and vascular endothelial cells. This may in part explain the suppression of immune reaction by UV irradiation.[47] The application of α-MSH or related peptides could offer a treatment option for inflammatory, autoimmune, or allergic diseases.[48]

References

1. Selkin BA, Reynolds RV, Selkin G. Cutaneous manifestations of internal malignancy. UptoDate® 2005 (www.utdol.com).
2. Mekhail TM, Markman M. Acanthosis nigricans with endometrial carcinoma: case report and review of the literature. Gynecol Oncol 2002; 84(2): 332–4.
3. Torley D, Bellus GA, Munro CS. Genes, growth factors and acanthosis nigricans. Br J Dermatol 2002; 147(6): 1096–101.
4. Garcia Hidalgo L. Dermatological complications of obesity. Am J Clin Dermatol 2002; 3(7): 497–506.
5. McPhaul MJ, Young M. Complexities of androgen action. J Am Acad Dermatol 2001; 45(3 Suppl): S87–94.
6. Gruber D, Sator M, Frigo P, Knogler W, Huber JC. Korrelation der Hautfaltendicke mit der Knochendichte, Östradiol, FSH und Prolactinspiegel bei 231 Frauen. Wien Klin Wochenschr 1995; 107(20): 622–5.
7. Denti L, Pasolini G, Sanfelici L et al. Aging-related decline of gonadal function in healthy men: correlation with body composition and lipoproteins. J Am Geriatr Soc 2000; 48(1): 51–8.
8. Öberg K. Carcinoid tumors, carcinoid syndrome, and related disorders. In: Larsen PR, Kronenberg HM, Melmed S, Polonsky KS, eds. Williams Textbook of Endocrinology, 10th edn. Saunders, St. Louis, MO; 2003: 1857–70.
9. Sitaraman SV, Goldfinger ST. The carcinoid syndrome. UptoDate June 2005. (www.utdol.com).
10. Freinkel RK, Freinkel N. Cutaneous manifestations of endocrine disorders. In: Fitzpatrick, Eisen AZ, Wolff K et al, eds. Dermatology in General Medicine. New York: McGraw Hill, 1987.
11. Stewart PM. The adrenal cortex. In: Larsen PR, Kronenberg HM, Melmed S, Polonsky KS, eds. Williams Textbook of Endocrinology, 10th edn, Saunders, St. Louis, MO, 2003: 491–551.
12. Ponec M. Hormone receptors in the skin. In: Fitzpatrick, Eisen AZ, Wolff K et al, eds. Dermatology in General Medicine. New York: McGraw Hill, 1987: 491–551.
13. Payne DN, Adcock IM. Molecular mechanisms of corticosteroid actions. Paediatr Respir Rev 2001; 2(2): 145–50.
14. Rosmond R. The glucocorticoid receptor gene and its association to metabolic syndrome. Obes Res 2002; 10(10): 1078–86.
15. Brazzini B, Pimpinelli N. New and established topical corticosteroids in dermatology: clinical pharmacology and therapeutic use. Am J Clin Dermatol 2002; 3(1): 47–58.
16. Morates AJ, Nolan JJ, Nelson JC, Yen SS. Effects of replacement dose of dehydroepiandrosterone in men and women of advancing age. J Clin Endocrinol Metab 1994; 78(6): 1360–7.
17. Baulieu EE, Thomas G, Legrain S et al. DHEA, DHEA sulfate and aging: contribution of the DHEAge Study to a sociobiomedical issue. PNAS 2000; 97: 4279–84.
18. Lee KS, Oh KY, Kim BC. Effects of dehydroepiandrosterone on collagen and collagenase gene expression by skin fibroblasts in culture. J Dermatol Sci 2000; 23(2): 103–10.
19. van Vollenhoven RF. Dehydroepiandrosterone for the treatment of systemic lupus erythematosus. Expert Opin Pharmacother 2002; 3(1): 23–31.

20. Wozniak KD, Bar M. Zur Bedeutung von Hautveranderungen beim Diabetes mellitus. Z Gesamte Inn Med 1990; 45(22): 669–73.

21. Richardson T, Kerr D. Skin-related complications of insulin therapy: epidemiology and emerging management strategies. Am J Clin Dermatol 2003; 4(10): 661–7.

22. Freinkel RK, Freinkel N. Cutaneous manifestations of endocrine disorders. In: Fitzpatrick, Eisen AZ, Wolff K et al, eds. Dermatology in General Medicine. New York: McGraw Hill, 1987.

23. Brownlee M, Aiello LP, Friedman E et al. Complications of diabetes mellitus. In: Larsen PR, Kronenberg HM, Melmed S, Polonsky KS, eds. Williams Textbook of Endocrinology, 10th edn, Saunders, St. Louis, MO, 2003: 1509–84.

24. Frykberg RG. An evidence-based approach to diabetic foot infections. Am J Surg 2003; 186(5A): 44–54S.

25. Robbins JM. Treatment of onychomycosis in the diabetic patient population. J Diabetes Comp 2003; 17(2): 98–104.

26. McCulloch DK. Evaluation of the diabetic foot. UptoDate® 2005 (www.utdol.com).

27. Raine-Fenning NJ, Brincat MP, Muscat-Baron Y. Skin aging and menopause: implications for treatment. Am J Clin Dermatol 2003; 4(6): 371–8.

28. Niewöhner CB, Nuttall RQ. Gynecomastia in a hospitalized male population. Am J Med 1984; 77: 633–8.

29. Rosenberg PM, Goldfinger ST. Glucagonoma and the glucagonoma syndrome. UptoDate® 2005 (www.utdol.com).

30. van Beek AP, de Haas ER, van Vloten WA et al. The glucagonoma syndrome and necrolytic migratory erythema: a clinical review. Eur J Endocrinol 2004; 151(5): 531–7.

31. Chastain MA. The glucagonoma syndrome: a review of its features and discussion of new perspectives. Am J Med Sci 2001; 321(5): 306–20.

32. Zhang M, Xu X, Shen Y et al. Clinical experience in diagnosis and treatment of glucagonoma syndrome. Hepatobiliary Pancreat Dis Int 2004; 3(3): 473–5.

33. Schwartz J, Huo JS, Piwien-Pilipuk G. Growth hormone regulated gene expression. Minerva Endocrinol 2002; 27(4): 231–41.

34. LeRoith D, Roberts CT Jr. The insulin-like growth factor system and cancer. Cancer Lett 2003; 195(2): 127–37.

35. Carroll PV, Christ ER, Bengtsson BA et al. Growth hormone deficiency in adulthood and the effects of growth hormone replacement: a review. Growth Hormone Research Society Scientific Committee. J Clin Endocrinol Metab 1998; 83(2): 382–95.

36. Larsen PR, Davies TF, Schlumberger MJ, Hay ID. Thyroid physiology and diagnostic evaluation of patients with thyroid disorders. In: Larsen PR, Kronenberg HM, Melmed S, Polonsky KS, eds. Williams Textbook of Endocrinology, 10th edn. Saunders, St. Louis, MO, 2003: 33–7.

37. Larsen PR, Davies TF. Hypothyreoidsm and thyreoditis. In: Larsen PR, Kronenberg HM, Melmed S, Polonsky KS, eds. Williams Textbook of Endocrinology, 10th edn. Saunders, St. Louis, MO, 2003: 423–56.

38. Davies TF, Larsen RP. Thyrotoxicosis. In: Larsen PR, Kronenberg HM, Melmed S, Polonsky KS, eds. Williams Textbook of Endocrinology, 10th edn, Saunders, St. Louis, MO, 2003: 374–422.

39. Stumpf WE. The endocrinology of sunlight and darkness. Complementary roles of vitamin D and pineal hormones. Naturwissenschaften 1988; 75(5): 247–51.

40. Bollinger Bollag W, Bollag RJ. 1,25-Dihydroxyvitamin D(3), phospholipase D and protein kinase C in keratinocyte differentiation. Mol Cell Endocrinol 2001; 177(1–2): 173–82.

41. Kira M, Kobayashi T, Yoshikawa K. Vitamin D and the skin. J Dermatol 2003; 30(6): 429–37.

42. Holick MF. Sunlight and vitamin D for bone health and prevention of autoimmune diseases, cancers, and cardiovascular disease. Am J Clin Nutr 2004; 80(6 Suppl): 1678–88S.

43. Njoo MD, Westerhof W. Vitiligo. Pathogenesis and treatment. Am J Clin Dermatol 2001; 2(3): 167–81.

44. Huang CL, Nordlund JJ, Boissy R. Vitiligo: a manifestation of apoptosis? Am J Clin Dermatol 2002; 3(5): 301–8.

45. Wankowicz-Kalinska A, Le Poole C, van den Wijngaard R, Storkus WJ, Das PK. Melanocyte-specific immune response in melanoma and vitiligo: two faces of the same coin? Pigment Cell Res 2003; 16(3): 254–60.

46. Kadekaro AL, Kanto H, Kavanagh R, Abdel-Malek ZA. Significance of the melanocortin 1 receptor in regulating human melanocyte pigmentation, proliferation, and survival. Ann NY Acad Sci 2003; 994: 359–65.

47. Luger TA, Schwarz T, Kalden H et al. Role of epidermal cell-derived α-melanocyte stimulating hormone in ultraviolet light mediated local immunosuppression. Ann NY Acad Sci 1999; 885: 209–16.

48. Luger TA, Scholzen TE, Brzoska T, Bohm M. New insights into the functions of α-MSH and related peptides in the immune system. Ann NY Acad Sci 2003; 994: 133–40.

CHAPTER 53

Skin disease caused by changes in the immune system and infection

Isaak Effendy and Karen Kuschela

Zoster

Zoster (shingles, Latin *cingulus* = belt; zoster, Greek *Zostrix* = belt) is a secondary infection with varicella zoster virus (VZV) usually in adults,[1] while varicella (chicken pox) provides the primary infection mostly in children. The primary infection with VZV leads to immunity, but the virus remains behind in neural ganglia which in the elderly or in immunosuppressed individuals, can be reactivated by certain local factors, e.g. trauma, radiation therapy, leading to involvement of a single sensory nerve and its dermatome.[2,3]

The crucial factor is immunosuppression, e.g. leukemia, lymphoma, or chemotherapy. However, in general the only risk factor is increasing age, and no certain triggering factor has been identified. Moreover, zoster does not provide a reliable marker of underlying malignancy in the normal elderly population.

Clinically, the patient experiences pain without any skin changes. Over a period of days, tense clear blisters develop in the erythematous ground area and new lesions spread throughout the involved dermatome (Fig. 1). The stable blisters may remain for 3–5 days before breaking followed by adherent crusts. Disseminated zoster reflects an immunosuppressed patient. Beside the intense acute pain, there may be persistent pain, known as postherpetic neuralgia (PHN), which may last for months to years and which may be disabling.

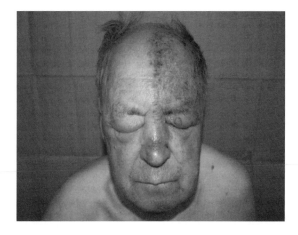

Figure 53.1 *Zoster on scalp involving* N. trigeminus *(first branch)*.

Up to 30% of elderly patients develop some degree of postherpetic neuralgia PHN.[4,5] The following clinical variants of zoster may occur:

- Ophthalmic zoster, associated with keratitis, uveitis, and muscle paralysis.[6] Ophthalmologic consultation is mandatory.
- Otic zoster (Ramsay Hunt syndrome), involving the tympanic membrane or the ear canal, with severe pain. Up to 30% of the patients may suffer from permanent hearing loss.
- Oral zoster: oral lesions may appear in the hard palate and maxilla (second branch) or tongue and mandible (third branch), when both branches of the *Nervus trigeminus* are involved.

VZV is much less sensitive to oral acyclovir than herpes simplex virus, so that a minimum regimen requires 800 mg five times daily for 1 week. However, the gastrointestinal absorption rate of acyclovir is rather low; hence, today oral valacyclovir or brivudine are more appropriate. However, intravenous therapy with acyclovir (375–500 mg three times daily) is required in elderly patients to ensure antiviral efficacy. Topical drying agents, e.g. zinc oxide lotion, and antibiotic ointment to prevent bacterial superinfection and loosen the crusts may also be helpful.[7]

Topical treatment for postherpetic neuralgia (PHN) is rather ineffective,[8,9] since postherpetic neuralgia may rather be dealing with central demyelination as well as neuronal destruction. Oral tricyclic antidepressants, antiepileptics, opioids are merely helpful.

Recently, the vaccine therapy for zoster is available. Both the vaccine against VZV (Varivax) and the newly released vaccine against herpes zoster (Zostavax) may lead to substantial reductions in morbidity from herpes zoster and PHN.[10–13]

WHO guidelines should be followed on the use of analgesics to treat acute pain. Gabapentin and other analgesic agents are recommended for weeks or months for postherpetic neuralgia. Topical treatment may not be useful in this case, as postherpetic neuralgia involves true nerve impairment.[8,9]

Yeast infections

Candida species, particularly Candida albicans, are the main pathogenic yeasts.[14] Candidosis is an infection with Candida species, mostly affecting moist skin areas (interdigital, anogenital, under the breasts). However, C. albicans may also be part of the normal flora in man, usually of the oral cavity, gastrointestinal tract, and external genitalia. Hence, the clinical correlation is essential for the diagnosis: if erythema and other inflammatory signs are present, the fungus is pathogenic. The identification of yeast in the blood reflects a sepsis.

The clinical types of candidosis are classified according to location:

- Oral candidosis. Immunosuppressed patients in particular may suffer from acute candidosis. Angular cheilitis or perlèche commonly occurs in children, and in older individuals who drool, whether from a stroke or poorly fitting dentures.[15,16]

- Genital candidosis. Almost every woman has at least one attack of vaginal candidosis in her lifetime. In contrast, men are less often infected. Nonetheless, in bed-ridden older individuals or in diabetic patients, candidal balanitis is a frequent problem.[17]

- Interdigital candidosis. In certain web spaces, retention of sweat, soap, and water leads to irritation and then secondary infection with C. albicans.

- Candidal intertrigo. Intertriginous areas, especially the groin, axillae, and beneath the breasts, are often secondarily affected by C. albicans. Immobile and overweight individuals are more frequently infected.

- Diaper candidosis. Secondary infection of diaper dermatitis occurs with C. albicans. Like infants, incontinent elderly patients are at high risk.

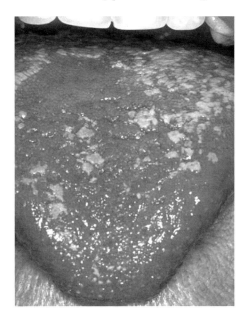

Figure 53.2 *Oral candidosis caused by* Candida albicans.

- Candidal sepsis. In immunosuppressed patients, particularly those undergoing chemotherapy or extensive antibiotic treatment, a candidemia may develop. Moreover, candidal sepsis should always be taken into account in the differential diagnosis of catheter-associated sepsis.[18–20]

Individuals with acquired or inherited defects in cellular or humoral immunity usually associated with endocrinopathy may develop chronic mucocutaneous candidosis, a very rare type. *C. albicans* can easily be identified by culture within 24–48 hours. Other *Candida* species can be identified on the basis of biologic assimilation and fermentation tests.[21]

Topical treatment for candidosis is achieved by the application of a polyene (nystatin, amphotericin B) as a cream, ointment, paste, or powder. Topical azoles (modern broad-spectrum antimycotics) are also applicable for candidosis. Both polyenes and azoles are available as troches and rinsing solutions for treating oral lesions.[21] In contrast, dyes such as gentian violet are less effective and no longer recommended. Reducing moisture and addressing predisposing factors are still major measures alongside the specific antifungal therapy.

The most widely used oral antifungal drug for candidosis is fluconazole. A single dose of 150 mg is usually effective for vaginal candidosis; other candidosis may need a longer treatment.[21] The drug is also used for antifungal prophylaxis in HIV/AIDS patients. However, fluconazole resistance has been known and is a major concern in certain patient groups.

Onychomycosis

Nail fungal infection (tinea unguium) is the most frequent nail disorder in man, primarily in the elderly.[22–25] It is mostly caused by the most common dermatophyte: *Trichophyton rubrum*. However, other dermatophytes, like *T. mentagrophytes* var. *interdigitale* and *Epidermophyton floccosum* can also be responsible for the infection.[26,27] In addition, yeasts, e.g. *Candida tropicalis*, and non-dermatophyte moulds, e.g. *Scopulariopsis brevicaulis*, *Hendersonula toruloidea*, and *Scytalidium hyalinum*, can occasionally affect the nails. The last-mentioned dimorphic fungi are rather unsusceptible to treatment, as they seem not to respond to azoles.

Toenails are far more often affected than fingernails, and elderly individuals are far more frequently infected than children or youths. Tinea pedis – and tinea manus – may be the real source of the infection. The fungi grow under the nail plate, mostly at the distal part, and eventually involve the nail bed.[28]

There are several different types of onychomycosis:[26,27]

- Distal and lateral subungual onychomycosis (DLSO), the most frequent type.
- Proximal subungual onychomycosis (PSO), rather rare in general, but much more frequent in HIV/AIDS patients.
- Superficial white onychomycosis (SWO), quite rare, and only seen on the toenails and usually caused by *T. mentagrophytes* var. *interdigitale*.
- Endonyx onychomycosis, isolated clumped fungal elements under the nail plate, which can hardly be reach by antifungal substances, explaining some treatment failures.
- Total dystrophic onychomycosis (TDO), the final stage of most nail fungal infection with extensive nail destruction, producing thickened discolored crumbly nail plates. Otherwise, TDO comprises the typical nail changes in chronic mucocutaneous candidosis.

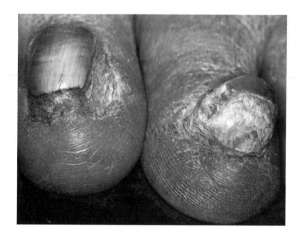

Figure 53.3 *Total dystropic onychomycosis due to* Trichophyton rubrum; *a final stage of fungal nail infection*.

Treatment for onychomycosis should best be chosen by the clinical type and extension of the nail involvement. Only minor distal subungual onychomycosis and SWO can effectively be cured by topical agents alone, the rest of the infection needs oral or combination antifungal therapy.[29] For topical treatment, a modern antifungal nail lacquer, e.g. 5% amorolfine, 8% ciclopirox, is appropriate. Surgical nail removal is rather obsolete, because of the potential matrix damage resulting in permanent dystrophic nails and other shortcomings. Instead, the thickened infected nail plates can be removed atraumatically by nail abrasion using electrical grinder or by mechanical removal employing urea paste 40% for days.[27,30] For oral treatment, terbinafin, itraconazole, and fluconazole are applicable.[31–33] Oral terbinafin (250 mg/day) seems to be the best substance for onychomycosis, so far. Griseofulvin is no longer recommended for treatment in adults, because of its limited efficacy. A sufficient topical as well as oral therapy for onychomycosis takes at least 3–6 months, depending on the course of healing in the patient.

Irritant dermatitis

Irritant contact dermatitis is far more common than allergic contact dermatitis.[34,35] Irritant (non-allergic) dermatitis (ID) is caused by skin exposure to agents that impair the skin barrier function.[36] This can be induced by one exposure to a highly toxic agent (TCA and other acids) or by repeated exposure to agents of low toxicity (intense wet work or a high frequency of daily hand washing). On the other hand, a chronic dry skin condition impairing the barrier function of the skin can also cause ID, and this is mostly seen in the elderly.[37–39]

Irritant dermatitis may be divided into three major groups:

* Acute irritant contact dermatitis. This is a mandatory skin reaction of any individual to a toxic substance. It occurs in particular in many work places, due to contact with physical agents (UV radiation, heat, cold, and mechanical factors) or chemical agents (alkaline and acid solutions). Thus this skin disease is mostly seen in young people. However, retired older individuals may also suffer from the disease, since toxic substances can also occur in the home and garden (acetone, soaps, detergents, croton oil, foodstuffs, airborne irritants (dust, plants)). The typical toxic skin reaction is tissue necrosis from a

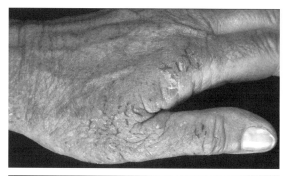
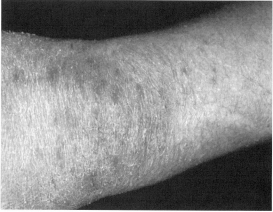

Figure 53.4 (a) Irritant contact dermatitis, typically located on the back of the hand, due to repeated exposure to irritant agents in daily work. (b) Dry skin eczema, usually on legs and arms.

concentrated acidic or basic solution within a minute. Topical corticosteroids are useful for the acute reaction for a short time, in order to reduce the skin inflammation (erythema, swelling, and blisters) following by skin care ointments.
* Cummulative irritant contact dermatitis. This is a chronic dermatitis resulting from repeated exposure to irritant agents mostly in work places, e.g. water, cutting oils, chemicals, and many others. So, occupational chronic hand dermatitis is a typical example of this skin disease – mostly seen in health-care workers, bakers, hairdressers, gardeners, cleaners, etc.[40] However, housewives are also at risk because of repeated exposure to water, soaps, soiled diapers, etc. ('housewives' dermatitis').[41] Not least, predisposing intrinsic factors, such as atopic diathesis, may promote chronic hand dermatitis. In

the elderly, other types of irritant dermatitis may occur which are associated with age-related problems (e.g. incontinence, etc.) such as diaper dermatitis, perianal dermatitis, intertrigo, and stomal dermatitis.[42–45]

- Chronic irritant non-contact dermatitis. This form occurs mostly in the elderly because of the age-related skin dryness.[37,38] Moreover, many older individuals are no longer able to take care of their skin, resulting in diffuse dryness with fine scaling (xerosis), and later in dry skin eczema (asteatotic dermatitis, exsiccation eczema), particularly in their legs.[39] Eczema craquelé provides a typical localized lesion of the dermatitis: the larger scales of deep inflamed fissures display the craquelé work seen on glazed china.[37,39] In general, the appropriate treatment for chronic irritant dermatitis is the removal and subsequent avoidance of the irritant agents.[46,47] In cases of irritant dermatitis caused by moist skin conditions (diaper dermatitis, intertrigo), drying measures are mandatory. After bathing or showering, the gentle use of a hairdryer is better than rubbing the skin dry. Dry skin eczema can be avoided by regular moisturizing skin care.[48,49] Initially, a short-term topical corticosteroid can rapidly reduce the skin inflammation, and this should be followed by the regular use of protecting agents (e.g. zinc oxide paste) in the intertriginous area or moisturizing agents (e.g. a urea-containing cream or lotion).

Psoriasis

Psoriasis is one of the most common skin diseases, with a prevalence of 2% in European populations. Onset of disease is usually from the second to the fourth decade. Psoriasis is primarily caused by a genetic predisposition rendering an imbalance in the immunologic network of the skin leading to an activation of T-cells.[50,51] As a consequence, proliferation and maturation of epidermal keratinocytes are enhanced, causing the clinical appearance of intense desquamation.

There are various clinical features of psoriasis. The chronic stationary plaque type is most frequent

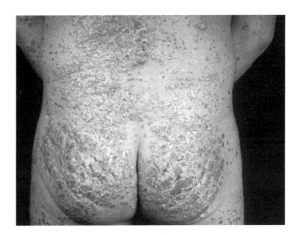

Figure 53.5 *Psoriasis, the chronic plaque type.*

and characterized by erythematosquamous plaques on the whole integument, but mainly in predisposed areas such as the elbows, knees, trunk, and scalp. As an autoimmune, genetic disorder, psoriasis is not limited to skin lesions but can induce severe arthritis. Most commonly the distal joints of fingers and toes are involved. The symptoms range from swelling and pain in the affected joints to incapacitating mutilations.[52]

Endogenous and exogenous factors have a great influence on the clinical course of psoriasis. In our clinical experience most patients who are hospitalized with severe psoriasis are in the age range of 40–70 years. This may be caused by an accumulation of trigger factors found in this age group, e.g. alcohol,[53] stress,[54] smoking, chronic bacterial infections (chronic streptococcal and staphylococcal infections such as tonsillitis),[55] and drugs (betablockers, lithium, and chloroquin).[56]

Psoriatic lesions can be accompanied by intense pruritus. The mechanical irritation caused by scratching itself can induce new lesions. This is known as the *koebner* phenomenon. Thus, pruritus should be taken seriously and treated with antihistamines if necessary. Topical treatment consists of desquamative agents (salicylic acid or urea preparations), vitamin D, analogon (e.g. calcipotriol), or dithranol paste. Corticosteroids should only be applied for intense inflammative lesions on a short-term basis. Ultraviolet light is another cornerstone of psoriasis therapy. UVA and narrow band UVB (311 nm) may be applied, as well as balneophotochemotherapy (psoralen + UVA).[57]

In severe cases unresponsive to topical therapy systemic treatment has to be addressed. Most systemic drugs are immunosuppressive – with potential liver or renal toxicity. Thus a careful, individual choice has to be made regarding the patient's medical condition, disease severity, and patient compliance. Retinoids, methotrexate, cyclosporine, fumaric acid esters, and TNF-alpha inhibitors (biologicals) are used.[58,59] Psoriatic arthritis is treated with non-steroidal anti-inflammatory drugs, methotrexate, leflunomide, and TNF-alpha inhibitors.[60]

Bullous diseases

Bullous diseases are a group of autoimmune dermatoses with the common feature of autoantibodies to components of the skin that lead to discontinuation of different skin layers. As a clinical consequence blisters develop. This section reviews the four most common diseases that are most likely to be encountered in elderly male patients.

Bullous pemphigoid

Bullous pemphigoid (BP) is the most common of all autoimmune blistering diseases. The incidence ranges between 7 and 10 cases per one million. There is an equal gender distribution with a median onset in the sixth to seventh decade.[61–63] Two different major antigens have been identified, which are corresponding hemidesmosomal glycoproteins.[64] Those antigens (BP 180 and BP 230) can be detected in the patients' sera and in skin biopsies by means of direct immunofluorescence. BP might be triggered by drugs such as betablockers and diuretics.[65] However, the correlation is controversial, since elderly BP patients have a high probability of being treated with such drugs. On the basis of clinical studies there is no correlation between BP and malignancies.[66]

Clinically tense blisters arise on either erythematous or normal-appearing skin accompanied by pruritus. Susceptible sites are the flexor surfaces of

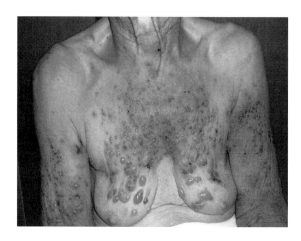

Figure 53.6 *Bullous pemphigoid, tense blisters in initially normal-appearing skin.*

the extremities. As a consequence of ruptured blisters, erosions and blood-tinged crusts might be present as well. Erythema or urticarial lesions, and sometimes intense itch, might precede blisters for months. Mild or localized cases can be effectively treated with topical high potency steroids only or in combination with antibiotics (tetracycline, doxycycline or erythromycin) and nicotinamide.[51,52] Topical tacrolimus may also be helpful.[67] Blisters should be aspirated and covered with a topical antibiotic-soaked gauze. In severe case, oral prednisolone (0.5–1 mg/kg/day) is applicable, if necessary in combination with azathioprine in term to reduce the dose of oral steriods.[62]

Mucous membrane pemphigoid

Mucous membrane pemphigoid (MP) is a disease of the elderly, with a predominance for the female gender and an incidence of one case per million. There are different target antigens of various components of the basal membrane. However, BP 180 provides the most common detectable antigen. In addition there seems to be a genetic predisposition for people expressing the HLA-DRQB*10301 allele.[67] Unlike bullous pemphigoid the histology might be non-specific.

Blisters that heal by scarring may appear on every mucous membrane and in 25% of the cases, on the skin as well. The oral cavity is most commonly involved, followed by the conjunctiva, nose, pharynx, genitalia, larynx, and esophagus. Ocular disease can result in symblepharon and trichiasis (scratching of eyelashes against the cornea), followed by corneal ulceration and blindness. Other complications of scarring include stricture of larynx, pharynx, and urethra as well as sexual dysfunction.[68]

When the oral mucosa alone is involved it may respond to topical steroid treatment only. With ocular, nasal, or genital involvement a high dose of oral prednisolone (1–2 mg/kg/day) should be initiated. In severe cases, additional treatment with oral or intravenous cyclophosphamide might be necessary. Due to the chronic course of the disease steroid-sparing agents such as azathioprine or mycophenolatmofetil may have to be introduced with long-term medication.[69]

Dermatitis herpetiformis

The incidence of dermatitis herpetiformis (DH) varies between different populations being the highest in northern Europe with 100 cases per million. Males are more often affected than women. The median age of onset lies between the second and the fourth decade.[70] All patients with DH have celiac disease. Whereas only about 10% of patients with DH experience clinical symptoms of celiac disease, in all cases serum antibodies to gliadin and tissue transglutaminase are detectable.[70]

The major characteristic symptom is intense pruritus and a burning sensation at the affected areas. Erythematous papules, plaques, and small tense blisters that are sometimes arranged in a herpetiform fashion typically arise at extensor sites of the arms and the lower back. DH is strongly associated with a number of other autoimmune diseases such as type-1 diabetes, autoimmune thyroiditis and gastritis, vitiligo, and lupus erythematosus.[71]

The treatment of choice is diaminodiphenylsulfone (DAPDS). With oral DAPDS given in a dosage of 1.5 mg/kg/day improvement in skin lesions and pruritus usually occurs after only a few days. Since DAPDS can cause methemoglobinemia, hemolysis, and agranulocytosis, methemoglobin levels and blood counts have to be closely monitored. Glucose-6-dehydrogenase deficiency has to be ruled out before initiating DADPS therapy. In addition patients should be advised to follow a gluten-free diet, which has a positive effect on skin lesions and reduces the required DADPS dose.

Pemphigus vulgaris

Pemphigus vulgaris (PV) is an intraepidermal blistering disease with an overall incidence of 1–5 cases per million, that occurs with a higher prevalence in Mediterranean and Jewish people. The mortality rate of 5–10% is the highest among all acquired autoimmune blistering diseases.[61] There is an equal gender distribution and median onset of disease lies between the fourth and sixth decades. PV patients express antibodies directed against desmoglein 3 and 1. Desmoglein proteins are adhesion molecules that are connected throughout the extracellular space of skin and mucosal epithelial tissue to ensure epidermal stability. As a result of loss of cohesion between desmoglein proteins, intraepidermal blistering occurs.[65]

The first symptoms of the disease are often very painful erosions of the oral mucosa. Later fragile blisters that easily turn into erosions are seen mainly on the trunk. The mucosal tissue of the nose, larynx, genitalia, and anus might be involved as well. Because of the loss of large epidermal areas, patients are prone to skin infections and even sepsis. The disease can also be induced by drugs or hematologic malignancies such as non-Hodgkin's lymphoma, chronic lymphatic leukemia or macroglobulinemia Waldenstrom. Drugs that cause PV are penicillamine, ACE inhibitors, piroxicam, penicilline, cephalosporines, pyrazolone derivates, and rifampicine.[63] PV has a chronic course in about two-thirds of cases. Those patients might need lifelong immunosuppressive medication, which raises the possibility of developing either serious infections or neoplasms.

Treatment consists of high-dose oral prednisolone (2 mg/kg/day), usually combined with steroid sparing agents such as azathioprine or cyclophosphamide. In unresponsive cases, intravenous steroid and cyclophosphamide pulse treatment or intravenous immunoglobulins might be neccesary.[71] An innovative therapy might be the TNF-alpha inhibitor infliximab, but the effectiveness suggested by case reports still has to be

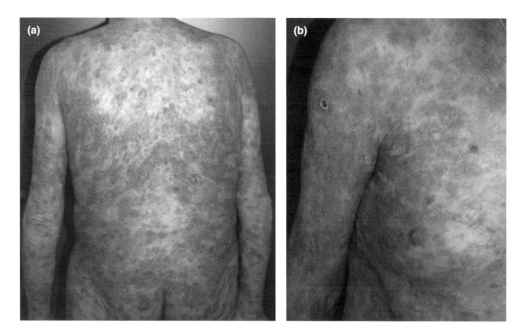

Figure 53.7 *(a) Cutaneous T-cell lymphoma (CTCL) in combination with Hodgkin's disease. (b) Cutaneous T-cell lymphoma (CTCL). A close up.*

evaluated in randomized studies.[72] Topical treatment of PV lesions is antiseptic to lower the risk of bacterial superinfection.

Cutaneous lymphoma

Cutaneous lymphomas are a rare group of malignancies consisting of more than 20 different entities with an estimated annual incidence of 1 in 100 000.[73] Cutaneous lymphomas can be divided into T-cell and B-cell derived malignancies, with T-cell lymphoma being far more common. Only the five most common lymphoma types that account for more than 95% of all clinical cases will be discussed here. The gender distribution shows a significantly higher percentage of males with T-cell lymphoma.[74]

Cutaneous T-cell lymphoma

Mycosis fungoides

Mycosis fungoides (MF) is the most common type of cutaneous T-cell lymphoma (CTCL). It is characterized by monoclonal proliferation of T-lymphocytes that accumulate in the epidermis. This phenomenon is known as epidermotropism. The median age at diagnosis is 55–60 years. The male-to-female ratio is 2:1.

The disease progresses through three clinical stages: patch, plaque, and tumor. In the first stage atropic, squamous small patches that can resemble eczema show mainly on the lateral trunk and flexural sides of the upper arms and thighs. MF is known to have a very wide range of possible clinical presentations including every kind of cutaneous efflorescence. Due to its relatively benign course, progression to the next stage can take years or even decades. Histologic changes in the very early stages of the disease are often non-specific and several biopsies taken over a period of months or years might be necessary to confirm the diagnosis.[75]

In the second stage more infiltrated plaques appear. The plaques are seperated by small spots of healthy skin known as nappes claires. The tumor stage is characterized by rapidly growing, often ulcerated tumors in combination with the above-mentioned lesions. Disseminated tumors without any other skin lesions are atypical and suggest other types of malignancies but usually in the plaque or tumor stage of MF, lymph nodes and internal organs may rarely become involved.

In the patch stage the treatment of choice consists of balneophotochemotherapy bathpuva and topical steroids. Aggressive treatment like systemic chemotherapy is not recommended and might even result in faster progession of the disease. In the later stages of MF combined treatment schedules are favored, including interferon-alpha, retinoids, extracorporal photopheresis, polychemotherapy, and radiotherapy.[75,76] The prognosis of MF is good due to the slow progression.

Primary cutaneous CD30 + lymphoproliferative disorders

This group accounts for 30% of CTCLs. It includes lymphomatoid papulosis (LP) and primary cutaneous anaplastic large cell lymphoma (PCALCL).[74] LP is characterized by disseminated papules and nodules that either spontaneously resolve or become necrotic and leave scars. The median age of onset is in the fourth to fifth decade.

The clinical course is chronic with occasional exacerbations over years or decades. Rarely LP patients develop other malignant lymphomas such as Hodgkin's disease or MF,[77] hence clinical staging should be performed at regular intervals. PCALCL presents with a solitary or only a few reddish nodular tumors that tend to ulceration. This group affects mostly elderly people or children.

LP responds well to psoralen + UVA (PUVA), often in combination with low-dose[76] methotrexate. PCALCL lesions can be excised or treated by radiotherapy. The prognosis of both diseases is excellent, with a 95% 5-year survival.[73]

Sezary syndrome

Sezary syndrome (SS) accounts for only 3% of CTCLs, but ranks in third position of the most common ones.[73] It is a disease of the elderly with a median onset in the sixth to seventh decade. SS is characterized by the clinical triad: T-cell leukemia with typical cerebriform sezary cells, generalized lymphadenopathy and erythrodermia. However, pruritus is one of the most disturbing symptoms.[75]

Treatment consists of PUVA combined with interferon, methotrexate, total skin electron beam irradiation, and chemotherapy with CHOP (cyclophosphamide hydroxydoxorubicin (Adriamycin[R]) vincristine (Oncovin[R])[75] and prednisolone.[26] The prognosis is poor, with a median survival of 2 to 4 years.[74,77,78]

Cutaneous B-cell lymphoma

Primary cutaneous B-cell lymphomas (PCBLs) are extremely rare. In most cases histologically proved cutaneous B-cell lymphoma lesions represent cutaneous infiltrations of a systemic disease. As a consquence a thorough staging has to be performed, including chest X-ray, abdominal ultrasound, bone marrow biopsy, and immunoelectrophoresis.

If systemic B-cell lymphoma can be excluded twice within 6 months the diagnosis of PCBL can be made.[78] PCBL follows an indolent clinical course, with the exception of diffuse large B-cell lymphoma of the leg, and the 5-year survival is close to 100%.[74]

Primary cutaneous follicle center lymphoma

Primary cutaneous follicle center lymphoma (PCFCL) accounts for 11% of all primary cutaneous lymphomas and occurs in elderly people.[72] Red, livid nodules and plaques with surrounding infiltrated erythema, sometimes only solitary lesions, develop on the susceptible sites of the head and neck.[74] If the anatomic position allows, surgical excision should be attempted. Other options are radiotherapy, CHOP chemotherapy, and systemic or intralesional application of the CD20 antibody rituximab.[79,80]

Primary cutaneous marginal zone B-cell lymphoma

Seven percent of primary cutaneous lymphomas are primary cutaneous marginal zone B-cell lymphomas (PCMZLs). An association of the disease with borreliosis in European populations has been shown.[74] Clinically, reddish, round nodules appear on the arms and trunk. The treatment is similar to that of

PCFCL. In case of positive borrelia serology an antibiotic therapy should be administered, before seeking other options.[74,79]

Cutaneous drug reactions

Around 5–15% of patients on a permanent medication experience adverse cutaneous drug reactions.[81] The clinical presentation of these reactions is diverse and can mimic a variety of idiopathic skin diseases. Drugs that frequently cause adverse skin reactions are antibiotics, mainly betalactames and sulfonamides, non-steroidal anti-inflammatory drugs, anticonvulsants, and cardiovascular drugs.[82]

The underlying immunologic mechanisms can be either classic allergic reactions or pseudoallergic in nature. Allergic reactions are categorized into four types after the classification of Coombs and Gell,[83] with types I, III, and IV causing skin changes. Type I reactions are mediated by specific IgE antibodies leading to angioedema, generalized urticaria, and anaphylactic shock usually within minutes after allergen exposure. Type III reactions cause vasculitis by binding of antigen–antibody complexes to vascular basal membranes. Vasculitis lesions develop within days after allergen intake. Type IV or delayed-type hypersensitivity is caused by sensitized T-cells that produce proinflammatory cytokines upon allergen encounter. As a clinical correlate, eczema or exanthema occurs usually within 2 to 3 days.[84] This classification is a simplified model. Thus clinical presentation and onset of reaction might widely vary, not fitting into any of the described types of allergy.

Pseudoallergy is a term used for reaction patterns similar to those of type I allergies that are not mediated by specific antibodies or T-cells. These reactions are dose-dependent and sometimes only occur during periods of intense activation of the immune system, such as bacterial or viral infections. Pseudoallergic reactions can often be observed after use of non-steroidal anti-inflammatory drugs, with acetyl salicylic acid being the most common trigger.[85]

There are some distinguishing clinical features of the cutaneous drug reaction:

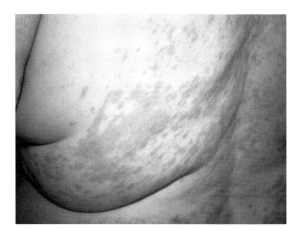

Figure 53.8 *Adverse skin reaction to drugs: maculopapular rash, frequently after antibiotics.*

- Maculopapular rash: this usually starts and is most intense on the trunk, but tends to generalize, accompanied by pruritus and fatigue. Antibiotics typically cause this type of drug reaction.
- Stevens–Johnson syndrome (SJS)/toxic epidermal necrolysis (TEN): SJS starts with a generalized maculopapular exanthema that progresses to an erythrodermic condition with widespread formation of blisters on the skin and mucosal tissues resembling second-degree burns. Primary lesions might also be annular, as the target lesions in erythema multiforme. If more than 30% of the body surface is covered with blisters a diagnosis of TEN has to be made.[86] TEN is a life-threatening condition; patients should be referred to a specialized burn unit immediately. The lethality of SJS is approximately 6%, but rises to 45% in TEN.[85]
- Angioedema/urticaria: this is characterized by swelling of the face and extremities and can become a life-threatening condition when the tongue and larynx become involved. Patients taking ACE inhibitors (ACEIs) can develop recurrent angioedema, which is most probably not an immunogenic effect, but rather a side-effect of its mechanism of action.[87] Angiotensin-II receptor blockers (ARBs) are commonly used to replace ACEIs in case of angioedema or other

drug reaction. After a few years of clinical experience with ARBs it seems that they have a similar profile regarding drug reactions and should therefore not be used as replacement for ACEIs.[88]

- Fixed drug eruption: this is a localized form of drug reaction and occurs on the same area of skin for a prolonged or repeated period of time. The clinical appearance can vary from erythema to bullae or eczema.
- Lichenoid exanthema: pruritic lichenoid papules and plaques delvelop in a localized or generalized fashion over a prolonged period of time without sites of predilection. Other lichenoid dermatoses such as lichen ruber planus have to be ruled out. Lichenoid drug eruptions are rare and mainly caused by beta-blockers, penicillamine, gold, and quinine.[89]
- Vasculitis: this drug reaction presents as disseminated petechial lesions, most prominent at the extremities. Vasculitic changes can involve not only the skin but also other internal organs. As a consequence, hepatic or renal failure may occur.[90]

The patient's medical history is usually not sufficient to make a diagnosis of drug allergy. In any case allergic tests including cutaneous-vascular testing and a double-blind placebo-controlled provocation are recommended.

All drug reactions are self-limiting diseases as long as the causative agent is withdrawn. Identifying the causative drug might be difficult, especially in elderly patients with several medications. Furthermore, adequate replacement treatment could prove difficult. Thus a thorough clinical investigation and the exclusion of other dermatoses should be undertaken, before medications are changed.

Mild cases of drug eruptions can be treated with topical steroids only, but severe cases might require systemic steroid use. Blisters should not be surgically removed, but aspirated with preservation of the blister roof to minimize epidermal loss. As stated above, TEN is an emergency situation. These patients need to be managed in the intensive care unit.

Complications of antineoplastic drug therapy

Skin changes in patients suffering from neoplastic diseases are quite common. The symptoms can be a direct effect of the underlying disease or can be related either to infections of the mostly immunosuppressed patients or to adverse reactions of the antineoplastic treatment, which is mostly conducted in elderly patients.

It can be very difficult to determine the cause of skin changes. In the case of suspected adverse drug reactions the physician often faces the dilemma of whether to reduce the dosage, change, or discontinue the necessary medication. These issues are considered here and the most common skin changes resulting from antineoplastic therapy are reviewed.

Hyperpigmentation

Hyperpigmentation is a harmless, but often disturbing and disfiguring skin change. Numerous cytostatic and immunosuppressive agents can induce hyperpigmentation not only of the skin, but also of the mucosal tissue, nails, and hair. The following list of causative substances includes only the most common drugs and should not regarded as complete: bleomycin, busulfan, carmustin, cisplatin, cyclophosphamide, daunorubicin, fluorouracil, hydroxyurea, methotrexate, paclitaxel, procarbazine, and vinca alkaloids.[91,92]

Hyperpigmentation usually occurs approximately one month after initiation of treatment and fades about 6 months after discontinuation. Sun screens and topical steroids can help to shorten the process.[93]

Neutrophil eccrine hidradenitis

Reddish infiltrated papules and plaques develop on the upper half of the trunk and face in neutrophil eccrine hidradenitis (NEH). The diagnosis is usually made through a skin biopsy, showing a neutrophilic infiltrate surrounding eccrine sweat glands and sweat gland necrosis.[94] The disease occurs mostly in patients with hematogenic malignancies who receive chemotherapy. The disease onset is 2 days to 3 weeks after application of the cytostatic drug. NEH is self-limiting, but can recur after each new therapy cycle. Non-steroidal anti-inflammatory drugs may have an ameliorating effect. Oral DADPS (dapson) 100 mg daily is used as a prophylaxis in recurring disease.[94]

Palmar plantar erythrodysesthesia

The so-called hand–foot syndrome constitutes a toxic, dose-dependent reaction to various cytostatics, mainly doxorubicin, cytarabin, docetaxel, and 5-fluorouracil. The incidence ranges from 6 to 64% depending on the treatment regimen. Clinically patients experience dysesthesia and a prickling sensation on palms and soles. Later blisters and desquamation accompanied by strong pain occur. In severe cases a dose reduction or even change of chemotherapy has to be considered.[95] Therapeutically, vitamin B6 100–300 mg daily and topical application of DMSO along with analgesic medications is used, but without consistent effects.[95]

Oral mucositis

Oral mucositis (OM) is another cytotoxic side-effect of chemotherapy and occurs in up to 40% of patients during the first days of treatment. It is often complicated by secondary candida or herpes infections. Antiseptic and analgesic mouth wash solutions are applicable, but treatment is mostly frustrating.[92] Experimental treatment options such as glutamine, keratinocyte growth factors, filgrastim, and TGF-beta3 are promising and are currently being evaluated in clinical studies.[96]

Hypersensitivity reactions

Type I allergic reactions with generalized urticaria, angioedema, and sometimes even anaphylactic shock are a common complication of asparginase, paclitaxel, and docetaxel chemotherapy. Similar symptons can be caused by a pseudoallergic mechanism as is known to occur with taxanes and platin derivatives. Prophylactic intravenous application of steroids and antihistamines 30 minutes before starting the chemotherapy is recommended in these cases.[97]

Skin reactions after radiation therapy

Some cytostatic agents can enhance the reaction to radiotherapy both in a positive sense of a better antineoplastic effect, but also in a negative sense of

more severe side-effects such as radiodermatitis. This phenomenon is known to occur with bleomycin, cisplatin, doxorubicin, fluorouracil, hydroxyurea, and methotrexate.

Another remarkable reaction is the radiation recall phenomenon. Upon administration of various cytostatic drugs an acute toxic dermatitis can occur at previously irradiated skin areas. The underlying mechanisms of this reaction are not fully understood yet. Nevertheless, cessation of the chemotherapeutic agent is not warranted as its benefits probably outweigh its risks. The dermatitis can be effectively treated with topical potent steroids.[98]

Extravasation

Extravasation of extremely toxic cytostatic agents is a common and severe complication of chemotherapy. Some reactions consist of self-limiting erythema that heals with scarring and hyperpigmentation. Other substances cause blisters, ulcerations, and skin necrosis with little healing tendency – these include doxorubicin, daunorubicin, taxanes, and mechlorethamin to name just a few. As soon as extravasation is noted the arm should be placed in a high position and should be cooled. Only after extravasation of vinka alkaloids should warmth be applied. If an antidote for the specific cytostatic agent is available, it should be injected immediately. However, all these measures can only aim at minimizing the tissue damage.[99]

Hydroxyurea-induced ulceration

Hydroxyurea can cause extremly painful, chronic leg ulcerations that do not respond to any kind of wound treatment. The only therapeutic option in this case is discontinuation of the therapy.[100]

References

1. Insinga RP, Itzler RF, Pellissier JM et al. The incidence of herpes zoster in a United States administrative database. J Gen Intern Med 2005; 8: 48–53.
2. Grose C. Varicella zoster virus: out of Africa and into the research laboratory. Herpes 2006; 2: 32–6.
3. Arvin AM. Varicella-zoster virus. Clin Microbiol Rev 1996; 3: 361–81.
4. Niv D, Maltsman-Tseikhin A, Lang E. Postherpectic neuralgia: what do we know and where are we heading? Pain Physician 2004; 2: 239–47.

5. Wassilew SW. Zoster-associated neuralgias. J Dtsch Dermatol Ges 2006; 10: 871–9; quiz 880–1.

6. Schoenlaub P, Grange F, Nasica X et al. Oculomotor nerve paralysis with complete ptosis in herpes zoster ophthalmicus: 2 cases. Ann Dermatol Venereol 1997; 5: 401–3.

7. Gross G, Schofer H, Wassilew S et al. Herpes zoster guideline of the German Dermatology Society (DDG). J Clin Viro 2003; 3: 277–89.

8. Khaliq W, Alam S, Puri N. Topical lidocaine for the treatment of postherpetic neuralgia. Cochrane Database Syst rev 2007; 2: CD004846.

9. Katz J, McDermott MP, Cooper EM et al. Psychosocial risk factors for postherpetic neuralgia: a prospective study of patients with herpes zoster. J Pain 2005; 12: 782–90.

10. Robinson DM, Perry CM. Zoster vaccine live (Oka/Merck). Drugs Aging 2006; 6: 525–31.

11. Holcomb K, Weinberg JM. A novel vaccine (Zostavax) to prevent herpes zoster and postherpetic neuralgia. J Drugs Dermatol 2006; 9: 863–6.

12. Oxman MN, Levin MJ, Johnson GR et al. A vaccine to prevent herpes zoster and postherpetic neuralgia in older adults. N Engl J Med 2005; 22: 271–84.

13. Hornberger J, Robertus K. Cost-effectiveness of a vaccine to prevent herpes zoster and postherpetic neuralgia in older adults. Ann Intern Med 2006; 5: 317–25.

14. Segal E. Candida, still number one–what do we know and where are we going from there? Mycoses 2005; Suppl 1: 3–11.

15. Zaremba ML, Daniluk T, Rozkiewicz D et al. Incidence rate of Candida species in the oral cavity of middle-aged and elderly subjects. Adv Med Sci 2006; Suppl 1: 233–6.

16. Paillaud E, Merlier I, Dupeyron C et al. Oral candidiasis and nutritional deficiencies in elderly hospitalised patients. Br J Nutr 2004; 5: 861–7.

17. Jobst D, Kraft K. Candida species in stool, symptoms and complaints in general practice–a cross-sectional study of 308 outpatients. Mycoses 2006; 5: 415–20.

18. Sandven P, Bevanger L, Digranes A et al. Candidemia in Norway (1991 to 2003): results from a nationwide study. J Clin Microbiol 2006; 6: 1977–81.

19. Nakamura T, Takahashi H. Epidemiological study of Candida infections in blood: susceptibilities of Candida spp. to antifungal agents, and clinical features associated with the candidemia. J Infect Chemother 2006; 3: 132–8.

20. Bader MS, Lai SM, Kumar V et al. Candidemia in patients with diabetes mellitus: epidemiology and predictors of mortality. Scand J Infect Dis 2004; 11–12: 860–4.

21. Seebacher C, Abeck D, Brasch J et al. Candidiasis of the skin. J Dtsch Dermatol Ges 2006; 7: 591–6.

22. Yalcin B, Tamer E, Toy GG et al. The prevalence of skin diseases in the elderly: analysis of 4099 geriatric patients. Int J Dermatol 2006; 6: 672–6.

23. Liao YH, Chen KH, Tseng MP et al. Pattern of skin diseases in a geriatric patient group in Taiwan: a 7-year survey from the outpatient clinic of a university medical center. Dermatology 2001; 4: 308–13.

24. Gupta AK. Onychomycosis in the elderly. Drugs Aging 2000; 6: 397–407.

25. Loo DS. Onychomycosis in the elderly: drug treatment options. Drug Aging 2007; 4:293.

26. Effendy I, Lecha M, Feuilhade de Chauvin M et al. Epidemiology and clinical classification of onychomycosis. J Eur Acad Dermatol Venereol 2005; Suppl 1: 8–12.

27. Seebacher C, Brasch J, Abeck D et al. Onychomycosis. J Dtsch Dermatol Ges 2007; 1: 61–6.

28. Saunte DM, Holgersen JB, Haedersdal M et al. Prevalence of toe nail onychomycosis in diabetic patients. Acta Derm Venereol 2006; 5: 425–8.

29. Lecha M, Effendy I, Feuihade de Cahuvin M et al. Treatment options - development of consensus guidelines. J Eur Acad Dermatol Venereol 2005; Suppl 1: 25–33.

30. Zhang AY, Camp WL, Elewski BE. Advances in topical and systemic antifungals. Dermatol Clin 2007; 2: 165–83.

31. Darkes MJ, Scott LJ, Goa KL. Terbinafine: a review of its use in onychomycosis in adults. Am J Clin Dermatol 2003; 1: 39–65.

32. Arca E, Tastan HB, Akar A et al. An open, randomized, comparative study of oral fluconazole, itraconazole and terbiinafine therapy in onychomycosis. J Dermatolog Treat 2002; 1: 3–9.

33. Baran R, Gupta AK, Pierard GE. Pharmacotherapy of onychomycosis. Expert Opin Pharmacother 2005; 4: 609–24.

34. Hanifin JM, Reed ML. A population-based survey of eczema prevalence in the United States. Dermatitis 2007; 2: 82–91.

35. Nedorost ST, Stevens SR. Diagnosis and treatment of allergic skin disorders in the elderly. Drugs Aging 2001; 11: 827–35.

36. Loffler H, Effendy I. Prevention of irritant contact dermatitis. Eur J Dermatol 2002; 1: 4–9.

37. Norman RA. Xerosis and pruritus in the elderly: recognition and management. Dermatol Ther 2003; 3: 254–9.

38. Thaipisuttikul Y. Pruritic skin diseases in the elderly. J Dermatol 1998; 3: 153–7.

39. Aoyama H, Tanaka M, Hara M et al. Nummular eczema: An addition of senile xerosis and unique cutaneous reactivities to environmental aeroallergens. Dermatology 1999; 2: 135–9.

40. Nettis E, Colanardi MC, Soccio AL et al. Occupational irritant and allergic contact dermatitis

among healthcare workers. Contact Dermatitis 2002; 2: 101–7.

41. Lazar AP, Lazar P. Dry skin, water, and lubrication. Dermatol Clin 1991; 1: 45–51.

42. Foureur N, Vanzo B, Meaume S et al. Prospective aetiological study of diaper dermatitis in the elderly. Br J Dermatol 2006; 5: 941–6.

43. de Wet PM, Rode H, van Dyk A et al. Perianal candidosis–a comparative study with mupirocin and nystatin. Int J Dermatol 1999; 8: 618–22.

44. Bauer A, Rodiger C, Grief C et al. Vulvar dermatoses–irritant and allergic contact dermatitis of the vulva. Dermatology 2005; 2: 143–9.

45. Uter W, Geier J, Pfahlberg A et al. The spectrum of contact allergy in elderly patients with and without lower leg dermatitis. Dermatology 2002; 4: 266–72.

46. Elsner P. Skin protection in the prevention of skin diseases. Curr Probl Dermatol 2007; 34: 1–10.

47. Lee JY, Effendy I, Maibach HI. Acute irritant contact dermatitis: recovery time in man. Contact Dermatitis 1997; 6: 285–90.

48. Loden M. Role of topical emolloents and moisturizers in the treatment of dry skin barrier disorders. Am J Clin Dermatol 2003; 11: 771–88.

49. Bikowski J. The use of therapeutic moisturizers in various dermatologic disorders. Cutis 2001; Suppl 1: 3–11.

50. Bos JD, de Rie MA, Teunissen MB et al. Psoriasis: dysregulation of innate immunity. Br J Dermatol 2005; 152: 1098–107.

51. Bowcock AM, Krueger JG. Getting under the skin: the immunogenetics of psoriasis. Nat Rev Immunol 2005; 5: 699–711.

52. Gladman DD, Antoni C, Mease P et al. Psoriatic arthritis: epidemiology, clinical features, course, and outcome. Ann Rheum Dis 2005; 64(Suppl 2): 4–7.

53. Gupta MA, Schork NJ, Gupta AK et al. Alcohol intake and treatment responsiveness of psoriasis: a prospective study. J Am Acad Dermatol 1993; 28: 730–2.

54. Rapp SR, Feldman SR, Exum ML et al. Psoriasis causes as much disability as other major medical diseases. J Am Acad Dermatol 1999; 41: 401–7.

55. Ockenfels HM. Trigger factors for psoriasis. Hautarzt 2003; 54: 215–23.

56. Tsankov N, Angelova I, Kazandjieva J. Drug-induced psoriasis. Recognition and management. Am J Clin Dermatol 2000; 1: 159–65.

57. Lebwohl M, Ali S. Treatment of psoriasis. Part 1. Topical therapy and phototherapy. J Am Acad Dermatol 2001; 45: 487–98.

58. Lebwohl M, Ali S. Treatment of psoriasis. Part 2. Systemic therapies. J Am Acad Dermatol 2001; 45: 649–61.

59. Sterry W, Barker J, Boehncke WH et al. Biological therapies in the systemic management of psoriasis:

international consensus conference. Br J Dermatol 2004; 151: 3–17.

60. Mease P, Goffe BS. Diagnosis and treatment of psoriatic arthritis. J Am Acad Dermatol 2005; 52: 1–19.

61. Khumalo N, Kirtschig G, Middleton P et al. Interventions for bullous pemphigoid. Cochrane Database Syst Rev 2005; (3): CD002292.

62. Patton T, Korman NJ. Bullous pemphigoid treatment review. Expert Opin Pharmacother 2006; 17: 2403–11.

63. Wojnarowska F, Kirtschig G, Highet AS et al. Guidelines for the management of bullous pemphigoid. Br J Dermatol 2002; 47: 214–21.

64. Schmidt E, Obe K, Brocker EB et al. Serum levels of autoantibodies to BP180 correlate with disease activity in patients with bullous pemphigoid. Arch Dermatol 2000; 136: 174–8.

65. Bastuji-Garin S, Joly P, Picard-Dahan C et al. Drugs associated with bullous pemphigoid. A case-control study. Arch Dermatol 1996; 132: 272–6.

66. Megahed M. Histopathology of Blistering Diseases. Springer Verlag Berlin, Heidelberg, New York: Springer 2004.

67. Ko MJ, Chu CY. Topical tacrolimus therapy for localized bullous pemphigoid. Br J Dermatol 2003; 5: 1079–81.

68. Fleming TE, Korman NJ. Cicatricial pemphigoid. J Am Acad Dermatol 2000; 43: 571–91.

69. Chan LS, Ahmed AR, Anhalt GJ et al. The first international consensus on mucous membrane pemphigoid: definition, diagnostic criteria, pathogenic factors, medical treatment and prognostic indicators. Arch Dermatol 2002; 138: 370–9.

70. Dieterich W, Laag E, Bruckner-Tuderman L et al. Antibodies to tissue transglutaminase as serologic markers in patients with dermatitis herpetiformis. J Invest Dermatol 1999; 113: 133–6.

71. Reunala T, Collin P. Diseases associated with dermatitis herpetiformis. Br J Dermatol 1997; 136: 315–18.

72. Toth GG, Jonkman MF. Therapy of pemphigus. Clin Dermatol 2001; 19: 761–7.

73. Pardo J, Mercader P, Mahiques L et al. Infliximab in the management of severe pemphigus vulgaris. Br J Dermatol 2005; 153: 222–3.

74. Willemze R, Jaffe ES, Burg G et al. WHO-EORTEC classification for cutaneous lymphomas. Blood 2005; 105: 3768–85.

75. Kim EJ, Hess S, Richardson SK et al. Immunopathogenesis and therapy of cutaneous T cell lymphoma. J Clin Invest 2005; 115: 798–812.

76. Whittaker SJ, Marsden JR, Spittle M et al. Joint British Association of Dermatologists and U.K. Cutaneous Lymphoma Group guidelines for the management of primary cutaneous T-cell lymphomas. Br J Dermatol 2003; 149: 1095–107.

77. Liu HL, Hoppe RT, Kohler S et al. CD30+ cutaneous lymphoproliferative disorders: the Stanford experience in lymphomatoid papulosis and primary cutaneous anaplastic large cell lymphoma. J Am Acad Dermatol 2003; 49: 1049–58.

78. Santucci M, Pimpinelli N. Primary cutaneous B-cell lymphomas. Current concepts. I. Haematologica 2004; 89: 1360–71.

79. El-Helw L, Goodwin S, Slater D et al. Primary B-cell lymphoma of the skin: the Sheffield Lymphoma Group Experience (1984–2003). Int J Oncol 2004; 25: 1453–8.

80. Gellrich S, Muche JM, Wilks A et al. Systemic eight-cycle anti CD 0 monoclonal antibody (rituximab) therapy in primary cutaneous B-cell lymphomas – an applicational observation. Br J Dermatol 2005; 153: 167–73.

81. Gruchalla R. Drug metabolism, danger signals, and drug-induced hypersensitivity. J Allergy Clin Immunol 2001; 108: 475–88.

82. Hunziker T, Kunzi UP, Braunschweig S et al. Comprehensive hospital drug monitoring (CHDM): adverse skin reactions, a 20-year survey. Allergy 1997; 52: 388–93.

83. Coombs RPA, Gell PGH. The classification of allergic reactions underlying disease. In Gell PGH and Coombs RPA, eds. Clinical Aspects of Immunology. Philadelphia, PA: Davis 1963; 317.

84. Gruchalla R. Understanding drug allergies. J Allergy Clin Immunol 2000; 105: 637–44.

85. Bastuji-Garin S, Rzany B, Stern RS et al. Clinical classification of cases of toxic epidermal necrolysis, Stevens–Johnson syndrome, and erythema multiforme. Arch Dermatol 1993; 129: 92–6.

86. Mockenhaupt M, Norgauer J. Cutaneous adverse drug reactions. ACI International 2002; 14: 143–9.

87. Torpet L, Kragelund C, Reibel J et al. Oral adverse drug reactions to cardiovascular drugs. Crit Rev Oral Biol Med 2004; 15: 28–46.

88. Nielsen EW. Hypotensive shock and angio-oedema from angiotensin II receptor blocker: a class effect in spite of tripled tryptase values. J Intern Med 2005; 258: 385–7.

89. Halevy S, Shai A. Lichenoid drug eruptions. J Am Acad Dermatol 1993; 29: 249–55.

90. Pichler WJ. Delayed drug hypersensitivity reactions. Ann Int Med 2003; 139: 683–93.

91. Pandya AG, Guevara IL. Disorders of hyperpigmentation. Dermatol Clin 2000; 18: 91–8.

92. De Spain JD. Dermatologic toxicity of chemotherapy. Semin Oncol 1992; 19: 501–7.

93. Bachmeyer C, Aractingi S. Neutrophilic eccrine hidradenitis. Clin Dermatol 2000; 18: 319–30.

94. Shear NH, Knowles SR, Shapiro L et al. Dapsone in prevention of recurrent neutrophilic eccrine hidradenitis. J Am Acad Dermatol 1996; 35: 819–22.

95. Nagore E, Insa A, Sanmartin O. Antineoplastic therapy-induced palmar plantar erythrodysesthesia ('hand–foot') syndrome. Incidence, recognition and management. Am J Clin Dermatol 2000; 1: 225–34.

96. Sharma R, Tobin P, Clarke SJ. Management of chemotherapy-induced nausea, vomiting, oral mucositis, and diarrhoea. Lancet Oncol 2005; 6: 93–102.

97. Alley E, Green R, Schuchter L. Cutaneous toxicities of cancer therapy. Curr Opin Oncol 2002; 14: 212–16.

98. Azria D, Magne N, Zouhait A et al. Radiation recall: a well recognized but neglected phenomenon. Cancer Treat Rev 2005; 31: 555–70.

99. Schrijvers DL. Extravasation: a dreaded complication of chemotherapy drugs: the art of consultation. Arch Dermatol 2003; 139: 77–81.

100. Weinlich G, Schuler G, Greil R et al. Leg ulcers associated with long-term hydroxyurea therapy. J Am Acad Dermatol 1998; 39: 372–4.

CHAPTER 54

Skin changes caused by venous diseases

Eberhard Rabe and Feliztas Pannier

Introduction

Chronic venous diseases like varicose veins and post-thrombotic syndrome are very common in the general population.[1] In earlier studies reported prevalences for varicose veins ranged from 1 to 73% in females and 2 to 56% in males and for chronic venous insufficiency from 1 to 40% in females and from 1 to 17% in males.[1-4] The results vary according to different geographic region, and also by the methods used for evaluation. In Western countries varicose veins are present in 25–33% of female and 10–20% of male adults. The incidence of varicose veins per year in the Framingham study was 2.6% in women and 1.9% in men.[5] The prevalence of skin changes was reported to vary between 3 and 13% in the population, and the prevalence of active and healed ulcers to vary between 1 and 2.7%.[1]

Chronic venous disorders are classified according to the CEAP classification.[6] This classification consists of different parts including clinical (C), etiologic (E), anatomic (A), and pathophysiologic (P) information (Table 54.1). The majority of the diseases are in the stages C1–C3. In the Bonn Vein Study,[7] telangiectases and reticular veins as the most severe finding were present in about 59% of the general population, almost equally in men and women. Varicose veins without skin changes and without edema were present in 12.4% of the male

Table 54.1 *CEAP classification[6]*

C_0 No visible or palpable signs of venous disease
C_1 Telangiectasies or reticular veins
C_2 Varicose veins; distinguished from reticular veins by a diameter of 3 mm or more
C_3 Edema
C_4 Changes in skin and subcutaneous tissue secondary to CVD, now divided into 2 subclasses to better define the differing severity of venous disease:
   C_{4a} Pigmentation or eczema
   C_{4b} Lipodermatosclerosis or atrophie blanche
C_5 Healed venous ulcer
C_6 Active venous ulcer

and 15.8% of the female population. C3, pitting edema caused by venous diseases, was present in 11.6% of the male and 14.9% of the female population. Skin changes start in stage C4a with eczema and pigmentation. Clinical stage C4b is defined by white atropy or dermatoliposclerosis. In C5 healed and in stage C6 active ulcer is present.

Definitions

Skin changes were defined in a consensus conference of the Union Internationale de Phlébologie in 2003 and adopted by the CEAP committee.[6,8]

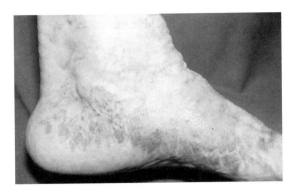

Figure 54.1 *Corona phlebectatica.*

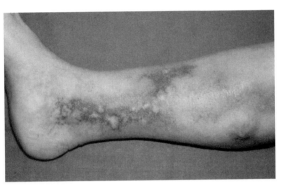

Figure 54.2 *Pigmentation.*

Eczema is erythematous dermatitis, which may progress to blistering, weeping, or scaling eruption of the skin of the leg. It is most often located near varicose veins, but may be located anywhere in the leg. Usually seen in uncontrolled chronic venous disorder (CVD), but may reflect sensitization to local therapy.

Edema in chronic venous disease is defined by a perceptible increase in the volume of fluid in the skin and subcutaneous tissue, characteristically indented with pressure. Venous edema usually occurs in the ankle region, but may extend to the leg and foot.

Corona phlebectatica is a fan-shaped pattern of numerous small intradermal veins on the medial or lateral aspects of the ankle and foot. It is commonly thought to be an early sign of advanced venous disease. Synonyms include malleolar flare and ankle flare (Figure 54.1).

Pigmentation is defined as a brownish darkening of the skin, resulting from extravasated blood. It usually occurs in the ankle region, but may extend to the leg and foot (Figure 54.2).

White atropy is localized, often circular, whitish and atropic skin areas surrounded by dilated capillaries and sometimes hyperpigmentation. It is a sign of severe CVD, not to be confused with healed ulcer scars. Scars of healed ulceration may also exhibit atropic skin with pigmentary changes, but they are distinguishable by a history of ulceration and their appearance from white atropy, and are excluded from this definition (Figure 54.3).

Lipodermatosclerosis (LDS) is defined as a localized chronic inflammation and fibrosis of the skin and subcutaneous tissues of the lower leg, sometimes associated with scarring or contracture of the Achilles tendon. LDS is sometimes preceded by diffuse inflammatory edema of the skin, which may be painful and which is often referred to as hypodermitis. LDS must be differentiated from lymphangitis, erysipelas, or cellulitis by their characteristically different local signs and systemic features. LDS is a sign of severe CVD (Figure 54.4).

Venous ulcer is a full-thickness defect of skin, most frequently in the ankle region, that fails to heal spontaneously and is sustained by CVD (Figure 54.5).

The clinical stages C3–C6 are defined as chronic venous insufficiency. This term was first used in 1957 by van der Molen.[9] He summarized clinical changes like edema, skin changes, corona phlebectatica paraplantaris, and skin ulcers caused by chronic venous diseases under the term chronic venous insufficiency.

Chronic venous insufficiency and gender

The risk for varicose veins is higher in the female population, with an odds ratio of 1.5 and a confidence interval of 1.25–1.79, whereas chronic venous insufficiency in the stages C4–C6 is almost equally distributed between men and women.[7]

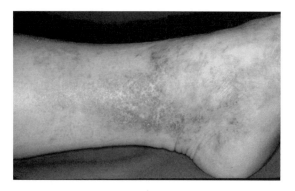

Figure 54.3 *White atropy.*

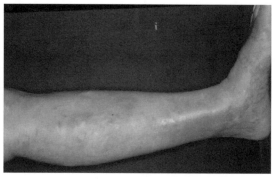

Figure 54.4 *Lipodermatosclerosis.*

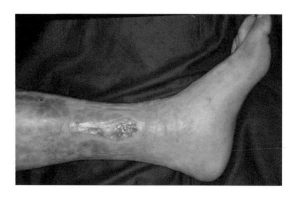

Figure 54.5 *Venous ulcer.*

Chronic venous insufficiency and age

The most important risk factor for venous disorders and also for chronic venous insufficiency is higher age. This has already been shown in different epidemiologic studies wordwide.[1,2,4] In the Bonn Vein Study the odds ratio for age as a risk factor increased to 15.5 (9.67–24.96) for varicose veins and up to 23.3 (12.26–44.24) for chronic venous insufficiency. Higher age is the most important risk factor for these diseases.

Skin changes such as pigmentation, dermatoliposclerosis, and venous ulcers increase severely with age (Table 54.2). As shown in the Bonn Vein Study, clinical stage C3 with edema starts to have a prevalence of more than 10% (12.9%) at the age of 40, increasing up to 25.6% in the 70–79 age group. Stage C4 shows a significant increase in prevalence, starting at the age of 50. Before this age, skin changes like eczema and white atropy are only present in less than 1% of the population. The prevalence rises from 3.4% in the 50–59-year-old population up to 8.5% in the 70–79 age range. Venous ulcers show an even later increase, from a prevalence less than 1% at ages below 60 years, increasing up to 2.4% in the 70–79 age range. The stages C4 to C6 show an equal distribution in prevalence between men and women.[7]

Table 54.2 *Prevalence of C of CEAP (mean, %) in the male and female population and in different age groups in the Bonn Vein Study[15]*

	C0		C1		C2		C3		C4		C5		C6		md		All
	n	%	n	%	n	%	n	%	n	%	n	%	n	%	n	%	n
Male	184	13.6	789	58.4	167	12.4	156	11.6	42	3.1	8	0.6	2	0.1	2	0.1	1350
Female	110	6.4	1025	59.5	272	15.8	256	14.9	46	2.7	11	0.6	1	0.1	1	0.1	1722
18–19	31	50.0	31	50.0		0.0		0.0		0.0		0.0		0.0		0.0	62
20–29	102	28.4	228	63.5	18	5.0	9	2.5	2	0.6		0.0		0.0		0.0	359
30–39	78	12.7	433	70.6	63	10.3	36	5.9	1	0.2	1	0.2	1	0.2		0.0	613
40–49	34	5.5	429	69.3	70	11.3	80	12.9	5	0.8	1	0.2		0.0		0.0	619
50–59	32	6.0	297	55.9	94	17.7	85	16.0	18	3.4	3	0.6	1	0.2	1	0.2	531
60–69	13	2.3	273	48.8	114	20.4	118	21.1	34	6.1	6	1.1		0.0	2	0.4	560
70–79	4	1.2	123	37.5	80	24.4	84	25.6	28	8.5	8	2.4	1	0.3		0.0	328
All	294	9.6	1814	59.0	439	14.3	412	13.4	88	2.9	19	0.6	3	0.1	3	0.1	3072

C of CEAP (max/participant)

md, missing data.
C0 to C6, clinical stages of the CEAP classification (as in Table 54.1).
Age range of males and females is 18–79 years.

Treatment

The majority of the population with CVD have varicose veins with a prevalence of 23% whereas a minority have post-thrombotic syndrome after deep venous thrombosis with a prevalence of 1.1%. The basic treatment of skin changes due to chronic venous insufficiency concerns physical measures like walking and leg elevation, and compression therapy with compression bandages or medical compression stockings.[10]

Radiofrequency treatment is a kind of endovenous procedure as is endovenous laser treatment.[11–16]

References

1. Beebe-Dimmer JL, Pfeifer J, Engle JS, Schottenfeld D. The epidemiology of chronic venous insufficiency and varicose veins. AEP 2005; 15: 175–84.
2. Carpentier PH, Maricq HR, Biro C, Poncot-Makinen CO, Franco A. Prevalence, risk factors and clinical patterns of chronic venous disorders of lower limbs: A population-based study in France. J Vasc Surg 2004; 40: 650–9.
3. Evans CJ, Fowkes FGR, Hajivassiliou CA, Harper DR, Ruckley C. Epidemiology of varicose veins – a review. Int Angiol 1994; 13: 263–70.
4. Jawien A, Grzela T, Ochwat A. Prevalence of chronic venous insufficiency in men and women in Poland: multicenter cross-sectional study in 40095 patients. Phlebology 2003; 18: 110–21.
5. Brand FN, Dannenberg AL, Abbott RD, Kannel WB. The epidemiology of varicose veins: the Framingham Study. Am J Prev Med 1988; 4: 96–101.
6. Eklof B, Rutherford RB, Bergan JJ et al. American Venous Forum International Ad Hoc Committee for Revision of the CEAP Classification. Revision of the CEAP classification for chronic venous disorders: consensus statement. J Vasc Surg 2004; 40: 1248–52.
7. Rabe E, Pannier-Fischer F, Bromen K et al. Bonner Venenstudie der Deutschen Gesellschaft für Phlebologie. Epidemiologische Untersuchung zur Frage der Häufigkeit und Ausprägung von chronischen Venenkrankheiten in der städtischen und ländlichen Wohnbevölkerung, Phlebologie 2003; 32(1): 1–14.
8. Allegra C, Antignani PL, Bergan JJ et al. The 'C' of CEAP: suggested definitions and refinements: an International Union of Phlebology conference of experts. J Vasc Surg 2003; 37: 129–31.
9. Molen van der HR. Über die chronische venöse Insuffizienz. Verhandlungen der Deutschen Gemeinschaft für Venenerkrankungen. Stuttgart: Schattauer, 1957: 41–57.
10. Kluess H, Noppeney T, Gerlach H et al. Leitlinie zur Diagnostik und Therapie des Krampfaderleidens. Phlebologie 2004; 32: 311–21.
11. Boné C. Tratamiento endoluminal de las varices con laser de Diodo. Estudio preliminary. Rev Patol Vasc 1999; 5: 35–46.
12. Lurie F, Creton D, Eklof B et al. Prospective randomised study of endovenous radiofrequency obliteration versus ligation and stripping in a selected patient population. Eur J Vasc Endovasc Surg 2005; 29: 67–73.
13. Min R, Zimmet S, Isaacs M, Forrestal M. Endovenous laser treatment of the incompetent greater saphenous vein. J Vasc Interv Radiol 2001; 12: 1167–71.
14. Noppeney T, Nüllem H. Gegenwärtiger Stand der operativen und endovaskulären Varizenchirurgie. Hautarzt 2006; 57: 33–9.
15. Pannier F, Rabe E. Endovenous laser therapy and radiofrequency ablation of saphenous varicose veins. J Cardiovasc Surg 2006; 47: 3–8.
16. Rabe E, Pannier-Fischer F, Gerlach H et al. Guidelines for sclerotherapy of varicose veins. Dermatol Surg 2004; 30: 687–93.

CHAPTER 55

Aging of hair

Ralph Trüeb and Rolf Hoffmann

Introduction

The appearance of hair plays an important role in people's overall physical appearance and self-perception. As early as can be traced in the history of human civilization, mankind has shown an interest to please by means of the natural ornament hair, given that its appearance is a feature of the body over which, unlike other hairy land mammals, we exert direct control. Hair length, color, and style play an important role in people's physical appearance and self-perception. We modify them according to how we wish to appear. The condition and style of hair play a role in how we discern the people we encounter, and how we are perceived by those we come upon. Our ancient preoccupation with hair is further heightened as our increasing life expectancy fuels our desire to preserve youthfulness. In today's world, physical appearance and the notion of looking young and energetic play a greater role than ever. Hair is not only intended to invoke male recognition of feminine appeal and desirability, but it has even become a predicate upon which social success and career opportunities are based. The hair care industry has become aware of this, and also more capable to deliver active products that are directed towards meeting this consumer demand. The discovery of pharmacologic targets and the development of safe and effective drugs also indicate strategies of the drug industry for maintenance of healthy and beautiful hair in the young and aged.

The different types of hair aging

Hair aging comprises weathering of the hair shaft, and aging of the hair follicle. The former involves progressive degeneration of the hair fiber from the tip to the root, while the latter manifests as a decrease in melanocyte function or graying, and a decrease in hair production in androgenetic and senescent alopecia. The scalp is also subject to intrinsic or physiologic aging, and extrinsic or premature aging due to external factors. Intrinsic factors are related to individual genetic and epigenetic mechanisms with interindividual variation. Prototypes are familial premature graying, and androgenetic alopecia. Extrinsic factors include ultraviolet radiation, air pollution, smoking, nutrition, and lifestyle. Experimental evidence supports the hypothesis that oxidative stress plays a major role in premature skin and probably also hair aging. It is the aim of this chapter to review the manifestations and management of aging hair.

Hair weathering

Weathering represents the wear and tear that mainly affects the free end of the growing hair fiber. Once the hair shaft leaves the skin and grows longer it undergoes some degree of degeneration depending on the extent of environmental and cosmetic damage. Since scalp hair has the longest hair growing phase, it is subject to more damage than hairs of other body sites. Given a hair growth rate of approximately 1 cm/month, the part of the hair fiber that is 12 cm from the scalp will reveal the accumulated physical and chemical trauma of one year of growth! In normal hair the damage is most prominent only near the tip of scalp hair, that often appears lusterless and paler than the more proximal growth, with varying degrees of split ends (trichoptilosis). The hair fiber with its normal surface structure of overlapping cuticular cells is potentially susceptible to friction damage from excessive combing and brushing, particularly when wet. Associated procedures may cause additional damage, in particular excessive heat 'blown' or from curling irons applied to the hair.

Chemical treatment of hair, i.e. bleaching, coloring, perming, and straightening, is a major cause of exaggerated hair weathering, since the cuticle becomes raised and softened in the course of these procedures, becoming more vulnerable to mechanical abrasion. Loss of cuticle leads to longitudinal fissures between exposed cortical cells, ultimately resulting in hair fractures at these sites.[1]

Abnormal hairs with inherent weakness are susceptible to excessive weathering. An example is pili annulati, a disorder characterized by air-filled spaces at regular intervals within the hair shaft. In these cases, hair fragility manifests itself after the onset of androgenetic alopecia, and trichorrhexis nodosa-like fracturing is exclusively limited to the androgenetic region. Thus, patients with androgenetic alopecia may be at special risk for developing the more severe weathering pattern. Besides minimizing chemical and physical trauma to the hair and special hair care measures (see below), specific and early treatment of androgenetic alopecia using appropriate systemic and/or topical therapy (see below) is of additional benefit for these patients.

Care of aging hair

While shampoos have been the most common form of cosmetic hair treatment, primarily aimed at cleansing the hair and scalp, today's consumer expects more options. With the cosmetic market being consumer driven, the industry has become aware of this, and at the same time capable to deliver active compounds towards meeting this consumer demand. The result are dermocosmetic agents that achieve cosmetic benefits by some degree of physiologic action. Current hair-care products are tailored to the variations associated with age, gender, hair quality, hair care habit, and specific problems related to the superficial condition of the scalp. Problems frequently associated with aging hair are hair thinning, dryness, and damage.

The mechanics of taking care of thin hair can be rewarding. The first thing to be recommended is to shampoo frequently, especially when hair is greasy. This will leave the hair fluffy and give the illusion of thicker hair. A parting in the hair should be avoided if possible, since it makes thin hair look more sparse. Individuals with thin hair should also avoid too-long hair styles, since the weight of the hair will drag it down. Permanent waves can make hair feel thicker and impart more body. Also, gray hair that has become thinner will feel thicker with hair color on it. Another technique is to get a hair cut that is layered. This technique cuts the hair on the top of the head shorter than the hair on the bottom.

Dry hair is hair which does not have enough moisture. It is difficult to style and has lost its shine. This is usually because the cuticle has become heavily weathered and porous, in damaged hair usually as a consequence of repeated cosmetic procedures. The hair cortex is exposed and cannot retain humidity. Treatment of dry and damaged hair consists of intensive conditioning. Conditioners protect the edges of the cuticle scales, although they cannot cure broken hairs where the cortex fibers have burst out (trichorrhexis and split ends). Hair-care products (conditioning shampoos, hair conditioners) designed for dry or damaged hair contain large molecules that collect on the edges of the damaged scales of the cuticle, helping to smooth over and fill in the fractures and fissures.[2] To dry hair they impart softness, easier grooming, and luster. To damaged hair they give back smoothness, gloss, and manageability. Cationic polymers, hydrolyzed proteins, and silicones, such as dimethicone, are useful in this process. In addition, panthenol is absorbed into the shaft and acts as a humefactant by providing moisture. Constant research to find new formulas is at the base of the progress achieved in the development of effective hair-care products. The recent identification of different amino acid profiles in normal and weathered hair, and the development of a system of amino acids lost from the hair shaft in the course of weathering and capable of being delivered from cosmetic formulations, is an example.[3]

Graying

Hair graying (canities) is a natural age-associated feature. The hair graying trait correlates closely with chronologic aging and occurs to varying degrees in all individuals. While the normal incidence of hair graying is 34 ± 9.6 years in Caucasians and 43.9 ± 10.3 years in Africans, it has been reported that, by 50 years of age, 50% of people have 50% gray hair. This graying incidence appears irrespective of sex and hair color. In men graying usually begins at the temples and in the sideburns. Gradually, the gray works its way back through the top, sides, and back of the hair. The rate at which an individual turns gray depends on genetics. It is not uncommon to observe kinships with marked early graying throughout. Hair is said to gray prematurely if it occurs before the age of 20 in Caucasians and before 30 in Africans. While premature canities more commonly appear without underlying pathology, presumably inherited in an autosomal dominant manner, it has also been associated with a similar cluster of autoimmune disorders as occurring in vitiligo (e.g. pernicious anemia, autoimmune thyroid disease) and several rare syndromes with premature aging (e.g. Werner's syndrome).

Although graying is understood as a loss of pigment in the shaft, its cellular and molecular origins are incompletely understood.[4] The color of hair mainly relies on the presence or absence of melanin pigment. Skin and hair melanins are formed in cytoplasmic organelles called melanosomes, produced by the melanocytes, and are the product of a complex biochemical pathway (melanogenesis) with tyrosinase being the rate-limiting enzyme. It has been shown that gray hair has undergone a marked reduction in melanogenically active melanocytes in the hair follicle.[5] The net effect of this reduction is that fewer melanosomes are incorporated into cortical keratinocytes of the hair shaft. In addition, there appears also to be a defect of melanosome transfer, as keratinocytes may not contain melanin despite their proximity to melanocytes with remaining melanosomes. This defect is further corroborated by the observation of melanin debris in and sometimes around the graying hair bulb. This anomaly is due to either defective melanosomal transfer to the cortical keratinocytes or melanin incontinence due to melanocyte degeneration. Eventually, no melanogenic melanocytes remain in the hair bulb. This decrease of melanin synthesis is associated with a decrease in tyrosinase activity, as indicated by a reduced DOPA reaction. Ultrastructural studies have shown that remaining melanocytes not only contain fewer melanosomes, but the residual melanosomes may be packaged within autophagolysosomes. This removal of melanosomes into autophagolysosomes suggests that they are defective, possibly with reactive melanin metabolites. This interpretation is supported by the observation that melanocytes in graying hair bulbs are frequently highly vacuolated, a common cellular response to increased oxidative stress. The extraordinary melanogenic activity of pigmented bulbar melanocytes, continuing for up to 10 years in some hair follicles, is likely to generate large amounts of reactive oxygen species via the hydroxylation of tyrosine and the oxidation of DOPA to melanin. If not adequately removed by an efficient antioxidant system, an accumulation of these reactive oxidative species will generate significant oxidative stress. It is possible that the antioxidant system becomes impaired with age, leading to damage to the melanocyte itself from its own melanogenesis-related oxidative stress. Since mutations occur at a higher rate in tissue exposed to high levels of oxidative stress, and these accumulate with age, the induction of replicative senescence with apoptosis is likely to be an important protective mechanism against cell transformation.

Possibilities for reversal of hair graying

Temporary hair darkening has been reported after ingestion of large doses of p-aminobenzoic acid or PABA. Sieve[6] gave 100 mg three times daily to 460 gray-haired individuals and noted a response in 82%. Darkening was obvious within 2–4 months of starting treatment. The hairs turned gray again

2–4 weeks after stopping therapy. Side-effects (gastrointestinal upset) at this high dosage of PABA limit its use. The mechanism of action has remained unclear.

In the absence of a natural way to reverse hair graying, hair colorants are the mainstay of covering lost hair color. Whether a person decides to color his hair depends on many factors. The first is whether the person is really too young to feel comfortable with premature gray hair; a second factor is whether the gray hair affects an individual's career opportunity; a third is cosmetics: gray hair may be unbecoming to a person's complexion, especially if he is pallid or sallow. There are several choices open to a person with gray hair:

- If hair is less than 10% gray, to pluck out the grays.
- To apply blond streaks to some of the hair, a procedure called highlightening.
- To color only the gray, especially in the beginning when the gray in men affects only the temples, or the perimeter in women.
- To color about half the hair by wrapping it with a lighter shade, producing a natural look.
- Finally, to color the entire head of hair, usually going two shades lighter than a person's natural color to prevent a harsh look.

The following major types of hair colors are currently used: temporary (textile dyes), natural coloring (henna), semipermanent (low molecular weight direct dyes), and permanent (aromatic amines). Temporary hair colorants consist of large complex organic structures that do not penetrate the cuticle. The colors are not intense but are capable of covering gray hair in a subtle way. This may be a good way for an individual to experiment with the coloring idea. The colorant washes out with the next shampoo. Henna, obtained form the plant *Lawsonia alba*, is a naturally occurring hair colorant. Its use dates back to ancient Egypt. Although the color can add red highlights to hair, occasionally on gray hair it may come out looking orange. Semipermanent colorants consist of small molecules that penetrate the cuticle. These compounds color gray hair very nicely, are easily applied in a lotion or foam at home, and last for six to ten shampoos. The most frequently used hair colorant is permanent hair dye. In permanent hair coloring the formation of colored molecules from their precursors occurs inside the hair fibers as a result of oxidation by hydrogen peroxide. The advantage of permanent color is that the color withstands normal hair washing. Because new growth comes out, the roots need to be touched up. Such products are used in a very gratifying manner and safely by millions of individuals worldwide. There have been studies that raised the possibility that long-term usage of permanent hair dyes (particularly black dyes) may be associated with an increased risk of developing certain cancers. However, taken together the evidence is insufficient to state with certainty whether there is a link between using hair dye and cancer. Nevertheless, it is recommended by Harvard Health Online[7] that those who use dark hair coloring and want to 'play safe' should try to use it as infrequently as possible, wear gloves when applying the dye, not leave it on the scalp any longer than necessary, and rinse the scalp thoroughly after using it. A small number of users may develop irritative and allergic contact reactions (commonly due to *p*-phenylenediamine) that may result in dermatitis and even hair loss.

Androgenetic alopecia

The clinical hallmark of androgenetic alopecia (AGA) in men is a patterned decrease in scalp hair density. As a rule AGA may start to develop with the onset of puberty in both men and women, although men tend to develop AGA earlier than females. AGA is distinct from the age-dependent thinning of scalp hair (senescent balding) that occurs in both sexes by the seventh or eighth decade of life. The first sign of AGA in men is usually a bitemporal recession, which can be seen in nearly all sexually mature Caucasian males, including those men not destined to develop further hair loss. However, balding of the vertex or diffuse thinning of hairs may also be seen. The prevalence of progressive AGA approaches 50% of Caucasian men beyond the age of 40, whereas in Asian, native American, and African-American men the prevalence is lower and AGA is less severe. All the hairs in an affected area may be involved in the miniaturization process and over the time the region may be covered with fine, hardly visible vellus hairs. Along with hair miniaturization the production of pigment ceases. There is still a controversy whether the total number of hair follicles decreases during AGA. However, it can be assumed that some hairs in AGA are definitely lost, but the majority of hair shafts are still present as tiny, barely visible vellus hairs.

Psychologic aspects of hair loss

The loss of hair is often trivialized, but hair loss may have profound effects on a patient´s well-being and quality of life.[8] Studies about the psychosocial impact on hair loss have shown that younger men are often concerned, at the onset of hair loss, about how they will look in the future, and virtually all men regard hair loss to be an unwanted, distressing experience that interferes with their body image. Physicians should therefore recognize that AGA goes well beyond the mere physical aspects of hair loss in the patient´s own perception. At times these symptoms may be exaggerated and it is essential to remember that a small but important minority of patients may have dysmorphophobia regarding their appearance.

Diagnosis and differential diagnosis

Only exceptionally are laboratory tests or scalp biopsies needed to confirm the diagnosis of AGA. The clinical assessment of AGA is largely a matter of common sense and practice. Therefore a thorough clinical examination and history is very important and will nearly always establish or exclude the diagnosis of AGA. In cases of doubt, histopathologic examination of scalp biopsies and some laboratory investigations are useful.

Pathogenesis

While the genetic involvement is pronounced but poorly understood and the changes within the androgen receptor have only recently been shown to be important for early-onset AGA in men, major advances have been achieved in understanding principal elements of the androgen metabolism involved in the pathogenesis of AGA.[9–11]

Androgen-dependent processes are predominantly due to the binding of dihydrotestosterone (DHT) to the androgen receptor (AR).

More than 60 years ago Hamilton observed that men who were castrated did not develop AGA.[12] Therefore it was concluded that the growth of hair follicles is in some areas androgen-dependent. At present it is unknown how androgens exert their paradoxic effect on the growth of hair follicles in different body sites, and which genes are involved. However, Hamilton had already shown that AGA can be triggered in castrated men by injecting testosterone. The androgen-dependent nature of AGA is furthermore demonstrated by the lack of frontal recession in androgen-insensitive men who lack functional androgen receptors and by the inducibility of AGA in the stump-tailed macaque by testosterone. DHT-dependent cell functions depend on the availability of weak androgens, their conversion to more potent androgens via the action of 5α-reductase, low enzymatic activity of androgen-inactivating enzymes, and functionally active ARs present in high numbers. The predisposed scalp exhibits high levels of DHT, and increased expression of the AR. Conversion of testosterone to DHT within the dermal papilla plays a central role, while androgen-regulated factors deriving from dermal papilla cells are believed to influence growth of other components of the hair follicle.

No or minimal beard growth or AGA is seen in pseudohermaphrodites who lack 5α-reductase, indicating that DHT, the 5α-reduced metabolite of testosterone, is the principal mediator of androgen-dependent hair loss. Interestingly, 5α-reduced metabolites of testosterone are increased in balding areas of the human scalp as well as in the scalp of the stump-tailed macaques. It is not yet clear whether DHT is derived from the local metabolism or from the circulation, but it can be assumed that under the influence of DHT hair loss is characterized by a shortening of the anagen phase and miniaturization of the hair follicle, which results in thinner and shorter hair.

Since many extrinsic hair growth-modulatory factors, such as androgens,[13] apparently operate at least in part via the dermal papilla, research is currently also focused on identifying androgen-regulated factors deriving from dermal papilla cells. Of the several factors that have been suggested to play a role in hair growth, so far only insulin-like growth factor (IGF-1) has been reported as altered in vitro by androgens,[14] and stem cell factor (SCF) has been found to be produced in higher amounts by androgen-dependent beard cells than in control non-balding scalp cells, presumably also in response to androgens.[15] Since SCF is the ligand for the cell surface receptor c-kit on melanocytes, this may also play a role in hair pigmentation. The limited success rate of treatment of AGA with hair growth promoters or modulators of androgen metabolism means that further pathogenic pathways may be taken into account.

The implication of microscopic follicular inflammation in the pathogenesis of AGA has emerged from several independent studies.[16,17] An early study referred to an inflammatory infiltrate of activated T-cells and macrophages in the upper third of the hair follicles, associated with an enlargement of the follicular dermal sheath composed of collagen bundles (perifollicular fibrosis), in regions of actively progressing alopecia. Horizontal section studies of scalp biopsies indicated that the perifollicular fibrosis is generally mild, consisting of loose, concentric layers of collagen that must be distinguished from cicatricial alopecia. The term 'microinflammation' has been proposed, because the process involves a slow, subtle, and indolent course, in contrast to the inflammatory and destructive process in the classical inflammatory scarring alopecias. An important question is how the inflammatory reaction pattern is generated around the individual hair follicle. Inflammation is regarded as a multistep process which may start from a primary event. The observation of a perifollicular infiltrate in the upper follicle near the infundibulum suggests that the primary causal event for the triggering of inflammation might occur near the infundibulum. On the basis of this localization and the microbial colonization of the follicular infundibulum with *Propionibacterium* sp., *Staphylococcus* sp., *Malassezia* sp., or other members of the transient flora, one could speculate that microbial toxins or antigens could be involved in the generation of the inflammatory response.

Alternatively, keratinocytes themselves may respond to chemical stress from irritants, pollutants, and UV irradiation, by producing radical oxygen species and nitric oxide, and by releasing intracellularly stored IL-1α. This pro-inflammatory cytokine by itself has been shown to inhibit the growth of isolated hair follicles in culture.[18] Moreover, adjacent keratinocytes, which express receptors for IL-1, start to engage the transcription of IL-1 responsive genes: mRNA coding for IL-1α, TNFα, and IL-1α, and for specific chemokine genes, such as IL-8, and monocyte chemoattractant protein-1 (MCP-1) and MCP-3, themselves mediators for the recruitment of neutrophils and macrophages, have been shown to be upregulated in the epithelial compartment of the human hair follicle. Besides, adjacent fibroblasts are also fully equipped to respond to such a pro-inflammatory signal. The upregulation of adhesion molecules for blood-borne cells in the capillary endothelia, together with the chemokine gradient, drive the transendothelial migration of inflammatory cells, which include neutrophils through the action of IL-8, T-cells, and Langerhans cells at least in part through the action of MCP-1. After processing of localized antigen, Langerhans cells, or alternatively keratinocytes, which may also have antigen-presenting capabilities, could then present antigen to newly infiltrating T lymphocytes and induce T-cell proliferation. The antigens are selectively destroyed by infiltrating macrophages, or natural killer cells. On the occasion that the causal agents persist, sustained inflammation is the result, together with connective tissue remodeling, where collagenases, such as matrix metalloproteinase (also transcriptionally driven by pro-inflammatory cytokines), play an active role. Collagenases are suspected to contribute to the tissue changes in perifollicular fibrosis. The significance of these findings has remained controversial. However, morphometric studies in patients with male pattern AGA treated with minoxidil showed that 55% of those with microinflammation had regrowth in response to treatment, in comparison to 77% in those patients without inflammation and fibrosis.

Treatment

The treatment of AGA is obscured by myths. Many products or procedures are advertized for the treatment of AGA, such as vitamins, trace elements, exotic herbs, amino acids, 'soft laser', scalp massage, etc. Most of these techniques or substances have never been verified in sound clinical trials. Because of the psychosocial impact of hair loss, it is important to explain the evaluation to the patient and to inform them on what they may expect in terms of continuing hair loss, and that response to any therapy may be slow and may include hair regrowth or only retardation of further thinning. A decision to have no treatment may be an appropriate option for certain patients. Nevertheless, patients with hair loss will often seek inappropriate or unproven therapies that are available in non-medical settings, that may be rather costly. This review will not list substances with doubtful efficacy but focus on proven medical treatment options. Surgical approaches or the detailed description of special wigs are beyond the scope of this review.

The aim of AGA treatment is to reverse or to stabilize the process of hair follicle miniaturization. This can be accomplished either by modifiers of the androgen signal transduction cascade or by other hair growth promoters. The first strategy tries to antagonize the androgen-induced processes within the hair follicles and is therefore a causative approach, whereas the latter strategy ignores the pathogenetic events leading to AGA.

Androgen receptor blockers (anti-androgens)

Anti-androgens are, in contrast to pure enzyme inhibitors, substances that prevent androgens from expressing their activity at target sites. They compete with DHT or testosterone for the specific AR, thus inhibiting androgen-mediated processes. AR blockers are used in the treatment of various diseases such as cancer of the prostate. Because AGA is an androgen-mediated process, AR blockers are a rational approach for treatment. For obvious reasons, however, this type of treatment is contraindicated in men.

Type 2 5α-reductase inhibitors

The first agent used for this purpose is finasteride, which is an orally active type 2 5α-reductase inhibitor. Clinical studies conducted to treat benign prostatic hyperplasia established the excellent safety profile of this drug. In theory, finasteride could be applied topically, but it should be noted that all lipophilic drugs will be absorbed. Dose-finding studies conducted to compare the efficacy of 5 mg versus 1 mg, 0.2 mg, and 0.01 mg finasteride to treat AGA in men indicated that 1 mg finasteride daily can be regarded as a safe and efficient approach for treatment. These preliminary data led to large-scale, phase III, placebo-controlled, cross-over designed clinical trials comprising 1879 men which showed that a 2-year trial of oral finasteride 1 mg/day promotes new hair growth in 66% (placebo 7%) and prevents further hair loss in 83% of patients.[19]

Finasteride 1 mg/day is well tolerated and is a 5α-reductase inhibitor which has in vivo a much higher affinity for the type 2 than the type 1 isoenzyme. In vitro, finasteride and testosterone appear to compete for the same binding site of 5α-reductase, but finasteride has no direct effect on the binding of testosterone or DHT to the androgen receptor. Even a single dose of 12.5 mg finasteride will lower systemic DHT levels by 56% for 72 hours. Hence it is understandable that finasteride 1 mg/day lowers DHT concentrations in the prostate and in the scalp. The serum DHT concentrations are lowered by approximately 68% with an associated slight increase in serum testosterone and estradiol levels, which is still within the normal range and is therefore clinically irrelevant. Finasteride does not influence the hypothalamic–pituitary–testicular axis, nor has it a significant effect on serum levels of prolactin, sex hormone-binding globulin, aldosterone, or cortisol.

Young rats fed with 20 to 80 mg/kg per day of finasteride first showed mild to moderate decreases in fertility after 12 weeks of treatment, whereas mature males (given only 80 mg/kg per day) did not show a similar decrease during 24 weeks of treatment. Finasteride in a dosage of 1 mg/day for men was not associated with any changes in sperm motility, morphology, or total sperm number. As a result of a diminished function of seminal glands the total volume of the ejaculate was slighly reduced but still within the normal range. Neither serum lipid levels nor bone metabolism are affected by finasteride. Finasteride 1 mg/day does, however, reduce slightly the mean prostate volume and PSA levels. Serum PSA levels higher than 40 ng/ml are suggestive of a cancer of the prostate and men harboring an unrecognized prostate cancer may, by taking 1 mg/day finasteride, lower their PSA levels, thus disguising their cancer in the serum test. Therefore, some authors suggest that in older men PSA levels should be monitored before finasteride is taken. Finasteride has no or only little effect on body hair; 7.7% of finasteride versus 7% of placebo recipients reported mild to moderate treatment-related adverse events (1.4% and 1.6%, respectively, withdrew). This difference was not statistically significant. The events reported more frequently on finasteride as compared to placebo treatment were decreased libido (1.8% vs 1.3%), ejaculation disturbances (1.2% vs 0.7%), and erectile dysfunction (1.3% vs 0.7%). These differences were slightly statistically significant but it should be noted that these effects resolved in most men still on drug therapy, and in all men who discontinued the treatment because of the adverse events.

Minoxidil

Minoxidil is a drug commonly leading to hypertrichosis in approximately 70% of patients treated systemically. This is apparent after a few weeks of systemic treatment and the hair will fall out 2 months after discontinuation of the drug. At present minoxidil is the only drug out of the list of drugs inducing hair that has been used topically to induce hair growth in AGA, and it was the first drug to be approved for the indication of AGA in both men and women. Minoxidil is a pyrimidine derivative (2,4-diamono-6-piperidinopyrimidine-3-oxide) initially developed as a potent antihypertensive agent. In addition to being a direct-acting vasodilator, it was unexpectedly found to stimulate hair growth in vivo, and this side effect led to its clinical use in AGA. It is so far unclear why minoxidil induces hair growth. It stimulates a time-dependent increase in 3[H]-thymidine and 35[S]-cysteine incorporation in mouse vibrissa follicles and it has been suggested that this effect is mediated via the K^+

channels and that a sulfated metabolite of M exerts this effect via M-sulfotransferase, which is present in hair follicles. One study showed that cutaneous blood flow increased after application of minoxidil, although a causal relationship has not been proven. Minoxidil has been shown to prolong anagen hair growth in vitro and some authors have considered that it may act via the inhibition of lysine hydroxylase, or via prostaglandin synthase-1.

Clinical trials of topical 2% and 5% minoxidil in male and female hair loss have all shown remarkably rapid increase in hair growth, measured by hair counts or hair weight.[20-26] The increase is evident within 6–8 weeks of treatment and has generally peaked by 12–16 weeks. However, topical minoxidil has not been studied in the specific perspective of aging and senescent alopecia. In a recent analysis of clinical trial data in 636 males a therapeutic benefit of topical 2 and 5% minoxidil solution was compared to age, duration of balding, and diameter of balding vertex area in males.[27] Age was found to be the denominator for predicting treatment success. The younger subjects experienced better efficacy than the older subjects, although clear treatment effects were noted also in the older age group. There was also an inverse relationship between effect and duration of balding. Males with duration of balding < 5 years showed a significantly better effect than those with duration of balding > 21 years. The diameter of vertex balding in men showed an inverse relationship with efficacy of minoxidil. Males with < 5 cm diameter vertex balding area showed a better effect of treatment than subjects with diameters > 15 cm. Finally, duration of hair loss less than 1 year compared to more than 10 years at onset of treatment resulted in a significantly more effective treatment with respect to stabilization of alopecia and new hair growth.

In sum, the treatment of AGA with minoxidil is able to induce some hair regrowth in a considerable number of patients. The exact rate of success is, however, controversial. Minoxidil treatment can be regarded as a safe therapy with side-effects restricted to local irritation and a rather low incidence of allergic contact dermatitis. Minoxidil must be used for life, because after discontinuation all regrown hair will be lost.

Autologous hair transplantation

Beside pharmacologic treatments, surgical procedures are becoming more and more popular. Ever since the invention of autologous hair transplantation, the transplants have become smaller and smaller to the stage that single hairs or follicular units are presently grafted. This delicate procedure produces very good clinical results, provided a talented hair surgeon undertakes the operation and a well-trained team cut the scalp tissues in a precise manner.

Senescent alopecia

Senile involutional or senescent alopecia has been defined as non-androgen-dependent hair thinning found in those over 50 years of age. Much like AGA, it involves a progressive decrease in the number of anagen follicles and hair diameter. It frequently occurs together with AGA, further complicating its delineation from the latter. Some authors have proposed that senescent alopecia may result from cumulative physiologic degeneration of selected hair follicles. In healthy murine skin they described clusters of perifollicular macrophages as perhaps indicating the existence of a physiologic program of immunologically controlled hair follicle degeneration by which malfunctioning follicles are removed by programmed organ deletion.[28] On the other hand, in his original description, Kligman proposed a pronounced inflammatory component in AGA (see above), but not in senescent alopecia. Moreover, Price et al[29] did not identify any 'drop-out' of follicles in senescent alopecia upon staining biopsies for elastin, whereas there was less 5α-reductase enzyme activity in comparison to AGA. Nevertheless, some forms of primary fibrosing alopecia may represent pathologic exaggeration of immune-mediated, programmed organ deletion, resulting in a follicular lichenoid reaction pattern, specifically postmenopausal frontal fibrosing alopecia,[30] and fibrosing alopecia in a pattern distribution.[31]

In their study on aging and hair cycles over an exceptionally long duration of 8 to 14 years, Courtois et al[32] found a reduction in the duration of hair growth and in the diameter of hair shafts, and a prolongation of the interval separating the loss of a hair in telogen and the emergence of a replacement hair in anagen (latency phase). These phenomena resembled those observed in the course of AGA, although their development was less marked, suggesting AGA is a premature aging phenomenon. This aging process was evidenced by a reduction in the number of hairs per unit area and a deterioration in the quality of scalp hair. The reduction in density was manifested to different degrees in different individuals. It amounted to less than 10% in 10 years in the individuals with the least alopecia, and was much more pronounced in the balding subjects. The maximal length of hair diminished as the subjects aged, and in parallel the hairs became finer. However, among non-balding subjects there was a tendency for the proportion of thicker hairs to increase. Finally, aging did not appear to follow a perfectly regular course over time. Periods of stability, or even partial remission, alternated with periods of more marked evolution, reflecting perhaps the influence of individual factors such as the subject's general health, lifestyle, and risk factors for accelerated aging.

Role of smoking and ultraviolet radiation

Besides being the single most preventable cause of significant morbidity and an important cause of death in the general population, tobacco smoking has been associated with adverse effects on the skin. Smoke-induced premature skin aging has attracted the attention of the medical community, while only recently an observational study indicated a relationship between smoking, graying of hair, and alopecia.[33] The mechanisms by which smoking causes hair loss are multifactorial, and probably related to effects of cigarette smoke on the microvasculature of the dermal hair papilla, smoke genotoxicants causing damage to DNA of the hair follicle, a smoke-induced imbalance in the follicular protease/antiprotease systems controlling tissue remodeling during the hair growth cycle, pro-oxidant effects of smoking leading to the release of pro-inflammatory cytokines resulting in follicular microinflammation and perifollicular fibrosis, and finally increased hydroxylation of estradiol creating a relative hypoestrogenic state. The fact that cigarette smoke-associated hair loss is of the androgenetic type again indicates that genetic factors contribute. Of course, variances between individuals also may result from patterns of conduct, in as much as persons exposed to one risk factor (smoking) are often exposed to others as well, such as intake of androgens and their precursors (such as DHEA in anti-aging protocols!), excessive ultraviolet exposure (see below), and stress, all of which have been implicated in one way or another in the pathogenesis of alopecia.

In view of the psychologic effects of hair loss on affected men, increasing public awareness of the association between smoking and alopecia offers an opportunity for health education against smoking, that may be more effective than the link between smoking and facial wrinkles or gray hair, since the latter can be effectively counteracted by current aesthetic dermatologic procedures, while treatment options for AGA have their limitations.

Progressive thinning of scalp hair in AGA results in a gradual decline in the natural protection of the scalp from ultraviolet radiation (UVR). While the consequences of sustained UVR on the unprotected scalp are obvious and well appreciated, specifically photocarcinogenesis and solar elastosis, the effects of UVR on hair loss have been widely ignored. However, clinical observations and theoretic considerations suggest that UVR may have negative effects:[34] acute telogen effluvium from UVR has been described,[35] and the production of porphyrins by *Propionibacterium* sp. in the pilosebaceous duct, with photoactivation of porphyrins[36] leading to oxidative tissue injury, may contribute to follicular microinflammation operative at the level of the follicular stem cells. Histopathologically elastosis is regularly found in scalp biopsies, especially in alopecic conditions. A recent study demonstrated a relationship between the degree of scalp elastosis and severity of AGA:[37] the scalp dermis was significantly thicker in AGA than in unaffected control subjects. The difference was due to more severe elastosis in baldness. The earliest signs of solar elastosis preceded hair thinning. When elastosis was thicker than 0.2 mm, a negative exponential correlation was found between the hair diameter and severity of solar elastosis.

As a consequence of increased leisure time with a growing popularity of outdoor activities and holidays in the sun, awareness of sun protection has become imperative. Topically applied chemicals that act as sun protectors are widely utilized and offer the most convenient means of protecting the glabrous skin against acute (sunburn) and chronic pathologic effects of UVR. Out of cosmetic reasons their use on the hair-bearing scalp is problematic, unless complete baldness is present. Although hats provide the best protection of the scalp from UVR, not all patients find it convenient or acceptable for this purpose. While protection of the hair against photodamage has been extensively studied, there are no data on photoprotection of the hair-bearing scalp. It has been found that hair dyes may protect hair against photodamage.[38] Cinnamidpropyltrimonium chloride, a quaternized UV absorber, delivered from a shampoo system, has been reported to be suitable for photoprotection of hair, while simultaneously providing an additional conditioning;[39] and solid lipid nanoparticles have been developed as novel carriers of UV blockers for use on skin and hair, while offering photoprotection on their own by reflecting and scattering UVR.[40]

Finally, systemic photoprotection has been the focus of more recent investigation, in as much as this would overcome some of the problems associated with the topical use of sunscreens. Preclinical studies have illustrated the photoprotective properties of supplemented antioxidants, particularly beta-carotene (provitamin A), alphatocopherol (vitamin E), and L-ascorbate (vitamin C). However, clinical evidence that these prevent, retard, or slow down solar skin damage is impending. The same applies to topical melatonin, which has been found to suppress UV-induced erythema and UV-induced reactive oxygen species in a dose-dependent manner.[41] Nevertheless, these results suggest the probable utility of combining these compounds with known sunscreens to maximize photoprotection.

Development of topical anti-aging compounds

Recent advances in the care of aging hair and scalp are topical anti-aging compounds. Due to water dilution and short contact time, neither topical hair growth stimulants nor anti-aging compound have any significant effect in shampoos. Antioxidants in shampoos, such as vitamins C and E, protect fatty substances in the shampoo from oxidation, and not the scalp. The rationale for the development of topical hair growth stimulants in the form of leave-on products is: effect on androgen metabolism (e.g. inhibition of 5α-reductase), effect on sebum production and microbial flora,[42] effect on microinflammation and fibrosis, and effect on vascularization and VEGF (e.g. minoxidil). Topical anti-aging compounds of current interest are green tea polyphenols, selenium, copper, phytoestrogens, melatonin, and as yet unidentified substances from Traditional Chinese Medicine and Ayurveda.

Future directions

There is an increasing interest in the hair follicular route for delivery of active compounds affecting the hair. Current research activities focus on using topical liposome targeting to selectively introduce melanins, genes, and proteins into hair follicles for therapeutic and cosmetic modification of the hair.[43] For example, selective delivery of topical liposomes to hair follicles has demonstrated the ability to color hair with melanin. Another line of research in the quest of new treatments for hair loss is tissue engineering cells of hair follicular origin with inductive properties.[44] Keeping in mind that thus far all medical treatments have only had limited success rates and that autologous hair transplants are time-consuming and costly, the use of adult hair follicle stem cells will be a future goal to treat androgenetic or senile balding.[45] By this approach hair follicle specific stem cells are isolated, grown in vitro, and injected into the scalp. This procedure works well in animal models and the future will show whether this becomes a treatment option for human hair loss.

References

1. Dawber R. Hair: its structure and response to cosmetic preparations. Clin Dermatol 1996; 14: 105–12.
2. Bouillon C. Shampoos. Clin Dermatol 1996; 14: 113–21.
3. Gummer CH, Schiel S. Amino acids – a potential solution for cosmetic hair problems. JDDG 2004; 2: 502.
4. Tobin DJ, Paus R. Graying: gerontobiology of the hair follicle pigmentary unit. Exp Gerontol 2001; 36: 29–54.
5. Commo S, Gaillard O, Bernard BA. Human hair greying is linked to a specific depletion of hair follicle melanocytes affecting both the bulb and the outer root sheath. Br J Dermatol 2004; 150; 435–43.
6. Sieve B. Darkening of gray hair following para-aminobenzoic acid. Science 1941; 94: 257–8.
7. Harvard Health Online. www.health.harvard.edn/medline/women/w801f.html.
8. Cash TF, Price VH, Savin RC. Psychological effects of androgenetic alopecia on women: comparisons with balding men and with female control subjects. J Am Acad Dermatol 1993; 29: 568–75.
9. Kaufman KD. Androgen metabolism as it affects hair growth in androgenetic alopecia. Dermatol Clin 1996; 14: 697–711.
10. Hoffmann R, Happle R. Current understanding of androgenetic alopecia I. Eur J Dermatol 2000; 10: 319–26.
11. Hoffmann R, Happle R. Current understanding of androgenetic alopecia II. Eur J Dermatol 2000; 10: 410–17.
12. Hamilton JB. Male hormone stimulation as a prerequisite and an incitement in common baldness. Am J Anat 1942; 71: 451–3.
13. Randall VA, Thornton MH, Messenger AG. Cultured dermal papilla cells from androgen-dependent human hair follicles (e.g. beard) contain more androgen receptors than those from non-balding areas of the scalp. J Endocrinol 1992; 133: 141–7.
14. Itami S, Kurata S, Takayasu S. Androgen induction of follicular epithelial cell growth mediated via insulin-like growth factor I from dermal papilla cells. Biochem Biophys Res Commun 1995; 221: 988–94.
15. Hibberts NA, Messenger AG, Randall VA. Dermal papilla cells derived from beard hair follicles secrete more stem cell factor (SCF) in culture than scalp cells or dermal fibroblasts. Biochem Biophys Res Commun 1996; 222: 401–5.
16. Mahé YF, Michelet JF, Billoni N et al. Androgenetic alopecia and microinflammation. Int J Dermatol 2000; 39: 576–84.
17. Whiting DA, Waldstreicher J, Sanchez M, Kaufman KD. Measuring reversal of hair miniaturization in androgenetic alopecia by follicular counts in horizontal sections of serial scalp biopsies: results of finasteride 1 mg treatment of men and postmenopausal women. J Invest Dermatol Symp Proc 1999; 4: 282–4.
18. Philpott MP, Sander DA, Bowen J, Kealey T. Effects of interleukins, colony stimulating factor and tumour necrosis factor on human hair follicle growth in vitro: a possible role for interleukin-1 and tumour necrosis factor-α in alopecia areata. Br J Dermatol 1996; 135: 942–8.

709

19. Kaufman KD, Olsen EA, Whiting D et al. Finasteride in the treatment of men with androgenetic alopecia. Finasteride Male Pattern Hair Loss Study Group. J Am Acad Dermatol 1998; 39: 578–89.

20. De Villez RL, Jacobs JP, Szpunar CA, Warner ML. Androgenetic alopecia in the female. Treatment with 2% topical minoxidil solution. Arch Dermatol 1994; 3: 303–7.

21. Lucky AW, Piacquadio DJ, Ditre CM et al. A randomized, placebo-controlled trial of 5% and 2% topical minoxidil solutions in the treatment of female pattern hair loss. J Am Acad Dermatol 2004; 50: 541–53.

22. Olsen EA, DeLong ER, Weiner MS. Long-term follow-up of men with male pattern baldness treated with topical minoxidil. J Am Acad Dermatol 1987; 16: 688–95.

23. Olsen EA, Dunlap FE, Funicella T et al. A randomized clinical trial of 5% topical minoxidil versus 2% topical minoxidil and placebo in the treatment of androgenetic alopecia in men. J Am Acad Dermatol 2002; 47: 377–85.

24. Olsen EA, Weiner MS, Delong ER et al. Topical minoxidil in early male pattern baldness. J Am Acad Dermatol 1985; 13: 185–92.

25. Olsen EA, Weiner MS, Amara IA, DeLong ER. Five-year follow-up of men with androgenetic alopecia treated with topical minoxidil. J Am Acad Dermatol 1990; 3–646.

26. Price VH, Menefee E. Quantitative estimation of hair growth I. Androgenetic alopecia in women: effect of minoxidil. J Invest Dermatol 1990; 95: 683–7.

27. Rundegren J. Pattern alopecia: what clinical features determine the response to topical minoxidil treatment? JDDG 2004; 2: 500.

28. Eichmüller S, van der Veen C, Mill I et al. Clusters of perifollicular macrophages in normal murine skin: physiological degeneration of selected hair follicles by programmed organ deletion. J Histochem Cytochem 1998; 46: 361–70.

29. Price V, Sawaya M, Headington J, Kibarian M. Histology and hormonal activity in senescent thinning in males (abstract 266). J Invest Dermatol 2001; 117: 434.

30. Kossard S. Postmenopausal frontal fibrosing alopecia. Arch Dermatol 1994; 130: 770–4.

31. Zinkernagel MS, Trüeb RM. Fibrosing alopecia in a pattern distribution. Patterned lichen planopilaris or androgenetic alopecia with a lichenoid tissue reaction pattern? Arch Dermatol 2000; 136: 205–11.

32. Courtois M, Loussouarn G, Hourseau C, Grollier JF. Ageing and hair cycles. Br J Dermatol 1995; 132: 86–93.

33. Mosley JG, Gibbs CC. Premature grey hair and hair loss among smokers: a new opportunity for health education? BMJ 1996; 313: 1616.

34. Trüeb RM. Association between smoking and hair loss: another opportunity for health education against smoking? Dermatology 2003; 206: 189–91.

35. Camacho F, Moreno JC, Garcia-Hernández. Telogen alopecia from UV rays. Arch Dermatol 1996; 132: 1398–9.

36. Johnsson A, Kjeldstad B, Melo TB. Fluorescence from pilosebaceous follicles. Arch Dermatol Res 1987; 279: 190–3.

37. Piérard-Franchimont C, Uhoda I, Saint-Léger D, Piérard GE. Androgenetic alopecia and stress-induced premature senescence by cumulative ultraviolet light exposure. Exog Dermatol 2001; 1: 203–6.

38. Pande CM, Albrecht L, Yang B. Hair photoprotection by dyes. J Cosmet Sci 2001; 52: 377–89.

39. Gao T, Bedell A. Ultraviolet damage on natural gray hair and ist photoprotection. J Cosmet Sci 2001; 52: 103–18.

40. Wissing SA, Muller RH. Solid lipid nanoparticles (SLN) – a novel carrier for UV blockers. Pharmazie 2001; 56: 783–6.

41. Bangha E, Elsner P, Kistler GS. Suppression of UV-induced erythema by topical treatment with melatonin (N-acetyl-5-methoxytryptamine). Arch Dermatol Res 1996; 288: 522–6.

42. Piérard GE, Piérard-Franchimont C, Nikkels-Tassoudji N et al. Improvement in the inflammatory aspect of androgenetic alopecia. A pilot study with an antimicrobial lotion. J Dermatol Treat 1996; 7: 153–7.

43. Hoffman RM. Topical liposome targeting of dyes, melanins, genes, and proteins electively to hair follicles. J Drug Target 1998; 5: 67–74.

44. Reynolds AJ, Lawrence C, Cserhalmi-Friedman PB, Christiano AM, Jahoda CAB. Trans-gender induction of hair follicles. Human follicle cells can be induced to grow in an incompatible host of the other sex. Nature 1999; 402: 33–4.

45. McElwee KJM, Wenzel E, Kissling S, Huth A, Hoffmann R. Cultured peribulbar dermal sheath cells can induce hair follicle development and contribute to the dermal sheath and dermal papilla. J Invest Dermatol 2003; 121(6): 1267–75.

Epilogue

Hormone treatments and preventative strategies in aging men: whom to treat, when to treat, and how to treat

Louis JG Gooren, Alvaro Morales, and Bruno Lunenfeld

Introduction

The field of hormonal alterations in the aging male has attracted the interest of the medical community and the public at large. The potential role of hormone replacement in the aging male is still a matter of debate and it will take many more years before hormone replacement therapy (HRT) will find its proper definitive place. It requires large-scale long-term studies, which are difficult to fund and execute but are in the planning stage. Apart from that, the attitude towards hormone replacement in the elderly has changed following the publication of the outcome of HRT in postmenopausal women of the Women's Health Initiative study, which found an excess of breast cancer and cardiovascular disease in the treatment group versus placebo.[1] Even though many methodologic questions still await answers, the approach to postmenopausal HRT has become more critical.[2] The approach to HRT in aging men has always been more cautionary than to HRT in women, and the outcome of the Women's Health Initiative study has added to this.[1,3] It is further recognized that the endocrinologic changes associated with aging, in both men and women, are not limited to sex hormones alone. Indeed, profound changes occur in other hormones such as growth hormone, dehydroepiandrosterone (DHEA), melatonin, while insulin levels tend to rise with aging. Plasma cortisol levels do not fall but the ratio of the catabolic corticosteroids to the anabolic androgens increases, with potentially deleterious effects. In patients receiving glucocorticoid treatment, simultaneous administration of testosterone appeared to ameliorate the catabolic effects of glucocorticoids on bone and muscle.[4]

The controversy over whether men show a decline in testosterone (T) levels with aging has been resolved. Several methodologically sound longitudinal studies in healthy men have shown that T, but particularly free or bioavailable levels of T, do decline with aging, though there is considerable interindividual variation and certainly not all aged men become hypogonadal. (For a review see reference 5.)

It is increasingly realized that androgens have a large number of non-reproductive effects; they are important anabolic factors in the maintenance of muscle mass and bone mass, glucose and lipid metabolism as constituents of the metabolic syndrome, and also in non-sexual psychologic functioning. The latter actions are important constituents of well-being in old age.

There is now growing consensus on the terminology of the age-related decline in testosterone. The suggestion of a male menopause was promptly dismissed by most scientists. Andropause might be a more acceptable term to describe the process of age-related changes in men, but as a term it is not very clear what it stands for. (Partial) androgen deficiency of the aging male has for a long time dominated the terminology, but has now been replaced by late onset hypogonadism.[6,7]

A small proportion of secreted androgens in the male are aromatized to estrogenic hormones. There are recent insights that these estrogens fulfill a significant role in the male body with regard to the state of the bones, the cardiovascular system, and the brain. Not only androgen production declines with aging, but also the secretion of growth hormone and adrenal androgens diminishes. The biologic actions of androgens and growth hormone are largely intertwined. Some anabolic effects of androgens have growth hormone-related factors as intermediaries.

Strategies have to be devised to allow the aging male to get the benefits from new medical insights into the aging process.[8,9] The track record of medical care for the aging male has been a poor one.[10] Up to the present day there is a considerable misuse of hormonal preparations in the medical care of aging men. The following contribution will address a number of pertinent issues in this area.[11,12] Only on the basis of sound scientific data will a consensus be reached on these controversial issues.

Quantitative aspects of the decline of androgen levels in aging

Several studies document that androgen levels decline with aging (for a review see reference 5). Longitudinal studies have documented a statistical decline of plasma testosterone by approximately 30% in healthy men between the ages of 25 and 75 years.[5] Since plasma levels of sex hormone-binding globulin (SHBG) increase with aging, plasma testosterone not bound to SHBG decreases even more – by about 50% – over that period.[5] Studies in twins have shown that genetic factors account for 63% of the variability in plasma T levels, and for 30% of the variability in SHBG levels.[13] In addition, systemic diseases, increasing with age, are a cause of declining plasma levels of T.[5] While it now has been shown, beyond doubt, that plasma T, and in particular bioavailable and FT, declines with aging, it remains uncertain what percentage of men actually becomes T deficient with aging in the sense that they will suffer the clinical consequences of T deficiency. Stringent criteria to diagnose T deficiency have not been formulated, either in the young or in the elderly male population. In a study of 300 healthy men between the ages of 20 and 100 years, Vermeulen,[14] defining the reference range of total T to be between 11 and 40 nmol/l, found one man with subnormal T in the age group between 20 and 40 years, but more than 20% above the age of 60 years, while 15% of men above the age of 80 years still had T values above 20 nmol/l. The implication is that only a certain proportion of men has lower than normal T values in old age. It is a group that is difficult to identify since symptoms of aging mimic symptoms of T deficiency.[6,7]

It has not become clear whether, for aging men, other criteria for T deficiency should be established than for younger men. Testosterone has a number of physiologic functions in the male. In adulthood it is responsible for maintenance of reproductive capacity and of secondary sex characteristics, it has positive effects on mood and libido, anabolic effects on bone and muscle, and it affects fat distribution and the cardiovascular system. Threshold plasma values of T for each of these functions are becoming established, but it remains uncertain whether these threshold values change over the life-cycle. Theoretically, it is possible that in old age androgen levels suffice for some but not for all androgen-related functions. Male sexual functioning in adulthood, for instance, can be maintained with lower than normal values,[15,16] especially in the younger adult. However, there are indications that the threshold required for behavioral effects of T increases with aging.[17] Bhasin et al[18] analyzed the dose–response relationships between plasma T and biologic effects, and showed that low to mid normal plasma levels of T suffice for most of its biologic actions. An exception is between plasma T and muscle mass, which shows a linear relationship.[18]

For androgen deficiency it is difficult to rely on clinical symptoms, particularly in elderly men. In adult persons who have previously been eugonadal, symptoms of T deficiency emerge only gradually. So, only the effects of long-standing T deficiency will be clinically recognized.

The laboratory reference values of T and FT show a wider range than those for most other hormones (for instance thyroid hormones), which makes it difficult to establish whether measured values of T in patients are normal or abnormal. Is a patient whose plasma levels of T fall from the upper to the lower range of normal (a drop of as much as 50%) T deficient? Levels may well remain within the reference range but may be inappropriate for that particular individual. In thyroid pathophysiology plasma TSH proves to be a better criterion of thyroid hyper/hypofunction than plasma T4 or T3, but it is uncertain whether plasma LH is a reliable indicator of hypogonadism in the elderly man.[5-7] With aging there are reductions in LH pulse frequency and amplitude. Several studies have found that LH levels are elevated in response to the decline of T levels with aging, but less so than is observed in younger men with similarly decreased T levels.[5] This may be due to a shift in the setpoint of the negative feedback of T on the hypothalamic/pituitary unit resulting in an enhanced negative feedback action, which consequently leads to a relatively lower LH output. Alternatively, it may be that the aging hypothalamus and pituitary fail to respond adequately to the feedback mechanisms.

Another variable that might be significant to assess the androgen status in old age is plasma levels of SHBG. Its levels increase even with healthy aging, possibly due to a decrease in growth hormone production and an increase in the ratio of free estradiol over FT.[5]

There are still a number of questions to be answered. Can reliable criteria of androgen deficiency in old age be formulated? Are there unequivocal laboratory criteria, such as levels of total and non-bound T, SHBG, and maybe LH? If yes, do we know threshold values for the diverse biologic actions of T, more specifically in elderly men? (For a review see reference 5.) On top of these questions there is the problem that measurements of serum T vary considerable from one laboratory to the other.[19-21]

Target tissues of androgens in aging men

While it can be shown statistically that plasma T levels drop with aging, the actual decrease is often only moderate and does not affect all men to the same degree. Set against the characteristics of aging reminiscent of androgen deficiency, such as loss of muscle and bone mass, deterioration of sexual functioning and vitality, plasma levels of androgens are often not correspondingly low. It must be remembered that the plasma level of a hormone merely provides information on the strength of the signal and not about receptor and postreceptor events, in other words how this hormonal signal will be translated into biologic action. It could be hypothesized that aging is associated with a decrease in androgen action through changes in receptor properties and/or postreceptor events, while plasma androgen levels remain rather normal or decline only marginally. A significant decrease in both T and dihydrotestosterone (DHT) concentrations has been found in different tissues with aging,[22] which may support this assumption. Aging might result in a reduction in androgen effect through a loss of sensitivity of target tissues to T via, for instance, alterations in receptor number or affinity, or in postreceptor mechanisms. The androgen receptor number and affinity are decreased in many organs of the aging rat.[23] In human pathophysiology a certain parallel might be drawn with X-linked spinal and bulbar muscular atrophy (Kennedy's disease), which is an abnormality of the androgen receptor. This genetic error of the androgen receptor manifests itself usually not earlier than the age of 20–40 years, but sometimes as late as 60. Patients frequently also show glucose intolerance or diabetes mellitus. The number of CAG triplets coding for glutamines in the androgen receptor, normally from 11–33, is approximately doubled in patients suffering from this condition.[24] That properties of the androgen receptor may be involved in the age-related decline of plasma androgen levels was recently documented. It could be demonstrated that the CAG repeat length was significantly associated with plasma T, albumin-bound T, and FT, when controlled for age, baseline hormone levels, and anthropometrics.

Follow-up levels of androgen measurements were inversely correlated with the number of CAG repeats.[25] In another study, certain types of age-related changes in aging men were associated with the length of the androgen receptor gene CAG repeat, suggesting that this parameter may play a role in setting different thresholds for the array of androgen actions in the male.[26]

If target organ sensitivity to androgens were to diminish with age, this would limit the potential benefit which androgen supplementation in aging men could have. Whether higher than normal dosages of androgens would be effective, as is the case in partial androgen sensitivity,[27] remains to be investigated.

The questions remain: Do plasma levels of androgens reliably reflect a subject's androgenic status, particularly in old age? Is there an impairment of the accumulation of androgens in target tissues or of the transcription of androgen action? Do the threshold levels for androgen to exert biologic effects change with aging?

A pragmatic approach to the issue of androgen deficiency in elderly men

The above has outlined the many unresolved questions as to the verification of deficiencies in the biologic action of androgens in old age and what plasma T levels conclusively represent androgen deficiency. Consequently, a pragmatic approach to this issue must be taken in order to let aging androgen-deficient men benefit from replacement therapy while these questions are resolved by clinical data. The question has received serious attention in the past years.[28,29] Vermeulen[30] argues that there is no generally accepted cut-off value of plasma T for defining androgen deficiency, and in the absence of convincing evidence for an altered androgen requirement in elderly men, he considers the normal range of FT levels in young males to be also valid for elderly men. In his healthy male, non-obese, population aged 20–40 years ($n = 150$), the mean of log transformed early morning T levels was 21.8 nmol/l (627 ng/dl); the mean minus 2 SD was 12.5 nmol/l (365 ng/dl) and the mean minus 2.5 SD

was 11 nmol/l (319 ng/dl). For FT, measured by equilibrium dialysis or calculated from T and SHBG levels,[14] the mean was 0.5 nmol/l (14 ng/dl), minus 2 SD 0.26 nmol/l (7.4 ng/dl), and minus 2.5 SD 0.225 nmol/l or 6.5 ng/dl. If one takes as the lower normal limit and threshold of partial androgen deficiency a conservative value of 11 nmol/l for T and 0.225 nmol/l for FT, which represent the lower 1% values for healthy young males, then it appears that more than 30% of men over 75 years have subnormal FT levels. It should be mentioned that direct FT assays using a T analog do not yield a reliable estimate of FT.[31] The age-associated decline in FT levels has both a testicular (decreased Leydig cell number) and central origin, the latter being characterized by a decrease in the amplitude of LH pulses in elderly men. Hence, many elderly men have normal LH levels and an increase in LH levels is unlikely to be required for the diagnosis of hypogonadism in elderly men.[5]

As already mentioned, in the absence of a reliable, clinically useful biologic parameter of androgen action these criteria of hypogonadism in the aging man are somewhat arbitrary but, for the time being, the best to provide guidance.[6,7]

Treatment should aim at restoring hormone levels to the normal range for young adults and, more importantly, at alleviating the symptoms associated with a diagnosis of hormone deficiency. The ultimate goals, however, are to maintain or regain the highest quality of life, to reduce disability, to compress major illnesses into a narrow age range, and to add life to years. A large number of authoritative reviews on the potentiality of T deficiency, the choice of a suitable T preparation, and the pitfalls of T replacement in aging men have appeared.[5–7,28–34] If the laboratory outcome is ambiguous but the clinical symptomatology is convincing, to initiate a 3–6-month trial of T treatment. This may provide the answer as to whether a man will benefit from restoring his T levels to normal.[35]

Cardiovascular aspects

The higher frequency of cardiovascular disease in men than in premenopausal women has usually been attributed to the atherogenic effects of androgens. It has become clear that both endogenous and exogenous T account for the lower high-density lipoprotein (HDL) cholesterol levels in men compared to women. However, this view turns out to be too narrow; both androgens and estrogens exert a wide range of favorable and unfavorable effects on laboratory variables related to cardiovascular disease, such as plasma endothelin, clotting factors, insulin sensitivity, homocysteine, and lipolysis (for review see references 36 and 37). There is no longer reason to believe that estrogen administration is a priori cardioprotective. The available evidence does not suggest that T exposure shortens the lifespan in either gender. Effects of androgens on biochemical variables related to cardiovascular disease do not explain the gender difference in age-specific cardiovascular death rates. It cannot be excluded that androgens are a factor in an earlier start of the atherosclerotic process in men compared to women, with a subsequent similar progression in men and women.[38] In cross-sectional studies of men relatively low levels of T appear to be associated with coronary disease and myocardial infarction.[39] A longitudinal study confirmed this observation. In a follow-up study over 13 years of 66 men, aged 41–61 years, the decline in endogenous T was associated with an increase in plasma triglycerides and a decrease in HDL cholesterol in multivariate analysis controlling for obesity and other lifestyle covariates.[40] There is some evidence that administration of androgens to middle-aged obese men improves their cardiovascular risk profile.[36,37,41]

Prostate disease and androgen supplementation in old age

A large number of authoritative reviews on the potentially harmful effects of T administration to the aging male have appeared.[28,42–45] An immediate concern of androgen supplementation in old age is whether there will be a development and/or progression of prostate diseases such as benign prostate hyperplasia (BPH) and prostate carcinoma. It is widely accepted that both conditions do not develop without T exposure early in life, up to early adulthood. The present position of experts in the field is that androgens do not truly cause BPH or prostate carcinoma but that they have a 'permissive' role, evidenced by the beneficial effects of treatment aiming to reduce the biologic effects of androgens on both conditions.[46] Several studies have found that the prevalence of microscopic prostate cancer and its precursor lesions increases strongly with aging, with a prevalence of 33–50% found in men between 60 and 70 years of age.[46–48] However, only a small subset of these men (4–5%) will go on to develop clinically detectable carcinomas.[46] The results of the Massachussets Male Aging Study showed convincingly that sex steroids only account for 11% of our current understanding of prostate cancer risks; 30% is related to nutrition and 40% to other factors largely not subject to change, such as height, weight, and family history.[49]

There is presently no evidence that those who do go on to develop carcinomas have higher androgen levels, but there is a great deal of controversy on this issue.[50] While the prevalence of microscopic prostate cancer is similar in different parts of the world, the progression to clinical cancer varies strongly, with the highest prevalence in those parts with a Western lifestyle.[51] Thus it is probable that lifestyle factors, such as nutrition, might play a role.[52] With regard to BPH, there is no evidence that androgen administration to hypogonadal or to eugonadal men increases the incidence of BPH over that observed in control eugonadal men. A number of studies of androgen supplementation in elderly men who were not hypogonadal have shown that, in the short term, there is only a modest increase in size and in levels of prostate-specific antigen (PSA).[53,54] So, it would seem that non-obstructive BPH is no contraindication for androgen administration, but obstructive BPH is.

Tissue concentrations of T and DHT in the prostate are substantially higher than serum concentrations; it could be that a modest increase in androgens in the peripheral circulation, as would be the aim of androgen supplementation in old age, has no large effect on prostate androgen levels. As to how far an androgen that can be aromatized to estradiol, but cannot be reduced to DHT by 5a-reductase, signifies progress with regard to safety for the prostate remains to be determined.[55,56] Thus, even if there are no reasons for immediate concern, T should be administered to aging men with caution. Recommendations for responsible administration of androgens to elderly men have been published.[5–7,28,54]

Other potential side-effects of androgen administration

The stimulatory effect of T on erythropoiesis is well documented. A moderate increase in hematocrit in elderly males is possibly beneficial, but hematocrit values should not go above 51%, which is the case in some studies. Available data suggest that the frequency of this side-effect is related to supraphysiologic T levels.[57–59]

Oral or transdermal patches yield T levels within the normal range; this may explain the reported lower frequency of polycythemia with this form of treatment, but polycythemia is still a possibility.[59] Whereas sleep apnea has been reported as a side-effect of testosterone treatment,[60,61] none of the reports on actual T supplementation in elderly males mentioned the development of sleep apnea, which itself is often associated with visceral obesity and lower testosterone levels.[62] Nevertheless, it is safe to consider obstructive pulmonary disease in overweight persons or heavy smokers as a relative contraindication.

As already discussed, T supplementation in physiologic doses does not seem to induce an atherogenic lipid profile, but, as mentioned, T also has non-lipid-mediated effects on the cardiovascular system which might even be beneficial.[36,37] Water and sodium retention generally do not cause a problem, except in patients with cardiac insufficiency, hypertension, or renal insufficiency. Gynecomastia is a benign complication of androgen supplementation, perhaps more frequent in elderly obese men than in young hypogonadal men. It is the consequence of the aromatization of T into estradiol in peripheral fat and muscle tissue.[63] A rare, but absolute contraindication is mammary carcinoma in the male as well as a prolactinoma, as their growth may be stimulated by testosterone and its aromatization products.[64]

Hepatotoxicity is rare, even after the long-term use of relatively high oral doses of testosterone undecanoate (TU),[65] but is relatively frequent when synthetic 17-alpha-alkylated anabolic-androgenic steroids are used.

Suitable testosterone preparations

If it turns out that some men benefit from androgen supplements, are there suitable T preparations available to treat them? The androgen deficiency of the aging male is only partial and consequently only partial substitution will be required. High doses of exogenous T will suppress the gonadotropin output of the hypothalamo-pituitary unit, but ideally T administration should leave the residual testicular androgen production intact.

Parenteral testosterone preparations

Conventional parenteral T preparations are far from ideal, even for young hypogonadal males. Plasma T levels fluctuate strongly following administration. The most widely used pharmaceutical forms are the intramuscularly administered hydrophobic, long-chain T-esters in oily depot, enanthate and cypionate, at a dose of 200–250 mg/2 weeks. They yield transient supraphysiologic levels the first 2–3 days after injection, followed by a steady decline to subphysiologic levels just prior to the next injection.[66] These fluctuations in T levels are experienced by some of the patients as unpleasant and accompanied by changes in energy, libido, and mood. The transient supraphysiologic levels might increase the frequency of side-effects.[66]

Parenteral TU is a new treatment modality for androgen replacement therapy. Several studies have documented its use in hypogonadal men.[67,68] In short: after two loading doses of 1000 mg TU at 0 and 6 weeks, repeated injections at 12-week intervals are sufficient to maintain T levels in the reference range of eugonadal men.[67,68] It has been argued that this preparation is less suitable for initiation of T treatment of aging men.[5] It is thought that the long duration of action might constitute a problem in case a prostate malignancy is diagnosed. Experienced urologists, however, reason that the delay between diagnosing prostate cancer and its treatment is usually much longer than 12 weeks, without an adverse effect on the outcome.[69,70] In addition, current recommendations advocate initial follow-up at 3-month intervals for the first year, which fits very well into the schedule of TU injections. In the highly hypothetic situation that a tumor is discovered, further treatment would be discontinued and the use of an anti-androgen might be considered. So, certainly after the first uneventful year of androgen administration, it seems reasonable to administer long-acting T preparations to elderly men.

Oral testosterone undecanoate

TU is T esterified in the 17β position with a long aliphatic sidechain, undecanoic acid, dissolved in oil and encapsulated in soft gelatin. Of the 40 mg capsule, 63% (25 mg) is T. After ingestion its route of absorption from the gastrointestinal tract is shifted from the portal vein to the thoracic duct.[71] For its adequate absorption from the gastrointestinal tract it is essential that oral TU is taken with a meal that contains dietary fat.[72] Without dietary fat the resorption and the resulting serum levels of T are minimal.[69] Maximum serum levels are reached 2 to 6 hours after ingestion. To increase shelf-life the preparation was recently reformulated and the oil in the capsule is now castor oil. Studies show that there is dose proportionality between serum T levels and the dose range of 20–80 mg.[72] With a dose of 120–240 mg per day over 80% of hypogonadal men showed plasma T levels in the normal range over 24 hours.[72]

TU, also on the basis of its flexible dosing, is probably best suited to supplement the reduced, but still present, endogenous testicular T production in the aging male with lower than normal, but not deeply hypogonadal, levels of T.[72,73] Long-term use has been proven to be safe, as demonstrated in a 10-year observation.[65]

Transbuccal testosterone administration
Transbuccal administration of T provides a means of oral administration of T. The resorption of T through the oral mucosa avoids intestinal absorption and subsequent hepatic inactivation of T. Two studies have

assessed the efficacy of transbuccal administration of T;[74,75] both found that administration of 30 mg of T formulated as a bioadhesive buccal tablet twice daily generated plasma T and DHT levels in the normal range in hypogonadal men.[74-76] Gum irritation was noted in approximately 3% of men.

Transdermal delivery
Testosterone can be delivered to the circulation through the intact skin, both genital and non-genital.[77] Transdermal administration delivers T at a controlled rate into the systemic circulation avoiding hepatic first pass and reproducing the diurnal rhythm of T secretion, without the peak and trough levels observed in long-acting T injections.

Transdermal patches
Scrotal patches were first designed to deliver T through the scrotal skin, where the permeability is 5 times greater than for other skin sites. It required weekly scrotal shaving, and was difficult for some patients to apply and maintain in position for 24 hours. Transdermal scrotal T administration is associated with high levels of DHT as a result of high concentrations of 5α-reductase in the scrotal skin.[71] The patch may be irritating and its use is not feasible if the scrotal surface is not adequate. To overcome these limitations, non-scrotal skin patches have been developed. These patches have a reservoir containing T with a permeation-enhancing vehicle and gelling agents.[78,79] Improvements have been reported in sexual function, libido, energy level, and mood.[79]

The most common adverse effects are local skin reactions. Fifty percent of men participating in a clinical trial reported transient, mild to moderate erythema at some time during therapy. However, most of these reactions were associated with the application of a patch over a bony prominence or on parts of the body that could have been subject to prolonged pressure during sleep or sitting.

Testosterone gel
Testosterone gel is also used for replacement therapy; it is hydro-alcoholic. Between 5 and 10 g of a 1% gel (10 mg T per gram gel) are administered per

day, amounting to between 50 and 100 mg T.[80] The pharmacokinetics of T gel has been extensively studied. It was reported that serum T levels rose 2–3 fold 2 hours after application, and rose further to 4–5 fold after 24 hours. Thereafter serum T remained steadily in the upper range of normal and returned to baseline within 4 days of termination of the application of the gel. Mean DHT levels followed the same pattern as T and were at or above the normal adult male range. Serum estradiol (E_2) levels rose and followed the same patterns as T. Application of the T gel at either one site or four sites did not have a substantial impact on the pharmacokinetic profile.[81] Later studies showed that 9–14% of the T administered is bioavailable. Steady-state T levels are achieved 48–72 hours after the first application. Serum T and FT are similar on days 30, 90, and 180 after the start of administration. The formulation of the T gel allows easy dose adjustments (50–75–100 mg T).[71,81–84]

The clinical efficacy of transdermal T gel on various androgen-dependent target organ systems has been very well documented.[80] The safety profile showed that PSA levels rose in proportion to the increase in T levels, but did not exceed normal values. Skin irritation was noted in 5.5% of patients in the study.[81–83] Later studies with a 2.5% T gel showed that 5 g of this gel achieved physiological serum T levels in men whose endogenous T production was pharmacologically suppressed. These levels were reached after approximately 10 days. Serum DHT and E_2 did not exceed normal levels. Remarkably, washing of the site of application 10 minutes after application of the gel did not affect pharmacokinetic profiles.[85] Transfer from one person to another was found to be insignificant. No increase of serum T was found after intense skin contact with persons whose endogenous testosterone levels had been suppressed.[85]

Recently, a new formulation of T gel has been introduced.[82,86]

Estrogens in men

Traditionally conceptualized as 'female hormones', estrogens appear to have significant effects in the male biologic system. Favorable effects have been noted on bone, brain, and cardiovascular physiology, while a potential role in the prostate pathology of the aging male has been seriously suspected (for review see references 87 and 88). Estrogens in the male are predominantly the products of peripheral aromatization of testicular and adrenal androgens. While the testicular and adrenal production of androgens declines with aging, levels of total plasma estradiol usually do not. This is to be ascribed to the common increase in fat mass with aging (the substrate of peripheral aromatization) and an increased aromatase activity with aging. But free or bioavailable estrogens may also decline due to an increase in SHBG.

Estrogens produce significant beneficial effects on skeletal growth and bone maturation. In old age estrogens are better predictors of bone fractures than androgens. Estrogens exert effects on the brain: on cognitive function, co-ordination of movement, pain, and the affective state, and may protect against Alzheimer's disease. Estrogenic effects on the cardiovascular system include those on lipid profiles, fat distribution, endocrine/paracrine factors produced by the vascular wall (such as endothelins, nitric oxide), blood platelets, inflammatory factors, and coagulation. Men who are devoid of estrogenic actions show severe signs and symptoms of the metabolic syndrome.

There may be potentially adverse effects of estrogens on the prostate due to a shift in the estrogen/androgen ratio with aging.[88]

Sources of estrogens in men are endogenous androgens or, in the case of androgen deficiency, exogenous androgens. Dietary phytoestrogens or selective estrogen receptor modulators may be significant as well. There is almost never an 'estrogen deficiency syndrome' in men. In other words, plasma levels of E_2 below which there are signs and symptoms of estrogen deficiency occur very rarely, mainly in men who are underweight and have too little fat mass to aromatize androgens to estrogens.[88]

Adrenal androgens

While it is now well documented that serum levels of adrenal androgens decline strongly with aging, it has not been definitively established whether this impressive fall of adrenal androgens has any (patho)physiologic significance. Theoretically, it could be a meaningful mechanism of adaptation to aging. There is no doubt that strong correlations can be established between the declining levels of adrenal androgens and ailments of aging, but whether these statistical associations are causally and pathophysiologically interrelated remains to be established. One way of establishing whether there is a relationship between the two is via intervention studies. Suppressing or elevating levels of adrenal androgens and monitoring the subsequent biologic effects could provide clues as to whether the falling levels of adrenal androgens with aging are a cause for concern. The effects in laboratory animals are impressive. Beneficial effects on processes such as atherosclerosis, type 2 diabetes, obesity, immune function/cancer prevention, and brain function have been reported, but it has to be remembered that laboratory animals, such as rats and rabbits, do not physiologically produce adrenal androgens in the quantities that the human species does.

So far, studies in humans are limited. While some studies have found correlations between circulating levels of adrenal androgens and age-related ailments, others have not. Intervention studies present an equally sober picture. One study has found a positive effect on well-being.[89] The effects of DHEA replacement on indices of sexual functioning in men and women with complete adrenal insufficiency, who are virtually devoid of adrenal androgens, are convincing.[90] It would seem that a total absence of adrenal androgens has negative effects on a woman's well-being and sexuality. A positive effect on self-esteem and perhaps on well-being was also found in men whose own adrenal androgen production was almost nil,[91] and this argues more in favor of an independent effect of DHEA on the brain, since the men were not testosterone deficient. Another group that might benefit from replacement with DHEA is men who receive glucocorticoid treatment and whose ACTH levels are suppressed and therewith their own production of both cortisol and adrenal androgens.[92] A consequence of the conversion of DHEA to androgens and estrogens is that the effects of

DHEA administration are not necessarily harmless. They may influence hormone-sensitive diseases such as breast or prostate cancer. So far there are no reports in the literature of any side-effects from self-administration of DHEA, which occurs on a massive scale with DHEA sold as a health product. Well-designed studies, investigating the effects of the deficiency of adrenal androgens and the results of replacement therapy in humans, are required to resolve the long-term effects of levels of adrenal androgens.[93]

A few studies published on the relevance of DHEA in endothelial function offer a perspective for potential benefits.[94–97]

Growth hormone

Signs associated with aging show a striking similarity with features observed in adults who are GH deficient, and therefore speculation has arisen that (some of the) features of aging must be ascribed to the age-related decline in GH, and can potentially be remedied with GH replacement (for review see reference 97).

The interrelationship between sleep and the somatotropic axis is well documented. This relationship is relevant since most aging subjects experience a deterioration in their sleep. During aging, slow-wave sleep and GH decline concurrently, raising the possibility that the age-related decline of GH is also a reflection of age-related alterations in sleep–wake patterns.

Unlike the situation in androgen physiology, it is much more difficult to establish who is GH deficient in adulthood. The pulsatile nature of GH secretion and the large number of factors determining circulating levels of GH complicate the matter considerably in the sense that a single measurement of GH does not provide meaningful information. A single measurement of insulin-like growth factor 1 (IGF-1) is a reasonable first indicator of GH status. In subjects over the age of 40 years an IGF-1 value of 15 nmol/l or higher excludes a deficiency of GH. The problem lies among patients with values below this level. Surprisingly, some patients with proven GH deficiency (on the basis of extensive testing such as insulin hypoglycemia, GHRH, and L-dopa stimulation tests) still have normal IGF-1 levels. Another useful index of the GH status is IGF-binding protein-3. For the time being, the combination of signs and symptoms potentially attributable to GH deficiency and an IGF-1 level and IGF-binding protein-3 in the lowest tertile provides a reasonable first indication of (relative) GH deficiency.[98] To confirm the diagnosis, a provocation test with growth hormone releasing hormone in combination with arginine or synthetic growth hormone releasing substance (GHS) is highly desirable.[97]

The starting dose of GH administration is not well established, but a dose of 0.05–0.1 U/kg subcutaneously seems reasonable. Once placed on GH administration, the patient's individual dose titration must be done on the basis of the IGF-1 levels resulting from GH administration and the occurrence of side-effects. The aim is to produce IGF-1 levels in the normal or only slightly above normal range (0–1 standard deviations above mean levels of IGF-1).[98] Secondly, if side-effects occur (flu-like symptoms, gynecomastia, myalgia, arthralgia, carpal tunnel syndrome, edema, impairment of glucose homeostasis) GH dosage is reduced in steps of 25%. Contraindications for GH use include type 1 diabetes, active (or a history of) cancer, intracranial hypertension, diabetic retinopathy or carpal tunnel syndrome, and severe cardiac insufficiency.

It seems there is a place for GH administration in aging subjects at this point in time, primarily to gather information as to whether there are groups that might benefit from its supplementation. In view of the narrow dose limits and potential side-effects, treatment should be reserved for patients with proven GH deficiency and it is not advisable at present to administer GH to aging patients outside the framework of a clinical trial that provides intensive guidance and safeguards to patients.[99]

Another important consideration is that the question has been raised whether the increase of rIGF-1 following GH administration might accelerate the development of neoplasia. Studies have found that high normal IGF-1 levels are associated with significantly increased risks of prostate[99] and colon cancer.[99]

Melatonin

Melatonin is a hormone produced in the pineal gland. It is synthesized from the amino acid tryptophan (derived from serotonin) by the enzyme 5-hydroxyindole-O-methyltransferase. Normally, production of melatonin by the pineal gland is inhibited by light and permitted by darkness. Melatonin and the pineal gland play a role in regulating sleep–wake cycles (circadian rhythms). Residents of nursing homes or others who are not exposed to daylight may experience sleeping problems on the basis of a disturbed light/dark cycle with an associated impaired melatonin rhythm.[100] Beta-blockers decrease nocturnal melatonin release and might have a negative effect on sleep.

In recent times, melatonin has become available as a medication and a dietary supplement. Because it does not have to be prescribed and is in the public domain, there have been few clinical trials conducted to determine its effectiveness in treating sleep disorders. Whether melatonin has some use against insomnia, jet lag, and other types of misalignments in circadian rhythms is still under debate. A recent meta-analysis found that melatonin is not helpful in treating sleep disorders or improving symptoms of jet lag,[101] but it was found to be safe, at least in the short term. However, other studies report more favorable effects.[102,103]

Melatonin is practically non-toxic and exhibits almost no side-effects, except for the occurrence of somnolence in most of the population at higher doses and sensations of chilliness due to its effects on thermogenesis. Individuals who experience orthostatic intolerance may experience a worsening of symptoms when taking melatonin. Exogenous melatonin normally does not affect the endogenous melatonin profile in the short or medium term.

The recommended dose is not well defined, but a dose of 0.3 mg was reported to be efficacious without side-effects.[102] Over-the-counter doses of melatonin can cause severe headaches, mental impairment, and mood changes. Melatonin pills sold as supplements contain 3 to 10 times the amount needed to produce the desirable physiologic nocturnal blood melatonin level for enhancement of night-time rest. It is at these elevated levels produced by typical over-the-counter dosage units that studies have found mental impairment and resultant headaches.

Oral melatonin has a short half-life and transdermal patches are being developed to prolong its action.

Thyroid disease in elderly men

The clinical presentation of thyroid disease in the aged differs from the typical clinical manifestation in the younger population. Further, laboratory test results should be interpreted with the age of the patient in mind. The use of drugs and the frequent occurrence of non-thyroidal disease in the elderly are factors in these age-related changes in laboratory parameters of thyroid function. The treatment of thyroid dysfunction in old age also requires more caution than in younger patients (for review see reference 104).

In elderly subjects there is a decrease in the production of T4 with a concomitant decrease in T4 clearance, so circulating levels do not change significantly. Since serious disease is not infrequent in old age, a thyroid hormone pattern may be present which has become known as the 'non-thyroid illness' (NTI), consisting of lowered T3 levels, and an insignificant reduction in T4.

Drugs may alter the profiles of thyroid hormone levels, which is relevant since the elderly subjects often take some form of medication over long periods. Long-term therapy with lithium may lead to hypothyroidism and patients should be screened for this complication. The iodine-containing cardiac drug amiodarone may produce both hyperthyroidism and hypothyroidism. Glucocorticoids inhibit the conversion of T4 to T3. Conversely, a state of hyperthyroidism or hypothyroidism affects the half-lives of certain drugs. In hypothyroidism the plasma half-lives of digoxin, morphine, glucocorticoids, and insulin are increased, with the consequence of a lower than normal maintenance dosage of these drugs. The reverse pattern is observed in hyperthyroidism.[105]

Hypothyroidism may be overlooked in the elderly since the symptoms may be less apparent.[106]

The symptoms themselves are often attributed to the aging process with its associated asthenia, effects of drug use, and loss of agility. These symptoms range from weakness, chronic fatigue, and decreased heart rate, to dry skin, hoarseness, and slower tendon reflexes. Intolerance to cold and weight gain may be less pronounced in the elderly. Hypothyroidism should be suspected if there are occurrences of unexplained high levels of cholesterol and creatinine phosphokinase, severe constipation, congestive heart failure with cardiomyopathy, and unexplained macrocytic anemia. Loss of weight due to anorexia may occur. Lethargy, memory loss, and depression may be the presenting symptoms. Long-term hypothyroidism will result in irreversible psychic symptoms.

The prevalence of hypothyroidism in the elderly lies somewhere between 1 and 7% for the fully fledged disease and 5 and 16% for subclinical hypothyroidism.[106] Patients who have been treated surgically with radioactive iodine may tip over to hypothyroidism later in their lives.

The best diagnostic test for primary hypothyroidism is an increased serum TSH level, although TSH levels in the elderly who have hypothyroidism are lower than in younger patients with the same disease. Levels of both T4 and free T3 are a less helpful indicator, since they are lower in cases of non-thyroidal illness.

Treatment of hypothyroidism in the elderly involves substitution with levothyroxine, the guiding principle being the normalization of TSH levels. An abrupt increase in circulating levels of T4 may provoke cardiac symptoms, therefore replacement should be carried out in a stepwise fashion.

Hyperthyroidism in the elderly may have a different presentation than in younger hyperthyroid subjects.[105] Patients with atrial fibrillation should be suspected of hyperthyroidism since the likelihood of thyroid hyperfunction is approximately 3 times higher. Conventional treatment of cardiac disease is less successful if hyperthyroidism lies at the basis of cardiac symptoms. Another complication of long-standing hyperthyroidism is osteoporosis. Bone resorption is increased, particularly in subjects with other etiologic factors. Unexplained osteoporosis must be a reminder of possible hyperthyroidism.

Erectile problems

Aging is the most robust factor predicting erectile difficulties. It is obvious that aging per se is associated with a deterioration of the biologic functions mediating erectile function: hormonal, vascular, and neural processes. This is often aggravated by intercurrent disease in old age, such as diabetes mellitus, cardiovacular disease, and use of medical drugs. There is still uneasiness with the aging population when it comes to discussing sexual dysfunction. It is essential that physicians make sexuality a conversation topic in their interaction with aging patients and provide an opportunity for patients to discuss the quality of their sex lives. It is a fact of life that lots of physicians themselves are not comfortable with bringing up these issues in their contact with patients and this conspiracy of silence is nonverbally communicated to patients. If embarrassment arises in a conversation on sexuality the doctor must give the patient 'permission' to use vernacular expressions to describe sexual complaints.

The availability of a highly efficacious and relatively safe compound such as the phosphodiesterase (PDE) type 5 inhibitor sildenafil has had a profound impact on diagnosis and treatment of erectile dysfunction (ED). Once the domain of the urologist attempting to define the precise etiology, ED is now largely treated by first-line physicians, without much of a diagnostic work-up. Despite the simplicity and safety of the present therapy of ED, approximately 50% of patients discontinue treatment. The reasons for discontinuation lie for a large part in an incomplete evaluation of the sexual problem. Hypogonadism, ejaculatory dysfunction, lower urinary tract symptoms (LUTS), depression, and, last but not least, partner issues may all be components of the sexual dysfunction of the patient, and apparently restoration of erectile function does not necessarily imply restoration of a happy sex life.[107] Nevertheless, the introduction of the PDE5 inhibitors has substantially enlarged the therapeutic options for ED.

The pharmacologic action of PDE5 inhibitors manifests itself only when a person is sexually aroused, which distinguishes this class of drugs from intracavernosal injections. This is also important information for the user.[108]

There are presently three PDE5 inhibitors available for prescription: sildenafil, vardenafil, and tadalafil. All are efficacious, but there are differences in pharmacokinetic profile, interactions with food and drugs, and possibly side-effects. Taking nitrate medications is an absolute contraindication to the use of PDE5 inhibitors since the latter increase the potential for excessively low blood pressure. Low blood pressure, though to a lesser degree, has also been observed with PDE5 inhibitors in men taking alpha-adrenoreceptor antagonists, which are used as antihypertensive agents or for symptomatic relief of LUTS, such as doxazosin, prazosin, terazosin, alfuzosin, or tamsulosin. The latter is relevant since sexual dysfunction is not rare in men with LUTS, both significantly increasing with age, and maybe sharing etiologic factors.[109]

Sildenafil and vardenafil work best if no (fatty) food has been taken within the last 2 hours, while tadalafil can be used without regard to food. Common adverse effects, attributable to vasodilatory effects, include headache, flushing, stuffy nose, stomach pain, back pain (tadalafil), and indigestion. Visual problems (for example, blurred vision, increased sensitivity to light, bluish haze, or temporary difficulty distinguishing between blue and green) may occur, more often with sildenafil since the latter is less selective in inhibiting phosphodiesterase 6 in the retina.

The prescribed tablet strength is swallowed 30–60 minutes before sexual activity. Tadalafil has a longer duration of increased sensitivity for developing an erection (up to 24–36 hours) compared with sildenafil and vardenafil (up to 4–12 hours). There is no convincing evidence that the three available PDE5 inhibitors differ significantly in their clinical efficacy. For sildenafil (50 and 100 mg) and tadalafil (10 and 20 mg) there is a dose–response relationship, which is not so much the case for vardenafil (10 and 20 mg).[110] In general, it is recommended to start with the lowest dose of PDE5 inhibitors.

The feature that distinguishes the three PDE5 inhibitors is their pharmacokinetic profile, which impacts on their clinical use in terms of the initiation of optimal pharmacologic effect and duration of pharmacologic action (for review see reference 111). The time to maximal plasma concentration (in minutes) is on average 60 (variation 30–120) for sildenafil, 120 (variation 30–720!) for tadalafil, and 60 (variation 30–120) for vardenafil. These are statistical data and individual patients may experience a faster onset of action. This information lets patients plan prospective sexual action. Another significant pharmacokinetic variable is the half-life of the drug, which provides an indication to how long the drug can be expected to be pharmacologically active after ingestion. The half-life of sildenafil 100 mg is 3–4 hours, for tadalafil 20 mg 17 hours, and for vardenafil 20 mg 3–6 hours. This information lets the patient make reasonable assumptions about the expected duration of the pharmacologic activity of the ingested compound.

It is not rare that patients wish to 'experiment' with the available PDE5 inhibitors to find the drug that suits them best. Patients do have distinctly different sexual habits with regard to timing of sexual activity. Another consideration is the 'readiness' of the patients when sexual activity is initiated by the partner.

Naturally, patients starting treatment with a PDE5 inhibitor will experience some anxiety about whether the new drug will indeed induce an erection. Anxiety may reduce sexual arousal, which is a necessary condition for the desired pharmacologic action of PDE5 inhibitors. Therefore, in cases where the patient recognizes this as a potential problem, it may be advisable to test the efficacy of the drug first with masturbation.

When the first PDE5 inhibitor sildenafil was introduced there was great concern about the cardiovascular safety of this class of drugs. In many patients the etiology of ED is (also) based on vascular disease. The availability of the drug prompted patients to resume sexual activity after prolonged periods of inactivity. The pharmacologic action of PDE5 inhibitors is vasodilatory. Fears arose that these elements would lead to myocardial ischemia or infarction when intercourse was attempted. Fortunately, these concerns have remained unsubstantiated. Placebo-controlled studies fail to show a higher cardiovascular morbidity/mortality in patients using PDE5 inhibitors.[112] Naturally, before starting PDE5 inhibitors, the cardiovascular risks of the patient must be assessed. A rule of thumb indicator is whether a patient can walk one kilometer in

10 minutes without cardiac symptoms, an equivalent of the physical exertion of sexual intercourse.[112]

Although it has been convincingly established that the main effect of androgens on male sexual functioning is on the central nervous system, additional evidence now suggests that they also affect nitric oxide synthase in the corpus cavernosum (nitric oxide induces smooth muscle relaxation of the penile vasculature, essential for penile erection) and that androgen administration may be helpful in men who respond poorly to treatment of ED with PDE5 inhibitors.[113] So there seems to be a point in treating men with low or low normal plasma T, who do not respond well to PDE5 inhibitors, with T. It has also been recommended and widely accepted that all men investigated for ED should have a serum T determination. To reserve this assessment to those who failed first-line treatment prevents many men from pursuing further evaluation and treatment of the dysfunction.

A fulfilling sex life is part of a good life. We need to educate our patients that, like any other human endeavor, human sexuality is not exempt from problems for which solutions must and often can be found. We have to tell our patients that aging has its impact on life and on sexuality, but it should not and need not defeat men. Erection and ejaculation become less dependable but there are also non-coital forms of sexual expression providing enjoyment and satisfaction. Sexual creativity is a must! The latter requires an open and playful relationship with one's own sexuality and one's sexual partner.

As indicated above, erectile potency is physiologically a complex interaction of vascular, neural, metabolic, endocrine, and, last but not least, psychologic factors. Erectile difficulties often provide a window into the presence of pathology of these areas. However, precisely the advent of successful treatment modalities of erectile difficulties has led to a concept of erectile failure as an entity in itself rather than an expression of underlying pathology of its constituents. In other words: it has opened the door to view diagnosis and treatment of underlying pathology of erectile failure as a redundancy. A holistic approach to the aging male requires, however, that all aspects of health are addressed and complaints of erectile difficulties provide an opportunity for a more thorough work-up of health problems of the aging man in question, who will find motivation to work on these health issues if the reward is an improvement in his sex life.

Nutrition and the epidemic of obesity

In industrialized countries outright nutritional deficiencies are rare nowadays unless in cases of severe gastrointestinal pathology or psychiatric disturbance. The oldest old may show deficiencies in intake of calcium, vitamin D, or iron. There is certainly room for improvement in the intake of water, fiber, and antioxidants, and for a larger consumption of fruit, etc. A simple rule for healthy eating is to ensure that the meal size is commensurate with energy expenditure, that fats, in particular animal fat, are avoided in the diet, and that there is a substantial fiber and fruit content to the daily food intake. A major problem is the management of overweight. Obesity is a condition that is reaching epidemic proportions in both the developed and the developing world.[114] In the USA, 63% of men and 55% of women are classified as overweight. Of these, 22% are deemed grossly overweight, with a body mass index above 30 kg/m^2, and the consequences of this rapid increase are serious. Approximately 80% of obese adults suffer from at least one, and 40% from two or more of the diseases associated with obesity, such as type 2 diabetes, hypertension, cardiovascular disease, gallbladder disease, cancers, and diseases of the locomotor system, such as arthrosis.

A significant role in the development of obesity is played by genetics, with studies in identical twins showing that 60–70% of overweight can be ascribed to genetic factors, with just 30–40% attributable to environmental influences.[115] The pathophysiology of obesity is poorly understood. In simple terms, obesity is a discrepancy between food intake on the one hand and energy expenditure on the other. However, the physiologic mechanisms involved, and how these can be influenced to redress obesity, are much more difficult questions.

The treatment of obesity and overweight is far from simple. Even more difficult is the maintenance of a reduced weight in the long term, after a successful weight loss. It is evident that a combination of reduced caloric intake and an increase in energy expenditure will lead to a reduction in weight. However, when placed on a calorie-restricted diet, the body responds by developing countermeasures to minimize the loss of weight, a system which evolved to enhance an individual's chance of survival during prolonged times of famine. Recent studies indicate that a weight loss of just 5–10% leads to clinically significant reductions in the risk factors associated with obesity, even if 'ideal' weight is not reached.[116] A reduction in weight of 10% in 6 months to 1 year can be considered good progress; however, it is estimated that over 80% of those who lose weight will gradually regain it. The addition of various pharmacotherapies to a weight-reducing diet can increase the degree of success.[117] However, it is difficult, even with pharmacotherapy, to achieve a weight reduction of more than 6–8% of initial body weight. Considering the amount of investment and expenditure directed towards weight reduction each year, the fight against obesity is largely unsuccessful. Indeed, it may be a difficult, if not impossible battle to win in the setting of clinical medicine. Eating patterns are very resistant to change.[118] Sometimes environmental clues may be helpful.[119] It will require extensive public health campaigns educating populations to eat sensibly and to be more physically active, from an early age on.[120,121] The food industry may play a significant role in view of the increasing consumption of convenience food. Marketing techniques of healthy food may have a large impact.

The current lack of success in the battle against obesity can lead to frustration for both patients and physicians alike. The medical profession has little to offer to the obese patient in terms of efficacious treatment. The physician is then inclined to leave the full responsibility for the loss of weight to the patient himself, implying more or less that the patient lacks willpower. Even if patients lack will power, the battle against the epidemic of obesity cannot be won.

Exercise and physical fitness

Technologic and socioeconomic developments have made a quantum leap in recent history in relation to the amount of physical exercise and energy expenditure required from our bodies on a daily basis. There are strong parallels with the situation of nutrition in modern times. These developments are very appealing to almost all people and must be considered as irreversible, durable products of Western civilization. The inevitable consequence is that many people are overfed and physically unfit. The outlook for an easy solution is not bright. Men should be advised to undertake regular physical exercise (aerobic exercise for maintaining cardiac function as well as anaerobic exercise targeted to specific muscle groups as well as stretching).[121,122] These exercises should be performed on a regular basis and tailored to the 'biologic age' and condition of the person.[123] Similar to the situation of overweight and restricted diet, people are of good will but lack the stamina to implement physical exercise in their daily lives far beyond a period of initial determination. In the lives of most people there are apparently too many intervening circumstances to allow regular exercise. The demands of daily life cause fatigue, which could in fact be remedied by recreational exercise if only people could muster the energy to do it. Again, similar to the situation with obesity, education seems to be a major factor and small steps must be encouraged.[124] Working out, albeit moderately, in the work place or with a group of friends may bolster tenacity of purpose. Nutrition and physical exercise with fitness as an outcome are pivotal for the health situation of the aging male and his quality of life, and therefore deserve a more prominent place in the medical curriculum. Their implementation can be left to health workers with a focused education exploring individual motivations and opportunities for a healthier lifestyle for which there is no substitute.[125]

Conclusions

Physicians who are educated about the value of preventative health care in prolonging lifespan and quality of life will be more likely to participate in health screening and become gate keepers for aging males. Men are not likely to consult a doctor until they have an (acute) illness. When a man comes to see his physician for a minor ailment the physician should, starting with the family history, body constitution, lifestyle, and risk factors, advise the patient on preventative strategies or refer him to consult the appropriate specialist. It is to be hoped that the next few years will enrich us with new evidence which will clarify the state of our present knowledge and will permit us to recognize some of the missing links and provide the tools and methodology to design and plan ways to understand the aging process of men. This will then permit us to improve their quality of life, prevent the preventable, and postpone and decrease the pain and suffering of the inevitable. For the time being, we have only unattractive advice to offer: healthy eating and exercise.

References

1. Rossouw JE, Anderson GL, Prentice RL et al. Risks and benefits of estrogen plus progestin in healthy postmenopausal women: principal results from the Women's Health Initiative randomized controlled trial. JAMA 2002; 288: 321–33.
2. Harman SM, Naftolin F. Is the estrogen controversy over? Deconstructing the Women's Health Initiative Study: a critical evaluation of the evidence. Ann NY Acad Sci 2005; 1052: 43–56.
3. Harman SM. Testosterone in older men after the Institute of Health Report: where do we go from here? Climacteric 2005; 8: 124–35.
4. Crawford BA, Liu PY, Kean MT et al. Randomized placebo-controlled trial of androgen effects on muscle and bone in men requiring long-term systemic glucocorticoid treatment. J Clin Endocrinol Metab 2003; 88: 3167–76.
5. Kaufman JM, Vermeulen A. The decline of androgen levels in elderly men and its clinical and therapeutic implications. Endocr Rev 2005; 26: 833–76.
6. Nieschlag E, Swerdloff R. Investigation, treatment and monitoring of late-onset hypogonadism in males: ISA, ISSAM, and EAU recommendations. Int J Androl 2005; 28: 125–7.
7. Nieschlag E, Swerdloff R. Investigation, treatment and monitoring of late-onset hypogonadism in males. Aging Male 2005; 8: 56–8.
8. Hijazi RA, Cunningham GR. Andropause: is androgen replacement therapy indicated for the aging male? Annu Rev Med 2005; 56: 117–37.

9. Lamberts SW, Romijn JA. The future endocrine patient. Reflections on the future of clinical endocrinology. Eur J Endocrinol 2003; 149: 169–75.

10. Schultheiss D, Jonas U. Some historical reflections on the ageing male. World J Urol 2002; 20: 40–4.

11. Vermeulen A. Androgen replacement therapy in the aging male – a critical evaluation. J Clin Endocrinol Metab 2001; 86: 2380–90.

12. Schubert M, Jockenhovel F. Late-onset hypogonadism in the aging male (LOH): definition, diagnostic and clinical aspects. J Endocrinol Invest 2005; 28(3 Suppl): 23–7.

13. Meikle AW, Bishop DT, Stringham JD et al. Quantitating genetic and nongenetic factors that determine plasma sex steroid variation in normal male twins. Metabolism 1986; 35: 1090–5.

14. Vermeulen A. Androgen replacement therapy in the aging male – a critical evaluation. J Clin Endocrinol Metab 2001; 86: 2380–90.

15. Gooren LJ. Androgen levels and sex functions in testosterone-treated hypogonadal men. Arch Sex Behav 1987; 16: 463–73.

16. Bagatell CJ, Heiman JR, Rivier JE et al. Effects of endogenous testosterone and estradiol on sexual behavior in normal young men. J Clin Endocrinol Metab 1994; 78: 711–16.

17. Gray PB, Singh AB. Dose-dependent effects of testosterone on sexual function, mood, and visuospatial cognition in older men. J Clin Endocrinol Metab 2005; 90: 3838–46.

18. Bhasin S, Woodhouse L, Casaburi R et al. Testosterone dose–response relationships in healthy young men. Am J Physiol Endocrinol Metab 2001; 281: E1172–81.

19. Wang C, Catlin DH. Measurement of total serum testosterone in adult men: comparison of current laboratory methods versus liquid chromatography-tandem mass spectrometry. J Clin Endocrinol Metab 2004; 89: 534–43.

20. Sikaris K, McLachlan RI, Kazlauskas R et al. Reproductive hormone reference intervals for healthy fertile young men: evaluation of automated platform assays. J Clin Endocrinol Metab 2005; 90: 5928–36.

21. Goncharov N, Katsya G, Dobracheva A et al. Serum testosterone measurement in men: evaluation of modern immunoassay technologies. Aging Male 2005; 8: 194–202.

22. Deslypere JP, Vermeulen A. Influence of age on steroid concentrations in skin and striated muscle in women and in cardiac muscle and lung tissue in men. J Clin Endocrinol Metab 1985; 61: 648–53.

23. Greenstein BD. Androgen receptors in the rat brain, anterior pituitary gland and ventral prostate gland: effects of orchidectomy and ageing. J Endocrinol 1979; 81: 75–81.

24. Sperfeld AD, Karitzky J, Brummer D et al. X-linked bulbospinal neuronopathy: Kennedy disease. Arch Neurol 2002; 59: 1921–6.

25. Krithivas K, Yurgalevitch SM, Mohr BA et al. Evidence that the CAG repeat in the androgen receptor gene is associated with the age-related decline in serum androgen levels in men. J Endocrinol 1999; 162: 137–42.

26. Harkonen K, Huhtaniemi I, Makinen J et al. The polymorphic androgen receptor gene CAG repeat, pituitary-testicular function and andropausal symptoms in ageing men. Int J Androl 2003; 26: 187–94.

27. Weidemann W, Peters B, Romalo G et al. Response to androgen treatment in a patient with partial androgen insensitivity and a mutation in the deoxyribonucleic acid-binding domain of the androgen receptor. J Clin Endocrinol Metab 1998; 83: 1173–6.

28. Morales A, Lunenfeld B. Investigation, treatment and monitoring of late-onset hypogonadism in males. Official recommendations of ISSAM. International Society for the Study of the Aging Male. Aging Male 2002; 5: 74–86.

29. Liu PY, Swerdloff RS, Veldhuis JD. Clinical review 171: the rationale, efficacy and safety of androgen therapy in older men: future research and current practice recommendations. J Clin Endocrinol Metab 2004; 89: 4789–96.

30. Vermeulen A. Androgen replacement therapy in the aging male – a critical evaluation. J Clin Endocrinol Metab 2001; 86: 2380–90.

31. Vermeulen A, Verdonck L, Kaufman JM. A critical evaluation of simple methods for the estimation of free testosterone in serum. J Clin Endocrinol Metab 1999; 84: 3666–72.

32. Krause W, Mueller U, Mazur A. Testosterone supplementation in the aging male: which questions have been answered? Aging Male 2005; 8: 31–8.

33. Lunenfeld B, Saad F, Hoesl CE. ISA, ISSAM and EAU recommendations for the investigation, treatment and monitoring of late-onset hypogonadism in males: scientific background and rationale. Aging Male 2005; 8: 59–74.

34. The Practice Committee of the American Society for Reproductive Medicine. Treatment of androgen deficiency in the aging male. Fertil Steril 2004; 82(Suppl 1): S46–50.

35. Black AM, Day AG. The reliability of clinical and biochemical assessment in symptomatic late-onset hypogonadism: can a case be made for a 3-month therapeutic trial? BJU Int 2004; 94: 1066–70.

36. Wu FC, von Eckardstein A. Androgens and coronary artery disease. Endocr Rev 2003; 24: 183–217.

37. Liu PY, Death AK, Handelsman DJ. Androgens and cardiovascular disease. Endocr Rev 2003; 24: 313–40.

38. Blouin K, Despres JP. Contribution of age and declining androgen levels to features of the metabolic syndrome in men. Metabolism 2005; 54: 1034–40.

39. Dubey RK, Oparil S, Imthurn B et al. Sex hormones and hypertension. Cardiovasc Res 2002; 53: 688–708.

40. Hak AE, Witteman JC, de Jong FH et al. Low levels of endogenous androgens increase the risk of atherosclerosis in elderly men: the Rotterdam study. J Clin Endocrinol Metab 2002; 87: 3632–9.

41. Kapoor D, Malkin CJ. Androgens, insulin resistance and vascular disease in men. Clin Endocrinol (Oxf) 2005; 63: 239–50.

42. Gaylis FD, Lin DW. Prostate cancer in men using testosterone supplementation. J Urol 2005; 174: 534–8; discussion 538.

43. Hsing AW. Hormones and prostate cancer: what's next? Epidemiol Rev 2001; 23: 42–58.

44. Matsumoto AM. Andropause: clinical implications of the decline in serum testosterone levels with aging in men. J Gerontol A Biol Sci Med Sci 2002; 57: M76–99.

45. Parsons JK, Carter HB. Serum testosterone and the risk of prostate cancer: potential implications for testosterone therapy. Cancer Epidemiol Biomarkers Prev 2005; 14: 2257–60.

46. De Marzo AM, Meeker AK, Zha S et al. Human prostate cancer precursors and pathobiology. Urology 2003; 62: 55–62.

47. Rhoden EL, Morgentaler A. Risks of testosterone-replacement therapy and recommendations for monitoring. N Engl J Med 2004; 350: 482–92.

48. Sengupta S, Duncan HJ. The development of prostate cancer despite late onset androgen deficiency. Int J Urol 2005; 12: 847–8.

49. Kalish LA, McDougal WS, McKinlay JB. Family history and the risk of prostate cancer. Urology 2000; 56: 803–6.

50. Stattin P, Lumme S, Tenkanen L et al. High levels of circulating testosterone are not associated with increased prostate cancer risk: a pooled prospective study. Int J Cancer 2004; 108: 418–24.

51. Mohr BA, Feldman HA, Kalish LA et al. Are serum hormones associated with the risk of prostate cancer? Prospective results from the Massachusetts Male Aging Study. Urology 2001; 57: 930–5.

52. Kolonel LN, Altshuler D, Henderson BE. The multiethnic cohort study: exploring genes, lifestyle and cancer risk. Nat Rev Cancer 2004; 4: 519–27.

53. Kaufman JM. The effect of androgen supplementation therapy on the prostate. Aging Male 2003; 6: 166–74.

54. Morales A. Androgen replacement therapy and prostate safety. Eur Urol 2002; 41: 113–20.

55. Anderson RA, Wallace AM, Sattar N, Kumar N, Sundaram K. Evidence for tissue selectivity of the synthetic androgen 7-alpha-methyl-19-nortestosterone in

56. Anderson RA, Martin CW, Kung AW et al. 7-Alpha-methyl-19-nortestosterone maintains sexual behavior and mood in hypogonadal men. J Clin Endocrinol Metab 1999; 84: 3556–62.

57. Calof OM, Singh AB, Lee ML et al. Adverse events associated with testosterone replacement in middle-aged and older men: a meta-analysis of randomized, placebo-controlled trials. J Gerontol A Biol Sci Med Sci 2005; 60: 1451–7.

58. Jockenhovel F, Vogel E. Effects of various modes of androgen substitution therapy on erythropoiesis. Eur J Med Res 1997; 2: 293–8.

59. Dobs AS, Meikle AW, Arver S et al. Pharmacokinetics, efficacy, and safety of a permeation-enhanced testosterone transdermal system in comparison with bi-weekly injections of testosterone enanthate for the treatment of hypogonadal men. J Clin Endocrinol Metab 1999; 84: 3469–78.

60. Luboshitzky R, Lavie L, Shen-Orr Z et al. Altered luteinizing hormone and testosterone secretion in middle-aged obese men with obstructive sleep apnea. Obes Res 2005; 13: 780–6.

61. Liu PY, Yee B, Wishart SM et al. The short-term effects of high-dose testosterone on sleep, breathing, and function in older men. J Clin Endocrinol Metab 2003; 88: 3605–13.

62. Vgontzas AN, Bixler EO, Chrousos GP. Metabolic disturbances in obesity versus sleep apnoea: the importance of visceral obesity and insulin resistance. J Intern Med 2003; 254: 32–44.

63. Bembo SA, Carlson HE. Gynecomastia: its features, and when and how to treat it. Cleve Clin J Med 2004; 71: 511–17.

64. Fentiman IS, Fourquet A, Hortobagyi GN. Male breast cancer. Lancet 2006; 367(9510): 595–604.

65. Gooren LJ. A ten-year safety study of the oral androgen testosterone undecanoate. J Androl 1994; 15: 212–15.

66. Schurmeyer T, Nieschlag E. Comparative pharmacokinetics of testosterone enanthate and testosterone cyclohexanecarboxylate as assessed by serum and salivary testosterone levels in normal men. Int J Androl 1984; 7: 181–7.

67. Harle L, Basaria S. Nebido: a long-acting injectable testosterone for the treatment of male hypogonadism. Expert Opin Pharmacother 2005; 6: 1751–9.

68. Schubert M, Minnemann T. Intramuscular testosterone undecanoate: pharmacokinetic aspects of a novel testosterone formulation during long-term treatment of men with hypogonadism. J Clin Endocrinol Metab 2004; 89: 5429–34.

69. Graefen M, Walz J. Reasonable delay of surgical treatment in men with localized prostate cancer – impact on prognosis? Eur Urol 2005; 47: 756–60.

729

70. Nam RK, Jewett MA. Delay in surgical therapy for clinically localized prostate cancer and biochemical recurrence after radical prostatectomy. Can J Urol 2003; 10: 1891–8.

71. Gooren LJ, Bunck MC. Androgen replacement therapy: present and future. Drugs 2004; 64: 1861–91.

72. Bagchus WM, Hust R, Maris F et al. Important effect of food on the bioavailability of oral testosterone undecanoate. Pharmacotherapy 2003; 23: 319–25.

73. Pechersky AV, Mazurov VI, Semiglazov VF. Androgen administration in middle-aged and ageing men: effects of oral testosterone undecanoate on dihydrotestosterone, oestradiol and prostate volume. Int J Androl 2002; 25: 119–25.

74. Wang C, Swerdloff R, Kipnes M et al. New testosterone buccal system (Striant) delivers physiological testosterone levels: pharmacokinetics study in hypogonadal men. J Clin Endocrinol Metab 2004; 89: 3821–9.

75. Ross RJ, Jabbar A, Jones TH et al. Pharmacokinetics and tolerability of a bioadhesive buccal testosterone tablet in hypogonadal men. Eur J Endocrinol 2004; 150: 57–63.

76. Korbonits M, Kipnes M. Striant SR: a novel, effective and convenient testosterone therapy for male hypogonadism. Int J Clin Pract 2004; 58: 1073–80.

77. Bhasin S, Bagatell CJ, Bremner WJ et al. Issues in testosterone replacement in older men. J Clin Endocrinol Metab 1998; 83: 3435–48.

78. Meikle AW, Mazer NA, Moellmer JF et al. Enhanced transdermal delivery of testosterone across nonscrotal skin produces physiological concentrations of testosterone and its metabolites in hypogonadal men. J Clin Endocrinol Metab 1992; 74: 623–8.

79. Dobs AS, Meikle AW, Arver S et al. Pharmacokinetics, efficacy, and safety of a permeation-enhanced testosterone transdermal system in comparison with bi-weekly injections of testosterone enanthate for the treatment of hypogonadal men. J Clin Endocrinol Metab 1999; 84: 3469–78.

80. Ebert T, Jockenhovel F. The current status of therapy for symptomatic late-onset hypogonadism with transdermal testosterone gel. Eur Urol 2005; 47: 137–46.

81. Wang C, Cunningham G, Dobs A et al. Long-term testosterone gel (AndroGel) treatment maintains beneficial effects on sexual function and mood, lean and fat mass, and bone mineral density in hypogonadal men. J Clin Endocrinol Metab 2004; 89: 2085–98.

82. McNicholas T, Ong T. Review of Testim gel. Expert Opin Pharmacother 2006; 7: 477–84.

83. Meikle AW, Matthias D, Hoffman AR. Transdermal testosterone gel: pharmacokinetics, efficacy of dosing and application site in hypogonadal men. BJU Int 2004; 93: 789–95.

84. Rolf C, Kemper S, Lemmnitz G et al. Pharmacokinetics of a new transdermal testosterone gel in gonadotrophin-suppressed normal men. Eur J Endocrinol 2002; 146: 673–9.

85. Rolf C, Knie U, Lemmnitz G. Interpersonal testosterone transfer after topical application of a newly developed testosterone gel preparation. Clin Endocrinol (Oxf) 2002; 56: 637–41.

86. McNicholas TA, Dean JD, Mulder H et al. A novel testosterone gel formulation normalizes androgen levels in hypogonadal men, with improvements in body composition and sexual function. BJU Int 2003; 91: 69–74.

87. Rochira V, Balestrieri A, Faustini-Fustini M et al. Role of estrogen on bone in the human male: insights from the natural models of congenital estrogen deficiency. Mol Cell Endocrinol 2001; 178: 215–20.

88. Gooren LJ, Toorians AW. Significance of oestrogens in male (patho)physiology. Ann Endocrinol (Paris) 2003; 64: 126–35.

89. Morales AJ, Nolan JJ, Nelson JC et al. Effects of replacement dose of dehydroepiandrosterone in men and women of advancing age. J Clin Endocrinol Metab 1994; 78: 1360–7.

90. Arlt W, Callies F, van Vlijmen JC et al. Dehydroepiandrosterone replacement in women with adrenal insufficiency. N Engl J Med 1999; 341: 1013–20.

91. Hunt PJ, Gurnell EM, Huppert FA et al. Improvement in mood and fatigue after dehydroepiandrosterone replacement in Addison's disease in a randomized, double blind trial. J Clin Endocrinol Metab 2000; 85: 4650–6.

92. Hampson G, Bhargava N, Cheung J et al. Low circulating estradiol and adrenal androgen concentrations in men on glucocorticoids: a potential contributory factor in steroid-induced osteoporosis. Metabolism 2002; 51: 1458–62.

93. Cameron DR, Braunstein GD. The use of dehydroepiandrosterone therapy in clinical practice. Treat Endocrinol 2005; 4: 95–114.

94. Martina V, Benso A. Short-term dehydroepiandrosterone treatment increases platelet cGMP production in elderly male subjects. Clin Endocrinol (Oxf) 2006; 64: 260–4.

95. Kawano H, Yasue H, Kitagawa A et al. Dehydroepiandrosterone supplementation improves endothelial function and insulin sensitivity in men. J Clin Endocrinol Metab 2003; 88: 3190–5.

96. Simoncini T, Mannella P, Fornari L et al. Dehydroepiandrosterone modulates endothelial nitric oxide synthesis via direct genomic and nongenomic mechanisms. Endocrinology 2003; 144: 3449–55.

97. Giordano R, Aimaretti G. Testing pituitary function in aging individuals. Endocrinol Metab Clin North Am 2005; 34: 895–906, viii–ix.

98. Mukherjee A, Monson JP, Jonsson PJ et al. Seeking the optimal target range for insulin-like growth factor I during the treatment of adult growth hormone disorders. J Clin Endocrinol Metab 2003; 88: 5865–70.

99. Harman SM, Blackman MR. Use of growth hormone for prevention or treatment of effects of aging. J Gerontol A Biol Sci Med Sci 2004; 59: 652–8.

100. Mishima K, Okawa M. Diminished melatonin secretion in the elderly caused by insufficient environmental illumination. J Clin Endocrinol Metab 2001; 86: 129–34.

101. Buscemi N, Vandermeer B. Efficacy and safety of exogenous melatonin for secondary sleep disorders and sleep disorders accompanying sleep restriction: meta-analysis. BMJ 2006; 332(7538): 385–93.

102. Zhdanova IV, Wurtman RJ. Melatonin treatment for age-related insomnia. J Clin Endocrinol Metab 2001; 86: 4727–30.

103. Kunz, D, Mahlberg R. Melatonin in patients with reduced REM sleep duration: two randomized controlled trials. J Clin Endocrinol Metab 2004; 89: 128–34.

104. Stan M, Morris JC. Thyrotropin-axis adaptation in aging and chronic disease. Endocrinol Metab Clin North Am 2005; 34: 973–92.

105. Toft AD. Clinical practice. Subclinical hyperthyroidism. N Engl J Med 2001; 345: 512–16.

106. Mohandas R, Gupta KL. Managing thyroid dysfunction in the elderly. Answers to seven common questions. Postgrad Med 2003; 113: 54–8.

107. Montorsi F, Althof SE. Partner responses to sildenafil citrate (Viagra) treatment of erectile dysfunction. Urology 2004; 63: 762–7.

108. Seftel AD. Phosphodiesterase type 5 inhibitor differentiation based on selectivity, pharmacokinetic, and efficacy profiles. Clin Cardiol 2004; 27: I14–19.

109. Rosen R, Altwein J, Boyle P et al. Lower urinary tract symptoms and male sexual dysfunction: the multinational survey of the aging male (MSAM-7). Eur Urol 2003; 44: 637–49.

110. Carson C, Giuliano F, Goldstein I et al. The 'effectiveness' scale – therapeutic outcome of pharmacologic therapies for ED: an international consensus panel report. Int J Impot Res 2004; 16: 207–13.

111. Porst H. Erectile dysfunction. New drugs with special consideration of the PDE 5 inhibitors. Urologe A 2004; 43: 820–8.

112. Jackson G, Rosen RC, Kloner RA et al. The second Princeton consensus on sexual dysfunction and cardiac risk: new guidelines for sexual medicine. J Sex Med 2006; 3: 28–36; discussion 36.

113. Aversa A, Isidori AM, Greco EA et al. Hormonal supplementation and erectile dysfunction. Eur Urol 2004; 45: 535–8.

114. Ogden CL, Carroll MD, Flegal KM. Epidemiologic trends in overweight and obesity. Endocrinol Metab Clin North Am 2003; 32: 741–60, vii.

115. Sorensen TI, Echwald SM. Obesity genes. BMJ 2001; 322: 630–1.

116. Mertens IL, Van Gaal LF. Overweight, obesity, and blood pressure: the effects of modest weight reduction. Obes Res 2000; 8: 270–8.

117. Mathys M. Pharmacologic agents for the treatment of obesity. Clin Geriatr Med 2005; 21: 735–46.

118. Tangney CC, Gustashaw KA. A review: which dietary plan is best for your patients seeking weight loss and sustained weight management? Dis Mon 2005; 51: 284–316.

119. Levitsky DA. The non-regulation of food intake in humans: hope for reversing the epidemic of obesity. Physiol Behav 2005; 86: 623–32.

120. Surtees PG, Wainwright NW, Khaw KT. Obesity, confidant support and functional health: cross-sectional evidence from the EPIC-Norfolk cohort. Int J Obes Relat Metab Disord 2004; 28: 748–58.

121. Darnton-Hill I, Nishida C, James WP. A life course approach to diet, nutrition and the prevention of chronic diseases. Pub Health Nutr 2004; 7: 101–21.

122. Mazzeo RS, Tanaka H. Exercise prescription for the elderly: current recommendations. Sports Med 2001; 31: 809–18.

123. Hogan M. Physical and cognitive activity and exercise for older adults: a review. Int J Aging Hum Dev 2005; 60: 95–126.

124. Brach JS, Simonsick EM, Kritchevsky S et al. The association between physical function and lifestyle activity and exercise in the health, aging and body composition study. J Am Geriatr Soc 2004; 52: 502–9.

125. Conn VS, Minor MA, Burks KJ et al. Integrative review of physical activity intervention research with aging adults. J Am Geriatr Soc 2003; 51: 1159–68.

Index

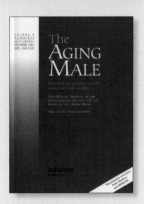

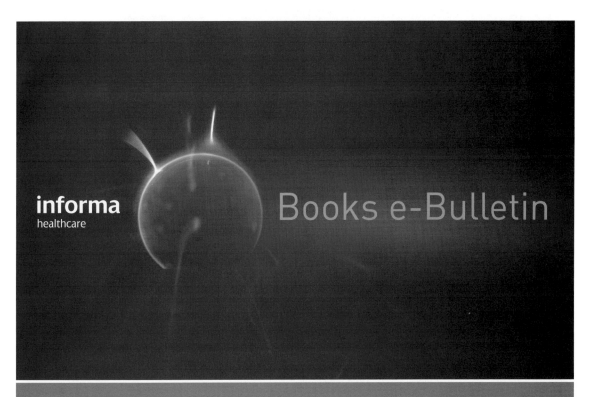
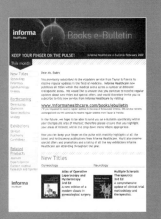